Third Edition

GRAFT-VS.-HOST DISEASE

Graft-vs.-Host Disease

Third Edition

edited by

James L. Ferrara
University of Michigan Cancer Center
Ann Arbor, Michigan, U.S.A.

Kenneth R. Cooke
University of Michigan Cancer Center
Ann Arbor, Michigan, U.S.A.

H. Joachim Deeg
Fred Hutchinson Cancer Research Center
Seattle, Washington, U.S.A.

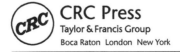

CRC Press
Taylor & Francis Group
Boca Raton   London   New York

CRC Press is an imprint of the
Taylor & Francis Group, an **informa** business

Graft-vs.-Host Disease

Third Edition

edited by

James L. Ferrara
University of Michigan Cancer Center
Ann Arbor, Michigan, U.S.A.

Kenneth R. Cooke
University of Michigan Cancer Center
Ann Arbor, Michigan, U.S.A.

H. Joachim Deeg
Fred Hutchinson Cancer Research Center
Seattle, Washington, U.S.A.

As part of our commitment to providing transplant professionals with the most up-to-date information available, we are pleased to supply you with this copy of *Graft-vs.-Host Disease, Third Edition*. We hope that you will find it informative and useful.

The opinions expressed in this handbook are those of the authors and do not necessarily reflect those of Fujisawa Healthcare, Inc.

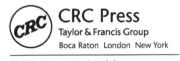

CRC Press
Taylor & Francis Group
Boca Raton London New York

CRC Press is an imprint of the
Taylor & Francis Group, an **informa** business

CRC Press
Taylor & Francis Group
6000 Broken Sound Parkway NW, Suite 300
Boca Raton, FL 33487-2742

First issued in paperback 2019

© 2005 by Taylor & Francis Group, LLC
CRC Press is an imprint of Taylor & Francis Group, an Informa business

No claim to original U.S. Government works

ISBN-13: 978-0-8247-5472-3 (hbk)
ISBN-13: 978-0-367-39347-2 (pbk)

Library of Congress Cataloging-in-Publication Data
A catalog record for this book is available from the Library of Congress.

**Visit the Taylor & Francis Web site at
http://www.taylorandfrancis.com**

**and the CRC Press Web site at
http://www.crcpress.com**

Foreword

More than 100,000 individuals in the United States owe their life to the successful treatment of potentially fatal diseases by hematopoietic cell transplantation. The technique of transplantation has evolved from a relatively crude procedure into an increasingly refined treatment strategy not only for lymphohematopoietic malignancies and genetic defects but also for certain solid tumors and autoimmune disorders. The most severe remaining problem is the development of graft-versus-host disease (GVHD), i.e., the manifestation of the alloreactivity of donor cells against the patient's tissues and organs. GVHD sets the stage for prolonged immunodeficiency, infections, chronic pulmonary disease, impaired growth and development and secondary malignancies.

The increasing use of mobilized peripheral blood cells (instead of marrow) results in an increase in chronic GVHD. The use of non-myeloablative or reduced intensity conditioning regimens has changed the kinetics of the development of GVHD. Acute symptoms may occur later than previously observed. Some of the older criteria for GVHD classification are now obsolete, and staging schemes that also consider the dynamics of GVHD must be developed. These changes appear to be related in part to activation of the transplanted cells by exposure of the donor to G-CSF for mobilization, with associated alterations in the cytokine profiles in monocytes and T-cells. Reduced intensity conditioning regimens also may have different effects on the host environment regarding antigen presentation, in particular by dendritic cells, and on the release of cytokines and chemokines. The regulation of apoptosis and the apparent differences in regards to proinflammatory and apoptotic pathways in different organs are also being studied.

There is evidence in murine models that manifestations of GVHD in target organs may be independent of the expression of MHC antigens. The role of cytokines such as interleukin-10, -15, -18 and others is only beginning to be understood, and a better understanding of these interactions may lead to more effective prophylactic and therapeutic strategies for GVHD. In clinical transplantation, the role of polymorphisms in the promoter regions of cytokine genes such as TNFα and IL-10 is coming into clearer focus, and should soon be able to define more precisely the risk of an individual patient for significant GVHD.

Since the second edition of this book, major advances have occurred in the area of histocompatibility. HLA typing has been refined to permit selection of unrelated individuals as donors on the basis of HLA identity at the DNA level for class I and class II antigens. As a result, outcome with unrelated donor transplants has approached or is identical to those achieved with HLA-identical siblings. Furthermore, HLA-C antigens have been identified as important components in the interaction between donor and host, in particular as targets for NK cells. While still controversial, there is evidence that differences between donor and host in regard to their killer inhibitory receptors (KIR) can be exploited for more effective eradication of a patient's leukemia without increasing the risk of GVHD. Similarly, considerable work has also been carried out on so-called minor antigens and their tissue specific expression, permitting donor cells to be directed at antigens present on hematopoietic (and leukemic) cells but not on other tissues.

Each refinement in histocompatibility typing makes it less likely that a perfect match can be found. Through the efforts of the National Marrow Donor Program, however, there are now more than 5 million HLA typed donors in the US registry and another 3 million in cooperative registries worldwide, making it increasingly possible to find a match.

Finally, several new pharmacological agents with anti-inflammatory, immuno-suppressive and mucosal protectant properties are being investigated in clinical trials. Results obtained with mycophenolate mofetil and with sirolimus, especially when used in combination regimens, are encouraging.

In the approximately 50 years since the work of Medawar and colleagues, we have known that it is possible to achieve a state of non-reactivity between incompatible donor and recipient cells. This state of tolerance, easily achieved during fetal life, has proved to be extremely difficult to achieve in later life. We continue to struggle with the consequences of this incompatibility between donor and host, graft rejection and GvHD. Numerous investigators have contributed their expertise to this third edition of the book to provide a comprehensive overview and update on recent developments in our understanding and the management of GVHD. It is reasonable to hope that we are nearing solutions to these problems and that the material presented here will hasten that process.

E. Donnall Thomas, M.D.

Preface to the Third Edition

Seven years have passed since the second edition of this textbook. The editors are gratified by the enthusiastic response of our readers who have often commented that the clear and clean writing in this volume makes it accessible to many who are new to the field.

We believe this book should be in the hands of every clinician caring for patients undergoing an allogeneic bone marrow transplant, as well as every scientist interested in the complex and fascinating immunologic phenomenon of GVHD. Because this text is used in over thirty countries throughout the world, we have made every effort in the third edition to maintain and enhance its accessibility. In order to keep this volume affordable to individuals, and particularly to young individuals at the early stages of their careers, we reduced its overall length. Because several new areas of investigation and expansion required inclusion, however, we decided to eliminate the introductory section of basic immunologic sciences. We have also emphasized the translational aspects of individual topics by including basic science and clinical perspectives in the same chapter wherever possible. We believe this fusion and streamlining will significantly enhance the utility of the book. Readers will note the rapid advance of certain topics. For example, in the second edition, there was not a single mention of regulatory or suppressive phenomena. Today, not only have regulatory cells become a hot topic in general immunology, they have been used very effectively to modulate GVHD in animal models. Our increased ability to identify these cells and isolate their molecular pathways leads us to hope that we will be able to manipulate these and other cells in ways that will benefit our patients in the years ahead.

Readers will also note that the editorship has changed. We are grateful to Steven Burakoff for his many contributions to the immunology of GVHD and for his help in earlier editions of this text. We are delighted to be joined by Kenneth Cooke, whose enthusiasm, energy and passion for excellence will help to make this third edition the best yet.

Finally we would like to dedicate this volume to our best teachers: our patients. It is our hope that by the time of the fourth edition, many of the insights illuminated in the following pages will have been translated into new therapies that will make allogeneic bone marrow transplantation a safer and more effective therapy for everyone who needs it.

James L. M. Ferrara
Kenneth R. Cooke
H. Joachim Deeg

Preface to the Second Edition

We begin this preface to the second edition of *Graft-vs.-Host Disease* with gratitude to our readership for the overwhelmingly positive response to the first edition, which required a second printing even while the revised volume was in progress. We appreciate the many thoughtful reviews and constructive suggestions, several of which have been incorporated into this new volume.

Many of our readers have specialty training in the fields of hematology and oncology, but relatively limited backgrounds in basic immunology, an area of investigation that has exploded in the past decade. Yet nowhere is transplantation immunology more complex than in a graft-vs.-host reaction, where the immune system is both effector and target. As a result, detailed discussions of graft-vs,-host disease (GVHD) are often dense and sometimes impenetrable to the very readers for whom this book was intended. We have therefore included, as introduction, a series of chapters that review important aspects of immunobiology necessary to the understanding of GVHD pathophysiology as well as the current efforts used to control this disease.

The first chapter in Part I reviews thymic ontogeny and summarizes the complex process of T-cell maturation and differentiation. The appreciation of the thymus as a target organ of GVHD helps to explain how the disease can have such devastating effects on the reconstitution of the immune system. Chapters on MHC Class I and Class II antigens review the structure and function of these molecules, which are responsible for activating $CD8^+$ and $CD4^+$ T cells, respectively. Overviews are presented on T-cell costimulation and anergy, molecular mechanisms of immunosuppression, and adhesion molecules critical to T-cell migration and traffic. One entire chapter is devoted to a detailed discussion of cytokine networks, an area of intense investigation that is central to multiple aspects of GVHD. Finally, reviews of target cell death by both cytolytic T lymphocytes and natural killer cells provide a context for mechanisms of specific target organ pathology.

The middle part of the book has been reorganized to bring together research from experimental models and clinical protocols into single chapters. The classic triad of target organs – skin, liver, and intestinal tract – is reviewed first, followed by other, less "classic" target organs such as the immune system, the hematopoietic system, and the lung. Mechanisms of graft-vs.-leukemia effects are explored in extensive detail, with a thorough discussion of the different cellular populations that participate in this process. This part concludes with two chapters that summarize recent contributions to GVHD patho-physiology: the role of endotoxin and infections and the functional interactions between lymphocytes from the perspective of their cytokine profiles.

The third and final part concentrates on clinical GVHD, its prevention and treatment. The first three chapters review the clinical spectra of GVHD after both allogeneic and autologous bone marrow transplantation (BMT), as well as transfusion-associated GVHD. Current strategies for preventing GVHD are summarized next: the matching of donor and host at HLA loci, the depletion of T cells from the donor marrow, the nonspecific immunosuppression of the host, and the use of cytokine antagonists. The following chapter reviews the emerging role of IL-10 in the induction and maintenance of donor–host tolerance after BMT. Alternative approaches to reducing GVHD are summarized next, including the selection of stem cells, adoptive immunotherapy, and the increasing efforts at genetic modification of hematopoietic cells and T cells. The last chapter serves as a sort of coda to the entire book, with contributions from 21 investigators reviewing the most recent advances in GVHD research, many of them still in press at this time.

An endeavor of this size and complexity requires the generous efforts of many contributors, whom we gratefully acknowledge. We would like to dedicate this volume to two groups of individuals who remain the bedrock of both experimental and clinical GVHD research: first, the outstanding animal care technicians and veterinarians without whose care and diligence the exploration of animal models would be impossible, and second, the nurses, residents, and fellows whose superb skills and compassion continue to offer hope to our patients for a brighter tomorrow. If this book can contribute in some small way to that hope, our efforts in bringing it forth will be more than amply rewarded.

James L. M. Ferrara
H. Joachim Deeg
Steven J. Burakoff

Preface to the First Edition

There are two major reasons for producing a broad overview of graft-vs.-host disease (GVHD). From a clinical standpoint, GVHD can be a devastating complication of bone marrow transplantation. Significant progress has been made; however, several obstacles remain in overcoming this problem, particularly in patients given histoincompatible grafts. Multiple approaches, discussed in the clinical sections of this book, have been taken, each with advantages and disadvantages. Frequently, those approaches were based on experimental models. Thus, it is only logical that the clinical sections are preceded by a description of preclinical studies. It is these animal models that have been critical in advancing our understanding of the physiology of GVHD. Control of genetic variables as well as the ability to produce GVHD in a variety of models have permitted insights not possible in a strictly clinical context. In addition, these systems have also provided models for understanding lymphocyte development and function in vivo irrespective of GVHD. The increasing sophistication and precision of cellular and molecular probes have initiated an analysis of cellular mechanisms in physiological environments rather than in a petri dish or test tube. The abnormalities of GVHD thus provide a perspective from which to understand the complexities of normal lymphocyte differentiation and activation. The insights from these studies should lead to improved understanding of fundamental lymphocyte biology and thus to new therapeutic strategies, not only in bone marrow transplantation, but in other areas, such as autoimmune diseases. It is our hope that future editions of this book will reflect this increased understanding and will witness further movement from experimental models to clinical realms.

The production of a book this size is a long and complex undertaking, and we are grateful to the many people who have given generously of their time and effort. We would like to thank particularly Joshua Hauser and Michele Fox for their labors in the preparation of the index. We also wish to acknowledge the continued support of our colleagues and teachers who have encouraged us over many years, especially David G. Nathan, Fred S. Rosen, Baruj Benacerraf, Rainer Storb, and E. Donnall Thomas.

Steven J. Burakoff
H. Joachim Deeg
James L. M. Ferrara
Kerry Atkinson

Contents

I. GRAFT-vs.-HOST DISEASE PATHOPHYSIOLOGY

Immune Activation and Dysregulation

Contents

Contributors

Görgün Akpek   University of Maryland Medical System, Baltimore, Maryland, U.S.A.

Joseph H. Antin   Harvard Medical School and Dana-Farber Cancer Institute, Boston, Massachusetts, U.S.A.

Anna Barbui   Ospedali Riuniti de Bergamo, Bergamo, Italy

Barbara E. Bierer   Harvard Medical School and Brigham and Women's Hospital, Boston, Massachusetts, U.S.A.

Bruce R. Blazar   University of Minnesota, Minneapolis, Minnesota, U.S.A.

Nelson J. Chao   Duke University, Durham, North Carolina, U.S.A.

Kenneth R. Cooke   University of Michigan Comprehensive Cancer Center, Ann Arbor, Michigan, U.S.A.

Lisette van de Corput   University Medical Center Utrecht and Wilhelmina Children's Hospital, Utrecht, The Netherlands

Daniel R. Couriel   The University of Texas M.D. Anderson Cancer Center, Houston, Texas, U.S.A.

James M. Crawford   University of Florida College of Medicine, Gainesville, Florida, U.S.A.

H. Joachim Deeg Fred Hutchinson Cancer Research Center and University of Washington, Seattle, Washington, U.S.A.

Frederik J. H. Falkenburg Leiden University Medical Center, Leiden, The Netherlands

James L. M. Ferrara University of Michigan Comprehensive Cancer Center, Ann Arbor, Michigan, U.S.A.

Daniel H. Fowler National Institutes of Health, Bethesda, Maryland, U.S.A.

Thea M. Friedman Kimmel Cancer Center, Thomas Jefferson University, Philadelphia, Pennsylvania, U.S.A.

Sergio Giralt The University of Texas M.D. Anderson Cancer Center, Houston, Texas, U.S.A.

Ronald E. Gress National Institutes of Health, Bethesda, Maryland, U.S.A.

Frances T. Hakim Pediatric Oncology Branch, Center for Cancer Research, National Cancer Institute, National Institutes of Health, Bethesda, Maryland, U.S.A.

Ernst Holler University of Regensburg, Regensburg, Germany

Stephen C. Jones Trudeau Institute, Inc., Saranac Lake, New York, U.S.A.

Hans-Jochem Kolb University of Munich, Munich, Germany

Robert Korngold Kimmel Cancer Center, Thomas Jefferson University, Philadelphia, Pennsylvania, U.S.A.

John E. Levine University of Michigan, Ann Arbor, Michigan, U.S.A.

Chen Liu University of Florida College of Medicine, Gainesville, Florida, U.S.A.

Crystal L. Mackall Pediatric Oncology Branch, Center for Cancer Research, National Cancer Institute, National Institutes of Health, Bethesda, Maryland, U.S.A.

Gerald F. Marshall Consultant, Niles, Michigan, U.S.A.

Jeffrey J. Molldrem The University of Texas, M. D. Anderson Cancer Center, Houston, Texas, U.S.A.

Allan Mowat University of Glasgow, Glasgow, Scotland

George F. Murphy Thomas Jefferson University, Philadelphia, Pennsylvania, and Harvard Medical School and Brigham and Women's Hospital, Boston, Massachusetts, U.S.A.

William J. Murphy Department of Microbiology and Immunology, University of Nevada, Reno, Nevada, U.S.A.

Effie W. Petersdorf University of Washington and Fred Hutchinson Cancer Research Center, Seattle, Washington, U.S.A.

David L. Porter University of Pennsylvania, Philadelphia, Pennsylvania, U.S.A.

Pavan Reddy University of Michigan Comprehensive Cancer Center, Ann Arbor, Michigan, U.S.A.

Takehiko Sasazuki Research Institute, International Medical Center of Japan, Tokyo, Japan

Jon S. Serody Departments of Medicine, Microbiology and Immunology, University of North Carolina at Chapel Hill, Chapel Hill, North Carolina, U.S.A.

Warren D. Shlomchik School of Medicine, Yale University, New Haven, Connecticut, U.S.A.

Gerard Socié Hospital St. Louis, Paris, France

Robert J. Soiffer Dana-Farber Cancer Institute, Boston, Massachusetts, U.S.A.

Patricia A. Taylor University of Minnesota, Minneapolis, Minnesota, U.S.A.

Takanori Teshima Department of Medicine II, Okayama University Graduate School of Medicine and Dentistry, Okayama, Japan

Andrea Velardi Department of Clinical and Experimental Medicine, Division of Hematology and Clinical Immunology, University of Perugia School of Medicine, Perugia, Italy

Charles S. Via University of Maryland Medical System, Baltimore, Maryland, U.S.A.

Georgia B. Vogelsang Johns Hopkins University School of Medicine, Baltimore, Maryland, U.S.A.

John L. Wagner Thomas Jefferson University, Philadelphia, Pennsylvania, and Harvard Medical School, Boston, Massachusetts, U.S.A.

Lisbeth A. Welniak Department of Microbiology and Immunology, University of Nevada, Reno, Nevada, U.S.A.

1

The Pathophysiology of Graft-vs.-Host Disease

JAMES L. M. FERRARA and KENNETH R. COOKE

University of Michigan Comprehensive Cancer Center, Ann Arbor, Michigan, U.S.A.

TAKANORI TESHIMA

Okayama University Graduate School of Medicine and Dentistry, Okayama, Japan

The graft-vs.-host (GVH) reaction was first noted more than a half century ago when irradiated mice were infused with allogeneic marrow and spleen cells. Although mice recovered from radiation injury and marrow aplasia, they subsequently died with "secondary disease," a syndrome consisting of diarrhea, weight loss, skin changes, and liver abnormalities (1). This phenomenon was subsequently recognized as GVH disease (GVHD). In 1966, Billingham formulated the three requirements necessary for GVHD. First, the transplanted graft must contain immunologically competent cells; second, the recipient must be incapable of rejecting the transplanted cells; third, the recipient must express tissue antigens that are not present in the transplant donor that could thus be recognized as foreign (2).

It is now known that mature T lymphocytes are the immunocompetent cells in the graft that fulfill the first precondition for GVHD (3). After allogeneic hematopoietic stem cell transplantation (SCT), the severity of GVHD correlates with the number of donor T cells transfused (4). Because experimental models have shown that the ability of marrow T cells to induce GVHD is much less potent than mature circulating T cells (5), the contamination of bone marrow with peripheral blood at the time of marrow harvest may contribute significantly to the development of GVHD.

The seond precondition for GVHD stipulates that the recipient must be immunocompromised. A normal immune system will usually reject T cells from a foreign donor. This requirement is found most commonly during allogeneic SCT, where

1

patients have traditionally received immunoablative doses of chemotherapy and/or radiation before stem cell infusion. Conditions are also met in other situations, such as during solid organ allografts and blood transfusion, where recipients are often immunosuppressed. There are, however, exceptions to this requirement. GVHD can occur in an immunocompetent recipient of tissues from a donor who is homozygous for one haplotype of the recipient (e.g., transfusion of blood from an HLA homozygous parent to a heterozygous child). This genetic situation prevents the recipient from rejecting the donor cells even though he or she is not immunocompromised (6).

The third precondition for GVHD, the expression of recipient tissue antigens not present in the donor, became the focus of intensive research with the discovery of the major histocompatibility complex (MHC). Human leukocyte antigens (HLA) are the gene products of the MHC. HLA are expressed on the cell surfaces of all nucleated cells in the human body and are essential to the activation of allogeneic T cells (7). During lymphocyte development, T cells are selected in the thymus to recognize self-MHC molecules, but when confronted with allogeneic (nonself) MHC molecules, the activated T cells mount a formidable attack that culminates in the destruction of the allogeneic tissues. In fact, MHC differences between donor and recipient are the most important risk factor for the induction of GVHD. In addition, there are minor histocompatibility antigens (mHAg) derived from the expression of polymorphic genes. Surprisingly, GVH reactions can occur between genetically identical strains and individuals (8,9). These rare observations have prompted a revision of the third postulate to include the inappropriate recognition of host self antigens.

GVHD can be considered both acute and chronic, given the timing of its occurrence. This chapter will focus on acute GVHD; chronic GVHD will be reviewed in Chapter 20.

I. ACUTE GVHD PATHIOPHYSIOLOGY: A THREE-STEP MODEL

The pathophysiology of acute GVHD can be considered as a three-step process where the innate and adaptive immune systems interact (Fig. 1). The three steps are 1) tissue damage to the recipient by the radiation/chemotherapy pretransplant conditioning regimen, 2) donor T-cell activation and clonal expansion, and 3) cellular and inflammatory factors. This schema underscores the importance of mononuclear phagocytes and other accessory cells to the development of GVHD after complex interactions with cytokines secreted by activated donor T cells. In step 1, the conditioning regimen (irradiation and/or chemotherapy) leads to damage and activation of host tissues throughout the body and the secretion of inflammatory cytokines tumor necrosis factor (TNF)-α and interleukin (IL)-1. These cytokines may enhance donor T-cell recognition of host alloantigens by increasing expression of MHC antigens and other molecules on host antigen-presenting cells (APCs). Inflammatory cytokines may also stimulate chemokine release, recuiting donor T cells into host target organs. In step 2, host APCs present alloantigen (an HLA-peptide complex) to the donor T cells. Costimulatory signals are required for T-cell activation, and these signals further activate APCs, which in turn enhance T-cell stimulation, characterized by cellular proliferation and the secretion of cytokines. IL-2 expands the T-cell clones and induces cytotoxic T cell (CTL) responses, whereas interferon (IFN)-γ has multiple effects, including the priming of mononuclear phagocytes to produce TNF-α and IL-1. In step 3, effector functions of mononuclear phagocytes and neutrophils are triggered through a secondary signal provided by mediators such as lipopolysaccharide (LPS) that leak through

(1) Conditioning

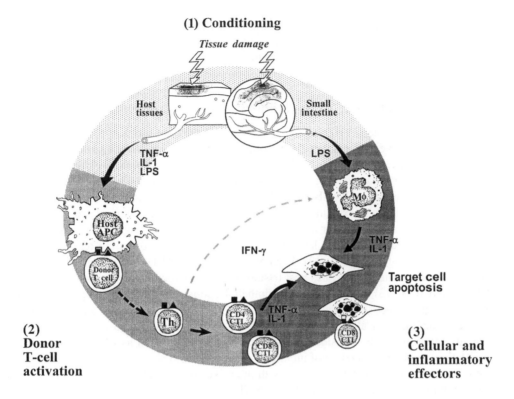

Figure 1 The pathophysiology of acute GVHD. GVHD pathophysiology can be summarized in a three-step process. In phase 1, the conditioning regimen (irradiation, chemotherapy, or both) leads to the damage and activation of host tissues, especially the intestinal mucosa. This allows the translocation of lipopolysaccharide (LPS) from the intestinal lumen to the circulation, stimulating the secretion of the inflammatory cytokines TNF-α and IL-1 from host tissues, particularly macrophages. These cytokines increase the expression of MHC antigens and adhesion molecules on host tissues, enhancing the recognition of MHC and minor histocompatibility antigens by mature donor T cells. Donor T-cell activation in phase 2 is characterized by the predominance of Th1 cells and the secretion of IFN-γ, which activates mononuclear phagocytes. In phase 3, effector functions of activated mononuclear phagocytes are triggered by the secondary signal provided by LPS and other stimulatory molecules that leak through the intestinal mucosa damaged during phases 1 and 2. Activated macrophages, along with CTL, secrete inflammatory cytokines that cause target cell apoptosis. CD8+ CTL also lyse target cells directly. Damage to the GI tract in this phase, principally by inflammatory cytokines, amplifies LPS release and leads to the "cytokine storm" characteristic of severe acute GVHD. This damage results in the amplification of local tissue injury, and it further promotes an inflammatory response.

the intestinal mucosa damaged during step 1. This inflammation, along with direct lysis of target cells by CTL, causes pathological changes in target organs.

It should be noted from the outset that not all these steps carry equal weight in the pathogenesis of acute GVHD. The pivotal interaction occurs in step 2, where host APCs activate allogeneic donor T cells. Although there is substantial evidence for inflammatory cytokines as major effectors of target organ damage, blockade of individual cytokines may not reverse established GVHD when other cellular effectors such as CTL are present.

GVHD can also occur when no conditioning of the host has occurred, e.g., transfusion-associated GVHD. This schema is not exhaustive and is intended to provide perspective on how the innate and adaptive immune systems interact in this complicated, inflammatory disease.

A. Step 1: Effects of SCT Conditioning

The first step of acute GVHD occurs before donor cells are infused. Prior to SCT, a patient's tissues have been damaged, sometimes profoundly, by several factors such as the underlying disease, its treatment, infection, and transplant conditioning. High-intensity chemoradiotherapy characteristic of SCT conditioning regimens can activate host APCs and help to recruit donor T cells infused in the stem cell inoculum. This inflammatory environment may help to explain a number of unique and seemingly unrelated aspects of GVHD. For example, a number of reports have noted increased risks of clinical GVHD associated with advanced-stage leukemia, certain intensive conditioning regimens, and histories of viral infections (10–12). Total body irradiation (TBI) is particularly important in this process because it activates host tissues to secrete inflammatory cytokines, such as TNF-α and IL-1 (13), and it induces endothelial apoptosis that leads to epithelial cell damage in gastrointestinal tract (14). After autologous SCT, injury to the gut is transient and self-limited. After allogeneic SCT, however, GVHD amplifies gastrointestinal (GI) damage by allowing the translocation of microbial products such as LPS into systemic circulation, increasing secretion of inflammatory cytokines. This scenario helps to explain the increased risk of GVHD associated with intensive conditioning regimens as observed both in animal models (15) and in clinical SCT (10,11).

B. Step 2: Donor T-Cell Activation and Cytokine Secretion

1.   Donor T-Cell Activation

Donor T-cell activation occurs during the second step of acute GVHD. Murine studies have demonstrated that host APCs alone are both necessary and sufficient to stimulate donor T cells (16,17). After allogeneic SCT, APCs derived from both the host and the donor are present in secondary lymphoid organs. T-cell receptors (TCRs) of donor T cells can recognize alloantigens either on host APCs (direct presentation) or donor APCs (indirect presentation). During direct presentation, donor T cells recognize either the peptide bound to allogeneic MHC molecules or the foreign MHC molecules themselves (18). During indirect presentation, T cells respond to the peptides generated by degradation of the allogeneic MHC molecules that are presented on self MHC (19). In GVHD to minor H antigens (mHAg), direct presentation is dominant because APCs derived from the host rather than from the donor are critical (16).

CD4 and CD8 proteins are coreceptors for constant portions of MHC class II and MHC class I molecules, respectively. MHC class I (HLA-A, B, C) differences stimulate CD8 + T cells, and MHC class II (HLA-DR, DP, DQ) differences stimulate CD4+ T cells (20). After HLA-identical SCT, GVHD is usually induced by mHAg, which are peptides derived from polymorphic cellular proteins presented on the cell surface by MHC molecules (21). Because the genes for these proteins are located outside of the MHC, two siblings will often have many different peptides in the same MHC that can be recognized by donor T cells and lead to GVHD. It remains unclear how many of these peptides behave as mHAg, although over 50 different minor histocompability genetic loci have been defined among inbred strains of mice (22). The actual number of so-called "major" minor antigens that can potentially induce GVHD is likely to be limited. In murine models, the protein H60 has been shown to be one such major minor (23). In humans, of five previously characterized mHAg (HA-1, 2, 3, 4, 5) recognized by T cells in association with HLA-A1 and A2, only mismatching of HA-1 significantly correlated with acute grade II–IV GVHD (24). Several minor histocompatibility antigens are encoded on the male-specific Y chromosome, and there is an increased risk of GVHD when male recipients are transplanted from female donors (25,26). mHAg with tissue expression limited to the hematopoietic system are potential target antigens of GVL reactivity (27), and separation of GVHD and GVL by using CTLs specific for such antigens is an area of intense research (28).

Signaling through the TCR after antigen recognition induces a conformational change in adhesion molecules, resulting in higher-affinity binding to the APC (29). Full T-cell activation also requires costimulatory signals provided by APCs in addition to TCR signals (Table 1). Two primary costimulatoty pathways signal through either CD28 or TNF receptors. Currently, there are four known CD28 superfamily members expressed on T cells: CD28, cytotoxic T-lymphocyte antigen 4 (CTLA-4), inducible costimulator (ICOS), and programmed death (PD)-1. In addition, there are four TNF receptor family members: CD40 ligand (CD154), 4-1BB (CD137), OX40, and HSV glycoprotein D for herpesvirus entry mediator (HVEM). The best-characterized costimulatory molecules, CD80 and CD86, deliver positive signals through CD28 that lower the threshold for T-cell activation and promote T-cell differentiation and survival, while signaling through CTLA-4 is inhibitory (30,31). This topic is reviewed in detail in Chapter 15.

Table 1 T Cell–APC Interactions

	T Cell	APC
Adhesion		
	ICAMs	LFA-1
	LFA-1	ICAMs
	CD2 (LFA-2)	LFA-3
Recognition		
	TCR/CD4	MHC II
	TCR/CD8	MHC I
Costimulation		
	CD28	CD80/86
	CD152 (CTLA-4)	CD80/86
	ICOS	B7H/B7RP-1
	PD-1	PD-L1, PD-L2
	unknown	B7-H3
	CD154 (CD40L)	CD40
	CD134 (OX40)	CD134L (OX40L)
	CD137 (4-1BB)	CD137L (4-1BBL)
	HVEM	LIGHT

HVEM, HSV glycoprotein D for herpesvirus entry mediator; LIGHT, homologous to lymphotoxins, shows inducible expression, and competes with herpes simplex virus glycoprotein D for herpesvirus entry mediator (HVEM), a receptor expressed by T lymphocytes.

The most potent APCs are dendritic cells (DCs); however, the relative contribution of DCs and other semiprofessional APCs such as monocytes/macrophages and B cells to the development of GVHD remains to be elucidated. DCs can be matured and activated during SCT by (1) inflammatory cytokines, (2) microbial products such as LPS and CpG entering systemic circulation from damaged intestinal mucosa, and (3) necrotic cells that are damaged by recipient conditioning. All of these stimuli may be considered "danger signals" (32) and may make the difference between an immune response and tolerance (33). When T cells are exposed to antigens in the presence of adjuvant such as LPS, the migration and survival of T cells are dramatically enhanced in vivo (34). Recent studies have shown that activation of DCs through Toll-like receptors that bind molecules such as LPS and CpG can induce an immune response and prevent the generation of tolerogenic T-regulatory cells (35).

The role of host APCs in acute GVHD is an area of intense current research. Enhanced allostimulatory activity of APCs in older hosts may also help explain the increased incidence of acute GVHD in older recipients (36). The distribution of APCs may help explain the unusual target organ distribution of GVHD. For example, selective removal of APCs from a specific organ may reduce GVHD in that target organ but not in others (37). The general elimination of host APCs by activated natural killer (NK) cells can prevent GVHD (38). This suppressive effect of NK cells on GVHD has been confirmed in humans: HLA class I differences driving donor NK-mediated alloreactions in the GVH direction mediate potent GVL effects and produce higher engraftment rates without causing severe acute GVHD (38,39).

2.   Cytokine Secretion by Donor T Cells

T-cell activation involves multiple, rapidly occurring intracellular biochemical pathways that in turn activate transcription of genes for cytokines, such as IL-2, IFN-γ, and their receptors. Cytokines secreted by activated T cells are generally classified as Th1 (secreting IL-2 and IFN-γ) or Th2 (secreting IL-4, IL-5, IL-10, and IL-13) (40). Several factors influence the ability of DCs to instruct naive CD4 + T cells to secrete Th1 or Th2 cytokines. These factors include the type and duration of DC activation along with the DC : T-cell ratio and the proportions of DC subsets present during T-cell interactions (41,42). Differential activation of Th1 or Th2 cells has been evoked in the immunopathogenesis of GVHD and the development of infectious and autoimmune diseases. In each setting, activated Th1 cells: (1) amplify T-cell proliferation by secreting IL-2, (2) lyse target cells by Fas/FasL interactions, (3) induce macrophage differentiation in the bone marrow by secreting IL-3 and GM-CSF, (4) activate monocytes and macrophages by secreting IFN-γ and by their CD40-CD40L interactions, (5) activate endothelium to induce macrophage binding and extravasation, and (6) recruit macrophages by secreting monocyte chemoattractant protein-1 (MCP-1) (43,44).

During step 2 of acute GVHD pathophysiology, IL-2 has a pivotal role in amplifying the immune response against alloantigens. IL-2 is secreted by donor CD4+ T cells in the first several days after GVHD induction (45). In some studies, the addition of low doses of IL-2 during the first week after allogeneic BMT enhanced the severity and mortality of GVHD (46,47). The precursor frequency of host-specific IL-2–producing cells (pHTL) predicts the occurrence of clinical acute GVHD, often preceding the onset of acute GVHD by approximately 2 weeks (48–50). Monoclonal antibodies (mAbs) against IL-2 or its receptor can prevent GVHD when administered shortly after the infusion of T cells (45,51,52), but this strategy was not particularly successful in reducing the incidence of severe GVHD (53,54). IL-15 is another critical cytokine in initiating allogeneic T-cell division in vivo (55), and elevated serum levels of IL-15 are associated with acute GVHD in humans (56). IL-15 may therefore also be important in the clonal expansion of donor T cells in step 2.

IFN-γ is a cytokine that can both amplify and suppress acute GVHD. In terms of amplification, increased levels of IFN-γ are associated with acute GVHD (15,57–59), and a large proportion of T-cell clones isolated from GVHD patients produce IFN-γ (60). In many experimental models of GVHD, IFN-γ levels peak between days 4 and 7 after transplant before clinical manifestations are apparent. CTLs that are specific for mHAgs and produce IFN-γ also correlate with the severity of GVH reaction in a skin-explant assay of human disease (28), but serum levels of IFN-γ were not significantly increased in a small series of patients with GVHD (61). IFN-γ modulates several aspects of the immune response of acute GVHD. First, IFN-γ increases the expression of numerous molecules, including adhesion molecules, chemokines, MHC antigens, and Fas, resulting in enhanced antigen presentation and the recruitment of effector cells into target organs (62–64). Second, IFN-γ alters target cells in the GI tract and in the skin, making them more vulnerable to damage; the administration of anti-IFN-γ mAbs prevents gastrointestinal GVHD (65), and high levels of both IFN-γ and TNF-α correlate with the most intense cellular damage in skin (66). Third, IFN-γ mediates the immunosuppression seen in several experimental GVHD systems in part by the induction of nitric oxide (NO) (67–72). Fourth, IFN-γ primes macrophages to produce pro-inflammatory cytokines and NO in response to LPS (73,74).

GVHD effector mechanisms can sometimes be inhibited if donor T cells produce fewer Th1 cytokines. Transplantation of Th2 cells into nonirradiated recipients results in reduced secretion of TNF-α and protection of recipient mice from LPS-induced, TNF-α– mediated lethality (75). Furthermore, cell mixtures of Th2 donor cells with otherwise lethal numbers of naïve T cells also protect recipient mice from LPS-induced lethality, demonstrating the ability of Th2 cells to modulate Th1 responses after allogeneic transplantation (76). Similarly, the injection of donor Th2 cells that have been polarized in an MLR with host stimulators in the presence of IL-4 fails to induce acute GVHD to MHC class I or class II antigens (77). Polarization of donor T cells toward a Th2 phenotype by pretreatment donors with granulocyte colony-stimulating factor (G-CSF) also results in less severe GVHD (78). Interestingly, GVHD still occurs if donor mice lack the signal transducer and activator of transcription (STAT) 4, which is crucial to a Th1 response, although GVHD is less severe than if the donor cells lacked STAT6, a molecule critical for Th2 polarization (79). These experiments support the concepts that Th1 cells induce GVHD more efficiently than Th2 cells and that the balance of Th1 and Th2 cytokines is critical in the development of a GVH reaction. It should be noted, however, that systemic administration of Th2 cytokines IL-4 or IL-10 as experimental prophylaxis of GVHD was either ineffective or toxic (80–82).

In this light it is surprising that administration of Th1 cytokines can also reduce GVHD. High doses of exogenous IL-2 early after bone marrow transplant (BMT) protect animals from GVHD mortality (83). IL-2 may mediate its protective effect via inhibition of IFN-γ (57). Furthermore, the injection of IFN-γ itself can prevent experimental GVHD (84), and neutralization of IFN-γ accelerates GVHD in lethally irradiated recipients (70). Interestingly, the use of TFN-γ–deficient donor cells can also accelerate GVHD in lethally irradiated recipients (85,86) but reduces GVHD in sublethally irradiated or unirradiated recipients (87,88). These paradoxes may be explained by the complex dynamics of donor T-cell activation, expansion, and contraction. Activation-induced cell death (AICD) is a major mechanism of clonal deletion and is largely responsible for the rapid contraction of activated T cells following an initial massive expansion (89). IFN-γ contracts the pool of activated CD4+ T cells by inducing AICD, and the complete absence of IFN-γ may result in an unrestrained expansion of activated donor T cells, leading to accelerated GVHD. This phenomenon may be of particular importance in recipients of intensified conditioning, which causes greater T-cell activation of host APCs (15). Similarly, administration of IFN-γ–inducing cytokines such as IL-12 or IL-18 early after BMT protects lethally irradiated recipients from GVHD in a Fas-dependent fashion (86,90,91). Thus, moderate amounts of Th1 cytokine production after donor T-cell expansion may amplify GVHD; extremes in production (either low or high), particularly early during T-cell expansion, may hasten the death of activated donor T cells, aborting T-cell expansion and reducing GVHD. Further consideration of Th1 and Th2 cytokines in this process is presented in Chapter 3.

Subpopulations of regulatory donor T cells can prevent GVHD. Repeated in vitro stimulation of donor CD4+ T cells with alloantigens results in the emergence of a population of regulatory T-cell clones (Treg cells) that secretes high amounts of IL-10 and TGF-β (92). The immunosuppressive properties of these cytokines are explained by their ability to inhibit APC function and to suppress proliferation of responding T cells directly. The addition of IL-10 or TGF-β to MLR cultures induces tolerance (93), with alterations in biochemical signaling similar to costimulatory blockade (94). So-called "Th3" cells that produce large amounts of TGF-β can also act as regulatory T cells. CD8+ suppressor cells have also been identified in both mice and humans (95–98). Natural suppressor (NS) cells reduce GVHD in a variety of experimental BMT models (99). NK1.1+ T cells (NKT) may possess such NS cell function (100), and both peripheral blood and marrow NKT cells can prevent GVHD by their IL-4 secretion (5,100,101). Recent research has also focused on CD4+CD25+ regulatory T cells that prevent lethal GVHD in several animal models (102). These topics are explored in detail in Chapter 4.

C.   Step 3: Cellular and Inflammatory Effectors

The pathophysiology of acute GVHD culminates in the generation of multiple cytotoxic effectors that contribute to target tissue injury. At a minimum, step 3 includes (1) several inflammatory cytokines, (2) specific antihost CTL activity using Fas and perforin pathways, (3) large granular lymphocytes (LGL) or NK cells, and (4) nitric oxide. Significant experimental and clinical data suggest that soluble inflammatory mediators act in conjunction with direct cell-mediated cytolysis by CTL and NK cells to cause the full spectrum of deleterious effects seen during acute GVHD. As such, the effector phase of GVHD involves aspects of both the innate and adaptive immune response and the synergistic interactions of cells and cytokines generated during step 1 and step 2.

1.   Cellular Effectors

The Fas/Fas ligand (FasL) and the perforin/granzyme (or granule exocytosis) pathways are the principal effector mechanisms used by CTLs and NK cells to lyse their target cells (103,104). Perforin is stored together with granzymes and other proteins in cytotoxic granules of CTLs and NK cells (105). Following recognition of a target cell through TCR-MHC interaction, perforin is secreted and inserts itself into the target cell membrane, forming "perforin pores" that allow granzymes to enter the cell and induce apoptosis through various downstream effector pathways (105). Ligation of Fas results in the formation of the death-inducing signaling complex (DISC) and the subsequent activation of caspases (106). A number of ligands on T cells also possess the capability to trimerize TNF receptor–like death receptors (DR) on their targets, such as TNF-related apoptosis-inducing ligand (TRAIL: DR4,5 ligand) and TNF-like weak inducer of apoptosis (TWEAK: DR3 ligand) (107–109).

The involvement of these pathways in GVHD has been tested by utilizing donor cells that are genetically deficient in each molecule. Transplantation of perforin-deficient T cells results in a marked delay in the onset of acute GVHD in transplants across mHAg (110), across both MHC and mHAg (111), and across isolated MHC I or II disparities (112,113). However, lethal GVHD occurs even in the absence of perforin-dependent killing, demonstrating that the perforin/granzyme pathway plays a significant, but not exclusive, role in target organ damage. CD4 + CTLs preferentially use the Fas/FasL pathway during acute GVHD, while CD8 + CTLs primarily use the perforin/granzyme pathway, consistent with other pathological onditions that involve cell-mediated cytolysis.

Fas is a TNF receptor (TNFR) family member that is expressed by many tissues, including GVHD target organs. Inflammatory cytokines such as IFN-γ and TNF-α can increase the expression of Fas during GVHD (114). FasL expression on donor T cells is increased during experimental GVHD (115–117), and elevated serum levels of soluble FasL and Fas have been observed in some patients with acute GVHD (118–121). FasL-defective donor T cells cause markedly reduced GVHD in the liver, skin, and lymphoid organs (110,122,123). The Fas-FasL pathway is particularly important in hepatic GVHD, consistent with the marked sensitivity of hepatocytes to Fas-mediated cytotoxicity in models of murine hepatitis (124). Fas-deficient recipients are protected from hepatic GVHD, but not from GVHD in other target organs (125). Administration of anti-FasL (but not anti-TNF) mAbs significantly blocked hepatic GVHD damage in one model (126), whereas the use of FasL-deficient donor T cells or the administration of neutralizing FasL mAbs had no effect on the development of intestinal GVHD in several studies (110,126,127).

Cytotoxic double-defficient (cdd) (absence of both perforin/granzyme and FasL pathways) donor T cells do not induce lethal GVHD across MHC class I and class II disparities after sublethal irradiation (111). However, the lack of acute GVHD was probably caused by the rejection of the donor cdd T cells because they lacked the effector mechanisms to eliminate host resistance to GVHD (128,129). When recipients were conditioned with a lethal dose of irradiation, cdd CD4+ T cells produced similar mortality to wild-type CD4+ T cells (129).

2. Inflammatory Effectors

In the effector phase of acute GVHD, inflammatory cytokines synergize with CTLs, resulting in the amplification of local tissue injury and the development of target organ dysfunction in the transplant recipient. The cytokines TNF-α and IL-1 are produced by an abundance of cell types involved in innate and adoptive immune responses, and they have synergistic and redundant roles during several phases of acute GVHD. A central role for inflammatory cytokines in acute GVHD was confirmed by a recent murine study using bone marrow chimeras in which alloantigens were not expressed on target epithelium but on APCs alone (17). GVHD target organ injury was induced in these chimeras even in the absence of epithelial alloantigens, and mortality and target organ injury were prevented by the neutralization of TNF-α and IL-1. These observations were particularly true for

CD4-mediated acute GVHD; in CD8-mediated disease, donor CTL effectors contributed to GVHD mortality.

A critical role for TNF-α in the pathophysiology of acute GVHD was first suggested almost 15 years ago when high levels of TNF-α mRNA were noted in GVHD tissues (130,131). Target organ damage could be inhibited by infusion of anti-TNF-α mAbs, and mortality could be reduced from 100% to 50% by the administration of the soluble form of the TNF-α receptor (sTNFR) (13). TNF-α plays a central role in intestinal GVHD (126,130,132) as well as in skin and lymphoid tissue (126,130,133,134) and to a lesser extent in the liver (17,135). TNF-α may be involved at many points within GVHD pathophysiology because TNF-α can (1) cause cachexia, a characteristic feature of GVHD, (2) induce maturation of DCs, thus enhancing alloantigen presentation, (3) recruit effector T cells, neutrophils, and monocytes into target organs through the induction of inflammatory chemokines, and (4) cause direct tissue damage by inducing apoptosis and necrosis (136). TNF-α is also involved in donor T-cell activation directly through its signaling via TNFR1 and TNFR2 on T cells; TNF-TNFR1 interactions promote alloreactive T-cell responses (137), whereas TNF-TNFR2 interactions are critical for intestinal GVHD (138).

An important role for TNF-α in clinical acute GVHD has also been suggested by multiple studies. Elevations of TNF-α protein (serum) and mRNA (peripheral blood mononuclear cells) have been measured in patients with acute GVHD and other endothelial complications, such as hepatic veno-occlusive disease (VOD) (139–142). Furthermore, a phase I/II trial using TNF-α receptor mAbs during the conditioning regimen as prophylaxis in patients at high risk for severe acute GVHD showed reduction in lesions of the intestine, skin, and liver, although GVHD flared after discontinuation of treatment (132). Collectively, these data might suggest that approaches to limit TNF-α secretion will be a very important avenue of investigation in allogeneic SCT.

IL-1 is the second major pro-inflammatory cytokine that contributes to acute GVHD toxicity. Secretion of IL-1 appears to occur predominantly during the effector phase of GVHD in the spleen and skin, two major GVHD target organs (143). A similar increase in mononuclear cell IL-1 mRNA has been shown during clinical acute GVHD (141). Although the use of an IL-1 receptor antagonist (IL-1RA) appeared promising in murine studies (144,145), a recent randomized trial of IL-1RA to prevent acute GVHD was not successful (146).

Finally, macrophages can produce significant amounts of NO as a result of activation during GVHD. Several studies have shown that NO contributes to the deleterious effects GVHD on target tissues and specifically to GVHD-induced immunosuppression (72,147). NO also inhibits repair mechanisms of target tissue by inhibiting proliferation of epithelial stem cells in the gut and skin (148). In humans and rats, development of GVHD is preceded by an increase in NO products in the serum (149,150).

3.   Lipopolysaccharide and Innate Immunity

During GVHD, cytokines (including IFN-γ) prime mononuclear cells. The secretion of inflammatory cytokines by these primed monocytes/macrophages occurs after stimulation by a second signal. This signal may be provided by LPS and other microbial products that have leaked though an intestinal mucosa damaged initially by SCT conditioning regimens during step 1. Since the GI tract is known to be particularly sensitive to the injurious effects of cytokines (130,151), damage to the GI tract incurred during the effector phase can lead to a positive feedback loop wherein increased translocation of LPS results in further cytokine production and progressive intestinal injury. Thus, the GI tract may be critical to propagating the "cytokine storm" characteristic of acute GVHD; increasing experimental and clinical evidence suggests that damage to the GI tract during acute GVHD plays a major role in the amplification of systemic disease (152).

This conceptual framework underscores the role of LPS in the development of acute GVHD, is suggested by several groups (74,151,153). LPS is a major structural component of gram-negative bacteria and is a potent stimulator of cellular activation and cytokine release (154,155). LPS shed from bacteria that comprise normal bowel flora can elicit a broad range of inflammatory responses from macrophages, monocytes, and neutrophils. In particular, LPS may stimulate gut-associated lymphocytes and macrophages (74). Following allogeneic SCT, LPS accumulates in both the liver and spleen of animals with GVHD prior to its appearance in the systemic circulation (153). Elevated serum levels of LPS have been shown to correlate directly with the degree of intestinal histopathology occurring after allogeneic SCT (151,156,157). The severity of GVHD also appears to be directly related to the level of macrophage priming (74). Injection of small, normally nonlethal amounts of LPS caused elevated TNF-α serum levels and death in animals with GVHD, which could be prevented with anti-TNF-α antiserum.

Mice known to be sensitive or resistant to LPS have been used as stem cell donors in order to determine the effect of donor responsiveness to LPS on the development of acute GVHD. C3Heb/Fej animals exhibit normal sensitivity to LPS challenge (LPS-s), whereas the receptor responsible for LPS signaling, a genetic mutation in the Toll-like receptor 4 of C3H/Hej mice, has made this strain resistant to LPS (LPS-r) (158–161). These defects are specific to LPS, and, importantly, T cells from LPS resistant mice respond normally to mitogen and alloantigen (162,163). In an irradiated parent (P) $\rightarrow$ F1 hybrid murine model of GVHD, SCT with LPS-r donor cells resulted in a significant reduction of TNF-α levels. GI tract histopathology, and systemic GVHD compared to animals receiving LPS-s SCT (151). Systemic neutralization of TNF-α further decreased the severity of intestinal and systemic GVHD in LPS-r SCT recipients (151).

Recent experiments using animals deficient in CD14 as SCT donors extend these observations. CD14, a cell surface protein on mononuclear cells and macrophages, is the principal receptor for the complex of LPS and its soluble LPS-binding protein (LBP) (164). The engagement of CD14 by LPS/LPB results in the association of the CD14 molecules with Toll-like receptors and subsequent intracellular signaling and cytokine synthesis during innate immune responses (49). Mononuclear cells from CD14-deficient (CD14−/−) animals are insensitive to LPS stimulation in vitro, and such mice are resistant to the lethal effects of LPS challenge in vivo (165). Transplantation of CD14−/− donor cells into irradiated allogeneic recipients reduces serum TNF-α levels and decreases gut histopathology compared to controls, resulting in less GVHD and improved long-term survival (166).

Data supporting a role for LPS in the GVH response are also provided by both experimental and clinical studies examining the effects of decontamination of the GI tract on the incidence of GVHD. Early animal studies showed that death from GVHD could be prevented if transplanted mice were given antibiotics to decontaminate the gut; normalization of the gut flora at or before day 20 abrogated this effect (167). After clinical SCT, endotoxemia is associated with biochemical parameters of intestinal injury, hepatic toxicity, acute GVHD, and fever in the absence of bacteremia (156,157). Further support is derived from studies where gram-negative gut decontamination during SCT reduces GVHD (168,169), and the degree of the decontamination predicts GVHD severity (170,171). Naturally occurring antibody titers to a rough-mutant strain of *Escherichia coli* J5 are also associated with a decreased incidence of acute GVHD after allogeneic SCT (172). Use of a polyclonal antiserum against *E. coli* J5 as prophylaxis for acute GVHD in a prospective, placebo-controlled trial reduced overall GVHD from 63% to 42%. The antiserum was particularly efficacious in a subset of patients with severe GVHD (173).

Blockade of cellular activation by LPS after allogeneic SCT has been studied using B975, a synthetic analog of *E. coli* lipid A that belongs to a family of potent antagonists of LPS-induced cellular activation (174). These molecules competitively inhibit LPS binding to its receptors and block NFκB activation and nuclear translocation. They are active both in vitro and in vivo and are devoid of agonistic activity even at high doses (174). Treatment of allogeneic BMT recipients with B975 for the first week after transplant blocked mononuclear cell responses to LPS and resulted in decreased inflammatory cytokine release and reduced GVHD severity. Importantly, LPS antagonism had no effect on donor T-cell responses to host antigens, and treatment with B975 did not diminish GVL effects and improved leukemia-free survival.

Collectively, the data outlined above demonstrate a critical role for LPS to the early inflammatory events responsible for GI toxicity and subsequent mortality from GVHD; LPS acts via a positive feedback mechanism to amplify intestinal injury by triggering cytokine release. These data provide the rationale for testing strategies that strengthen the mucosal lining of the GI tract in order to reduce or prevent GVHD. Hypothetically, such an approach would block immune dysregulation before the inflammatory cytokine cascade is initiated, maintain the integrity of the GI mucosal barrier, and limit translocation of immunostimulatory molecules (including endogenous LPS) into the circulation. Because direct shielding of the GI tract is not feasible, this effort would utilize pharmacological agents that provide a "cytokine shield" to reduce gut mucosal injury incurred initially by the effects of SCT conditioning regimens and ultimately by the direct effects of GVHD.

Keratinocyte growth factor (KGF) is a member of the fibroblast growth factor family (FGF-7) that stimulates growth of cells that express its receptors such as gut epithelial cells, hepatocytes, keratinocytes, and alveolar type II cells (175–177). KGF has been studied extensively for its cytoprotective properties against chemotherapeutic and radiation toxicity to a variety of tissues including the bowel, lung, and bladder (178–181). KGF administration prior to autologous SCT in mice protected the GI tract from damage resulting from lethal conditioning (178) and may do so by promoting potent trophic effects on intestinal epithelium and enhancing crypt stem cell survival (175,182). The mechanism of action of KGF is believed to involve regulation of genes that reduce oxidative damage and enhance DNA repair (175,183).

Several recent studies have examined the effects of human recombinant KGF alter experimental allogeneic SCT (184–188). Administration of KGF prior to lethal SCT conditioning significant reduced GVHD mortality and the severity of target organ damage in surviving animals (184,185). Extension of the dosing schedule from day −3 to day +7 abrogated GVHD of the GI tract early after SCT and resulted in further improvement in long-term survival (184). Consistent with the hypothesis that protection of the GI mucosa could block the inflammatory cascade of GVHD, KGF prevented the translocation of LPS into the circulation and resulted in a significant reduction in systemic TNF-α. Thus the protection afforded by KGF was attributed directly to its trophic effects on the intestinal epithelium, aborting the destructive and atrophic phase of GI GVHD, and indirectly to a significant reduction in systemic cytokine dysregulation. KGF has also been shown to attenuate glutathione depletion and organ injury from reactive oxygen species and upregulate the secretion of anti-inflammatory cytokines after experimental SCT (186–188). Moreover, KGF has also been shown to facilitate alloengraftment and ameliorate GVHD in mice by a mechanism that is independent of a reparative response to conditioning-induced tissue damage (186). Importantly, KGF administration does not protect malignant cell lines from chemoradiotherapy and preserved donor cytolytic T-cell responses and allospecific GVL effects after SCT (184).

Based upon these preclinical data, two phase I/II clinical trials are underway to determine the safety and efficacy of KGF when administered along with methotrexate and tacrolimus or cyclosporine prior to either matched related or mismatched related/unrelated donor SCT. In the mismatched related/unrelated donor setting, KGF is administered 3 consecutive days prior to the conditioning regimen and then for 3 consecutive days each week starting at day 0, with a dose escalation planned at 2-week intervals to a total of 36 possible injections of KGF (9 weeks of therapy). Preliminary data from this schedule escalation trial suggest that KGF can be administered safely and that its potential efficacy in preventing GVHD may be schedule dependent; of 9 evaluable patients, all 4 receiving 6 doses of KGF developed grade II–IV acute GVHD compared to 1 of 5 patients receiving 12–18 doses of KGF (189). These early results at higher KGF doses compare favorably to historical controls in whom the incidence of acute GVHD is 50–75% in this high-risk group of patients. Taken together, experimental and preliminary clinical results suggest that KGF may hold promise as a non–cross-reactive adjunct to standard GVHD prophylaxis and as a novel strategy to effectively separate the toxicity of GVHD from the desirable GVL effects.

4. Inflammatory Chemokines

Regulation of effector cell migration into target tissues during the development of GVHD occurs in a complex milieu of chemotactic signals where several chemokine receptors may be triggered simultaneously or successively. Inflammatory chemokines expressed in inflamed tissues are specialized to recruit effector cells such as T cells, neutrophils, and monocytes (190). Chemokine receptors are differentially expressed on subsets of activated/effector T cells. Upon stimulation, T cells can rapidly switch chemokine receptor expression, acquiring new migratory capacity (34,191). The involvement of inflammatory chemokines and their receptors in GVHD has been recently investigated in mouse models of GVHD. MIP-1α recruits CCR5+ CD8+ T cells into the liver, lung, and spleen during GVHD (192,193), and levels of several chemokines are elevated in GVHD-associated lung injury (194). Chemokine gradients may play a role in the unusual target organ distribution of GVHD; a recent paper showed that CCR5 appears essential for donor T-cell homing to Peyer's patches and the subsequent development of lethal GVHD (195). Further studies will help to determine whether expression of specific chemokines and their receptors control the homing of effector cells to GVHD target organs (skin, gut, and liver), and whether these molecules will prove to be potential targets for modulation of GVHD. This topic is reviewed in detail in Chapter 5.

II. GVHD PREVENTION AND TREATMENT: TRANSLATION TO CLINICAL SCT

In general, strategies to prevent and treat GVHD have been based on an "oncological" model of the disease, i.e., the notion that since GVHD is dangerous and life-threatening, management requires the utilization of high-dose immunosuppressant regimens. High doses of multiple immunosuppressive agents have been used much like we use combination chemotherapy to treat malignancies. While there is often reasonable control of the clinical manifestations of GVHD, this broadly aggressive approach is often associated with opportunistic infections, lymphoproliferative disorders, or relapse of the underlying malignancy. Indeed, infection often results in mortality while GVHD is in remission.

The three-phase model of GVHD presented here suggests that the disease is an exaggerated and dysregulated response of a normal immune system to tissue damage that is intrinsic to transplantation. The donor's immune system reacts as if there is a massive and uncontrolled infection, and its attempts to deal with this injury result in the clinical manifestations of GVHD. The tissue injury intrinsic to the administration of high-dose chemoradiotherapy initiates the breakdown of mucosal barriers, allowing endotoxin into the tissues. Toll-like receptors on dendritic cells bind to endotoxin and activate signal transduction pathways that lead to dendritic cell maturation and induce inflammation (196). The upregulation of co-stimulatory molecules, MHC molecules, adhesion molecules, cytokines, chemokines, prostanoids, and other inflammatory mediators prime and trigger attack on target tissues, fueling the fire. It is likely that components of a cytokine storm (197), the danger hypothesis (32), and more traditional notions of adaptive and innate immunity (198) all apply to the disease process.

A. Step 1: Reduced Intensity Conditioning Regimens

The three cardinal organs affected by GVHD are skin, intestinal tract, and liver. One common thread linking the three would seem to be exposure to the environment. Skin and gut have very obvious barrier functions and a well-developed reticuloendothelial system. Similarly, the liver is the first line of defense downstream of the gut. One would expect the lung to be a similar target, and we argue elsewhere in this volume (Chapter 11) that it should be considered as such. It may be that less intense exposure to organisms, particularly gram-negative rods, reduces the manifestations of acute GVHD in the lung. All of these organs are rich in dendritic cells, a probable prerequisite for antigen presentation and the generation of injurious cytokines. They are all subject to injury from conditioning, and breaches of the barrier would allow organisms or endotoxin into the circulation.

One prediction of this model is that less intense conditioning regimens would be associated with less GVHD. For example, when donor lymphocyte infusions were administered without pharmacological GVHD prophylaxis, the resultant GVHD has been less frequent and severe than would be expected in the absence of immunosuppressive drugs (reviewed in Chapter 19). Similarly, the GVHD expected after reduced-intensity conditioning regimens might be less severe both through less cellular injury per se and through a reduction in endotoxin exposure by virtue of less mucosal injury (see also Chapter 18). Thus, while data on reducing both colonization with bacteria and reducing tissue injury with less intense regimens are suggestive and support the basic concepts described above, the effect is insufficient to control GVHD adequately in human transplantation.

B.   Step 2: Modulation of Donor T Cells

1.   Reduced T-Cell Numbers

Elimination of T cells with monoclonal antibodies, immunotoxins, lectins, CD34 columns, or physical techniques is effective at reducing GVHD. T-cell depletion of marrow is relatively straightforward because the number of T cells in the marrow is low compared with the total nucleated cell count, making it relatively easy to manipulate in the laboratory. As the use of peripheral blood stem cells has become more prevalent, the 10-fold increase in number of T cells is a technical challenge. A typical unmanipulated marrow transplant entails the infusion of $\sim 10^7$ T cells per kg of recipient weight. A T-cell dose of $\leq 10^5$ per kg has been associated with complete control of GVHD (4). More recently, the combination of very high stem cell numbers and CD3 T cell numbers $<3 \times 10^4$ per kg allowed haploidentical transplantation without GVHD (199).

Depletion of all T cells from the marrow using a broad panel of monoclonal antibodies has been largely abandoned because of the risk of graft failure (200). However, it is clear that even depletion of T-cell subsets must be undertaken with caution. Depletion of CD8+ T cells alone may be associated with a high graft failure rate (201–202). However, depletion of CD5+ or CD6+ T cells seems to be associated with a low graft failure rate (203,204). Presumably host immune cells that survive the initial conditioning are responsible for graft rejection. When the stem cell source is rich in T cells, the GVH reaction further reduces the residual population capable of alloreactivity, thus decreasing graft rejection. To some degree the higher graft failure rates may be controlled by increasing the intensity of the immunosuppression of the conditioning regimen (201,205) or by adding back T cells (206). Additional problems associated with T-cell depletion include a higher incidence of Epstein-Barr virus–induced lymphoproliferative disorders, loss of the graft-vs.-leukemia effect and a consequent increase in relapses, and slower immunological recovery due to reduced transfer of donor immunocompetent donor T cells. These issues are reviewed in detail in Chapter 17. In no case has there been an improvement in survival that can be definitively attributed to T-cell depletion.

Since activated T cells contribute to GVHD and resting T cells presumably have other, potentially useful specificities, selective elimination of activated populations might be of some interest. Treatment of established GVHD with specific T-cell antibodies has produced mixed results. While antithymocyte globulin has definite activity in established GVHD, the nonspecific clearance of T cells may result in increased opportunistic infections and no improvement in survival (207–209). More specific therapies such as the humanized anti-IL-2 receptor antibody daclizumab (210,211) or the humanized anti-CD3 antibody visilizumab (212) are promising because they offer the potential selectively removing the activated T cells. However, an increased risk of infection may still be observed (213).

2.   Reduced T-Cell Activation

The introduction of cyclosporine in the late 1970s was a significant advance in GVHD prevention. More recently, a similar agent, tacrolimus, has been shown to provide similar control of GVHD. Both drugs inhibit T-lymphocyte activation, and they are reviewed in detail in Chapter 15.

As a single agent, cyclosporine was about as effective as methotrexate (214). However, in combination with methotrexate, there was a significant reduction in the incidence of GVHD and an improvement in survival (215). Subsequent trials of tacrolimus and methotrexate compared with cyclosporine and methotrexate showed no advantage for either combination (216,217). The addition of prednisone to the conventional two-drug regimen resulted in similar rates of GVHD and no improvement in survival (218).

Dendritic cells appear to be critical to the development of acute GVHD (16,195), and interference with dendritic cell function may be a prophylactic strategy. DC2 seem to foster Th2 responses, which are less likely to result in GVHD. Preliminary data suggest that extracorporeal photopheresis (ECP) may result in attenuation of Th1-mediated cytokine secretion, a shift in the DC1/DC2 ratio favoring plasmacytoid rather than monocytoid dendritic cell profiles, and a decrease in antigen responsiveness by dendritic cells (219,220). Campath, an anti-CD52 monoclonal antibody, targets all white blood cells: B cells, T cells, monocytes, and DCs. When the drug was administered prior to transplantation, host DCs were selectively depleted and the donor DCs repopulated the recipient (221). These observations are difficult to separate from concomitant T-cell depletion, but they are consistent with the theme that facilitation of DC turnover may ameliorate GVHD. Finally, flt3 ligand therapy has shown similar effects on DC function and reduced GVHD in mice (222). Human trials should be very interesting.

3.   Reduced T-Cell Proliferation

The first generally prescribed GVHD-preventive regimen was the administration of intermittent low-dose methotrexate as developed in a dog model by Thomas and Storb (223). The principle of this approach was to administer a cell cycle–specific chemo-therapeutic agent immediately after transplant, when donor T cells have started to divide after stimulation by exposure to allogeneic antigens. Subsequently, the addition of anti-thymocyte globulin, prednisone, or both resulted in incremental improvement in the GVHD rate but no improvement in survival (224,225). Ultimately the course of methotrexate was abbreviated and combined with a T-cell activation inhibitor, such as cyclosporine or tacrolimus.

More recently, mycophenolate mofetil (MMF), the prodrug of mycophenolic acid (MPA), has been used to inhibit inosine monophosphate dehydrogenase, an enzyme critical to the de novo synthesis of guanosine nucleotide. Since T lymphocytes are more dependent on such synthesis than myeloid or mucosal cells, MPA preferentially inhibits proliferative responses of T cells and may be useful in the prevention of GVHD (226).

Sirolimus (rapamycin) is a macrocyclic lactone immunosuppressant that is similar in structure to tacrolimus and cyclosporine. All three drugs bind to immunophilins; however, sirolimus complexed with FKBP12 inhibits T-cell proliferation by interfering with signal transduction and cell cycle progression. The sirolimus:FKBP12 complex binds to mammalian target of rapamycin (mTOR), which blocks IL-2–mediated signal transduction pathways that prevent G1 → S phase transition (227). The drug has similar effects on proliferation of T cells induced by IL-2, IL-4, IL-7, IL-12, and IL-15. In addition, sirolimus contributes to massive T-cell apoptosis if signals 1 and 2 of T-cell activation are blocked—an effect that is not seen with cyclosporine (228). Sirolimus has excellent antirejection activity in organ transplantation (229), and combination therapy with sirolimus and tacrolimus appears to be extremely effective in preventing rejection of human organ allografts (230,231) and in preventing GVHD in murine models (232,233). Because sirolimus acts through a separate mechanism from the tacrolimus-FKBP complex (and cyclosporine-cyclophilin complex), it is synergistic with both tacrolimus and cyclosporine.

C. Step 3: Blockade of Inflammatory Stimulation and Effectors

1. Reduced Exposure to Organisms

Another hypothesis that flows from the three-step model of acute GVHD is that reduction of intestinal colonization with bacteria could prevent GVHD. Animal studies in germ-free environments support this notion, where GVHD was not observed until mice were colonized with gram-negative organisms (167). Later, gut decontamination and use of a laminar air flow environment was associated with less GVHD and better survival in patients with severe aplastic anemia (168). Similarly, studies of intestinal decontamination in patients with malignancies have shown less GVHD in some (170,171) but not all studies (234). As noted above, drugs that enhance the proliferation of GI mucosa such as KGF can prevent the systemic translocation of these inflammatory stimuli and prevent GVHD in preclinical models. Early phase I/II trials of this drug are currently in progress.

2. Blockade of Inflammatory Effectors

An important role for TNF-α in clinical acute GVHD was suggested by observations of elevated levels of TNF-α in the serum of patients with acute GVHD and other endothelial complications such as veno-occlusive disease (139,140,235). Importantly, the first appearance of the increased levels predicted the severity of complications and overall survival. Patients with higher serum TNF-α levels during the conditioning regimen had a 90% incidence of grade II or greater acute GVHD and an overall mortality of 70%, compared with a mortality of 20% in patients without TNF-α elevations (140). Murine monoclonal antibodies or F(ab)$_2'$ fragments directed at TNF-α have been studied either as therapy for steroid-resistant GVHD (132) or as prophylaxis (236). There were no complete responses in the patients with uncontrolled GVHD, but some partial responses were observed. Recently, therapy of GVHD with humanized anti-TNF-α (infliximab) (237,238) or a dimeric fusion protein consisting of the extracellular ligand-binding portion of the human TNF-α receptor (TNFR) linked to the Fc portion of human IgG1 (etanercept) (239) have shown some promise.

The second major proinflammatory cytokine that appears to play an important role in the effector phase of acute GVHD is IL-1. This cytokine is produced mainly by activated mononuclear phagocytes, and it shares with TNF-α a wide variety of biological activities (240). In a murine model, secretion of IL-1 occurred predominantly during the effector phase of GVHD in the spleen and skin, two major GVHD target organs (143). IL-1 receptor antagonist (IL-1RA) is a naturally occurring pure competitive inhibitor of IL-1 that is produced by monocytes/macrophages and keratinocytes. Interestingly, the IL-1RA gene is polymorphic, and the presence in the donor of the allele that is linked to higher secretion of IL-1RA was associated with less acute GVHD (241). In a murine model of GVHD to multiple mHAgs, intraperitoneal administration of recombinant IL-1RA for 10 days after BMT prevented the development of GVHD in the majority of animals (242). Two phase I/II clinical trials of IL-1RA showed promise and resulted in remissions in 50–60% of patients with steroid-resistant GVHD (243,244). However, a subsequent randomized trial of the addition of IL-1RA or placebo to cyclosporine and methotrexate beginning at the time of conditioning and continuing through day 14 after stem cell infusion did not show any protective effect of the drug (146). Thus, at least as administered in that study, IL-1 inhibition by IL-1RA was insufficient to prevent GVHD in humans. IL-11 was also able to protect the GI tract in animal models and prevent GVHD (245,246), but it did not prevent clinical GVHD (219). Thus, not all preclinical data successfully translates to new therapies.

IL-6 might be expected to play a role in the pathophysiology of GVHD, particularly since it is known to have inflammatory properties and is induced in monocytes after stimulation by IFN-γ and TNF-α. Little experimental work has been done in animal models, but there are reports of elevated serum IL-6 levels in patients with acute GVHD and hepatorenal syndrome (247) and in patients with transplant-related toxicities after autologous BMT (248). However, IL-6 levels may respond to many stimuli and the lack of specificity may limit the utility of blood measurements. IL-8, also called neutrophil-activating peptide (NAP-1), may also play a role in GVHD. IL-8 is produced in response to inflammatory mediators such as endotoxin, IL-1, and TNF-α, and its systemic administration inhibits the adhesion of leukocytes to endothelial surfaces. A recent study reported that among patients receiving BMT for β-thalassemia, those with GVHD showed significantly elevated IL-8 blood levels compared to those without GVHD (249). An interesting implication of this observation is that granulocytes and macrophages may contribute to GVHD pathology, and in fact most GVHD occurs after leukocyte recovery. These kinetics are typically interpreted as a reflection of the time necessary for lymphocytes to expand to a critical mass. However, it might equally suggest that the inflammatory cytokine network also activates and recruits neutrophils, and that these newly produced myeloid cells follow chemotactic signals to injured epithelium, where they contribute to tissue injury by releasing activated oxygen metabolites as well as cytotoxic and proteolytic enzymes.

III. SYNGENEIC GRAFT-VS.-HOST DISEASE

In experimental models, pathological changes of GVHD have been observed in animals receiving marrow transplants from genetically identical donors (or even autologous marrow transplants), findings that substantiate the reports of GVHD occurring in recipients of transplants from their identical twin donors, described over a decade ago (250). This syngeneic GVHD appears to be mediated by autoreactive lymphocytes directed at MHC class II proteins (251). Autoreactive T cells are thought to develop in a severely damaged thymic medulla where MHC class II–bearing cells are deficient or absent. T cells thus escape the usual negative selection (clonal deletion) within the thymus and migrate to the periphery, where they trigger or mediate target organ damage. Other regulatory lymphocytes, which would normally inactivate or eliminate such autoreactive cells, have themselves been eliminated by total body irradiation (as part of the preparative regimen). The experimental transfer of normal lymphocytes to these irradiated hosts restores the regulatory mechanism and prevents the autoaggressive process. The effects of cyclosporine are important in these models, both in preventing the reestablishment of regulatory cells and in allowing the development of autoreactive cells; these two processes seem related to the damage that cyclosporine inflicts on the thymic medulla (252).

These findings have recently been confirmed in a different model where the lack of MHC class II expression on thymic APCs prevented negative selection and caused an autoimmune disease that was indistinguishable from acute GVHD and that could be reduced by blockade of inflammatory cytokines (253). Thus, syngeneic GVHD can be seen as an imbalance between autoreactive and autoregulatory lymphocytes, an imbalance that results from thymic dysfunction. In experimental animals, cutaneous pathological findings of syngeneic and chronic GVHD are similar, and it appears that the efferent arms of syngeneic and chronic GVHD may be similar if not identical. In humans the development of chronic GVHD after syngeneic transplantation has not been convincingly demonstrated.

IV. CONCLUSIONS

Complications of BMT, particularly GVHD, remain major barriers to the wider application of allogeneic BMT for a variety of diseases. Recent advances in the understanding of cytokine networks as well as the direct mediators of cellular cytotoxicity have led to improved understanding of this complex disease process. GVHD can be considered an exaggerated, undesirable manifestation of a normal inflammatory mechanism in which donor lymphocytes encounter foreign antigens in a milieu that fosters inflammation. Tissue injury related to the conditioning regimen or infection is then amplified by direct cytotoxicity via perforin-granzyme and Fas-FasL pathways, through direct cytokine-induced damage, and by recruitment of secondary effectors such as granulocytes and monocytes. Cytokine dysregulation may further result in the production of secondary mediators such as nitric oxide. The net effects of this complex system are the severe inflammatory manifestations that we recognize as clinical GVHD.

REFERENCES

1. Barnes D, Loutit J. Treatment of murine leukaemia with x-rays and homologous bone marrow. Br J Haematol 1957; 3:241–252.
2. Billingham RE. The biology of graft-versus-host reactions. Harvey Lec 1966; 62:21–78.
3. Korngold R, Sprent J. T cell subsets in graft-vs.-host disease. In: Burakoff SJ, Deeg HJ, Ferrara J, Atkinson K, eds. Graft-vs.-Host Disease: Immunology, Pathophysiology, and Treatment. New York: Marcel Dekker, 1990:31–50.
4. Kernan NA, Collins NH, Juliano L, Cartagena T, Dupont B, O'Reilly RJ. Clonable T lymphocytes in T cell-depleted bone marrow transplants correlate with development of graft-v-host disease. Blood 1986; 68:770–773.
5. Zeng D, Lewis D, Dejbakhsh-Jones S, Lan F, Garcia-Ojeda M, Sibley R, Strober S. Bone marrow NK1.1(−) and NK1.1(+) T cells reciprocally regulate acute graft versus host disease. J Exp Med 1999; 189:1073–1081.
6. Anderson KC. Transfusion-associated graft-versus-host disease. In: Ferrara JLM, Deeg HJ, Burakoff SJ, eds. Graft-vs.-Host Disease. New York: Marcel Dekker, 1997:587–605.
7. Krensky AM, Weiss A, Crabtree G, Davis MM, Parham P. T-lymphocyte-antigen interactions in transplant rejection. N Engl J Med 1990; 322:510–517.
8. Rappaport H, Khalil A, Halle-Pannenko O, Pritchard L, Dantchev D, Mathe G. Histopathologic sequence of events in adult mice undergoing lethal graft-versus-host reactions developed across H-2 and/or non H-2 histocompatbility barriers. Am J Pathol 1979; 96:121–142.
9. Hess AD, Fischer AC. Immune mechanisms in cyclosporine-induced syngeneic graft-versus-host disease. Transplantation 1989; 48:895–900.
10. Fefer A, Sullivan K, Weiden P. Graft versus leukemia effect in man: the relapse rate of acute leukemia is lower after allogeneic than after syngeneic marrow transplantation. In: Truitt R, Gale R, Bortin M, eds. Cellular Immunotherapy of Cancer. New York: AR Liss, 1987:401–408.
11. Clift RA, Buckner CD, Appelbaum FR, Bearman SI, Petersen FB, Fisher LB, Anasetti C, Beatty P, Bensigner WI, Doney K, Hill RS, McDonald GB, Martin P, Sanders J, Singer J, Stewart P, Sullivan KM, Witherspoon R, Storb R, Hansen JA, Thomas ED. Allogeneic marrow transplantation in patients with acute myeloid leukemia in first remission: a randomized trial of two irradiation regimens. Blood 1990; 76: 1867–1871.

12. Ringden O. Viral infections and graft-vs.-host disease. In: Burakoff SJ, Deeg HJ, Ferrara J, Atkinson K, eds. Graft-vs.-Host Disease. New York: Marcel Dekker, 1990:467.
13. Xun CQ, Thompson JS, Jennings CD, Brown SA, Widmer MB. Effect of total body irradiation, busulfan-cyclophosphamide, or cyclophosphamide conditioning on inflammatory cytokine release and development of acute and chronic graft-versus-host disease in H-2-incompatible transplanted SCID mice. Blood 1994; 83:2360–2367.
14. Paris F, Fuks Z, Kang A, Capodieci P, Juan G, Ehleiter D, Haimovitz-Friedman A, Cordon-Cardo C, Kolesnick R. Endothelial apoptosis as the primary lesion initiating intestinal radiation damage in mice. Science 2001; 293:293–297.
15. Hill GR, Crawford JM, Cooke KJ, Brinson YS, Pan L, Ferrara JLM. Total body irradiation and acute graft versus host disease. The role of gastrointestinal damage and inflammatory cytokines. Blood 1997; 90:3204–3213.
16. Shlomchik WD, Couzens MS, Tang CB, McNiff J, Robert ME, Liu J, Shlomchik MJ, Emerson SG. Prevention of graft versus host disease by inactivation of host antigen-presenting cells. Science 1999; 285:412–415.
17. Teshima T, Ordemann R, Reddy P, Gagin S, Liu C, Cooke KR, Ferrara JL. Acute graft-versus-host disease does not require alloantigen expression on host epithelium. Nat Med 2002; 8:575–581.
18. Newton-Nash DK. The molecular basis of allorecognition. Assessment of the involvement of peptide. Hum Immunol 1994; 41:105–111.
19. Sayegh MH, Perico N, Gallon L, Imberti O, Hancock WW, Remuzzi G, Carpenter CB. Mechanisms of acquired thymic unresponsiveness to renal allografts. Thymic recognition of immunodominant allo-MHC peptides induces peripheral T cell anergy. Transplantation 1994; 58:125–132.
20. Sprent J, Schaefer M, Gao EK, Korngold R. Role of T cell subsets in lethal graft-versus-host disease (GVHD) directed to class I versus class II H-2 differences. I. L3T4+ cells can either augment or retard GVHD elicited by Lyt-2 + cells in class I different hosts. J Exp Med 1988; 167:556–569.
21. Goumy L, Ferran C, Merite S, Bach J-F, Chatenoud L. In vivo anti-CD3-driven cell activation. Transplantation 1996; 61:83–87.
22. Doolittle DP, Davission MT, Guidi JN, Green MC. Catalog of mutant genes and polymorphic loci. In: Lyon MF, Tastan S, Brown SDM, eds. Genetic Variants and Strains of Laboratory Mouse. New York: Oxford University Press, 1996:17–854.
23. Choi EY, Christianson GJ, Yoshimura Y, Jung N, Sproule TJ, Malarkannan S, Joyce S, Roopenian DC. Real-time T-cell profiling identifies H60 as a major minor histocompatibility antigen in murine graft-versus-host disease. Blood 2002; 100:4259–4265.
24. Goulmy E, Schipper R, Pool J, Blokland E, Falkenburg F. Mismatches of minor histo-compatibility antigens between HLA-identical donors and recipients and the development of graft-versus-host disease after bone marrow transplantation. N Engl J Med 1996; 334:281–285.
25. Nash A, Pepe MS, Storb R, Longton G, Pettinger M, Anasetti C, Appelbaum FR, Bowden RA, Deeg HJ, Doney K, Martin PJ, Sullivan KM, Sanders J, Witherspoon R. Acute graft-versus-host disease analysis of risk factors after allogeneic marrow transplantation and prophylaxis with cyclosporine and methotrexate. Blood 1992; 80:1838–1845.
26. Hansen JA, Gooley TA, Martin PJ, Appelbaum F, Chauncey TR, Clift RA, Petersdorf EW, Radich J, Sanders JE, Storb RF, Sullivan KM, Anasetti C. Bone marrow transplants from unrelated donors for patients with chronic myeloid leukemia. N Engl J Med 1998; 338:962–968.
27. Goulmy E. Human minor histocompatibility antigens: new concepts for marrow transplantation and adoptive immunotherapy. Immunol Rev 1997; 157:125–140.
28. Dickinson AM, Wang XN, Sviland L, Vyth-Dreese FA, Jackson GH, Schumacher TN, Haanen JB, Mutis T, Goulmy E. In situ dissection of the graft-versus-host activities of cytotoxic T cells specific for minor histocompatibility antigens. Nat Med 2002; 8:410–414.

29. Dustin ML, Springer TA. T-cell receptor cross-linking transiently stimulates adhesiveness through LFA-1. Nature 1989; 341:619–624.

30. Alegre ML, Frauwirth KA, Thompson CB. T-cell regulation by CD28 and CTLA-4. Nat Rev Immunol 2001; 1:220–228.

31. Slavik JM, Hutchcroft JE, Bierer BE. CD28/CTLA-4 and CD80/CD86 families: signaling and function. Immunol Res 1999; 19:1–24.

32. Matzinger P. The danger model: a renewed sense of self. Science 2002; 296:301–305.

33. Roncarolo MG, Levings MK, Traversari C. Differentiation of T regulatory cells by immature dendritic cells. J Exp Med 2001; 193:F5–F9.

34. Reinhardt RL, Khoruts A, Merica R, Zell T, Jenkins MK. Visualizing the generation of memory CD4 T cells in the whole body. Nature 2001; 410:101–105.

35. Pasare C, Medzhitov R. Toll pathway-dependent blockade of CD4+CD25+ T cell mediated suppression by dendritic cells. Science 2003; 299:1033–1036.

36. Ordemann R, Hutchinson R, Friedman J, Burakoff SJ, Reddy P, Duffner U, Braun TM, Liu C, Teshima T, Ferrara JL. Enhanced allostimulatory activity of host antigen-presenting cells in old mice intensifies acute graft-versus-host disease. J Clin Invest 2002; 109: 1249–1256.

37. Zhang Y, Shlomchik WD, Joe G, Louboutin JP, Zhu J, Rivera A, Giannola D, Emerson SG. APCs in the liver and spleen recruit activated allogeneic CD8+ T cells to elicit hepatic graft-versus-host disease. J Immunol 2002; 169:7111–7118.

38. Ruggen L, Capanni M, Urbani E, Perruccio K, Shlomchik WD, Tosti A, Posati S, Rogaia D, Frassoni F, Aversa F, Martelli MF, Velardi A. Effectiveness of donor natural killer cell alloreactivity in mismatched hematopoietic transplants. Science 2002; 295:2097–2100.

39. Ruggeri L, Capanni M, Martelli MF, Velardi A. Cellular therapy: exploiting NK cell alloreactivity in transplantation. Curr Opin Hematol 2001; 8:355–359.

40. Mosmann TR, Cherwinski H, Bond MW, Giedlin MA, Coffman RL. Two types of murine helper T cell clone. I. Definition according to profiles of lymphokine activities and secreted proteins. J Immunol 1986; 136:2348–2357.

41. Rissoan M, Soumelis V, Kadowaki N, Grouard G, Briere F, de Waal M, Liu Y. Reciprocal control of T helper cell and dendritic cell differentiation. Science 1999; 5405:1183–1186.

42. Reid SD, Penna G, Adonni L. The control of T cell responses by dendritic cell subsets. Curr Opin Immunol 2000; 12:114–121.

43. Carvalho-Pinto CE, Garcia MI, Mellado M, Rodriguez-Frade JM, Martin-Caballero J, Flores J, Martinez AC, Balomenos D. Autocrine production of IFN-gamma by macrophages controls their recruitment to kidney and the development of glomerulonephritis in MRL/lpr mice. J Immunol 2002; 169:1058–1067.

44. Lalor PF, Shields P, Grant A, Adams DH. Recruitment of lymphocytes to the human liver. Immunol Cell Biol 2002; 80:52–64.

45. Via CS, Finkelman FD. Critical role of interleukin-2 in the development of acute graft-versus-host disease. Int Immunol 1993; 5:565–572.

46. Jadus MR, Peck AB. Lethal murine graft-versus-host disease in the absence of detectable cytotoxic T lymphocytes. Transplantation 1983; 36:281–289.

47. Malkovsky M, Brenner MK, Hunt R, et al. T cell-depletion of allogeneic bone marrow prevents acceleration of graft-versus-host disease induced by exogenous interleukin-2. Cell Immunol 1986; 103:476–480.

48. Theobald M, Nierle T, Bunjes D, Arnold R, Heimpel H. Host-specific interleukin-2-secreting donor T-cell precursors as predictors of acute graft-versus-host disease in bone marrow transplantation between HLA-identical siblings. N Engl J Med 1992; 327: 1613–1617.

49. Nierle T, Bunjes D, Arnold R, Heimpel H, Theobald M. Quantitative assessment of posttransplant host-specific interleukin-2-secreting T-helper cell precursors in patients with and without acute graft-versus-host disease after allogeneic HLA-identical sibling bone marrow transplantation. Blood 1993; 81:841–848.

50. Schwarer AP, Jiang YZ, Brookes PA, Barrett AJ, Batchelor JR, Goldman JM, Lechler RI. Frequency of anti-recipient alloreactive helper T-cell precursors in donor blood and graft-versus-host disease after HLA-identical sibling bone-marrow transplantation. Lancet 1993; 341:203–205.

51. Ferrara JLM, Cooke KR, Pan L, Krenger W. The immunopathophysiology of acute graft-versus-host disease. Stem Cells 1996; 14:473–489.

52. Herve P, Wijdenes J, Bergerat JP, Bordigoni P, Milpied N, Cahn JY, Clement C, Beliard R, Morel-Fourrier B, Racadot E, Troussard X, Benz-Lemoine F, Gaud C, Legros M, Attal M, Kloft M, Peters A. Treatment of corticosteroid-resistant acute graft-versus-host disease by in vivo administration of anti-interleukin-2 receptor monoclonal antibody (B-B10). Blood 1990; 75:1017–1023.

53. Anasetti C, Martin PM, Hansen JA, Appelbaum FR, Beatty PG, Doney K, Harkonen S, Jackson A, Reichert T, Stewart P, Storb R, Sullivan K, Donnall Thomas E, Warner N, Witherspoon RP. A phase I–II study evaluating the murine anti-IL-2 receptor antibody 2A3 for treatment of acute graft-versus-host disease. Transplantation 1990; 50:49–54.

54. Belanger C, Esperou-Bourdeau H, Bordigoni P, Jouet JP, Souillet G, Milpied N, Troussard X, Kuentz M, Herve P, Reiffers J, et al. Use of an anti-interleukin-2 receptor monoclonal antibody for GVHD prophylaxis in unrelated donor BMT. Bone Marrow Transplant 1993; 11:293–297.

55. Li XC, Demirci G, Ferrari-Lacraz S, Groves C, Coyle A, Malek TR, Strom TB. IL-15 and IL-2: a matter of life and death for T cells in vivo. Nat Med 2001; 7:114–118.

56. Kumaki S, Minegishi M, Fujie H, Sasahara Y, Ohashi Y, Tsuchiya S, Konno T. Prolonged secretion of IL-15 in patients with severe forms of acute graft-versus-host disease after allogeneic bone marrow transplantation in children. Int J Hematol 1998; 67:307–312.

57. Szebeni J, Wang MG, Pearson DA, Szot GL, Sykes M. IL-2 inhibits early increases in serum gamma interferon levels associated with graft-versus-host disease. Transplantation 1994; 58:1385–1393.

58. Wang MG, Szebeni J, Pearson DA, Szot GL, Sykes M. Inhibition of graft-versus-host disease by interleukin-2 treatment is associated with altered cytokine production by expanded graft-versus-host-reactive CD4+ helper cells. Transplantation 1995; 60:481–490.

59. Troutt AB, Maraskovsky E, Rogers LA, Pech MH, Kelso A. Quantitative analysis of lymphokine expression in vivo and in vitro. Immunol Cell Biol 1992; 70(pt 1):51–57.

60. Velardi A, Varese P, Terenzi A, Dembech C, Albi N, Grossi CE, Moretta L, Martelli MF, Grignani F, Mingari MC. Lymphokine production by T-cell clones after human bone marrow transplantation. Blood 1989; 74:1665–1672.

61. Niederwieser D, Herold M, Woloszczuk W, Aulitsky W, Meister B, Tilg H, Gastl G, Bowden R, Huber C. Endogenous IFN-gamma during human bone marrow transplantation. Transplantation 1990; 50:620–625.

62. Dufour JH, Dziejman M, Liu MT, Leung JH, Lane TE, Luster AD. IFN-gamma-inducible protein 10 (IP-10; CXCL10)-deficient mice reveal a role for IP-10 in effector T cell generation and trafficking. J Immunol 2002; 168:3195–3204.

63. de Veer MJ, Holko M, Frevel M, Walker E, Der S, Paranjape JM, Silverman RH, Williams BR. Functional classification of interferon-stimulated genes identified using microarrays. J Leukoc Biol 2001; 69:912–920.

64. Mohan K, Ding Z, Hanly J, Issekutz TB. IFN-gamma-inducible T cell alpha chemoattractant is a potent stimulator of normal human blood T lymphocyte transendothelial migration: differential regulation by IFN-gamma and TNF-alpha. J Immunol 2002; 168: 6420–6428.

65. Mowat A. Antibodies to IFN-gamma prevent immunological mediated intestinal damage in murine graft-versus-host reactions. Immunology 1989; 68:18–24.

66. Dickinson AM, Sviland L, Dunn J, Carey P, Proctor SJ. Demonstration of direct involvement of cytokines in graft-versus-host reactions using an in vitro skin explant model. Bone Marrow Transplant 1991; 7:209–216.

67. Holda JH, Maier T, Claman NH. Evidence that IFN-g is responsible for natural suppressor activity in GVHD spleen and normal bone marrow. Transplantation 1988; 45:772–777.

68. Wall DA, Hamberg SD, Reynolds DS, Burakoff SJ, Abbas AK, Ferrara JL. Immunodeficiency in graft-versus-host disease. I. Mechanism of immune suppression. J Immunol 1988; 140:2970–2976.

69. Klimpel GR, Annable CR, Cleveland MG, Jerrels TR, Patterson JC. Immunosuppression and lymphoid hypoplasia associated with chronic graft-versus-host disease is dependent upon TFN-g production. J Immunol 1990; 144:84–93.

70. Wall DA, Sheehan KC. The role of tumor necrosis factor-alpha and interferon gamma in graft-versus-host disease and related immunodeficiency. Transplantation 1994; 57:273–279.

71. Huchet R, Bruley-Rosset M, Mathiot C, Grandjon D, Halle-Pannenko O. Involvement of IFN-gamma and transforming growth factor-beta in graft-vs-host reaction-associated immuno-suppression. J Immunol 1993; 150:2517–2524.

72. Krenger W, Falzarano G, Delmonte J, Snyder KM, Byon JCH, Ferrara JLM. Interferon-γ suppresses T-cell proliferation to mitogen via the nitric oxide pathway during experimental acute graft-versus-host disease. Blood 1996; 88:1113–1121.

73. Gifford GE, Lohmann-Matthes M-L. Gamma interferon priming of mouse and human macrophages for induction of tumor necrosis factor production by bacterial lipopolysacchar-ide. J Natl Cancer Inst 1987; 78:121–124.

74. Nestel FP, Price KS, Seemayer TA, Lapp WS. Macrophage priming and lipopolysaccharide-triggered release of tumor necrosis factor alpha during graft-versus host disease. J Exp Med 1992; 175:405–413.

75. Fowler DH, Kurasawa K, Husebekk A, Cohen PA, Gress RE. Cells of the Th2 cytokine phenotype prevent LPS-induced lethality during murine graft-versus-host reaction. J Immunol 1994; 152:1004–1011.

76. Fowler DH, Kurasawa K, Smith R, Eckhaus MA, Gress RE. Donor CD4-enriched cells of Th2 cytokine phenotype regulate graft-versus-host disease without impairing allogeneic engraftment in sublethally irradiated mice. Blood 1994; 84:3540.

77. Krenger W, Snyder KM, Byon CH, Falzarano G, Ferrara JLM. Polarized type 2 alloreactive CD4+ and CD8+ donor T cells fail to induce experimental acute graft-versus-host disease. J Immunol 1995; 155:585–593.

78. Pan L, Delmonte J, Jalonen C, Ferrara J. Pretreatment of donor mice with granulocyte colony-stimulating factor polarizes donor T-lymphocytes toward type-2 cytokine production and reduces severity of experimental graft-versus-host disease. Blood 1995; 86: 4422–4429.

79. Nikolic B, Lee S, Bronson RT, Grusby MJ, Sykes M. Th1 and Th2 mediate acute graft-versus-host disease, each with distinct end-organ targets. J Clin Invest 2000; 105: 1289–1298.

80. Atkinson K, Matias C, Guiffre A, Seymour R, Cooley M, BIggs J, Munro V, Gillis S. In vivo administration of granulocyte colony-stimulating factor (G-CSF), granulocyte-macrophage CSF, interleukin-1 (IL-1), and IL-4, alone and in combination, after allogeneic murine hematopoietic stem cell transplantation. Blood 1991; 77:1376–1382.

81. Krenger W, Snyder K, Smith S, Ferrara JLM. Effects of exogenous interleukin-10 in a murine podel of graft-versus-host disease to minor histocompatibility antigens. Transplantation 1994; 58:1251–1257.

82. Blazar BR, Taylor PA, Smith S, Vallera DA. Interleukin-10 administration decreases survival in murine recipients of major histocompatibility complex disparate donor bone marrow grafts. Blood 1995; 85:842–851.

83. Sykes M, Romick ML, Hoyles KA, Sachs DH. In vivo administration of interleukin 2 plus T cell-depleted syngeneic marrow prevents graft-versus-host disease mortality and permits alloengraftment. J Exp Med 1990; 171:645–658.

84. Brok HPM, Heidt PJ, van der Meide PH, Zurcher C, Vossen JM. Interferon-γ prevents graft-versus-host disease after allogeneic bone marrow transplantation in mice. J Immunol 1993; 151:6451–6459.

85. Gorham JD, Guler ML, Fenoglio D, Gubler U, Murphy KM. Low dose TGF-beta attenuates IL-12 responsiveness in murine Th cells. J Immunol 1998; 161:1664–1670.

86. Dey BR, Yang YG, Szot GL, Pearson DA, Sykes M. Interleukin-12 inhibits graft-versus-host disease through an Fas-mediated mechanism associated with alterations in donor T-cell activation and expansion. Blood 1998; 91:3315–3322.

87. Ellison CA, Fischer JM, HayGlass KT, Gartner JG. Murine graft-versus-host disease in an F1-hybrid model using IFN-gamma gene knockout donors. J Immunol 1998; 161: 631–640.

88. Welniak LA, Blazar BR, Anver MR, Wiltrout RH, Murphy WJ. Opposing roles of interferon-gamma on CD4+ T cell-mediated graft-versus-host disease: effects of conditioning. Biol Blood Marrow Transplant 2000; 6:604–612.

89. Li XC, Strom TB, Turka LA, Wells AD. T cell death and transplantation tolerance. Immunity 2001; 14:407–416.

90. Sykes M, Szot GL, Nguyen PL, Pearson DA. Interleukin-12 inhibits murine graft-versus-host disease. Blood 1995; 86:2429–2438.

91. Reddy P, Teshima T, Kukuruga M, Ordemann R, Liu C, Lowler K, Ferrara JL. Interleukin-18 regulates acute graft-versus-host disease by enhancing Fas-mediated donor T cell apoptosis. J Exp Med 2001; 194:1433–1440.

92. Jonuleit H, Schmitt E, Schuler G, Knop J, Enk AH. Induction of interleukin 10-producing, nonproliferating CD4(+) T cells with regulatory properties by repetitive stimulation with allogeneic immature human dendritic cells. J Exp Med 2000; 192:1213–1222.

93. Zeller JC, Panoskaltsis-Mortari A, Murphy WJ, Ruscetti FW, Narula S, Roncarolo MG, Blazar BR. Induction of CD4+ T cell alloantigen-specific hyporesponsiveness by IL-10 and TGF-beta. J Immunol 1999; 163:3684–3691.

94. Boussiotis VA, Chen ZM, Zeller JC, Murphy WJ, Berezovskaya A, Narula S, Roncarolo MG, Blazar BR. Altered T-cell receptor + CD28-mediated signaling and blocked cell cycle progression in interleukin 10 and transforming growth factor-beta-treated alloreactive T cells that do not induce graft-versus-host disease. Blood 2001; 97:565–571.

95. Rolink AG, Gleichmann E. Allosuppressor- and allohelper-T cells in acute and chronic graft-versus-host (GVH) disease. III. Different Lyt subsets of donor T cells induce different pathological syndromes. J Exp Med 1983; 158:546–558.

96. Hurtenbach U, Shearer GM. Analysis of murine T lymphocyte markers during the early phases of GvH-associated suppression of cytotoxic T lymphocyte responses. J Immunol 1983; 130:1561–1566.

97. Autran B, Leblond V, Sadat-Sowti B, Lefranc E, Got P, Sutton L, Binet JL, Debre P. A soluble factor released by CD8+CD57+ lymphocytes from bone marrow transplanted patients inhibits cell-mediated cytolysis. Blood 1991; 77:2237–2241.

98. Tsoi MS, Storb R, Dobbs S, Kopecky K, Santos E, Wieden P, Thomas ED. Nonspecific suppressor cells in patients with chronic graft-versus-host disease after marrow grafting. J Immunol 1979; 123:1970–1973.

99. Strober S. Natural suppressor (NS) cells, neonatal tolerance, and total lymphoid irradiation: exploring obscure relationships. Annu Rev Immunol 1984; 2:219–237.

100. Lan F, Zeng D, Higuchi M, Huie P, Higgins JP, Strober S. Predominance of NK1.1+TCR alpha beta+ or DX5+TCR alpha beta+ T cells in mice conditioned with fractionated lymphoid irradiation protects against graft-versus-host disease: "natural suppressor" cells. J Immunol 2001; 167:2087–2096.

101. Eberl G, MacDonald HR. Rapid death and regeneration of NKT cells in an anti-CD3epsilon- or IL-12-treated mice: a major role for bone marrow in NKT cell homeostasis. Immunity 1998; 9:345–353.

102. Hoffmann P, Ermann J, Edinger M, Fathman CG, Strober S. Donor-type CD4(+)CD25(+) regulatory T cells suppress lethal acute graft-versus-host disease after allogeneic bone marrow transplantation. J Exp Med 2002; 196:389–399.

103. Kagi D, Vignaux F, Ledermann B, Burki K, Depraetere V, Nagata S, Hengartner H, Golstein P. Fas and perforin pathways as major mechanisms of T cell-mediated cytotoxicity. Science 1994; 265:528–530.

104. Lowin B, Hahne M, Mattmann C, Tschopp J. Cytolytic T-cell cytotoxicity is mediated through perforin and Fas lytic pathways. Nature (London) 1994; 370:650–620.

105. Shresta S, Pham C, Thomas D, Braubert T, Ley T. How do cytotoxic lymphocytes kill their targets? Curr Opin Immunol 1998; 10:581–587.

106. Krammer PH. CD95's deadly mission in the immune system. Nature 2000; 407:789–795.

107. Chinnaiyan A, O'Rourke K, Yu G, Lyons R, Garg M, Duan D, Xing L, Gentz R, Ni J, Dixit V. Signal transduction by DR3, a death domain-containing receptor related to TNFR-1 and CD95. Science 1996; 274:990–992.

108. Chicheportiche Y, Bourdon PR, Xu H, Hsu YM, Scott H, Hession C, Garcia I, Browning JL. TWEAK, a new secreted ligand in the tumor necrosis factor family that weakly induces apoptosis. J Biol Chem 1997; 272:32401–32410.

109. Pan G, O'Rourke K, Chinnaiyan AM, Gentz R, Ebner R. The receptor for the cytotoxic ligand TRAIL. Science 1997; 276:111–113.

110. Baker MB, Altman NH, Podack ER, Levy RB. The role of cell-mediated cytotoxicity in acute GVHD after MHC-matched allogeneic bone marrow transplantation in mice. J Exp Med 1996; 183:2645–2656.

111. Braun YM, Lowin B, French L, Acha-Orbea H, Tschopp J. Cytotoxic T cells deficient in both functional Fas ligand and perforin show residual cytolytic activity yet lose their capacity to induce lethal acute graft-versus-host disease. J Exp Med 1996; 183:657–661.

112. Graubert TA, DiPersio JF, Russell JH, Ley TJ. Perforin/granzyme-dependent and independent mechanisms are both important for the development of graft-versus-host disease after murine bone marrow transplantation. J Clin Invest 1997; 100:904–911.

113. Blazar BR, Taylor PA, Vallera DA. CD4+ and CD8+ T cells each can utilize a perforin-dependent pathway to mediate lethal graft-versus-host disease in major histocompatibility complex-disparate recipients. Transplantation 1997; 64:571–576.

114. Ueno Y, Ishii M, Yahagi K, Mano Y, Kisara N, Nakamura N, Shimosegawa T, Toyota T, Nagata S. Fas-mediated cholangiopathy in the murine model of graft versus host disease. Hepatology 2000; 31:966–974.

115. Shustov A, Nguyen P, Finkelman F, Elkon KB, Via CS. Differential expression of Fas and Fas ligand in acute and chronic graft-versus-host disease: up-regulation of Fas and Fas ligand requires CD8+ T cell, activation and IFN-gamma production. J Immunol 1998; 161:2848–2855.

116. Lee S, Chong SY, Lee JW, Kim SC, Min YH, Hahn JS, Ko YW. Difference in the expression of Fas/Fas-ligand and the lymphocyte subset reconstitution according to the occurrence of acute GVHD. Bone Marrow Transplant 1997; 20:883–888.

117. Wasem C, Frutschi C, Arnold D, Vallan C, Lin T, Green DR, Mueller C, Brunner T. Accumulation and activation-induced release of preformed Fas (CD95) ligand during the pathogenesis of experimental graft-versus-host disease. J Immunol 2001; 167:2936–2941.

118. Liem LM, van Lopik T, van Nieuwenhuijze AEM, van Houwelingen HC, Aarden L, Goulmy E. Soluble fas levels in sera of bone marrow transplantation recipients are increased during acute graft-versus-host disease but not during infections. Blood 1998; 91:1464–1468.

119. Das H, Imoto S, Murayama T, Kajimoto K, Sugimoto T, Isobe T, Nakagawa T, Nishimura R, Koizumi T. Levels of soluble FasL and FasL gene expression during the development of graft-versus-host disease in DLT-treated patients. Br J Haematol 1999; 104:795–800.

120. Kanda Y, Tanaka Y, Shirakawa K, Yatomi T, Nakamura N, Kami M, Saito T, Izutsu K, Asai T, Yuji K, Ogawa S, Honda H, Mitani K, Chiba S, Yazaki Y, Hirai H. Increased soluble

Fas-ligand in sera of bone marrow transplant recipients with acute graft-versus-host disease. Bone Marrow Transplant 1998; 22:751–754.

121. Kayaba H, Hirokawa M, Watanabe A, Saitoh N, Changhao C, Yamada Y, Honda K, Kobayashi Y, Urayama O, Chihara J. Serum markers of graft-versus-host disease after bone marrow transplantation. J Allergy Clin Immunol 2000; 106:S40–S44.

122. Baker MB, Riley RL, Podack ER, Levy RB. GVHD-associated lymphoid hypoplasia and B cell dysfunction is dependent upon donor T cell-mediated Fas-ligand function, but not perforin function. Proc Natl Acad Sci USA 1997; 94:1366–1371.

123. Via CS, Nguyen P, Shustov A, Drappa J, Elkon KB. A major role for the Fas pathway in acute graft-versus-host disease. J Immunol 1996; 157:5387–5393.

124. Kondo T, Suda T, Fukuyama H, Adachi M, Nagata S. Essential roles of the Fas ligand in the development of hepatitis. Nat Med 1997; 4:409–413.

125. van den Brink M, Moore E, Horndasch E, Crawford J, Hoffman J, Murphy G, Burakoff S. Fas-deficient *lpr* mice are more susceptible to graft-versus-host disease. J Immunol 2000; 164:469–480.

126. Hattori K, Hirano T, Miyajima H, Yamakawa N, Tateno M, Oshimi K, Kayagaki N, Yagita H, Okumura K. Differential effects of anti-Fas ligand and anti-tumor necrosis factor-α antibodies on acute graft-versus-host disease pathologies. Blood 1998; 91:4051–4055.

127. Stuber E, Buschenfeld A, von Freier A, Arendt T, Folsch UR. Intestinal crypt cell apoptosis in murine acute graft versus host disease is mediated by tumour necrosis factor alpha and not by the FasL-Fas interaction: effect of pentoxifylline on the development of mucosal atrophy. Gut 1999; 45:229–235.

128. Martin PJ, Akatsuka Y, Hahne M, Sale G. Involvement of donor T-cell cytotoxic effector mechanisms in preventing allogeneic marrow graft rejection. Blood 1998; 92:2177–2181.

129. Jiang Z, Podack E, Levy RB. Major histocompatibility complex-mismatched allogeneic bone marrow transplantation using perform and/or Fas ligand double-defective CD4(+) donor T cells: involvement of cytotoxic function by donor lymphocytes prior to graft-versus-host disease pathogenesis. Blood 2001; 98:390–397.

130. Piguet PF, Grau GE, Allet B, Vassalli PJ. Tumor necrosis factor/cachectin is an effector of skin and gut lesions of the acute phase of graft-versus-host disease. J Exp Med 1987; 166:1280–1289.

131. Piguet PF, Grau GE, Collart MA, Vassalli P, Kapanci Y. Pneumopathies of the graft-versus-host reaction. Alveolitis associated with an increased level of tumor necrosis factor MRNA and chronic interstitial pneumonitis. Lab Invest 1989; 61:37–45.

132. Herve P, Flesch M, Tiberghien P, Wijdenes J, Racadot E, Bordigoni P, Plouvier E, Stephan JL, Bourdeau H, Holler E, Lioure B, Roche C, Vilmer E, Demeocq F, Kuentz M, Cahn YJ. Phase I–II trial of a monoclonal anti-tumor necrosis factor alpha antibody for the treatment of refractory severe acute graft-versus-host disease. Blood 1992; 81:1993–1999.

133. Murphy GF, Sueki H, Teuscher C, Whitaker D, Korngold R. Role of mast cells in early epithelial target cell injury in experimental acute graft-vs-host disease. J Invest Dermatol 1994; 102:451–461.

134. Gilliam AC, Whitaker-Menezes D, Korngold R, Murphy GF. Apoptosis is the predominant form of epithelial target cell injury in acute experimental graft-versus-host disease. J Invest Dermatol 1996; 107:377–383.

135. Cooke KR, Hill GR, Gerbitz A, Kobzik L, Martin TR, Crawford JM, Brewer JP, Ferrara JL. Tumor necrosis factor-alpha neutralization reduces lung injury after experimental allogeneic bone marrow transplantation. Transplantation 2000; 70:272–279.

136. Laster SM, Wood JG, Gooding LR. Tumor necrosis factor can induce both apoptic and necrotic forms of cell lysis. J Immunol 1988; 141:2629–2634.

137. Hill GR, Teshima T, Rebel VI, Krijanovski OI, Cooke KR, Brinson YS, Ferrara JL. The p55 TNF-alpha receptor plays a critical role in T cell alloreactivity. J Immunol 2000; 164:656–663.

138. Brown GR, Lee E, Thiele DL. TNF-TNFR2 interactions are critical for the development of intestinal graft-versus-host disease in MHC class II-disparate (C57BL/6J → C57BL/6J × bm12)F1 mice. J Immunol 2002; 168:3065–3071.

139. Holler E, Kolb HJ, Moller A, Kempeni J, Lisenfeld S, Pechumer H, Lehmacher W, Ruckdeschel G, Gleixner B, Riedner C, Ledderose G, Brehm G, Mittermuller J, Wilmanns W. Increased serum levels of tumor necrosis factor alpha precede major complications of bone marrow transplantation. Blood 1990; 75:1011–1016.

140. Holler E, Kolb HJ, Hintermeier-Knabe R, Mittermuller J, Thierfelde S, Kaul M, Wilmanns W. The role of tumor necrosis factor alpha in acute graft-versus-host disease and complications following allogeneic bone marrow transplantation. Transplant Proc 1993; 25:1234–1236.

141. Tanaka J, Imamura M, Kasai M, Masauzi N, Matsuura A, Ohizumi H, Morii K, Kiyama Y, Naohara T, Saitho M, et al. Cytokine gene expression in peripheral blood mononuclear cells during graft-versus-host disease after allogeneic bone marrow transplantation. Br J Haematol 1993; 85:558–565.

142. Tanaka J, Imamura M, Kasai M, Masauzi N, Watanabe M, Matsuura A, Morii K, Kiyama Y, Naohara T, Higa T, Honke K, Gasa S, Sakurada K, Miyazaki T. Rapid analysis of tumor necrosis factor-alpha mRNA expression during venooclusive disease of the liver after allogeneic bone marrow transplantation. Transplantation 1993; 55:430–432.

143. Abhyankar S, Gilliland DG, Ferrara JLM. Interleukin 1 is a critical effector molecule during cytokine dysregulation in graft-versus-host disease to minor histocompatibility antigens. Transplantation 1993; 56:1518–1523.

144. Eisenberg SP, Evans RJ, Arend WP, Verderberr E, Brewer MT, Hannum CH, Thompson RC. Primary structure and functional expression from complementary DNA of a human interleukin-1 receptor antagonist. Nature 1990; 343:341.

145. Hannum CH, Wilcox CJ, Arend WP, Joslin FG, Dripps DJ, Heimdal PL, Armes LG, Sommer A, Eisenberg SP, Thompson RC. Interleukin-1 receptor antagonist activity of a human interleukin-1 inhibitor. Nature 1990; 343:336–340.

146. Antin JH, Weisdorf D, Neuberg D, et al. In press Interleukin-1 blockade does not prevent acute graft-versus-host disease. Results of a randomized, double blinded, placebo-controlled trial of interleukin 1 receptor antagonist in allogeneic bone marrow transplantation. Blood 2002; 100:3479–3482.

147. Falzarano G, Krenger W, Snyder KM, Delmonte J, Karandikar M, Ferrara JLM. Suppression of B cell proliferation to lipopolysaccharide is mediated through induction of the nitric oxide pathway by tumor necrosis factor-a in mice with acute graft-versus-host disease. Blood 1996; 87:2853–2860.

148. Nestel FP, Greene RN, Kichian K, Ponka P, Lapp WS. Activation of macrophage cytostatic effector mechanisms during acute graft-versus-host disease: release of intracellular iron and nitric oxide-mediated cytostasis. Blood 2000; 96:1836–1843.

149. Weiss G, Schwaighofer H, Herold M. Nitric oxide formation as predictive parameter for acute graft-versus-host disease after human allogeneic bone marrow transplantation. Transplantation 1995; 60:1239–1244.

150. Langrehr JM, Murase N, Markus PM, Cai X, Neuhaus P, Schraut W, Simmons RL, Hoffmann RA. Nitric oxide production in host-versus-graft and graft-versus-host reactions in the rat. J Clin Invest 1992; 90:679–683.

151. Cooke K, Hill G, Crawford J, Bungard D, Brinson Y, Delmonte Jr. J, Ferrara J. Tumor necrosis factor-a production to lipopolysaccharide stimulation by donor cells predicts the severity of experimental acute graft versus host disease. J Clin Invest 1998; 102:1882–1891.

152. Hill G, Ferrara J. The primacy of the gastrointestinal tract as a target organ of acute graft-versus-host disease: rationale for the use of cytokine shields in allogeneic bone marrow transplantation. Blood 2000; 95:2754–2759.

153. Price KS, Nestel FP, Lapp WS. Progressive accumulation of bacterial lipopolysaccharide in vivo during murine acute graft-versus-host disease. Scand J Immunol 1997; 45:294–300.

154. Morrison DC, Ryan JL. Endotoxins and disease mechanisms. Annu Rev Med 1987; 38:417–432.
155. Raetz C. Biochemistry of endotoxins. Annu Rev Biochem 1990; 59:129–170.
156. Fegan C, Poynton CH, Whittaker JA. The gut mucosal barrier in bone marrow transplantation. Bone Marrow Transplant 1990; 5:373–377.
157. Jackson SK, Parton J, Barnes RA, Poynton CH, Fegan C. Effect of IgM-enriched intravenous immunoglobulin (Pentaglobulin) on endotoxaemia and anti-endotoxin antibodies in bone marrow transplantation. Eur J Clin Invest 1993; 23:540–545.
158. Glode LM, Rosenstreich DL. Genetic control of B cell activation by bacterial lipopolysaccaride is mediated by multiple distinct genes or alleles. J Immunol 1976; 117: 2061–2066.
159. Watson J, Kelly K, Largen M, Taylor BA. The genetic mapping of a defective LPS response gene in C3H/Hej mice. J Immunol 1978; 120:422–424.
160. Sultzer BM, Castagna R, Bandeakar J, Wong P. Lipopolysaccharide nonresponder cells: the C3H/HeJ defect. Immunobiology 1993; 187:257–271.
161. Poltorak A, Ziaolong H, Smirnova I, Liu M-Y, Van Huffel C, Du X, Birdwell D, Alejos E, Silva M, Galanos C, Freudenberg M, Ricciardi-Castagnoli P, Layton B, Beutler B. Defective LPS signaling in C3H/HeJ and C57BL/20ScCr mice: mutations in Tlr4 gene. Science 1998; 282:2085–2088.
162. Sultzer BM, Goodman GW. Endotoxin protein: a B cell mitogen and polyclonal activator of C3H/Hej lymphocytes. J Exp Med 1976; 144:821–827.
163. Sultzer BM. Lymphocyte activation by endotoxin and endotoxin protein: the role of the C3H/ Hej mouse. In: Nowotny A, ed. Beneficial Effects of Endotoxin. New York: Plenum Press, 1983:227–245.
164. Ulevitch Ri, Tobias PS. Receptor-dependent mechanisms of cell stimulation by bacterial endotoxin. Annu Rev Immunol 1995; 13:437–457.
165. Haziot A, Ferrero E, Kontgen F. Resistance to endotoxin shock and reduced dissemination of gram-negative bacteria in CD14-deficient mice. Immunity 1996; 4:407–414.
166. Cooke K, Olkiewicz K, Clouthier S, Liu C, Ferrara J. Critical role for CD14 and the innate immune response in the induction of experimental acute graft-versus-host disease. Blood 2001; 98:776a.
167. van Bekkum DW, Roodenburg J, Heidt PJ, van der Waaij D. Mitigation of secondary disease of allogeneic mouse radiation chimeras by modification of the intestinal microflora. J Natl Cancer Inst 1974; 52:401–404.
168. Storb R, Prentice RL, Buckner CD, Clift RA, Appelbaum F, Deeg J, Doney K, Hansen JA, Mason M, Sanders JE, Singer J, Sullivan KM, Witherspoon RP, Thomas ED. Graft-versus-host disease and survival in patients with aplastic anemia treated by marrow grafts from HLA-identical siblings. Beneficial effect of a protective environment. N Engl J Med 1983; 308:302–307.
169. Moller J, Skirhoj P, Hoiby N, Peterson FB. Protection against graft versus host disease by gut sterilization? Exp Haematol 1982; 10:101–102.
170. Beelen DW, Haralambie E, Brandt H, Linzenmcicr G, Muller K-D, Quabeck K, Sayer HG, Graeven U, Mahmoud HK, Schaefer UW. Evidence that sustained growth suppression of intestinal anaerobic bacteria reduces the risk of acute graft-versus-host disease after sibling marrow transplantation. Blood 1992; 80:2668–2676.
171. Beelen D, Elmaagacli A, Muller K, Hirche H, Schaefer U. Influence of intestinal bacterial decontamination using metronidazole and ciprofloxacin or ciprofloxacin alone on the development of acute graft-versus-host disease after marrow transplantation in patients with hematologic malignancies: final results and long term follow-up of an open-label prospective randomized trial. Blood 1999; 93:3267–3275.
172. Cohen JL, Boyer O, Salomon B, Onclerq R, Charlotte F. Prevention of graft-versus-host disease in mice using a suicide gene expressed in T lymphocytes. Blood 1997; 89: 4636–4645.

173. Bayston K, Baumgartner J, Clark P, Cohen J. Anti-endotoxin antibody for prevention of acute GVHD. Bone Marrow Transplantation 1991; 8:426–427.

174. Christ W, Asano O, Robidoux A, Perez M, Wang Y, Dubuc G, Gavin W, Hawkins L, McGuinness P, Mullarkey M, Lewis M, Kishi Y, Kawata T, Bristol J, Rose J, Rossignol D, Kobayashi S, Hishinuma I, Kimura A, Asakawa N, Katayama K, Yamatsu I. E5531, a pure endotoxin antagonist of high potency. Science 1995; 268:80–83.

175. Housley R, Morris C, Boyle W, Ring B, Biltz R, Tarpley J, Aukerman S, Devin P, Whitehead R, Pierce G. Keratinocyte growth factor induces proliferation of hepatocytes and epithelial cells throughout the rat gastrointestinal tract. J Clin Invest 1994; 94: 1764–1777.

176. Pierce G, Yanagihara D, Klopchin K, Danilenko D, Hsu E, Kenny W, Morris C. Stimulation of all epithelial elements during skin regeneration by keratinocyte growth factor. J Exp Med 1994; 179:831–840.

177. Panos R, Rubin J, Aaronson S, Mason R. Keratinocyte growth factor scatter factor are heparin-binding growth factors for alvealar type II cells in fibroblast-conditioned medium. J Clin Invest 1993; 92:969–977.

178. Farrell C, Bready J, Rex K, Chen J, Dipalma C, Whitcomb KL, Yin S, Hill D, Wiemann B, Starnes C, Havill A, Lu Z, Aukerman S, Pierce G, Thomasen A, Potten CS, Ulich T, Lacy D. Keratincyte growth factor protects mice from chemotherapy and radiation-induced gastrointestinal injury and mortality. Cancer Res 1998; 58:933–939.

179. Ulich TR, Whitcomb L, Tang W, O'Conner Tressel P, Tarpley J, Yi ES, Lacey D. Keratinocyte growth factor ameliorates cyclophosphamide-induced ulcerative hemorrhagic cystitis. Cancer Res 1997; 57:472–475.

180. Yi ES, Williams ST, Lee H, Malicki DM, Chin EM, Yin S, Tarpley J, Ulich TR. Keratinocyte growth factor ameliorates radiation- and bleomycin-induced lung injury and mortality. Am J Pathol 1996; 149:1963–1970.

181. Danilenko DM. Preclinical and early clinical development of keratinocyte growth factor, an epithelial-specific tissue growth factor. Toxicol Pathol 1999; 27:64–71.

182. Frank S, Muna B, Werner S. The human homologue of a bovine-none-selenium glutathione peroxidase is a novel keratinocyte growth factor-regulated gene. Oncogene 1997; 14: 915–921.

183. Takeoka M, Ward WF, Pollack H, Kamp DW, Panos RJ. KGF facilitates repair of radiation-induced DNA damage in alveolar epithelial cells. Am J Physiol 1997; 276:L1174–L1180.

184. Krijanovski OI, Hill GR, Cooke KR, Teshima T, Crawford JM, Brinson YS, Ferrara JL. Keratinocyte growth factor separates graft-versus-leukemia effects from graft-versus-host disease. Blood 1999; 94:825–831.

185. Panoskaltsis-Mortari A, Lacey DL, Vallera DA, Blazer BR. Keratinocyte growth factor administered before conditioning ameliorates graft-versus-host disease after allogeneic bone marrow transplantation in mice. Blood 1998; 92:3960–3967.

186. Panoskaltsis-Mortari A, Taylor PA, Rubin JS, Uren A, Welniak LA, Murphy WJ, Farrell CL, Lacey DL, Blazar BR. Keratinocyte growth factor facilitates alloengraftment and ameliorates graft-versus-host disease in mice by a mechanism independent of repair of conditioning-induced tissue injury. Blood 2000; 96:4350–4356.

187. Panoskaltsis-Mortari A, Ingbar DH, Jung P, Haddad JY, Bitterman PB, Wangensteen OD, Farrell CL, Lacey DL, Blazar BR. KGF pretreatment decreases B7 and granzyme B expression and hastens repair in lungs of mice after allogeneic BMT. Am J Physiol Lung Cell Mol Physiol 2000; 278:L988–999.

188. Ziegler TR, Panoskaltsus-Mortari A, Gu LH, Jonas CR, Farrell CL, Lacey DL, Jones DP, Blazar BR. Regulation of glutathione redox status in lung and liver by conditioning regimens and keratinocyte growth factor in murine allogeneic bone marrow transplantation. Transplantation 2001; 72:1354–1362.

189. Reynolds C, Ferrara JLM, Hutchinson R, Braun T, Ratanatharathorn V, Ayash L, Levine J, Yanik G, Cooke KR, Silver S, Reddy P, Becker M, Uberti J. A phase I/II study of recombinant human keratinocyte growth factor (KGF) in patients with high risk hematopoietic malignacies undergoing mismatched related or unreleated donor transplant. Biol Blood Marrow Transplant 2003; 9:67.

190. Moser B, Loetscher P. Lymphocyte traffic control by chemokines. Nat Immunol 2001; 2:123–128.

191. Sallusto F, Lenig D, Forster R, Lipp M, Lanzavecchia A. Two subsets of memory T lymphocytes with distinct homing potentials and effector functions. Nature 1999; 401:708–712.

192. Murai M, Yoneyama H, Harada A, Yi Z, Vestergaard C, Guo B, Suzuki K, Asakura H, Matsushima K. Active participation of CCR5(+)CD8(+) T lymphocytes in the pathogenesis of liver injury in graft-versus-host disease. J Clin Invest 1999; 104:49–57.

193. Serody JS, Burkett SE, Panoskaltsis-Mortari A, Ng-Cashin J, McMahon E, Matsushima GK, Lira SA, Cook DN, Blazar BR. T-lymphocyte production of macrophage inflammatory protein-1alpha is critical to the recruitment of CD8(+) T cells to the liver, lung, and spleen during graft-versus-host disease. Blood 2000; 96:2973–2980.

194. Panoskaltsis-Mortari A, Striter RM, Hermanson JR, Fegeding KV, Murphy WJ, Farrell CL, Lacey DL, Blazar BR. Induction of monocyte- and T-cell-attracting chemokines in the lung during the generation of idiopathic pneumonia syndrome following allogeneic murine bone marrow transplantation. Blood 2000; 96:834–839.

195. Murai M, Yoneyama H, Ezaki T, Suematsu M, Terashima Y, Harada A, Hamada H, Asakura H, Ishikawa H, Matsushima K. Peyer's patch is the essential site in initiating murine acute and lethal graft-versus-host reaction. Nat Immunol 2003; 4:154–160.

196. Schnare M, Barton GM, Holt AC, Takeda K, Akira S, Medzhitov R. Toll-like receptors control activation of adaptive immune responses. Nat Immunol 2001; 2:947–950.

197. Antin JH, Ferrara JLM. Cytokine dysregulation and acute graft-versus-host disease. Blood 1992; 80:2964–2968.

198. Medzhitov R, Janeway CA, Jr. Decoding the patterns of self and nonself by the innate immune system. Science 2002; 296:298–300.

199. Aversa F, Tabilio A, Velardi A, Cunningham I, Terenzi A, Falzetti F, Ruggeri L, Barbabietola G, Aristei C, Latini P, Reisner Y, Martelli MF. Treatment of high-risk acute leukemia with T-cell-depleted stem cells from related donors with one fully mismatched HLA haplotype. N Engl J Med 1998; 339:1186–1193.

200. Martin P, Hansen J, Buckner C. Effects of in vitro depletion of T cells in HLA-identical allogeneic marrow grafts. Blood 1985; 66:664–672.

201. Champlin R. T-cell depletion to prevent graft-versus-host disease after bone marrow transplantation. Hematol Oncol Clin North Am 1990; 4:687.

202. Martin T, Goodman R. The role of chemokines in the pathophysiology of the acute respiratory distress syndrome (ARDS). In: Hebert C, ed. Chemokines in Disease. Totowa, NJ: Humana Press, 1999:81–110.

203. Soiffer RJ, Weller E, Alyea EP, Mauch P, Webb IL, Fisher DC, Freedman AS, Schlossman RL, Gribben J, Lee S, Anderson KC, Marcus K, Stone RM, Antin JH, Ritz J. CD6+ donor marrow T-cell depletion as the sole form of graft-versus-host disease prophylaxis in patients undergoing allogeneic bone marrow transplant from unrelated donors. J Clin Oncol 2001; 19:1152–1159.

204. Antin J, Bierer B, Smith B. Selective depletion of bone marrow T lymphocytes with anti-CD5 monoclonal antibodies: effective prophylaxis for graft-versus-host disease in patients with hematologic malignancies. Blood 1991; 78:2139–2149.

205. Papadopoulos EB, Carabasi MH, Castro-Malaspina H, Childs BH, Mackinnon S, Boulad F, Gillio AP, Kernan NA, Small TN, Szabolcs P, Taylor J, Yahalom J, Collins NH, Bleau SA, Black PM, Heller G, O'Reilly RJ, Young JW. T-cell-depleted allogeneic bone marrow

transplantation as postremission therapy for acute myelogenous leukemia: freedom from relapse in the absence of graft-versus-host disease. Blood 1998; 91:1083–1090.

206. Wagner J, Santos G, Noga S. Bone marrow graft engineering by counterflow centrifugal elutration: results of a phase I–II clinical trial. Blood 1990; 75:1370–1377.

207. Martin PJ, Schoch G, Fisher L, et al. A retrospective analysis of therapy for acute graft-versus-host disease: secondary treatment. Blood 1991; 77:1821–1828.

208. Martin P, Schoch G, Fisher L, Byers V, Anasetti C, Applebaum F, Beatty P, Doney K, McDonald G, Sanders J, Sullivan K, Storb R, Thomas E, Witherspoon R, Lomen P, Hannigan J, Hansen J. A retrospective analysis of therapy for acute graft-versus-host diesase: initial treatment. Blood 1990; 76:1464–1472.

209. Cragg L, Blazar BR, Defor T, Kolatker N, Miller W, Kersey J, Ramsay M, McGlave P, Filipovich A, Weisdorf D. A randomized trial comparing prednisone with antithymocyte globulin/prednisone as an initial systemic therapy for moderately severe acute graft-versus-host disease. Biol Blood Marrow Transplant 2000; 6:441–447.

210. Anasetti C, Hansen JA, Waldmann TA, Applebaum FR, Davis J, Deeg HJ, Doney K, Martin PJ, Nash R, Storb R, Sullivan KM, Witherspoon RP, Binger M, Chizzonite R, Hakimi J, Mould D, Satoh H, Light SE. Treatment of acute graft versus host disease with humanized anti-Tac: an antibody that binds to the interleukin-2 receptor. Blood 1994; 84:1320–1327.

211. Przepiorka D, Kernan NA, Ippoliti C, Papadopoulos EB, Giralt S, Khouri I, Lu JG, Gajewski J, Durett A, Cleary K, Champlin R, Andersson BS, Light S. Daclizumab, a humanized anti-interleukin-2 receptor alpha chain antibody, for treatment of acute graft-versus-host disease. Blood 2000; 95:83–89.

212. Carpenter PA, Appelbaum FR, Corey L, Deeg HJ, Doney K, Gooley T, Krueger J, Martin P, Pavlovic S, Sanders J, Slattery J, Levitt D, Storb R, Woolfrey A, Anasetti C. A humanized non-FcR-binding anti-CD3 antibody, visilizumab, for treatment of steroid-refractory acute graft-versus-host disease. Blood 2002; 99:2712–2719.

213. Willenbacher W, Basara N, Blau IW, Fauser AA, Kiehl MG. Treatment of steroid refractory acute and chronic graft-versus-host disease with daclizumab. Br J Haematol 2001; 112: 820–823.

214. Storb R, Thomas ED. Graft-versus-host disease in dog and man: the Seattle experience. Immunol Rev 1985; 88:215–238.

215. Storb R, Deeg HJ, Pepe M, Appelbaum F, Anasetti C, Beatty P, Bensinger W, Berenson R, Buckner CD, Clift R, et al. Methotrexate and cyclosporine versus cyclosporine alone for prophylaxis of graft-versus-host disease in patients given HLA-identical marrow grafts for leukemia: long-term follow-up of a controlled trial. Blood 1989; 73:1729–1734.

216. Nash RA, Antin JH, Karanes C, Fay JW, Avalos BR, Yeager AM, Przepiorka D, Davies S, Petersen FB, Bartels P, Buell D, Fitzsimmons W, Anasetti C, Storb R, Ratanatharathorn V. Phase 3 study comparing methotrexate and tacrolimus with methotrexate and cyclosporine for prophylaxis of acute graft-versus-host disease after marrow transplantation from unrelated donors. Blood 2000; 96:2062–2068.

217. Ratanatharathorn V, Nash RA, Przepiorka D, Devine SM, Klein JL, Weisdorf D, Fay JW, Nademanee A, Antin JH, Christiansen NP, van der Jagt R, Herzig RH, Litzow MR, Wolff SN, Longo WL, Petersen FB, Karanes C, Avalos B, Storb R, Buell DN, Maher RM, Fitzsimmons WE, Wingard JR. Phase III study comparing methotrexate and tacrolimus (prograf, FK506) with methotrexate and cyclosporine for graft-versus-host disease prophylaxis after HLA-identical sibling bone marrow transplantation. Blood 1998; 92:2303–2314.

218. Chao NJ, Snyder DS, Jain M, Wong RM, Niland JC, Negrin RS, Long GD, Hu WW, Stockerl-Goldstein KE, Johnston U, Amylon MD, Tierney DK, O'Donnell MR, Nademanee AP, Parker P, Stein A, Molina A, Fung H, Kashyap A, Kohler S, Spielberger R, Krishnan A,

Rodriguez R, Forman SJ, Bluzme KG. Equivalence of 2 effective graft-versus-host disease prophylaxis regimens: results of a prospective double-blind randomized trial. Biol Blood Marrow Transplant 2000; 6:254–261.

219. Gorgun G, Miller KB, Foss FM. Immunologic mechanisms of extracorporeal photo-chemotherapy in chronic graft-versus-host disease. Blood 2002; 100:941–947.

220. Foss FM, Gorgun G, Miller KB. Extracorporeal photopheresis in chronic graft-versus-host disease. Bone Marrow Transplant 2002; 29:719–725.

221. Klangsinsirikul P, Carter GI, Byrne JL, Hale G, Russell NH. Campath-1G causes rapid depletion of circulating host dendritic cells (DCs) before allogeneic transplantation but does not delay donor DC reconstitution. Blood 2002; 99:2586–2591.

222. Teshima T, Reddy P, Lowler KP, KuKuruga MA, Liu C, Cooke KR, Ferrara JL. Flt3 ligand therapy for recipients of allogeneic bone marrow transplants expands host CD8 alpha(+) dendritic cells and reduces experimental acute graft-versus-host disease. Blood 2002; 99:1825–1832.

223. Storb R, Epstein RB, Graham TC, Thomas ED. Methotrexate regimens for control of graft-versus-host disease in dogs with allogeneic marrow grafts. Transplantation 1970; 9:240–246.

224. Ramsay NK, Kersey JH, Robison LL, McGlave PB, Woods WG, Krivit W, Kim TH, Goldman AL, Nesbit ME, Jr. A randomized study of the prevention of acute graft-versus-host disease. N Engl J Med 1982; 306:392–397.

225. Blume K, Beutler E, Bross K. Bone marrow ablation and allogeneic marrow transplantation in acute leukemia. N Engl J Med 1980; 302:1041–1046.

226. Allison AC, Eugui EM. Mycophenolate mofetil and its mechanisms of action. Immunopharmacology 2000; 47:85–118.

227. Sehgal SN. Rapamune (RAPA, rapamycin, sirolimus): mechanism of action immunosuppressive effect results from blockade of signal transduction and inhibition of cell cycle progression. Clin Biochem 1998; 31:335–340.

228. Li Y, Li XC, Zheng XX, Wells AD, Turka LA, Strom TB. Blocking both signal 1 and signal 2 of T-cell activation prevents apoptosis of alloreactive T cells and induction of peripheral allograft tolerance. Nat Med 1999; 5:1298–1302.

229. Groth CG, Backman L, Morales JM, Calne R, Kreis H, Lang P, Touraine JU, Claesson K, Campistol JM, Durand D, Wramner U, Brattstrom C, Charpentier B. Sirolimus (rapamycin)-based therapy in human renal transplantation: similar efficacy and different toxicity compared with cyclosporine. Sirolimus European Renal Transplant Study Group. Transplantation 1999; 67:1036–1042.

230. Shapiro AM, Lakey JR, Ryan EA, Korbutt GS, Toth E, Wamock GL, Kneteman NM, Rajotte RV. Islet transplantation in seven patients with type 1 diabetes mellitus using a glucocorticoid-free immunosuppressive regimen. N Engl J Med 2000; 343:230–238.

231. Longoria JM, Turner NH, Philips BU, Jr. Community leaders help increase response rates in AIDS survey. Am J Public Health 1991; 81:654–655.

232. Blazar BR, Taylor PA, Panoskaltsis-Mortari A, Sehgal S, Vallera DA. In vivo inhibition of cytokine responsiveness and graft-versus-host disease mortality by rapamycin leads to a clinical-pathological syndrome discrete from that observed with cyclosporin A. Blood 1996; 87:4001–4009.

233. Blazar BR, Korngold R, Vallera DA. Recent advances in graft-versus-host disease (GVHD) prevention. Immunol Rev 1997; 157:79–109.

234. Passweg JR, Rowlings PA, Atkinson KA, Barrett AJ, Gale RP, Gratwohl A, Jacobsen N, Klein JP, Ljungman P, Russell JA, Schaefer UW, Sobocinski KA, Vossen JM, Zhang MJ, Horowitz MM. Influence of protective isolation on outcome of allogeneic bone marrow transplantation for leukemia. Bone Marrow Transplant 1998; 21:1231–1238.

235. Huang XJ, Wan J, Lu DP. Serum TNFalpha levels in patients with acute graft-versus-host disease after bone marrow transplantation. Leukemia 2001; 15:1089–1091.

236. Holler E, Kolb HJ, Mittermueller J, Kaul M, Ledderose G, Duell T, Seeber B, Schleuning M, Hintermeier-Knabe R, Ertl B, Kempeni J, Wilmanns W. Modulation of acute graft-versus-host disease after allogeneic bone marrow transplantation by tumor necrosis factor α (TNFα) release in the course of pretransplant conditioning: role of conditioning regimens and prophylactic application of a monoclonal antibody neutralizing human TNFα (MAK 195F). Blood 1995; 86:890–899.

237. Kobbe G, Schneider P, Rohr U, Fenk R, Neumann F, Aivado M, Dietze L, Kronenwett R, Hunerliturkoglu A, Haas R. Treatment of severe steroid refractory acute graft-versus-host disease with infliximab, a chimeric human/mouse antiTNFalpha antibody. Bone Marrow Transplant 2001; 28:47–49.

238. Couriel DR, Hicks K, Giralt S, Champlin RE. Role of tumor necrosis factor-alpha inhibition with inflixiMAB in cancer therapy and hematopoietic stem cell transplantation. Curr Opin Oncol 2000; 12:582–587.

239. Chiang KY, Abhyankar S, Bridges K, Godder K, Henslee-Downey JP. Recombinant human tumor necrosis factor receptor fusion protein as complementary treatment for chronic graft-versus-host disease. Transplantation 2002; 73:665–667.

240. Dinarello CA. Interleukin-1 and interleukin-1 antagonism. Blood 1991; 77:1627–1652.

241. Cullup H, Dickinson AM, Jackson GH, Taylor PR, Cavet J, Middleton PG. Donor interleukin 1 receptor antagonist genotype associated with acute graft-versus-host disease in human leucocyte antigen-matched sibling allogeneic transplants. Br J Haematol 2001; 113:807–813.

242. McCarthy PL, Abhyankar S, Neben S, Newman G, Sieff C, Thompson RC, Burakoff SJ, Ferrara JLM. Inhibition of interleukin-1 by an interleukin-1 receptor antagonist prevents graft-versus-host disease. Blood 1991; 78:1915–1918.

243. McCarthy PL, Williams L, Harris-Bacile M, Yen J, Przepiorka D, Ippoliti C, Champlin R, Fay J, Blosch C, Jacobs C, Anascetti C. A clinical phase I/II study of recombinant human interleukin-1 receptor in glucocorticoid-resistant graft-versus-host disease. Transplantation 1996; 62:626–631.

244. Antin JH, Weinstein HJ, Guinan EC, McCarthy P, Bierer BE, Gilliland DG, Parsons SK, Ballen KK, Rimm IJ, Falzarano G, Bloedow DC, Abate L, Lebsack M, Burakoff SJ, Ferrara JLM. Recombinant human interleukin-1 receptor antagonist in the treatment of steroid-resistant graft-versus-host disease. Blood 1994; 84:1342–1348.

245. Hill GR, Cooke KR, Teshima T, Crawford JM, Keith JC, Bnnson YS, Bungard D, Ferrara JLM. Interleukin-11 promotes T cell polarization and prevents acute graft-versus-host disease after allogeneic bone marrow transplantation. J Clin Invest 1998; 102:115–123.

246. Antin JH, Lee SJ, Neuberg D, Alyea E, Soiffer RJ, Sonis S, Ferrara JL. A phase I/II double-blind, placebo-controlled study of recombinant human interleukin-11 for mucositis and acute GVHD prevention in allogeneic stem cell transplantation. Bone Marrow Transplant 2002; 29:373–377.

247. Symington FW, Symington BE, Liu PY, Viguet H, Santhanam U, Sehgal PB. The relationship of serum IL-6 levels to acute graft-versus-host disease and hepatorenal disease after human bone marrow transplantation. Transplantation 1992; 54:457–462.

248. Rabinowitz J, Petros WP, Stuart AR, Peters WP. Characterization of endogenous cytokine concentrations after high-dose chemotherapy with autologous bone marrow support. Blood 1993; 81:2452–2459.

249. Uguccioni M, Meliconi R, Nesci S, Lucarelli G, Ceska M, Gasbarrini G, Facchini A. Elevated interleukin-8 serum concentrations in beta-thalassemia and graft-versus-host disease. Blood 1993; 81:2252–2256.

250. Einsele H, Quabeck K, Muller KD, Hebart H, Rothenhofer I, Loffler J, Schaefer UW. Prediction of invasive pulmonary aspergillosis from colonisation of lower respiratory tract before marrow transplantation. Lancet 1998; 352:1443.

251. Hess AD, Horwitz L, Beschorner WE, Santos GW. Development of graft-vs.-host disease-like syndrome in cyclosporine-treated rats after syngeneic bone marrow transplantation. I. Development of cytotoxic T lymphocytes with apparent polyclonal anti-Ia specificity, including autoreactivity. J Exp Med 1985; 161:718–730.
252. Fischer AC, Beschomer WE, Hess AD. Requirements for the induction and adoptive transfer of cyclosporine-induced syngeneic graft-versus-host disease. J Exp Med 1989; 169:1031–1041.
253. Teshima T, Reddy P, Liu C, Williams D, Cooke KR, Ferrara J. Impaired thymic negative selection causes autoimmime graft-versus-host disease. Blood 2003; 102:429–435.

2

Animal Models of Graft-vs.-Host Disease

ROBERT KORNGOLD and THEA M. FRIEDMAN

Thomas Jefferson University, Philadelphia, Pennsylvania, U.S.A.

STEPHEN C. JONES

Trudeau Institute, Inc., Saranac Lake, New York, U.S.A.

I. INTRODUCTION

In the last decade, immunotherapeutic strategies have gained recognition as viable alternatives to more conventional therapeutic modalities for the treatment of cancer. The ability to provide both therapeutic benefit as well as curative potential has moved the efforts to develop immunotherapeutic approaches into the forefront of cancer research. In this regard, adoptive T cell therapy through allogeneic hematopoietic stem cell transplantation (HSCT) has offered the first evidence that antitumor effects could be achieved against hematological malignancies (1,2). Theoretically, allogeneic HSCT also represents one of the few potentially curative treatments for advanced solid tumors, metabolic and autoimmune disorders, as well as immunodeficiencies. However, donor T-cell–mediated graft-vs.-host disease (GVHD) continues to be the principal complication of allogeneic HSCT, along with graft rejection, leukemic relapse, and opportunistic infections. The depletion of T cells from donor stem cell inocula, while significantly reducing the development of GVHD, has been clearly associated with increased incidence of the other risk factors, probably due to slow immunological reconstitution in the recipients (3–6). Thus, the key to successful allogeneic HSCT lies in the ability to ameliorate GVHD while still promoting the beneficial T-cell responses of graft-vs.-leukemia (GVL) effects, enhanced stem cell engraftment, and the capacity to resist infections.

Historically, the development of histocompatability matching has made a significant contribution to the advancement of HSCT by decreasing the incidence of severe GVHD. Histocompatability recognition is one of the essential features of T-cell specificity. T cells

35

typically expressing an $\alpha\beta$ T-cell receptor (TCR) molecule specifically engage antigenic peptide fragments bound by class I and class II molecules of the major histocompatibility complex (MHC), comprising the H2 system in mice, RT1 in rats, human leukocyte antigen (HLA) in humans, and dog leukocyte antigen (DLA) in dogs (7,8). A more detailed understanding of MHC molecules can be found in Chapter 14. Thymic selection processes result in the establishment of a $\alpha\beta^+$ T-cell repertoire that is tolerant to self MHC molecules and the various self peptides bound to these molecules, but display reactivity to self MHC molecules complexed to foreign peptides, such as viral and bacterial antigens (9,10). In the context of allogeneic HSCT, donor T-cell specificities encompass reactivity both to foreign, nonself (allo) MHC molecules as well as minor histocompatibility antigens (miHA), which are host polymorphic peptides presented by self MHC molecules in MHC-matched situations. The high precursor frequency of T cells directed against allo-MHC molecules is largely responsible for the intense level of GVHD pathology in MHC-mismatched HSCT. The severity of GVHD directed to MHC differences could also be attributed to the high level of MHC antigen concentration in the target tissues, either constitutively expressed or induced by inflammatory cytokines.

There are two subsets of $\alpha\beta^+$ T cells, as defined by the presence of the membrane-bound CD8 or CD4 coreceptors (11). The CD8 and CD4 proteins act as adhesion molecules binding to nonpolymorphic regions of the two different classes of MHC molecules termed class I and class II (12). MHC class I molecules are found on most nucleated cells and are recognized by $CD8^+$ T cells. MHC class II molecules exhibit a more restricted tissue expression and are recognized by $CD4^+$ T cells. The binding of the CD4 and CD8 coreceptors to their appropriate MHC molecules both enhances the avidity of the TCR/antigen-MHC interaction (11) and contributes to the specificity of T-cell binding. Thus, $CD8^+$ T cells react more effectively with antigen presented by class I molecules, while $CD4^+$ cells show specificity for class II. The restricted recognition by T cells for their respective MHC class molecules has implications for the immunopathological development of GVHD by dictating the level of participation of each cell subset.

T-cell activation of unprimed T cells depends on contact with MHC-associated peptide expressed on specialized antigen-presenting cells (APC), such as macrophages and dendritic cells (9,12). These cells tend to reside in the T-dependent areas of the lymphoid tissues, i.e., the periarteriolar lymphocyte sheaths of the splenic white pulp and the paracortical areas of the lymph nodes. Thus, following HSCT, the entering donor T cells initially encounter host alloantigens expressed constitutively on host APCs in the T-dependent areas of the recipient's lymphoid tissue. After contact and activation by alloantigen on APC, T cells proliferate extensively, release various cytokines, and differentiate into effector cells; this chain of events constitutes a GVH reaction, which may or may not progress to the overt pathological GVHD state. Whereas resting T cells are usually confined to the recirculating lymphocyte pool (between blood and the lymphatic system), antigen-activated T cells have the capacity to extravasate through the walls of capillary blood vessels and disseminate throughout the body's tissues. Activated and/or effector T cells show a particular propensity for homing to the gut, liver, lung, and skin, sites commonly affected by GVHD. When activated T cells reencounter antigen expressed on local APC or target tissue cells in these organs, the cells express their various effector functions.

The relationships between T-cell effector functions and GVHD pathogenesis are very complex and difficult to classify (12). The direct activity of cytotoxic T lymphocytes (CTL), which include mostly the $CD8^+$ subset, in killing host cells via perforin/granzyme release is probably the dominant cause of the pathology seen in GVHD. On the other hand,

T cells, primarily of the CD4$^+$ type, are able to release large quantities of various inflammatory cytokines that can attract a variety of blood mononuclear cells or cause direct tissue destruction [e.g., tumor necrosis factor-alpha (TNF-α)]. In addition, the effector functions of CD4$^+$ and CD8$^+$ cells may not be as distinct as once thought, since CD8$^+$ cells can also release cytokines and some CD4$^+$ cells can exhibit CTL activity (12).

Much of the elucidation of the pathophysiology and immunobiology of GVHD has been derived through the use of several experimental animal systems such as canine, rat, and murine transplantation models. The canine systems largely involve the use of random-bred species, whereas both the murine and rat systems are comprised of more highly inbred strains. In addition, murine models afford the use of numerous transgenic and knockout strains that can be utilized to examine not only the pathogenesis, but also the underlying effector mechanisms of GVHD. Nevertheless, canine HSCT models have played an important role in the study of different pretransplant conditioning regimens involving the use of total body irradiation (13) and immunosuppressive reagents (14). The treatment and prevention of GVHD with drugs such as methotrexate (15), cyclosporin (16), and antithymocyte serum (17) have also been investigated in canine models, and several of these studies have been directly translated to clinical HSCT settings. On the other hand, rat models have proven useful in several studies designed to minimize GVHD by transplanting graded numbers of donor T cells (18) or by introducing suicide genes that could allow for the in vivo elimination of alloreactive T cells (19). For the most part, however, largely due to their relative ease of breeding, relative cost, and genetic versatility, studies using murine models have played a pivotal role in contributing to our understanding of GVHD directed to MHC and miHA alloantigens and the relative contributions of CD4$^+$ and CD8$^+$ T cells to pathological development. Thus, investigations with murine models will be the focus of this chapter.

II. HOST RESISTANCE TO DONOR CELL ENGRAFTMENT

In order to develop GVHD, certain criteria have to be met, the first of which is that the donor T cells have to overcome any host immune resistance to their engraftment. In the clinical setting, host-vs.-graft (HVG) reactions are a complicating factor for successful allogeneic HSCT, especially if the host has been presensitized to donor alloantigens as the result of blood transfusions. In mice, normal adult mice transplanted with large doses of allogeneic T cells generally do not develop GVHD because the recipients mount a powerful immune response directed toward the donor alloantigens expressed on the incoming cells. Three cell types can be involved in normal HVG reactions: T cells, B cells, and natural killer (NK) cells (20–23). The simplest approach for inactivating them in adult mice is to expose the host to total body irradiation (TBI), which is effective at eliminating the highly radiosensitive resting T and B cells. Therefore, irradiation is commonly used as a conditioning regimen for HSCT models, but even here, depending upon the exposure intensity, there are host immune elements that may still be able to survive and reject donor cells. Host T cells, particularly CTL, specific for donor MHC antigens or presensitized to donor miHA differences, can mediate rejection utilizing an array of cytolytic effector mechanisms, including perforin/granzymes and pathways involving TRAIL, TNF, or Fas ligand activity, and possibly other more obscure means (24).

NK cell–mediated HVG reactions can occur a very short time after donor cell transfer and can be quite intense (21,22). Evidence suggests that the specificity of NK cells participating in HVG reactions is directed to cells that lack self class I molecules (23).

There are no NK-mediated HVG reactions generated during transfer of heterozygous F_1 cells into its homozygous parental strain because the parental host strain class I molecules are fully represented on the F_1 donor cells. HVG reactions in this situation are solely mediated by alloreactive T and B cells responding to the other parental MHC molecules expressed by the donor cells. In contrast, homozygous parental cells transplanted into an F_1 recipient can elicit host "hybrid resistance," where the host NK cells reject the parental cells (21). The absence of the other parental F_1 MHC haplotype on the donor cells is responsible for this rejection, and the intensity of hybrid resistance varies considerably according to the particular class I disparity involved. In practice, hybrid resistance is only a problem when there is heterozygosity involving the H2D^b class I molecule, e.g., when [C57BL × CBA (K^{k}D^k)]F$_1$ are transplanted with C57BL (K^{b}D^b) cells. More robust NK-mediated HVG reactions termed "allogeneic resistance," occur when cells are transplanted between two fully MHC mismatched or haploidentical strains, where the donor cells do not express the same or the complete set of class I molecules of the host (25). In attempts to avoid NK cell–mediated HVG responses, inactivation of host NK cells by increased irradiation is often difficult because these cells are highly radioresistant; injection of anti-NK antibodies can be effective, but this is a cumbersome and expensive procedure. In practice, the optimum way to overcome the problem is simply either to inject a larger dose of donor HSC and lymphoid cells or to use parent → F_1 combinations that avoid the recipient H2D^b heterozygosity. It is also worth noting that NK-mediated HVG reactions do not operate in miHA-different combinations since the donor and host are H2 identical.

III. GVHD DIRECTED TO MHC ANTIGENS

The robust proliferative response in vitro following the co-culture of MHC disparate lymphocyte populations (the mixed lymphocyte response) is a reflection of the aggressive nature of the GVHD that follows the transfer of even small numbers of parental strain (H2^x) T cells into irradiated F_1 (H2^{xy}) mice. Whole T-cell–mediated GVHD is especially severe when the host expresses combined H2 class I and II differences. In this scenario, GVHD involves CD8$^+$ or CD4$^+$ T cells responding to MHC class I and class II differences, respectively. As will be seen below, however, either population alone is able to induce lethal GVHD (26–29). The nature of the TCR-MHC interaction responsible for driving alloactivation is an area of active research. Crystallization of an alloreactive TCR bound to its cognate MHC class I–peptide ligand suggests an interaction much like that seen during TCR interaction with a foreign peptide bound to self MHC (30). These observations agree with data demonstrating a requirement for MHC class I–bound peptide during alloactivation (31,32). Class II–restricted alloactivation is not as well understood. However, it also appears that interaction with the allogeneic class II molecule in itself (independent of peptide) is not sufficient to drive T-cell activation (33). Determining the relative importance of either class I or II antigens in eliciting acute GVHD is most directly studied by using donor/host combinations differing solely at class I or II loci.

A. GVHD to MHC Class I Antigens

Mice express H2K and H2D MHC class I molecules, both of which can be involved in severe lethal GVHD development. The most straightforward approach for studying anti-class I GVHD is to use class I mutant mice, e.g., the series of bm mutant mice (34). As determined by skin graft rejection, investigators have isolated more than a dozen different bm mutant strains of mice exhibiting small mutations (1–4 amino acid substitutions) of the H2K molecules of the B6 (H2^b) strain. The immunogenicity of these mutant molecules for wild-type B6 T cells is quite variable. By measuring proliferative and CTL responses generated in vitro, some mutants (e.g., bm1) were found to be strongly stimulatory, whereas others (e.g., bm9) elicited only low responses (35). Detailed information on the capacity of the various class I mutants to elicit GVHD is not yet available. The observations discussed below were formulated based on the B6 → bm1 combination, using (B6 × bm1)F$_1$ mice as hosts.

Purified B6 CD8$^+$ T cells give spectacularly high proliferative and CTL responses to bm1 stimulators in vitro in the absence of CD4$^+$ T cells or their products despite the view that CD8$^+$ cells function poorly without exogenous help (35). Helper-independent responses of CD8$^+$ cells are also seen in vivo (27,35). Thus, when purified B6 CD8$^+$ cells are transferred to irradiated bm1 F$_1$ mice, the donor cells proliferate extensively in the lymphoid tissues in the absence of CD4$^+$ cells and then disseminate throughout the body to mediate their effector functions resulting in GVHD. It should be mentioned that B6 CD4$^+$ cells respond very poorly to bm1, and even large doses of B6 CD4$^+$ cells fail to elicit GVHD in bm1 F$_1$ hosts (36).

B. CD8-Mediated GVHD with Donor Marrow

In the class I-different B6/bm1 combination injecting irradiated (B6 × bm1)F$_1$ hosts with B6 CD8$^+$ I cells plus B6 marrow cells causes significant mortality regardless of whether the hosts are conditioned with heavy irradiation (10 Gy) or light irradiation (6 Gy) (36). Mortality rates approaching 100% are seen with a wide range of T-cell numbers, i.e., from 2×10^7 down to 1×10^5 cells. These results stand out in contrast to those observed in the class II-different combination of B6 and bm12, as mentioned below, where B6 CD4$^+$ cells plus donor marrow fail to cause lethal GVHD in clean mice unless the hosts receive heavy irradiation. Most interestingly, GVHD induced by B6 CD8$^+$ T cells → bm1 tends to be chronic rather than acute. Except for mild weight loss, most of the recipients appear reasonably healthy for the first month after transfer, but later develop diarrhea, marked weight loss, and hunched posture. The condition of the mice worsens progressively, and deaths occur between 5 and 8 weeks after transfer. Autopsies of the mice show typical signs of GVHD with lymphohemopoietic atrophy and lymphocytic infiltrations in various organs. Skin lesions are observed and can be severe, although this is variable. Gut damage is evident but is much less severe than in class II-different combinations (37,38).

C. CD8-Mediated GVHD with Host Marrow

When B6 CD8$^+$ T cells are transferred with host rather than donor marrow cells, they cause marked aplasia in bm1 hosts (36). Presumably to CTL activity directed toward the hematopoietic stem cells, the mice rapidly develop profound marrow aplasia and die within 2 weeks. However, with a mixture of both donor and host marrow cells, hematopoietic failure is avoided and the hosts exhibit the typical pattern of progressive chronic GVHD.

D. Effect of CD4$^+$ Cells on CD8-Mediated GVHD

Although in vitro CD8$^+$ T cells have been shown to mediate helper-independent responses, in vivo GVHD elicited to class I antigens could reflect help from radioresistant host CD4$^+$ T cells. However, this does not seem to be the case because purified $CD8^+$ T cells cause lethal GVHD in hosts given multiple injections of anti-CD4 antibody (36). Nevertheless, supplementing the injected $CD8^+$ T cells with small doses of donor $CD4^+$ T cells causes a marked alteration in the pattern of GVHD; instead of developing progressive chronic GVHD, the hosts develop acute GVHD and die 2–3 weeks after transfer. This finding implies that although $CD8^+$ cells function well in the absence of exogenous help in vivo, adding help significantly increases their potency. The capacity of $CD4^+$ T cells to augment CD8-mediated GVHD is only observed when $CD4^+$ T cells are injected in small numbers ($\leq 1 \times 10^6$). When high numbers of $CD4^+$ cells are transferred, marked protection occurs (36). Thus, if an inoculum of 2×10^6 B6 $CD8^+$ cells is supplemented with 2×10^7 B6 $CD4^+$ cells, death rates in irradiated (B6 × bm1)F_1 hosts drop from 100% to 0%. Mortality rates are also very low when a large dose of 1×10^8 unseparated B6 spleen cells is transferred.

E. GVHD to MHC Class II Antigens

The mouse homologs of the HLA-DQ and HLA-DR molecules are the I-A and I-E molecules, respectively, which are expressed by most mouse strains. In general, the severity of GVHD is dependent upon the strength of the antigenic disparity between strain combinations, and of the two, I-E alloantigens are less immunogenic. This is reflected by relatively weak and generally nonlethal GVHD elicited by I-E differences. In contrast, I-A antigens are potent inducers of GVHD, as demonstrated by the extensively studied C57BL/6 (B6) → B6.C-H2^{bm12} model (27). Here, although alloreactivity is generated by only a 3-amino-acid difference in the β chain of the I-A molecule, upon transplant into lethally irradiated bm12 recipients, B6 T cells respond with vigor and generate a response as strong as with an allelic (nonmutant) I-A difference (35). As one would expect, GVHD in this strain combination is strictly dependent upon $CD4^+$ I cells, with little to no contribution from the $CD8^+$ subset (27,39). This is because, as mentioned earlier, the specificity of $CD8^+$ T cells is strongly skewed to recognition of class I antigens, apparently even in the context of allorecognition. Thus, whereas under defined conditions (see below), even small numbers of B6 (or bm12) $CD4^+$ T cells can mediate rapidly lethal GVHD upon transfer into irradiated (B6 × bm12)F_1 recipients, even large doses of highly $CD4^+$-depleted $CD8^+$ T cells from the same donor strains are incapable of causing GVHD mortality in this model. This is also reflected in vitro by the extremely weak proliferative response of purified B6 $CD8^+$ T cells to bm12 APCs (35).

Upon transplant of B6 $CD4^+$ T cells into irradiated (B6 × bm12)F_1 recipients, donor T cells home to the host lymphoid compartment, where they first encounter allogeneic class II antigens expressed on host APCs. This results in a powerful proliferative response (27) that is followed by the migration of large numbers of activated, blast-like donor cells out into the peripheral circulation. Tissue injury as a result of preconditioning generates chemokine gradients and the increased expression of adhesion molecules such as ICAM-1 and VCAM-1 (40); both help to recruit circulating alloreactive donor cells to the skin, gut, and liver, among other sites, where the cells' effector functions cause GVHD. The type and severity of GVHD are, however, dependent upon a number of factors other than simple allorecognition. Some of the other factors that contribute to the overall pathogenesis of GVHD are discussed in detail below.

F. CD4-Mediated GVHD with Donor Marrow

As discussed above for $CD8^+$ T-cell–mediated GVHD, the most commonly studied GVHD model involves injecting F_1 host mice with a mixture of donor $CD4^+$ T cells and donor bone marrow cells (39). Under these conditions, the pathogenesis of GVHD can be clearly studied, as the donor $CD4^+$ T cells selectively attack host alloantigen-expressing tissue and do not impair hematopoietic cell reconstitution. Nevertheless, GVHD severity can be quite variable and can be profoundly affected by the general health of the animal colony. Thus, if the animals are kept in a clean environment and are free from infection, a conditioning dose of irradiation of 10 Gy is required for acute GVHD to develop. Significant mortality within 2 weeks of injection occurs and is preceded by marked weight loss, mild atrophy of the lymphohemopoietic system, and a distended small intestine. Acute exudative enteropathy is apparent, and death is most likely a reflection of gut damage leading to nutrient loss, dehydration, and acute infection (37,38,41). As discussed in other chapters, inflammatory cytokine dysregulation plays a key role in gut injury during GVHD. This is apparent from the finding that mice can be protected against gut damage (and death) by injecting anti-TNF-α antibodies early after GVHD induction (42).

CD4$^+$ T-cell–mediated GVHD in heavily irradiated recipients requires surprisingly few cells. In fact, close to 100% mortality can be achieved with doses of 1×10^5 CD4$^+$ cells, and even 10-fold fewer can cause significant mortality. If the health of the colony is suboptimal, acute lethal GVHD is seen with much lower doses of irradiation, e.g., 7 Gy; in contrast, in a healthy colony a TBI dose of 8 Gy will generate only low mortality with minimal and transient GVHD pathology.

Interestingly, in the F_1 model, the few mice that do survive acute disease after transfer of a large number of CD4$^+$ T cells generally show very rapid recovery, with only sporadic chronic GVHD. Chronic GVHD instead is generally seen only when very low numbers of CD4$^+$ T cells are transferred and is characterized by prolonged weight loss, lymphoid atrophy, and evidence of infection; however skin lesions are rarely seen.

G. CD4-Mediated GVHD with Host Marrow

Compared to transplant with donor marrow and CD4$^+$ cells, when donor CD4$^+$ cells are transferred with host marrow cells a very different pattern of GVHD occurs (39,41). In this scenario, the alloreactive donor CD4$^+$ T cells attack all of the F_1 host stem cells, including those in the bone marrow graft, preventing stem cell engraftment, and causing death from hematopoietic failure. Although stem cell engraftment is apparent at one week posttransplant, by day 14 the entire lymphohemopoietic system, including the marrow, shows near total aplasia; death occurs by 3 weeks. Here, mortality rates approach 100% over a wide range of the irradiation conditioning doses (6–10 Gy) and donor T-cell numbers (1×10^5–2×10^7).

The specificity of this reaction is underscored by the observation that lethal marrow aplasia does not occur when a mixture of donor and host bone marrow is injected along with donor CD4$^+$ T cells. In this scenario, despite destruction of host-derived stem cells, the donor bone marrow is spared from attack and can go on to engraft the host hematopoietic compartment. It is important to note that since semi-purified or enriched CD4$^+$ cells are often contaminated with stem cells, especially when harvested from the spleen. Therefore, demonstrating marrow aplasia by this mechanism requires a highly purified CD4$^+$ population, lest there is unintended hematopoietic stem engraftment from the T-cell injection.

H. High Doses of Donor CD4$^+$ T Cells

In the context of the observations described above, paradoxical results are observed when much higher doses of donor CD4$^+$ cells are injected into heavily irradiated recipients; the incidence of GVHD mortality actually drops significantly. Whereas a dose of 1×10^6 $CD4^+$ cells generally causes nearly 100% mortality, increasing the number of $CD4^+$ cells to 2×10^7 reduces the mortality rate to less than 40% (39). This protection is augmented when bulk populations of $CD4^+$ cells and B cells are injected; lethally irradiated (10 Gy) $(B6 \times bm12)F_1$ recipients that are injected with 1×10^8 unseparated B6 spleen cells ($CD4^+$ and $CD8^+$ cells, B cells, and stem cells) go through a "crisis" about 2 weeks after injection (animals show runting and lethargy) but then experience less than 10% mortality. To fully appreciate the mechanism likely responsible for this protection, it must first be revealed that mice kept under sterile conditions are much less susceptible to lethal GVHD (43), suggesting that mortality is, at least in part, a consequence of infection. Indeed, irradiation preconditioning and the GVH response effectively ablate the host's immune system and at the same time cause epithelial tissue damage (normally the most significant barrier to pathogens), enhancing the risk of infection. Therefore, protection from lethality by large doses of $CD4^+$ T cells and B cells may work by restoring an immune compartment that is competent enough to protect the host from opportunistic bacteriemia, thus allowing for survival. Such a mechanism would therefore limit the consequences but not prevent the initial GVHD reaction itself.

IV. GVHD IN NONIRRADIATED HOSTS

Some GVHD models are carried out with nonirradiated hosts. Here, results tend to vary according to the age of the recipients. When neonatal hosts are used in P → F_1 models, large doses of either donor $CD4^+$ or $CD8^+$ T cells result in lethal GVHD by 2–3 weeks. Disease is characterized by prominent lymphocytic infiltrations in various target organs, especially the liver (27,44). Enlargement of the spleen is also common in this GVHD model, and measuring its size has long been a popular indicator of GVHD severity; splenomegaly is most pronounced at about 10 days postinjection (44). Splenomegaly is usually attributed to the action of $CD4^+$ T cells; however, in the MHC class I disparate B6 → bm1 model, purified $CD8^+$ T cells also mediate considerable spleen enlargement (27).

When nonirradiated adult mice are used as hosts, two distinct patterns of GVHD pathology are seen, dependent upon the T-cell subsets responsible for mediating disease (45,46). When purified B6 $CD4^+$ T cells are transferred to nonirradiated adult $(B6 \times bm12)F_1$ mice, the $CD4^+$ cells mount a prolonged response against host class II antigens. This drives a chronic "proliferative" form of sublethal GVHD characterized, in part, by splenomegaly. Prominent autoantibody production is also noted and is presumably secondary to aberrant donor $CD4^+$ T-cell responses to alloantigens on host B cells, which drive the B cells to undergo polyclonal activation. Such a syndrome is not specific to the $(B6 \times bm12)F_1$ model, as a similar proliferative type of nonlethal GVHD is also seen when purified $CD4^+$ cells are transferred across whole MHC barriers (47).

A quite different type of GVHD occurs upon transplant of unseparated T cells across a combined MHC class I and II barrier, for instance, when whole B6 T cells are transferred to nonirradiated $(bm1 \times bm12)F_1$ mice (45). Here the GVH reaction involves both $CD4^+$ and $CD8^+$ cells and begins with the host mice exhibiting the proliferative form of GVHD discussed above. This is succeeded after a few weeks by a phase of acute GVHD associated with bone marrow aplasia that leads to death in many recipients. In this model, aplastic GVHD is known to require the presence of donor $CD8^+$ T cells, although the mechanism of aplasia is poorly understood. Although some investigators argue that the $CD8^+$ cells play a suppressor role (48,49), the simplest explanation is that progressive tissue damage caused by

CTL activity of donor $CD8^+$ cells eventually overwhelms the recipient. Importantly, help from allostimulated $CD4^+$ cells seems to be essential, as only minimal disease occurs when the donor cells are depleted of $CD4^+$ cells or when unseparated donor T cells are injected into hosts expressing only a class I difference. The inability of purified $CD8^+$ T cells to cause lethal GVHD applies only to nonirradiated hosts. As discussed earlier, $CD8^+$ cells alone are highly potent at causing an aplastic form of lethal GVHD in irradiated hosts.

An interesting case is one using nonirradiated (B6 × DBA/2)F_1 mice ($H2^b$ × $H2^d$) as recipients of unseparated DBA/2 T cells ($CD4^+$ and $CD8^+$). GVHD in this P → F_1 model also occurs across an MHC class I and II mismatch, but in contrast to the aplastic form of GVHD discussed above, these recipients develop chronic proliferative GVHD (49). In stark contrast, the injection of either B6 or B10.D2 T cells leads to acute aplastic GVHD. These models have been used to examine the mechanistic differences between the development of acute vs. chronic GVHD. Importantly, in this situation, the divergence of the two responses appears to be dependent upon the failure of DBA/2 $CD8^+$ T cells to expand in the host following engraftment (50). Indeed, aside from being important for the cytopathic stage of the GVHD response, donor $CD8^+$ T cells are also hypothesized to have a modulatory function in this model, possibly by influencing the cytokine secretion profile of donor $CD4^+$ T cells such that Th1-like cytokines are produced (50). Th1-like cytokines are more associated with acute GVHD, and accordingly, increased levels of IFN-γ (a classic Th1-like cytokine) are observed when B6 donor T cells are used compared to lower levels after the injection of DBA/2 T cells. Therefore, although transplant of unseparated T cells across a combined class I and II difference generally leads to an aplastic form of GVHD in unirradiated recipients, this finding is not invariable and may vary based upon inherent differences, either qualitative or quantitative, in donor T-cell populations.

V. GVHD TO MINOR HISTOCOMPATIBILITY ANTIGENS

HSCT in humans is primarily restricted to donor/host combinations between HLA-compatible siblings or matched unrelated donors; therefore, mouse models for GVHD directed to minor H antigens (miHA) are of obvious clinical relevance. As discussed in Chapter 14, GVHD in HLA-compatible combinations can be very severe. GVHD is probably directed largely, and perhaps entirely, to miHA. In this regard, several human miHA have been identified, some of which are ubiquitously expressed by host tissues in the context of appropriate MHC molecules, whereas others have more tissue-restricted expression such as HA-1 on hematopoietic cells (51).

Studies in which untreated marrow cells were transferred to irradiated H2-compatible hosts expressing a variety of non-H2 differences provided the first evidence that miHA were targets for GVHD (52,53). When the donor and host differed at three or more minor H loci, a high incidence of lethal GVHD was seen. Difference at other loci (e.g., Ly or Mls loci) failed to cause GVHD. The evidence that T cells mediated GVHD came from the finding that depleting the marrow inoculum of contaminating mature T cells with anti-Thy1 antibody plus complement abolished GVHD (52). It should be noted that, in contrast to human marrow, mouse marrow contains only small numbers of mature T cells (1–2%).

A. MiHA Target Antigens

While it is clear that lethal GVHD in non–H2-different combinations requires miHA incompatibility, which particular miHA provide the targets for GVHD is still unclear.

Studies with available congeneic strains of mice differing selectively at defined miHA have shown that none of these isolated miHA differences elicit lethal GVHD (54,55). Currently, a single class I–restricted miHA that can cause GVHD has been identified in only one strain combination, C3H.SW → B6 (56). It is likely that only a very limited number of immunodominant miHA may be responsible for GVHD in particular strain combinations that are known to differ at dozens of minor H loci (54,57–60). Why some miHA are more potent than others in inducing GVHD is unclear. Experiments using B6 → BALB.B and CXB recombinant inbred strains have indicated that the miHA that act as targets for GVHD do not necessarily correspond with strong in vitro CTL responses (61). In addition, several strong miHA have now been fully characterized molecularly and genetically in these strain combinations (62–64), but they have been shown not to correlate with the development of GVHD (54,55,61). In addition, a curious form of immunodominance, whereby in vitro CTL responses to weak antigens are suppressed by responses to stronger antigens (65), does not seem to apply to GVHD (see $V\beta$ analyses below). Instead, it appears that GVHD pathology is caused by a limited number of miHA in each donor/recipient combination that satisfy the criteria of being (1) expressed in appropriate target tissue and (2) capable of stimulating a large enough T-cell response. Theoretically, all of these miHA could contribute to the development of disease, and given enough responding T cells, each may be capable of inducing GVHD pathology in their own right.

B. Features of Anti-miHA GVHD

Utilizing several strain combinations expressing three or more minor H antigen differences, studies have shown that transferring a mixture of purified unprimed donor T cells plus T-depleted donor marrow cells to mice given an intermediate dose of irradiation (7.5–8 Gy) causes significant mortality in each combination (66). The most detailed information has come from the CBA → B10.BR combination (52,67,68) in which lethal GVHD approaches 100% even with very small numbers of T cells ($<1 \times 10^5$). Based on experiments in which donor T cells were negatively selected to class I–or class II–restricted miHA by blood to lymph passage through irradiated H2 recombinant intermediate hosts, the T cells mediating GVHD in the CBA → B10.BR combination respond to miHA presented by host class I rather than class II molecules (67,68). These cells comprise a mixture of H2D- and H2K-restricted T cells.

The dose of T cells injected determines the patterns of GVHD elicited by miHA, whereby large numbers of T cells produce early-onset GVHD and deaths and smaller numbers of T cells lead to late-onset GVHD and mortality (52). Histopathology of mice with chronic GVHD involves lymphoid atrophy, weight loss, and lymphocyte infiltration of the skin, liver, and lungs (69–73); involvement of the gut is mild, although some mice develop chronic diarrhea. Symptoms of GVHD tend to be more severe in hosts conditioned with heavy irradiation (8–10 Gy), rather than light irradiation (6–8 Gy), and when the general health of the colony is suboptimal. With regard to the marrow inoculum, using host rather than donor marrow has little effect in potentiating GVHD (74). This contrasts with anti-H2 GVHD where reconstitution with host marrow leads to marked marrow aplasia (see above). It is worth mentioning that the capacity of large doses of $CD4^+$ cells to protect against lethal GVHD does not seem to apply to GVHD directed to minor H antigens (74). The reason for this difference is obscure.

C. Role of CD8$^+$ Cells

GVHD to miHA is mediated largely, though not exclusively, by CD8$^+$ cells (66). This was apparent from the above finding that the effector cells in the CBA → B10.BR combination were H2 class I restricted. In this and several other combinations, either depleting CD4$^+$ cells from the donor T-cell inoculum (67) injecting the host mice with anti-CD4 antibody (74) generally has little or no effect in reducing the intensity of GVHD. As discussed earlier, these findings imply that the capacity of CD8$^+$ cells to mediate GVHD to miHA does not necessarily require help from CD4$^+$ cells. Yet, in some strain combinations like B6 → BALB.B, the CD8$^+$ cells will only mediate GVHD in the presence of CD4$^+$ cells (75) (Table 1). Host APC expression of 4-1BB ligand, which binds to its counterpart (4-1BB; CD137) on the CD8$^+$ T cells and serves as a costimulatory molecule for activation and survival (76), appears to dictate CD8$^+$ cell dependency on exogenous help.

The repertoire of the responding CD8$^+$ T cells in the B6 → BALB.B (8.25 Gy) GVHD model analyzed by TCR Vβ CDR3-size spectratype analysis in an effort to investigate the heterogeneity of T-cell responses in a multidisparate miHA donor/recipient strain combination. This response was found to involve T cells from seven Vβ families (77) (Table 2). With the exception of a single Vβ family, these responses were also found after transplantation of B6 CD8$^+$ T cells into irradiated CXBE mice. CXBE is a recombinant inbred strain that is derived from a cross between B6 and BALB/c mice and therefore expresses a subset of the minor H antigens found in the BALB.B strain. This overlap in the CD8$^+$ T-cell response repertoire suggested that the phenomenon of competitive immunodominance was not a factor in the recognition of miHA involved in the development of GVHD. In addition, lethal GVHD could be induced by the transplantation of a single purified B6 CD8$^+$ Vβ family into either an irradiated BALB.B or CXBE recipient strain, supporting the involvement of a single purified Vβ family in disease pathogenesis and suggesting a hierarchy of GVHD-mediating specificities within the responding T-cell population (77).

Table 1 GVHD Across Minor Histocompatability Antigen Barriers Mediated by CD4$^+$ and CD8$^+$ T Cells

Donor → Recipient[a]	H2	GVHD severity[b]		
		Whole T	CD4$^+$	CD8$^+$
C3H.SW → B6	H2	++	−	+++
DBA/2 → B10.D2	H2	+	−	+++
B10.BR → CBA/J	H2	+++	+	+++
B10.S → SJL	H2	+++	−	+++
B10.D2 → DBA/2	H2	+++	+++	++
B10.D2 → BALB/C	H2	+++	+++	+++
B6 → BALB.B	H2	+++	+++	+++[c]
B6 → CXBE	H2	+++	−	+++[c]

[a]Lethally irradiated (7.5–8.25 Gy) hosts were injected i.v. with T-cell–depleted donor bone marrow and the respective T-cell subset.
[b]% mortality: +++, ≥70; ++, 40–70; +, 15–40; −, ≤15. Recipients given T-cell–depleted bone alone served as negative controls and had nearly 100% survival.
[c]CD8$^+$ T-cell–mediated GVHD is CD4$^+$ helper T-cell dependent.
Source: Refs. 66, 75.

Table 2 Summary of T-Cell Receptor Vβ Usage from B6 Anti-BALB.B and Anti-CXBE CD8$^+$ and CD4$^+$ Responses[a]

Vβ	CD8$^+$		CD4$^+$	
	BALB.B	CXBE	BALB.B	CXBE
1	+[b]	+	−[c]	−
2	−	−	+	−
3	−	−	−	−
4	+	−	+	+
5$_{1,2}$	−	−	−	−
6	+	+	+	+
7	−	−	+	+
8$_{1,2,3}$	+	+	+	+
9	+	+	+	+
10	+	+	+	+
11	−	−	+	+
12	−	−	+	+
13	−	−	+	+
14	+	+	−	+
15	−	−	−	−
16	−	−	−	+
18	ND	ND	−	+
20	−	−	−	−

ND, Not determined.
[a]Lethally irradiated BALB.B and CXBE hosts were injected i.v. with T-cell–depleted donor bone marrow 1.7×10^7 host-presensitized B6 donor T cells and cannulated 5 days later. CD8$^+$ and CD4$^+$ T cells were isolated, and CDR3-size spectratype analysis performed.
[b] + indicates that the area under the band peak was significantly increased over the corresponding peak in normal B6 splenic CD8$^+$ or CD4$^+$ T cell spectratype. P = 0.05 by student's t-test.
[c] − indicates that the area under the band peak was not increased over the corresponding peak in normal B6 splenic CD8$^+$ and CD4$^+$ T-cell spectratype.
Source: Refs. 77, 79.

D. Role of CD4$^+$ Cells

It is clear that in certain strain combinations CD4$^+$ T cells do not play a significant role in the pathogenesis of GVHD. However, when assessing the potential of T-cell subsets to mediate GVHD across a panel of six H2-matched strain combinations, it was determined that purified CD4$^+$ T cells caused a high incidence of lethal GVHD in two of these combinations, namely B10.D2 → BALB/c and B10.D2 → DBA/2 (78). This is also true in the B6 → BALB.B combination, in which CD4$^+$ T cells are required for CD8-mediated GVHD and are potent mediators of lethal GVHD themselves (75). Overall, the capacity of CD4$^+$ T cells to mediate lethal GVHD is variable compared to CD8$^+$ cells (66). Insight into why CD4$^+$ cells mediate GVHD in only a limited number of miHA-disparate strain combinations has been obtained by studying the B6 CD4$^+$-mediated GVHD response in lethally irradiated BALB.B vs. CXBE recipients. Here, despite sharing multiple miHA, BALB.B, but not CXBE recipients succumb to lethal CD4$^+$ T-cell–mediated GVHD.

Using spectratype analysis, a comparison of early B6 CD4$^+$ anti-BALB.B and anti-CXBE responses was made and revealed that 11 different Vβ families were involved in the B6 $\rightarrow$ BALB.B response (79) (Table 2). The finding of increased numbers of some of these Vβ families in GVHD target tissue lesions, along with the loss of lethality after the removal these Vβ families from the B6 CD4$^+$ inoculation, provided direct evidence that these Vβ families were important for the severity of GVHD in the BALB.B recipients (79).

Interestingly, out of the 11 different Vβ families found involved in the CD4$^+$ anti-BALB.B reaction, 9 were also implicated in the anti-CXBE response, demonstrating a large degree of overlap between the two responses (79). The pathological significance of the two BALB.B-specific Vβ families was assessed by injecting enriched preparations of each into irradiated BALB.B mice; both Vβ families and they were capable of producing GVHD lethality similar to that of unseparated CD4$^+$ T cells (124). This supports the hypothesis that GVHD across a multiple miHA barrier may depend upon the response to a limited number of miHA. Also of significance, two Vβ families were implicated in the B6 $\rightarrow$ CXBE GVH reaction that were not involved in the anti-BALB.B response. This result may hint at immunodominant effects, since one would have expected these responses to also be present in the B6 $\rightarrow$ BALB.B strain combination (79).

An interesting question with regard to the development of GVHD is whether or not the scope of the miHA-driven alloresponse changes during the progression of the disease. To address this concept, spectratype analysis was again used to assess the involvement of individual Vβ families at early, intermediate, and later time points posttransplant. Analysis of both CD8- and CD4-mediated B6 $\rightarrow$ BALB.B GVHD revealed that while the majority of Vβ families present early post-SCT persisted throughout the period of observation, the pattern of response broadened at later time points to include Vβ families that were not involved at earlier timepoints. The reasons for the delayed appearance of these Vβ families is unclear, but may be secondary to interactions with antigens (miHA or bacterial) released as a consequence of ongoing GVHD-associated tissue injury. In support of this hypothesis, reducing early injury by transplanting a CD4 population depleted of the Vβ families consistently involved in GVHD further delayed the appearance of the second layer of Vβ responses (125).

One further aspect of the Vβ research that remains unclear is the capacity of a single miHA to drive the response of multiple Vβ families. Insight into this issue will provide clues as to the minimum number of miHA required to elicit GVHD in an MHC-matched combination. Nevertheless, the study of Vβ representation in a heterogeneously responding T-cell population has provided valuable information regarding the scope and plasticity of the allogeneic T-cell response when challenged by multiple miHA targets and, most importantly, how this correlates with the development of acute GVHD.

VI. STRATEGIES TO SEPARATE GVHD FROM GVL EFFECTS

The ultimate application of the knowledge gained about the biology of allogeneic HSCT and GVHD is to design approaches that minimize GVHD without sacrificing the beneficial GVL effect or the more generalized graft-vs.-tumor (GVT) effect. Some of these approaches have included the depletion of selective lymphocyte subsets (CD4$^+$, CD8$^+$, or NK1.1$^+$) (80–82) in vivo cytokine manipulation (83–87), treatments based upon effector phenotype differences between GVHD and GVL mediating T-cell populations (88–91) and in vivo posttransplant T-cell depletion (92,93). Additional strategies are discussed in this section.

Administration of donor lymphocyte infusion (DLI) after SCT has recently emerged as a potentially powerful tool to separate GVHD from GVL effects. The strength of this approach is underscored by the observation in mice that the administration of a DLI to stable mixed hematopoietic chimeras can convert the recipients to full donor chimerism without the development of GVHD (94,95). Importantly, the use of DLI to achieve an effective GVL effect without concomitant significant GVHD has also been effectively demonstrated (96–98). In one report, effective DLI-mediated GVL was shown to depend upon donor-host mixed chimerism (presumably for maximal DLI alloactivation by residual host APC), as indicated by a complete loss of GVL activity upon DLI infusion into full donor chimeras (98). The reason why the DLI GVH response does not progress beyond the lymphohematopoietic compartment in this model is not completely clear but may involve the activity of de novo–derived donor regulatory T cells (99,100). A contributing factor to the absence of GVHD after DLI is also the time interval between the delayed infusion and the original host-preconditioning regimen. As discussed earlier, the inflammatory environment generated by the preconditioning potentiates the development of GVHD (40); the delay between preconditioning and DLI most likely allows the inflammatory environment to return to near basal levels, thus reducing the likelihood of acute GVHD.

Noting the important role that host preconditioning–induced tissue damage plays in the pathogenesis of GVHD, two soluble factors, IL-11 and keratinocyte growth factor (KGF), which are known to have valuable tissue protection and wound repair properties, have been utilized in allogeneic HSCT. Both factors reduce GVHD severity when administered either before or shortly after allogeneic HSCT (85,86,101) by reducing conditioning-related gut injury and preventing the release of lipopolysaccharide (LPS) into the systemic circulation. In addition, the treatments did not abrogate a potent GVL effect, thus demonstrating that by reducing conditioning-related toxicity, GVHD can be minimized without the loss of a GVL response (85,86).

A more targeted strategy to GVHD/GVL separation is to promote specific antihost responses against putative leukemia-related antigens. To this end, CDR3-size spectratype analysis has been used to identify TCR Vβ families involved in the antitumor but not the antihost allogeneic response and successfully transfer T cells capable of mediating GVL effects without GVHD (102). Spectratype analysis has also been used to identify the Vβ utilization of those T cells involved in GVHD at different target tissue sites (T. M. Friedman and R. Korngold, unpublished data). Removal of these cells from the original donor stem cell inoculum may reduce specific target tissue injury, allowing for investigation of the hypothesis that preventing particular target organ GVHD involvement (e.g., gut) will reduce the severity of GVHD without the loss of GVL effects.

An approach distinct from those discussed above involves allowing an initial, unrestricted GVH reaction to begin for the benefit of a more effective GVL effect. This tactic is based upon clinical observations suggesting that the most successful GVL response occurs within the context of GVHD (103–105). The conceptual advance here would be to induce a transient GVHD reaction that is subsequently controlled prior to the development of full-blown disease. Such an approach is supported by a number of studies where a greater GVL effect and more complete donor engraftment were noted using protocols targeted for GVHD therapy rather than prevention (92,93). In a recent study, the capacity of $CD4^+CD25^+$ T cells to achieve this regulation posttransplant was assessed (126). $CD4^+CD25^+$ T cells are known to have potent immunoregulatory properties and are important for the maintenance of peripheral self-tolerance and the prevention of autoimmunity (106–108). In the context of allogeneic HSCT, a number of groups have demonstrated that when added to the donor stem cell inoculum, freshly isolated or ex vivo expanded donor type CD4$^+$CD25$^+$ T cells ameliorate GVHD severity and extend survival (109–111). In the miHA-disparate B10.BR → CBA model, freshly isolated donor CD4$^+$CD25$^+$ T cells were also highly capable of suppressing ongoing GVHD when injected as late as 10 days post-HSCT. Following regulation, GVHD lethality was significantly ameliorated for the duration of the experiment (Fig. 1). Importantly, regulation of GVHD did not abrogate donor engraftment or a potent GVL effect.

VII. IMMUNOPATHOLOGY

The effector mechanisms involved in both anti-MHC and anti-miHA driven GVHD are still not fully understood; questions regarumg CTL effector mechanisms in disease pathogenesis remain unanaswered. While it appears that both perforin and FasL can play a role in overcoming host resistance to donor engraftment, their role as effector mechanisms during GVHD seems variable (112–115). Furthermore, it was recently demonstrated that although tumor necrosis factor-related apoptosis inducing ligand (TRAIL) is important for GVT reactions, it does not play a significant role in GVHD pathogenesis (116). Further investigation utilizing increasingly more intricate in vivo models should improve our understanding of T cell effector mechanisms during GVHD.

Nevertheless, investigation in a number of different models of GVHD across miHA barriers has led to a number of valuable observations. For example, while the overall

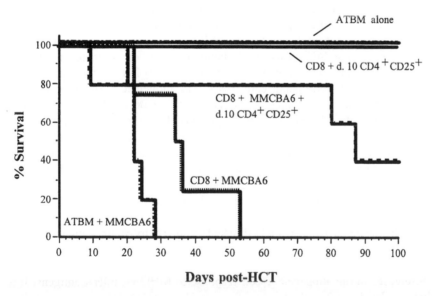

Figure 1 Infusion of donor CD4$^+$CD25$^+$ T cells day 10 post-HCT reduces lethal GVHD across a minor antigen barrier while allowing sufficient GVL effect. CBA (H2^k) mice were challenged i.p. with 1.5×10^5 MMCBA6 leukemia cells (a CBA-derived myeloid leukemia cell line) or left untreated, and in both cases were lethally irradiated the following day (13 Gy, split dose) and injected with B10.BR (H2^k) ATBM (anti-T-cell–depleted bone marrow) alone or in combination with $3–15 \times 10^6$ B10.BR CD8 + T cells. On day 10 post-HCT, recipients were either left untreated or infused with 1×10^6 freshly isolated B10.BR CD4$^+$CD25$^+$ T cells.

histopathology of GVHD mediated by CD4$^+$ and CD8$^+$ T-cell subsets is similar in the major tissues of the skin, liver, and intestinal tract, there are some interesting differences. Gut pathology is more prominent in recipients of CD4$^+$ T cells (73). Epidermal cytotoxicity in the skin is induced by both subsets, albeit by different pathways, whereas dermal fibrosis seems to be a unique aspect of CD8-mediated GVHD. Interestingly, skin injury sometimes appears prior to comparative levels of T-cell infiltration. This may be due to mast cell activity, as degranulation of these cells occurs in the skin early after transplantation and before lymphocyte infiltration is detected (117). Although TNF-α (from mast cells or T cells) does not appear to play a role in the initial keratinocyte damage associated with GVHD, it is involved in subsequent CD4-mediated pathology observed after the cells have infiltrated into the epidermal layers. In the case of CD8$^+$ cells, damage to the skin primarily reflects direct CTL activity. Apoptosis has a central role in epithelial injury in acute skin GVHD (118), and the follicular stem cells are the primary targets of attack (119,120). An interesting observation in GVHD across the BALB.C $\rightarrow$ B6 MHC barrier is the separation of target organ injury based upon the cytokine expression profile of the effector T cells; T cells producing Th2-like cytokines are required for hepatic and skin GVHD, whereas T cells producing either Th1- or Th2-like cytokines are capable of causing intestinal pathology (121).

The induction of GVHD fundamentally depends upon the recognition of foreign host antigens by donor T cells. Recently it has been suggested that the thorough depletion of host APC prior to transplant would be an effective means to prevent GVHD (122). This suggestion is based upon experiments demonstrating loss of CD8$^+$ T-cell–mediated GVHD lethality using recipients that specifically lack MHC class I expression on cells of the hematopoietic compartment (e.g., B cells, professional APC), while expressing normal levels on all other tissues (epithelium, endothelium, and parenchyma) (122). This restricted expression was accomplished by generating bone marrow chimera, which left the recipient with either a MHC class I$^{-/-}$ hematopoietic compartment or one that expressed only class I molecules syngeneic to the donor. This line of investigation was extended by a subsequent study using chimeras where allogeneic MHC class I and II expression was restricted to the hematopoietic compartment only, which demonstrated that either CD4$^+$ or CD8$^+$ T-cell–mediated lethal GVHD across MHC barriers does not require alloantigen expression anywhere but on host APC (123). It is important to understand, however, that this observation does not necessarily apply to the MHC-matched miHA-disparate situation. Indeed, earlier bone marrow chimera studies across the B10.BR $\rightarrow$ CBA MiHA barrier clearly demonstrated that miHA expression on host APC alone was insufficient to elicit CD8-mediated lethal GVHD (68). More recently, investigations involving the H2-matched B6 $\rightarrow$ BALB.B system have also revealed that for CD4$^+$ T-cell–mediated lethal GVHD directed to miHA to occur, antigen must be expressed by nonhematopoietic tissues. In fact, GVHD in this context can be elicited even when recipients have a hematopoietic compartment syngeneic to the donor (127). Clearly there are differences in the allogeneic T-cell response to MHC vs. miHA antigens. It is possible that smaller donor T cell precursor frequencies to miHA differences result in a less robust alloresponse to antigens presented by the hematopoietic compartment. By contrast, T-cell responses to MHC differences are large in comparison and much more likely to generate inflammatory cytokine levels capable of acute tissue damage early after SCT. Second, whereas in the context of an MHC mismatch the only difference between hematopoietic and all other tissues is likely to be the level of MHC expression, in a miHA mismatch scenario epithelial tissues might be a source for novel miHAs not expressed by the hematopoietic compartment. Such an antigen could be directly presented by class I or II molecules on the epithelial cells or picked up and presented exogenously by professional APC, thus increasing the immunogenicity of hematopoietic cells to levels required for a more aggressive alloresponse. In all, the course and kinetics of pathogenesis in GVHD may depend on several variables, including the strength of the individual CD4 and CD8 cell responses, the levels of expression of antigens in target tissues, and the fluctuations of cytokines, both local and systemically.

VII. SUMMARY

The use of animal SCT models and murine systems in particular has been instrumental to our understanding of the pathophysiology and immunobiology of GVHD. The generation of numerous transgenic and knockout strains has enabled investigators not only to examine the pathogenesis of GVHD but also to gain insights into the underlying effector mechanisms used by T-cell subsets involved in this process. Current and future studies will ultimately provide the knowledge necessary to develop novel immunotherapeutic strategies that will selectively reduce the risk of GVHD while promoting curative GVL effects and protection from infectious pathogens.

REFERENCES

1. Riddell SR, Murata M, Bryant S, Warren EH. T-cell therapy of leukemia. Cancer Control 2002; 9:114–122.
2. Kolb HJ, Schattenberg A, Goldman JM, Hertenstein B, Jacobsen N, Arcese W, Ljungman P, Ferrant A, Verdonck L, Niederwieser D. Graft-versus-leukemia effect of donor lymphocyte transfusions in marrow grafted patients. Blood 1995; 86:2041–2050.
3. Franceschini F, Butturini A, Gale RP. Clinical trials of T-cell depletion in bone marrow transplantation. In: Gale RP, Champlin R, eds. Progress in Bone Marrow Transplantation. New York: Alan R Liss, 1987:323–340.
4. Henslee PJ, Thompson JS, Romond EH, Doukas MA, Metcalfe M, Marshall ME, MacDonald JS. T cell depletion of HLA and haploidentical marrow reduces graft-versus-host disease but it may impair a graft-versus-leukemia effect. Transplant Proc 1987; 19:2701–2706.
5. Gale RP, Champlin RE. How does bone marrow transplantation cure leukemia? Lancet 1984; 2:28–30.
6. Weiner RS, Dicke KA. Risk factors for interstitial pneumonitis following allogeneic bone marrow transplantation for severe apiastic anemia: a preliminary report. Transplant Proc 1987; 19:2693–2642.
7. Bakonyi A, Berho M, Ruiz P, Misiakos E, Carreno M, de Faria W, Sommariva A, Inverardi L, Miller J, Ricordi C, Tzakis AG. Donor and recipient pretransplant conditioning with nonlethal radiation and antilymphocyte serum improves the graft survival in a rat small bowel transplantation model. Transplantation 2001; 72:983–988.
8. Ladiges WC, Storb R, Thomas ED. Canine models of bone marrow transplantation. Lab Animal Sci 1990; 40:11–15.
9. Sprent J. T lymphocytes and the thymus. In: Paul WE, ed. Fundamental Immunology. 3rd ed. New York: Raven Press, 1993:75–110.
10. von Boehmer H. Developmental biology of T cells in T-cell receptor transgenic mice. Annu Rev Immunol 1990; 8:531–556.
11. Shevach EM. Accessory molecules. In: Paul WE, ed. Fundamental Immunology. 3rd ed. New York: Raven Press, 1993:531–576.

12. Sprent J, Webb SR. Function and specificity of T-cell subsets in the mouse. Adv Immunol 1987; 41:39–133.

13. Storb R, Thomas ED. Bone marrow transplantation in randomly bred animal species an in man. Proceedings of the Sixth Leukocyte Culture Conference. New York: Academic Press, 1972:805–840.

14. Santos GW, Owens AH. Bull Johns Hosp 1965; 116:327.

15. Thomas ED, Collins JA, Herman EC, et al. Marrow transplants in lethally irradiated dogs given methotrexate. Blood 1962; 19:217–228.

16. Storb R, Deeg HJ, Atkinson K, Weiden PL, Sale G, Colby R, Thomas ED. Cyclosporin A abrogates transfusion-induced sensitization and prevents marrow graft rejection in DLA-identical canine littermates. Blood 1982; 60:524–526.

17. Kolb HJ, Storb R, Graham TC, Kolb H, Thomas ED. Antithymocyte serum and methotrexate for control of graft-versus-host disease in dogs. Transplantation 1973; 16:17–23.

18. Kloosterman TC, Tielemans MJC, Martens ACM, van Bekkum DW, Hagenbeek A. Quantitative studies on graft-versus-leukemia after allogeneic bone marrow transplantation in rat models for acute myelocytic and lymphocytic leukemia. Bone Marrow Transplant 1994; 14:15–22.

19. Weijtens M, Spronsen A, Hagenbeek A, Braakman E, Martens A. Reduced graft-versus-host disease-inducing capacity of T cells after activation, culturing, and magnetic cell sorting selection in an allogeneic bone marrow transplantation model in rats. Hum Gene Therapy 2002; 13:187–198.

20. Sprent J, Korngold R. A comparison of lethal graft-versus-host disease to minor-versus-major differences in mice: implications for marrow transplantation in man. Progr Immunol 1983; 5:1461–1475.

21. Bennett M. Biology and genetics of hybrid resistance. Adv Immunol 1987; 41:333–445.

22. Murphy WJ, Kumar V, Bennett M. Rejection of bone marrow allografts by mice with severe combined immunodeficiency (SCID): Evidence that natural killer (NK) cells can mediate the specificity of marrow graft rejection. J Exp Med 1987; 165:1212–1217.

23. Bix M, Liao NS, Zijlstra M, Loring J, Jaenisch R, Raulet D. Rejection of class I MHC-deficient hematopoietic cells by irradiated MHC-matched mice. Nature 1991; 349: 329–331.

24. Jones M, Komatsu M, Levy RB. Cytotoxically impaired transplants recipients can efficiently resist MHC matched BM allografts. Biol Blood Marrow Transplant 2000; 6:456–464.

25. Moller G, Ed. Elimination of allogeneic lymphoid cells. Immunol Rev 1983; 73:1–126.

26. Korngold R, Sprent J. Surface markers of T cells causing lethal graft-versus-host disease to class I vs. class II H-2 differences. J Immunol 1985; 135:3004–3010.

27. Sprent J, Schaefer M, Lo D, Korngold R. Properties of purified T-cell subsets. II. In vivo responses to class I vs. class II H-2 differences. J Exp Med 1986; 163:998–1011.

28. Korngold R, Sprent J. Purified T-cell subsets and lethal graft-versus-host disease in mice. In: Gale RP, Champlin R, eds. Progress in Bone Marrow Transplantation. New York: Liss, 1987:213–218.

29. Cobbold S, Martin G, Waldmann H. Monoclonal antibodies for the prevention of graft-versus-host disease and marrow graft rejection. Transplantation 1986; 42:239–247.

30. Reiser JB, Darnault C, Guimezanes A, Gregoire C, Mosser T, Schmitt AM, Camps JC, Malissen B, Housset D, Mazza G. Crystal structure of a T cell receptor bound to an allogeneic MHC molecule. Nature Immunol 2000; 1:291–297.

31. Crumpacker DB, Alexander J, Cresswell P, Engelhard V. Role of endogenous peptides in murine allogeneic cytotoxic T cell responses assessed using transfectants of the antigen processing mutant 174 × CEM.T2. J Immmunol 1992; 148:3004–3011.

32. Smith KD, Huczko E, Engelhard VH, Li Y, Lutz CT. Alloreactive cytotoxic T lymphocytes focus on specific major histocompatability complex-bound peptides. Transplantation 1997; 64:351–359.

33. Demotz S, Sette A, Sakaguchi K, Buchner R, Appella E, Grey HM. Self peptide requirement for class II major histocompatability complex recognition. Proc Natl Acad Sci 1991; 88:8730–8734.

34. Nathenson SG, Geliebter J, Pfaffenbach GM, Zeff RA. Murine major histocompatability complex class-I mutants: molecular analysis and structure-function implications. Ann Rev Immunol 1986; 4:471–502.

35. Sprent J, Schaefer M, Lo D, Korngold R. Function of purified L3T4$^+$ and Lyt-2$^+$ cells in vitro and in vivo. Immunol Rev 1986; 91:195–218.

36. Sprent J, Schaefer M, Gao E-K, Korngold R. Role of T-cell subsets in lethal graft-vs.-host disease (GVHD) directed to class I versus class II H-2 differences. I. L3T4$^+$ cells can either augment or retard GVHD elicited by Lyt-2$^+$ cells in class I-different hosts. J Exp Med 1988; 167:556–569.

37. Guy-Grand D, Vassalli P. Gut injury in mouse graft-versus-host reactions. J Clin Invest 1986; 77:1584–1595.

38. Mowat AM, Sprent J. Induction of intestinal graft-versus-host reactions across mutant major histocompatability antigens by T lymphocyte subsets in mice. Transplantation 1989; 47:857–863.

39. Sprent J, Schaeler M, Korngold R. Role of T-cell subsets in lethal graft-versus-host disease (GVHD) directed to class I versus class II H-2 differences. II. Protective effects of L3T4$^+$ cells in anti-class II H-2 differences. J Immunol 1990; 144:2946–2954.

40. Krenger W, Ferrara J. Graft-versus-host disease and the Th1/Th2 paradigm. Immunol Res 1996; 15:50–73.

41. Piguet P-F. GVHR elicited by products of class I or class II loci of the MHC: analysis of the response of mouse T lymphocytes to products of class I and class II loci of the MHC in correlation with GVHR-induced mortality, medullary aplasia, and enteropathy. J Immunol 1985; 135:1637–1643.

42. Piguet P-F, Grau GE, Allet B, Vassalli P. Tumor necrosis factor/cachectin is an effector of skin and gut lesions of the acute phase of graft-vs.-host disease. J Exp Med 1987; 166:1280–1289.

43. Vossen JM, Heidt PJ. Gnotobiotic measures for prevention of acute graft-versus-host disease. In: Burakoff SJ, Deeg HJ, Ferrara JLM, Atkinson K, eds. Graft-vs.-Host Disease: Immunology, Pathophysiology and Treatment. New York: Marcel Dekker, 1990:403–413.

44. Simonsen M. Graft-versus-host reactions. Their natural history and applicability as tools of research. Progr Allergy 1962; 6:349–467.

45. Rolink AG, Pals ST, Gleichmann E. Allosuppressor and allohelper T cells in acute and chronic graft-vs.-host disease. II. F1 recipients carrying mutations at H-2K and/or I-A. J Exp Med 1983; 157:755–771.

46. Gleichmann E, Pals ST, Rolink AG, Radaszkiewicz T, Gleichmann H. Graft-versus-host reactions: clues to the etiopathology of a spectrum of immunological diseases. Immunol Today 1984; 5:324–332.

47. Rolink AG, Gleichmann E. Allosuppressor and allohelper T cells in acute and chronic graft-vs.-host disease. III. Different Lyt subsets of donor T cells induce different pathologic syndromes. J Exp Med 1983; 158:546–558.

48. Rolink AG, Radaszkiewicz T, Pals ST, van der Meer WGJ, Gleichmann E. Allosuppressor and allohelper T cells in acute and chronic graft-vs.-host disease. I. Alloreactive suppressor cells rather than killer T cells appear to be the decisive cells in lethal graft-vs.-host disease. J Exp Med 1982; 155:1501–1522.

49. van Elven EH, Rolink AG, van der Veen F, Gleichmann E. Capacity of genetically different T lymphocytes to induce lethal graft-versus-host disease correlates with their capacity to generate suppression but not with their capacity to generate anti-F1 killer cells. A non-H-2 locus determines the inability to induce lethal graft-versus-hosts disease. J Exp Med 1981; 153:1474–1488.

50. Rus V, Svetic A, Nguyen P, Gause WC, Via CS. Kinetics of Th1 and Th2 cytokine production during the early course of acute and chronic murine graft-versus-host disease. Regulatory role of donor CD8$^+$ T Cells. J Immunol 1995; 155:2396–2406.

51. Goulmy E. Minor histocompatability antigens: from T cell recognition to peptide identification. Hum Immunol 1997; 54:8–14.

52. Korngold R, Sprent J. Lethal graft-versus-host disease after bone-marrow transplantation across minor histocompatibility barriers in mice. Prevention by removing mature T cells from marrow. J Exp Med 1978; 148:1687–1698.

53. Hamilton BL, Bevan MJ, Parkman R. Anti-recipient cytotoxic T lymphocyte precursors are present in the spleens of mice with acute graft-versus-host disease due to minor histocompatibility antigens. J Immunol 1981; 126:621–625.

54. Korngold R, Leighton C, Mobraaten LE, Berger MA. Inter-strain graft-versus-host disease T cell responses to immunodominant minor histocompatibility antigens. Biol Blood Marrow Transplant 1997; 3:57–64.

55. Blazar BR, Roopenian DC, Taylor PA, Christianson GJ, Panoskaltsis-Mortari A, Vallera DA. Lack of GVHD across classical, single minor histocompatibility (miH) locus barriers in mice. Transplantation 1996; 61:619–624.

56. Perreault C, Jutras J, Roy DC, Filep JG, Brochu S. Identification of an immunodominant mouse minor histocompatibility antigen (MiHA). T cell response to a single dominant MiHA causes graft-versus-host disease. J Clin Invest 1996; 98:622–628.

57. Berger MA, Korngold R. Immunodominant CD4$^+$ T cell receptor Vβ repertoire involved in graft-versus-host disease responses to minor histocompatibility antigens. J Immunol 1997; 159:77–85.

58. Howell CD, Li J, Roper E, Kotzin BL. Biased liver T cell receptor Vβ repertoire in a murine graft-versus-host disease model. J Immunol 1995; 155:2350–2358.

59. Brochu S, Baron C, Hetu F, Roy DC, Perreault C. Oligoclonal expansion of CTLs directed against a restricted number of dominant minor histocompatibility antigens in hemopoietic chimeras. J Immunol 1995; 155:5104–5114.

60. Perreault C, Roy DC, Fortin C. Immunodominant minor histocompatibility antigens: the major ones. Immunol Today 1998; 19:69–74.

61. Korngold R, Wettstein PJ. Immunodominance in the graft-vs.-host disease T-cell response to minor histocompatibility antigen. J Immunol 1990; 145:4079–4088.

62. Nevala WK, Wettstein PJ. H4 and CTT-2 minor histocompatibility antigens: concordant genetic linkage and migration in two-dimensional peptide separation. Immunogenetics 1996; 44:400–404.

63. Malarkannan S, Shih PP, Eden PA, Horng T, Zuberi AR, Christianson G, Roopenian D, Shastri N. The molecular and functional characterization of a dominant minor H antigen, H60. J Immunol 1998; 161:3501–3509.

64. Malarkannan S, Horng T, Eden P, Gonzalez F, Shih P, Brouwenstijn N, Klinge H, Christianson G, Roopenian D, Shastri N. Differences that matter: major cytotoxic T cell-stimulating minor histocompatibility antigens. Immunity 2000; 3:333–344.

65. Wettstein PJ. Immunodominance in the T-cell response to multiple non-H-2 histocompatibility antigens. II. Observation of a hierarchy among dominant antigens. Immunogenetics 1986; 24:24–31.

66. Korngold R, Sprent J. Variable capacity of L3T4$^+$ T cells to cause lethal graft-versus-host disease across minor histocompatibility bamers in mice. J Exp Med 1987; 165:1522–1564.

67. Korngold R, Sprent J. Lethal GVHD across minor histocompatibility barriers: nature of the effector cells and role of the H-2 complex. Immunol Rev 1983; 71:5–29.

68. Korngold R, Sprent J. Features of T cells causing H-2-restricted lethal graft-versus-host disease across minor histocompatibility barriers. J Exp Med 1982; 155:872–883.

69. Jaffee BD, Claman HN. Chronic graft-versus-host disease (GVHD) as a model for scleroderma. I. Description of model systems. Cell Immunol 1983; 77:1–12.

70. Ferrara J, Guillen FJ, Sleckman B, Burakoff SJ, Murphy GF. Cutaneous acute graft-versus-host disease to minor histocompatibility antigens in a murine model: histologic analysis and correlation to clinical disease. J Invest Dermatol 1986; 123:401–406.

71. Rappaport H, Khalil A, Halle-Pannenko O, Pritchard L, Dantcher D, Mathe G. Histopathologic sequence of events in adult mice undergoing lethal graft-vs.-host reaction developed across H-2 and/or non H-2 histocompatibility barriers. Am J Pathol 1979; 96:121–143.

72. Charley MR, Bangert JL, Hamilton BL, Gilliam JN, Sontheimer RD. Murine graft-versus-host skin disease: a chronologic and quantitative analysis of two histologic patterns. J Invest Dermatol 1983; 81:412–417.

73. Murphy GF, Whitaker D, Sprent J, Korngold R. Characterization of target injury of murine acute graft-versus-host disease directed to multiple minor histocompatibility antigens elicited by either CD4$^+$ or CD8$^+$ effector cells. Am J Path 1991; 138:983–990.

74. Korngold R. Lethal graft-versus-host disease in mice directed to multiple minor histocompatibility antigens: features of CD8$^+$ and CD4$^+$ T-cell responses. Bone Marrow Transplant 1992; 9:355–364.

75. Berger M, Wettstein PJ, Korngold R. T cell subsets involved in lethal graft-versus-host disease directed to immunodominant minor histocompatability antigens. Transplantation 1994; 57:1095–1102.

76. Kwon B, Moon CH, Kang S, Seo SK, Kwon BS. 4-1BB: still in the midst of darkness. Mol Cells 2000; 10:119–126.

77. Friedman TM, Gilbert M, Briggs C, Korngold R. Repertoire analysis of CD8$^+$ T cell responses to minor histocompatability antigens involved in graft-versus-host disease. J Immunol 1998; 161:41–48.

78. Hamilton BL. L3T4-positive T cells in the induction of graft-versus-host disease in response to minor histocompatability antigens. J Immunol 1987; 139:2511–2515.

79. Friedman TM, Statton D, Jones SC, Berger MA, Murphy GF, Korngold R. Vβ spectratype analysis reveals heterogeneity of CD4$^+$ T cell responses to minor histocompatability antigens involved in graft-versus-host disease: correlations with epithelial tissue infiltrate. Biol Blood Marrow Transplant 2001; 7:2–13.

80. Johnson BD, Truitt RL. A decrease in graft-vs.-host disease without loss of graft-vs.-leukemia reactivity after MHC-matched bone marrow transplantation by selective depletion of donor NK cells in vivo. Transplantation 1992; 54:104–112.

81. Korngold R, Leighton C, Manser T. Graft-versus-myeloid responses following sygeneic and allogeneic bone marrow transplantation. Transplantation 1994; 58:278–287.

82. Aizawa S, Kamisaku H, Sado T. An MHC-compatible allogeneic bone marrow donor with a distinct role of T cell subsets in graft-versus-leukemia effect and lethal graft-versus-host disease. Bone Marrow Transplant 1995; 16:603–609.

83. Sykes M, Harty MW, Szot GL, Pearson DA. Interleukin-2 inhibits graft-versus-host disease-promoting activity of CD4$^+$ T cells while preserving CD4- and CD8-mediated graft-versus-leukemia effects. Blood 1994; 83:2560–2569.

84. Yang YG, Sykes M. The role of interleukin-12 in preserving the graft-versus-leukemia effect of allogeneic CD8 T cells independently of GVHD. Leukemia and Lymphoma 1999; 33:409–420.

85. Krijanovski OI, Hill GR, Cooke KR, Teshima T, Crawford JM, Brinson YS, Ferrara JL. Keratinocyte growth factor separates graft-versus-leukemia effects from graft-versus-host disease. Blood 1999; 94:825–831.

86. Teshima T, Hill GR, Pan L, Brinson YS, van den Brink MR, Cooke KR, Ferrara JL. IL-11 separates graft-versus-leukemia effects from graft-versus-host disease after bone marrow transplant. J Clin Invest 1999; 104:317–325.

87. Leshem B, Vourka-Karussis U, Slavin S. Correlation between enhancement of graft-vs.-leukemia effects following allogeneic bone marrow transplantation by rIL-2 and increased frequency of cytotoxic T-lymphocyte-precursors in murine myeloid leukemia. Cytokines Cell Mol Ther 2000; 6:141–147.

88. Fowler DH, Breglio J, Nagel G, Hirose C, Gress RE. Allospecific CD4$^+$, Th1/Th2 and CD8$^+$ Tc1/Tc2 populations in murine GVL: type I cells generate GVL and type II cells abrogate GVL. Biol Blood Marrow Transplant 1996; 2:118–125.
89. Tsukada N, Kobata T, Aizawa Y, Yagita H, Okumura K. Graft-versus-leukemia effect and graft-versus-host disease can be differentiated by cytotoxic mechanisms in a murine model of allogeneic bone marrow transplantation. Blood 1999; 93:2738–2747.
90. Schmaltz C, Alpdogan O, Horndasch KJ, Muriglan SJ, Kappel BJ, Teshima T, Ferrara JL, Burakoff SJ, Van den Brink MR. Differential use of fas ligand and perforin cytotoxic pathways by donor T cells in graft-versus-host disease and graft-versus-leukemia effect. Blood 2001; 97:2886–2895.
91. Hseih MH, Varadi G, Flomenberg N, Korngold R. Leucyl-leucine methyl ester-treated haploidentical donor lymphocyte infusions can mediate graft-versus-leukemia activity with minimal graft-versus-host disease risk. Biol Blood Marrow Transplant 2002; 8:303–315.
92. Johnson BD, McCabe C, Hanke CA, Truitt RL. Use of anti-CD3e F(ab')$_2$ fragments in vivo modulate graft-versus-host disease without loss of graft-versus-leukemia reactivity alter MHC-matched bone marrow transplantation. J Immunol 1995; 154:5542–5554.
93. Drobyski WR, Morse HC III, Burns WH, Casper JT, Sanford G. Protection from lethal murine graft-versus-host disease without compromise of alloengraftment using transgenic donor T cells expressing a thymidine kinase suicide gene. Blood 2001; 97:2506–2513.
94. Sykes M, Sheard MA, Sachs DH. Graft-versus-host-related immunosuppression is induced in mixed chimeras by alloresponses against either host or donor lymphohematopoietic cells. J Exp Med 1988; 168:2391–2396.
95. Pelot MR, Pearson DA, Swenson K, Zhao G, Sachs J, Yang YG, Sykes M. Lymphohematopoietic graft-vs.-host reactions can be induced without graft-vs.-host disease in murine mixed chimeras established with a cyclophosphamide-based non-myeloablative conditioning regimen. Biol Blood Marrow Transplant 1999; 5:133–143.
96. Johnson BD, Drobyski WR, Truitt RL. Delayed infusion of normal donor cells after MHC-matched bone marrow transplantation provides anti-leukemia reaction without graft-versus-host disease. Bone Marrow Transplant 1993; 11:329–336.
97. Johnson BD, Truitt RL. Delayed infusion of immunocompetent donor cells after bone marrow transplantation breaks graft-host tolerance and allows for persistent antileukemic reactivity without severe graft versus host disease. Blood 1995; 85:3302–3312.
98. Mapara MY, Kim YM, Wang S-P, Bronson R, Sachs DH, Sykes M. Donor lymphocyte infusions mediate superior graft-versus-leukemia effects in mixed compared to fully allogeneic chimeras: a critical role for host antigen-presenting cells. Blood 2002; 100:1903–1909.
99. Johnson BD, Becker EE, LaBelle JL, Truitt RL. Role of immunoregulatory donor T cells in suppression of graft-versus-host disease following donor leukocyte infusion therapy. J Immunol 1999; 163:6479–6487.
100. Blazar BR, Lees CJ, Martin PJ, Noelle RJ, Kwon B, Murphy W, Taylor PA. Host T cells resist graft-versus-host disease mediated by donor leukocyte infusions. J Immunol 2000; 165:4901–4909.
101. Panskaltsis A-M, Lacey DL, Vallera DA, Blazar BR. Keratinocyte growth factor administered before conditioning ameliorates graft-versus-host disease after allogeneic bone marrow transplantation in mice. Blood 1998; 92:3960–3967.
102. Patterson AE, Korngold R. Infusion of select leukemia-reactive TCR Vβ^+ T cells provides graft-versus-leukemia responses with minimization of graft-versus-host disease following murine hematopoietic stem cell transplantation. Biol Blood Marrow Transplant 2001; 7:187–196.
103. Weiden PL, Sullivan KM, Flournoy N, Storb R, Thomas ED. Antileukemic effect of chronic graft-versus-host disease: contribution to improved survival after allogeneic marrow transplants. N Engl J Med 1981; 304:1529–1533.

104. Storb R. Graft rejection and graft-versus-host disease in marrow transplantation. Transplant Proc 1989; 21:2915–2918.
105. Slavin S, Ackerstein A, Naparstek E, Or R, Weiss L. The graft-versus-leukemia phenomenon: is GVL separable from GVHD? Bone Marrow Transplant 1990; 6:155–161.
106. Asano M, Toda M, Sakaguchi N, Sakaguchi S. Autoimmune disease as a consequence of developmental abnormality of a T cell subpopulation. J Exp Med 1996; 184:387–396.
107. Kuniyasu Y, Takahashi T, Itoh M, Shimizu J, Toda G, Sakaguchi S. Naturally anergic and suppressive CD4$^+$CD25$^+$ T cells as a functionally and phenotypically distinct immunoregulatory T cell subpopulation. Int Immunol 2000; 12:1145–1155.
108. Read S, Powrie F. CD4(+) regulatory T cells. Curr Opin Immunol 2001; 13:644–649.
109. Taylor PA, Lees CJ, Blazar BR. The infusion of ex vivo activated and expanded CD4$^+$CD25$^+$ immune regulatory cells inhibits graft-versus-host disease lethality. Blood 2002; 99:3493–3499.
110. Hoffmann P, Ermann J, Edinger M, Fathmman CG, Strober S. Donor-type CD4$^+$CD25$^+$ regulatory T cells suppress lethal acute graft-versus-host disease after allogeneic bone marrow transplantation. J Exp Med 2002; 196:389–399.
111. Cohen JL, Trenado A, Vasey D, Klatzmann D, Salomon BL. CD4$^+$CD25$^+$ immunoregulatory T cells: new therapeutics for graft-versus-host disease. J Exp Med 2002; 196:401–406.
112. Blazar BR, Taylor PA, Vallera DA. CD4$^+$ and CD8$^+$ T cells each can utilize a perforin-dependent pathway to mediate lethal graft-versus-host disease in major histocompatibility complex-disparate recipients. Transplantation 1997; 64:571–576.
113. Graubert TA, DiPersio JF, Russell JH, Ley TJ. Perforin/granzyme-dependent and independent mechanisms are both important for the development of graft-versus-host disease after murine bone marrow transplantation. J Clin Invest 1997; 100:904–911.
114. Baker MB, Altman NH, Podack ER, Levy RB. The role of cell-mediated cytotoxicity in acute GVHD after MHC-matched allogeneic bone marrow transplantation in mice. J Exp Med 1996; 183:2645–2656.
115. Jiang Z, Podack E, Levy RB. MHC-mismatched allogeneic bone marrow transplantation using perforin and/or Fas ligand double defective CD4$^+$ donor T cells: involvement of cytotoxic function by donor lymphocytes prior to GVHD pathogenesis. Blood 2001; 98:390–397.
116. Schmaltz C, Alpdogan O, Kappel B, Muriglan S, Rotolo J, Ongchin J, Willis L, Greenberg A, Eng J, Crawford J, Murphy G, Yagita H, Walczak H, Peschon J, van den Brink M. T cells require TRAIL for optimal graft-versus-tumor activity. Nat Immunol 2002; 8:1433–1437.
117. Murphy GF, Sueki H, Teuscher C, Whitaker D, Korngold R. Role of mast cells in early epithelial target cell injury in experimental acute graft-versus-host disease. J Invest Dermatol 1994; 102:451–461.
118. Gilliam AC, Whitaker-Menezes D, Korngold R, Murphy GF. Apoptosis is the predominant form of epithelial target cell injury in acute expenmental graft-versus-host disease. J Invest Dermatol 1996; 107:377–383.
119. Murphy GF, Lavker RM, Whitaker D, Korngold R. Cytotoxic folliculitis in acute graft-versus-host disease: evidence of follicular stem cell injury and recovery. J Cutan Pathol 1991; 18:309–314.
120. Sale GE, Beauchamp M. The parafollicular hair bulge in human GVHD: a stem cell rich primary target. Bone Marrow Transplant 1993; 11:223–225.
121. Nikolic B, Lee S, Bronson RT, Grusby MJ, Sykes M. Th1 and Th2 mediate acute graft-versus-host disease, each with distinct end-organ targets. J Clin Invest 2000; 105:1289–1298.
122. Shlomchik WD, Couzens MS, Tang CB, McNiff J, Robert ME, Liu J, Shlomchik MJ, Emerson SG. Prevention of graft versus host disease by inactivation of host antigen-presenting cells. Science 1999; 285:412–415.
123. Teshima T, Ordemann R, Reddy P, Gagin S, Liu C, Cooke KR, Ferrara JLM. Acute graft-versus-host disease does not require alloantigen expression on host epithelium. Nat Med 2002; 8:575–581.

124. Jones SC, Friedman TM, Murphy GF, Korngold R. Specific donor Vβ-associated CD4$^+$ T cell responses correlate with severe acute graft-versus-host disease directed to multiple minor histocompatibility antigens. Biology of Blood and Marrow Transplantation. In press.

125. Friedman TM, Jones SJ, Statton D, Murphy GF, Korngold R. Evolution of responding CD4$^+$ and CD8$^+$ T cell repertoires during the development of graft-versus-host disease directed to minor histocompatibility antigens. Biology of Blood and Marrow Transplantation. In press.

126. Jones SC, Murphy GF, Korngold R. Post-hematopoietic cell transplant control of graft-versus-host disease by donor CD4+25+ T cells to allow an effective graft-versus-leukemia response. Biology of Blood and Marrow Transplantation 2003; 9:243–256.

127. Jones SC, Murphy GF, Friedman TM, Korngold R. Importance of minor histocompatibility antigen expression by non-hematopoietic tissues in a CD4+ T-cell-mediated graft-versus-host disease model. J Clin Invest 2003; 112:1880–1886.

3

Graft-vs.-Host Disease as a Th1-Type Process: Regulation by Th2-Type Cells

DANIEL H. FOWLER and RONALD E. GRESS

National Institutes of Health, Bethesda, Maryland, U.S.A.

I. INTRODUCTION

Donor T lymphocytes, because they protect against infection, mediate antitumor effects, and prevent graft rejection, yet cause graft-vs.-host disease (GVHD), represent a double-edged sword as a cell component of bone marrow or peripheral blood allografts. An ability to augment or preserve beneficial allogeneic T-cell effects, while limiting detrimental GVHD, is an essential requirement for further optimization of allogeneic hematopoietic stem cell transplantation (SCT). One emerging area of immunology relevant to this challenge involves the study of T-cell cytokine phenotypes. In this chapter we provide an update on current Th1/Th2 research, review this biology as it relates to GVHD pathogenesis, and consider how this insight may provide an opportunity for modulating allogeneic T-cell immune responses and effects.

II. Th1/Th2 BIOLOGY

The origins of Th1/Th2 research began when Mosmann and colleagues described dichotomous murine CD4$^+$ T-cell clones that were antigen specific, yet responded to antigen with a restricted pattern of either IL-2 or IL-4 cytokine secretion (1). In subsequent years, Th1/Th2 research rapidly increased. Cytokines were discovered that controlled Th1/Th2 development, further defined their secretion profiles, or were downstream mediators of their disparate effects. Th1/Th2 research evolved to include in vivo murine disease models, leading to an early understanding that Th1/Th2 subsets were cross-regulatory and modulated infectious disease natural history (2). Further efforts extended the research focus from CD4$^+$ T cells to (1) cells that differentially promote Th1 or Th2 cells, such as natural killer cell NK1/NK2 subsets and dendritic cell DC1/DC2 subsets and (2) cells that are differentially promoted by Th1 or Th2 cells, such as $CD8^+$ Tc1/Tc2 subsets. Th1/Th2 investigations have therefore expanded from a modest evaluation of clonal CD4 cell cytokine secretion patterns in vitro to an in vivo assessment of cellular effector networks that promote or otherwise effect Th1/Th2 responses. Finally, human cells and disease states appear to follow the Th1/Th2 paradigm, suggesting that Th1/Th2 modulation may have therapeutic benefit in multiple disease processes, including GVHD.

Cytokine noncommitted ("Th0") $CD4^+$ T cells may obtain instruction for Th1 vs. Th2 differentiation via innate immunity (through MHC-nonrestricted NK cells) or acquired immunity [through MHC-restricted interaction with antigen-presenting cells (APC)]. In some instances, IL-4, which is not only secreted by Th2 cells but also paramount for initial induction of Th0 $\Rightarrow$ Th2 differentiation (3), may link innate and acquired immunity with respect to Th1/Th2 polarity. For example, a specific NK subset elaborating IL-4 can promote initial CD4 polarization towards Th2 type (4). Once NK-generated IL-4 primes for Th2 polarity, CD4 cells may then secrete IL-4 in an antigen-restricted manner and thereby dictate type II differentiation of downstream cellular effectors, including $CD8^+$ T cells, towards a Tc2 phenotype. NK cells, in addition to providing an initial IL-4 burst, also secrete IL-13, which is closely related to IL-4; both cytokines bind a common IL-4Rα/IL-13Rα heterodimeric receptor and signal via the STAT6 pathway (5). However, murine data indicate that T cells express the dedicated IL-4 receptor but not this common IL-4/IL-13 heterodimer (6). Because the murine IL-4R binds only IL-4, NK secretion of IL-4, but not IL-13, likely directs Th2 differentiation.

The nature of the interactions between dendritic cells and CD4 cells can also promote Th2 polarity. The molecular basis for DC promotion of Th2 cells is not entirely clear, as DC do not secrete significant IL-4. MHC-restricted Th2 promotion may occur through a suboptimal DC dose, reduced DC antigen expression, or antigen presentation on non-DC APC (7). In addition to these TCR-associated "signal 1" effects (8), the nature of APC expression of co-stimulatory "signal 2" molecules can influence Th1/Th2 polarity. The initially described CD28/B7 signal 2 interaction appeared to promote either Th1 or Th2 responses in an unbiased manner, and the ultimate outcome was largely a function of the cytokine microenvironment (e.g., the presence of IL-4 or IL-12) (9,10). It should be noted, however, that limited CD28 signaling, "co-stimulation light," may preferentially promote a Th2 response (11). The mechanism whereby CD28 co-stimulation can promote either Th1 or Th2 responses likely resides in the primary function of this molecule; CD28 provides a T-cell survival signal through upregulation of bc1-xL (12) and other molecules (13).

Alternatively, non-CD28 co-stimulatory pathways may play a larger role in Th1/Th2 polarization. An inducible co-stimulatory molecule (ICOS), working downstream in the immune system from CD28, primarily co-stimulates effector T cells. Importantly, ICOS may preferentially maintain type II effector T-cell responses (14), although not all studies have reached this conclusion (15). Effector T-cell expression of 4-1BB (CD137) can also promote effector T-cell responses in vivo (16), and 4-1BB may preferentially augment Th1-type effector cells (17). In sum, the primary afferent co-stimulatory pathway, CD28, appears to be truly unbiased with respect to Th1/Th2 development, whereas more downstream co-stimulatory pathways such as ICOS and 4-1BB may act to promote cytokine polarity by maintaining effector Th2 or Th1 responses, respectively.

Th2 cells may also be promoted by their interaction with a specific dendritic cell population, the DC2 subset. DC2 cells may arise from a lymphoid precursor cell distinct from myeloid-derived DC1 cells and can be identified by their co-expression of classical

DC surface markers and the IL-3 receptor (CD123). Such DC2 cells promote Th2 differentiation by an undefined mechanism that does not appear to involve IL-4 signaling (18). Other investigators have generated DC2-type cells that are defined not by lineage-specific criteria, but simply by their ability to functionally promote Th2 differentiation. A DC2 functional phenotype can be induced from myeloid precursors either by incubation with prostaglandin E_2 (19) or calcium ionophore (20). In each case, the DC2-type myeloid cells express greatly reduced IL-12, suggesting that a functional DC2 cell may be more clearly defined by an absence of T1-promoting IL-12 than by the presence of some currently unidentified non–IL-4 T2-promoting factor.

If the factors leading to Th2 polarization can be simplified to IL-4 exposure during signal 1/signal 2 activation, then Th1 polarization can be distilled to IL-12 exposure during co-stimulation. This critical IL-4 vs. IL-12 influence may be dictated at an innate level via NK cells, as both IL-4– and IL-12–secreting NK cells, the NK1/NK2 subsets, have been described (21). Such IL-12–secreting NK cells may be promoted by another Th1-promoting innate cytokine, IL-18 (22). This IL-12/IL-18 axis is complex, however, since some studies demonstrate that IL-18 promotes Th2 responses (23). In addition to NK sources of IL-12, DC1 cells promote Th1 immunity at least in part through IL-12 secretion. The evidence that IL-12 is the primary cytokine influencing Th1 promotion has been solidified by studies demonstrating preferential IL-12 receptor expression on Th1 cells (24).

$CD4^+$ T cells represent an afferent or "helper" arm of immunity, with Th1 cells facilitating primarily cell-mediated immunity and Th2 cells facilitating antibody-mediated immunity. Although this generalization has some utility, it breaks down in several important aspects: Th1 and Th2 cells can function as effectors, and both Th1 and Th2 populations promote $CD8^+$ cytotoxic T-cell differentiation (cell-mediated immunity). The existence of $CD8^+$ cytotoxic T cells secreting type II cytokines was initially not appreciated, as alloreactive murine $CD8^+$ CTL were defined as exclusive secretors of Th1-type cytokines (25). However, it was soon reported that IL-4–secreting $CD8^+$ T cells were readily isolated from humans with inadequate immunity to infectious diseases (26) and that IL-12 and IL-4 can polarize $CD8^+$ CTL towards Th1- or Th2-type cytokine production, respectively, thereby prompting the Tc1/Tc2 nomenclature (27,28).

Differential cytokine secretion by Th1/Th2 and Tc1/Tc2 cells is certainly the initial and most studied feature of these subsets. In some respects, the most important cytokines that define T1/T2 biology are IL-2 and IL-4. IL-2 primarily accounts for the afferent nature of the Th1-type helper response, as it promotes not only Th1 autocrine growth but also paracrine expansion of a Tc1-type response. Within CD8 cells, the Tc1 subset can secrete IL-2, typically with a magnitude 1 log less than $CD4^+$ Th1 cells (27). $CD8^+$ T-cell IL-2 secretion may allow such cells to operate without the assistance of $CD4^+$ T cells in a helper-independent manner (29). On the other hand, by definition, Th2 and Tc2 cells do not secrete IL-2, and as a result, their expansion is dependent upon other growth factor sources, such as autocrine IL-4 (30) or utilization of IL-2 secreted by Th1- or Tc1-type cells. This biology of IL-2 production (Th1-type cells) and IL-2 utilization (Th2-type cells) may help determine the dominant nature of Th2-type cells in conditions having mixed Th1/Th2 components. Whereas T-cell secretion of IL-2 denotes a T1 phenotype, T-cell secretion of IL-4 is the hallmark of T2 cells. The presence of IL-4 secretion from T cells implies prior IL-4 priming (31) and is thus not consistent with a highly enriched T1 phenotype. Indeed, exposure of even highly committed T1 cells to IL-4 can induce a partial T1 $\rightarrow$ T2 shift (32).

The role of other type I and type II cytokines in defining cytokine polarity is well described, but perhaps not quite as restricted as the role of IL-2 and IL-4. For example, although IFN-γ is a hallmark of effector Th1 and Tc1 cytokine secretion, Th2 cells, and in particular Tc2 cells, tend to express a measurable albeit reduced level of IFN-γ (27). Nonetheless, IFN-γ has been shown to promote T1 responses, most recently through its induction of t-bet transcription factor, with subsequent upregulation of IL-12 receptor (24). IL-10 is a cytokine clearly associated with murine Th2 and Tc2 cells and can cross-regulate Th1-type responses through multiple mechanisms (33). However, studies using human T cells have found significant IL-10 secretion from Th1-type cells (34) and diminished IL-10 production in mature Th2-type effector cells (35). Given these apparently disparate observations, it is important to note that Th1/Th2 immunity is a network of cellular regulation and that attributing a specific effect to a particular cytokine may not best reflect this biology. To further this point, studies using mRNA expression profiling of Th1/Th2 and Tc1/Tc2 cells have identified a wide range of differentially expressed genes, each of which may act alone or in concert to mediate T1 or T2 cellular effects (36).

T1 and T2 populations differ not only in their cytokine secretion profile, but also in their utilization of cytolytic effector molecules. This difference is particularly striking with respect to the CD4$^+$ subsets, as only Th1-type cells have been commonly associated with lytic function. Interestingly, Th1-mediated cytolysis is affected primarily through fas ligand (fasL), with little contribution from the other primary lytic mechanism, the perforin/granzyme pathway. This Th1/Th2 dichotomy extends as well to the fas receptor, as the Th1 population is preferentially sensitive to fas-mediated death (37). This combined Th1 expression of fasL and sensitivity to fas signaling highlights the role for this pathway in Th1 effector function and in autoregulation. By contrast, Th2 cells are relatively inefficient at eliminating fas targets and have greatly reduced susceptibility to fas autoregulation, in part based on the role of IL-4 in reducing fas receptor expression and signaling (38).

Differential T1/T2 cytolytic function also exists within the CD8$^+$ Tc1 and Tc2 subsets. In contrast to CD4$^+$ Th2 cells, which have nominal cytolytic function, CD8$^+$ type II cytokine-secreting cells (Tc2 cells) have potent cytolytic function. Importantly, although the total cytolytic capacity of Tc2 cells is comparable to type I cytokine-secreting Tc1 cells, Tc1 and Tc2 subsets appear to utilize distinct pathways of cytolysis. Similar to their Th1 counterpart, Tc1 cells utilize primarily fasL; in contrast, Tc2 cells primarily utilize a perforin/granzyme-mediated killing mechanism (39). Because both fas- and perforin-based mechanisms contribute to antitumor and anti-infection responses and to immune regulation (40), the differential lytic mechanisms of Tc1 and Tc2 cells appear to broaden immunity in a nonredundant manner. Of the two pathways, some literature indicates that the fas pathway may be most essential for mediation of curative antitumor responses (41), which would suggest that T1-type immunity is most crucial.

In addition to cytokine and cytolytic functions, the Th1/Th2 subsets also differ with respect to chemokine receptor expression (42), and the rapid expansion of chemokine biology has furthered our understanding of Th1/Th2 biology (reviewed in Ref. 43). Type I T cells may exist in a positive feedback loop with IP-10, MIG, and RANTES; these chemokines are released during DTH-type immune responses and attract type I T cells and monocytes via the expression of the corresponding chemokine receptors (CXCR3, CCR5, and CCR1). The resultant local secretion of T1 cell IFN-γ induces further IP-10, MIG, and RANTES production. In contrast, type II T cells may exist in a positive feedback loop with eotaxin, MDC, and TARC released during allergic inflammatory responses. These chemokines attract type II T cells, eosinophils, and basophils by binding to CCR3 and

CCR4. The resultant local secretion of IL-4 or IL-13 induces further eotaxin, MDC, and TARC production. This differential Th1/Th2 chemokine biology may have important in vivo consequences. For example, in a model of viral pneumonia, specific chemokine receptor expression on Tc1 cells correlated with improved trafficking into lung tissue and enhanced Tc1 antiviral effect relative to Tc2 cells (44). Chemokine receptor expression, in addition to dictating T-cell homing pattern, may also help diagnose T1 vs. T2 immunity in vivo. For example, patients with type II associated pathology, such as atopic dermatitis or progression of HIV infection, have increased Th2 and Tc2 cell expression of CRTh2, a newly identified, type II–associated, chemokine receptor (45).

When considering the Th1/Th2 paradigm, it is necessary not only to address the differential effect of various APC functional subsets on Th1/Th2 differentiation, but also to delineate the subsequent effect of the Th1/Th2 subsets back on APC. A key T-cell molecule contributing to this APC cross-talk is CD40 ligand (CD40L), which binds to CD40 on B cells and DC (46). Such CD40L/CD40 interaction increases antigen presentation, CD80 and CD86 co-stimulatory molecule expression, and IL-12 production, and is therefore thought to be a major mechanism of $CD4^+$ T-cell helper function. In this context it is interesting and predictable that CD40L expression is increased in Th1 cells (47), thereby providing a positive feedback loop between Th1 cells and IL-12–secreting DC1 cells. Although Th2 cells express reduced CD40L, this level of expression is likely sufficient to modulate APC function and maturation (48). In addition to APC modulation, T-cell CD40L expression may beneficially induce leukemia or solid tumor cell acquisition of APC characteristics (49,50).

Recent advances in Th1/Th2 biology have additionally occurred at the molecular level, with the understanding that t-bet and GATA-3 transcription factors differentially control Th1 and Th2 cell function, respectively (51). For Th1 cells, t-bet is a transcription factor that induces stable chromatin remodeling (DNA demethylation) in the IFN-γ allele, which increases IFN-γ production and expression of the IL-12 receptorβ_2 chain (24). T-bet thereby confers sensitivity of Th1 cells to exogenous IL-12, which results in STAT4 signaling and further increases IFN-γ levels and Th1 cell survival (52). These findings support the concept that t-bet, and not IL-12, truly controls Th1 cell phenotype, with IL-12 acting primarily as a survival and amplification factor. Importantly, the t-bet effect on Th1 cells may be long lasting, as the DNA demethylation pattern can be passed to progeny (53). This set of observations may help explain the persistence of a polarized T-cell phenotype remote from the initial polarizing condition. Interestingly, the t-bet pathway does not appear to involve $CD8^+$ T cells, and research is underway to identify transcription factors that may control Tc1 vs. Tc2 polarization (54). For Th2 cells, GATA-3 is a transcription factor that increases Th2 cytokine expression while limiting IL-12 Rβ expression. Importantly, GATA-3 expression is greatly augmented by CD28 signaling, which may help explain the association of CD28 signaling with Th2 differentiation (55). The mechanism of IL-4–mediated Th2 polarization is also better understood; IL-4–induced STAT6 activation upregulates a newly identified GFI-1 transcription factor that provides Th2 cells a survival signal during GATA-3–induced differentiation (56). It is important to note that these transcription factor–based definitions of Th1/Th2 biology have primarily been carried out in the murine system, although initial studies involving human CD4 cells have been relatively corroboratory (57).

In summary, the past few years have witnessed great advances in the field of Th1/Th2 cell biology. The concept that certain functional subsets promote Th1 vs. Th2 differentiation, such as the NK1/NK2 and DC1/DC2 cell populations, has been better characterized. The nature of the originally defined CD4$^+$ Th1/Th2 subsets has been further refined, with new definitions expanding to include specific patterns of transcription factor and chemokine receptor expression. The Th1 and Th2 paradigm has clearly been extended to CD8$^+$ T cells with delineation of Tc1 and Tc2 populations that differ not only in cytokine secretion, but also in cytolytic mechanism. The extent of these advances underscores the complexity of type I vs. type II immunity, and therefore represents both a challenge and an opportunity to better understand and modulate T-cell function in the transplant setting.

III. Th1/Th2 BIOLOGY IN VIVO IN HEALTH AND DISEASE

Although the Th1/Th2 framework was initiated from studies of murine T-cell clones in vitro, this biology has clear relevance in vivo. Studies involving polarized murine CD4 (58) and CD8 cells (59) have shown that antigen-specific Th1/Th2 or Tc1/Tc2 cells can persist long term in vivo. Furthermore, upon restimulation with relevant antigen, such T cells secrete cytokines in a polarized pattern consistent with the initial T1/T2 phenotype. Generally, in states of health the immune system likely exists in a state of Th1/Th2 balance. In situations requiring increased Th1 immunity, for example, control of infection or malignancy, a curative Th1 response may appropriately escalate, only then to be downmodulated by a Th2 response or another regulatory pathway (e.g., Th1 auto-regulation or T-regulatory cell involvement). In contrast, states of disease can be associated with a disproportionate Th1 or Th2 response, which may be the result of a deficiency or overactivity of a particular subset.

An in vivo immune system with a Th1 shift, either on the basis of an overactive Th1 response or an insufficient Th2 response, can result in a wide range of inflammatory conditions, many of which resemble aspects of acute GVHD. The best example of such a Th1-mediated condition is inflammatory bowel disease (IBD). Murine models clearly demonstrate that IBD is caused by Th1-type cells that are unopposed by either Th2-type cells (60) or type II cytokine-secreting T-regulatory cells (61). Type II counterbalance of Th1-driven IBD has been mechanistically attributed to IL-10; mice genetically deficient in IL-10 develop IBD (62), which can then be alleviated with IL-10 therapy (63). Importantly, the predictive value of these findings for human disease is substantial, as IBD patients appear to have local Th1 pathology and reduced IL-10 expression (64), and early attempts to treat clinical IBD with exogenous IL-10 have shown promise (65). In addition to IBD, murine and clinical data indicate that certain autoimmune diseases, in particular rheumatoid arthritis (66) and multiple sclerosis (67), are associated with Th1 pathology and an insufficient Th2 counterregulatory response.

Although Th2 responses reduce Th1-mediated inflammation involving monocytes and macrophages, unchecked Th2 processes mediate inflammation driven by eosinophils and basophils. In murine models, Th2-associated IL-13 production is the most common mechanism proposed for Th2-driven disorders, including liver fibrosis (68) and pulmonary inflammation (69). Another Th2 cytokine, IL-5, is associated with eosinophil-based inflammation, including intestinal infiltration (70). Although most data indicate that IL-5 and IL-13 are the primary type II cytokines generating inflammation, Th2 cells capable of IL-4 secretion and incapable of IL-5 and IL-13 secretion can mediate inflammation as well, albeit with slower kinetics than wild-type cells (71). Further research indicates that IL-4, IL-5, and IL-13 likely work in concert to cause Th2 cell-involved inflammation (72).

While Th2 cells can clearly contribute to inflammation, Th2-biased immune systems are associated with a lack of protective immunity against malignancy. In this setting, the Th2 bias is typically noninflammatory and therefore likely results more from a deficiency in Th1 elements than from an overproduction of Th2 elements. In humans, cancer patients in remission and normal volunteers have a balanced Th1/Th2 or skewed Th1 response to tumor antigen, whereas cancer patients with active disease demonstrate a Th2 biased antitumor immunity (73). In experimental studies Th1 responses associate with optimal antitumor immunity (74,75), although some tumors may be susceptible to both Th1 and Th2 responses (76). In mouse models evaluating $CD8^+$ antitumor immunity, both Tc1 and Tc2 cells generally result in significant antitumor effects, although the Tc1 phenotype is typically more potent (77,78). In conclusion, type II immunity, in particular that restricted to $CD4^+$ Th2 cells, is associated with reduced antitumor effects in the syngeneic setting; $CD8^+$ Tc2 cells, even though they have potent cytolytic function in vitro, generally mediate reduced antitumor effects in vivo. Suboptimal Tc2 antitumor immunity may result from a relative deficiency in IFN-γ and fasL, a chemokine receptor pattern not associated with optimal cell migration (44) or, as we have found in recent studies, reduced antigen-driven clonal expansion (44a).

IV. PATHOGENESIS OF GVHD AS A Th1-TYPE PROCESS

Using this current understanding of Th1/Th2 biology, the pathogenesis of acute GVHD is best described primarily as a Th1-type process. Donor $CD4^+$ T cells are known to initiate acute GVHD (79), and such CD4 reactivity is typically of Th1 phenotype. In murine studies, the key afferent Th1 cytokine IL-2 is elaborated early during GVHD (80) and appears to play a role in GVHD natural history (81). Furthermore, in human clinical transplantation, early studies demonstrated a strong correlation between the precursor frequency of donor CD4 cells capable of secreting IL-2 in response to alloantigen and the incidence and severity of acute GVHD (82). Advances in the understanding of effector mechanisms mediating Th1 effects further implicate this population in acute GVHD. CD40L, a molecule preferentially expressed on Th1 cells that mediates helper capacity via APC activation, has been clearly linked to GVHD (83). In addition, Th1 cell preferential expression of fasL links Th1 cells to fas-mediated GVHD (84,85), an effector pathway associated with target cell injury in the skin, liver, and gut (86–89). As such, Th1-type CD4 cells can contribute to GVHD pathogenesis through multiple mechanisms, including type I cytokine secretion, CD40L expression, and fasL cytolytic function.

Donor CD8 cells, in particular those of Tc1 phenotype, are also tightly linked to GVHD. Of the CD8 cytolytic mechanisms known to contribute to GVHD, the fasL pathway, which the Tc1 subset preferentially utilizes, is perhaps most contributory. It should be noted that although Th1 and Tc1cell expression of fasL contributes to GVHD, T-cell fasL can also dampen GVHD via autoregulation or elimination of host APC (90), and as such, a deficiency in fasL may paradoxically increase GVHD. From the cytokine standpoint, Th1 and Tc1 cells are an abundant source of the type I cytokine IFN-γ that is essential for initial priming of monocytes and macrophages for pro-inflammatory cytokine secretion (91). Although most studies correlate such Th1- and Tc1-mediated IFN-γ secretion with acute GVHD, this association has not been absolute. IFN-γ, in addition to its APC activation and inflammatory cytokine functions, also can downregulate immunity (92,93). Not unexpectedly, in this context, murine studies demonstrate that donor T cells deficient in IFN-γ can actually cause increased GVHD (94). Interestingly, the absence of donor T-cell IFN-γ is deleterious in the setting of ablative host preparation, yet protective in sublethally prepared hosts (95). Although these data forbid strict interpretation of a Th1/Th2 paradigm in acute GVHD, most observations indicate that T-cell mediation of acute GVHD utilizes type I effector pathways, including IL-2 and IFN-γ secretion, CD40L-mediated APC activation, and fasL-mediated cytolysis. This association was confirmed in studies utilizing adoptively transferred polarized donor T cells; Th1 and Tc1 cells mediated increased GVHD relative to Th2 and Tc2 cells (96–98).

CD4$^+$ and CD8$^+$ T cells can directly mediate target cell injury, but a large body of data, some of it recent (99), indicates that a significant component of GVHD tissue damage is mediated indirectly through non-T-cell–generated inflammatory cytokines, including IL-1α and TNF-α. The association of TNF-α to murine intestinal GVHD (100) and human clinical GVHD (101) can be viewed as a downstream Th1-type process, since IL-2 and IFN-γ both prime monocytes and macrophages for TNF-α secretion (102). This linkage of proximal IFN-γ and distal TNF-α was carefully detailed in murine GVHD (91), with bacterial LPS providing the environmental stimulus for macrophage TNF release. The distal phase of non–T-cell cytokine release also involves IL-1, which led to the description of cytokine storm GVHD (80). In murine studies involving intensified host preparative regimens, the contribution of IL-1-β to GVHD pathogenesis is relatively comparable to that mediated by TNF-α (103). Furthermore, data using donor or host DNA polymorphism analysis for TNF-α or IL-1 receptor antagonist alleles is consistent with a role for the cytokine storm in human GVHD (104–106).

To further evaluate the potential role of IL-1α and TNF-α pathways after clinical allogeneic PBSCT, we have monitored monocyte intracellular expression of these cytokines post-SCT. As Figure 1 shows, patients who developed more severe gut GVHD had modestly increased monocyte IL-1α and markedly increased TNF-α relative to patients with nominal or absent gut GVHD. Monocyte cytokine elevations typically occurred after the second week post-SCT. Although attempts to modulate the TNF or IL-1 pathways for clinical benefit have not yet proven efficacious (107,108), our data suggests that cytokine inhibitor therapy may need to extend beyond the peri-transplant interval.

V. Th2-TYPE MODULATION OF GVHD

Because type I T cells induce IL-1α and TNF-α during GVHD, modulation of the cytokine storm may be achieved either through specific or general inhibition of inflammatory cytokines (109) or through increasing the more proximal Th2 immunity. The latter has been demonstrated in murine models where donor T-cell strategies that polarize towards Th2 reduce distal inflammatory cytokine levels (96,110).

Treatment of donor mice with IL-4 polarizes CD4$^+$ splenic T cells towards a Th2 phenotype and reduces lethal graft-versus-host disease induced by unmanipulated donor T cells (110). Supplementation of allogeneic stem cell inocula with donor Th2 cells modulated GVHR by reducing donor CD8$^+$ T-cell expansion, T1 cytokines, and TNF-α in vivo. The ability of Th2 cells to modulate naïve donor T cells in the bone marrow allograft is reminiscent of infectious tolerance, a process that has now been attributed to Th2-type or Th2 cytokine secreting T-regulatory cells (111,112). In other studies (113) we utilized IL-4–generated Th2 cells to modulate GVHD in the setting of MHC-disparate allotransplantation and observed that Th2 cells reduced GVHD without impairing engraftment. Similar observations were made in MHC class I, class II, and minor

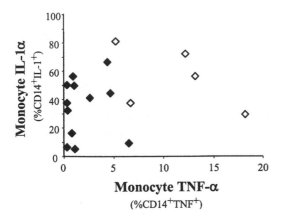

Figure 1 Correlation of monocyte IL-1-α and TNF-α with clinical acute gut GVHD. Patients with refractory hematological malignancy received reduced-intensity, HLA-matched sibling allogeneic PBSCT (see Refs. 135, 136). Cyclosporin A GVHD prophylaxis was initiated on day -1 prior to PBSCT. Complete donor lymphoid and myeloid chimerism, as assessed by VNTR-PCR analysis, was achieved in most patients by day 14 post-SCT and in all patients by day 28 post-SCT. Of $n = 19$ patients receiving this regimen (without Th2 cells), acute GVHD severity was grade 0–I ($n = 7$), grade II ($n = 6$), and grade III ($n = 6$). Peripheral blood was harvested and cultured overnight in X-Vivo 20 media supplemented with 10% FCS and monensin A (Golgi-Stop; PharMingen). After 16–24 hours cells were harvested, surface stained with anti-CD14, permeabilized, and stained intracellularly with anti-IL-1α or anti-TNF-α. Two-color flow cytometry identified the percentage of cytokine-secreting monocytes. Monocytes evaluated in the second week post-SCT were typically quiescent, with median $CD14^+IL-1^+$ of 2.0% and median $CD14^+TNF^+$ of 0.1%. Samples evaluated proximal to peak clinical GVHD onset, which occurred at a median of 31 days post-SCT, are identified in the figure. The open diamond identifies patients having significant gut GVHD (stage 2–3), whereas the closed diamond identifies patients with nominal gut GVHD (stage 0–1). Relative to patients with stage 0–1 gut GVHD ($n = 12$), patients with stage 2–3 gut GVHD ($n = 5$) had an increase in both monocyte IL-1α ($\%CD14^+IL-1^+$: 36.4 $\pm$ 6.0 vs. 57.4 $\pm$ 9.9; $p < 0.05$) and monocyte TNF-α ($\%CD14^+TNF^+$: 1.8 $\pm$ 0.6 vs. 10.9 $\pm$ 2.2; $p < 0.05$).

HC-disparate systems (96,114). As such, strategies that increase allograft T2 immune function can reduce GVHD while preserving a beneficial component of the donor T cells.

In vitro allosensitization of purified $CD4^+$ or $CD8^+$ T cells in the presence of either T1 (IL-12)– or T2 (IL-4)–promoting conditions has also been used to generate allospecific donor T cells of $CD4^+$ Th1/Th2 or $CD8^+$ Tc1/Tc2 phenotype (97,98). Strikingly, although $CD8^+$ Tc2 cells mediated potent cytolysis in vitro, their infusion resulted in greatly reduced GVHD in vivo. Relative to Tc1 cells, the capacity of the Tc2 cells to mediate a GVL effect against bcr/abl-transfected CML-type cells was attenuated, however, the Tc2 cells were still uniquely capable of mediating a GVL effect without inducing severe ongoing GVHD. This result is consistent with findings from syngeneic tumor models, wherein antigen-specific Tc2 cells have typically been less efficacious than Tc1 cells in mediating antitumor effects (44,77,115,116). Our studies also indicated that the capacity of Tc2 cells to mediate a GVL effect was inversely related to the level of IL-10 secretion. Of particular interest, $CD4^+$ Th2 cells downregulated GVHD but had no GVL capacity in their own right and fully abrogated Tc1-mediated GVL effects (98). As such, although Th2 and Tc2 cells were clearly associated with reduced GVHD, a highly skewed Th2 response appeared to have deleterious effects with respect to GVL mediation. This cautionary note regarding donor T2 cell administration does not, however, extend to the abrogation of rejection across MHC barriers; Tc2 cells are actually more potent at preventing graft rejection than Tc1 cells in models not involving donor antihost alloreactivity (117). In sum, donor T-cell cytokine phenotype, determined through in vitro culture under T1- or T2-promoting conditions, can differentially modulate allogeneic transplantation responses. SCT with Th2 and Tc2 cells reduces GVHD and abrogates graft rejection, and Tc2 cells can preserve some component of a GVL response, although utilization of T1 immunity is optimal for antitumor effects.

Other methods of generating T2-shifted allogeneic immunity have been studied. Granulocyte colony-stimulating factor (G-CSF), a cytokine used for stem cell mobilization, also has important effects on both murine (118) and human (119) T cells and facilitates a shift towards Th2 cytokine secretion. In murine studies, SCT with G-CSF–generated T2 cells greatly reduced GVHD and maintained a GVL effect against P815 leukemia (120). It is interesting to note that G-CSF–generated T2 cells mediated GVL effects through a perforin-dependent mechanism, a pathway classically associated with T2 biology. Administration of IL-11 after SCT also skewed donor T-cell differentiation towards the T2 phenotype in vivo, subsequently reducing T1 cytokine production, APC IL-12 secretion, systemic TNF-α levels and GVHD severity (121). Importantly, IL-11 administration reduced GVHD yet preserved a perforin-dependent GVL effect against P815 tumor cells (122). In sum, these data demonstrate that (1) multiple cytokine therapies can induce T2-shifted donor T-cell immunity, (2) allospecific or polyclonal T2 populations are associated with reduced GVHD, and (3) T2 cells can mediate a significant GVL effect, particularly when the tumor target is sensitive to the perforin lytic pathway.

In addition to these studies involving conventional CD4$^+$ or CD8$^+$ T cells secreting type II cytokines, strategies using DC, NK, or CD4$^+$ T-regulatory (T reg) cells have also demonstrated a T2-associated modulation of GVHD. A CD3$^+$NK1.1$^+$ population, characterized as having a T2 cytokine phenotype, abrogated GVHD induced by unmanipulated donor T cells; this effect was dependent upon NK1.1$^+$ cell IL-4 secretion (123). In another study, a CD4$^+$CD25$^+$ T reg population abrogated GVHD, with this effect dependent upon T-regulatory cell IL-10 secretion (124). Finally, the Th2-inducing dendritic cells (DC2 subset) may also play a role in GVHD modulation (125,126).

In recent murine studies (127), we have developed alternative, CD28-based methods of generating donor T2 cells and evaluated their GVT effects in murine allogeneic SCT models for epithelial malignancy. CD28 is a co-stimulatory pathway that yields efficient T-cell expansion in vitro and also facilitates Th2-type effector function, particularly in the presence of IL-4. In addition, CD3, CD28-generated T cells express a polyclonal T-cell receptor repertoire (128), which may be advantageous in the setting of MHC-matched allogeneic transplantation where in vitro stimulation with relevant minor histocompatibility antigens is less feasible. Consistent with previous results, stimulation of murine CD4$^+$ or CD8$^+$ T cells under T1 (IL-12) or T2 (IL-4) conditions expands Th1/Tc1 or Th2/Tc2 populations, respectively. The T1-polarized T cells secreted the type I cytokines IL-2 and IFN-γ, whereas the T2-polarized populations secreted primarily the type II cytokines IL-4 and IL-10 (Fig. 2A–D). Differential cytolytic function of the T-cell subsets was also apparent, as the T1 cells mediated primarily fasL-based cytolysis, whereas the T2 cells killed primarily by perforin-based cytolysis. Similar to prior results, co-stimulated

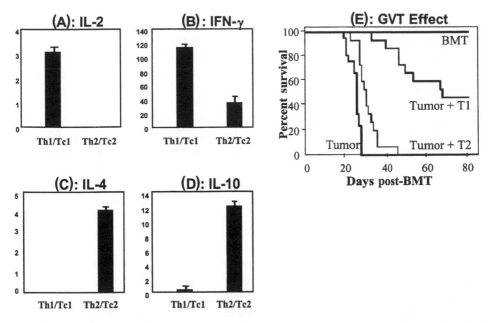

Figure 2 CD28 co-stimulated murine T1 vs. T2 cells: GVT effect. Murine Th1/Tc1 (T1) or Th2/Tc2 (T2) cells were generated by stimulation of splenic CD4$^+$ and CD8$^+$ T cells with anti-CD3, anti-CD28 coated magnetic beads in the presence of either T1- or T2-polarizing conditions (IL-12, anti-IL-4, IL-2, IL-7 or IL-4, IL-2, IL-7). After 5 days in culture, donor CD4 and CD8 cells expanded ~100-fold in either T1 or T2 conditions. Cells were restimulated with anti-CD3, anti-CD28, and the supernatant was evaluated for cytokine content by ELISA (A–D); cytokine values listed are in ng/mL/0.5 × 10^6 T cells per mL/24 hr. Th1/Tc1 and Th2/Tc2 effectors were generated from parental C57B1/6 mice (H-2^b) and transplanted into allogeneic CB6F$_1$ hosts (Allo; H-2$^{b/d}$) that were inoculated with the host-type mammary breast cancer cell line TS/A (H-2^d). (E) Recipients of tumor and allogeneic SCT alone ($n = 21$) died within a month post-BMT. Recipients of allogeneic Th1/Tc1 cells ($n = 15$) or Th2/Tc2 cells ($n = 15$) benefited from a GVT effect, although the T1 GVT effect was much greater than the T2 GVT effect. Death in T1 recipients was due to GVHD, whereas death in T2 recipients was due to tumor.

donor T2 cells mediated significantly less GVHD than co-stimulated T1 cells, with reduced weight loss, histological lesions of GVHD, and lethality. Both T1 and T2 populations also mediated a significant GVT effect (Fig. 2E), but only the T1 effect was associated with long-term tumor-free survival. Donor T1 cells from *gld* mice mediated a GVT effect, indicating that the T1-associated GVT effect was not dependent on fasL.

Determination of the mechanism(s) whereby T1 cells mediate a GVT effect will require further study. Although T1 cells do not utilize perforin/granzyme lysis to a significant degree in vitro, it is possible that this pathway may be operational in vivo. Alternatively, T1 cells may generate antitumor effects primarily via cytokine-mediated pathways. The lack of involvement of T1 cell fasL in the GVT effect suggests that, at least in some tumor settings, abrogation of T1 cell fasL may represent a strategy for allowing a potent GVT effect with reduced GVHD. The development of such strategies may be required to optimally utilize T1/T2 immune modulation in allogeneic SCT for aggressive malignancy. Such strategies might include abrogation of T1-associated GVHD by T1 suicide gene insertion or specific molecule blockade (fasL), generation of mixed T1/T2 immunity post-SCT, or use of sequential T1 → T2 therapy.

This body of work demonstrates that Th2 cell modulation of GVHD represents a form of allograft engineering. As a benchmark for success, graft engineering strategies should reduce GVHD without increasing the risk of graft rejection or reducing a GVL or GVT effect. It should be noted that data exist that challenge the application of the Th1/Th2 paradigm to GVHD. In the first scenario, the experimental methods employed involve abrogation of a T2 mechanism in unmanipulated donor T cells, and therefore differ from each of the successful T2 strategies whereby activated T2 cells supplement the allograft. For example, ablation of IL-4– or IL-2–secreting, transgenic T cells after SCT can downmodulate GVHD (129). Similarly, experiments using IL-4–deficient mice as SCT donors resulted in reduced GVHD (94). In another example, both STAT 4 (T1-associated) and STAT6 (T2-associated) signaling pathways in donor T cells contributed to GVHD (130). Collectively, these findings show that IL-4–secreting (T2) cells can contribute to GVHD and are consistent with the known inflammatory capacity of T2 cells. It is interesting to note that human studies diverge from these murine results, since an increased precursor frequency of IL-4–secreting alloreactive donor T cells associates with reduced GVHD (131). Nonetheless, it is likely that both T1 and T2 immunity can contribute to GVHD pathogenesis, but in situations where the T2 component is amplified and administered in an augmented manner at the time of transplantation, reduced GVHD severity is observed.

Second, it has been difficult to reduce GVHD via administration of a single T2-associated cytokine. This observation may relate to the fact that Th2 biology is a cellular phenomenon and that Th2 activity likely represents complex molecular interactions that operate in a cellular microenvironment and involve other T cells and APC. Having said this, the molecule best characterized as having a Th2 influence has been IL-10. Initial murine studies demonstrated that IL-10 administration was initially not associated with reduced GVHD (132), but subsequent attempts found that more physiological dosing of IL-10 could yield a protective effect. In humans, IL-10 serum levels have been associated with a favorable GVHD profile (133,134); furthermore, an IL-10 gene polymorphism has been associated with reduced GVHD risk (105). With these results in hand, investigators will likely evaluate single or multiple cytokine strategies for T2 modulation of transplantation as a potential alternative to existing T2 cellular approaches.

VI. CO-STIMULATED Th2 CELLS: CLINICAL EVALUATION

Given data that Th2 cells can favorably modulate GVHD, we have developed a clinical protocol to evaluate the use of donor CD4$^+$ Th2 cells as a form of allograft engineering and chose a strategy where a T-cell–replete allograft would be supplemented with additional donor CD4$^+$ Th2 cells. In this approach, the donor Th2 cells are intended to modulate the GVHD-inducing nature of the unmanipulated donor CD4$^+$ and CD8$^+$ T cells contained in the allograft.

In an attempt to achieve rapid donor alloengraftment with reduced regimen-related toxicity and potentially reduced acute GVHD (103), we pursued our evaluation of donor Th2 cells in the setting of a new reduced-intensity preparative regimen. In this approach, host CD4$^+$ and CD8$^+$ T cells were depleted to levels considered immunoablative, initially with outpatient chemotherapy (fludarabine with EPOCH) and subsequently with inpatient chemotherapy (fludarabine with cyclophosphamide) (135,136). Based on murine studies

(137), such host immunoablation should more completely abrogate the host-vs.-graft rejection response and thus allow for more rapid and complete donor engraftment. Indeed, we did observe rapid donor T lymphoid and myeloid engraftment with this approach, with most recipients having complete donor elements by day 14 post-SCT with unmanipulated, G-CSF–mobilized peripheral blood stem cells. As illustrated in Figure 3F, acute GVHD using this regimen occurred with kinetics, incidence, and severity reminiscent of standard myeloablative transplantation using similar GVHD chemoprophylaxis (single agent cyclosporine) (138). These results suggest that in humans, clinical GVHD is more closely linked to the kinetics of donor lymphoid engraftment than to the nature of the preparative regimen and that further therapeutic advances using this immunoablative approach will require an ability to modulate GVHD.

With respect to this strategy of Th2 graft augmentation, one immediate consideration relates to the safety/feasibility of the isolation, generation, characterization of the Th2 cells and their administration during allogeneic SCT. Although advances in Th2 biology indicate that specific receptor expression or transcription factor utilization may help define Th2 cells, a functional definition of Th2 cells based upon polarity of cytokine secretion remains the standard criterion. To generate donor Th2 cells in clinical grade and scale, we utilized an artificial APC system developed by Bruce Levine and Carl June that is based upon T-cell stimulation with magnetic beads coated with anti-CD3 and anti-CD28 (128). This co-stimulation method, in the absence of polarizing cytokines in vitro, generates primarily Th0- or Th1-type CD4 cells that have been evaluated clinically for their capacity to modulate immunity in the setting of HIV or cancer (139,140). Given the role of CD28 signaling and IL-4 exposure in the promotion of Th2 responses, we reasoned that this APC-free system might generate a polyclonal population of human CD4 cells that were Th2 biased and therefore capable of modulating GVHD after allogeneic PBSCT.

Input $CD4^+$ T cells ("Th0") from SCT donors secreted high levels of IL-2 and modest amounts of IFN-γ, with markedly nominal variation in the cytokine secreting capacity between donors (Fig. 3A). Co-stimulation in T2-polarizing conditions containing both recombinant human IL-4 (1000 IU/mL), and recombinant human IL-2 (20 IU/mL) resulted in a dramatic expansion of donor CD4 cells of 4–5 log over 20 days of culture. After one round (12 days) of co-stimulation in the T2 culture condition, we observed an induction of T2 cytokines, a reduction in IL-2 capacity, but an actual increase in IFN-γ secretion. These data are consistent with an incomplete Th0 → Th2 state of differentiation or a mixed Th1/Th2 effector pattern. However, after a second round of costimulation, we observed elimination of IL-2 secretion, a dramatic reduction in IFN-γ secretion, and maintenance of T2 cytokine secretion.

Donor Th2 cells expanded in T2 polarizing conditions after CD3, CD28 co-stimulation have multiple phenotypic characteristics of potential significance to their modulation of transplantation responses. With respect to cytokine secretion, the complete loss of IL-2 and diminished IFN-γ secretion are consistent with a cell population with reduced capacity for GVHD induction. In fact, we have found that the day 20 Th2 population actually consumes high levels of IL-2 upon restimulation, and thereby may possess a mechanism for regulating IL-2–driven expansion of unmanipulated donor T cells. Interleukin-13 was the predominant type II cytokine secreted from Th2 cells after tertiary CD3, CD28 co-stimulation, with additional Th2 cell secretion of IL-4, IL-5, and IL-10 observed. In addition to cytokine phenotype, other effector molecules, in particular CD40L, can contribute to GVHD pathogenesis. To this extent it is important to note that expanded donor Th2 cells did express CD40L (albeit reduced relative to control Th1

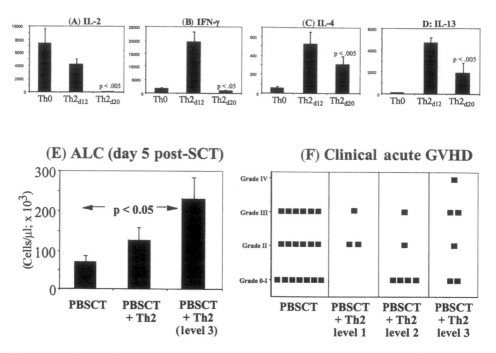

Figure 3 Phase I clinical trial of CD28 co-stimulated donor Th2 cells. Donor CD4$^+$ T cells were isolated from PBSCT donors prior to G-CSF treatment. CD4 enrichment was by negative selection using anti-CD19, anti-CD20, anti-CD22, and anti-CD8 antibodies with sheep antimouse bead depletion. Th2 cell generation was by CD4 cell stimulation with anti-CD3, anti-CD28–coated tosylated Dynal beads in a CD4 : bead ratio of 1 : 3 in X-Vivo 20 media supplemented with 5% human serum albumin, recombinant human IL-4 (1000 IU/mL), and recombinant human IL-2 (20 IU/mL). On day 12 of culture, CD4 cells were harvested and restimulated with anti-CD3, anti-CD28–coated beads (1 : 3 ratio) and expanded in media containing IL-4 and IL-2 through day 20 of culture. Supernatant was harvested after anti-CD3, anti-CD28 stimulation on day 0 of culture (Th0), at day 12 of culture (Th2$_{d12}$), and at day 20 of culture (Th2$_{d20}$) and tested for cytokine content by ELISA. (A–D) Data are expressed as pg of cytokine secreted/0.5×10^6 CD4 cells per mL/24 hr and represent median values for $n = 11$ donor cultures. (E) The absolute lymphocyte count (ALC) on day 5 after HLA-matched allogeneic PBSCT with or without Th2 cells. The PBSCT group represent median ALC value from recipients of PBSCT without Th2 cells ($n = 19$), whereas PBSCT + Th2 represents median ALC value of all recipients on the phase I Th2 study ($n = 15$). PBSCT + Th2 level 3 represents median ALC value for patients that received high-dose Th2 cells (125×10^6 Th2/kg; $n = 6$). (F) The clinical acute GVHD grade for the control group not receiving Th2 cells (PBSCT; $n = 19$) and for the treatment groups receiving dose level 1 (5×10^6 Th2/kg; $n = 3$), dose level 2 (25×10^6 Th2/kg; $n = 6$), or dose level 3 (125×10^6 Th2/kg; $n = 6$).

cells), thereby providing one mechanism whereby co-stimulated Th2 cells might augment alloreactivity through host APC interaction. Efforts are underway to identify methods to generate more highly polarized human CD4 cells. For example, we have found that initiation of Th2 cultures with CD4$^+$ T cells of naïve CD45RA phenotype significantly increases the polarity of the Th2/Th1 cytokine ratio (141). In sum, polarization of donor CD4$^+$ T cells can proceed from a Th0 → Th2 pattern of differentiation via CD28-driven expansion under T2-promoting conditions, thereby allowing an evaluation of donor Th2 cells after allogeneic PBSCT.

Using the immunoablative host preparative regimen, co-stimulated donor Th2 cells were administered on day 1 post-SCT in a phase I study, with patients receiving 5×10^6 Th2 cells/kg ($n = 3$ patients), 25×10^6 Th2 cells/kg ($n = 6$), or 125×10^6 Th2 cells/kg ($n = 6$). There were no transfusion-related side effects from the Th2 infusion. All patients in the phase I cohort had rapid and complete donor lymphoid and myeloid chimerism at day 14 post-SCT (15/15 patients). Figure 3E shows that by day 5 post-SCT, Th2 recipients, in particular those receiving the highest dose of Th2 cells, had a dramatic increase in the absolute lymphocyte count that was comprised of both $CD4^+$ and $CD8^+$ T cells. Because the Th2 infusion typically contained $<0.1\%$ $CD8^+$ cells, this early lymphocyte expansion is likely derived from both the infused $CD4^+$ Th2 cells and the unmanipulated $CD4^+$ and $CD8^+$ T cells in the allograft.

These reconstituting $CD4^+$ and $CD8^+$ T cells secreted both T1 and T2 cytokines (142). This result indicates that the co-stimulated Th2 cells may have escaped the T-cell inhibition typically associated with cyclosporine administration and promoted a mixed Th1/Th2 and Tc1/Tc2 pattern of differentiation in vivo. Given this apparent immune activation in Th2 recipients, it is not surprising that Th2 recipients had an increase in monocyte IL-1α is a more general immune activation cytokine post-SCT, with TNF-α being more closely associated with gut GVHD.

As Figure 3F demonstrates, the rate and severity of acute GVHD at Th2 dose levels 1 and 3 was similar to the control group receiving cyclosporine without Th2 cells. However, because four of six patients at Th2 cell dose level 2 did not develop acute GVHD, this cohort is currently being expanded to obtain further experience at this intermediate Th2 cell dose. Importantly, the majority of patients in this phase I study, most of whom had refractory lymphoma, achieved a complete remission of tumor, typically within the first 100 days post-SCT. These results indicate that donor Th2 cells are feasible to generate, safe to administer, do not abrogate engraftment, enhance donor T-cell numbers early post-SCT, and secrete both T1 and T2 of cytokines post-SCT. Further trials involving Th2 cells will be required to evaluate whether the observed Th2-induced immune activation can be utilized for therapeutic benefit through modulation of GVHD, enhancement of an allogeneic GVL or GVT effect, and acceleration of immune reconstitution.

VII. Th1/Th2 MODULATION OF GVHD: FUTURE DIRECTIONS

Inclusion of allogeneic T cells within stem cell grafts mediates both beneficial and detrimental effects post-SCT. Use of donor T cells has therefore been referred to as a double-edged sword. Unfortunately, the sword is too often dull on the side mediating antitumor effects and sharp on the GVHD aspect. Much therefore remains to be solved regarding optimization of allogeneic SCT, particularly when used as therapy for aggressive malignancy. This clinical requirement to both enhance antitumor immunity and limit GVHD is a conundrum that may have some resolution through approaches that modulate Th1/Th2 biology.

In the future, Th1/Th2 biology post-SCT might be individualized to enhance the therapeutic index of donor T cells. In MHC-matched transplantation for nonmalignant conditions, reliance upon alloreactivity for successful transplant outcome is relatively low, and as such, infusion of populations primarily capable of eliciting Th2/Tc2 immunity may be preferable. On the other hand, transplantation therapy for aggressive malignancy may require a stronger alloreactive effect resulting from a balanced T1/T2 immunity or a sequential T1 → T2 approach. For patients with indolent malignancy or nonmalignant conditions, transfer of allogeneic populations enriched for Tc2 function may represent a strategy for ensuring engraftment with less risk of GVHD. Further research should develop the understanding and clinical methodologies that will allow for this type of improved control over T1/T2 biology. Such research foci include refinements in the functional definition of T1 vs. T2 effectors, a better understanding of factors that control stability of cytokine polarity, and development of methods that allow more extreme T-cell polarization, particularly in humans. The influence of immunosuppressive agents on T1/T2 effectors post-SCT has been a relatively neglected topic. Along these lines, the development of T1/T2 modulation strategies that allow allogeneic T-cell transfer with little or no immunosuppressive drug therapy should be a goal of future studies. Finally, allogeneic T1/T2 research will need to incorporate advances in tumor biology such that effector mechanisms required for immunological cure of different types of malignancy can be optimized.

REFERENCES

1. Mosmann TR, Cerwinski H, Bond MW, Giedlin MA, Coffman RI. Two types of murine helper T cell clone. I. Definition according to profiles of lymphokine activities and secreted proteins. J Immunol 1986; 136:2348–2357.
2. Sher A, Gazzinelli RT, Oswald IP, Clerici M, Kullberg M, Pearce EJ, Berzofsky JA, Mosmann TR, James SL, Morse HC 3rd. Role of T-cell derived cytokines in the downregulation of immune responses in parasitic and retroviral infection. Immunol Rev 1992; 127:183–204.
3. Le Gros G, Ben-Sasson SZ, Seder R, Finkelman FD, Paul WE. Generation of interleukin 4 (IL-4)-producing cells in vivo and in vitro: IL-2 and IL-4 are required for in vitro generation of IL-4-producing cells. J Exp Med 1990; 172:921–929.
4. Yoshimoto T, Bendelac A, Watson C, Hu-Li J, Paul WE. Role of NK1.1⁺ T cells in a TH2 response and in immunoglobulin E production. Science 1995; 270:1845–1847.
5. Terabe M, Matsui S, Noben-Trauth N, Chen H, Watson C, Donaldson DD, Carbone DP, Paul WE, Berzofsky JA. NKT cell-mediated repression of tumor immunosurveillance by IL-13 and the IL-4R-STAT6 pathway. Nat Immunol 2000; 1:515–520.
6. Guo L, Hu-Li J, Zhu J, Pannetier C, Watson C, McKenzie GJ, McKenzie AN, Paul WE. Disrupting IL-13 impairs production of IL-4 specified by the linked allele. Nat Immunol 2001; 2:461–466.
7. Constant SL, Bottomly K. Induction of Th1 and Th2 CD4⁺ T cell responses: the alternative approaches. Ann Rev Immunol 1997; 15:297–322.
8. Mueller DL, Jenkins MK, Schwartz RH. An accessory cell-derived costimulatory signal acts independently of protein kinase C activation to allow T cell proliferation and prevent the induction of unresponsiveness. J Immunol 1989; 142:2617–2628.
9. Thompson CB, Lindsten T, Ledbetter JA, Kunkel SL, Young HA, Emerson SG, Leiden JM, June CH. CD28 activation pathway regulates the production of multiple T-cell-derived lymphokines/cytokines. Proc Natl Acad Sci USA 1989; 86:1333–1337.
10. Brown DR, Green JM, Moskowitz NH, Davis M, Thompson CB, Reiner SL. Limited role of CD28-mediated signals in T helper subset differentiation. J Exp Med 1996; 184:803–810.
11. Broeren CP, Gray GS, Carreno BM, June CH. Costimulation light: activation of CD4⁺ T cells with CD80 or CD86 rather than anti-CD28 leads to a Th2 cytokine profile. J Immunol 2000; 165:6908–6914.

12. Boise LH, Minn AJ, Noel PJ, June CH, Accavitti MA, Lindsten T, Thompson CB. CD28 costimulation can promote T cell survival by enhancing the expression of Bc1-XL. Immunity 1995; 3:87–98.

13. Okkenhaug K, Wu L, Garza KM, La Rose J, Khoo W, Odermatt B, Mak TW, Ohashi PS, Rottapel R. A point mutation in CD28 distinguishes proliferative signals from survival signals. Nat Immunol 2001; 2:325–332.

14. Tafuri A, Shahinian A, Bladt F, Yoshinaga SK, Jordana M, Wakeham A, Boucher LM, Bouchard D, Chan VS, Duncan G, Odermatt B, Ho A, Itie A, Horan T, Whoriskey JS, Pawson T, Penninger JM, Ohashi PS, Mak TW. ICOS is essential for effective T-helper-cell responses. Nature 2001; 409:105–109.

15. Kopf M, Coyle AJ, Schmitz N, Barner M, Oxenius A, Gallimore A, Gutierrez-Ramos JC, Bachmann MF. Inducible costimulator protein (ICOS) controls T helper cell subset polarization after virus and parasite infection. J Exp Med 2000; 192:53–61.

16. DeBenedette MA, Wen T, Bachmann MF, Ohashi PS, Barber BH, Stocking KL, Peschon JJ, Watts TH. Analysis of 4-1BB ligand (4-1BBL)-deficient mice and of mice lacking both 4-1BBL and CD28 reveals a role for 4-1BBL in skin allograft rejection and in the cytotoxic T cell response to influenza virus. J Immunol 1999; 163:4833–4841.

17. Kim YJ, Kim SH, Mantel P, Kwon BS. Human 4-1BB regulates CD28 co-stimulation to promote Th1 cell responses. Eur J Immunol 1998; 28:881–890.

18. Rissoan MC, Soumelis V, Kadowaki N, Grouard G, Briere F, de Waal Malefyt R, Liu YJ. Reciprocal control of T helper cell and dendritic cell differentiation [comment]. Science 1999; 283:1183–1186.

19. Kalinski P, Hilkens CM, Snijders A, Snijdewint FG, Kapsenberg ML. IL-12-deficient dendritic cells, generated in the presence of prostaglandin E2, promote type 2 cytokine production in maturing human naive T helper cells. J Immunol 1997; 159:28–35.

20. Faries MB, Bedrosian I, Xu S, Koski G, Roros JG, Moise MA, Nguyen HQ, Engels FH, Cohen PA, Czerniecki BJ. Calcium signaling inhibits interleukin-12 production and activates CD82(+) dendritic cells that induce Th2 cell development. Blood 2001; 98:2489–2497.

21. Loza MJ, Perussia B. Final steps of natural killer cell maturation: a model for type 1-type 2 differentiation? [comment]. Nat Immunol 2001; 2:917–924.

22. Smeltz RB, Chen J, Hu-Li J, Shevach EM. Regulation of interleukin (IL)-18 receptor alpha chain expression on CD4(+) T cells during T helper (Th)1/Th2 differentiation. Critical downregulatory role of IL-4. J Exp Med 2001; 194:143–153.

23. Hoshino T, Wiltrout RH, Young HA. IL-18 is a potent coinducer of IL-13 in NK and T cells: a new potential role for IL-18 in modulating the immune response. J Immunol 1999; 162:5070–5077.

24. Afkarian M, Sedy JR, Yang J, Jacobson NG, Cereb N, Yang SY, Murphy TL, Murphy KM. T-bet is a STAT1-induced regulator of IL-12R expression in naive CD4[+] T cells [comment]. Nat Immunol 2002; 3:549–557.

25. Fong TA, Mosmann TR. Alloreactive murine CD8[+] T cell clones secrete the Th1 pattern of cytokines. J Immunol 1990; 144:1744–1752.

26. Salgame P, Abrams JS, Clayberger C, Goldstein H, Convit J, Modlin RL, Bloom BR. Differing lymphokine profiles of functional subsets of human CD4 and CD8 T cell clones. Science 1991; 254:279–282.

27. Croft M, Carter L, Swain SL, Dutton RW. Generation of polarized antigen-specific CD8 effector populations: reciprocal action of interleukin (IL)-4 and IL-12 in promoting type 2 versus type 1 cytokine profiles. J Exp Med 1994; 180:1715–1728.

28. Sad S, Marcotte R, Mosmann TR. Cytokine-induced differentiation of precursor mouse CD8[+]. T cells into cytotoxic CD8[+] T cells secreting Th1 or Th2 cytokines. Immunity 1995; 2:271–279.

29. Klarnet JP, Kern DE, Dower SK, Matis LA, Cheever MA, Greenberg PD. Helper-independent CD8[+] cytotoxic T lymphocytes express IL-1 receptors and require IL-1 for secretion of IL-2. J Immunol 1989; 142:2187–2191.

30. Wang LH, Kirken RA, Yang XY, Erwin RA, DaSilva L, Yu CR, Farrar WL. Selective disruption of interleukin 4 autocrine-regulated loop by a tyrosine kinase inhibitor restricts activity of T-helper 2 cells. Blood 2000; 95:3816–3822.

31. Seder RA, Paul WE, Davis MM, Fazekas de St Groth B. The presence of interleukin 4 during in vitro priming determines the lymphokine-producing potential of $CD4^+$ T cells from T cell receptor transgenic mice. J Exp Med 1992; 176:1091–1098.

32. Sad S, Li L, Mosmann TR. Cytokine-deficient $CD8^+$ Tc1 cells induced by IL-4: retained inflammation and perforin and Fas cytotoxicity but compromised long term killing of tumor cells. J Immunol 1997; 159:606–613.

33. Moore KW, de Waal Malefyt R, Coffman RL, O'Garra A. Interleukin-10 and the interleukin-10 receptor. Ann Rev Immunol 2001; 19:683–765.

34. Windhagen A, Anderson DE, Carrizosa A, Williams RE, Hafler DA. IL-12 induces human T cells secreting IL-10 with IFN-gamma. J Immunol 1996; 157:1127–1131.

35. Cousins DJ, Lee TH, Staynov DZ. Cytokine coexpression during human Th1/Th2 cell differentiation: direct evidence for coordinated expression of Th2 cytokines. J Immunol 2002; 169:2498–2506.

36. Chtanova T, Kemp RA, Sutherland AP, Ronchese F, Mackay CR. Gene microarrays reveal extensive differential gene expression in both CD4(+) and CD8(+) type 1 and type 2 T cells. J Immunol 2001; 167:3057–3063.

37. Hahn S, Stalder T, Wernli M, Burgin D, Tschopp J, Nagata S, Erb P. Down-modulation of $CD4^+$ T helper type 2 and type 0 cells by T helper type 1 cells via Fas/Fas-ligand interaction. Eur J Immunol 1995; 25:2679–2685.

38. Foote LC, Howard RG, Marshak-Rothstein A, Rothstein TL. IL-4 induces Fas resistance in B cells. J Immunol 1996; 157:2749–2753.

39. Carter LL, Dutton RW. Relative perforin- and Fas-mediated lysis in T1 and T2 CD8 effector populations. J Immunol 1995; 155:1028–1031.

40. Kagi D, Ledermann B, Burki K, Zinkernagel RM, Hengartner H. Molecular mechanisms of lymphocyte-mediated cytotoxicity and their role in immunological protection and pathogenesis in vivo. Ann Rev Immunol 1996; 14:207–232.

41. Owen-Schaub LB, van Golen KL, Hill LL, Price JE. Fas and Fas ligand interactions suppress melanoma lung metastasis. J Exp Med 1998; 188:1717–1723.

42. Sallusto F, Lenig D, Mackay CR, Lanzavecchia A. Flexible programs of chemokine receptor expression on human polarized T helper 1 and 2 lymphocytes. J Exp Med 1998; 187:875–883.

43. Sallusto F, Mackay CR, Lanzavecchia A. The role of chemokine receptors in primary, effector, and memory immune responses. Ann Rev Immunol 2000; 18:593–620.

44. Cerwenka A, Morgan TM, Harmsen AG, Dutton RW. Migration kinetics and final destination of type 1 and type 2 CD8 effector cells predict protection against pulmonary virus infection. J Exp Med 1999; 189:423–434.

44a. Jung U, Foley JE, Erdmann AE, Eckhaus MA, Fowler DH. CD3, CD28 Co-stimulated T1 vs. T2 subsets: differential in vivo allosensitization generates distinct GVT and GVHD effects. Blood 2003; 102(9):3439–3446.

45. Cosmi L, Annunziato F, Galli MIG, Maggi RME, Nagata K, Romagnani S. CRTH2 is the most reliable marker for the detection of circulating human type 2 Th and type 2 T cytotoxic cells in health and disease. Eur J Immunol 2000; 30:2972–2979.

46. van Kooten C, Banchereau J. CD40-CD40 ligand. J Leuk Biol 2000; 67:2–17.

47. Lee BO, Haynes L, Eaton SM, Swain SL, Randall TD. The biological outcome of CD40 signaling is dependent on the duration of CD40 ligand expression: reciprocal regulation by interleukin (IL)-4 and IL-12. J Exp Med 2002; 196:693–704.

48. Gilliet M, Liu YJ. Generation of human CD8 T regulatory cells by CD40 ligand-activated plasmacytoid dendritic cells. J Exp Med 2002; 195:695–704.

49. Wierda WG, Cantwell MJ, Woods SJ, Rassenti LZ, Prussak CE, Kipps TJ. CD40-ligand (CD154) gene therapy for chronic lymphocytic leukemia [comment]. Blood 2000; 96:2917–2924.

50. Tong AW, Papayoti MH, Netto G, Armstrong DT, Ordonez G, Lawson JM, Stone MJ. Growth-inhibitory effects of CD40 ligand (CD154) and its endogenous expression in human breast cancer. Clin Cancer Res 2001; 7:691–703.

51. Glimcher LH. Lineage commitment in lymphocytes: controlling the immune response. J Clin Invest 2001; 108:s25–s30.

52. Mullen AC, High FA, Hutchins AS, Lee HW, Villarino AV, Livingston DM, Kung AL, Cereb N, Yao TP, Yang SY, Reiner SL. Role of T-bet in commitment of TH1 cells before IL-12-dependent selection. Science 2001; 292:1907–1910.

53. Mullen AC, Hutchins AS, High FA, Lee HW, Sykes KJ, Chodosh LA, Reiner SL. Hlx is induced by and genetically interacts with T-bet to promote heritable T(H)1 gene induction. Nat Immunol 2002; 3:652–658.

54. Szabo SJ, Sullivan BM, Stemmann C, Satoskar AR, Sleckman BP, Glimcher LH. Distinct effects of T-bet in TH1 lineage commitment and IFN-gamma production in CD4 and CD8 T cells. Science 2002; 295:338–342.

55. Rodriguez-Palmero M, Hara T, Thumbs A, Hunig T. Triggering of T cell proliferation through CD28 induces GATA-3 and promotes T helper type 2 differentiation in vitro and in vivo. Eur J Immunol 1999; 29:3914–3924.

56. Zhu J, Guo L, Min B, Watson CJ, Hu-Li J, Young HA, Tsichlis PN, Paul WE. Growth factor independent-1 induced by IL-4 regulates Th2 cell proliferation. Immunity 2002; 16:733–744.

57. Lantelme E, Mantovani S, Palermo B, Campanelli R, Sallusto F, Giachino C. Kinetics of GATA-3 gene expression in early polarizing and committed human T cells. Immunology 2001; 102:123–130.

58. Swain SL. Generation and in vivo persistence of polarized Th1 and Th2 memory cells. Immunity 1994; 1:543–552.

59. Cerwenka A, Carter LL, Reome JB, Swain SL, Dutton RW. In vivo persistence of CD8 polarized T cell subsets producing type 1 or type 2 cytokines. J Immunol 1998; 161:97–105.

60. Powrie F, Leach MW, Mauze S, Menon S, Caddle LB, Coffman RL. Inhibition of Th1 responses prevents inflammatory bowel disease in scid mice reconstituted with CD45RBhi CD4$^+$ T cells. Immunity 1994; 1:553–562.

61. Asseman C, Mauze S, Leach MW, Coffman RL, Powrie F. An essential role for interleukin 10 in the function of regulatory T cells that inhibit intestinal inflammation. J Exp Med 1999; 190:995–1004.

62. Davidson NJ, Fort MM, Muller W, Leach MW, Rennick DM. Chronic colitis in IL-10-/- mice: insufficient counter regulation of a Th1 response. Int Rev Immunol 2000; 19:91–121.

63. Steidler L, Hans W, Schotte L, Neirynck S, Obermeier F, Falk W, Fiers W, Remaut E. Treatment of murine colitis by *Lactococcus lactis* secreting interleukin-10. Science 2000; 289:1352–1355.

64. Autschbach F, Braunstein J, Helmke B, Zuna I, Schurmann G, Niemir ZI, Wallich R, Otto HF, Meuer SC. In situ expression of interleukin-10 in noninflamed human gut and in inflammatory bowel disease. Am J Pathol 1998; 153:121–130.

65. Schreiber S, Heinig T, Thiele HG, Raedler A. Immunoregulatory role of interleukin 10 in patients with inflammatory bowel disease. Gastroenterology 1995; 108:1434–1444.

66. Gerli R, Bistoni O, Russano A, Fiorucci S, Borgato L, Cesarotti ME, Lunardi C. In vivo activated T cells in rheumatoid synovitis. Analysis of Th1- and Th2-type cytokine production at clonal level in different stages of disease. Clin Exp Immunol 2002; 129:549–555.

67. Youssef S, Stuve O, Patarroyo JC, Ruiz PJ, Radosevich JL, Hur EM, Bravo M, Michell DJ, Sobel RA, Steinman L, Zanvil SS. The HMG-CoA reductase inhibitor, atorvastatin, promotes

a Th2 bias and reverses paralysis in central nervous system autoimmune disease. Nature 2002; 420(6911):78–84.

68. Chiaramonte MG, Donaldson DD, Cheever AW, Wynn TA. An IL-13 inhibitor blocks the development of hepatic fibrosis during a T-helper type 2-dominated inflammatory response. J Clin Invest 1999; 104:777–785.

69. Lanone S, Zheng T, Zhu Z, Liu W, Lee CG, Ma B, Chen Q, Homer RJ, Wang J, Rabach LA, Rabach ME, Shipley JM, Shapiro SD, Senior RM, Elias JA. Overlapping and enzyme-specific contributions of matrix metalloproteinases-9 and -12 in IL-13-induced inflammation and remodeling. J Clin Invest 2002; 110:463–474.

70. Mishra A, Hogan SP, Brandt EB, Rothenberg ME. IL-5 promotes eosinophil trafficking to the esophagus. J Immunol 2002; 168:2464–2469.

71. Fallon PG, Jolin HE, Smith P, Emson CL, Townsend MJ, Fallon R, McKenzie AN. IL-4 induces characteristic Th2 responses even in the combined absence of IL-5, IL-9, and IL-13. Immunity 2002; 17:7–17.

72. Webb DC, McKenzie AN, Koskinen AM, Yang M, Mattes J, Foster PS. Integrated signals between IL-13, IL-4, and IL-5 regulate airways hyperreactivity. J Immunol 2000; 165:108–113.

73. Tatsumi T, Kierstead LS, Ranieri E, Gesualdo L, Schena FP, Finke JH, Bukowski RM, Mueller-Berghaus J, Kirkwood JM, Kwok WW, Storkus WJ. Disease-associated bias in T helper type 1 (Th1)/Th2 CD4(+) T cell responses against MAGE-6 in HLA-DRB10401(+) patients with renal cell carcinoma or melanoma. J Exp Med 2002; 196:619–628.

74. Zitvogel L, Mayordomo JI, Tjandrawan T, DeLeo AB, Clarke MR, Lotze MT, Storkus WJ. Therapy of murine tumors with tumor peptide-pulsed dendritic cells: dependence on T cells, B7 costimulation, and T helper cell 1-associated cytokines. J Exp Med 1996; 183:87–97.

75. To WC, Seeley BM, Barthel SW, Shu S. Therapeutic efficacy of Th1 and Th2 L-selectin-CD4$^+$ tumor-reactive T cells. Laryngoscope 2000; 110:1648–1654.

76. Nishimura T, Iwakabe K, Sekimoto M, Ohmi Y, Yahata T, Nakui M, Sato T, Habu S, Tashiro H, Sato M, Ohta A. Distinct role of antigen-specific T helper type 1 (Th1) and Th2 cells in tumor eradication in vivo. J Exp Med 1999; 190:617–627.

77. Dobrzanski MJ, Reome JB, Dutton RW. Therapeutic effects of tumor-reactive type 1 and type 2 CD8$^+$ T cell subpopulations in established pulmonary metastases. J Immunol 1999; 162:6671–6680.

78. Dobrzanski MJ, Reome JB, Dutton RW. Type 1 and type 2 CD8$^+$ effector T cell subpopulations promote long-term tumor immunity and protection to progressively growing tumor. J Immunol 2000; 164:916–925.

79. Korngold R, Sprent J. Graft-versus-host disease in experimental allogeneic bone marrow transplantation. Proc Soc Exp Biol Med 1991; 197:12–18.

80. Abhyankar S, Gilliland DG, Ferrara JL. Interleukin-1 is a critical effector molecule during cytokine dysregulation in graft versus host disease to minor histocompatibility antigens. Transplantation 1993; 56:1518–1523.

81. Via CS, Finkelman FD. Critical role of interleukin-2 in the development of acute graft-versus-host disease. Int Immunol 1993; 5:565–572.

82. Schwarer AP, Jiang YZ, Brookes PA, Barrett AJ, Batchelor JR, Goldman JM, Lechler RI. Frequency of anti-recipient alloreactive helper T-cell precursors in donor blood and graft-versus-host disease after HLA-identical sibling bone-marrow transplantation. Lancet 1993; 341:203–205.

83. Blazar BR, Taylor PA, Panoskaltsis-Mortari A, Buhlman J, Xu J, Flavell RA, Korngold R, Noelle R, Vallera DA. Blockade of CD40 ligand-CD40 interaction impairs CD4$^+$ T cell-mediated alloreactivity by inhibiting mature donor T cell expansion and function after bone marrow transplantation. J Immunol 1997; 158:29–39.

84. Via CS, Nguyen P, Shustov A, Drappa J, Elkon KB. A major role for the Fas pathway in acute graft-versus-host disease. J Immunol 1996; 157:5387–5393.

85. Schmaltz C, Alpdogan O, Horndasch KJ, Murigian SJ, Kappel BJ, Teshima T, Ferrara JL, Burakoff SJ, van den Brink MR. Differential use of Fas ligand and perforin cytotoxic pathways by donor T cells in graft-versus-host disease and graft-versus-leukemia effect. Blood 2001; 97:2886–2895.

86. Wasem C, Frutschi C, Arnold D, Vallan C, Lin T, Green DR, Mueller C, Brunner T. Accumulation and activation-induced release of preformed Fas (CD95) ligand during the pathogenesis of experimental graft-versus-host disease. J Immunol 2001; 167:2936–2941.

87. Kataoka Y, Iwasaki T, Kuroiwa T, Seto Y, Iwata N, Hashimoto N, Ogata A, Hamano T, Kakishita E. The role of donor T cells for target organ injuries in acute and chronic graft-versus-host disease. Immunology 2001; 103:310–318.

88. Baker MB, Altman NH, Podack ER, Levy RB. The role of cell-mediated cytotoxicity in acute GVHD after MHC-matched allogeneic bone marrow transplantation in mice. J Exp Med 1996; 183:2645–2656.

89. Lin T, Brunner T, Tietz B, Madsen J, Bonfoco E, Reaves M, Huflejt M, Green DR. Fas ligand-mediated killing by intestinal intraepithelial lymphocytes. Participation in intestinal graft-versus-host disease. J Clin Invest 1998; 101:570–577.

90. van Den Brink MR, Moore E, Horndasch KJ, Crawford JM, Hoffman J, Murphy GF, Burakoff SJ. Fas-deficient lpr mice are more susceptible to graft-versus-host disease. J Immunol 2000; 164:469–480.

91. Nestel FP, Price KS, Seemayer TA, Lapp WS. Macrophage priming and lipopolysaccharide-triggered release of tumor necrosis factor alpha during graft-versus-host disease. J Exp Med 1992; 175:405–413.

92. Trinchieri G. Regulatory role of T cells producing both interferon gamma and interleukin 10 in persistent infection. J Exp Med 2001; 194:F53–F57.

93. Refaeli Y, Van Parijs L, Alexander SI, Abbas AK. Interferon gamma is required for activation-induced death of T lymphocytes. J Exp Med 2002; 196:999–1005.

94. Murphy WJ, Welniak LA, Taub DD, Wiltrout RH, Taylor PA, Vallera DA, Kopf M, Young H, Longo DL, Blazar BR. Differential effects of the absence of interferon-gamma and IL-4 in acute graft-versus-host disease after allogeneic bone marrow transplantation in mice. J Clin Invest 1998; 102:1742–1748.

95. Welniak LA, Blazar BR, Anver MR, Wiltrout RH, Murphy WJ. Opposing roles of interferon-gamma on CD4$^+$ T cell-mediated graft-versus-host disease: effects of conditioning. Biol Blood Marrow Transplant 2000; 6:604–612.

96. Krenger W, Snyder KM, Byon JC, Falzarano G, Ferrara JL. Polarized type 2 alloreactive CD4$^+$ and CD8$^+$ donor T cells fail to induce experimental acute graft-versus-host disease. J Immunol 1995; 155:585–593.

97. Fowler DH, Breglio J, Nagel G, Eckhaus MA, Gress RE. Allospecific CD8$^+$ Tc1 and Tc2 populations in graft-versus-leukemia effect and graft-versus-host disease. J Immunol 1996; 157:4811–4821.

98. Fowler DH, Breglio J, Nagel G, Hirose C, Gress RE. Allospecific CD4$^+$, Th1/Th2 and CD8$^+$, Tc1/Tc2 populations in murine GVL: type I cells generate GVL and type II cells abrogate GVL. Biol Blood Marrow Transplant 1996; 2:118–125.

99. Teshima T, Ordemann R, Reddy P, Gagin S, Liu C, Cooke KR, Ferrara JL. Acute graft-versus-host disease does not require alloantigen expression on host epithelium [comment][erratum appears in Nat Med 2002; 8(9):1039]. Nat Med 2002; 8:575–581.

100. Piguet PF, Grau GE, Allet B, Vassalli P. Tumor necrosis factor/cachectin is an effector of skin and gut lesions of the acute phase of graft-vs.-host disease. J Exp Med 1987; 166:1280–1289.

101. Holler E, Kolb HJ, Moller A, Kempeni J, Liesenfeld S, Pechumer H, Lehmacher W, Ruckdeschel G, Gleixner B, Riedner C, et al. Increased serum levels of tumor necrosis factor alpha precede major complications of bone marrow transplantation [comment]. Blood 1990; 75:1011–1016.

102. Cox GW, Melillo G, Chattopadhyay U, Mullet D, Fertel RH, Varesio L. Tumor necrosis factor-alpha-dependent production of reactive nitrogen intermediates mediates IFN-gamma plus IL-2-induced murine macrophage tumoricidal activity. J Immunol 1992; 149:3290–3296.
103. Hill GR, Teshima T, Gerbitz A, Pan L, Cooke KR, Brinson YS, Crawford JM, Ferrara JL. Differential roles of IL-1 and TNF-alpha on graft-versus-host disease and graft versus leukemia. J Clin Invest 1999; 104:459–467.
104. Takahashi H, Furukawa T, Hashimoto S, Suzuki N, Yuroha T, Yamazaki F, Inano K, Takahashi M, Aizawa Y, Koike T. Contribution of TNF-alpha and IL-10 gene polymorphisms to graft-versus-host disease following allo-hematopoietic stem cell transplantation. Bone Marrow Transplant 2000; 26:1317–1323.
105. Cavet J, Middleton PG, Segall M, Noreen H, Davies SM, Dickinson AM. Recipient tumor necrosis factor-alpha and interleukin-10 gene polymorphisms associate with early mortality and acute graft-versus-host disease severity in HLA-matched sibling bone marrow transplants. Blood 1999; 94:3941–3946.
106. Cullup H, Dickinson AM, Jackson GH, Taylor PR, Cavet J, Middleton PG. Donor interleukin 1 receptor antagonist genotype associated with acute graft-versus-host disease in human leucocyte antigen-matched sibling allogeneic transplants. Br J Haematol 2001; 113:807–813.
107. Holler E, Kolb HJ, Mittermuller J, Kaul M, Ledderose G, Duell T, Seeber B, Schleuning M, Hintermeier-Knabe R, Ertl B, et al. Modulation of acute graft-versus-host-disease after allogeneic bone marrow transplantation by tumor necrosis factor alpha (TNF alpha) release in the course of pretransplant conditioning: role of conditioning regimens and prophylactic application of a monoclonal antibody neutralizing human TNF alpha (MAK 195F). Blood 1995; 86:890–899.
108. Antin JH, Weisdorf D, Neuberg D, Nicklow R, Clouthier S, Lee SJ, Alyea E, McGarigle C, Blazar BR, Sonis S, Soiffer RJ, and Ferrara JL. Interleukin 1 blockade does not prevent acute graft versus host disease: results of a randomized, double-blind, placebo-controlled trial of IL-1 receptor antagonist in allogeneic bone marrow transplantation. Blood 2002; 100(10):3479–3482.
109. Cooke KR, Gerbitz A, Crawford JM, Teshima T, Hill GR, Tesolin A, Rossignol DP, Ferrara JL. LPS antagonism reduces graft-versus-host disease and preserves graft-versus-leukemia activity after experimental bone marrow transplantation [comment]. J Clin Invest 2001; 107:1581–1589.
110. Fowler DH, Kurasawa K, Husebekk A, Cohen PA, Gress RE. Cells of Th2 cytokine phenotype prevent LPS-induced lethality during murine graft-versus-host reaction. Regulation of cytokines and CD8$^+$ lymphoid engraftment. J Immunol 1994; 152:1004–1013.
111. Zelenika D, Adams E, Humm S, Lin CY, Waldmann H, Cobbold SP. The role of CD4$^+$ T-cell subsets in determining transplantation rejection or tolerance. Immunol Rev 2001; 182:164–179.
112. Zelenika D, Adams E, Humm S, Graca L, Thompson S, Cobbold SP, Waldmann H. Regulatory T cells overexpress a subset of Th2 gene transcripts. J Immunol 2002; 168:1069–1079.
113. Fowler DH, Kurasawa K, Smith R, Eckhaus MA, Gress RE. Donor CD4-enriched cells of Th2 cytokine phenotype regulate graft-versus-host disease without impairing allogeneic engraftment in sublethally irradiated mice. Blood 1994; 84:3540–3549.
114. Krenger W, Cooke KR, Crawford JM, Sonis ST, Simmons R, Pan L, Delmonte J, Jr., Karandikar M, Ferrara JL. Transplantation of polarized type 2 donor T cells reduces mortality caused by experimental graft-versus-host disease. Transplantation 1996; 62:1278–1285.
115. Helmich BK, Dutton RW. The role of adoptively transferred CD8 T cells and host cells in the control of the growth of the EG7 thymoma: factors that determine the relative effectiveness and homing properties of Tc1 and Tc2 effectors. J Immunol 2001; 166:6500–6508.

116. Kemp RA, Ronchese F. Tumor-specific Tc1, but not Tc2, cells deliver protective antitumor immunity. J Immunol 2001; 167:6497–6502.

117. Fowler DH, Whitfield B, Livingston M, Chrobak P, Gress RE. Non-host-reactive donor $CD8^+$ T cells of Tc2 phenotype potently inhibit marrow graft rejection. Blood 1998; 91:4045–4050.

118. Pan L, Delmonte J, Jr., Jalonen CK, Ferrara JL. Pretreatment of donor mice with granulocyte colony-stimulating factor polarizes donor T lymphocytes toward type-2 cytokine production and reduces severity of experimental graft-versus-host disease. Blood 1995; 86:4422–4429.

119. Sloand EM, Kim S, Maciejewski JP, Van Rhee F, Chaudhuri A, Barrett J, Young NS. Pharmacologic doses of granulocyte colony-stimulating factor affect cytokine production by lymphocytes in vitro and in vivo. Blood 2000; 95:2269–2274.

120. Pan L, Teshima T, Hill GR, Bungard D, Brinson YS, Reddy VS, Cooke KR, Ferrara JL. Granulocyte colony-stimulating factor-mobilized allogeneic stem cell transplantation maintains graft-versus-leukemia effects through a perforin-dependent pathway while preventing graft-versus-host disease. Blood 1999; 93:4071–4078.

121. Hill GR, Cooke KR, Teshima T, Crawford JM, Keith JC, Jr., Brinson YS, Bungard D, Ferrara JL. Interleukin-11 promotes T cell polarization and prevents acute graft-versus-host disease after allogeneic bone marrow transplantation. J Clin Invest 1998; 102:115–123.

122. Teshima T, Hill GR, Pan L, Brinson YS, van den Brink MR, Cooke KR, Ferrara JL. IL-11 separates graft-versus-leukemia effects from graft-versus-host disease after bone marrow transplantation. J Clin Invest 1999; 104:317–325.

123. Lan F, Zeng D, Higuchi M, Huie P, Higgins JP, Strober S. Predominance of $NK1.1^+$ TCR alpha beta$^+$ or $DX5^+$ TCR alpha beta$^+$ T cells in mice conditioned with fractionated lymphoid irradiation protects against graft-versus-host disease: "natural suppressor" cells. J Immunol 2001; 167:2087–2096.

124. Hoffmann P, Ermann J, Edinger M, Fathman CG, Strober S. Donor-type CD4(+)CD25(+) regulatory T cells suppress lethal acute graft-versus-host disease after allogeneic bone marrow transplantation. J Exp Med 2002; 196:389–399.

125. Arpinati M, Green CL, Heimfeld S, Heuser JE, Anasetti C. Granulocyte-colony stimulating factor mobilizes T helper 2-inducing dendritic cells. Blood 2000; 95:2484–2490.

126. Waller EK, Rosenthal H, Jones TW, Peel J, Lonial S, Langston A, Redei I, Jurickova I, Boyer MW. Larger numbers of CD4(bright) dendritic cells in donor bone marrow are associated with increased relapse after allogeneic bone marrow transplantation. Blood 2001; 97:2948–2956.

127. Jung U, Foley JE, Coppins JL, Eckhaus MA, Fowler DH. Co-stimulated allogeneic Tc1 cells mediate a curable GVT effect against murine breast cancer cells in a fasL-independent manner. Abstract presented at the annual meeting of the American Society of Hematology, Dec. 9, 2001.

128. Levine BL, Bernstein WB, Connors M, Craighead N, Lindsten T, Thompson CB, June CH. Effects of CD28 costimulation on long-term proliferation of $CD4^+$ T cells in the absence of exogenous feeder cells. J Immunol 1997; 159:5921–5930.

129. Liu J, Anderson BE, Robert ME, McNiff JM, Emerson SG, Shlomchik WD, Shlomchik MJ. Selective T-cell subset ablation demonstrates a role for T1 and T2 cells in ongoing acute graft-versus-host disease: a model system for the reversal of disease. Blood 2001; 98:3367–3375.

130. Nikolic B, Lee S, Bronson RT, Grusby MJ, Sykes M. Th1 and Th2 mediate acute graft-versus-host disease, each with distinct end-organ targets. J Clin Invest 2000; 105:1289–1298.

131. Imami N, Brookes PA, Lombardi G, Hakooz B, Johns M, Goldman JM, Batchelor JR, Lechler RI, Ritter MA. Association between interleukin-4-producing T lymphocyte frequencies and reduced risk of graft-versus-host disease. Transplantation 1998; 65:979–988.

132. Blazar BR, Taylor PA, Panoskaltsis-Mortari A, Narula SK, Smith SR, Roncarolo MG, Vallera DA. Interleukin-10 dose-dependent regulation of $CD4^+$ and $CD8^+$ T cell-mediated graft-versus-host disease. Transplantation 1998; 66:1220–1229.

133. Bacchetta R, Bigler M, Touraine JL, Parkman R, Tovo PA, Abrams J, de Waal Malefyt R, de Vries JE, Roncarolo MG. High levels of interleukin 10 production in vivo are associated with tolerance in SCID patients transplanted with HLA mismatched hematopoietic stem cells. J Exp Med 1994; 179:493–502.

134. Holler E, Roncarolo MG, Hintermeier-Knabe R, Eissner G, Ertl B, Schulz U, Knabe H, Kolb HJ, Andreesen R, Wilmanns W. Prognostic significance of increased IL-10 production in patients prior to allogeneic bone marrow transplantation. Bone Marrow Transplant 2000; 25:237–241.

135. Fowler DH, Hou J, Foley J, Hakim F, Odom J, Castro K, Carter C, Read EJ, Gea-Benacloche J, Kasten-Sportes CKL, Wilson W, Levine B, June C, Gress R, Bishop MR. Phase I clinical trial of donor Th2 cells after immunoablative reduced intensity allogeneic PBSCT. Cytotherapy 2002; 4:429–430.

136. Bishop MRHJ, Wilson WH, Steinberg SM, Odom J, Castro K, Kasten-Sportes C, Gea-Banacloche J, Marchigiani D, Gress RE, Fowler DH. Establishment of early donor engraftment after reduced-intensity allogeneic hematopoietic stem cell transplantation to potentiate the graft-versus-lymphoma effect against refractory lymphomas. Biol Blood Marrow Transplant 2003; 9:162–169.

137. Petrus MJ, Williams JF, Eckhaus MA, Gress RE, Fowler DH. An immunoablative regimen of fludarabine and cyclophosphamide prevents fully MHC-mismatched murine marrow graft rejection independent of GVHD. Biol Blood Marrow Transplant 2000; 6:182–189.

138. Deeg HJ, Lin D, Leisenring W, Boeckh M, Anasetti C, Appelbaum FR, Chauncey TR, Doney K, Flowers M, Martin P, Nash R, Schoch G, Sullivan KM, Witherspoon RP, Storb R. Cyclosporine or cyclosporine plus methylprednisolone for prophylaxis of graft-versus-host disease: a prospective, randomized trial. Blood 1997; 89:3880–3887.

139. Garlie NK, LeFever AV, Siebenlist RE, Levine BL, June CH, Lum LG. T cells coactivated with immobilized anti-CD3 and anti-CD28 as potential immunotherapy for cancer. J Immunother 1999; 22:336–345.

140. Levine BL, Bernstein WB, Aronson NE, Schlienger K, Cotte J, Perfetto S, Humphries MJ, Ratto-Kim S, Birx DL, Steffens C, Landay A, Carroll RG, June CH. Adoptive transfer of costimulated $CD4^+$ T cells induces expansion of peripheral T cells and decreased CCR5 expression in HIV infection. Nat Med 2002; 8:47–53.

141. Hou J, Levine B, June C, Fowler DH. Naive ($CD45RA^+$) vs. memory ($CD45RO^+$) status of human CD4 cells greatly influences Th1/Th2 polarization potential. Abstract at the 2002 Meeting of the American Society of Hematology, 2002.

142. Fowler DH, Odom J, Castro K, Kasten-Sportes C, Gea-Banacloche J, Dean R, Wilson W, Foley J, Hou J, Hakim F, Leitman S, Read EJ, Carter C, Levine B, June C, Gress R, Bishop MR. Co-stimulated Th2 cells for modulation of acute GVHD: phase I clinical trial results. Abstract at the 2002 Meeting of the American Society of Hematology, 2002.

4

Role of T-Cell Costimulation and Regulatory Cells in Allogeneic Hematopoietic Cell Transplantation

BRUCE R. BLAZAR and PATRICIA A. TAYLOR

University of Minnesota, Minneapolis, Minnesota, U.S.A.

I. TOLERANCE INDUCTION BY REGULATING ANTIGEN-SPECIFIC T-CELL RESPONSES

The concept that T cells require two distinct signals for full activation was offered more than three decades ago. The first signal, antigen recognition, is provided by the interaction between an MHC/peptide complex on an antigen-presenting cell (APC) and the T-cell receptor (TCR). The second, or costimulatory, signal is provided by the ligation of accessory molecules expressed on the surface of APC (among other cell types) to counterreceptors expressed on T cells. T-cell costimulation stabilizes cytokine mRNA, facilitates cell cycle progression, and induces antiapoptotic proteins, resulting in productive and sustained T-cell responses (1–3). In the absence of positive costimulatory signals, TCR ligation by the MHC/peptide complex induces the T cell to become specifically nonresponsive (tolerant) to subsequent MHC/peptide engagement. Jenkins and Schwartz demonstrated that interference with costimulation of T-cell activation in antigen-activated murine T-cell clones can render these cells incapable of proliferating in response to the relevant antigen even though the clones retain proliferative capacity to polyclonal activators (4). This state has been termed anergy. A hallmark of anergy induction is a defect in IL-2 transcription. Anergic T cells fail to produce sufficient IL-2 to permit a fully productive immune response to occur upon restimulation with their relevant antigen (4,5). Antigen-specific nonresponsiveness can be prevented by supplying an exogenous source of IL-2; anergic T cells reexposed to relevant antigen in the presence of IL-2 acquire the capability of mounting a productive proliferative response to that antigen (4,5).

Although anergy induction was initially believed to be a passive process in which T cells fail to receive sufficient signals to divide, it now is viewed as an active process; T cells must receive appropriate TCR signaling, in the absence of costimulation, to be rendered nonresponsibe to the relevant MHC/peptide complex. In vivo costimulatory pathway blockade could be an effective strategy to prevent graft-vs.-host disease (GVHD) since donor T cells that have a high likelihood of encountering abundant host alloantigens/ peptides would be tolerized. In contrast, antiviral or antitumor immune responses may be preserved if the viral or tumor antigen density is too low to engage the appropriate TCR during the in vivo costimulatory blockade. Such may be the case early after stem cell transplantation (SCT) when, in many patients, host alloantigens would likely be available in higher concentrations than viral antigens. Because the frequency of alloreactive T cells is small (estimated to be $\leq 0.1\%$ in many SCT settings), the vast majority of T cells would be available to mount effective responses while alloreactive T cells would be rendered tolerant. Such is the promise and hope of new strategies aimed at regulating T-cell responses via targeting costimulatory pathways.

II. OVERVIEW OF IMMUNE RESPONSE REGULATION

Most members of T-cell costimulatory pathways belong to the immunoglobulin (Ig) supergene or tumor necrosis factor (TNF) nerve growth factor (NGF) receptor gene families (Table 1). Although redundancy exists in the biological functions of these pathways that may provide safeguards for the immune system, each pathway has unique functions that can directly or indirectly regulate the specific type [e.g., naïve vs. effector/ memory cells; Th1/Tc1 (IFN-γ, IL-2) vs. Th2/Tc2 (IL-4, -5, -10, -13); CD4 vs. CD8] or location (e.g., lymphohematopoietic or nonlymphoid tissues) of T-cell responses. The existence of several costimulatory pathways that have some redundant features increases the likelihood that a productive response can occur if needed. Importantly, despite considerable redundancy and the contribution of numerous costimulatory pathways to the pathogenesis of GVHD and graft rejection, many investigators have demonstrated significant therapeutic benefits by the targeting of a single pathway.

Although an increasing number of known costimulatory pathways facilitate immune responses against foreign pathogens, injured tissues, or dying cells, the immune system also has safeguards to prevent uncontrolled T-cell activation and proliferation. Such mechanisms serve several purposes, including limiting severe immune-mediated tissue destruction as might occur during viral infections or the likelihood of autoimmunity due to the uncontrolled immune response to autoantigens. Costimulation was initially thought to provide only positive signals to activated T cells, but it now well known that certain pathways result in the delivery of negative signals that limit T-cell responses. In addition to modifying T-cell signals by altering costimulation, immune responses can be dampened or suppressed by a variety of cell types, collectively termed regulatory or suppressor cells. Regulatory cells, an important component of immune homeostasis, represent a naturally occurring, phenotypically diverse population of cells.

This chapter will focus upon the in vivo role of several costimulatory pathways and regulatory cell populations as they specifically relate to GVHD, graft-vs.-leukemia (GVL) effects, and bone marrow (BM) graft rejection. Although cell surface adhesion molecules (e.g., LFA-1/ICAM, CD2/CD48) can support and modify T-cell responses, these pathways will not be discussed here.

Table 1 Costimulatory Pathways Operating During GVHD

	Function	Expression	Ligand	Other names	Expression
Ig superfamily					
CD28	Costimulation	T and NK cells	CD80 CD86	B7-1	Activated APC and activated T cells
CTLA-4 (CD152)	Inhibition	Activated T cells	CD80	B7-2	Activated APC and activated T cells
			CD86	B7-2	APC (upregulated) and activated T cells
ICOS	Costimulation	Activated T cells	B7RP-1	ICOSL, GL50, B7-H2, B7h	B cells, monocytes, small fraction of T cells
Inhibitory molecules					
PD-1	Inhibition	Activated T and B cells	PD-L1	B7-H1	Dendritic cells, activated T cells, stimulated monocytes and keratinocytes, skeletal muscle, heart
			PD-L2	B7-DC	Monocytes, macrophages, DC, lung, liver, pancreas, skeletal muscle, heart
CTLA-4 (CD152)	Inhibition	Activated T cells	CD80	B7-1	Activated APC and activated T cells
			CD86	B7-2	APC (upregulated) and activated T cells
TNRF family					
CD30	Costimulation	Activated T, NK, and B cells, Reed-Sternberg cells in Hodgkin's disease	CD153	CD30L	Neutrophils, activated B and T cells

(Continued)

Table 1 *Continued*

	Function	Expression	Ligand	Other names	Expression
CD40	Costimulation	APC, T subset, endothelium, some epithelial cells	CD40L	CD154, gp39	Activated CD4+ cells, small fraction of activated B cells and CD8+ T cells, platelets
4-1BB (CD137)	Costimulation	Activated T cells, NK cells	4-1BBL	CD137L	Activated B, DC, peritoneal cells, monocytes/macrophages
OX40 (CD134)	Costimulation	Activated T cells	OX40L	CD134L	Activated B cells, macrophages, endothelial cells, microglial cells, T cells
LIGHT	Costimulation	Peripheral blood mononuclear cells, dendritic cells	HVEM, lymphotoxin β receptor, DcR3/TR6		T cells, B cells, NK cells, endothelium

III. COSTIMULATORY PATHWAYS AND MODULATION OF ALLOGENEIC T-CELL RESPONSES

A. The CD28/CTLA-4 (CD152):B7-1 (CD80)/B7-2 (CD86) Pathway

The first pathway formally shown to be necessary and sufficient for T-cell costimulation involved the signaling of CD28 by B7 ligands (6–10). CD28 and CD152 exist as homologous counterreceptors that compete for the binding of two distinct B7 ligands (7–9,11,12). CD28 is constitutively expressed on T cells and NK cells. CD152 is upregulated on T cells during activation and has a higher affinity for B7 ligands than CD28 (7–9,11,13,14). Binding of B7 to CD28 results in the delivery of a positive costimulatory signal to antigen-activated T cells (7–10). In contrast, the binding of B7 to CD152 results in the delivery of a negative or inhibitory costimulatory signal (9,14–21). The two known natural ligands for CD28 and CD152, CD80 and CD86, are expressed on APC (7–9,11,22–29). CD86 is expressed constitutively at a low level on APCs but is inducible, whereas CD80 expression requires induction (27,30,31). We found that pro-inflammatory signals from TBI conditioning and alloreactivity upregulate CD80 and CD86 expression in GVHD target organs early post-BMT (32). This finding set the stage for studies directed toward interrupting CD28/B7 interactions as a strategy to prevent GVHD. Early studies to block this pathway were made possible by the construction of CTLA4-Ig, a protein consisting of the high-avidity B7 ligand–binding extracellular domain of CTLA-4 fused to the $C\gamma1$ moiety of Ig, designed to prolong in vivo half-life of this recombinant protein (33,34). Data from us and other groups indicated that CTLA4-Ig infusions reduce but do not eliminate GVHD in recipients of fully allogeneic, semi-allogeneic, or minor histocompatibility (miH) antigen disparate donor grafts conditioned with lethal or sublethal irradiation doses (32,35–40). Thus, the partial efficacy of CTLA4-Ig infusion in preventing GVHD was not secondary to the unique biology of a given GVHD model or to whether CD4+ or CD8+ T cells were the major mediators of GVHD (40).

CTLA4-Ig fusion proteins have a relatively short in vivo half-life, suggesting that incomplete GVHD inhibition might be due to inadequate CD28/B7 blockade (32). With the availability of anti-B7 monoclonal antibodies (mAb), a higher and more prolonged degree of blockade of the CD28/CD152:B7 pathway could be achieved. In comparison to studies using CTLA4-Ig to reduce GVHD, the effect achieved with anti-B7 antibody treatment was superior (41), anti-B7 mAb infusion reproducibly led to survival rates ranging from approximately 40 to 60%, in contrast to the more variable and generally lower survival rates (typically ≤25%) following CTLA4-Ig infusion (B. R. Blazar and P. A. Taylor, unpublished data). We found that the infusion of anti-CD80 and anti-CD86 mAb inhibited donor CD4+ and CD8+ T-cell expansion by almost 100-fold (41). Despite this high degree of inhibition, approximately one half of lethally irradiated mice receiving a high dose of allogeneic T cells succumbed to GVHD lethality, and survivors were not GVHD-free (41).

Although the lack of uniform GVHD prevention may have been the result of other costimulatory pathways not blocked by anti-B7 mAb (discussed below), it is important to emphasize that CTLA4-Ig and anti-B7 mAb should block both the stimulatory CD28/B7 and the inhibitory CD152/B7 pathways. CD152/B7 inhibits cell cycle entry, reduces IL-2 secretion, and is necessary for tolerance induction (42). Indirect proof for the hypothesis that preservation of CD152/B7 interactions would be beneficial in downregulating GVHD lethality was derived from our studies using anti-CD152 mAb infusions in a lethally irradiated model in which MHC class I and class II disparate donor grafts are given (43).

Under these conditions, anti-CD152 mAb enhanced in vivo donor T-cell expansion and GVHD lethality. To maintain the downregulatory capacity of CD152:B7 on alloreactive T-cell responses, several groups have used CD28−/− donor mice as a source of GVHD-causing T cells (43–46). A critical role for the B7:CD28 pathway was demonstrated by the markedly reduced expansion of CD28−/− T cells and diminished GVHD lethality when limited numbers of purified CD4+ or CD8+ CD28−/− T cells were infused (43,44). In vitro, alloresponses of CD28−/− T cells are markedly lower than controls. In sub-lethally irradiated recipients of purified CD28−/−CD4+ or CD8+ T cells, GVHD lethality was reduced by more than 10-fold and more than 3-fold, respectively, as compared to CD28+/+ cells (43). Additionally, the administration of anti-B7 mAb into heavily irradiated recipients of CD28−/− donor splenocytes augmented the hemato-logical and histological manifestations of GVHD, again suggesting that CD152:B7 signaling downregulates GVHD responses (46). Importantly, many studies have shown that CD28−/− T cells can mediate lethal GVHD if large numbers are infused into lethally irradiated mice, indicating that the requirement for CD28:B7 interaction is not absolute. The recent discovery that CD4+CD25+ regulatory cells that suppress GVHD (discussed in detail below) are present in low numbers in CD28−/− mice (47) further complicates the interpretation of these studies. In an entirely different approach, Anasetti's group showed that anti-CD28 mAb modulated the CD28 receptor in vivo, selectively inhibiting donor antihost alloreactive T-cell expansion and reducing GVHD (38). Interestingly, CD152 signaling was necessary for this effect because treatment with CTLA4-Ig (which blocks both CD28/B7 and CD152/B7 interactions) did not prevent GVHD as effectively as anti-CD289 mAb (38).

Although B7 molecules are expressed on APCs, CD86 is also constitutively expressed on T cells, and both CD80 and CD86 are upregulated on activated T cells in mice with GVHD (41). Using CD80/CD86-deficient mice (B7 DKO) (22) and mice overexpressing CD86 on all T cells [CD86 transgenic (Tg)] (48) as T-cell donors, we showed that T cells from B7 DKO mice result in significant GVHD acceleration compared to wild-type (WT) T cells (49). Conversely, BMT with CD86 Tg donor T cells results in reduced GVHD mortality compared to WT controls. Additional studies indicated that B7 expression on T cells downregulates alloresponses through CD152 ligation. These data, which demonstrate the importance of T-cell–associated B7 as a negative regulator of GVHD, along with other data suggesting the existence of a third B7 ligand, add to the complexity of the CD28/CD152:B7 pathway in regulating GVHD lethality (50).

Allogeneic donor T cells also can eliminate host leukemia cells in vivo via a GVL effect. Potential mechanisms for a GVL effect include the expression of allogeneic MHC or miH antigens on host leukemia cells, cross-presentation of leukemia antigens by host APC, or nonspecific amplification of antileukemia T-cell responses via the elaboration of soluble factors from bona fide donor antihost reactive T cells. Inhibiting donor T-cell alloresponses may have detrimental effects post-BMT. Anti-B7 mAb completely eliminated both GVHD and the GVL effect mediated by delayed lymphocyte infusions (DLI) given to recipients of AML cells. By contrast, the forced expression of B7 ligands on AML cells by gene transfer techniques markedly augmented GVL effects (51). Conversely, anti-CD152 mAb treatment was strikingly advantageous in facilitating the GVL effects after DLI, but GVHD was also augmented (51). It should be noted that our data indicating that anti-B7 mAb eliminate a GVL effect contradict those of Ohata et al., who showed that anti-B7 mAb administered beginning on the day of BMT diminished GVHD but did not eliminate GVL effect against a B leukemia cell line (52).

The importance of the CD28:B7 pathway on inducing optimal GVHD and GVL effects suggested that blockade of this pathway could be exploited to dampen host antidonor alloreactive T-cell responses, which can result in BM graft rejection. Recently, investigators have focused upon the use of nonmyeloablative conditioning regimens that result in a high propensity toward host cell recovery without evidence of donor cell engraftment. Sukes et al. showed that mice conditioned with 3 Gy TBI and given anti-CD4 and anti-CD8 mAb along with CTLA4-Ig developed high levels of stable multilineage chimerism, with specific tolerance to skin grafts and deletion of donor-reactive CD4+ cells in the peripheral blood, spleen, and thymus (53). Storb and colleagues have shown that CTLA4-Ig can permit the reduction of TBI dose from 2 to 1 Gy in a large animal model wherein canine recipients are given cyclosporin A and mycophenolate along with DLA-matched donor hematopoietic cells (54). In our rodent studies using low-dose TBI (1 or 2 Gy TBI), anti-B7 mAb alone did not promote donor engraftment in mice given modest BM cell doses (40×10^6) in contrast to anti-CD154 (CD40L) mAb, which did facilitate donor chimerism (55). However, anti-B7 mAb did increase engraftment under some conditions when combined with anti-CD154 mAb (55). Finally, recent data indicate that targeting B7 ligands with proteins such as CTLA4-Ig may alter the APC and not simply block T-cell:APC interactions (56). Regardless of the reagents used to target the CD28/CD152:B7 pathway, preclinical and clinical trials should be designed with knowledge of the separate functions and complexities of the CD28/B7 and CD152/B7 pathways.

B. The CD40L (CD154):CD40 Pathway

CD40 is a member of the TNF/NGF receptor family and is expressed on nonprofessional and professional APC, endothelial cells, and some epithelial cells (57–61). The T-cell counterreceptor for CD40, CD40 ligand (CD40L, gp39, CD154), is transiently expressed on antigen-activated CD4+ T cells and a small fraction of activated CD8+ T cells and B cells (62–67). CD154 transduces a signal to CD40-expressing B cells to upregulate molecules involved in T-cell costimulation, including CD80 and CD86 (68–71). Although both CD28-dependent and -independent pathways are involved in the induction of CD154 expression on activated T cells, the kinetics and density of CD154 expression are increased by CD28:B7-mediated costimulation (72,73). T cells can be rendered tolerant when exposed to antigen presented by CD40-deficient B cells in vivo, indicating a critical role of the CD154/CD40 pathway signaling in preventing tolerance induction (74,75). Noelle and colleagues first showed that in vivo administration of anti-CD154 mAb inhibits the acute and chronic forms of nonlethal GVHD in nonirradiated F1 recipients of parental donor splenocytes (76). Similarly, studies by Stuber et al. demonstrated that intestinal GVHD induced in nonirradiated recipients of parental donor grafts is inhibited by CD154/CD40 pathway blockade (77).

CD154/CD40 interactions result in the induction of proinflammatory cytokines and nitric oxide generation (78–81). Irradiation has been shown to contribute to the generation of these mediators early after the infusion of allogeneic donor cells (82–84). Thus, we asked whether anti-CD154 mAb would be as effective in inhibiting GVHD lethality in irradiated recipients as had been reported in nonirradiated recipients and whether the induction of proinflammatory cytokine mRNA was downregulated by anti-CD154 mAb administration. We observed that anti-CD154 mAb resulted in a long-term survival rate of 60% vs. 0% in controls (85). Early donor T-cell expansion was reduced by more than 2.5-fold, and T cells from anti-CD154 mAb-treated allogeneic BMT recipients had a greater than 2-fold reduction in antihost proliferative responses upon secondary restimulation in vitro (85). Additionally, the frequency of T cells from mAb-treated recipients expressing Th1 (IL-2, IL-12, and IFN-γ) cytokine mRNA was markedly diminished as compared to controls, indicating that Th1-associated GVHD responses were highly susceptible to CD154:CD40 blockade.

In studies involving the infusion of purified T-cell populations into sublethally irradiated recipients, anti-CD154 mAb was effective in reducing GVHD lethality mediated by CD4+ but not CD8+ T cells, consistent with the known upregulation of CD154 expression on activated CD4+ but not on most CD8+ T cells (85). CD154 expression on alloreactive CD4+ T cells was also critical for optimal expansion and antihost cytolytic T-cell (CTL) capacity of donor alloreactive CD8+ T cells (86). Therefore, the inhibition of CD8+ T-cell alloresponses by anti-CD154 mAb likely occurred by either a reduction in CD4+ support of CD8+ T-cell expansion or by a preferential augmentation of regulatory CD4+ T cells that can suppress CD8+ T cell function. To determine if host B-cell regulation of donor T-cell function was critical for the effects of anti-CD154 mAb, B6 severe combined immuno-deficient (B6-SCID) mice were used as recipients of allogeneic CD4+ T cells (85). Anti-CD154 mAb infusion protected a similar proportion of wild-type and SCID recipients indicating that anti-CD154 mAb did not mediate its protective effect strictly by interrupting T-B cognate interaction.

In studies directly comparing the blockade of the CD154/CD40 versus the CD28/CD152:B7 pathway in lethally irradiated recipients of allogeneic donor splenocytes, anti-CD154 mAb was significantly more effective than anti-B7 mAb in reducing GVHD lethality (87). Interestingly, the combined administration of anti-CD154 and anti-B7 mAb was no more effective than anti-CD154 mAb alone. However, these results do not necessarily imply a greater role for the CD154/CD40 pathway than the CD28/CD152-B7 pathway in the regulation of GVHD. Rather, these data may reflect the limitations of targeting complex pathways by mAb therapy. For example, in addition to blockade of CD28/B7 interactions, anti-B7 mAb also block the inhibitory CD152/B7 pathway, prevent downregulatory T-cell–associated B7 interactions, and possibly inhibit CD4+CD25+ regulatory cell function (8). Consistent with this hypothesis, the additive benefits of combined CD28/B7 and CD154/CD40 blockade can be seen in settings in which CD152/B7 interactions are preserved; in vivo blockade of the CD154/CD40 pathway significantly improved the clinical manifestations of GVHD (weight loss) and reduced antihost proliferative responses of reisolated donor T cells in heavily irradiated recipients of allogeneic CD28−/− splenocytes (46). We also found that the median survival time (MST) was significantly extended from 9 to 35 days by the administration of anti-CD154 mAb to allogeneic recipients of a high dose of CD28−/−. T cells demonstrating the benefits of CD28/B7 and CD154/CD40 coblockade (P. A. Taylor and B. R. Blazar, unpublished data). In addition to the blockade of positive costimulatory signals, anti-CD154 mAb infusion can lead to an active suppression of the immune response. Waldmann's group has shown that anti-CD154 mAb can result in a process of linked suppression in vivo (88). Tolerance induction to a given alloantigen (e.g., H2b/d on donor skin grafts) achieved during mAb infusion resulted in the subsequent failure of immune response to a different antigen co-expressed with one of the original alloantigens (e.g., H2b/k on third-party skin grafts). Our data indicate that the ex vivo blockade of CD154/CD40 during an MLR culture not only renders CD4+ T cells nonresponsive upon alloantigen restimulation, but also resulted in the generation of a potent regulatory T cell that inhibits naïve alloresponses both in vitro and in vivo (89–92). Thus, blockade of the CD154/CD40 pathway may preferentially preserve or even augment the function of regulatory T cells that serve to actively dampen the immune response.

With respect to the role of the CD154:CD40 pathway in regulating GVL effects, Ohata et al. showed that, in contrast to anti-B7 mAb, treatment with anti-CD154 mAb beginning on the day of BMT diminished GVHD lethality as well as GVL effects against a B-cell leukemia line (52). These authors showed that IL-12 mRNA expression was preferentially inhibited by anti-CD154 rather than anti-B7 mAb, a finding that may explain the loss of GVL effects. We found that anti-CD154 mAb eliminated the GVL effect of DLI against an AML cell line (P. A. Taylor and B. R. Blazar, unpublished data). These two studies indicate that anti-CD154 mAb can interfere with GVL effects, possibly due to its known inhibitory effects on Th1/Tc1 cells (85,93).

Perhaps the most prominent use of anti-CD154 mAb in allogeneic SCT has been in the area of chimerism induction. As a single agent used to promote alloengraftment in nonmyeloablative recipients, we observed that anti-CD154 mAb inhibited graft rejection such that sublethally irradiated (6.25–6.5 Gy TBI) recipients of pan-T-cell–depleted (TCD), fully allogeneic, donor BM (10^7 cells) had significantly higher mean levels of donor engraftment as compared to irrelevant mAb-treated controls (mean donor levels 90% vs. 60%, respectively) (85). Sykes and colleagues extended this work and demonstrated that anti-CD154 mAb permitted the induction of high levels of stable mixed chimerism and donor-specific tolerance when given to recipients treated with anti-CD4 and anti-CD8 Ab along with 3 Gy TBI and subsequently rescued with conventional BM cell doses (53). This approach was also sufficient to completely overcome CD4+ T-cell–mediated resistance to allogeneic BM engraftment and to rapidly induce CD4+ T-cell tolerance, but did not reliably overcome CD8+ CTL-mediated alloresistance (94). Furthermore, substitution of anti-T-cell mAb (95) with CTLA4 Ig resulted in similar outcomes. Chimerism was preceded by progressive deletion of host antidonor reactive T cells within the thymus and subsequently in the periphery. Similarly, Larsen's group has shown that a single dose of busulfan, which was less myelosuppressive than 3 Gy TBI, results in engraftment of a conventional dose of TCD BM if CTLA4-Ig and anti-CD154 mAb are co-administered (96). Chimerism levels were sufficient to correct mice with hemoglobinopathies (97) and were also associated with intrathymic clonal deletion of most antidonor reactive T cells.

Our group has analyzed the engraftment-promoting effects of anti-CD154 mAb given to recipients of a single, fully allogeneic, modestly high (40×10^6) BM cell dose and conditioned solely with ≤ 2 Gy TBI (55). Such conditioning resulted in a $\leq 5\%$ reduction in BM cellularity on day 7 or 14 post-BMT and was associated with a partial and transient reduction in peripheral T cells. Whereas engraftment was not detectable in irrelevant antibody-treated controls, donor chim/erism was observed in 91% of anti-CD154 mAb-treated recipients, and the mean donor engraftment level in these mice as 48% $\pm$ 19% 6 weeks after BMT. Chimerism was multilineage and increased over time. Long-term chimeras had permanent donor skin graft acceptance with prompt rejection of third-party skin grafts. Host CD4+ T cells were required for the engraftment-promoting effect of anti-CD154 mAb. Interestingly, although CD8+ T cells participate in BM graft rejection in this strain combination, donor engraftment was not increased when CD8+ cells were depleted in conjunction with anti-CD154 mAb administration (55). These data, which used high amounts of anti-CD154 mAb for a prolonged time period post-BMT contrast those of Sykes and colleagues, who showed a beneficial effect on engraftment when anti-CD8 mAb were administered short-term to anti-CD154 mAb–treated allogeneic recipients (94). Our data suggest that CD8-mediated rejection may be indirectly impaired by prolonged anti-CD154 mAb administration through the interference of requisite CD4+ T-cell help or the generation of regulatory/suppressor CD4+ T cells. Alternatively, anti-CD154 may induce regulatory CDD4+ cells that suppress CD8+ T-cell rejection. Consistent with this more speculative hypothesis, anti-CD154 mAb significantly, and unexpectedly, increased donor chimerism in a class I disparate engraftment model in which rejection is mediated by only CD8+ T cells (55). Additionally, in contrast to anti-CD154 mAb–treated wild-type (WT) mice, CD154−/− recipients conditioned with 200 cGy and infused with 40 million class I disparate BM did not engraft (55).

It is important to note that engraftment was BM cell dose dependent in recipients conditioned with 200 cGy TBI; only 20% of mice engrafted if the BM cell dose was reduced from 40 to 20 million (55). The inclusion of anti-CD154 mAb in the content of 200 cGy TBI resulted in an equivalent engraftment promoting effect as would be observed by increasing TBI doses to 450-500 cGy and was far more effective and permanent than the in vivo infusion of pan-TCD mAb (55). At lower dose TBI, 80% of anti-CD154 mAb–treated recipients given 50 cGy engrafted (mean donor % = 10%), while 90% of mice given 100 cGy engrafted (mean donor % = 24%) (55). These data are in agreement with those reported by Quesenberry et al. (98).

In an attempt to further improve engraftment rates after very low dose TBI (100 cGy), an abbreviated course of anti-CD154 mAb was combined with anti-B7 mAb (98). Engraftment was reproducibly and significantly increased over either agent alone or as compared to a more prolonged course of anti-CD154 mAb. However, some of the benefits of anti-B7 mAb may not have been fully realized since, as previously discussed, both the CD28/B7 and CD152/B7 pathways were concurrently blocked. Specifically, anti-CD152 mAb administration prevented alloengraftment in anti-CD154 mAb–treated recipients given TBI doses of 2 Gy, consistent with the requirements of CD152/B7 interactions for tolerance induction (98).

Data combining costimulatory pathway blockade approaches with calcineurin inhibitors such as FK506 (Tacrolimus) or cyclosporin A (CsA) or rapamycin (Sirolimus), which binds to the molecular target of rapamycin (mTOR), are of particular clinical interest. Calcineurin inhibitors blunt TCR signaling and may therefore antagonize tolerance induction induced by costimulatory pathway blockade by (1) precluding T cell activation, a necessary step in tolerance induction, or (2) specifically inhibiting the upregulation of costimulatory molecules such as CD154 that are targets of mAb-based strategies (99). Rapamycin blocks a late stage of T-cell activation (downstream of both TCR engagement and costimulation) and mediates immunosuppression at least in part by inhibiting IL-2 responsiveness. This predicted that rapamycin could be combined with costimulatory blockade to increase alloengraftment by preventing the expansion of alloreactive T cells that might escape costimulatory blockade and/or by promoting the apoptosis of alloreactive T cells by IL-2 withdrawal.

Experimental data indicate that rapamycin is a potent facilitator of alloengraftment when used with anti-CD154 alone (100) or with anti-CD154 mAb and CTLA4-Ig (101). Because CsA and tacrolimus block TCR signaling at an early stage in T-cell activation, it is not surprising that some (but not all) studies indicate that these agents may antagonize tolerance induction when used in combination with costimulatory blockade strategies (102,103). We hypothesize that calcineurin inhibitors may be beneficial in some costimulatory blockade strategies by reducing the potency of TCR signaling to levels that will more readily permit tolerance induction. In other instances, calcineurin inhibitors may antagonize tolerance induction by blunting TCR signals to levels below which the active process of tolerance induction can occur. Thus, rapamycin, rather than calcineurin inhibitors, may be the preferred pharmacological agent to improve the tolerance-inducing effects of costimulatory blockade.

The potency of costimulatory blockade strategies to induce donor chimerism is particularly evident in those studies using completely nonconditioned murine recipients. Sykes et al. administered CTLA-4Ig and anti-CD154 to nonconditioned mice receiving very high BM cell dose (200×10^6) and achieved long-term, low-level multilineage chimerism (104). Larsen et al. showed that multilineage chimerism (6–12% donor) could be achieved in recipients given repetitive BM (totaling 160×10^6) and anti-CD154 mAb infusions over the first 3 months after transplantation (105). In our studies, anti-CD154 mAb as a single agent was ineffective in achieving engraftment in nonconditioned allogeneic recipients given one or two modestly high BM cell doses (up to 80×10^6) (100). Although the combination of rapamycin and anti-CD154 did induce chimerism in 30 of 30 recipients, donor T-cell levels were very low and mice were not tolerant of donor skin grafts (100). In conclusion, anti-CD154 mAb has proven to be an important approach to engraftment promotion in numerous models wherein mice are given nonmyeloablative conditioning or no conditioning at all along with megadose BM infusions.

C. The 4-1BB (CD137):4-1BBL (CD137L) Pathway

CD137 is a member of the TNF/NGFR family and is expressed on activated CD8+ and CD4+ T cells as well as NK cells (106–108). The ligand for CD137 is CD137L and is expressed on APCs including B cells, macrophages, and DC (109,110). Signals delivered to the T cell by CD137 can induce T cells to produce IL-2, proliferate, and differentiate, as well as protect T cells from activation-induced cell death (ACID) (107,110–116). Despite equivalent kinetics and degree of expression of CD137 on both activated CD4+ and CD8+ T cells, initial data suggested that the CD137:CD137L pathway plays a more prominent role in CD8+ T-cell responses than in CD4+ T-cell responses (116–119). For example, agonistic anti-CD137 mAb enhanced the in vitro proliferative responses of CD8+ T cells to suboptimal anti-CD3 doses to a greater degree than those of CD4+ T cells (119). The importance of the CD137/CD137L pathway in regulating GVH responses was first demonstrated by Shuford et al., who showed that the in vivo infusion of an agonistic anti-CD137 mAb along with parental splenocytes into nonconditioned F1 recipients resulted in increased donor CD8+ T-cell expansion and enhanced CTL activity (117). These data were extended by Nozawa et al., who found that an antagonistic anti-CD137L mAb significantly reduced GVHD-induced mortality in a lethally irradiated model of acute GVHD (120). Expansion of donor CD8+ T cells, but not CD4+ T cells, was inhibited in anti-CD137L mAb–treated mice.

Although the T-cell–activating effects of CD137 signaling are less robust for CD4+ cells (117), we found that CD137:CD137L interaction play an important role in GVHD mediated by either CD4+ or CD8+ donor T cells (121). We infused a normally sublethal dose of CD4+ T cells with donor BM into lethally irradiated MHC class II disparate recipients and found that the administration of agonistic anti-CD137 mAb increase mortality from 0 to 100%. Recipients of MHC class II disparate CD137−/−CD4 T cells also had significantly reduced GVHD mortality compared to recipients of CD137 +/+CD4 T cells (121). Likewise, the infusion of MHC class II disparate CD4+ cells resulted in reduced lethality in CD137L−/− recipients compared to +/+ recipients. The effects of CD137 ligation on CD4+ T-cell–mediated GVHD was only partially CD28 dependent, revealing both redundant and nonredundant roles of the CD137/CD137L and CD28/B7 pathways (121). Finally, enhanced mortality from GVHD was also observed in sublethally and lethally irradiated recipients given MHC class II disparate CD4+ T cells and *agonistic* anti-CD137 mAb, indicating that this pathway regulates alloresponses under low and high proinflammatory conditions.

In lethally irradiated recipients of fully MHC disparate donor splenocytes in which both CD4+ and CD8+ T cells contribute to GVHD-induced mortality, a 3-fold lower incidence of GVHD lethality was observed when infusing CD137−/− versus CD137+/+ splenocytes. Using T-cell dose titration studies in sublethally irradiated MHC class I or class II disparate GVHD models, we determined that the magnitude of this effect on GVHD lethality was equivalent to an approximate 3-fold difference in the number of CD8+ or CD4+ T cells infused, respectively.

Azuma's group has investigated the potential differential effects of CD137/CD137L pathway on acute GVHD using a blocking anti-CD137L mAb (120). The reduction in GVHD lethality seen after the administration of anti-CD137L mAb was associated with diminished donor CD8+ T-cell expansion and IFN-γ production without significant effects on CD4+ T-cell expansion. In a chronic GVHD model, anti-CD137L treatment resulted in enhanced autoantibody formation and a higher frequency of IL-4–expressing CD4+ T cells as compared to controls (120) consistent with the effects of CD137/CD137L blockade on skewing T-cell responses to a Th2 phenotype in some systems.

To determine whether an *agonist* anti-CD137 mAb could be used to increase GVL activity via its effects on facilitating CD8+ T-cell expansion and the induction of CTL effectors, donor splenocytes were given 3 weeks after transplantation to lethally irradiated, BM-reconstituted allogeneic recipients (121). Mice were treated with control or anti-CD137 mAb and challenged with a lethal dose of acute myeloid leukemia cells at 4 weeks post-BMT. Whereas control-treated recipients given DLI all died with acute leukemia, anti-CD137 mAb–treated recipients of DLI had a 70% survival rate. Leukemia dose-response curves showed that the combined approach of DLI and anti-CD137 mAb resulted in a reduction in leukemia-associated mortality equivalent to infusing a >100-fold lower leukemia cell dose. However, anti-CD137 mAb also significantly increased the mortality from DLI-mediated GVHD that became evident at higher DLI doses.

In engraftment studies conducted in sublethally irradiated recipients, we have observed that the infusion of agonistic anti-CD137 mAb augments allogeneic MHC class I or II disparate BM rejection mediated by either CD4+ or CD8+ host T cells, respectively (121). Phenotyping of peripheral blood leukocytes 4 months after transplantation revealed decreased donor chimerism in anti-CD137 mAb–treated mice compared to irrelevant mAb–treated mice (66% vs. 97% donor for MHC class I disparate and 38% vs. 84% donor for MHC class II disparate recipients). Collectively the data indicate that blockade of the CD137:CD137L pathway may be beneficial for the reduction of GVHD and donor BM rejection while *agonistic* anti-CD137 mAb given later post-SCT may enhance GVL effects and reduce leukemic relapse.

D. The OX40 (CD134):OX40L (CD134L) Pathway

CD134 is a member of the TNF/NGFR family which is expressed on activated CD4+ and CD8+ T cells in rodents and humans (122–127). CD134L is expressed predominantly on activated DC, B cells, and macrophages (128–130) and also on endothelial cells, microglial cells, and T cells (131–134). Provision of signals delivered via engagement of the CD134 receptor promotes CD4+ T cells to produce Th1 and Th2 cytokines, as well as antiapoptotic proteins and to clonally expand, survive, and develop into memory cells (133,135–151).

Although Chen et al. showed comparable MR responses using CD134L−/− and CD134+/+ DC as stimulators of allogeneic CD4+ T cells (137), Pippig and coworkers demonstrated that CD134−/− T cells have a blunted allogeneic MLR response (133). Tittle and colleagues observed that increased numbers of alloreactive CD4$^+$ T cells that co-expressed CD134 were present in the peripheral blood, lymphohematopoietic organs, and liver of rats with GVHD (152). Furthermore, blocking CD134/CD134L interactions with either a CD134-Ig fusion protein or CD134L mAb has been shown to diminish intestinal GVHD (153) and to ameliorate GVHD-mediated lethality (154,155) in non-irradiated and irradiated BMT models, respectively. Similarly, GVHD lethality is also reduced when CD134−/− splenocytes are infused into lethally irradiated, NHC disparate recipients and when CD134L−/− recipients are lethally irradiated and given fully allogeneic BM and T cells. Consistent with these findings, we have observed that an agonistic anti-CD134 mAb given in the peri-BMT period significantly increases GVHD-induced mortality in heavily irradiated recipients of fully MHC disparate donor splenocytes.

Despite the fact that CD134 is upregulated on both CD4+ and CD8+ T cells obtained from mice with acute GVHD (155), much of the published literature indicates that CD134:CD134L interactions may play a more critical role in CD4+ T-cell responses than in CD8 T-cell responses. In our studies, optimal CD4+ T-cell–mediated GVHD lethality is dependent upon the CD134/CD134L pathway (155). The infusion of CD134−/− CD4+ T cells results in significantly lower acute GVHD-induced mortality in either sublethally or lethally irradiated MHC class II disparate recipients. In addition, the administration of blocking anti-CD134L mAb to sublethally irradiated recipients of MHC class II disparate CD4+ T cells significantly reduced GVHD-induced mortality, whereas agonistic anti-CD134 mAb markedly accelerated mortality in this system. In contrast, CD134 does not appear to be a major regulator of alloreactive CD8+ T cells in sublethally irradiated MHC class I disparate recipients; agonistic anti-CD134 did not increase mortality from GVHD, and the use of CD134−/− and CD134+/+ CD8+ T cells resulted in equivalent survival after BMT.

Some studies have proposed that CD134 ligation preferentially supports Th2 differentiation, while others demonstrate that Th1 responses are also affected (133,135, 139,156). To determine how CD134 ligation affects Th1/Tc1- or Th2/Tc2-mediated GVHD lethality, donor splenocytes from STAT-4−/− (Th1/Tc1-defective) or STAT-6−/− (Th2/Tc2-defective) were infused into lethally irradiated recipients that were treated with an antagonistic anti-CD134L mAb (155). Results of these studies indicate that the inhibitory effect of CD134/CD134L blockade does not depend upon the expression of STAT4 or STAT6 expression. Consistent with these data, an agonistic anti-CD134 mAb accelerated GVHD lethality in STAT 4−/− as well as STAT 6−/− recipients. Thus, the regulation of GVHD lethality by the CD134/CD134L pathway does not involve a simple shift in the balance of Th1/Tc1 or Th2/Tc2 subsets. Finally, although CD134L also has been reported to be expressed on activated T cells (134), we could find no convincing evidence that CD134L expression on donor T cells regulates GVHD lethality as determined in a series of GVHD experiments in which donor T cells were derived from CD134L+/+ vs. CD134L−/− mice and infused into a variety of recipients using several conditioning regimens (155).

To determine whether the anti-GVHD effects of CD134/CD134L blockade were fully redundant with other costimulatory pathways, studies were performed to co-block either the CD28/B7 or CD154/CD40 pathways. To assess the former, donor T cells obtained from CED28−/− or CD28+/+ mice were infused into lethally irradiated allogeneic recipients along with irrelevant, agonistic anti-CD134, or blocking anti-CD134L mAb (155). In each case, GVHD lethality was either accelerated by anti-CD134 mAb or completely inhibited by anti-CD134L mAb. In other studies, the infusion of purified CD28−/− T cells into lethally irradiated fully allogeneic CD134L−/− recipients resulted in a significant survival advantage as compared to CD134L+/+ controls (155). To assess the potential utility of co-blocking CD154/CD40 along with CD134/CD134L pathways, irrelevant, anti-CD154 and/or CD134L mAb were administered to lethally irradiated recipients of MHC-disparate donor grafts. Individual mAb resulted in MSTs of 12, 45, and 27 days, respectively, the latter two groups surviving significantly longer than controls (87), whereas the combined administration of anti-CD154 + anti-CD134L mAb resulted in an MST of >100 days. This MST was significantly longer than any of the other groups and longer than recipients that received anti-CD154 + anti-B7 mAb (MST of 44 days). Taken together, these data indicate that neither the CD28/B7 nor CD154/CD40 pathway is fully redundant with the CD134/CD134L pathway and that the co-blockade of the CD154/CD40 and the CD134/CD134L pathways is a highly effective approach in inhibiting GVHD mortality in lethally irradiated recipients of full MHC disparate donor grafts.

Given the potent effects of anti-CD134 mAb in augmenting alloresponses when administered early post-BMT, we performed studies in our DLI model to determine whether *agonistic* anti-CD134 mAb could be utilized to increase the DLI-GVL effect without inducing lethal GVHD (155). TBI can cause the release of pro-inflammatory cytokines that upregulate CD134/CD134L expression and lower the threshold for T-cell responses. In addition, TBI-induced tissue injury may predispose GVHD target organs to further injury. Therefore, studies were performed to determine whether the delayed administration of an agonistic anti-CD134 mAb could be used to generate a GVL effect of DLI administered at a time when TBI injury has largely subsided. Despite delaying mAb for 3 weeks post-SCT, allogeneic recipients given DLI and anti-CD134 mAb rapidly succumbed to GVHD before antileukemia immune responses could be evaluated.

Augmenting CD134/CD134L interactions clearly accelerates GVHD induction mediated preferentially by CD4+ donor T cells. To determine whether CD134 signaling regulates host CD4+ or CD8+ T cells that can reject donor BM cells, we tested agonistic anti-CD134 or blocking anti-CD134L mAb administration for effects on alloengraftment (155). Anti-CD134 mAb resulted in a marked reduction in engraftment in sublethally irradiated recipients of donor MHC class II disparate TCD BM, whereas anti-CD134L mAb increased alloengraftment at two different TBI doses. Consistent with the lack of pronounced effects of CD134/CD134L interactions on modifying CD8+ T-cell−mediated GVHD lethality, anti-CD134 mAb administration had only subtle effects on alloengraftment in a CD8+ T-cell−mediated rejection model, while anti-CD134L mAb had no engraftment promoting properties in this setting.

In sum, these data demonstrate a more pronounced role for the CD134/CD134L pathway in regulating CD4+ as compared to CD8+ T-cell alloresponses in vivo. Specifically, the CD134 pathway is a major regulator of CD4+ T-cell−mediated GVHD and host T-cell−mediated graft rejection and has lesser effects on CD8+ T-cell−mediated responses in each context. Co-blockade of the CD28/CD152:B7 and CD154/CD40 pathways are at least additive with blockade of the CD134/CD134L pathway, indicating that these pathways are not fully redundant and providing a strategy to optimize GVHD prevention and potentially to promote alloengraftment.

E. The Inducible Costimulator (ICOS)/ICOSL Pathway

ICOS, a member of the Ig supergene family, is expressed on CD4+ and CD8+ T cells within 24–48 hours after activation (157–160). The ligand for ICOS [ICOS-L, also termed B7 homolog (B7h), B7-related protein-1 (B7RP-1), B60H2, and GL50] is a B7 family member that has 20% homology to CD80 and CD86 and is constitutively expressed by B cells, monocytes, and about 15% of T cells (160–167). Much but not all of the literature indicates that ICOS/ICOS-L ligation has a preferential effect on inducing IL-4 and IL-10 (Th2) rather than IFN-γ (Th1) cytokine production (157,158,160,166–177). In the absence of ICOS, a Th1 response is favored and IL-12 downregulates ICOS expression (158,168,170–172,178). ICOS is critical for immunoglobulin isotype switching and germinal center formation as well as the activation and function of Th2 effector cells and in particular IL-4 and IL-13 production (157,160,167,168,170–172,179–181).

While interplay exists between the CD28 and ICOS pathways, these pathways have overlapping and nonoverlapping functions (159,169,170,178,182). For example, inhibition of B7-mediated signaling to T cells reduces ICOS expression, and ICOS−/− CD4+ T cells are stimulated less by B7−/− versus B7+/+ APCs, indicating that ICOS can have a CD28/CD152:B7-independent costimulatory effect on CD4+ T-cell proliferation (170). CD28 and ICOS regulate Th2 cell generation and synergize for effects on IL-4 generation (159,170,183). CD28 regulates IL-2 production while ICOS regulates TNF-α production (159,162,183).

In the presence of CD28/B7 signaling, ICOS appears to preferentially regulate the Th2 pathway (159,166), whereas in the absence of CD28/B7 interaction, ICOS can regulate both Th1 and Th2 pathways. While CD28/CD152:B7 signaling regulates anergy induction, ICOS/ICOS-L may not (159,170,183). CD28/B7 is largely responsible for the initial T-cell response, while ICOS/ICOSL affects subsequent T-cell expansion and the effector phase of the immune response in a predominantly CD28-independent fashion (158,159,166,168,170,183).

Consistent with the effects of ICOS on Th2 differentiation, Ogawa and coworkers showed that the in vivo administration of an anti-ICOS mAb inhibited chronic (Th2-dominated) GVHD in a parent-into-F1 model (184). In contrast, in a Th1-dominated system, anti-ICOS mAb did not inhibit acute GVHD (184). However, interpretation of the data may be complicated by the fact that both donor and host T cells are likely to be affected by mAb infusion in these nonirradiated GVHD recipients. Therefore, to determine whether ICOS/ICOSL blockade could affect GVHD after lethal TBI when host antidonor effects would be minimized, we administered an irrelevant or a blocking anti-ICOS mAb to recipients of fully allogeneic donor grafts (185). Our results indicate that anti-ICOS mAb initiated at the time of SCT was highly effective in inhibiting GVHD mortality, with 75% of anti-ICOS mAb–treated recipients surviving long term vs. 10% of irrelevant mAb–treated controls.

The inducible expression of ICOS shortly after T-cell activation suggests that ICOS may be particularly important in providing costimulatory signals to activated T cells and in the subsequent generation of memory cells. For example, ICOS expression has been reported to be higher on activated Th2 effector cells, which require 3–4 rounds of division for their induction vs. resting or activated Th1, which require fewer divisions (158,166, 169,170). ICOS signaling does not appear to be required for naïve T-cell responses with the exception of those involved in superantigen-induced expansion (183). There are a significantly higher number of CD4+ ICOS−/− T cells that retain the naïve phenotype (CD62Lbright) after activation, consistent with a defect in memory cell generation in ICOS−/− mice (170,176). In contrast to CTLA4-Ig, which is dominant in inhibiting primary responses (158,166), the infusion of ICOS-Ig results in more pronounced effects when given during induction of the secondary rather than the primary immune response.

The requirement for T-cell activation to induce ICOS expression in combination with the preferential effects of the ICOS/ICOS-L pathway on activated T cells, led us to examine the effects of anti-ICOS mAb initiated on day 5 after BMT (P. A. Taylor and B. R. Blazar, unpublished data). This is a time when donor T-cell expansion has increased 50- to 100-fold, donor antihost effector T cells have been generated, and GVHD is evident in target organs (41,85). In comparison to irrelevant mAb, anti-ICOS mAb significantly extended the MST (30 vs. 11 days post-BMT) and time to uniform lethality (33 vs. 19 days post-SCT). In contrast, anti-CD154 mAb, which is highly protective when initiated at time of transplantation, had no effect when mAb infusion was delayed until 5 days after transplantation. Survival was significantly improved by combining anti-ICOS and anti-CD154 mAb when compared to the infusion of anti-CD154 or anti-ICOS mAb alone, although all mice still died by day 47 post-BMT.

These data indicate that the ICOS/ICOSL and the CD154/CD40 pathways are not fully redundant, although each pathway is known to affect the function of the other. For example, ICOS −/− and CD40 −/− mice each have defective germinal center formation and Th responses (170,171,180,186), and CD40 signaling can partially restore the switching defect seen in ICOS −/− mice (170). ICOS costimulation induces CD40L expression on T cells. Moreover, Hancock and colleagues showed that anti-CD40L mAb suppress the induction of ICOS within transplanted cardiac allografts (187). Consistent with our findings that these pathways have some nonredundant functions, anti-ICOS mAb prevents atherosclerosis, which occurs in anti-CD40L mAb-treated cardiac allograft recipients (187). Importantly, studies indicate that the expansion of memory T cells is regulated by ICOS but not CD40L. Our data and that of the literature suggest that co-blockade of these two pathways may be particularly advantageous in blocking alloresponses in vivo. This pathway clearly warrants additional investigation in studies designed to prevent and treat GVHD and to promote alloengraftment by impairing host anti-donor T-cell responses.

F. The LIGHT-HVEM Pathway

LIGHT [homologous to lymphotoxins, exhibits inducible expression, and competes with herpesvirus glycoprotein D for herpesvirus entry mediator (HVEM) expressed on T lymphocytes] is an inducible member of the TNF superfamily (188). LIGHT RNA is expressed in most activated peripheral blood mononuclear cells and on mouse DC and immature but not mature human DC (189–191). HVEM is expressed on T cells, B cells, NK cells, and endothelial cells (190,192). Although LIGHT has three receptors—HVEM, lymphotoxin β receptor (LTBR), and DcR3/TR6—HVEM is the primary receptor for T-cell costimulation by LIGHT since LTβR is not expressed on T cells and DcR3/TR6 protein is found only in soluble form (188,193–195).

LIGHT provides potent T-cell costimulation resulting in enhanced proliferation and Th1 cytokine production, independent of the CD28/B7 pathway (191,196). Blockade of LIGHT-HVEM interactions inhibits, and engagement of HVEM enhances, allogeneic MLR proliferation (190,191,196). Ligation of LIGHT can costimulate CD28$-/-$ T cells, indicating that these pathways are not fully redundant (196). Alloreactive CTL generation is inhibited in vivo by blocking LIGHT-HVEM interactions with either an anti-LIGHT antibody or a soluble LTβR-Ig that competes with HVEM for binding to LIGHT and results in a significant increase in survival after allogeneic SCT (196,197).

To determine whether LIGHT-HVEM blockade had differential effects on inhibiting CD4+ vs. CD8+ T-cell–mediated GVHD, sublethally irradiated recipients of MHC class II or I disparate T cells were treated with irrelevant or LTβR-Ig fusion protein. CD8+ but not CD4+ T-cell–mediated GVHD lethality could be inhibited by LTβR-Ig fusion protein (197). Since CD4+ T-cell–mediated GVHD appeared to be refractory to LTβR-Ig inhibition, anti-CD154 mAb were co-administered to block CD4+ T-cell expansion (197) and Th1/Tc1 induction. Although anti-CD154 mAb prevented GVHD lethality in about 40% of recipients, combined LTβR-Ig and anti-CD154 mAb resulted in 100% survival. In this model, donor antihost CTL generation, which was associated with acute GVHD, was unaffected by anti-CD154 mAb, reduced by LTβR-Ig, and further reduced by the administration of LTBR-Ig and anti-CD154 mAb. The combination of anti-CD154 and LTBR-Ig did not preclude donor CD8+ T-cell reconstitution or activation or the generation of donor CTL responses to nominal antigens not present in the recipient during mAb or protein administration. Donor antihost specific CTL generation could be restored in vitro by exogenous IL-2, consistent with the induction of anergy in donor T cells. Finally, Chen and colleagues have also shown that antitumor CD8+ CTL are induced by transfection of tumor cells with a LIGHT plasmid (196). The antitumor responses induced by LIGHT overexpression were abolished by CD8+ T-cell depletion and only partially inhibited by CD4+ T-cell depletion (196).

In conclusion, the combined administration of LTβR-Ig and anti-CD154 mAb represents a highly effective approach that target CD8+ and CD4+ T cells, resulting in the induction of anergy. Future studies on the effects of the LIGHT-HVEM pathway alone and in conjunction with the CD154/CD40 pathway in GVL and alloengraftment models are indicated.

G. The CD30/CD30L Pathway

CD30, a TNF/NGFR family member, is expressed on Reed-Sternberg cells in Hodgkin's disease, B cells, and mitogen-stimulated T cells (98–200). CD30+ T cells produce both Th1/Tc1 and Th2/Tc2 cytokines (201–203). CD28 ligation enhances CD30 expression and CD30 signals augment proliferation of T cells after TCR ligation has occurred (204). Alloantigen activation induces CD30 on CD8+ and to a lesser extent CD4+ T cells (199,205,206). Consistent with effects on CD8+ T cells, CD30 signaling regulates CTL generation and also renders T cells sensitive to cell death (207–211). CD30 ligand (CD30L, CD153) is a member of the TNF family. CD30L, which is expressed on activated T cells, primarily CD4+ T cells of both Th1 and Th2 phenotype, can provide signals for B-cell growth and differentiation (199,200,212,213).

To determine whether the CD30/CD30L pathway may play a role in GVHD, we performed studies in which sublethally or heavily irradiated recipients were given CD30$-/-$ or CD30+/+ MHC class II disparate CD4+ T cells (214). In each case, recipients of CD30$-$/$-$ cells had significantly higher survival rates compared to animals receiving wild-type ($+$/$+$) cells. Consistent with this finding, the administration of an antagonistic anti-CD30L mAb also reduced mortality after BMT with MHC class II disparate CD30$+$/$+$ CD4$+$ T cells similar to findings in CD30L$-$/$-$ recipients given irrelevant mAb. In contrast, no survival advantage was seen in sublethally irradiated recipients of MHC class I disparate CD30$-$/$-$ CD8$+$ T cells as compared to recipients of CD30$+$/$+$ cells (214). Thus, data available to date suggest that the CD30/CD30L pathway is more critical for CD4$+$ rather than CD8$+$ T-cell–mediated GVHD lethality.

H.   The PD-1/PD-L1,-2 Pathway

Programmed death-1 (PD-1), a recently described member of the Ig superfamily, has two known ligands: PD-L1 and PD-L2 (215–223). PD-1 is induced on mature peripheral T cells, B cells, and myeloid cells upon activation (215,217,224). PD-1 and CD152 have structural similarities, and PD-1 has an immunoreceptor tyrosine-based inhibitory motif (ITIM) in its cytoplasmic tail, suggesting an inhibitory function of PD-1 signaling (9,215,225–227). PD-1$-$/$-$ mice develop splenomegaly, a lupus-like glomerulone-phritis, and destructive arthritis with aging (218). Thus, PD-1 ligation appears necessary to prevent autoimmunity.

PD-1 ligand, PD-L1, also termed B7-H1, is a member of the B7 family. PD-L1 is constitutively expressed on DC, some activated CD3$+$ cells, and IFN-γ–stimulated monocytes and keratinocytes (228). PD-L2, also termed B7-DC, is constitutively expressed on resting monocytes (221,222). PD-L1 and PD-L2 mRNA is expressed in lymphohematopoietic tissues and activated keratinocytes (221,222,228). Some tissues (lung, liver, pancreas) express PD-L2 but not PD-L1, while others (heart, skeletal muscle) express both. Because PD-L1 is upregulated during a Th1 response and PD-L2 during a Th2 response, these ligands may regulate Th1 and Th2 responses, respectively.

Experimental data suggest that the function of the PD-1/PD-L pathway is to modulate T-cell responses (219,221,222,228). Despite the fact that conflicting in vitro data exist as to whether signaling via the PD1 pathway provides positive or negative costimulatory signals, the phenotype of the PD-1$-$/$-$ mouse indicates that the dominant in vivo role of the PD-1 pathway is to inhibit T-cell response (218,229,230). Nishimura et al. have studied the effects of introducing the PD-1 null mutation into the 2C-TCR (anti H-2L^d) transgenic mouse in which the CD8$+$ T cells are potentially autoreactive (231). When 2C-TCR mice are cross-bred with PD-1$-$/$-$ mice backcrossed to the BALB/c background, the 2C-TCR $\times$ PD-1$-$/$-$ H-2^{bxd} mice develop a GVHD-like syndrome that is associated with a markedly increased CD8$+$ T-cell proliferative response to H-2^d allogeneic cells in vitro. These data suggest that potentially autoreactive peripheral T cells can become activated in the absence of PD-1.

To determine if this pathway may be involved in GVHD, GVHD target tissues were examined for the presence of PD-1$+$ cells. In lethally irradiated recipients of full MHC disparate donor T cells, PD-1 infiltrating cells were found in increased frequency in multiple GVHD target organs (spleen, colon, liver) as compared to BMT controls (232). To block the PD-1 pathway, anti-PD-1 mAb or a PDL1:Fc fusion protein was administered to lethally irradiated recipients of MHC disparate cells (232). In each case, blockade of the PD-1 pathway resulted in a significant increase in GVHD-induced mortality. Since PD-L1.Fc and anti-PD-1 mAb infusion could either provide a positive or preclude a negative costimulatory signal to donor T cells, experiments were performed comparing the GVHD lethality effects of PD-1+/+ or PD-1−/− splenocytes (232). Our results demonstrated that PD-1−/− splenocytes had a markedly enhanced capacity to induce lethal GVHD as compared to WT cells, and PD-1 expression was a major regulator of GVHD mediated by both CD4+ and CD8+ T cells.

The downregulatory effects of the PD-1/PD-L pathway on GVHD are similar to previous observations reported for the CD152/B7 pathway under these same conditions. To determine whether these pathways are fully redundant, lethally irradiated recipients of MHC disparate donor cells were given irrelevant mAb or anti-PD-1, anti-CD152, or both blocking antibodies (232). Whereas anti-CD152 mAb did not significantly accelerate GVHD lethality, anti-PD-1 mAb did. Importantly, the combined administration of both mAb was significantly more potent than either alone in accelerating GVHD mortality, indicating that the PD-1/PD-L and CD152/B7 pathways are not fully redundant. Finally, whereas the lack of either perforin or FasL (CD95L) expression by donor T cells did not modify the GVHD-potentiating effects of the anti-PD-1 mAb, donor T-cell IFN-γ production was critical (232). Moreover, blockade of the PD-1/PD-L pathway markedly increased IFN-γ production as measured from MLR culture supernatants and from sera of anti-PD-1 mAb–treated allogeneic SCT recipients with GVHD. Thus, the PD-1/PD-L pathway is a major regulator of GVHD lethality and IFN-γ production. Hence, blockade of the PD-1/PD-L pathway may be beneficial in those situations in which a Th1/Tc1 immune response is desirable (i.e., augmenting the DLI-GVL effects in patients that are typically refractory to DLI). Conversely, reagents that may provide an agonistic signal to PD-1+ T cells may be of benefit in inhibiting GVHD and host T-cell–mediated graft rejection.

I. Tolerance Induction by Ex Vivo Approaches

The prior discussions have focused on the in vivo administration of antibodies peri-SCT. However, tolerance induction by ex vivo costimulatory blockade is a potential therapeutic strategy for the prevention of clinical GVHD. An ex vivo tolerization approach involves the culturing of donor T cells with host alloantigen in the presence of mAb or proteins capable of blocking T-cell costimulation. Such a procedure has several conceptual advantages over in vivo tolerization attempts that include: (1) a higher likelihood of tolerance induction by ensuring costimulatory pathway blockade is delivered to the site of T cell–APC interactions, (2) the ability to achieve tolerance induction prior to in vivo infusion into an inflammatory milieu, (3) the capacity to monitor the depth of tolerance induction by in vitro assays prior to T-cell infusion, and (4) avoidance of potential in vivo toxicities of mAb or proteins used to induce tolerance.

We have described an ex vivo approach wherein the blockade of CD154/CD40, using anti-CD154 mAb added to a 7- to 10-day culture of CD4+ T cells and irradiated MHC class II disparate stimulators, induces tolerance (89–92). Tolerant CD4+ T cells are hyporesponsive to initial alloantigen challenge and to restimulation in vitro. More importantly, tolerized T cells do not mediate GVHD upon their in vivo transfer to alloantigen-bearing recipient mice. Despite a profound reduction in GVHD capacity, T cells had intact in vitro responses to antigens not present during the tolerization culture (89). In vivo, tolerance was long-lived and not readily reversible (89). Tolerance induction also resulted in the generation of a potent immunoregulatory cell that could inhibit both naïve and primed alloresponses as assessed by in vitro and in vivo assays (92). With respect to the latter, the separate co-infusion of tolerized cells with an otherwise uniformly lethal dose of naïve CD4+ cells (1 : 1 ratio) prevented GVHD mortality in 75% of mice. Thus, the generation of regulatory cells during tolerization may provide a fail-safe mechanism to control alloreactive T cells that may have escaped tolerization.

Although most of our work has focused on blockade of CD154/CD40 interactions, ex vivo blockade of CD28/CD152-B7 pathway in the same type of allo-MLR culture is highly effective in inhibiting primary and secondary T-cell responses in vitro and GVHD lethality after adoptive transfer of tolerized CD4+ T cells in vivo (91). In an initial human trial, Guinan et al. cocultured donor BM with irradiated cells from the recipient for 36 hours in the presence of CTLA4Ig to block CD28/CTLA-4:B7 costimulation (233). Most donor-recipient pairs had several HLA disparities, and large numbers of T cells were infused. They found a dramatic reduction in the frequency of T cells capable of recognizing alloantigen of the recipient. The incidence and severity of acute GVHD appeared to be reduced given what might be expected after taking into account the degree of HLA disparity and the number of mature T cells infused, suggesting that this approach may be of clinical benefit.

In a different ex vivo approach, we have also shown that CD4+ T cells can be rendered tolerant to MHC class II disparate alloantigens when exposed to immuno-regulatory cytokines (i.e., IL-10 and TGF-β) ex vivo (234–236). Such tolerization profoundly inhibits primary and secondary alloantigenic responses while preserving responses to nominal antigens not present during the tolerization process (235). Tolerization is sufficient to prevent GVHD in the majority of recipients and to induce suppressor cells that have the capacity to potently inhibit GVHD induced by naïve T cells (235,236). In humans, IL-10 alone is sufficient to induce alloantigen-specific hyporesponsiveness in vitro because of the subsequent induction of TGFβ production in human, but not murine, tolerization cultures (237). A clinical trial is underway in a haploidentical SCT setting using IL-10 to tolerize donor T cells to host alloantigens in vitro before infusing these cells approximately 5–6 weeks post-BMT (238).

IV. REGULATORY CELLS AND ALLOGENEIC IMMUNE RESPONSES

A. Overview

A variety of murine cells that display regulatory function in vitro or in vivo have been described. These cells can be subdivided based upon their surface antigen expression, the types of cytokines produced, and the mechanisms of regulation employed (239–241). At least eight distinct subpopulations of regulatory cells have been identified, including five that express the CD4 antigen, CD8+ T cells that produce IFN-γ, TCR-γ/δ+ T cells that produce TGF-β and IL-10, and T cells that co-express NK determinants (NKT cells) (239). Some of these subsets, particularly those that are CD4+, have overlapping characteristics. We will review the biology of two distinct types of T-regulatory (Treg) cells that have well-defined phenotypic and functional properties and have been shown to be potent inhibitors of acute GVHD (NKT cells; CD4+CD25+ cells).

B. NKT Cells

NKT cells are thymus- or BM-derived, natural suppressor cells that co-express $\alpha\beta$ TCR and NK receptors [e.g., NK1.1 (CD161), DX5, Ly49] and are reactive to CD1d molecules in mice and humans (242,243). Most NKT cells have a highly skewed TCR repertoire, characterized by a single invariant TCR encoded by Vα14 and Jα281 gene segments in mice and the homologous Vα24-JaQ segments in humans, which are associated with a limited set of Vβ genes (242,244). Such NKT cells recognize a glycosphingolipid, α-galactosyl ceramide, presented by the nonpolymorphic MHC class I–like molecule CD1d (242–246). A smaller subset of NKT cells has a diverse TCR repertoire and functions in a CD1-independent fashion. The majority of NKT are CD4CD8−, although some co-express D8 or CD4 antigens or both (242–244). CD1-dependent Vα14-Jα281 expressing NKT cells are located mainly in the thymus, liver, spleen, and BM, while murine CD1-independent NKT cells can be present in the spleen, lymph node, and thymus (242–244).

NKT cells have an immunosuppressive role; a BM-derived NKT cell line that suppressed the GVHD response of allogeneic donor cells has been described (247). BM NKT cells are approximately equally distributed between CD4−CD8− and CD4+ and/ or CD8+ cells (248,249). Strober's group has shown that BM TCRα/β + CD4+ CD8+ cells, the majority of which are NKT cells, are markedly impaired in their GVHD capacity (248). In contrast, the infusion of an equal number of NK-depleted TCRα/β + CD4+ CD8+ cells resulted in GVHD lethality in a high proportion of recipients. In addition to failing to cause GVHD, NKT cells suppressed GVHD lethality by NK-TCRα/ β + CD4+/CD8+ BM T cells, fulfilling the in vivo definition of suppressor cells (248,250). A distinct difference between conventional naïve TCRα/β + T cells and NKT cells is the rapid, high-level production of IL-4 and IFN-γ by the latter (243,248,250,251). Indeed, IL-4 production by NKT cells is required both for their impaired capacity to mediate GVHD lethality and for their suppressor effects on conventional T-cell–mediated GVHD lethality (248,250).

While the frequency of NKT cells in BM and peripheral lymphoid organs is low, Strober's group has shown that fractionated total lymphoid irradiation (TLI) given with marrow shields markedly increases the frequency of splenic NKT cells (1% → 66% of TCRα/β + cells co-expressed NK determinants) (250). The majority of these splenic NKT co-expressed CD4. As compared to non-manipulated control splenocytes, TCRα/ β+ splenocytes obtained from recipients given fractionated TLI made significant amounts of IL-4 and resulted in a marked reduction in GVHD lethality when infused alone or with splenic T cells obtained from control donors (250). Furthermore, GVHD protection by NKT cells was IL-4 dependent. Preliminary human studies indicate that peripheral blood NKT cells are substantially increased in patients receiving fractionated TLI prior to hematopoietic cell infusion as compared to peripheral blood cells obtained from these patients analyzed prior to TLI. It will be of considerable interest to correlate the frequency of NKT cells in peripheral blood of patients receiving fractionated TLI as part of their pretransplant conditioning regimen and the subsequent incidence and severity of GVHD.

C. Regulatory T(CD4+/CD25+) Cells

In both rodents and humans, a subpopulation of thymus-derived naïve CD4+ T cells that co-express the IL-2Rα chain, CD25, has potent suppressor activity (240,241,252–261). In rodents, this population comprises 8–12% of lymph node CD4+ T cells in most strains, whereas in humans, CD4+CD25bright cells are present in lower frequencies in the blood (1–3%). Despite the relatively low frequency, CD4+CD25+ cells play a vital role in the induction and maintenance of peripheral self-tolerance. Specifically, these professional regulatory cells prevent the activation and proliferation of potentially autoreactive T cells that have escaped thymic deletion or recognize extrathymic antigens. Sakaguchi first observed that the transfer of a subpopulation of CD4+ T cells that were CD25− into nude mice led to the development of organ-specific and systemic autoimmune disorders, which could be prevented by the co-transfer of CD4+CD25+ T cells (259). Other studies have demonstrated that transfer of CD4+CD25+ T cells prevent autoimmunity resulting from neonatal thymectomy (240,241,258), inhibit the effector function of autoreactive T cell clones, and regulate the development of autoimmune gastrointestinal inflammation and autoimmune diabetes in diabetes-prone [nonobese diabetes (NOD)] mice (8,47,240,241,252,253,258,262–266). CD25-deficient mice develop a profound peripheral lymphadenopathy associated with numerous multisystemic autoimmune disorders (267). Collectively, these data indicate that CD4+CD25+ cells are essential for self-tolerance.

To determine whether CD4+CD25+ cells were required for tolerance induction to alloantigen, we used an in vitro MLR culture in which CD4+ T cells or CD4+CD25− T cells were incubated with alloantigen in the presence of anti-CD154 or anti-B7 mAb (91). In control cultures, CD4+CD25− T cells were hyperresponsive to alloantigens as compared to CD4+ T cells that were not CD25 depleted, and adding back a graded number of CD4+CD25+ T cells resulted in a dose-response reduction in proliferation to alloantigen. In cultures containing only CD4+CD25− T cells, tolerance to alloantigen (assessed by primary or secondary proliferative responses or by GVHD lethality generation) could not be achieved by adding either anti-CD154 or anti-B7 mAb. While these studies demonstrated the critical role of CD4+CD25+ cells in inducing tolerance via costimulatory pathway blockade ex vivo, it should be noted that costimulatory blockade in vivo can inhibit GVHD in recipients that receive CD25-depleted donor T cells. Furthermore, IL-10/TGFβ–induced tolerization does not require the presence of CD4+CD25+ responder cells (236).

Many studies have also elucidated the vital in vivo role of CD4+CD25+ cells in T-cell homeostasis, immune regulation, and self-tolerance (268,269). However, fewer studies have addressed their role in regulating in vivo alloresponses. Sakaguchi et al. found that nude mice rejected allogeneic skin grafts faster if transferred lymphocytes were first depleted of CD25+ cells, indicating that CD25+ cells suppress alloresponses (259). Our initial studies demonstrated that freshly isolated CD4+CD25+ did not induce GVHD and that the co-infusion of these cells (1 : 1 ratio) with CD4+CD25− T cells modestly diminished GVHD lethality (91). Furthermore, the depletion of CD4+CD25+ cells from the donor T-cell inoculum prior to its infusion or in vivo CD25 depletion of the recipient before BMT resulted in accelerated GVHD severity, indicating that CD4+CD25+ cells play a role in the regulation of GVHD (270). Notably, CD25 depletion of donor inocula prior to BMT accelerated GVHD lethality in several strain combinations irrespective of the conditioning regimen and whether GVHD was mediated only by CD4+ T cells or both CD4+ and CD8+ T cells (270).

We hypothesized that the infusion of higher numbers of CD4+CD25+ cells would inhibit GVHD to a greater degree than observed by simply preserving the small number of CD4+CD25+ present in a nonmanipulated donor allograft. Because of the relatively low frequency of these cells in vivo and the relatively modest effect of freshly purified CD25+ cells on GVHD suppression in early studies, we elected to test ex vivo expanded CD4+CD25+ cells for the suppression of GVHD (270). CD4+CD25+ T cells are hyporesponsive to TCR stimulation as compared to CD4+25− cells, and high concentrations of exogenous IL-2 are required to drive the expansion of TCR ligated CD4+25+ cells in vitro and promote T-cell survival in vivo (271,272). Additionally, data from Thornton and Shevach indicated that CD4+CD25+ cells become more potent suppressor cells after activation and expansion with anti-CD3 mAb and IL-2 (271). We therefore tested a variety of protocols to activate CD4+CD25+ T cells in which the TCR was triggered by either anti-CD3 mAb or allogeneic APC in the presence of exogenous IL-2 (270). While different ex vivo activation protocols led to varying degrees of CD4+CD25+ cell expansion, all protocols resulted in cells that significantly inhibited GVHD. Specifically, the infusion of ex vivo activated and expanded CD4+CD25+ cells increased the MST from 10 days to 72 days in nonirradiated SCID mice receiving allogeneic CD4+ T cells (270). In lethally irradiated recipients of allogeneic BMT, two infusions of ex vivo expanded CD4+CD25+ cells on days 0 and 4 post-BMT resulted in a 88% long-term survival rate in contrast to 0% survival in control mice by day 38 (P. A. Taylor and B. R. Blazar, unpublished data). Because of the known potential deficits of activated cultured cells in homing, migration, survival, and function in vivo, it is particularly notable that the GVHD suppression function of these ex vivo activated and expanded Treg cells was maintained and, in fact, likely augmented. Since CD4+CD25+ cells do not require activation by alloantigen per se to inhibit alloreactive CD25− T cells, it may be desirable to achieve maximal activation and expansion by polyclonal inducers of TCR signaling as long as ACID does not completely mitigate the beneficial effect. We believe that activation and expansion protocols can be modified to optimize expansion, in vivo survival, and homing and suppressor function.

   Similarly, Cohen et al. also demonstrated that the removal of CD4+CD25+ Treg cells from the donor cell inoculum accelerated GVHD (273). They further showed that the addition of freshly isolated CD4+CD25+ Treg cells to the donor inoculum delayed GVHD onset and protected some recipients from GVHD-induced lethality (273). Treg cells sorted for expression of high levels of CD62L could be expanded up to 100-fold in 4 weeks with only partial loss of CD62L by repetitive stimulation with allogeneic APC in the presence of IL-2. Such activated and cultured CD4+CD25+ cells had strong regulatory activity in vitro and could suppress GVHD lethality in vivo. Strober's group also showed that freshly isolated CD4+CD25+ T cells markedly inhibit the capacity of co-infused T cells to cause GVHD in irradiated allogeneic recipients (274). This protective effect depended in part on the ability of the transferred CD4+CD25+ Treg cells to secrete IL-10. Only donor and not host CD4+CD25+ T cells were capable of inhibiting GVHD lethality, suggesting that donor CD4+CD25+ T cells were activated in vivo by host alloantigens at a sufficient magnitude and kinetics to downregulate the GVHD lethality mediated by naïve T cells. Regardless of the suppressive capacity of freshly isolated CD4+CD25+ Treg cells in rodent systems, clinical studies using CD4+CD25+ cells to prevent or treat GVHD will likely require ex vivo expansion due to the lower frequency of this population in humans. Ex vivo expansion of CD4+CD25+ Treg cells may activate these cells to become more potent suppressor cells and allow the possibility of multiple infusions, which can be a highly effective strategy in rodent systems (P. A. Taylor and B. R. Blazar, unpublished data).

   Although IL-10 production by donor CD4+CD25+ T cells appears to contribute to their GVHD inhibitory capacity in one GVHD model tested (274), elucidation of additional mechanisms by which activated CD25+ cells inhibit GVHD remains to be determined. The literature suggests several possibilities that are not necessarily mutually exclusive. In vitro suppression is dependent upon cell-cell contact. While data from Nakamura et al. suggested that cell surface−bound TGF-β was responsible for the cell contact−dependent immunosuppression mediated by CD4+CD25+ cells, other mechanisms may be operative (275,276). Thornton and Shevach showed that CD4+CD25+

T cells block the induction of IL-2 production by the CD4+CD25− cells at the level of RNA transcription (257). The relative paucity of IL-2 could inhibit the activation, proliferation, and effector function of both CD4+CD25− and CD8+ T cells. Other data indicate that the expression of CD152, glucocorticoid-induced TNF receptor (GITR), or the transcription factor, FoxP3, by CD4+CD25+ cells or the activation of CD4+CD25+ cells by signaling of Toll-like receptors also contributes to their regulatory function (266,277–284).

An interesting issue raised by these studies is whether current strategies that deplete alloreactive CD25+ T cells in order to prevent or treat GVHD may have a more limited beneficial effect than might be expected due to the simultaneous depletion of beneficial CD4+CD25+ regulatory cells (285–292). We do not know the answer to this question. Although studies indicate that the infusion of anti-CD25 mAb clearly has efficacy in regulating GVHD, we hypothesize that CD4+CD25+ cells are a minority population in vivo such that the depletionary effect of anti-CD25 mAb is primarily directed against the dominant, non-Treg, activated T-cell population. Alternatively these clinical mAb may be less efficacious in depleting the CD4+CD25+ Treg-cell population as compared to the non-Treg cells.

CD4+CD25+ cells are capable of suppressing both CD4+ and CD8+ T cells (271). Therefore, it is reasonable to presume that CD4+CD25+ cells may be beneficial in suppressing host antidonor responses that can cause BM graft rejection. Data by Levy's group indicate that CD4+CD25+ cells can facilitate engraftment in 7 Gy TBI-conditioned (a nonmyeloablative TBI dose) fully allogeneic recipient (293). Preliminary data from our laboratory also demonstrate that ex vivo expanded CD4+CD25+ cells have engraftment facilitating potential when infused into 4.25 Gy TBI-conditioned allogeneic recipients (P. A. Taylor and B. R. Blazar, unpublished data).

Since donor CD4+CD25+ cells can suppress GVHD and graft rejection, it also is reasonable to presume that GVL effects may be adversely affected by these cells. In a recent study, Korngold and coworkers examined the GVHD and GVL effects of CD4+CD25+ cells in a miH disparate model (294). In this setting, even delayed infusions of fresh CD4+CD25+ Treg cells (up to 10 days) could still prevent GVHD. Importantly, the delayed infusion of CD4+CD25+ cells did not block effective in vivo GVL responses to a myeloid leukemia. The Negrin laboratory has reported a similar separation of GVHD from GVL that may be secondary to preferential homing of CD4+CD25+ Treg cells to the mesenteric lymph nodes (295,296).

In summary, CD4+CD25+ cells play an important role in alloresponses in vivo and in the generation of GVHD. Fresh and ex vivo expanded Treg cells significantly inhibit rapidly lethal GVHD and enhance donor cell engraftment in a number of experimental models. Fortunately, however, GVL activity is not eliminated by CD4+CD25+ cell infusions. Because human CD4+CD25+ Treg cells can inhibit in vitro alloresponses of both naïve and memory CD4+ T cells and can be expanded ex vivo with maintenance of suppressor function, insights gained in the laboratory should now be tested in the clinic.

V. CONCLUSION

Positive and negative forces regulate the immune system and ultimately contribute to the generation of balanced immunological responses. Costimulatory pathways, initially believed to deliver only positive signals, now are known to transmit both positive and negative signals that allow the immune system to respond to foreign peptides including alloantigens, viral antigens, or tumor antigens in such a way as to prevent widespread tissue destruction. In addition to these cell surface events, specific cellular effectors can mediate vigorous responses to these foreign antigens or can dampen the immune reaction in order to control tissue injury and prevent detrimental side effects to the whole organism. Understanding the complexity of these responses and harnessing those aspects that are most beneficial for a given purpose are required to achieve the most desired outcome. Such efforts aimed at reducing the complications of SCT including GVHD, graft rejection, and tumor relapse have been initiated in preclinical animal models and are now poised to progress to human trials with the goal of making allogeneic SCT a more safe and efficacious therapy for eligible patients.

ACKNOWLEDGMENT

Supported in part by NIH grants R01 AI 34495, 2R37 HL56067, R01 HL63452, and R01 CA72669.

REFERENCES

1. Schwartz RH. A cell culture model for T lymphocyte clonal anergy. Science 1990; 248:1349–1356.
2. Schwartz RH. Costimulation of T lymphocytes: the role of CD28, CTLA-4, and B7/BB1 in interleukin-2 production and immunotherapy. Cell 1992; 71:1065–1068.
3. Schwartz RH. Models of T cell anergy: is there a common molecular mechanism? J Exp Med 1996; 184:1–8.
4. Jenkins MK, Schwartz RH. Antigen presentation by chemically modified splenocytes induces antigen-specific T cell unresponsiveness in vitro and in vivo. J Exp Med 1987; 165:302–319.
5. Jenkins MK, Pardoll DM, Mizuguchi J, Chused TM, Schwartz RH. Molecular events in the induction of a nonresponsive state in interleukin 2-producing helper T-lymphocyte clones. Proc Natl Acad Sci USA 1987; 84:5409.
6. Bluestone JA. Costimulation and its role in organ transplantation. Clin Transplant 1996; 10:104–109.
7. Lenschow DJ, Walunas TL, Bluestone JA. CD28/B7 system of T cell costimulation. Annu Rev Immunol 1996; 14:233–258.
8. Salomon B, Bluestone JA. Complexities of CD28/B7: CTLA-4 costimulatory pathways in autoimmunity and transplantation. Annu Rev Immunol 2001; 19:225–252.
9. Sharpe AH, Freeman GJ. The B7-CD28 superfamily. Nat Rev Immunol 2002; 2:116–126.
10. Linsley PS, Brady W, Grosmaire L, Aruffo A, Damle NK, Ledbetter JA. Binding of the B cell activation antigen B7 to CD28 costimulates T cell proliferation and interleukin 2 mRNA accumulation. J Exp Med 1991; 173:721–730.
11. Linsley PS, Greene JL, Brady W, Bajorath J, Ledbetter JA, Peach R. Human B7-1 (CD80) and B7-2 (CD86) bind with similar avidities but distinct kinetics to CD28 and CTLA-4 receptors. Immunity 1994; 1:793–801.
12. Linsley PS, Greene JL, Tan P, Bradshaw J, Ledbetter JA, Anasetti C, Damle NK. Coexpression and functional cooperation of CTLA-4 and CD28 on activated T lymphocytes. J Exp Med 1992; 176:1595–1604.
13. Linsley PS, Brady W, Urnes M, Grosmaire LS, Damle NK, Ledbetter JA. CTLA-4 is a second receptor for the B cell activation antigen B7. J Exp Med 1991; 174:561–569.
14. Oosterwegel MA, Greenwald RJ, Mandelbrot DA, Lorsbach RB, Sharpe AH. CTLA-4 and T cell activation. Curr Opin Immunol 1991; 11:294–300.

15. Bluestone JA. Is CTLA-4 a master switch for peripheral T cell tolerance? J Immunol 1997; 158:1989–1993.

16. Karandikar NJ, Vanderlugt CL, Walunas TL, Miller SD, Bluestone JA. CTLA-4: a negative regulator of autoimmune disease. J Exp Med 1996; 184:783–788.

17. Kearney ER, Walunas TL, Karr RW, Morton PA, Loh DY, Bluestone JA, Jenkins MK. Antigen-dependent clonal expansion of a trace population of antigen-specific CD4+ T cells in vivo is dependent on CD28 costimulation and inhibited by CTLA4. J Immunol 1995; 155:1032–1036.

18. Walunas TL, Lenschow DJ, Bakker CY, Linsley PS, Freeman GJ, Green JM, Thompson CB, Bluestone JA. CTLA-4 can function as a negative regulator of T cell activation. Immunity 1994; 1:405–413.

19. Walunas TL, Bakker CY, Bluestone JA. CTLA-4 ligation blocks CD28-dependent T cell activation. J Exp Med 1996; 183:2541–2550.

20. Tivol EA, Borriello F, Schweitzer AN, Lynch WP, Bluestone JA, Sharpe AH. Loss of CTLA-4 leads to massive lymphoproliferation and fatal multiorgan tissue destruction, revealing a critical negative regulatory role of CTLA-4. Immunity 1995; 3:541–547.

21. Waterhouse P, Penninger JM, Timms E, Wakeham A, Shahinian A, Lee KP, Thompson CB, Griesser H, Mak TW. Lymphoproliferative disorders with early lethality in mice deficient in CTLA4. Science 1995; 270:985–988.

22. Borriello F, Sethna MP, Boyd SD, Schweitzer AN, Tivol EA, Jacoby D, Strom TB, Simpson EM, Freeman GJ, Sharpe AH. B7-1 and B7-2 have overlapping, critical roles in immunoglobulin class switching and germinal center formation. Immunity 1997; 6:303–313.

23. Freeman GJ, Borriello F, Hodes RJ, Reiser H, Gribben JG, Ng JW, Kim J, Goldberg JM, Hathcock KS, Laszlo G, Lombard DB, Wang S, Gray GS, Nadler LM, Sharpe AH. Murine B7-2, an alternative CTLA4 counter-receptor that costimulates T cell proliferation and interleukin 2 production. J Exp Med 1993; 178:2185–2192.

24. Freeman GJ, Borriello F, Hodes RJ, Reiser H, Hathcock KS, Laszlo G, McKnight AJ, Kim J, Du L, Lomberd DB, Gray G, Nadler LM, Sharpe AH. Uncovering of functional alternative CTLA-4 counter-receptor in B7-deficient mice. Science 1993; 262:907–909.

25. Schweitzer AN, Sharpe AH. Studies using antigen-presenting cells lacking expression of both B7-1 (CD80) and B7-2 (CD86) show distinct requirements for B7 molecules during priming versus restimulation of Th2 but not Th1 cytokine production. J Immunol 1998; 161:2762–2771.

26. Lenschow DJ, Su GH, Zuckerman LA, Nabavi N, Jellis CL, Gray GS, Miller J, Bluestone JA. Expression and functional significance of an additional ligand for CTLA-4. Proc Natl Acad Sci USA 1993; 90:11054–11058.

27. Hathcock KS, Laszlo G, Pucillo C, Linsley P. Hodes RJ. Comparative analysis of B7-1 and B7-2 costimulatory ligands: expression and function. J Exp Med 1994; 180:631–640.

28. Hathcock KS, Laszlo G, Dickler HB, Bradshaw J, Linsley P, Hodes RJ. Identification of an alternative CTLA-4 ligand costimulatory for T cell activation. Science 1993; 262:905–907.

29. Azuma M, Ito D, Yagita H. B70 antigen is a Second Ligand for CTLA4 and CD28. Nature 1993; 366:76–79.

30. Freeman GJ, Gribben JG, Boussiotis VA, Ng JW, Restivo Jr VA, Lombard LA, Gray GS, Nadler LM. Cloning of B7-2: A CTLA-4 counter-receptor that costimulates human T cell proliferation. Science 1993; 262:909–911.

31. Freeman GJ, Boussiotis VA, Anumanthan A, Bernstein GM, Ke X-Y, Rennert PD, Gray GS, Gribben JG, Nadler LM. B7-1 and B7-2 do not deliver identical costimulatory signals, since B7-2 but not B7-1 preferentially costimulates the initial production of IL-4. Immunity 1995; 2:523–532.

32. Blazar BR, Taylor PA, Linsley PS, Vallera DA. In vivo blockade of CD28/CTLA4: B7/BB1 interaction with CTLA4-Ig reduces lethal murine graft-versus-host disease across the major histocompatibility complex barrier in mice. Blood 1994; 83:3815–3825.

33. Linsley PS, Wallace PM, Johnson J, Gibson MG, Greene JL, Ledbetter JA, Singh C, Tepper MA. Immunosuppression in vivo by a soluble form of the CTLA-4 T cell activation molecule. Science 1992; 257:792–795.

34. Lenschow DJ, Zeng Y, Thistlethwaite R, Montag A, Brady W, Gibson MG, Linsley PS, Bluestone JA. Long-term survival of xenogeneic pancreatic islet grafts induced by CTLA4Ig. Science 1992; 257:789–792.

35. Wallace PM, Johnson JS, MacMaster JF, Kennedy KA, Gladstone P, Linsley PS. CTLA4Ig ameliorates the lethality of murine graft-versus-host disease across major histocompatibility complex barriers. Transplantation 1994; 58:602–610.

36. Via CS, Rus V, Nguyen P, Linsley P, Gause WC. Differential effect of CTLA4Ig on murine graft-versus-host disease (GVHD) development: CTLA4Ig prevents both acute and chronic GVHD development but reverses only chronic GVHD. J Immunol 1996; 157:4258–4267.

37. Hakim FT, Cepeda R, Gray GS, June CH, Abe R. Acute graft-versus-host reaction can be aborted by blockade of costimulatory molecules. J Immunol 1995; 155:1757–1766.

38. Yu XZ, Bidwell SJ, Martin PJ, Anasetti C. CD28-specific antibody prevents graft-versus-host disease in mice. J Immunol 2000; 164:4564–4568.

39. Blazar BR, Taylor PA, Panoskaltsis-Mortari A, Gray GS, Vallera DA. Coblockade of the LFA1:ICAM and CD28/CTLA4:B7 pathways is a highly effective means of preventing acute lethal graft-versus-host disease induced by fully major histocompatibility complex-disparate donor grafts. Blood 1995; 85:2607–2618.

40. Blazar BR, Taylor PA, Gray GS, Vallera DA. The role of T cell subsets in regulating the in vivo efficacy of CTLA4-Ig in preventing graft-versus-host disease in recipients of fully MHC or multiple minor histocompatibility-disparate donor inocula. Transplantation 1994; 58:1422–1426.

41. Blazar BR, Sharpe AH, Taylor PA, Panoskaltsis-Mortari A, Gray GS, Korngold R, Vallera DA. Infusion of anti-B7.1 (CD80) and anti-B7.2 (CD86) monoclonal antibodies inhibits murine graft-versus-host disease lethality in part via direct effects on CD4+ and CD8+ T cells. J Immunol 1996; 157:3250–3259.

42. Greenwald RJ, Boussiotis VA, Lorsbach RB, Abbas AK, Sharpe AH. CTLA-4 regulates induction of anergy in vivo. Immunity 2001; 14:145–155.

43. Blazar BR, Taylor PA, Panoskaltsis-Mortari A, Sharpe AH, Vallera DA. Opposing roles of CD28:B7 and CTLA-4:B7 pathways in regulating in vivo alloresponses in murine recipients of MHC disparate T cells. J Immunol 1999; 162:6368–6377.

44. Yu XZ, Martin PJ, Anasetti C. Role of CD28 in acute graft-versus-host disease. Blood 1998; 92:2963–2970.

45. Speiser DE, Bachmann MF, Shahinian A, Mak TW, Ohashi PS. Acute graft-versus-host disease without costimulation via CD28. Transplantation 1997; 63:1042–1044.

46. Saito K, Sakurai J, Ohata J, Kohsaka T, Hashimoto H, Okumura K, Abe R, Azuma M. Involvement of CD40 ligand-CD40 and CTLA4-B7 pathways in murine acute graft-versus-host disease induced by allogeneic T cells lacking CD28. J Immunol 1998; 160:4225–4231.

47. Salomon B, Lenschow DJ, Rhee L, Ashourian N, Singh B, Sharpe A, Bluestone JA. B7/CD28 costimulation is essential for the homeostasis of the CD4+CD25+ immunoregulatory T cells that control autoimmune diabetes. Immunity 2000; 12:431–440.

48. Fournier S, Rathmell JC, Goodnow CC, Allison JP. T cell-mediated elimination of B7.2 transgenic B cells. Immunity 1997; 6:327–339.

49. Taylor PA, Lees CJ, Fournier S, Allison JP, Sharpe AH, Blazar BR. B7 expression on T cells down-regulates immune responses via T-T interactions. J Immunol 2004; 172:34–39.

50. Mandelbrot DA, Oosterwegel MA, Shimizu K, Yamada A, Freeman GJ, Mitchell RN, Sayegh MH, Sharpe AH. B7-dependent T-cell costimulation in mice lacking CD28 and CTLA4. J Clin Invest 2001; 107:881–887.

51. Blazar BR, Taylor PA, Boyer MW, Panoskaltsis-Mortari A, Allison JP, Vallera DA. CD28/B7 interactions are required for sustaining the graft-versus-leukemia effect of delayed post-bone marrow transplantation splenocyte infusion in murine recipients of myeloid or lymphoid leukemia cells. J Immunol 1997; 159:3460–3473.

52. Ohata J, Sakurai J, Saito K, Tani K, Asano S, Azuma M. Differential graft-versus-leukaemia effect by CD28 and CD40 co-stimulatory blockade after graft-versus-host disease prophylaxis. Clin Exp Immunol 2002; 129:61–68.

53. Wekerle T, Sayegh MH, Ito H, Hill J, Chandraker A, Pearson DA, Swenson KG, Zhao G, Sykes M. Anti-CD154 or CTLA4Ig obviates the need for thymic irradiation in a non-myeloablative conditioning regimen for the induction of mixed hematopoietic chimerism and tolerance. Transplantation 1999; 68:1348–1355.

54. Storb R, Yu C, Zaucha JM, Deeg HJ, Georges G, Kiem HP, Nash RA, McSweeney PA, Wagner JL. Stable mixed hematopoietic chimerism in dogs given donor antigen, CTLA4Ig, and 100 cGy total body irradiation before and pharmacologic immunosuppression after marrow transplant. Blood 1999; 94:2523–2529.

55. Taylor PA, Lees CJ, Waldmann H, Noelle RJ, Blazar BR. Requirements for the promotion of allogeneic engraftment by anti-CD154 (anti-CD40L) monoclonal antibody under nonmyeloablative conditions. Blood 2001; 98:467–474.

56. Grohmann U, Orabona C, Fallarino F, Vacca C, Calcinaro F, Falomi A, Candeloro P, Belladonna ML, Bianchi R, Fioretti MC, Puccetti P. CTLA-4-Ig regulates tryptophan catabolism in vivo. Nat Immunol 2002; 3:1097–1101.

57. Stamenkovic I, Clark EA, Seed B. A B-lymphocyte activation molecule related to the nerve growth factor receptor and induced by cytokines in carcinomas. EMBO J 1989; 8:1403–1410.

58. Clark EA, Ledbetter JA. Activation of human B cells mediated through two distinct cell surface differentiation antigens, Bp35 and Bp50. Proc Natl Acad Sci USA 1986; 83:4494–4498.

59. Hart DN, McKenzie JL. Isolation and characterization of human tonsil dendritic cells. J Exp Med 1988; 168:157–170.

60. Schriever F, Freedman AS, Freeman G, Messner E, Lee G, Daley J, Nadler LM. Isolated human follicular dendritic cells display a unique antigenic phenotype. J Exp Med 1989; 169:2043–2058.

61. Galy AH, Spits H. CD40 is functionally expressed on human thymic epithelial cells. J Immunol 1992; 149:775–782.

62. Hollenbaugh D, Grosmaire LS, Kullas CD, Chalupny NJ, Braesch-Andersen S, Noelle RJ, Stamenkovic I, Ledbetter JA, Aruffo A. The human T cell antigen gp39, a member of the TNF gene family, is a ligand for the CD40 receptor: expression of a soluble form of gp39 with B cell co-stimulatory activity. EMBO J 1992; 11:4313–4321.

63. Armitage RJ, Fanslow WC, Strockbine L, Sato TA, Clifford KN, Macduff BM, Anderson DM, Gimpel SD, Davis-Smith T, Maliszewski CR, et al. Molecular and biological characterization of a murine ligand for CD40. Nature 1992; 357:80–82.

64. Noelle RJ, Roy M, Shepherd DM, Stamenkovic I, Ledbetter JA, Aruffo A. A 39-kDa protein on activated helper T cells binds CD40 and transduces the signal for cognate activation of B cells. Proc Natl Acad Sci USA 1992; 89:6550–6554.

65. Lederman S, Yellin MJ, Inghirami G, Lee JJ, Knowles DM, Chess L. Molecular interactions mediating T-B lymphocyte collaboration in human lymphoid follicles. Roles of T cell-B-cell-activating molecule (5c8 antigen) and CD40 in contact-dependent help. J Immunol 1992; 149:3817–3826.

66. Hermann P, Van-Kooten C, Gaillard C, Banchereau J, Blanchard D. CD40 ligand-positive CD8+ T cell clones allow B cell growth and differentiation. Eur J Immunol 1995; 25:2972–2977.

67. Grammer AC, Bergman MC, Miura Y, Fujita K, Davis LS, Lipsky PE. The CD40 ligand expressed by human B cells costimulates B cell responses. J Immunol 1995; 154:4996–5010.

68. Ranheim EA, Kipps TJ. Activated T cells induce expression of B7/BB1 on normal or leukemic B cells through a CD40-dependent signal. J Exp Med 1993; 177:925–935.

69. Kennedy MK, Mohler KM, Shanebeck KD, Baum PR, Picha KS, Otten-Evans CA, Janeway CA, Jr., Grabstein KH. Induction of B cell costimulatory function by recombinant murine CD40 ligand. Eur J Immunol 1994; 24:116–123.

70. Klaus SJ, Pinchuk LM, Ochs HD, Law CL, Fanslow WC, Armitage RJ, Clark EA. Costimulation through CD28 enhances T cell-dependent B cell activation via CD40-CD40L interaction. J Immunol 1994; 152:5643–5652.

71. Roy M, Aruffo A, Ledbetter J, Linsley P, Kehery M, Noelle R. Studies on the interdependence of gp39 and B7 expression and function during antigen-specific immune responses. Eur J Immunol 1995; 25:596–603.

72. Ding L, Green JM, Thompson CB, Shevach EM. B7/CD28-dependent and -independent induction of CD40 ligand expression. J Immunol 1995; 155:5124–5132.

73. Jaiswal AI, Dubey C, Swain SL, Croft M. Regulation of CD40 ligand expression on naive CD4 T cells: a role for TCR but not co-stimulatory signals. Int Immunol 1996; 8:275–285.

74. Hollander GA, Castigli E, Kulbacki R, Su M, Burakoff SJ, Gutierrez-Ramos JC, Geha RS. Induction of alloantigen-specific tolerance by B cells from CD40-deficient mice. Proc Natl Acad Sci USA 1996; 93:4994–4998.

75. Buhlmann JE, Foy TM, Aruffo A, Crassi KM, Ledbetter JA, Green WR, Xu JC, Shultz LD, Roopesian D, Flavell RA, et al. In the absence of a CD40 signal, B cells are tolerogenic. Immunity 1995; 2:645–653.

76. Durie FH, Aruffo A, Ledbetter J, Crassi KM, Green WR, Fast LD, Noelle RJ. Antibody to the ligand of CD40, gp39, blocks the occurrence of the acute and chronic forms of graft-vs-host disease. J Clin Invest 1994; 94:1333–1338.

77. Stuber E, von Freier A, Folsch UR. The effect of anti-gp39 treatment on the intestinal manifestations of acute murine graft-versus-host disease. Clin Immunol 1999; 90:334–339.

78. Wagner DH, Jr., Stout RD, Suttles J. Role of the CD40-CD40 ligand interaction in CD4+ T cell contact-dependent activation of monocyte interleukin-1 synthesis. Eur J Immunol 1994; 24:3148–3154.

79. Tao X, Stout RD. T cell-mediated cognate signaling of nitric oxide production by macrophages. Requirements for macrophage activation by plasma membranes isolated from T cells. Eur J Immunol 1993; 23:2916–2921.

80. Stout RD, Suttles J, Xu J, Grewal IS, Flavell RA. Impaired T cell-mediated macrophage activation in CD40 ligand-deficient mice. J Immunol 1996; 156:8–11.

81. Tian L, Noelle RJ, Lawrence DA. Activated T cells enhance nitric oxide production by murine splenic macrophages through gp39 and LFA-1. Eur J Immunol 1995; 25:306–309.

82. Ferrara JL. Cytokines other than growth factors in bone marrow transplantation. Curr Opin Oncol 1994; 6:127–134.

83. Antin JH, Ferrara JL. Cytokine dysregulation and acute graft-versus-host disease. Blood 1992; 80:2964–2968.

84. Xun CQ, Thompson JS, Jennings CD, Brown SA, Widmer MB. Effect of total body irradiation, busulfan-cyclophosphamide, or cyclophosphamide conditioning on inflammatory cytokine release and development of acute and chronic graft-versus-host disease in H-2-incompatible transplanted SCID mice. Blood 1994; 83:2360–2367.

85. Blazar BR, Taylor PA, Panoskaltsis-Mortari A, Buhlman J, Xu J, Flavell RA, Korngold R, Noelle R, Vallera DA. Blockade of CD40 ligand-CD40 interaction impairs CD4+ T cell-mediated alloreactivity by inhibiting mature donor T cell expansion and function after bone marrow transplantation. J Immunol 1997; 158:29–39.

86. Buhlmann JE, Gonzalez M, Ginther B, Panoskaltsis-Mortari A, Blazar BR, Greiner DL, Rossini AA, Flavell R, Noelle RJ. Cutting edge: sustained expansion of CD8+ T cells requires CD154 expression by Th cells in acute graft versus host disease. J Immunol 1999; 162:4373–4376.

87. Taylor PA, Lees CJ, Noelle RJ, Yagita H, Killeen N, Sharpe AH, Blazar BR. Superior GVHD prevention by combined costimulatory blockade: comparison of single and combined pathway blockade of CD28/CTLA-4:B7, CD40L:CD40 and OX40:OX40L pathways. Blood 2002; 100:818a.
88. Graca L, Honey K, Adams E, Cobbold SP, Waldmann H. Cutting edge: anti-CD154 therapeutic antibodies induce infectious transplantation tolerance. J Immunol 2000; 165:4783–4786.
89. Blazar BR, Taylor PA, Noelle RJ, Vallera DA. CD4(+) T cells tolerized ex vivo to host alloantigen by anti-CD40 ligand (CD40L:CD154) antibody lose their graft-versus-host disease lethality capacity but retain nominal antigen responses. J Clin Invest 1998; 102:473–482.
90. Taylor PA, Panoskaltsis-Mortari A, Noelle RJ, Blazar BR. Analysis of the requirements for the induction of CD4+ T cell alloantigen hyporesponsiveness by ex vivo anti-CD40 ligand antibody. J Immunol 2000; 164:612–622.
91. Taylor PA, Noelle RJ, Blazar BR. CD4(+)CD25(+) immune regulatory cells are required for induction of tolerance to alloantigen via costimulatory blockade. J Exp Med 2001; 193:1311–1318.
92. Taylor PA, Friedman TM, Korngold R, Noelle RJ, Blazar BR. Tolerance induction of alloreactive T cells via ex vivo blockade of the CD40:CD40L costimulatory pathway results in the generation of a potent immune regulatory cell. Blood 2002; 99:4601–4609.
93. Blazar BR, Taylor PA, Panoskaltsis-Mortari A, Vallera DA. Rapamycin inhibits the generation of graft-versus-host disease- and graft-versus-leukemia-causing T cells by interfering with the production of Th1 or Th1 cytotoxic cytokines. J Immunol 1998; 160:5355–5365.
94. Ito H, Kurtz J, Shaffer J, Sykes M. CD4 T cell-mediated alloresistance to fully MHC-mismatched allogeneic bone marrow engraftment is dependent on CD40-CD40 ligand interactions, and lasting T cell tolerance is induced by bone marrow transplantation with initial blockade of this pathway. J Immunol 2001; 166:2970–2981.
95. Wekerle T, Sayegh MH, Hill J, Zhao Y, Chandraker A, Swenson KG, Zhao G, Sykes M. Extrathymic T cell deletion and allogeneic stem cell engraftment induced with costimulatory blockade is followed by central T cell tolerance. J Exp Med 1998; 187:2037–2044.
96. Adams AB, Durham MM, Kean L, Shirasugi N, Ha J, Williams MA, Rees PA, Cheung MC, Mittelstaedt S, Bingaman AW, Archer DR, Pearson TC, Waller EK, Larsen CP. Costimulation blockade busulfan, and bone marrow promote titratable macrochimerism, induce transplantation tolerance, and correct genetic hemoglobinopathies with minimal myelosuppression. J Immunol 2001; 167:1103–1111.
97. Kean LS, Durham MM, Adams AB, Hsu LL, Perry JR, Dillehay D, Pearson TC, Waller EK, Larsen CP, Archer DR. A cure for murine sickle cell disease through stable mixed chimerism and tolerance induction after nonmyeloablative conditioning and major histocompatibility complex-mismatched bone marrow transplantation. Blood 2002; 99:1840–1849.
98. Quesenberry PJ, Zhong S, Wang H, Stewart M. Allogeneic chimerism with low-dose irradiation, antigen presensitization, and costimulator blockade in H-2 mismatched mice. Blood 2001; 97:557–564.
99. Smiley ST, Csizmadia V, Gao W, Turka LA, Hancock WW. Differential effects of cyclosporine A, methylprednisolone, mycophenolate, and rapamycin on CD154 induction and requirement for NFkappaB: implications for tolerance induction. Transplantation 2000; 70:415–419.
100. Taylor PA, Lees CJ, Wilson JM, Ehrhardt MJ, Campbell MT, Noelle RJ, Blazar BR. Combined effects of calcineurin inhibitors or sirolimus with anti-CD40L mAb on alloengraftment under nonmyeloablative conditions. Blood 2002; 100:3400–3407.
101. Blaha P, Bigenzahn S, Koporc Z, Schmid M, Langer F, Selzer E, Bergmeister H, Wrba F, Kurtz J, Kiss C, Roth E, Muehlbacher F, Sykes M, Wekerle T. The influence of immunosuppressive drugs on tolerance induction through bone marrow transplantation with costimulation blockade. Blood 2003; 101:2886-2893.

102. Li Y, Li XC, Zheng XX, Wells AD, Turka LA, Strom TB. Blocking both signal 1 and signal 2 of T-cell activation prevents apoptosis of alloreactive T cells and induction of peripheral allograft tolerance. Nat Med 1999; 5:1298–1302.

103. Li Y, Zheng XX, Li XC, Zand MS, Strom TB. Combined costimulation blockade plus rapamycin but not cyclosporine produces permanent engraftment. Transplantation 1998; 66:1387–1388.

104. Wekerle T, Kurtz J, Ito H, Ronquillo JV, Dong V, Zhao G, Shaffer J, Sayegh MH, Sykes M. Allogeneic bone marrow transplantation with co-stimulatory blockade induces macrochimerism and tolerance without cytoreductive host treatment. Nat Med 2000; 6:464–469.

105. Durham MM, Bingaman AW, Adams AB, Ha J, Waitze SY, Pearson TC, Larsen CP. Cutting edge: administration of anti-CD40 ligand and donor bone marrow leads to hemopoietic chimerism and donor-specific tolerance without cytoreductive conditioning. J Immunol 2000; 165:1–4.

106. Kwon BS, Weissman SM. cDNA sequences of two inducible T-cell genes. Proc Natl Acad Sci USA 1989; 86:1963–1967.

107. Pollok KE, Kim YJ, Zhou Z, Hurtado J, Kim KK, Pickard RT, Kwon BS. Inducible T cell antigen 4-1BB. Analysis of expression and function. J Immunol 1993; 150:771–781.

108. Melero I, Johnston JV, Shufford WW, Mittler RS, Chen L. NK1.1 cells express 4-1BB (CDw137) costimulatory molecule and are required for tumor immunity elicited by anti-4-1BB monoclonal antibodies. Cell Immunol 1998; 190:167–172.

109. Pollok KE, Kim YJ, Hurtado J, Zhou Z, Kim KK, Kwon BS. 4-1BB T-cell antigen binds to mature B cells and macrophages, and costimulates anti-mu-primed splenic B cells. Eur J Immunol 1994; 24:367–374.

110. DeBenedette MA, Shahinian A, Mak TW, Watts TH. Costimulation of CD28- T lymphocytes by 4-1BB ligand. J Immunol 1997; 158:551–559.

111. Goodwin RG, Din WS, Davis-Smith T, Anderson DM, Gimpel SD, Sato TA, Maliszewski CR, Brannan CI, Copeland NG, Jenkins NA, et al. Molecular cloning of a ligand for the inducible T cell gene 4-1BB: a member of an emerging family of cytokines with homology to tumor necrosis factor. Eur J Immunol 1993; 23:2631–2641.

112. Alderson MR, Smith CA, Tough TW, Davis-Smith T, Armitage RJ, Falk B, Roux E, Baker E, Sutherland GR, Din WS. Molecular and biological characterization of human 4-1BB and its ligand. Eur J Immunol 1994; 24:2219–2227.

113. Hurtado JC, Kim SH, Pollok KE, Lee ZH, Kwon BS. Potential role of 4-1BB in T cell activation. Comparison with the costimulatory molecule CD28. J Immunol 1995; 155:3360–3367.

114. Saoulli K, Lee SY, Cannons JL, Yeh WC, Santana A, Goldstein MD, Bangia N, DeBenedette MA, Mak TW, Choi Y, Watts TH. CD28-independent, TRAF2-dependent costimulation of resting T cells by 4-1BB ligand. J Exp Med 1998; 187:1849–1862.

115. Hurtado JC, Kim YJ, Kwon BS. Signals through 4-1BB are costimulatory to previously activated splenic T cells and inhibit activation-induced cell death. J Immunol 1997; 158:2600–2609.

116. Takahashi C, Mittler RS, Vella AT. Cutting edge: 4-1BB is a bona fide CD8 T cell survival signal. J Immunol 1999; 162:5037–5040.

117. Shuford WW, Klussman K, Tritchler DD, Loo DT, Chalupny J, Siadak AW, Brown TJ, Emswiler J, Raecho H, Larsen CP, Pearson TC, Ledbetter JA, Aruffo A, Mittler RS. 4-1BB costimulatory signals preferentially induce CD8+ T cell proliferation and lead to the amplification in vivo of cytotoxic T cell responses. J Exp Med 1997; 186:47–55.

118. Tan JT, Whitmire JK, Ahmed R, Pearson TC, Larsen CP. 4-1BB ligand, a member of the TNF family, is important for the generation of antiviral CD8 T cell responses. J Immunol 1999; 163:4859–4868.

119. Tan JT, Ha J, Cho HR, Tucker-Burden C, Hendrix RC, Mittler RS, Pearson TC, Larsen CP. Analysis of expression and function of the costimulatory molecule 4-1BB in alloimmune responses. Transplantation 2000; 70:175–183.

120. Nozawa K, Ohata J, Sakurai J, Hashimoto H, Miyajima H, Yagita H, Okumura K, Azuma M. Preferential blockade of CD8(+) T cell responses by administration of anti-CD137 ligand monoclonal antibody results in differential effect on development of murine acute and chronic graft-versus-host diseases. J Immunol 2001; 167:4981–4986.

121. Blazar BR, Kwon BS, Panoskaltsis-Mortari A, Kwak KB, Peschon JJ, Taylor PA. Ligation of 4-1BB (CDw137) regulates graft-versus-host disease, graft-versus-leukemia, and graft rejection in allogeneic bone marrow transplant recipients. J Immunol 2001; 166:3174–3183.

122. Mallett S, Fossum S, Barclay AN. Characterization of the MRC OX40 antigen of activated CD4 positive T lymphocytes—a molecule related to nerve growth factor receptor. EMBO J 1990; 9:1063–1068.

123. Calderhead DM, Buhlmann JE, van den Eertwegh AJ, Claassen E, Noelle RJ, Fell HP. Cloning of mouse Ox40: a T cell activation marker that may mediate T-B cell interactions. J Immunol 1993; 151:5261–5271.

124. Baum PR, Gayle RB, 3rd, Ramsdell F, Srinivasan S, Sorensen RA, Watson ML, Seldin MF, Baker E, Sutherland GR, Clifford KN, et al. Molecular characterization of murine and human OX40/OX40 ligand systems: identification of a human OX40 ligand as the HTLV-1-regulated protein gp34. EMBO J 1994; 13:3992–4001.

125. Baum PR, Gayle RB, 3rd, Ramsdell F, Srinivasan S, Sorensen RA, Watson ML, Seldin MF, Clifford KN, Grabstein K, Alderson MR, et al. Identification of OX40 ligand and preliminary characterization of its activities on OX40 receptor. Circ Shock 1994; 44:30–34.

126. Latza U, Durkop H, Schnittger S, Ringeling J, Eitelbach F, Hummel M, Fonatsch C, Stein H. The human OX40 homolog: cDNA structure, expression and chromosomal assignment of the ACT35 antigen. Eur J Immunol 1994; 24:677–683.

127. Birkeland ML, Copeland NG, Gilbert DJ, Jenkins NA, Barclay AN. Gene structure and chromosomal localization of the mouse homologue of rat OX40 protein. Eur J Immunol 1995; 25:926–930.

128. Stuber E, Neurath M, Calderhead D, Fell HP, Strober W. Cross-linking of OX40 ligand, a member of the TNF/NGF cytokine family, induces proliferation and differentiation in murine splenic B cells. Immunity 1995; 2:507–521.

129. Ohshima Y, Tanaka Y, Tozawa H, Takahashi Y, Maliszewski C, Delespesse G. Expression and function of OX40 ligand on human dendritic cells. J Immunol 1997; 159:3838–3848.

130. Brocker T, Gulbranson-Judge A, Flynn S, Riedinger M, Raykundalia C, Lane P. CD4 T cell traffic control: in vivo evidence that ligation of OX40 on CD4 T cells by OX40-ligand expressed on dendritic cells leads to the accumulation of CD4 T cells in B follicles. Eur J Immunol 1999; 29:1610–1616.

131. Imura A, Hori T, Imada K, Ishikawa T, Tanaka Y, Maeda M, Imamura S, Uchiyama T. The human OX40/gp34 system directly mediates adhesion of activated T cells to vascular endothelial cells. J Exp Med 1996; 183:2185–2195.

132. Weinberg AD, Wegmann KW, Funatake C, Whitham RH. Blocking OX-40/OX-40 ligand interaction in vitro and in vivo leads to decreased T cell function and amelioration of experimental allergic encephalomyelitis. J Immunol 1999; 162:1818–1826.

133. Pippig SD, Pena-Rossi C, Long J, Godfrey WR, Fowell DJ, Reiner SL, Birkeland ML, Locksley RM, Barclay AN, Killeen N. Robust B cell immunity but impaired T cell proliferation in the absence of CD134 (OX40). J Immunol 1999; 163:6520–6529.

134. Miura S, Ohtani K, Numata N, Niki M, Ohbo K, Ina Y, Gojobori T, Tanaka Y, Tozawa H, Nakamura M, et al. Molecular cloning and characterization of a novel glycoprotein, gp34, that is specifically induced by the human T-cell leukemia virus type I transactivator p40tax. Mol Cell Biol 1991; 11:1313–1325.

135. Flynn S, Toellner KM, Raykundalia C, Goodall M, Lane P. CD4 T cell cytokine differentiation: the B cell activation molecule, OX40 ligand, instructs CD4 T cells to express interleukin 4 and upregulates expression of the chemokine receptor, B1r-1. J Exp Med 1998; 188:297–304.

136. Ohshima Y, Yang LP, Uchiyama T, Tanaka Y, Baum P, Sergerie M, Hermann P, Delespesse G. OX40 costimulation enhances interleukin-4 (IL-4) expression at priming and promotes the differentiation of naive human CD4(+) T cells into high IL-4-producing effectors. Blood 1998; 92:3338–3345.

137. Chen AI, McAdam AJ, Buhlmann JE, Scott S, Lupher ML, Jr., Greenfield EA, Baum PR, Fanslow WC, Calderhead DM, Freeman GJ, Sharpe AH. Ox40-ligand has a critical costimulatory role in dendritic cell:T cell interactions. Immunity 1999; 11:689–698.

138. Kopf M, Ruedl C, Schmitz N, Gallimore A, Lefrang K, Ecabert B, Odermatt B, Bachmann MF. OX40-deficient mice are defective in Th cell proliferation but are competent in generating B cell and CTL responses after virus infection. Immunity 1999; 11:699–708.

139. Akiba H, Miyahira Y, Atsuta M, Takeda K, Nohara C, Futagawa T, Matsuda H, Aoki T, Yagita H, Okumura K. Critical contribution of OX40 ligand to T helper cell type 2 differentiation in experimental leishmaniasis. J Exp Med 2000; 191:375–380.

140. Gramaglia I, Jember A, Pippig SD, Weinberg AD, Killeen N, Croft M. The OX40 costimulatory receptor determines the development of CD4 memory by regulating primary clonal expansion. J Immunol 2000; 165:3043–3050.

141. Murata K, Ishii N, Takano H, Miura S, Ndhlovu LC, Nose M, Noda T, Sugamura K. Impairment of antigen-presenting cell function in mice lacking expression of OX40 ligand. J Exp Med 2000; 191:365–374.

142. Bansal-Pakala P, Jember AG, Croft M. Signaling through OX40 (CD134) breaks peripheral T-cell tolerance. Nat Med 2001; 7:907–912.

143. Evans DE, Prell RA, Thalhofer CJ, Hurwitz AA, Weinberg AD. Engagement of OX40 enhances antigen-specific CD4(+) T cell mobilization/memory development and humoral immunity: comparison of alphaOX-40 with alphaCTLA-4. J Immunol 2001; 167:6804–6811.

144. Rogers PR, Song J, Gramaglia I, Killeen N, Croft M. OX40 promotes Bcl-xL and Bcl-2 expression and is essential for long-term survival of CD4 T cells. Immunity 2001; 15:445–455.

145. Weatherill AR, Maxwell JR, Takahashi C, Weinberg AD, Vella AT. OX40 ligation enhances cell cycle turnover of Ag-activated CD4 T cells in vivo. Cell Immunol 2001; 209:63–75.

146. De Smedt T, Smith J, Baum P, Fanslow W, Butz E, Maliszewski C. Ox40 costimulation enhances the development of T cell responses induced by dendritic cells in vivo. J Immunol 2002; 168:661–670.

147. Weinberg AD. OX40: targeted immunotherapy—implications for tempering autoimmunity and enhancing vaccines. Trends Immunol 2002; 23:102–109.

148. Rogers PR, Croft M. CD28, Ox-40, LFA-1, and CD4 modulation of Th1/Th2 differentiation is directly dependent on the dose of antigen. J Immunol 2000; 164:2955–2963.

149. Gramaglia I, Weinberg AD, Lemon M, Croft M. Ox-40 ligand: a potent costimulatory molecule for sustaining primary CD4 T cell responses. J Immunol 1998; 161:6510–6517.

150. Weinberg AD, Vella AT, Croft M. OX-40: life beyond the effector T cell stage. Semin Immunol 1998; 10:471–480.

151. Weinberg AD, Rivera MM, Prell R, Morris A, Ramstad T, Vetto JT, Urba WJ, Alvord G, Bunce C, Shields J. Engagement of the OX-40 receptor in vivo enhances antitumor immunity. J Immunol 2000; 164:2160–2169.

152. Tittle TV, Weinberg AD, Steinkeler CN, Maziarz RT. Expression of the T-cell activation antigen, OX-40, identifies alloreactive T cells in acute graft-versus-host disease. Blood 1997; 89:4652–4658.

153. Stuber E, Von Freier A, Marinescu D, Folsch UR. Involvement of OX40-OX40L interactions in the intestinal manifestations of the murine acute graft-versus-host disease. Gastroenterology 1998; 115:1205–1215.

154. Tsukada N, Akiba H, Kobata T, Aizawa Y, Yagita H, Okumura K. Blockade of CD134(OX40)-CD134L interaction ameliorates lethal acute graft-versus-host disease in a murine model of allogeneic bone marrow transplantation. Blood 2000; 95:2434–2439.

155. Blazar BR, Sharpe AH, Chen AI, Panoskaltsis-Mortari A, Lees C, Akiba H, Yagita H, Killeen N, Taylor PA. Ligation of OX40 (CD134) regulates graft-versus-host disease (GVHD) and graft rejection in allogenic bone marrow transplant (SCT) recipients. Blood 2003.

156. Jember AG, Zuberi R, Liu FT, Croft M. Development or allergic inflammation in a murine model of asthma is dependent on the costimulatory receptor OX40. J Exp Med 2001; 193:387–392.

157. Hutloff A, Dittrich AM, Beier KC, Eljaschewitsch B, Kraft R, Anagnostopoulos I, Kroczek RA. ICOS is an inducible T-cell co-stimulator structurally and functionally related to CD28. Nature 1999; 397:263–266.

158. Coyle AJ, Lehar S, Lloyd C, Tian J, Delaney T, Manning S, Nguyen T, Burwell T, Schneider H, Gonzalo JA, Gosselin M, Owen LR, Rudd CE, Gutierrez-Ramos JC. The CD28-related molecule ICOS is required for effective T cell- dependent immune responses. Immunity 2000; 13:95–105.

159. Kopf M, Coyle AJ, Schmitz N, Barner M, Oxenius A, Gallimore A, Gutierrez-Ramos JC, Bachmann MF. Inducible costimulator protein (ICOS) controls T helper cell subset polarization after virus and parasite infection. J Exp Med 2000; 192:53–61.

160. Sperling AI, Bluestone JA. ICOS costimulation: it's not just for TH2 cells anymore. Nat Immunol 2001; 2:573–574.

161. Aicher A, Hayden-Ledbetter M, Brady WA, Pezzutto A, Richter G, Magaletti D, Buckwalter S, Ledbetter JA, Clark EA. Characterization of human inducible costimulator ligand expression and function. J Immunol 2000; 164:4689–4696.

162. Swallow MM, Wallin JJ, Sha WC. B7h, a novel costimulatory homolog of B7.1 and B7.2, is induced by TNFalpha. Immunity 1999; 11:423–432.

163. Wang S, Zhu G, Chapoval AI, Dong H, Tamada K, Ni J, Chen L. Costimulation of T cells by B7-H2, a B7-like molecule that binds ICOS. Blood 2000; 96:2808–2813.

164. Ling V, Wu PW, Finnerty HF, Bean KM, Spaulding V, Fouser LA, Leonard JP, Hunter SE, Zollner R, Thomas JL, Miyashiro JS, Jacobs KA, Collins M. Cutting edge: identification of GL50, a novel B7-like protein that functionally binds to ICOS receptor. J Immunol 2000; 164:1653–1657.

165. Ling V, Wu PW, Miyashiro JS, Marusic S, Finnerty HF, Collins M. Differential expression of inducible costimulator-ligand splice variants: lymphoid regulation of mouse GL50-B and human GL50 molecules. J Immunol 2001; 166:7300–7308.

166. Gonzalo JA, Tian J, Delaney T, Corcoran J, Rottman JB, Lora J, Al-garawi A, Kroczek R, Gutierrez-Ramos JC, Coyle AJ. ICOS is critical for T helper cell-mediated lung mucosal inflammatory responses. Nat Immunol 2001; 2:597–604.

167. Yoshinaga SK, Whoriskey JS, Khare SD, Sarmiento U, Guo J, Horan T, Shi, G, Zhang M, Coccia MA, Kohno T, Tafuri-Bladt A, Brankow D, Campbell P, Chang D, Chiu L, Dai T, Duncan G, Elliott GS, Hui A, McCabe SM, Scully S, Shahinian A, Shaklee CL, Van G, Mak TW, et al. T-cell co-stimulation through B7RP-1 and ICOS. Nature 1999; 402:827–832.

168. Coyle AJ, Gutierrez-Ramos JC. The expanding B7 superfamily: increasing complexity in costimulatory signals regulating T cell function. Nat Immunol 2001; 2:203–209.

169. McAdam AJ, Chang TT, Lumelsky AE, Greenfield EA, Boussiotis VA, Duke-Cohan JS, Chernova T, Malenkovich N, Jabs C, Kuchroo VK, Ling V, Collins M, Sharpe AH, Freeman GJ. Mouse inducible costimulatory molecule (ICOS) expression is enhanced by CD28 costimulation and regulates differentiation of CD4(+) T cells. J Immunol 2000; 165:5035–5040.

170. McAdam AJ, Greenwald RJ, Levin MA, Chernova T, Malenkovich N, Ling V, Freeman GJ, Sharpe AH. ICOS is critical for CD40-mediated antibody class switching. Nature 2001; 409:102–105.

171. Dong C, Juedes AM, Temann U-A, Shresta S, Allison JP, Ruddle NH, Flavell RA. ICOS co-stimulatory receptor is essential for T-cell activation and function. Nature 2001; 409:97–101.

172. Tafuri A, Shahinian A, Bladt F, Yoshinaga SK, Jordana M, Wakeham A, Boucher L-M, Bouchard D, Chan VSF, Duncan G, Odermatt B, Ho A, Itie A, Horan T, Whoriskey JS, Pawson T, Penninger JM, Ohashi PS, Mak TW. ICOS is essential for effective T-helper-cell responses. Nature 2001; 409:105–109.

173. Tesciuba AG, Subudhi S, Rother RP, Faas SJ, Frantz AM, Elliot D, Weinstock J, Matis LA, Bluestone JA, Sperling AI. Inducible costimulator regulates Th2-mediated inflammation, but not Th2 differentiation, in a model of allergic airway disease. J Immunol 2001; 167:1996–2003.

174. Khayyamian S, Hutloff A, Buchner K, Grafe M, Henn V, Kroczek RA, Mages HW. ICOS-ligand, expressed on human endothelial cells, costimulates Th1 and Th2 cytokine secretion by memory CD4+ T cells. Proc Natl Acad Sci USA 2002; 99:6198–6203.

175. Yoshinaga SK, Zhang M, Pistillo J, Horan T, Khare SD, Miner K, Sonnenberg M, Boone T, Brankow D, Dai T, Delaney J, Han H, Hui A, Kohno T, Manoukian R, Whoriskey JS, Occia MA. Characterization of a new human B7-related protein: B7RP-1 is the ligand to the co-stimulatory protein ICOS. Int Immunol 2000; 12:1439–1447.

176. Dong C, Juedes AE, Temann UA, Shresta S, Allison JP, Ruddle NH, Flavell RA. ICOS co-stimulatory receptor is essential for T-cell activation and function. Nature 2001; 409:97–101.

177. Tamura H, Dong H, Zhu G, Sica GL, Flies DB, Tamada K, Chen L. B7-H1 costimulation preferentially enhances CD28-independent T-helper cell function. Blood 2001; 97:1809–1816.

178. Riley JL, Blair PJ, Musser JT, Abe R, Tezuka K, Tsuji T, June CH. ICOS costimulation requires IL-2 and can be prevented by CTLA-4 engagement. J Immunol 2001; 166:4943–4948.

179. Greenwald RJ, McAdam AJ, Van der Woude D, Satoskar AR, Sharpe AH. Cutting edge: inducible costimulator protein regulates both Th1 and Th2 responses to cutaneous leishmaniasis. J Immunol 2002; 168:991–995.

180. Dong C, Temann UA, Flavell RA. Cutting edge: critical role of inducible costimulator in germinal center reactions. J Immunol 2001; 166:3659–3662.

181. Rottman JB, Smith T, Tonra JR, Ganley K, Bloom T, Silva R, Pierce B, Gutierrez-Ramos JC, Ozkaynak E, Coyle AJ. The costimulatory molecule ICOS plays an important role in the immunopathogenesis of EAE. Nat Immunol 2001; 2:605–611.

182. Tamura H, Dong H, Zhu G, Sica GL, Flies DB, Tamada K, Chen L. B7-H1 costimulation preferentially enhances CD28-independent T-helper cell function. Blood 2001; 97:1809–1816.

183. Gonzalo JA, Delaney T, Corcoran J, Goodearl A, Gutierrez-Ramos JC, Coyle AJ. Cutting edge: the related molecules CD28 and inducible costimulator deliver both unique and complementary signals required for optimal T cell activation. J Immunol 2001; 166:1–5.

184. Ogawa S, Nagamatsu G, Watanabe M, Watanabe S, Hayashi T, Horita S, Nitta K, Nihei H, Tezuka K, Abe R. Opposing effects of anti-activation-inducible lymphocyte-immunomodulatory molecule/inducible costimulator antibody on the development of acute versus chronic graft-versus-host disease. J Immunol 2001; 167:5741–5748.

185. Taylor PA, Lees CJ, Noelle RJ, Yagita H, Killeen N, Sharpe AH, Blazar BR. Superior GVHD prevention by combined costimulatory blockade: comparison of single and combined blockade of CD28/CTLA4:B7, CD40L:CD40, and OX40:OX40L pathways. Blood. In press.

186. Tafuri A, Shahinian A, Bladt F, Yoshinaga SK, Jordana M, Wakeham A, Boucher LM, Bouchard D, Chan VS, Duncan G, Odermatt B, Ho A, Itie A, Horan T, Whoriskey JS, Pawson T, Penninger JM, Ohashi PS, Mak TW. ICOS is essential for effective T-helper-cell responses. Nature 2001; 409:105–109.

187. Ozkaynak E, Gao W, Shemmeri N, Wang C, Gutierrez-Ramos JC, Amaral J, Qin S, Rottman JB, Coyle AJ, Hancock WW. Importance of ICOS-B7RP-1 costimulation in acute and chronic allograft rejection. Nat Immunol 2001; 2:591–596.
188. Mauri DN, Ebner R, Montgomery RI, Kochel KD, Cheung TC, Yu GL, Ruben S, Murphy M, Eisenberg RJ, Cohen GH, Spear PG, Ware CF. LIGHT, a new member of the TNF superfamily, and lymphotoxin alpha are ligands for herpesvirus entry mediator. Immunity 1998; 8:21–30.
189. Zhai Y, Guo R, Hsu TL, Yu GL, Ni J, Kwon Bs, Jiang GW, Lu J, Tan J, Ugustus M, Carter K, Rojas L, Zhu F, Lincoln C, Endress G, Xing L, Wang S, Oh KO, Gentz R, Ruben S, Lippman ME, Hsieh SL, Yang D. LIGHT, a novel ligand for lymphotoxin beta receptor and TR2/HVEM induces apoptosis and suppresses in vivo tumor formation via gene transfer. J Clin Invest 1998; 102:1142–1151.
190. Harrop JA, McDonnell PC, Brigham-Burke M, Lyn SD, Minton J, Tan KB, Dede K, Spampanato J, Silverman C, Hensley P, DiPrinzio R, Emery JG, Deen K, Eichman C, Chabot-Fletcher M, Truneh A, Young PR. Herpesvirus entry mediator ligand (HVEM-L), a novel ligand for HVEM/Tr2, stimulates proliferation of T cells and inhibits HT29 cell growth. J Biol Chem 1998; 273:27548–27556.
191. Tamada K, Shimozaki K, Chapoval AI, Zhai Y, Su J, Chen SF, Hsieh SL, Nagata S, Ni J, Chen L. LIGHT, a TNF-like molecule, costimulates T cell proliferation and is required for dendritic cell-mediated allogeneic T cell response. J Immunol 2000; 164:4105–4110.
192. Kwon BS, Tan KB, Ni J, Oh KO, Lee ZH, Kim KK, Kim YJ, Wang S, Gentz R, Yu GL, Harrop J, Lyn SD, Silverman C, Porter TG, Truneh A, Young PR. A newly identified member of the tumor necrosis factor receptor superfamily with a wide tissue distribution and involvement in lymphocyte activation. J Biol Chem 1997; 272:14272–14276.
193. Browning JL, Sizing ID, Lawton P, Bourdon PR, Rennert PD, Majeau GR, Ambrose CM, Hession C, Miatkowski K, Griffiths DA, Ngam-ek A, Meier W, Benjamin CD, Hochman PS. Characterization of lymphotoxin-alpha beta complexes on the surface of mouse lymphocytes. J Immunol 1997; 159:3288–3298.
194. Yu KY, Kwon B, Ni J, Zhai Y, Ebner R, Kwon BS. A newly identified member of tumor necrosis factor receptor superfamily (TR6) suppresses LIGHT-mediated apoptosis. J Biol Chem 1999; 274:13733–13736.
195. Pitti RM, Marsters SA, Lawrence DA, Roy M, Kischkel FC, Dowd P, Huang A, Donahue CJ, Sherwood SW, Baldwin DT, Godowski PJ, Wood WI, Gurney AL, Hillan KJ, Cohen RL, Goddard AD, Botstein D, Ashkenazi A. Genomic amplification of a decoy receptor for Fas ligand in lung and colon cancer. Nature 1998; 396:699–703.
196. Tamada K, Shimozaki K, Chapoval AI, Zhu G, Sica G, Flies D, Boone T, Hsu H, Fu YX, Nagata S, Ni J, Chen L. Modulation of T-cell-mediated immunity in tumor and graft-versus-host disease models through the LIGHT co-stimulatory pathway. Nat Med 2000; 6:283–289.
197. Tamada K, Tamura H, Flies D, Fu YX, Celis E, Pease LR, Blazar BR, Chen L. Blockade of LIGHT/LTbeta and CD40 signaling induces allospecific T cell anergy, preventing graft-versus-host disease. J Clin Invest 2002; 109:549–557.
198. Durkop H, Latza U, Hummel M, Eitclbach F, Seed B, Stein H. Molecular cloning and expression of a new member of the nerve growth factor receptor family that is characteristic for Hodgkin's disease. Cell 1992; 68:421–427.
199. Bowen MA, Lee RK, Miragliotta G, Nam SY, Podack ER. Structure and expression of murine CD30 and its role in cytokine production. J Immunol 1996; 156:442–449.
200. Shanebeck KD, Maliszewski CR, Kennedy MK, Picha KS, Smith CA, Goodwin RG, Grabstein KH. Regulation of murine B cell growth and differentiation by CD30 ligand. Eur J Immunol 1995; 25:2147–2153.
201. Alzona M, Jack HM, Fisher RI, Ellis TM. CD30 defines a subset of activated human T cells that produce IFN-gamma and IL-5 and exhibit enhanced B cell helper activity. J Immunol 1994; 153:2861–2867.

202. Nakamura T, Lee RK, Nam SY, Al-Ramadi BK, Koni PA, Bottomly K, Podack ER, Flavell RA. Reciprocal regulation of CD30 expression on CD4+ T cells by IL-4 and IFN-gamma. J Immunol 1997; 158:2090–2098.

203. Harlin H, Podack E, Boothby M, Alegre ML. TCR-independent CD30 signaling selectively induces IL-13 production via a TNF receptor-associated factor/p38 mitogen-activated protein kinase-dependent mechanism. J Immunol 2002; 169:2451–2459.

204. Gilfillan MC, Noel PJ, Podack ER, Reiner SL, Thompson CB. Expression of the costimulatory receptor CD30 is regulated by both CD28 and cytokines. J Immunol 1998; 160:2180–2187.

205. Martinez OM, Villanueva J, Abtahi S, Beatty PR, Esquivel CO, Krams SM. CD30 expression identifies a functional alloreactive human T-lymphocyte subset. Transplantation 1998; 65:1240–1247.

206. Chan KW, Hopke CD, Krams SM, Martinez OM. CD30 expression identifies the predominant proliferating T lymphocyte population in human alloimmune responses. J Immunol 2002; 169:1784–1791.

207. Duckett CS, Thompson CB. CD30-dependent degradation of TRAF2: implications for negative regulation of TRAF signaling and the control of cell survival. Genes Dev 1997; 11:2810–2821.

208. Telford WG, Nam SY, Podack ER, Miller RA. CD30-regulated apoptosis in murine CD8 T cells after cessation of TCR signals. Cell Immunol 1997; 182:125–136.

209. Amakawa R, Hakem A, Kundig TM, Matsuyama T, Simard JJ, Timms E, Wakeham A, Mittruecker HW, Griesser H, Takimoto H, Schmits R, Shahinian A, Ohashi P, Penninger JM, Mak TW. Impaired negative selection of T cells in Hodgkin's disease antigen CD30-deficient mice. Cell 1996; 84:551–562.

210. Kurts C, Carbone FR, Krummel MF, Koch KM, Miller JF, Heath WR. Signalling through CD30 protects against autoimmune diabetes mediated by CD8 T cells. Nature 1999; 398:341–344.

211. Chiarle R, Podda A, Prolla G, Podack ER, Thorbecke GJ, Inghirami G. CD30 overexpression enhances negative selection in the thymus and mediates programmed cell death via a Bcl-2-sensitive pathway. J Immunol 1999; 163:194–205.

212. Shimozato O, Takeda K, Yagita H, Okumura K. Expression of CD30 ligand (CD153) on murine activated T cells. Biochem Biophys Res Commun 1999; 256:519–526.

213. Wiley SR, Goodwin RG, Smith CA. Reverse signaling via CD30 ligand. J Immunol 1996; 157:3635–3639.

214. Blazar BR, Levy RB, Mak TW, Panoskaltsis-Mortari A, Muta H, Jones M, Yagita H, Podack E, Taylor PA. CD30/CD30 ligand (CD153) interaction regulates CD4+ T cell-mediated graft-versus-host-disease (GVHD). Submitted.

215. Ishida Y, Agata Y, Shibahara K, Honjo T. Induced expression of PD-1, a novel member of the immunoglobulin gene superfamily, upon programmed cell death. EMBO J 1992; 11:3887–3895.

216. Shinohara T, Taniwaki M, Ishida Y, Kawaichi M, Honjo T. Structure and chromosomal localization of the human PD-1 gene (PDCD1). Genomics 1994; 23:704–706.

217. Agata Y, Kawasaki H, Nishimura H, Ishida Y, Tsubata T, Yagita H, Honjo T. Expression of the PD-1 antigen on the surface of stimulated mouse T and B lymphocytes. Int Immunol 1996; 8:765–772.

218. Nishimura H, Nose M, Hiai H, Minato N, Honjo T. Development of lupus-like autoimmune diseases by disruption of the PD-1 gene encoding an ITIM motif-carrying immunoreceptor. Immunity 1999; 11:141–151.

219. Dong H, Zhu G, Tamada K, Chen L. B7-H1, a third member of the B7 family, co-stimulates T cell proliferation and interleukin-10 secretion. Nature Medicine 1999; 5:1365–1369.

220. Freeman GJ, Long AJ, Iwaii Y, Bourque K, Chernova T, Nishimura H, Fitz LJ, Malenkovich N, Okazaki T, Byrne MC, Horton HF, Fouser L, Carter L, Ling V, Bowman MR, Carreno BM, Collins M, Wood CR, Honjo T. Engagement of the PD-1 immunoinhibitory receptor by a novel B7 family member leads to negative regulation of lymphocyte activation. J Exp Med 2000; 192:1027–1034.

221. Latchman Y, Wood C, Chernova T, Chaudhary D, Borde M, Chernova I Iwai Y, Long A, Brown J, Nunes R, Greenfield E, Bourque K, Boussiotis V, Carter L, Carreno B, Malenkovich N, Nishimura H, Honjo T, Freeman G, Sharpe A. PD-L2 is a second ligand for PD-1 and inhibits T cell activation. Nat Immunol 2001; 2:261–268.

222. Tseng SY, Otsuji M, Gorski K, Huang X, Slansky JE, Pai SI, Shalabi A, Shin T, Pardoll DM, Tsuchiya H. B7-DC, a new dendritic cell molecule with potent costimulatory properties for T cells. J Exp Med 2001; 193:839–846.

223. Kingsbury GA, Feeney LA, Nong Y, Calandra SA, Murphy CJ, Corcoran JM, Wang Y, Prabhu Das MR, Busfield SJ, Fraser CC, Villeval JL. Cloning, expression, and function of BLAME, a novel member of the CD2 family. J Immunol 2001; 166:5675–5680.

224. Vibhakar R, Juan G, Traganos F, Darzynkiewicz Z, Finger LR. Activation-induced expression of human programmed death-1 gene in T-lymphocytes. Exp Cell Res 1997; 232:25–28.

225. Coyle AJ, C G-RJ. The expanding B7 superfamily: increasing complexity in costimulatory signals regulating T cell function. Nat Immunol 2001; 2:203–209.

226. Shinohara T, Taniwaki M, Ishida Y, Kawaichi M, Honjo T. Structure and chromosomal localization of the human PD-1 gene (PPCP1). Genomics 1994; 23:704–706.

227. Vivier E, Daeron M. Immunoreceptor tyrosine-based inhibition motifs. Immunol Today 1997; 18:286–291.

228. Freeman G, Long A, Iwai Y, Bourque K, Chernova T, Nishimura H, Fitz L, Malenkovich N, Okazaki T, Byrne M, Horton H, Fouser L, Carter L, Ling V, Bowman M, Carreno B, Collins M, Wood C, Honjo T. Engagement of the PD-1 Immunoinhibitory receptor by a novel B7 family member leads to negative regulation of lymphocyte activation. J Exp Med 2000; 192:1–9.

229. Nishimura H, Minato N, Nakano T, Honjo T. Immunological studies on PD-1 deficient mice: implication of PD-1 as a negative regulator for B cell responses. Int Immunol 1998; 10:1563–1572.

230. Nishimura H, Okazaki T, Tanaka Y, Nakatani K, Hara M, Matsumori A, Sasayama S, Mizoguchi A, Hiai H, Minato N, Honjo T. Autoimmune dilated cardiomyopathy in PD-1 receptor deficient mice. Science 2001; 291;319–322.

231. Nishimura H, Nose M, Hiai H, Minato N, Honjo T. Development of lupus-like autoimmune diseases by disruption of the PD-1 gene encoding an ITIM motif-carrying immunoreceptor. Immunity 1999; 11:141–151.

232. Blazar BR, Carreno BM, Panoskaltsis-Mortari A, Carter L, Iwai Y, Yagita H, Nishimura H, Taylor PA. Blockade of programmed death-1 engagement accelerates graft-versus-host disease lethality by an IFN-gamma dependent mechanism. J Immunol 2003; 171:1272–1277.

233. Guinan EC, Boussiotis VA, Neuberg D, Brennan LL, Hirano N, Nadler LM, Gribben JG. Transplantation of anergic histoincompatible bone marrow allografts. N Engl J Med 1999; 340:1704–1714.

234. Boussiotis VA, Chen ZM, Zeller JC, Murphy WJ, Berezovskaya A, Narula S, Roncarolo MG, Blazar BR. Altered T-cell receptor + CD28-mediated signaling and blocked cell cycle progression in interleukin 10 and transforming growth factor-beta-treated alloreactive T cells that do not induce graft-versus-host disease. Blood 2001; 97:565–571.

235. Zeller JC, Panoskaltsis-Mortari A, Murphy WJ, Ruscetti FW, Narula S, Roncarolo MG, Blazar BR. Induction of CD4+ T cell alloantigen-specific hyporesponsiveness by IL-10 and TGF-beta. J Immunol 1999; 163:3684–3691.

236. Chen ZM, O'Shaughnessy MJ, Gramaglia I, Panoskaltsis-Mortari A, Murphy WJ, Narula S, Roncarolo MG, Blazar BR. IL-10 and TGF-{beta} induce alloreactive CD4+CD25− T cells to acquire regulatory cell function. Blood 2003.

237. Groux H, Bigler M, de Vries JE, Roncarolo MG. Interleukin-10 induces a long-term antigen-specific anergic state in human CD4+ T cells. J Exp Med 1996; 184:19–29.

238. Bacchetta R, Zappone E, Zino E, Fleischhauer K, Blazar B, Narula S, Bordignon C, Roncarolo MG. Use of IL-10 anergized T cells in haploidentical bone marrow transplantation. Blood 2000; 96:580a.

239. Battaglia M, Blazar BR, Roncarolo MG. The puzzling world of murine T regulatory cells. Microbes Infect 2002; 4:559–566.

240. Shevach EM, McHugh RS, Piccirillo CA, Thornton AM. Control of T-cell activation by CD4+CD25+ suppressor T cells. Immunol Rev 2001; 182:58–67.

241. Sakaguchi S, Sakaguchi N, Shimizu J, Yamazaki S, Sakihama T, Itoh M, Kuniyasu Y, Nomura T, Toda M, Takahashi T. Immunologic tolerance maintained by CD25+CD4+ regulatory T cells: their common role in controlling autoimmunity, tumor immunity, and transplantation tolerance. Immunol Rev 2001; 182:18–32.

242. Elewaut D, Kronenberg M. Molecular biology of NK T cell specificity and development. Semin Immunol 2000; 12:561–568.

243. Bendelac A, Rivera MN, Park SH, Roark JH. Mouse CD1-specific NK1 T cells: development, specificity, and function. Annu Rev Immunol 1997; 15:535–562.

244. Raulet DH, Vance RE, McMahon CW. Regulation of the natural killer cell receptor repertoire. Annu Rev Immunol 2001; 19:291–330.

245. Kawano T, Cui J, Koezuka Y, Toura I, Kaneko Y, Motoki K, Ueno H, Nakagawa R, Sato H, Kondo E, Koseki H, Taniguchi M. CD1d-restricted and TCR-mediated activation of valpha14 NKT cells by glycosylceramides. Science 1997; 278:1626–1629.

246. Burdin N, Brossay L, Koezuka Y, Smiley ST, Grusby MJ, Gui M, Taniguchi M, Hayakawa K, Kronenberg M. Selective ability of mouse CD1 to present glycolipids: alpha-galactosylceramide specifically stimulates V alpha 14 + NK T lymphocytes. J Immunol 1998; 161:3271–3281.

247. Sykes M, Hoyles KA, Romick ML, Sachs DH. In vitro and in vivo analysis of bone marrow-derived CD3+, CD4−, CD8−, NK1.1+ cell lines. Cell Immunol 1990; 129:478–493.

248. Zeng D, Lewis D, Dejbakhsh-Jones S, Lan F, Garcia-Ojeda M, Sibley R, Strober S. Bone marrow NK1.1(−) and NK1.1(+) T cells reciprocally regulate acute graft versus host disease. J Exp Med 1999; 189:1073–1081.

249. Zeng D, Gazit G, Dejbakhsh-Jones S, Balk SP, Snapper S, Taniguchi M, Strober S. Heterogeneity of NK1.1+ T cells in the bone marrow: divergence from the thymus. J Immunol 1999; 163:5338–5345.

250. Lan F, Zeng D, Higuchi M, Huie P, Higgins JP, Strober S. Predominance of NK1.1+ TCR alpha beta+ or DX5+TCR alpha beta+ T cells in mice conditioned with fractionated lymphoid irradiation protects against graft-versus-host disease: "natural suppressor" cells. J Immunol 2001; 167:2087–2096.

251. Bendelac A. Positive selection of mouse NK1+ T cells by CD1-expressing cortical thymocytes. J Exp Med 1995; 182:2091–2096.

252. Shevach EM. CD4+CD25+ suppressor T cells: more questions than answers. Nat Rev Immunol 2002; 2:389–400.

253. Shevach EM. Certified professionals: CD4(+)CD25(+) suppressor T cells. J Exp Med 2001; 193:F41–F46.

254. Levings MK, Sangregorio R, Roncarolo MG. Human cd25(+)cd4(+) t regulatory cells suppress naÿve and memory T cell proliferation and can be expanded in vitro without loss of function. J Exp Med 2001; 193:1295–1302.

255. Dieckmann D, Plottner H, Berchtold S, Berger T, Schuler G. Ex vivo isolation and characterization of CD4(+)CD25(+) T cells with regulatory properties from human blood. J Exp Med 2001; 193:1303–1310.

256. Jonuleit H, Schmitt E, Stassen M, Tuettenberg A, Knop J, Enk AH. Identification and functional characterization of human CD4(+)CD25(+) T cells with regulatory properties isolated from peripheral blood. J Exp Med 2001; 193:1285–1294.

257. Thornton AM, Shevach EM. CD4+CD25+ immunoregulatory T cells suppress polyclonal T cell activation in vitro by inhibiting interleukin 2 production. J Exp Med 1998; 188:287–296.

258. Suri-Payer E, Amar AZ, Thornton AM, Shevach EM. CD4+CD25+ T cells inhibit both the induction and effector function of autoreactive T cells land represent a unique lineage of immunoregulatory cells. J Immunol 1998; 160:1212–1218.

259. Sakaguchi S, Sakaguchi N, Asano M, Itoh M, Toda M. Immunologic self-tolerance maintained by activated T cells expressing IL-2 receptor alpha-chains (CD25). Breakdown of a single mechanism of self-tolerance causes various autoimmune diseases. J Immunol 1995; 155:1151–1164.

260. Baecher-Allan C, Brown JA, Freeman GJ, Hafler DA. CD4+CD25high regulatory cells in human peripheral blood. J Immunol 2001; 167:1245–1253.

261. Jonuleit H, Schmitt E, Kakirman H, Stassen M, Knop J, Enk AH. Infectious tolerance: human CD25(+) regulatory T cells convey suppressor activity to conventional CD4(+) T helper cells. J Exp Med 2002; 196:255–260.

262. Chatenoud L, Salomon B, Bluestone JA. Suppressor T cells—they're back and critical for regulation of autoimmunity! Immunol Rev 2001; 182:149–163.

263. Asano M, Toda M, Sakaguchi N, Sakaguchi S. Autoimmune disease as a consequence of developmental abnormality of a T cell subpopulation. J Exp Med 1996; 184:387–396.

264. Bonomo A, Kehn PJ, Payer E, Rizzo L, Cheever AW, Shevach EM. Pathogenesis of post-thymectomy autoimmunity. Role of syngeneic MLR-reactive T cells. J Immunol 1995; 154:6602–6611.

265. Suri-Payer E, Kehn PJ, Cheever AW, Shevach EM. Pathogenesis of post-thymectomy autoimmune gastritis. Identification of anti-H/K adenosine triphosphatase-reactive T cells. J Immunol 1996; 157:1799–1805.

266. Read S, Malmstrom V, Powrie F. Cytotoxic T lymphocyte-associated antigen 4 plays an essential role in the function of CD25(+)CD4(+) regulatory cells that control intestinal inflammation. J Exp Med 2000; 192:295–302.

267. Suzuki H, Kundig TM, Furlonger C, Wakeham A, Timms E, Matsuyama T, Schmits R, Simard JJ, Ohashi PS, Griesser H, et al. Deregulated T cell activation and autoimmunity in mice lacking interleukin-2 receptor beta. Science 1995; 268:1472–1476.

268. Willerford DM, Chen J, Ferry JA, Davidson L, Ma A, Alt FW. Interleukin-2 receptor alpha chain regulates the size and content of the peripheral lymphoid compartment. Immunity 1995; 3:521–530.

269. Takahashi T, Kuniyasu Y, Toda M, Sakaguchi N, Itoh M, Iwata M, Shimizu J, Sakaguchi S. Immunologic self-tolerance maintained by CD25+CD4+ natural anergic and suppressive T cells: induction of autoimmune disease by breaking their anergic/suppressive state. Int Immunol 1998; 10:1969–1980.

270. Taylor PA, Lees CJ, Blazar BR. The infusion of ex vivo activated and expanded CD4(+)CD25(+) immune regulatory cells inhibits graft-versus-host disease lethality. Blood 2002; 99:3493–3499.

271. Thornton AM, Shevach EM. Suppressor effector function of CD4+CD25+ immunoregulatory T cells is antigen nonspecific. J Immunol 2000; 164:183–190.

272. Lenardo MJ. Interleukin-2 programs mouse alpha beta T lymphocytes for apoptosis. Nature 1991; 353:858–861.

273. Cohen JL, Trenado A, Vasey D, Klatzmann D, Salomon BL. CD4(+)CD25(+) immunoregulatory T cells: new therapeutics for graft-versus-host disease. J Exp Med 2002; 196:401–406.

274. Hoffmann P, Ermann J, Edinger M, Fathman CG, Strober S. Donor-type CD4(+)CD25(+) regulatory T cells suppress lethal acute graft-versus-host disease after allogeneic bone marrow transplantation. J Exp Med 2002; 196:389–399.

275. Nakamura K, Kitani A, Strober W. Cell contact-dependent immunosuppression by CD4(+)CD25(+) regulatory T cells is mediated by cell surface-bound transforming growth factor beta. J Exp Med 2001; 194:629–644.

276. Piccirillo CA, Letterio JJ, Thornton AM, McHugh RS, Mamura M, Mizuhara H, Shevach EM. CD4(+)CD25(+) regulatory T cells can mediate suppressor function in the absence of transforming growth factor beta1 production and responsiveness. J Exp Med 2002; 196:237–246.

277. McHugh RS, Whitters MJ, Piccirillo CA, Young DA, Shevach EM, Collins M, Byrne MC. CD4(+)CD25(+) immunoregulatory T cells: gene expression analysis reveals a functional role for the glucocorticoid-induced TNF receptor. Immunity 2002; 16:311–323.

278. Shimizu J, Yamazaki S, Takahashi T, Ishida Y, Sakaguchi S. Stimulation of CD25(+)CD4(+) regulatory T cells through GITR breaks immunological self-tolerance. Nat Immunol 2002; 3:135–142.

279. Hori S, Nomura T, Sakaguchi S. Control of regulatory T cell development by the transcription factor Foxp3. Science 2003; 299:1057–1061.

280. Takahashi T, Tagami T, Yamazaki S, Uede T, Shimizu J, Sakaguchi N, Mak TW, Sakaguchi S. Immunologic self-tolerance maintained by CD25(+)CD4(+) regulatory T cells constitutively expressing cytotoxic T lymphocyte-associated antigen 4. J Exp Med 2000; 192:303–310.

281. Powrie F, Maloy KJ. Immunology. Regulating the regulators. Science 2003; 299:1030–1031.

282. Sakaguchi S. Control of immune responses by naturally arising CD4(+) regulatory T cells that express Toll-like receptors. J Exp Med 2003; 197:397–401.

283. Pasare C, Medzhitov R. Toll pathway-dependent blockade of CD4+CD25+ T cell-mediated suppression by dendritic cells. Science 2003; 299:1033–1036.

284. Caramalho I, Lopes-Carvalho T, Ostler D, Zelenay S, Haury M, Demengeot J. Regulatory T cells selectively express Toll-like receptors and are activated by lipopolysaccharide. J Exp Med 2003; 197:403–411.

285. Herve P, Wijdenes J, Bergerat JP, Bordigoni P, Milpied N, Cahn JY, Clement C, Beliard R, Morel-Fourrier B, Racadot E, et al. Treatment of corticosteroid resistant acute graft-versus-host disease by in vivo administration of anti-interleukin-2 receptor monoclonal antibody (B-B10). Blood 1990; 75:1017–1023.

286. Cuthbert RJ, Phillips GL, Barnett MJ, Nantel SH, Reece DE, Shepherd JD, Klingemann HG. Anti-interleukin-2 receptor monoclonal antibody (BT 563) in the treatment of severe acute GVHD refractory to systemic corticosteroid therapy. Bone Marrow Transplant 1992; 10:451–455.

287. Anasetti C, Hansen JA, Waldmann TA, Appelbaum FR, Davis J, Deeg HJ, Doney K, Martin PJ, Nash R, Storb R, et al. Treatment of acute graft-versus-host disease with humanized anti-Tac: an antibody that binds to the interleukin-2 receptor. Blood 1994; 84:1320–1327.

288. Przepiorka D, Kernan NA, Ippoliti C, Papadopoulos EB, Giralt S, Khouri I, Lu JG, Gajewski J, Durett A, Cleary K, Champlin R, Andersson BS, Light S. Daclizumab, a humanized anti-interleukin-2 receptor alpha chain antibody, for treatment of acute graft-versus-host disease. Blood 2000; 95:83–89.

289. Mavroudis DA, Jiang YZ, Hensel N, Lewalle P, Couriel D, Kreitman RJ, Pastan I, Barrett AJ. Specific depletion of alloreactivity against haplotype mismatched related individuals by a recombinant immunotoxin: a new approach to graft-versus-host disease prophylaxis in haploidentical bone marrow transplantation. Bone Marrow Transplant 1996; 17:793–799.

290. Fehse B, Goldmann M, Frerk O, Bulduk M, Zander AR. Depletion of alloreactive donor T cells using immunomagnetic cell selection. Bone Marrow Transplant 2000; 25(suppl) 2:S39–S42.

291. van Dijk AM, Kessler FL, Stadhouders-Keet SA, Verdonck LF, de Gast GC, Otten HG. Selective depletion of major and minor histocompatibility antigen reactive T cells: towards prevention of acute graft-versus-host disease. Br J Haematol 1999; 107:169–175.

292. Blaise D, Olive D, Hirn M, Viens P, Lafage M, Attal M, Stoppa AM, Gabert J, Gastaut JA, Camerlo J, et al. Prevention of acute GVHD by in vivo use of anti-interleukin-2 receptor monoclonal antibody (33B3.1): a feasibility trial in 15 patients. Bone Marrow Transplant 1991; 8:105–111.

293. Hanash A, Levy R. Donor CD4+CD25+ regulatory T-cells can support engraftment in the absence of GVHD during noon-myeloablative allogeneic murine bone marrow transplantation. Blood 2002; 100:213a.

294. Jones SC, Murphy GF, Korngold R. Post-hematopoietic cell transplant control of graft-versus-host disease by donor CD4+25+ T cells allow for an effective graft-versus-leukemia response. Biol Blood Marrow Transplant 2003; 9:243–256.

295. Edinger M, Hoffman P, Ermann J, Drago K, Beihack A, Fathman CG, Strober SS, Negrin RS. CD4+CD25+ regulatory T cells preserve graft-versus-tumor activity while inhibiting graft-versus-host disease after bone marrow transplantation. Nat Med 2003; 9:1144–1150.

296. Hoffman P, Edinger M, Negrin RS, Fathman CG, Strober S, Ermann J. CD4+CD25+ regulatory T cells act in secondary lymphoid organs to protect against lethal GVHD. Blood 2002; 100:143a.

5

Chemokines and Graft-vs.-Host Disease

KENNETH R. COOKE

University of Michigan Comprehensive Cancer Center, Ann Arbor, Michigan, U.S.A.

JON S. SERODY

University of North Carolina at Chapel Hill, Chapel Hill, North Carolina, U.S.A.

LISBETH A. WELNIAK and WILLIAM J. MURPHY

University of Nevada, Reno, Nevada, U.S.A.

I. INTRODUCTION

Graft-vs.-host disease (GVHD) is a complex process that affects multiple tissues and involves a variety of cell types in both its generation and subsequent pathological manifestations. At the core of GVHD is an immune response involving donor T cells and the genetically disparate recipient. From this seemingly simple immune interaction, the GVH response intensifies and ultimately involves a vast array of cellular effectors that are linked by the actions of immunoregulatory cytokines. Chemokines, a subset of cytokines traditionally defined by their ability to mediate immune cell chemotaxis, may contribute to this process. Our understanding of chemokine biology has expanded from considering these molecules solely as promoters of chemotaxis to factors that can affect leukocyte activation and differentiation during an emerging immune response. Our ability to delineate the precise role(s) of chemokines in a GVH response is hampered by the pleotropic effects these molecules have and by the differences that exist in the animal models used to study GVHD. This review will attempt to survey and reconcile the sometimes contradictory literature in this area of research, at times drawing on studies that have examined the role of chemokines in other models of transplantation and disease. Importantly, since hematopoietic stem cell transplantation (SCT) is often used as a treatment for cancer, assessing the role of chemokines in tumor progression as well as GVHD may provide insight as to how the function of chemokines may be exploited to provide maximal therapeutic benefit after SCT.

II. THE CHANGING PARADIGM OF GVHD AND ITS STUDY

In order to assess the role of a particular cytokine or chemokine in the development of GVHD, the model used must accurately reflect the disease. Unfortunately, the clinical spectrum of GVHD has changed in recent years and is significantly influenced by the use of reduced-intensity conditioning regimens and the administration of donor leukocyte infusions (DLI). Furthermore, the development of animal models that employ a variety of endpoints to study the pathogenesis of GVHD has made the evaluation and comparison of data from different laboratories challenging at times. Although the GVH reaction is still initiated by the interaction between donor T cells and host antigen-presenting cells (APCs) in each scenario, modification of several other parameters can significantly influence the role a particular cytokine or chemokine has in the evolution of GVHD. In this light, several key factors must be considered when comparing data generated from the various in vivo models used to study this process.

The intensity of conditioning that is applied prior to SCT is one of the most important variables to consider. The majority of animal models use some degree of total body irradiation (TBI). TBI serves at least two important functions: it reduces (or ablates) host hematopoiesis and immunosuppresses the recipient to facilitate the engraftment of donor stem cells. Administration of "lethal" conditioning results in death from hematopoietic failure if the recipient is not given a SCT, whereas host hematopoiesis recovers (and may in fact be a target of the GVH response) when "sublethal" conditioning is applied. Several studies have clarified, however, that intense conditioning results in much more than immunosuppression; a plethora of inflammatory cytokines, including tumor necrosis factor (TNF)-α, interferon (IFN)-γ, interleukin (IL)-1 and IL-6, is released from the diffuse, nonspecific damage that occurs to host tissues. The tissues affected by SCT conditioning, notably the gut, are weakened and primed for eventual immune attack. Alteration of TBI intensity directly correlates with the extent of intestinal injury, the degree of macrophage priming, and the severity of systemic GVHD that occurs after allogeneic SCT (1). Subsequent inflammatory cytokine release and tissue destruction result in GVHD pathology and kinetics similar to that seen after conventional clinical SCT conditioning. Cytokines such as TNF-α directly upregulate chemokine expression (2–4) and therefore represent a link between the inflammatory signals induced by conditioning and enhanced chemokine expression observed after SCT. By contrast, some murine GVHD models use sublethal conditioning regimens or no conditioning whatsoever. These models do not include a SCT but instead involve the transfer of large number of donor T cells or splenocytes. Obviously, the kinetics and pathology of GVHD can be significantly altered in this scenario. Since chemokines can be upregulated by inflammatory cytokine release, the expression of chemokines and their specific contribution to the development of GVHD after SCT with low or absent conditioning may also be greatly affected.

The extent to which inbred mice used for SCT experiments are genetically "matched" or "mismatched" is another important variable that affects the kinetics of GVHD induction and the ultimate severity of disease. The degree of antigenic disparity between donor and host can range from totally allogeneic (complete MHC mismatch) to differences at MHC class I or class II only, to strain combinations that are MHC matched but differ at multiple minor antigens and perhaps most closely reflect the situation that exists in a matched unrelated donor SCT in the clinical setting. In addition, other models utilize a haploidentical "parent into F1" system that is unidirectional with regard to T-cell recognition. Other variables in GVHD models include the amount and purity of donor T cells administered, the presence of subclinical infections in the mouse colony (i.e., heliobacter, parvovirus), and the presence of tumors when graft-vs.-tumor (GVT) effects are evaluated in the context of GVHD. Ultimately, all of these variables need to be considered when attempting to reconcile the literature on chemokines and GVHD; a specific chemokine may have one effect in a lethal TBI model of GVHD and the opposite effect in a model using no conditioning.

III. CHEMOKINES AND THE PATHOGENESIS OF ACUTE GVHD

A. GVHD Pathophysiology

The pathophysiology of GVHD is complex and involves aspects of the adaptive and the innate immune responses. GVHD can occur in acute or chronic forms that differ in their kinetics, pathophysiology, and underlying immune mechanisms (see also Chapters 1, 2, and 20). Clinical and experimental data demonstrate that GVHD target organs are vulnerable to injury from both soluble and cellular effectors. The GI tract is critical to the propagation of early inflammatory events that are the hallmark of acute GVHD, and it is also the target of an immunological feedback loop involving synergistic interactions between cells of lymphoid and myeloid lineages (5,6). Infiltrating alloreactive lymphocytes not only contribute to mucosal damage, which facilitates the translocation of lipopolysaccharide (LPS) into the systemic circulation, but also produce IFN-γ, which greatly enhances the sensitivity of mononuclear cells to LPS stimulation (5). When triggered by LPS, IFN-γ-"primed" mononuclear cells release cytopathic amounts of TNF-α and other cytokines that exacerbate intestinal injury and increase mucosal permeability to LPS (7). These early events create a systemic pro-inflammatory environment that directly enhances chemokine expression in target organs (8) and may therefore contribute to the recruitment of donor derived T cells, monocytes/macrophages, and neutrophils to sites of inflammation.

Th1/Th1 T-cell effectors present in host target tissue contribute to tissue damage by direct cytotoxic killing via either the perforin-granzyme or the Fas-Fas ligand (FasL) pathway. T cells utilizing the Fas-FasL pathway are critical to the damage of host hematopoietic cells, skin, liver, and lung during GVHD (9–13), whereas cytotoxic T-lymphocyte (CTL) activity mediated by perforin contributes to GVHD-associated cachexia and the kinetics of systemic disease severity (14,15). The role of monocytes and neutrophils appears directly related to the effects of both TNF-α and LPS, two inflammatory mediators that can greatly enhance chemokine production. The responsiveness of donor accessory cells to LPS stimulation has been shown to predict the severity of experimental GVHD (7,16). Furthermore, the presence of donor-derived, TNF-α-producing, CD14+ cells in the peripheral blood correlates directly with the development of grade II–IV GI GVHD after clinical SCT; the number of these cells is significantly increased at disease onset and returns to baseline after successful treatment (D. Fowler, personal communication).

If the development of GVHD is divided into discrete stages, it is relatively easy to speculate where chemokines may play a role in the evolution of this disease. The first stage of GVHD involves the effects of SCT conditioning regimens on host tissues. Stage 2 focuses upon the recognition of host antigens by donor T cells. Data suggest that host APCs play an important role in this initial response (17). The alloantigen-specific donor T-cell clones expand, migrate to GVHD target organs, and ultimately secrete cytokines (and

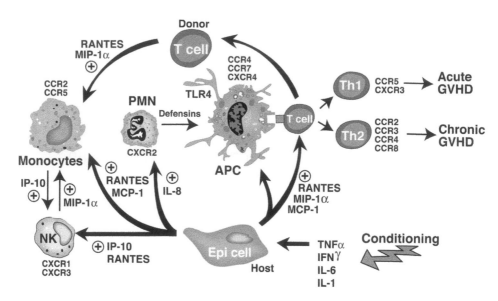

Figure 1 Chemokine cascades after SCT: Chemokines are pleiotropic cytokines that can function in many aspects of GVHD pathophysiology. SCT preparative regimens cause diffuse injury to a variety of tissues and induce pro-inflammatory cytokine secretion that upregulates chemokine expression. This proinflammatory environment enhances the ability of host antigen-presenting cells (APC) to interact with mature donor T cells by (1) enhancing APC maturation, (2) facilitating the migration of APC to secondary lymphoid tissue (via upregulation of CCR7, CCR4, and CXCR4), and (3) upregulating MHC, adhesion, and costimulatory molecules. Once engaged, donor T cells become activated and differentiate into T1 (acute) or T2 (chronic) GVHD effector cells and preferentially express specific chemokine receptors. Thus, the expression of the cognate ligands for these receptors may result in different outcomes in chronic or acute GVHD. Chemokines including MIP-1α, RANTES, and MCP-1 can have a direct effect on APC : T-cell interactions and along with IP-10 and IL-8 can affect the activation, recruitment, and function of other immune cell types including monocytes, NK cells, and neutrophils. A growing amount of data supports the interplay between the adaptive and innate immune responses during GVHD. Not only are monocytes and macrophages "primed" by T-cell–generated IFN-γ to secrete cytopathic cytokines during the effector phase of GVHD, but neutrophils may contribute to T-cell activation via the release of defensins, which, via Toll-like receptors, can affect APC maturation and function.

presumably chemokines) that recruit other cells, including granulocytes, natural killer (NK) cells, and monocytes to these sites. Inflammatory cytokine release, in combination with direct cell-mediated killing, contributes to the third and final effector phase of GVHD that culminates in target tissue injury and dysfunction (Fig. 1). It is reasonable to assume that chemokines may potentially play a role in all of these stages.

B. Chemokine Biology

Although the role of cellular effectors in the development of GVHD is clear, the mechanisms by which activated white blood cells (WBCs) traffic to target organs and cause inflammation after allogeneic SCT remain unresolved. Leukocyte trafficking to sites of inflammation is a complex process involving interactions between WBCs and endothelial cells that is facilitated by adhesion molecules, chemoattractants, and their receptors (18). Chemoattractants are fundamental to leukocyte migration, and chemokines are an important subset of these regulatory proteins; substantial evidence suggests that the accumulation of various effector cells within inflamed tissue is a dynamic process orchestrated by the regulated expression of chemokines and their receptors. Chemokines (a hybrid of "chemotactic cytokines") are a large family of 8–10 kDa polypeptide molecules that regulate many aspects of the immune response. Chemokines have well-defined roles in directing the movements of lymphocytes, monocytes, and neutrophils directly via their chemoattractant properties (i.e., by providing "directional clues") and indirectly via integrin activation (19). Like cytokines, a chemokine response (a) can be elicited by nearly any stimulus that disrupts immunological homeostasis and (b) results in a robust recruitment of inflammatory cells. When that stimulus is potent and long lasting, an injurious rather than protective chemokine response may ensue and foster progressive leukocyte-mediated tissue damage and organ dysfunction.

Although originally defined by their ability to control leukocyte chemotaxis (19,20), chemokines can also regulate the differentiation (Th1 and Th2) of effector T-cell subsets and the activation status of myeloid cells (21). In each case, chemokines can have both inductive and repressive effects. Thus, cellular responsiveness to chemoattractant signals can be tightly coupled to signals that regulate cell activation or differentiation (19,20). The 50+ chemokines (Table 1) that have been identified to date are classified structurally into four main groups according to the configuration of cysteine residues near the NH_2 terminus (CC, CXC, C, and CX_3C). The CC, or "αchemokines," and CXC, or "β chemokines," are the two largest subsets (19), and members of each will be the primary focus of this chapter. CC chemokines have either four or six cysteines in highly conserved positions where the first two cysteines are juxtaposed, whereas the CXC chemokines are characterized by four cysteine residues at the N terminus, the first two of which are separated by a nonconserved amino acid (20). CXC chemokines are classified further by the presence or the absence of the AA sequence glutamic acid–leucine–arginine (the ELR motif) that immediately precedes the CXC sequence. ELR+ chemokines have been shown to promote angiogenesis, whereas ELR- chemokines inhibit it (22). Nearly all of the known ELR-CXC chemokines also promote neutrophil chemotaxis (22).

Actions of chemokines are mediated through a large family of seven-trans-membrane-spanning, serpentine, G-protein–coupled receptors. To date, approximately 20 chemokine receptors have been identified (Table 1). Each receptor has ligand specificity and a restricted expression on subclasses of leukocytes. However, ligand specificities can overlap; some chemokines bind to several receptors, and some receptors bind multiple ligands (23). Chemokines and their receptors can be functionally divided into two broad categories. Inducible or inflammatory chemokines, which are regulated by pro-inflammatory stimuli, help orchestrate innate and adaptive immunity and recruit leukocytes to sites of inflammation in response to physiological stress. Constitutive or homeostatic chemokines are responsible for basal leukocyte migration during immune surveillance and formation of the architectural framework of secondary lymphoid organs. Inducible or inflammatory chemokines classically include RANTES (CCL5), MIP-1α (CCL3), IP-10 (CXCL10), Mig (CXCL9), I-TAC (CXCL11), MCP-1 (CCL2), and KC/ MIP2 (CXCL2), are produced by a variety of cell types, and are induced to high levels of expression by inflammatory stimuli such as LPS, IL-1, and TNF-α (18). The corresponding inflammatory chemokine receptors include CCR5, CCR1, CXCR3, CCR2, and CXCR2. Generally, these receptors have more promiscuous or redundant ligand binding interactions compared to homeostatic receptors and tend to be expressed on cells

Table 1   Chemokine Superfamily

Chemokine	Human ligand and alternate names	Mouse ligand and alternate names	Receptor
C family			
XCL1	Lymphotactinα, SCM-1α, ATAC	Lymphotactin	XCR1
XCL2	Lymphotactinβ		XCR1
CC family			
CCL1	I-309	TCA-3	CCR8
CCL2	MCP-1, MCAF	JE?	CCR2
CCL3	MIP-1α, LD78α	MIP-1α	CCR1, 5
CCL4	MIP-1β	MIP-1β	CCR5, 8
CCL5	RANTES	RANTES	CCR1, 3, 5
CCL6		C10, MRP-1	Unknown
CCL7	MCP-3, FIC, MARC	MARC?	CCR1, 2, 3
CCL8	MCP-2, HC-14	MCP-2?	CCR1, 2, 3, 5
CCL9/10		MRP-2, MIP-1γ	CCR1
CCL11	Eotaxin	Eotaxin	CCR3
CCL12		MCP-5	CCR2
CCL13	MCP-4		CCR1, 2, 3
CCL14	HCC-1		CCR11, 5
CCL15	HCC-2, lkn-1, MIP-5, MIP-1δ		CCR1, 3
CCL16	HCC-4, monotactin-1, LEC		CCR1
CCL17	TARC, ABCD-2	TARC, ABCD-2	CCR4, 8
CCL18	PARC, DC-CK-1, MIP-4		Unknown
CCL19	MIP-3β, ELC, exodus-3, ckβ11	MIP-3β, ELC	CCR7
CCL20	MIP-3α, LARC, exodus-1	MIP-3α, LARC	CCR6
CCL21	6ckine, SLC, exodus-2	6ckine, SLC	CCR7, CXCR3
CCL22	MDC, ABCD-1, Dctactin-1	MDC, ABCD-1	CCR4
CCL23	MPIF-1, ckβ8		CCR1
CCL24	eotaxin-2, MPIF-2, ckβ6	MPIF-2	CCR3
CCL25	TECK	TECK	CCR9
CCL26	Eotaxin-3, MIP-4α		CCR3, 10
CCL27	CTACK, Eskine	CTACK, ALP	CCR10
CCL28	MEC	CCL28/MEC	CCR10
CXC family			
CXCL1	Groα, MGSA-α	N51/KC, MIP-2	CXCR2 > 1
CXCL2	Groβ, MIP-2α	Gro/KC	CXCR2
CXCL3	Groγ, MIP-2β	Gro/KC	CXCR2
CXCL4	Platelet factor-4		Unknown
CXCL5	ENA-78, AMCF-11	GCP-2, LIX?	CXCR2
CXCL6	GCP-2, Ckβ3	GCP-2, LIX?	CXCR1, 2
CXCL7	PBP, CTAP-III, β-TG, NAP-2		CXCR2
CXCL8	IL-8		CXCR1, 2
CXCL9	Mig	Mig	CXCR3
CXCL10	IP-10	CRG-2, IP-10	CXCR3
CXCL11	I-TAC	I-TAC	CXCR3
CXCL12	SDF-1α, SDF-1βPBSF	SDF-1α, SDF-1β	CXCR4
CSCL13	BCA-1, BLC	BLC	CXCR5

Table 1 Continued

Chemokine	Human ligand and alternate names	Mouse ligand and alternate names	Receptor
CXCL14	BRAK, BMAC	BRAK, BMAC	Unknown
CXCL15		Lungkine	Unknown
CXCL16	CXCL16	CXCL16	CXCR6
CX$_3$C family			
CX$_3$CL1	Fractalkine, ABCD-3	Neurotactin	CX3CR1

with an effector phenotype. Although simplistic, the functional division provides insight into how specific chemokine interactions orchestrate leukocyte movements during development, how they orchestrate antigen-driven differentiation and migration to sites of inflammation, and how they ultimately contribute to disease (24).

To date, the study of chemokine biology has largely focused on the correlation of protein or mRNA levels with a functional event, the administration of neutralizing antibodies in vivo and in vitro, or the use of genetically targeted knockout mice that lack a particular chemokine or receptor. All of these approaches have advantages and disadvantages. Surprisingly, despite the very nature of GVHD lending itself as a prime candidate disease for the study of chemokines, very little work has actually been published in this area (Table 2). A significant amount of data using chemokine-neutralizing antibodies and knockout mice has, however, been generated using either solid organ transplantation (skin, trachea, and cardiac) or infectious disease models. These models, while different from those used to study GVHD, may still provide insight into how chemokines may affect GVH reactions.

IV. CHEMOKINES AND LEUKOCYTE TRAFFICKING DURING GVHD

A. Stem Cell Homing

The success of hematopoietic SCT fundamentally depends upon the ability of the transplanted donor stem cells to home to the bone marrow microenvironment and recapitulate the hematopoietic and peripheral immune elements of the recipient. Homing is a complex process that involves (a) the migration of hematopoietic stem cells (HSC) through the bone marrow vascular endothelium followed by (b) the localization into the appropriate stem cell "niche," which is facilitated by adhesive interactions with the bone marrow stroma and extracellular matrix. Although some of the components responsible for stem cell homing have been elucidated, the overall process remains poorly understood.

Pertinent to this chapter, interactions between CXCR4 and its primary ligand, SDF-1α (CXCL12), may significantly contribute to HSC homing and engraftment (25). CXCR4 is expressed on HSC, and SDF-1α is a chemoattractant for HSC in vitro (26). SDF-1α upregulates surface adhesion molecules that are critical to the arrest and transmigration of CD34+ cells through vascular endothelial cells (27,28). Moreover, animals lacking SDF-1α or CXCR4 do not successfully transition from fetal liver to bone marrow hematopoiesis and die in the perinatal period (29). Recent studies that have focused upon mechanisms of chemokine receptor ligand interactions in stem cells homing have also underscored the

Table 2   Murine GVHD Models and Chemokine Assessment

Strain	Conditioning	Cells transferred	Organ pathology	Chemokine role in GVHD
B6 → bm1 [CD8]	6 Gy	Purified T cells or splenocytes	(acute) Liver, gut, skin, lungs	T cells; MIP-1α KO protect from CD8-mediated disease
B6 → bm12 [CD4]				
B6 → B6D2F1	None	Splenocytes	(acute) Liver	CCR5 antibodies protect
B6 → B6D2F1	None	Splenocytes	(acute) Liver	CCR5-deficient donor cell protect
B6 → BALB/c (major and minor MHC mismatch)	Lethal TBI (8–10 Gy)	Splenocytes	(acute) Liver, gut, skin	CCR5-deficient donor cell accelerate disease and C cell expansion
B10 → B10.BR (major MHC mismatch)				
DBA/2 → B6D2F1	None	Splenocytes	(chronic) Host B-cell expansion and autoantibody production	CCL21 antagonism protect
B10.D2 → BALB/c	Lethal TBI (7 Gy)	Splenocytes	(chronic) Skin	Elevated MCP-1, MIP-1 situ

role of SDF-1α in this process (30,31). Adams and colleagues found that co-infused CD8+ T cells augment CD34+ cell homing to the bone marrow by altering the phosphotyrosine-mediated signaling of CD34+ cells in response to SDF-1α (31). Furthermore, Christopherson et al. demonstrated that cleavage of the N-terminus region of SDF-1α by the membrane-bound peptidase CD26/dipeptidylpeptidase IV may represent a novel regulatory mechanism in the migration, homing, and mobilization of HSC (30).

The role SDF-1α/CXCR4 interactions in HSC homing has been challenged by data demonstrating that CXCR4−/− fetal liver cells can home and engraft in the BM compartment of wild-type mice (32) and specific inhibitors of CXCR4 function do not significantly disrupt HSC engraftment (33). These findings suggest that SDF-1α/CXCR4 interactions may act in conjunction with other factors to facilitate HSC homing and engraftment. In this context, other candidate molecules that many compensate for SDF-1α/CXCR4 include CCL25 (TECK), via its interactions with CCR9, and any of the ligands of CCR3 since mRNA for CCR3 and CCR9 is expressed on purified HSC (34). However, the role of CCR3 and CCR9 receptors in HSC homing has yet to be fully elucidated; HSC fail to migrate to the ligands for these receptors, and it is not known if these receptors are constitutively expressed (34).

Once HSC have successfully homed to the bone marrow microenvironment, they must begin the processes of self-renewal and lineage specific repopulation of the host bone marrow and peripheral blood. As hematopoietic precursors mature and become more restricted in proliferative and lineage potential, there is a differential expression of chemokine receptors on the cell surface. In this context, CXCR4 expression is again important and has been shown to regulate the retention of granulocyte precursors in the bone marrow (32). The inflammatory processes of GVHD can suppress myelopoiesis directly through production of inflammatory cytokines and through induction of chemokines, many of which can inhibit proliferation of myeloid progenitors (35–38). Furthermore, although "mature" donor T cells contaminating the stem cell inoculum are responsible for initiating the GVH response, marrow-derived donor cells of the myeloid lineage also have a significant role in systemic inflammation and target tissue injury from GVHD. Recent data suggest that the effector functions of myeloid and lymphoid cells synergize to cause target organ damage (39), and the contribution of donor myeloid or "accessory" cells consists primarily of the secretion of inflammatory cytokines and chemokines (7,39). Thus, the effects of chemokines on hematopoietic reconstitution may influence SCT outcomes via both GVHD-independent and -dependent mechanisms.

B.   Antigen Presentation and T-Cell Activation

The second stage of GVHD is fundamentally dependent upon the recognition of host alloantigens by donor T cells. Recent data suggest that chemokines play a direct role in this complex set of interactions and may therefore have profound effects on GVHD during the initiation phase of this process. For example, the pro-inflammatory environment established early after SCT can facilitate the maturation of host dendritic cells (DCs) or APCs. DC maturation results in complete reprogramming of the cell with down-regulation of endocytic activity and upregulation of MHC, adhesion and co-stimulatory molecules. In addition, a switch in chemokine receptor usage occurs involving the downregulation of "inflammatory" chemokine receptors and an upregulation of receptors for "lymphoid" chemokines such as CXCR4, CCR4, and CCR7. This pivotal switch makes the DCs more sensitive to the CCR7 ligands SLC and ELC (expressed by lymphatic endothelial cells and in T-cell zones of lymphoid organs) and guides the recently matured DCs from the site of antigen capture back to the lymph node or site of antigen presentation (40). Recent studies suggest that CCR7 may be necessary for an optimal alloimmune response. CCR7 KO mice have delayed T- and B-cell responses, and the mice have severe defects in their lymphoid architecture (41).

Data also suggest that chemokines may contribute to donor T-cell activation and differentiation. Chemokines such as CXCL12 (SDF-1α) have also been shown to promote CD4+ T-cell responses (42), and recent studies suggest that T-cell clones can be directly stimulated by RANTES (CCL5) and other chemokines in vitro (43–45). Specifically, RANTES and MIP-1α play a significant role in the polyclonal as well as antigen-specific activation of helper and cytotoxic T cells and can upregulate APC functions (44). Additional studies using knock-out mice have underscored the importance of RANTES for the generation of optimal T-cell responses (46). MIP-1α may also have a direct effect on T-cell differentiation; addition of MIP-1α to antigen or anti-TCR stimulated T cells in vitro results in the generation of IFN-γ–producing cells via a mechanism independent of IFN-γ or IL-12 (21). Consistent with this finding, polyclonal activation of T cells from MIP-1α–deficient mice produce 50% less IFN-γ compared to wild-type (wt) controls (21).

MCP-1 is also known to have a significant role in T-cell polarization. Specifically, MCP-1 has been shown to contribute to the development of Th2 responses and may do so by decreasing IL-12 and enhancing IL-4 production (21). Administration of MCP-1 during CD4+ T-cell activation via either antigen-pulsed APCs or TCR cross-linking leads to increased IL-4 but not IFN-γ secretion (47). Consistent with this result, MCP-1$-/-$ mice have diminished T-cell responses, are functionally Th2 deficient, and are resistant to lethal infection by *Leishmania major* (48). However, using an in vitro system with DNA immunogen constructs, Kim and coworkers generated contrasting data; MCP-1 was determined to be a potent activator of CD8+ CTL activity, a finding associated with the increased expression of IFN-γ and TNF-α (49).

Chemokines have also been shown to directly affect the activation and function of other immune cells types (i.e., NK cells, monocytes, neutrophils) that are operative during the effector phase of GVHD. Chemokines such as MIP-1α (CCL3), IP-10 (CXCL10), RANTES (CCL5), and MCP-1 (CCL2) can increase NK cell activity (50–52), and IL-8 (CXCL8) is known to enhance neutrophil degranulation (53,54). Furthermore, chemokines known as defensins, via interactions with Toll-like receptors, can enhance dendritic cell maturation and function and thereby directly affect T-cell–mediated immune responses (55)

C. Cellular Recruitment to GVHD Target Organs

1. Overview

The regulation of leukocyte migration into target tissues during the development of GVHD occurs in a complex milieu of chemotactic signals where several chemokine receptors may be triggered simultaneously or consecutively. Resident epithelial cells and macrophages that are present in organs such as the gut, lung, and liver possess significant chemokine-producing capability that likely contribute to the mucosal, peri-bronchiolar, and bile duct–associated inflammation observed during GVHD. Because of their positive charge, secreted chemokines bind to extracellular matrix and cell surface heparin sulfate proteoglycans and are retained locally, thereby establishing a concentration gradient around the inflammatory stimulus and on the surface of the overlying endothelium (56). The migrating leukocyte must therefore distinguish between a hierarchy of signals within the tissue in order to successfully reach the site of inflammation. Chemokine receptors are differentially expressed on subsets of activated/effector T cells, and upon stimulation T cells can rapidly switch chemokine receptor expression, acquiring new migratory capacity (57,58). Thus, despite the relative paucity of published data regarding the role of chemokines in the development of GVHD, it is quite likely that these molecules and their respective receptors significantly contribute to target organ injury that occurs in this proinflammatory disorder. The remainder of this section will focus on specific "inflammatory" chemokine receptor: ligand interactions and their potential contribution to the recruitment of T-cell effectors, monocytes, and neutrophils to GVHD target tissues after allogeneic SCT.

2. Recruitment of T-Cell Effectors

Once activated, allospecific T-cell clones differentiate and subsequently migrate to GVHD target tissue, where they significantly contribute to target tissue injury and facilitate the recruitment of other cellular effectors. Effector T cells are characterized by their responsiveness to numerous inflammatory chemokines produced at the site of tissue injury. Under conditions of stress or antigen challenge, most inflammatory chemokines are upregulated in nonlymphoid tissue and facilitate the recruitment of effector T cells that are typically activated. The cell surface receptors that bind the inflammatory chemokine ligands are upregulated on newly generated effector T cells in secondary lymphoid organs. In vitro studies have demonstrated that receptor expression and response to inflammatory chemokines are very dependent on IL-2, a cytokine that links the acquisition of migratory responsiveness to T-cell expansion (59). "Tissue-specific" recruitment and retention of activated lymphocytes enhance the likelihood that antigen-specific lymphocytes will encounter their cognate antigen and reduce the exposure of an expanded, activated lymphocyte population to potentially cross-reactive antigens in other tissues.

Both CXCR3 and CCR5 appear to mark a subset of T cells with the capacity to migrate to sites of inflammation; both are expressed on a high proportion of T cells associated within inflammatory lesions compared to T cells in the peripheral blood or lymph node (60,61). CXCR3+ and CCR5+ T cells in the blood generally have a phenotype consistent with previous activation: $\beta_1$integrin^{hi}, CD45RO+, and CD45RA^{low}. Similarly, after alloantigen stimulation in an MLR, CD4+ T cells with an activated phenotype (CD45RO+, CD45RA−, CD69+, CD25+) upregulate CXCR3 (62). Although CXCR3 and CCR5 can be expressed on both Th1 and Th2 effectors, the expression of each is believed to be more of a marker for Th1 cells (60) (Fig. 1), whereas Th2 cells preferentially express CCR3, CCR4, and CCR8. Immunohistochemical staining of inflamed tissues from patients with rheumatoid arthritis and multiple sclerosis (two Th1 diseases) demonstrated that virtually all infiltrating cells express CCR5 and CXCR3 (63). These findings suggest that CXCR3 and CCR5 are not only markers for T cells associated with certain Th1 inflammatory responses, but also appear to identify subsets of T cells with a predilection for homing to these corresponding sites of inflammation (60). Since much recent data suggest that the effector T cells that contribute to acute GVHD are primarily of the T1 phenotype, the potential contribution of CXCR3 and CCR5 expression to the development of the GVH response will be discussed in detail.

Receptor : Ligand Interactions Involving CXCR3 with Mig (CXCL9), IP-10 (CXCL10), and I-TAC (CXCL11). Effector T cells that are involved in the development of acute GVHD are believed to be primarily of the T1 phenotype; therefore, the potential contribution of CXCR3- and CCR5-expressing lymphocytes will be discussed in detail. CXCR3 is highly expressed on activated T cells and is believed to be critical to the recruitment of these cells to sites of inflammation and allograft rejection (60,64–66). It is also found on a proportion of circulating NK cells but not on monocytes, neutrophils, or resting T cells (60). CXCR3 mediates chemotaxis in response to its ligands IP-10 (IFN-γ–inducible protein-10), Mig (monokine induced by IFN-γ), and I-TAC (IFN-inducible T-cell α chemoattractant), and is not known to recognize other CXC or CC chemokines. Conversely, Mig, IP-10, and I-TAC are CXC chemokines that are potent chemoattractants for activated T cells (67–69). Each can be produced by endothelium, macrophages, and neutrophils (64), and, as their names imply, the expression of each is enhanced by IFN-γ.

A significant role for CXCR3 and its ligands has been demonstrated in models of solid organ transplantation. For example, Mig expression appears to significantly contribute to skin allograft rejection; administration of Mig antibodies to recipients of MHC class II, but not class I disparate skin grafts prevents T-cell infiltration resulting in long-term allograft survival (70). Furthermore, the administration of rMig directly to the skin graft can overcome the inability of alloantigen-primed T cells from IFN-γ−/− recipients to cause acute rejection (70). The expression of CXCR3 and its ligands has also been shown to contribute to the development of cardiac allograft vasculopathy and rejection in both clinical and preclinical studies (64–66,71). In a fully mismatched mouse model, Hancock and colleagues showed progressive intragraft mRNA expression of CXCR3 along with IP-10, Mig, and I-TAC in the days leading up to end-stage rejection (65). Use of CXCR3$-/-$ mice as recipients resulted in a significant improvement in allograft survival. By day 7, CXCR3$-/-$ recipients had a decreased number of infiltrating CD4+, CD8+ cells, a reduced infiltration of macrophages, and the absence of CD25+ (IL-2R+) cells. Addition of CSA at a dose that had minimal effect on allograft survival in wild-type mice resulted in permanent engraftment of the fully mismatched graft (65).

A subsequent study determined that Mig, rather than IP-10, is the dominant factor responsible for recruiting alloantigen-primed T cells into cardiac allografts during rejection; treatment of allograft recipients with polyclonal antibodies to Mig resulted in a marked reduction in T-cell infiltration and significantly prolonged allograft survival (64). Further investigation revealed that anti-Mig antibodies impaired the recruitment but not the priming of CXCR3+ T cells responsible for rejection. In these studies, Mig was produced by the allograft endothelium and also by infiltrating macrophage and neutrophils, indicating a potential novel role for these cells in effector T-cell recruitment during acute rejection (64). Collectively, these experimental data directly correlated with clinical findings; expression of CXCR3 and its ligands in endomyocardial biopsies from heart transplant recipients is increased during acute rejection (66,71). Furthermore, immunohistochemistry and in situ hybridization techniques showed that CXCR3 mRNA was localized to the both vascular and infiltrating mononuclear cells.

Interactions involving CXCR3 and its ligands (Mig, IP-10, and ITAC) may also be important to the infiltration of donor T cells to sites of target tissue inflammation during the development of GVHD. Although the expression of IP-10, Mig, and CXCR3 is increased in the lung after allogeneic SCT (72) (K. R. Cooke, unpublished observation), the significance of these findings with respect to the development of pulmonary injury is under investigation. Using a system in which GVHD develops to multiple minor HC antigens (C57BL/6 → C3H.SW), Duffner and colleagues have found that the expression of CXCR3 is important for the migration of CD8+ cells to the GI tract (73). Mice receiving allogeneic SCT from CXCR3$-/-$ donors had significantly fewer donor CD8+ lymphocytes in lamina propria and intraepithelial compartments compared to animals receiving CXCR3+/+ cells (Table 3). CXCR3$-/-$ SCT recipients also had improved survival and lower clinical GVHD scores compared to allogeneic controls. In another GVHD model, CXCR3 expression was also found to be increased on CD8+ cells infiltrating the liver one week after the transfer of allogeneic spleen cells (74). Taken together, these data suggest that the expression of CXCR3 on infiltrating CD8+ lymphocytes may contribute to both target tissue and systemic GVHD.

Receptor: Ligand Interactions Involving CCR5 and CCR1 with RANTES (CCL5) and MIP-1α (CCL3).   Many groups have studied the expression patterns of CCR1 and CCR5 and their ligands MIP-1αand RANTES (21,75). RANTES and MIP-1α can be produced by a number of activated cell types, including macrophages, DCs, lymphocytes, and endothelial cells (ECs). In particular, RANTES can be expressed by fibroblasts, ECs, and epithelial cells within minutes of stimulation by TNF-α, IL-1, and LPS, and also by T lymphocytes days after activation (76). RANTES and MIP-1 can attract a variety of cell types, including activated T cells, monocytes, macrophages, NK cells, immature DCs, and neutrophils (via CCR1 expression in the mouse) (77–79). Whereas the interactions of Mig, IP-10, and I-TAC with CXCR3 are primarily related to chemotaxis of cellular

Table 3 SCT with CXCR3$-/-$ Donors Results in Decreased Systemic and Target Organ GVHD

Group	Spleen CD8 + cells [$\times 10^6$]	Lamina propria CD8 + cells [$\times 10^6$]	Intraepithelial CD8 + cells [$\times 10^6$]	Survival day 35 (%)	Clinical score day 35
Syngeneic	0.3 ± 0.01	0.1 ± 0.01	0.2 ± 0.04	100	0.1 ± 0.01
Allo wild type	3.6 ± 0.5	1.8 ± 0.2	4.5 ± 0.7	5	6.4 ± 0.5
Allo CXCR3$-/-$	$7.4 \pm 0.5^*$	$1.0 \pm 0.3^*$	$1.0 \pm 0.2^*$	63^*	$4.3 \pm 0.4^*$

Lethally irradiated C3H.SW mice received allogeneic SCT from either MHC-matched, C57BL/6 wild-type, or CXCR3-deficient (CXCR3$-/-$) donors. Irradiated C3H.SW recipients of syngeneic (C3H.SW) SCT served as negative GVHD controls. Animals were monitored daily for survival and assessed weekly using a clinical GVHD scoring system that evaluates weight change, fur texture, skin integrity, hunching, and activity. In parallel experiments, SCT recipients were sacrificed on day +14 and CD8+ T cells were isolated from the spleen and the lamina propria and intraepithelial compartments of the small bowel. Data are expressed as mean $\pm$SEM and represent one of two similar experiments. *p < 0.05.

effectors, both RANTES and MIP-1α have been shown to play a significant role in both antigen-specific activation of helper and cytotoxic T cells and their subsequent recruitment to sites of inflammation (21,44). In addition to their effects on T cells, RANTES and MIP-1α have been shown to mediate macrophage influx in the lung, pulmonary capillary leak, and early mortality during endotoxemia (80,81). The ability of chemokine receptor : ligand interactions involving CCR5 to modulate aspects of both the adaptive and innate immune response is consistent with reports that such interactions play a significant role in acute GVHD induction (6,74,82)

In mice, CCR5 is found on both CD4+ and CD8+ T cells and NK cells and is weakly detectable on monocytes (83), whereas CCR1 can be expressed on monocytes, macrophages, and neutrophils (75). CCR5 expression is enhanced during T-cell activation and differentiation of monocytes to macrophages, which could explain the co-localization of these cells with effector T cells in the organs of animals with GVHD (84). As noted above, CCR5 is also expressed at high levels on Th1 but not Th2 lymphocytes (74,79). CCR5 appears, however, to be a marker of, but is not essential for, the development of Th1 responses in humans; individuals homozygous for the Δ32 mutation (and who lack CCR5 expression) are healthy and have adequate numbers of IFN-γ- and IL-2–producing cells (85,86).

A role for CCR5/CCR1 interactions in allograft rejection is underscored by several recent studies. RANTES is increased in the bronchoalveolar lavage (BAL) fluid of patients and rodents undergoing lung transplant rejection and is associated with migration of CCR1+ and CCR5+ mononuclear cells in this context. In vivo neutralization of RANTES in a tracheal transplant model decreased mononuclear cell infiltration and reduced the severity of acute allograft rejection (87). RANTES expression increases during kidney rejection in humans and in rodent models and localizes to infiltrating leukocytes and tubular epithelial cells. The administration of the chemokine antagonist Met-RANTES significantly reduced acute renal allograft rejection in rats (88). Infiltration of CCR5+ cells occurs during both acute and chronic renal transplant rejection, and the distribution of CCR5+ cells matches the intragraft expression of RANTES (23).

The functional importance of CCR5 in transplantation immunology is exemplified by examining a cohort of patients that underwent renal allografting and were genetically deficient in CCR5; only 1 of 21 CCR5-deficient patients had evidence for transplant rejection and loss of renal function during follow-up (89). $CCR1-/-$ mice are permissive to prolonged cardiac allograft survival and permanently accept class II mismatched grafts without immunosuppression (90). Furthermore, administration of BX 471, a CCR1 antagonist, results in a reduction of monocytic graft infiltration and subsequent prolonged cardiac allograft survival (91).

Recently, several investigators have used mouse SCT models to study the role of CCR5 and its ligands in the development of GVHD (Table 4). Not only is the expression of RANTES, MIP-1α, and MIP-1β increased in the lung after allogeneic SCT (72), but MIP-1α significantly contributes to the recruitment of CCR5+ and CD8+ T cells into the lung, liver, and spleen in this setting (74,82). Using strain combinations in which donor and host differ by either class I or class II MHC antigens, Serody and colleagues (82) showed that MIP1-α expression was increased in multiple organs within the first 2 weeks after allogeneic SCT. The majority of MIP-1α produced within the first week in the liver, lung, and spleen was of donor T-cell origin; transfer of splenocytes from MIP-1α-deficient donors resulted in a decrease in MIP-1α expression in these organs, but not in the GI tract. In the MHC class I system, this reduction in MIP-1α was associated with decreased recruitment of CD8+ cells to the liver and lung and resulted in reduced mortality from GVHD (82). These experiments used relatively low-dose radiation and transferred donor splenocytes only to SCT recipients. Hence, how these data would reflect conditions in other SCT systems where host somatic cells (in response to higher doses of TBI and a systemic pro-inflammatory environment) and donor monocytes and macrophages (from the BM graft) may also contribute to chemokine production is not clear. In this regard, Panoskaltsis-Mortari and colleagues (92) used a fully allogeneic SCT model with extensive conditioning and found that SCT with MIP-1$\alpha-/-$ donor cells resulted in increased mortality from GVHD. In these experiments, MIP-1$\alpha-/-$ SCT was also associated with an accelerated influx of cytolytic, granzyme B+ cells into the lungs of recipient mice at day 3 after transfer compared to SCT with MIP-1$\alpha+/+$ cells. However,

Table 4 Selected Chemokines and Possible Role in Cancer and GVT

Chemokine	Receptor	Possible role in cancer and GVT
CC family		
CCL1	CCR8	Induces tumor immune response
CCL2	CCR2	Angiogenesis
CCL5	CCR1, 3, 5	Promotes late stage of tumor growth
CCL11	CCR3	Angiogenesis
CCL21	CCR7, CXCR3	Promotes antitumor immunity
CXC family		
CXCL1	CXCR2	Angiogenesis
CXCL2	CXCR2	Autocrine tumor growth factor
CXCL4	Unknown	Inhibits angiogenesis
CXCL8	CXCR1	Angiogenesis
CXCL9		Promotes tumor immune response
CXCL10	CXCR3	Inhibits angiogenesis
CXCL12	CXCR4	Angiogenesis inhibits immune function, promotes metastasis

the impact this finding had on survival was unclear since recipients of MIP-1α−/− and wild-type donor cells had the same degree of pulmonary dysfunction as measured by wet/dry lung weight ratios, pulmonary function, and donor cell infiltration by day 7 (92).

The initial work by Serody was extended by studies showing that CCR5+,CD8+ donor lymphocytes significantly contribute to liver GVHD in an unirradiated P → F1 model. In this study, CCR5 expression was increased on CD8+ cells infiltrating the liver, and the administration of anti-CCR5 antibodies reduced the severity of hepatic GVHD. Furthermore, MIP-1α was critical for the recruitment of donor T cells; to the liver; MIP-1 mRNA levels were significantly increased in the liver after the infusion of donor splenocytes, and antibodies to MIP-1α reduced the influx of CCR5+,CD8+ donor T cells to this organ (74). In addition, CCR5 significantly contributes to the migration of CD8+ cells to the subepithelial dome (SED) of gut Peyer's patches, which has recently been shown to be a pivotal anatomical site for the generation of anti-host CTL and the subsequent induction of systemic GVHD (6). In these studies the secretion of RANTES rather than MIP-1α by CD11c+ dendritic cells was the dominant CCR5 ligand responsible for the recruitment of T cells to the Peyer's patch. The infusion of allogeneic splenocytes deficient in CCR5 resulted not only in a reduction in the percentage of donor lymphocytes in the SED, spleen, and mesenteric lymph nodes, but also in the complete absence of hepatic injury in recipient mice (6).

In stark contrast to these findings, the use of CCR5 knockout (KO) mice as SCT donors has also resulted in greater GVHD lethality. These data were generated using models in which lethal conditioning was administered and total MHC mismatch combinations were utilized (93) (J. R. Serody, manuscript submitted, W. J. Murphy, unpublished observation). Increases in donor CD8 T-cell expansion were also observed in the recipients of CCR5−/− SCT, suggesting that CCR5 may play a role in downregulating CD8 T-cell expansion. This finding is supported by reports demonstrating increased delayed-type hypersensitivity and CD4-mediated antiviral responses in CCR5-deficient mice (94,95) and by the recent observation that CCR5 is expressed on CD4+/CD25+ T-regulatory (T-reg) cells, which are known to have suppressive effects on T-cell proliferation in GVHD models (96,97). Studies have also shown that APCs can recruit T-reg cells by the elaboration of the CCR5 ligand MIP-1β (CCL4) (98) (J. S. Serody, unpublished observation). Interestingly, MIP-1α−/− mice also produce less MIP-1β, suggesting that enhanced systemic GVHD seen after SCT with MIP-1α−/− cells in an MHC disparate system could be due to alterations in the activity or recruitment of T-regs.

Collectively, these results demonstrate that the role of CCR5 in GVHD can be significantly influenced by the experimental model used. As data showing protection from GVHD using CCR5 KO donor cells used a parent-into-F1 model with no conditioning, it is possible that conditioning may be particularly important in this scenario. Additionally, the parent-into-F1 model primarily resulted in liver pathology, whereas the lethal TBI models can (and often do) involve other organ sites (gut, skin, lung) and can predispose to infection. Since chemokines may also play a role in resistance to infection, particularly through actions on neutrophils and monocytes, the ability to discern a dominant role for a particular chemokine receptor or its ligands in pathogenesis of GVHD may be thwarted by the complexity and redundancy of the accompanying immune response. Indeed, the use of small molecule antagonists of chemokine receptors can increase mucositis and staphylococcal infections in mice undergoing GVHD (W. J. Murphy et al., unpublished observations). Clearly, additional studies need to be completed in order to (a) improve our understanding of how chemokine ligands and their receptors contribute to GVHD and (b) help decipher the paradoxical findings reported after inhibition of these proteins in experimental models.

3. Monocyte Recruitment and CCR2 : MCP (CCL2) Interactions

Once recruited to sites of inflammation, effector T cells can be restimulated to secrete additional chemokines and through this mechanism may contribute to the recruitment of monocytes, neutrophils, and additional Th1 cells (21). Donor accessory cells contribute to the pathogenesis of acute GVHD and are believed to do so via the secretion of soluble inflammatory mediators like TNF-α and IL-1 (7,99,100). Mononuclear cell infiltration is a consistent histopathological finding of GVHD of the gut, liver, and lung, and it is likely that chemokine receptor : ligand interactions involving CCR2 and perhaps CCR5 facilitate the recruitment of these cells to GVHD target organs.

CR2 is highly expressed on monocytes, DCs, NK cells, and activated T cells of both the Th1 and Th2 phenotype but not on naïve T cells, neutrophils, or eosinophils (83). CCR2, a major regulator of induced macrophage trafficking in vivo (101), is critical to the arrest of rolling monocytes during flow conditions (102) and also appears to have a role in the generation of Th1 versus Th2 responses. CCR2$-/-$ animals develop normally but exhibit significant defects in monocyte/macrophage recruitment to sites of inflammation (101,103,104). They also have diminished IFN-γ response in vivo and in vitro, although the mechanism for this defect is not completely understood (105,106). MCP-1 (CCL2) is perhaps the best-studied ligand for CCR2 (107). MCP-1 (murine JE) is a member of the CC chemokine family that has chemoattractant activity for monocytes, T cells, mast cells, and basophils. MCP-1 is produced by a variety of hematopoietic and nonhematopoietic cells, and LPS, TNF-α, IL-1, and IL-4 can enhance its expression (108). MCP-1 is believed to influence innate immunity by its effects on monocytes and adaptive immunity through its regulatory effects on effector T-cell differentiation (48). In addition to its chemoattractant effects on monocytes, MCP-1 is believed to have pro-inflammatory activity via direct activation of specific macrophage and CTL effector functions (49,108).

A role for CCR2 and MCP-1 in allogeneic immune reactions has been suggested by several studies. Upregulation of MCP-1 expression has been observed during renal allograft rejection in humans and in mouse cardiac, skin, and orthotopic tracheal transplant models (109,110). A mixed inflammatory infiltrate comprised of monocytes and neutrophils along with a concurrent increase in MCP-1, MIP-2, and KC is also observed in response to early ischemia-reperfusion injury in heart and skin transplant models. Increased MCP-1 expression persists and is accompanied by the appearance of ligands for both CXCR3 and CCR5 as allograft rejection progresses (24). In this context, the use of CCR2$-/-$ recipients increases cardiac graft survival time by 100% in the absence of additional immunosuppression. A critical role for receptor : ligand interactions between CCR2 and MCP-1 has also been reported in the pathogenesis of bronchiolitis obliterans (BrOb) that occurs during lung allograft rejection (111). Belperio and coworkers (111) found that elevated levels of biologically active MCP-1 in human BAL fluid correlated with the progression of acute to chronic rejection in lung transplant recipients. Translation studies using a murine model of BrOb demonstrated that enhanced expression of MCP-1 and CCR2 paralleled the influx of mononuclear cells into tracheal allografts. Importantly, attenuation of MCP-1/CCR2 signaling by using CCR2$-/-$ transplant recipients or neutralizing antibodies to MCP-1 significantly reduced monocyte/macrophage infiltration and the severity of BrOb.

Finally, enhanced MCP-1 expression has been observed in the liver and lung within the first 2 weeks after allogeneic SCT (8,72). In a murine model of IPS, Panoskaltsis-Mortari and colleagues found that increases in MCP-1 levels in the lung preceded the influx of host macrophages, whereas increases in MIP-1α expression accompanied donor T-cell infiltration (72). These findings were extended by recent work showing that pulmonary MCP-1 and CCR2 mRNA levels are increased during the development of IPS and that the absence of CCR2 on donor cells results in decreased lung pathology and a reduction of donor CD8+ lymphocytes and macrophages in the bronchoalveolar space after allogeneic SCT (112) (see Chapter 11).

4. Neutrophil Recruitment and Interactions Between CXCR2, MIP-2 and KC

The role of neutrophils in the development of GVHD target tissue damage is poorly understood but is likely related to the effects of LPS and inflammatory cytokine release (113). Neutrophilic infiltrates are observed in development of acute and chronic GVHD of the lung in both humans and mice and are also consistently identified in intestine and liver of animals with GVHD (113–115). Unlike lymphocytes, neutrophils are not capable of tissue-specific migration or immunological memory but can contribute to proteolytic and oxidative tissue damage when recruited to GVHD target organs. In this light, neutrophils may represent an important link between innate and adaptive immune responses occurring after allogeneic SCT.

As noted above, the chemotactic activity of CXC family members is based upon the presence of a three-amino-acid "ELR" (glutamic acid–leucine–arginine) motif. ELR+ CXC chemokine ligands are potent chemoattractants for and activators of neutrophils (116–119), whereas the major targets of non-ELR members are T and B cells. The two best studied murine ELR+ CXC chemokines, MIP-2 and KC, are the functional homologues of human IL-8 and GRO-chemokines (120,121). ELR+ CXC chemokines are produced by a variety of cells including pulmonary epithelium, vascular endothelium, neutrophils, and macrophages, and their expression is enhanced by inflammatory mediators like LPS, TNF-α, and IL-1β (122). Two receptors for ELR+ CXC chemokines have been identified in humans: CXCR1 and CXCR2 (123). Mice, however, express only CXCR2, which, like the human homologue, is believed to bind nearly all of the ELR+ CXC chemokines (124). CXCR2 is abundantly expressed on neutrophils and to a lesser extent on the surface of T cells and monocytes, myeloid precursors and some non-hematopoietic cells, including synovial fibroblasts, epithelial cells, and hepatocytes (75). Neutrophil recruitment in CXCR2-deficient mice is markedly impaired in both allergic and non-allergic models of inflammation (125–127) and specifically in response to KC and MIP-2, demonstrating the exclusive utilization of CXCR2 by these two chemokines (126).

A potential role for CXCR2 and its ligand in damage incurred during alloimmune responses has been suggested by several studies. In both human heart and kidney allografts, mRNA and protein expression of IL-8 and CINC (the rat homolog of human Gro-a and murine KC) correlated with organs undergoing rejection, and these levels decreased if the rejection episode responded to immunosuppression (128). Enhanced mRNA expression of CINC and the accumulation of neutrophils are also characteristic of acute rejection of liver transplants (129). In this setting, immunohistochemistry revealed that CINC was expressed predominantly by mononuclear cells and neutrophils infiltrating the portal areas (130). Interestingly, hepatic allograft recipients treated with FK506 expressed lower levels of CINC mRNA and had less neutrophil infiltration (130). A critical role for KC has been observed in the early inflammatory events associated with cardiac allograft rejection. Increased KC expression was present early after transplantation, peaked within 6 hours, and was followed by increases in MCP-1 and then MIP-1α and MIP-1β and the subsequent progression of graft rejection. Administration of a polyclonal anti-KC antibody early after graft placement attenuated subsequent expression of T-cell chemoattractants, cellular infiltration into the graft, and graft rejection (131). These findings suggest that the temporal expression of neutrophil and macrophage chemoattractants early after transplant is required for optimal recruitment of T cells into the graft and suggest a link between innate and acquired immunity during the development of acute rejection. The development of bronchiolitis obliterans syndrome (BOS) during chronic lung allograft rejection is also associated with increased neutrophil infiltration into the bronchial walls and bronchoalveolar space and with increased BAL fluid IL-8 levels (132). In this setting, IL-8 is believed to be produced initially by bronchial epithelial cells and may mediate airway inflammation and subsequent fibroproliferation and obliteration, which are hallmarks of this disease process (133,134).

Accordingly, increased CXCR2 and MIP-2 mRNA levels have been observed in the liver (MIP-2) and lung (CXCR2 and MIP-2) after allogeneic SCT in mice (8,72)

(K. R. Cooke, unpublished observation). In particular, KC and MIP-2 appear to significantly contribute to the amplification of lung GVHD seen after the administration of LPS (113). BAL fluid MIP-2 levels increased dramatically after LPS challenge, and this response was completely blunted when animals were treated with rhTNFR:Fc (K. R. Cooke, unpublished observation). Similar changes were observed in BAL fluid levels of KC, suggesting that neutrophil chemoattractant effects of LPS are regulated by TNF-α and the downstream release of MIP-2 and KC. Despite these associations, a causal relationship between CXCR2:MIP-2 receptor:ligand interactions, neutrophil influx, and GVHD severity has yet to be determined.

5.   Tissue-Specific Homing and the Migration of Th2 Effector Cells

The potential role of other chemokine receptor-ligand interactions in the development of GVHD, and particularly those involved in tissue-selective trafficking of memory and effector T cells, deserves mention. Interactions between CCR9 and TECK (CCL25) specifically contribute to intestinal homing of T lymphocytes. CCR9 is expressed at high levels by essentially all T lymphocytes in the small intestine, whereas lymphocytes from a variety of other secondary lymphoid and nonlymphoid tissue are universally CCR9 negative (75). TECK is selectively expressed by endothelial cells of gut-associated tissues and, via CCR9, attracts a subset of intestinal ($\alpha4\beta7^{hi}$) memory cells but not cutaneous or other systemic memory cells (135). Similarly, effector T cells with a predilection for inflamed skin can be identified by their coexpression of cutaneous lymphocyte antigen (CLA) and CCR4 (102). Two ligands for CCR4, TARC and CTACK, are expressed on the endothelium of inflamed skin (TARC) or by keratinocytes (CTACK) and are involved in firm adhesion of and extravasation of CLA+ T cells. Furthermore, CCR4 (via TARC) may play a role in the pathogenesis of liver injury induced by LPS administration (136) and perhaps lung inflammation through interactions with a third ligand monocyte-derived chemokine (MDC) (137). Although CCR9/TECK and CCR4/TARC may have important implications in the development of acute GVHD of the gut and skin, respectively, the significance of these receptor ligand interactions in these settings has yet to be established in vivo.

Finally, this section has focused sharply on the role of Th1 effectors in the development of acute GVHD. However, Th2 cells can also contribute to target organ injury in the acute and chronic setting (138,139). As noted above, Th1 cells preferentially express CCR5 and CXCR3, whereas CCR3, CCR4, and CCR8 are generally displayed on Th2 cells (23) (Fig. 2). In particular, CCR3 is expressed on eosinophils, basophils, and polarized Th2 lymphocytes, all of which are recruited to sites of allergic inflammation by the effects of eotaxin. Eotaxin is believed to be one of the most relevant chemokines in the pathophysiology of allergic conditions, but its expression is also increased in the skin, liver, and lung during the induction of acute GVHD. However, what role, if any, eotaxin plays in the recruitment of CCR3-expressing cells to GVHD target organs as well as

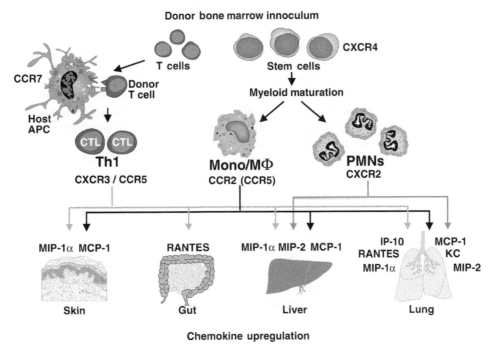

Figure 2 Chemokines and leukocyte trafficking after allogeneic SCT: Leukocyte trafficking after allogeneic SCT is a complex process. After the infusion of the donor marrow or peripheral blood inoculum, HSC must home to the bone marrow microenvironment to recapitulate elements of the hematopoietic and peripheral immune systems in the SCT recipient. Recent studies support a role for CXCR4 in both HSC homing and myeloid maturation. Upregulation of CCR7 on the surface of host APC occurs in parallel and facilitates the migration of these cells to secondary lymphoid tissue where they interact with mature donor T cells. Once engaged, donor T cells become activated and differentiate into T1 effectors. Significant experimental data have shown that cells of the lymphoid and myeloid lineages synergize to cause systemic inflammation and target organ damage characteristic of acute GVHD. The recruitment of cellular effectors to GVHD target tissue is dependent, in part, upon the upregulation of chemokine receptors on donor leukocytes including CXCR3 and CCR5 on T1 CTL, CCR2 (and possibly CCR5) on cells of the monocyte/macrophage lineage, and CXCR2 on neutrophils. Donor leukocytes that have been released from secondary lymphoid tissues or the bone marrow are recruited to GVHD target organs by the respective chemokine ligands that have been upregulated by a proinflammatory environment present early after SCT.

potential roles in chronic GVHD remains to be determined. A recent study demonstrated that analogues of SLC (secondary lymphoid tissue chemokine/CCRL21) block responses by CCR7-expressing cells and reduce the autoimmune component of chronic GVHD (host B-cell expansion, presence of anti-DNA antibodies) in an unirradiated murine model (140). These data are suggestive that chemokine antagonism may be of benefit in chronic GVHD, but the impact of this strategy acute GVHD severity was not addressed.

V. CHEMOKINES AND GVT RESPONSES

Allogeneic SCT is used extensively in the treatment of cancer. While GVHD remains a significant cause of morbidity following allogeneic SCT, relapse from the original malignancy also remains a serious concern. The therapeutic potential of allogeneic SCT resides in the presence of GVT effects, which are closely linked to acute GVHD. Not surprisingly, chemokines have been shown to play a role in tumorigenesis, and these interactions must be taken into consideration when attempting to clinically exploit the actions of chemokines after SCT. In particular, chemokines are known to play a significant role in tumor angiogenesis (Table 4), and chemokine neutralization strategies have been used in an attempt to generate antitumor effects. It is therefore attractive to envision an approach wherein the neutralization of select chemokine receptor-ligand interactions would reduce GVHD and enhance GVT effects. However, recent work suggests that the redundancy of chemokine expression on tumor cells can make selective inhibition problematic (141). This is illustrated by data using human monoclonal antibodies to IL-8. Using a xenograft model of human breast cancer, administration of antibodies to MCP-1 was initially found to result in significant tumor regression in vivo (142). Although many human tumors also make IL-8, attempts to demonstrate antitumor effects by using anti-IL-8 antibodies were unsuccessful. However, when the antibodies to IL-8 and MCP-1 were used in combination, much greater antitumor effects were achieved (143). This suggests that neutralization of multiple chemokines may be necessary for significant and sustained in vivo antitumor effects. It will be of interest to use such an approach in tumor-bearing mice receiving an allogeneic SCT in order to develop strategies that will successfully separate the toxicity of GVHD from the beneficial GVT effect.

VI. CONCLUSIONS

The migration of leukocytes from secondary lymphoid tissue to the blood stream and ultimately into target organs is an essential component of the graft-vs.-host reaction. Diffuse injury to host tissues incurred by SCT conditioning regimens results in a pro-inflammatory milieu that sets the stage for chemokine upregulation and early leukocyte infiltration and activation. This is followed in turn by the recruitment of additional effector cells and the progression of acute GVHD. Chemokines are critical extracellular messengers that facilitate leukocyte trafficking and migration to sites of inflammation. They also appear to directly modulate the immune response due to their ability to act as co-stimulatory molecules for all of the immune cells involved in GVHD pathology. Despite the complexity of the chemokine microenvironment at sites of tissue injury and the redundancy that exists with respect to chemokine receptor ligand specificities, emerging data suggest that these molecules will play a significant role in recruitment of activated lymphocytes, monocytes, and neutrophils to GVHD target organs (Fig. 2). However, it is clear that differences among the in vivo models used to study GVHD process can have dramatic effects on outcome. This confounding factor can complicate our ability to draw definitive conclusions about the role of chemokines in the GVH response. Future studies will determine whether expression of chemokines and their receptors can explain the unusual cluster of GVHD target organs (skin, gut, and liver), and whether these molecules will prove to be potential targets for modulation of GVHD. Finally, in light of the effects that chemokines have on tumorigenesis, strategies that disrupt specific chemokine receptor ligand interactions may provide a means to dissociate GVHD from GVT responses when allogeneic SCT is used for cancer.

ACKNOWLEDGMENT

Supported by grants CA 58233 and 89961 from the National Cancer Institute (JSS) and HL 072258 from the NHLBI (KRC).

REFERENCES

1. Hill GR, Crawford JM, Cooke KJ, Brinson YS, Pan L, Ferrara JLM. Total body irradiation and acute graft versus host disease. The role of gastrointestinal damage and inflammatory cytokines. Blood 1997; 90:3204–3213.
2. DeVries ME, Hosiawa KA, Cameron CM, Bosinger SE, Persad D, Kelvin AA, Coombs JC, Wang H, Zhong R, Cameron MJ, Kelvin DJ. The role of chemokines and chemokine receptors in alloantigen-independent and alloantigen-dependent transplantation injury. Semin Immunol 2003; 15:33–48.
3. Yan SF, Fujita T, Lu J, Okada K, Shan Zou Y, Mackman N, Pinsky DJ, Stern DM. Egr-1, a master switch coordinating upregulation of divergent gene families underlying ischemic stress. Nat Med 2000; 6:1355–1361.
4. Ben-Ari Z, Hochhauser E, Burstein I, Papo O, Kaganovsky E, Krasnov T, Vamichkim A, Vidne BA. Role of anti-tumor necrosis factor-alpha in ischemia/reperfusion injury in isolated rat liver in a blood-free environment. Transplantation 2002; 73:1875–1880.
5. Hill G, Ferrara J. The primacy of the gastrointestinal tract as a target organ of acute graft-versus-host disease: rationale for the use of cytokine shields in allogeneic bone marrow transplantation. Blood 2000; 95:2754–2759.
6. Murai M, Yoneyama H, Ezaki T, Suematsu M, Terashim Y, Harada A, Hamada H, Asakura H, Ishikawa H, Matsushima K. Peyer's patch is the essential site in initiating murine acute and lethal graft-versus-host reaction. Nat Immunol 2003; 4.
7. Cooke K, Hill G, Crawford J, Bungard D, Brinson Y, Delmonte Jr. J, Ferrara J. Tumor necrosis factor-α production to lipopolysaccharide stimulation by donor cells predicts the severity of experimental acute graft versus host disease. J Clin Invest 1998; 102:1882–1891.
8. Mapara MY, Kim Y-M, Nikolic B, Bronson R, Luster AD, Sykes M. Expression of chemokines in GVHD target organs following lethal irradiation and syngeneic or allogeneic bone marrow transplantation: possible role of MCP-1 and eotaxin as initiating chemokines in liver and skin GVHD. Blood 2000; 96:771a.
9. Baker MB, Riley RL, Podack ER, Levy RB. GVHD-associated lymphoid hypoplasia and B cell dysfunction is dependent upon donor T cell-mediated Fas-ligand function, but not perforin function. Proc Natl Acad Sci USA 1997; 94:1366–1371.
10. Mori T, Nishimura T, Ikeda Y, Hotta T, Yagita H, Ando K. Involvement of Fas-mediated apoptosis in the hematopoietic progenitor cells of graft-versus-host reaction-associated myelosuppression. Blood 1998; 92:101–107.
11. Via CS, Nguyen P, Shustov A, Drappa J, Elkon KB. A major role for the Fas pathway in acute graft-versus-host disease. J Immunol 1996; 157:5387–5393.

12. Hattori K, Hirano T, Miyajima H, Yamakawa N, Tateno M, Oshimi K, Kayagaki N, Yagita H, Okumura K. Differential effects of anti-Fas ligand and anti-tumor necrosis factor-α antibodies on acute graft-versus-host disease pathologies. Blood 1998; 91:4051–4055.

13. Cooke K, Kobzik L, Teshima T, Lowler K, Clouthier S, Ferrara J. A role for Fas-Fas ligand but not perforin mediated cytolysis in the development of experimental idiopathic pneumonia syndrome. Blood 2000; 96:768a.

14. Blazar BR, Taylor PA, Vallera DA. CD4+ and CD8+ T cells each can utilize a perforin-dependent pathway to mediate lethal graft-versus-host disease in major histocompatibility complex-disparate recipients. Transplantation 1997; 64:571–576.

15. Baker MB, Altman NH, Podack ER, Levy RB. The role of cell-mediated cytotoxicity in acute GVHD after MHC-matched allogeneic bone marrow transplantation in mice. J Exp Med 1997; 183:2645–2656.

16. Cooke K, Olkiewicz K, Clouthier S, Liu C, Ferrara J. Critical role for CD14 and the innate immune response in the induction of experimental acute graft-versus-host disease. Blood 2001; 98:776a.

17. Shlomchik WD, Couzens MS, Tang CB, McNiff J, Robert ME, Liu J, Shlomchik MJ, Emerson SG. Prevention of graft versus host disease by inactivation of host antigen-presenting cells. Science 1999; 285:412–415.

18. Mackay CR. Chemokines: immunology's high impact factors. Nat Immunol 2001; 2:95–101.

19. Luster AD. Chemokines—chemotactic cytokines that mediate inflammation. N Engl J Med 1998; 338:436–445.

20. Rollins BJ. Chemokines. Blood 1997; 90:909–928.

21. Luther SA, Cyster JG. Chemokines as regulators of T cell differentiation. Nat Immunol 2001; 2:102–107.

22. Strieter RM, Polverini PJ, Kunkel SL, Arenberg DA, Burdick MD, Kasper J, Dzuiba J, Van Damme J, Walz A, Marriott D, et al. The functional role of the ELR motif in CXC chemokine-mediated angiogenesis. J Biol Chem 1995; 270:27348–27357.

23. Nelson PJ, Krensky AM. Chemokines, chemokine receptors, and allograft rejection. Immunity 2001; 14:377–386.

24. Gerard C, Rollins BJ. Chemokines and disease. Nat Immunol 2001; 2:108–115.

25. Peled A, Petit I, Kollet O, Magid M, Ponomaryov T, Byk T, Nagler A, Ben-Hur H, Many A, Shultz L, Lider O, Alon R, Zipori D, Lapidot T. Dependence of human stem cell engraftment and repopulation of NOD/SCID mice on CXCR4. Science 1999; 283:845–848.

26. Mohle R, Bautz F, Rafii S, Moore MA, Brugger W, Kanz L 1998 The chemokine receptor CXCR-4 is expressed on CD34+ hematopoietic progenitors and leukemic cells and mediates transendothelial migration induced by stromal cell-derived factor-1. Blood 1998; 91:4523–4530.

27. Peled A, Grabovsky V, Habler L, Sandbank J, Arenzana-Seisdedos F, Petit I, Ben-Hur H, Lapidot T, Alon R. The chemokine SDF-1 stimulates integrin-mediated arrest of CD34(+) cells on vascular endothelium under shear flow. J Clin Invest 1999; 104:1199–1211.

28. Peled A, Kollet O, Ponomaryov T, Petit I, Franitza S, Grabovsky V, Slav MM, Nagler A, Lider O, Alon R, Zipori D, Lapidot T. The chemokine SDF-1 activates the integrins LFA-1, VLA-4, and VLA-5 on immature human CD34(+) cells: role in transendothelial/stromal migration and engraftment of NOD/SCID mice. Blood 2000; 95:3289–3296.

29. Nagasawa T, Hirota S, Tachibana K, Takakura N, Nishikawa S, Kitamura Y, Yoshida N, Kikutani H, Kishimoto T. Defects of B-cell lymphopoiesis and bone-marrow myelopoiesis in mice lacking the CXC chemokine PBSF/SDF-1. Nature 1996; 382:635–638.

30. Christopherson KW, 2nd, Hangoc G, Broxmeyer HE. Cell surface peptidase CD26/dipeptidylpeptidase IV regulates CXCL12/stromal cell-derived factor-1 alpha-mediated chemotaxis of human cord blood CD34+ progenitor cells. J Immunol 2002; 169:7000–7008.

31. Adams GB, Chabner KT, Foxall RB, Weibrecht KW, Rodrigues NP, Dombkowski D, Fallon R, Poznansky MC, Scadden DT. Heterologous cells cooperate to augment stem cell migration, homing, and engraftment. Blood 2003; 101:45–51.

32. Ma Q, Jones D, Springer TA. The chemokine receptor CXCR4 is required for the retention of B lineage and granulocytic precursors within the bone marrow microenvironment. Immunity 1999; 10:463–471.

33. Wiesmann A, Spangrude GJ. Marrow engraftment of hematopoietic stem and progenitor cells is independent of Galphai-coupled chemokine receptors. Exp Hematol 1999; 27:946–955.

34. Wright DE, Bowman EP, Wagers AJ, Butcher EC, Weissman IL. Hematopoietic stem cells are uniquely selective in their migratory response to chemokines. J Exp Med 2002; 195:1145–1154.

35. Hromas R, Gray PW, Chantry D, Godiska R, Krathwohl M, Fife K, Bell GI, Takeda J, Aronica S, Gordon M, Cooper S, Broxmeyer HE, Klemsz MJ. Cloning and characterization of exodus, a novel beta-chemokine. Blood 1997; 89:3315–3322.

36. Broxmeyer HE, Cooper S, Cacalano G, Hague NL, Bailish E, Moore MW. Involvement of interleukin (IL) 8 receptor in negative regulation of myeloid progenitor cells in vivo: evidence from mice lacking the murine IL-8 receptor homologue. J Exp Med 1996; 184:1825–1832.

37. Reid S, Ritchie A, Boring L, Gosling J, Cooper S, Hangoc G, Charo IF, Broxmeyer HE. Enhanced myeloid progenitor cell cycling and apoptosis in mice lacking the chemokine receptor, CCR2. Blood 1999; 93:1524–1533.

38. Broxmeyer HE, Sherry B, Cooper S, Lu L, Maze R, Beckmann MP, Cerami A, Ralph P. Comparative analysis of the human macrophage inflammatory protein family of cytokines (chemokines) on proliferation of human myeloid progenitor cells. Interacting effects involving suppression, synergistic suppression, and blocking of suppression. J Immunol 1993; 150:3448–3458.

39. Hill GR, Ferrara JL. The primacy of the gastrointestinal tract as a target organ of acute graft-versus-host disease: rationale for the use of cytokine shields in allogeneic bone marrow transplantation. Blood 2000; 95:2754–2759.

40. Kunkel EJ, Butcher EC. Chemokines and the tissue-specific migration of lymphocytes. Immunity 2002; 16:1–4.

41. Forster R, Schubel A, Breitfeld D, Kremmer E, Renner-Muller I, Wolf E, Lipp M. CCR7 coordinates the primary immune response by establishing functional microenvironments in secondary lymphoid organs. Cell 1999; 99:23–33.

42. Nanki T, Lipsky PE. Cutting edge: stromal cell-derived factor-1 is a costimulator for CD4+ T cell activation. J Immunol 2000; 164:5010–5014.

43. Makino Y, Cook DN, Smithies O, Hwang OY, Neilson EG, Turka LA, Sato H, Wells AD, Danoff TM. Impaired T cell function in RANTES-deficient mice. Clin Immunol 2002; 102:302–309.

44. Taub DD, Ortaldo JR, Turcovski-Corrales SM, Key ML, Longo DL, Murphy WJ. Beta chemokines costimulate lymphocyte cytolysis, proliferation, and lymphokine production. J Leukoc Biol 1996; 59:81–89.

45. Taub DD, Murphy EJ, Asai O, Genton RG, Peltz G, Ky ML, Turcovski-Corrales S, Longo DL. Induction of alloantigen-specific T-cell tolerance through the treatment of human T lymphocytes with wortmannin. J Immunol 1997; 158. In press.

46. Wong MM, Fish EN. Chemokines: attractive mediators of the immune response. Semin Immunol 2003; 15:5–14.

47. Karpus WJ, Lukacs NW, Kennedy KJ, Smith WS, Hurst SD, Barrett TA. Differential CC chemokine-induced enhancement of T helper cell cytokine production. J Immunol 1997; 158:4129–4136.

48. Gu L, Tseng S, Horner RM, Tam C, Loda M, Rollins BJ. Control of TH2 polarization by the chemokine monocyte chemoattractant protein-1. Nature 2000; 404:407–411.

49. Kim JJ, Nottingham LK, Sin JI, Tsai A, Morrison L, Oh J, Dang K, Hu Y, Kazahaya K, Bennett M, Dentchev T, Wilson DM, Chalian AA, Boyer JD, Agadjanyan MG, Weiner DB. CD8 positive T cells influence antigen-specific immune responses through the expression of chemokines. J Clin Invest 1998; 102:1112–1124.

50. Maghazachi AA, al-Aoukaty A, Schall TJ. C-C chemokines induce the chemotaxis of NK and IL-2-activated NK cells. Role for G proteins. J Immunol 1994; 153:4969–4977.

51. Robertson MJ. Role of chemokines in the biology of natural killer cells. J Leukoc Biol 2002; 71:173–183.

52. Taub DD, Sayers TJ, Carter CR, Ortaldo JR. Alpha and beta chemokines induce NK cell migration and enhance NK- mediated cytolysis. J Immunol 1995; 155:3877–3888.

53. Taub DD, Anver M, Oppenheim JJ, Longo DL, Murphy WJ. T lymphocyte recruitment by interleukin-8 (IL-8). IL-8-induced degranulation of neutrophils releases potent chemoattractants for human T lymphocytes both in vitro and in vivo. J Clin Invest 1996; 97:1931–1941.

54. Willems J, Joniau M, Cinque S, van Damme J. Human granulocyte chemotactic peptide (IL-8) as a specific neutrophil degranulator: comparison with other monokines. Immunology 1989; 67:540–542.

55. Biragyn A, Ruffini PA, Leifer CA, Klyushnenkova E, Shakhov A, Chertov O, Shirakawa AK, Farber JM, Segal DM, Oppenheim JJ, Kwak LW. Toll-like receptor 4-dependent activation of dendritic cells by beta-defensin 2. Science 2002; 298:1025–1029.

56. Moser B, Loetscher P. Lymphocyte traffic control by chemokines. Nat Immunol 2001; 2:123–128.

57. Sallusto F, Lenig D, Forster R, Lipp M, Lanzavecchia A. Two subsets of memory T lymphocytes with distinct homing potentials and effector functions. Nature 1999; 401:708–712.

58. Reinhardt RL, Khoruts A, Merica R, Zell T, Jenkins MK. Visualizing the generation of memory CD4 T cells in the whole body. Nature 2001; 410:101–105.

59. Loetscher M, Gerber B, Loetscher P, Jones SA, Piali L, Clark-Lewis I, Baggiolini M, Moser B. Chemokine receptor specific for IP10 and mig: structure, function, and expression in activated T-lymphocytes. J Exp Med 1996; 184:963–969.

60. Qin S, Rottman JB, Myers P, Kassam N, Weinblatt M, Loetscher M, Koch AE, Moser B, Mackay CR. The chemokine receptors CXCR3 and CCR5 mark subsets of T cells associated with certain inflammatory reactions. J Clin Invest 1998; 101:746–754.

61. Kunkel EJ, Boisvert J, Murphy K, Vierra MA, Genovese MC, Wardlaw AJ, Greenberg HB, Hodge MR, Wu L, Butcher EC, Campbell JJ. Expression of the chemokine receptors CCR4, CCR5, and CXCR3 by human tissue-infiltrating lymphocytes. Am J Pathol 2002; 160:347–355.

62. Ebert LM, McColl SR. Coregulation of CXC chemokine receptor and CD4 expression on T lymphocytes during allogeneic activation. J Immunol 2001; 166:4870–4878.

63. von Andrian UH, Mackay CR. T-cell function and migration. Two sides of the same coin. N Engl J Med 2000; 343:1020–1034.

64. Miura M, Morita K, Kobayashi H, Hamilton TA, Burdick MD, Strieter RM, Fairchild RL. Monokine induced by IFN-gamma is a dominant factor directing T cells into murine cardiac allografts during acute rejection. J Immunol 2001; 167:3494–3504.

65. Hancock WW, Lu B, Gao W, Csizmadia V, Faia K, King JA, Smiley ST, Ling M, Gerard NP, Gerard C. Requirement of the chemokine receptor CXCR3 for acute allograft rejection. J Exp Med 2000; 192:1515–1520.

66. Melter M, Exeni A, Reinders ME, Fang JC, McMahon G, Ganz P, Hancock WW, Briscoe DM. Expression of the chemokine receptor CXCR3 and its ligand IP-10 during human cardiac allograft rejection. Circulation 2001; 104:2558–2564.

67. Liao F, Rabin RL, Yannelli JR, Koniaris LG, Vanguri P, Farber JM. Human Mig chemokine: biochemical and functional characterization. J Exp Med 1995; 182:1301–1314.

68. Murdoch C, Finn A. Chemokine receptors and their role in inflammation and infectious diseases. Blood 2000; 95:3032–3043.

69. Taub DD, Lloyd AR, Conlon K, Wang JM, Ortaldo JR, Harada A, Matsushima K, Kelvin DJ, Oppenheim JJ. Recombinant human interferon-inducible protein 10 is a chemoattractant for human monocytes and T lymphocytes and promotes T cell adhesion to endothelial cells. J Exp Med 1993; 177:1809–1814.

70. Koga S, Auerbach MB, Engeman TM, Novick AC, Toma H, Fairchild RL. T cell infiltration into class II MHC-disparate allografts and acute rejection is dependent on the IFN-gamma-induced chemokine Mig. J Immunol 1999; 163:4878–4885.

71. Zhao DX, Hu Y, Miller GG, Luster AD, Mitchell RN, Libby P. Differential expression of the IFN-gamma-inducible CXCR3-binding chemokines, IFN-inducible protein 10, monokine induced by IFN, and IFN-inducible T cell alpha chemoattractant in human cardiac allografts: association with cardiac allograft vasculopathy and acute rejection. J Immunol 2002; 169:1556–1560.

72. Panoskaltsis-Mortari A, Strieter RM, Hermanson JR, Fegeding KV, Murphy WJ, Farrell CL, Lacey DL, Blazar BR. Induction of monocyte- and T-cell-attracting chemokines in the lung during the generation of idiopathic pneumonia syndrome following allogeneic murine bone marrow transplantation. Blood 2000; 96:834–839.

73. Duffner U, Lu B, Teshima T, Williams D, Hildebrandt G, Reddy P, Ordemann R, Lowler K, Liu C, Cooke KR, Ferrara JLM. CXCR3 dependent donor T cell migration during acute GVHD. 2003; Submitted.

74. Murai M, Yoneyama H, Harada A, Yi Z, Vestergaard C, Guo B, Suzuki K, Asakura H, Matsushima K. Active participation of CCR5(+)CD8(+) T lymphocytes in the pathogenesis of liver injury in graft-versus-host disease. J Clin Invest 1999; 104:49–57.

75. Horuk R. Survey: chemokine receptors. Cytokine Growth Factor Rev 2001; 12:313–335.

76. Song A, Nikolcheva T, Krensky AM. Transcriptional regulation of RANTES expression in T lymphocytes. Immunol Rev 2000; 177:236–245.

77. Alam R, Stafford S, Forsythe P, Harrison R, Faubion D, Lett-Brown MA, Grant JA. RANTES is a chemotactic and activating factor for human eosinophils. J Immunol 1993; 150:3442–3448.

78. Bischoff SC, Krieger M, Brunner T, Rot A, von Tscharner V, Baggiolini M, Dahinden CA. RANTES and related chemokines activate human basophil granulocytes through different G protein-coupled receptors. Eur J Immunol 1993; 23:761–767.

79. Schall TJ, Bacon K, Toy KJ, Goeddel DV. Selective attraction of monocytes and T lymphocytes of the memory phenotype by cytokine RANTES. Nature 1990; 347:669–671.

80. VanOtteren GM, Strieter RM, Kunkel SL, Paine R, 3rd, Greenberger MJ, Danforth JM, Burdick MD, Standiford TJ. Compartmentalized expression of RANTES in a murine model of endotoxemia. J Immunol 1995; 154:1900–1908.

81. Standiford TJ, Kunkel SL, Lukacs NW, Greenberger MJ, Danforth JM, Kunkel RG, Strieter RM. Macrophage inflammatory protein-1 alpha mediates lung leukocyte recruitment, lung capillary leak, and early mortality in murine endotoxemia. J Immunol 1995; 155:1515–1524.

82. Serody JS, Burkett SE, Panoskaltsis-Mortari A, Ng-Cashin J, McMahon E, Matsushima GK, Lira SA, Cook DN, Blazar BR. T-lymphocyte production of macrophage inflammatory protein-1alpha is critical to the recruitment of CD8(+) T cells to the liver, lung, and spleen during graft-versus-host disease. Blood 2000; 96:2973–2980.

83. Mack M, Cihak J, Simonis C, Luckow B, Proudfoot AE, Plachy J, Bruhl H, Frink M, Anders HJ, Vielhauer V, Pfirstinger J, Stangassinger M, Schlondorff D. Expression and characterization of the chemokine receptors CCR2 and CCR5 in mice. J Immunol 2001; 166:4697–4704.

84. Kaufmann A, Salentin R, Gemsa D, Sprenger H. Increase of CCR1 and CCR5 expression and enhanced functional response to MIP-1 alpha during differentiation of human monocytes to macrophages. J Leukoc Biol 2001; 69:248–252.

85. Odum N, Bregenholt S, Eriksen KW, Skov S, Ryder LP, Bendtzen K, Van Neerven RJ, Svejgaard A, Garred P. The CC-chemokine receptor 5 (CCR5) is a marker of, but not essential for the development of human Th1 cells. Tissue Antigens 1999; 54:572–577.

86. Libert F, Cochaux P, Beckman G, Samson M, Aksenova M, Cao A, Czeizel A, Claustres M, de la Rua C, Ferrari M, Ferrec C, Glover G, Grinde B, Guran S, Kucinskas V, Lavinha J, Mercier B, Ogur G, Peltonen L, Rosatelli C, Schwartz M, Spitsyn V, Timar L, Beckman L, Vassart G, et al. The deltaccr5 mutation conferring protection against HIV-1 in Caucasian populations has a single and recent origin in northeastern Europe. Hum Mol Genet 1998; 7:399–406.

87. Belperio JA, Burdick MD, Keane MP, Xue YY, Lynch JP, 3rd, Daugherty BL, Kunkel SL, Strieter RM. The role of the CC chemokine, RANTES, in acute lung allograft rejection. J Immunol 2000; 165:461–472.

88. Grone HJ, Weber C, Weber KS, Grone EF, Rabelink T, Klier CM, Wells TN, Proudfood AE, Schlondorff D, Nelson PJ. Met-RANTES reduces vascular and tubular damage during acute renal transplant rejection: blocking monocyte arrest and recruitment. FASEB J 1999; 13:1371–1383.

89. Fischereder M, Luckow B, Hocher B, Wuthrich RP, Rothenpieler U, Schneeberger H, Panzer U, Stahl RA, Hauser IA, Budde K, Neumayer H, Kramer BK, Land W, Schlondorff D. CC chemokine receptor 5 and renal-transplant survival. Lancet 2001; 357:1758–1761.

90. Gao W, Topham PS, King JA, Smiley ST, Csizmadia V, Lu B, Gerard CJ, Hancock WW. Targeting of the chemokine receptor CCR1 suppresses development of acute and chronic cardiac allograft rejection. J Clin Invest 2000; 105:35–44.

91. Horuk R, Clayberger C, Krensky AM, Wang Z, Grone HJ, Weber C, Weber KS, Nelson PJ, May K, Rosser M, Dunning L, Liang M, Buckman B, Ghannam A, Ng HP, Islam I, Bauman JG, Wei GP, Monahan S, Xu W, Snider RM, Morrissey MM, Hesselgesser J, Perez HD. A non-peptide functional antagonist of the CCR1 chemokine receptor is effective in rat heart transplant rejection. J Biol Chem 2001; 276:4199–4204.

92. Panoskaltsis-Mortari A, Hermanson JR, Taras E, Wangensteen OD, Serody JS, Blazar BR. Acceleration of idiopathic pneumonia syndrome (IPS) in the absence of donor MIP-1{alpha} (CCL3) post-allogeneic BMT in mice. Blood 2003; 2:2.

93. Murphy WJ, Wang Z, Welniak LA, Kuziel W, Blazar BR. T cells from CCR5 knockout mice induce accelerated acute graft-versus-host disease lethality after allogeneic BMT in mice. BBMT 2002; 8:66–67.

94. Zhou Y, Kurihara T, Ryseck RP, Yang Y, Ryan C, Loy J, Warr G, Bravo R. Impaired macrophage function and enhanced T cell-dependent immune response in mice lacking CCR5, the mouse homologue of the major HIV-1 coreceptor. J Immunol 1998; 160:4018–4025.

95. Nansen A, Christensen JP, Andreasen SO, Bartholdy C, Christensen JE, Thomsen AR; The role of CC chemokine receptor 5 in antiviral immunity. Blood 2002; 99:1237–1245.

96. Hoffmann P, Ermann J, Edinger M, Fathman CG, Strober S. Donor-type CD4(+)CD25(+) regulatory T cells suppress lethal acute graft-versus-host disease after allogeneic bone marrow transplantation. J Exp Med 2002; 196:389–399.

97. Cohen JL, Trenado A, Vasey D, Klatzmann D, Salomon BL. CD4(+)CD25(+) immunoregulatory T cells: new therapeutics for graft-versus-host disease. J Exp Med 2002; 196:401–406.

98. Bystry RS, Aluvihare V, Welch KA, Kallikourdis M, Betz AG. B cells and professional APCs recruit regulatory T cells via CCL4. Nat Immunol 2001; 2:1126–1132.

99. Nestel FP, Price KS, Seemayer TA, Lapp WS. Macrophage priming and lipopolysaccharide-triggered release of tumor necrosis factor alpha during graft-versus-host disease. J Exp Med 1992; 175:405–413.

100. Cooke K, Hill G, Gerbitz A, Kobzik L, Martin T, Crawford J, Brewer J, Ferrara J. Hyporesponsiveness of donor cells to LPS stimulation reduces the severity of experimental idiopathic pneumonia syndrome: potential role for a gut-lung axis of inflammation. J Immunol 2000; 165:6612–6619.

101. Kuziel WA, Morgan SJ, Dawson TC, Griffin S, Smithies O, Ley K, Maeda N. Severe reduction in leukocyte adhesion and monocyte extravasation in mice deficient in CC chemokine receptor 2. Proc Natl Acad Sci USA 1997; 94:12053–12058.

102. Sallusto F, Mackay CR, Lanzavecchia A. The role of chemokine receptors in primary, effector, and memory immune responses. Annu Rev Immunol 2000; 18:593–620.

103. Traynor TR, Kuziel WA, Toews GB, Huffnagle GB. CCR2 expression determines T1 versus T2 polarization during pulmonary *Cryptococcus neoformans* infection. J Immunol 2000; 164:2021–2027.

104. Kurihara T, Warr G, Loy J, Bravo R. Defects in macrophage recruitment and host defense in mice lacking the CCR2 chemokine receptor. J Exp Med 1997; 186:1757–1762.

105. Sato N, Kuziel WA, Melby PC, Reddick RL, Kostecki V, Zhao W, Maeda N, Ahuja SK, Ahuja SS. Defects in the generation of IFN-gamma are overcome to control infection with *Leishmania donovani* in CC chemokine receptor (CCR) 5-, macrophage inflammatory protein-1 alpha-, or CCR2-deficient mice. J Immunol 1999; 163:5519–5525.

106. Peters W, Dupuis M, Charo IF. A mechanism for the impaired IFN-gamma production in C-C chemokine receptor 2 (CCR2) knockout mice: role of CCR2 in linking the innate and adaptive immune responses. J Immunol 2000; 165:7072–7077.

107. Kurihara T, Bravo R. Cloning and functional expression of mCCR2, a murine receptor for the C-C chemokines JE and FIC. J Biol Chem 1996; 271:11603–11607.

108. Zisman DA, Kunkel SL, Strieter RM, Tsai WC, Bucknell K, Wilkowski J, Standiford TJ. MCP-1 protects mice in lethal endotoxemia. J Clin Invest 1997; 99:2832–2836.

109. Robertson H, Morley AR, Talbot D, Callanan K, Kirby JA. Renal allograft rejection: beta-chemokine involvement in the development of tubulitis. Transplantation 2000; 69:684–687.

110. Boehler A, Bai XH, Liu M, Cassivi S, Chamberlain D, Slutsky AS, Keshavjee S. Upregulation of T-helper 1 cytokines and chemokine expression in post-transplant airway obliteration. Am J Respir Crit Care Med 1999; 159:1910–1917.

111. Belperio JA, Keane MP, Burdick MD, Lynch JP, 3rd, Xue YY, Berlin A, Ross DJ, Kunkel SL, Charo IF, Strieter RM. Critical role for the chemokine MCP-1/CCR2 in the pathogenesis of bronchiolitis obliterans syndrome. J Clin Invest 2001; 108:547–556.

112. Hildebrandt GC, Duffner UA, Olkiewicz K, Willimarth NE, Corrion LA, Clouthier SG, Williams DL, Reddy PR, Moore BB, Liu C, Cooke KR. A critical role for CCR2 in the development of idiopathic pneumonia syndrome after allogeneic bone marrow transplantation. 2003; Submitted.

113. Cooke KR, Hill GR, Gerbitz A, Kobzik L, Martin TR, Crawford JM, Brewer JP, Ferrara JL. Tumor necrosis factor-alpha neutralization reduces lung injury after experimental allogeneic bone marrow transplantation. Transplantation 2000; 70:272–279.

114. Cooke KR, Kobzik L, Martin TR, Brewer J, Delmonte J, Crawford JM, Ferrara JLM. An experimental model of idiopathic pneumonia syndrome after bone marrow transplantation. I. The roles of minor H antigens and endotoxin. Blood 1996; 8:3230–3239.

115. Krijanovski OI, Hill GR, Cooke KR, Teshima T, Crawford JM, Brinson YS, Ferrara JL. Keratinocyte growth factor separates graft-versus-leukemia effects from graft-versus-host disease. Blood 1999; 94:825–831.

116. Mehrad B, Strieter R, Standiford T. Role of TNFα in pulmonary host defense in murine invasive aspergillosis. J Immunol 1999; 162:1633–1640.

117. Crawford S, Longton G, Storb R. Acute graft versus host disease and the risks for idiopathic pneumonia after marrow transplantation for severe aplastic anemia. Bone Marrow Transplant 1993; 12:225.

118. Kantrow SP, Hackman RC, Boeckh M, Myerson D, Crawford SW. Idiopathic pneumonia syndrome: changing spectrum of lung injury after marrow transplantation. Transplantation 1997; 63:1079–1086.

119. Keane MP, Belperio JA, Moore TA, Moore BB, Arenberg DA, Smith RE, Burdick MD, Kunkel SL, Strieter RM. Neutralization of the CXC chemokine, macrophage inflammatory protein-2, attenuates bleomycin-induced pulmonary fibrosis. J Immunol 1999; 162:5511–5518.

120. Tekamp-Olson P, Gallegos C, Bauer D, McClain J, Sherry B, Fabre M, van Deventer S, Cerami A. Cloning and characterization of cDNAs for murine macrophage inflammatory protein 2 and its human homologues. J Exp Med 1990; 172:911–919.

121. Rovai LE, Herschman HR, Smith JB. The murine neutrophil-chemoattractant chemokines LIX, KC, and MIP-2 have distinct induction kinetics, tissue distributions, and tissue-specific sensitivities to glucocorticoid regulation in endotoxemia. J Leukoc Biol 1998; 64:494–502.

122. Martin T, Goodman R 1999 The role of chemokines in the pathophysiology of the acute respiratory distress syndrome (ARDS). In Hebert C (ed) Chemokines in Disease. Humana Press, Totowa, pp 81–110.

123. Lee J, Horuk R, Rice GC, Bennett GL, Camerato T, Wood WI. Characterization of two high affinity human interleukin-8 receptors. J Biol Chem 1992; 267:16283–16287.

124. Lee J, Cacalano G, Camerato T, Toy K, Moore MW, Wood WI. Chemokine binding and activities mediated by the mouse IL-8 receptor. J Immunol 1995; 155:2158–2164.

125. De Sanctis GT, MacLean JA, Qin S, Wolyniec WW, Grasemann H, Yandava CN, Jiao A, Noonan T, Stein-Streilein J, Green FH, Drazen JM. Interleukin-8 receptor modulates IgE production and B-cell expansion and trafficking in allergen-induced pulmonary inflammation. J Clin Invest 1999; 103:507–515.

126. Cacalano G, Lee J, Kikly K, Ryan AM, Pitts-Meek S, Hultgren B, Wood WI, Moore MW. Neutrophil and B cell expansion in mice that lack the murine IL-8 receptor homolog. Science 1994; 265:682–684.

127. Godaly G, Hang L, Frendeus B, Svanborg C. Transepithelial neutrophil migration is CXCR1 dependent in vitro and is defective in IL-8 receptor knockout mice. J Immunol 2000; 165:5287–5294.

128. DeVries ME, Ran L, Kelvin DJ. On the edge: the physiological and pathophysiological role of chemokines during inflammatory and immunological responses. Semin Immunol 1999; 11:95–104.

129. Hancock WW, Gao W, Faia KL, Csizmadia V. Chemokines and their receptors in allograft rejection. Curr Opin Immunol 2000; 12:511–516.

130. Yamaguchi Y, Ichiguchi O, Matsumura F, Akizuki E, Matsuda T, Okabe K, Yamada S, Liang J, Mori K, Ogawa M. Enhanced expression of cytokine-induced neutrophil chemoattractant in rat hepatic allografts during acute rejection. Hepatology 1997; 26:1546–1552.

131. Morita K, Miura M, Paolone DR, Engeman TM, Kapoor A, Remick DG, Fairchild RL. Early chemokine cascades in murine cardiac grafts regulate T cell recruitment and progression of acute allograft rejection. J Immunol 2001; 167:2979–2984.

132. Zheng L, Walters EH, Ward C, Wang N, Orsida B, Whitford H, Williams TJ, Kotsimbos T, Snell GI. Airway neutrophilia in stable and bronchiolitis obliterans syndrome patients following lung transplantation. Thorax 2000; 55:53–59.

133. Elssner A, Jaumann F, Dobmann S, Behr J, Schwaiblmair M, Reichenspurner H, Furst H, Briegel J, Vogelmeier C. Elevated Levels of Interleukin-8 and Transforming Growth Factor-beta in Bronchoalveolar Lavage Fluid from Patients with Bronchiolitis Obliterans Syndrome: Proinflammatory Role of Bronchial Epithelial Cells. Munich Lung Transplant Group. Transplantation 2000; 70:362–367.

134. Elssner A, Vogelmeier C. The role of neutrophils in the pathogenesis of obliterative bronchiolitis after lung transplantation. Transpl Infect Dis 2001; 3:168–176.

135. Zabel BA, Agace WW, Campbell JJ, Heath HM, Parent D, Roberts AI, Ebert EC, Kassam N, Qin S, Zovko M, LaRosa GJ, Yang LL, Soler D, Butcher EC, Ponath PD, Parker CM, Andrew DP. Human G protein-coupled receptor GPR-9-6/CC chemokine receptor 9 is selectively expressed on intestinal homing T lymphocytes, mucosal lymphocytes, and thymocytes and is required for thymus-expressed chemokine-mediated chemotaxis. J Exp Med 1999; 190:1241–1256.

136. Yoneyama H, Harada A, Imai T, Baba M, Yoshie O, Zhang Y, Higashi H, Murai M, Asakura H, Matsushima K. Pivotal role of TARC, a CC chemokine, in bacteria-induced fulminant hepatic failure in mice. J Clin Invest 1998; 102:1933–1941.

137. Gonzalo JA, Pan Y, Lloyd CM, Jia GQ, Yu G, Dussault B, Powers CA, Proudfoot AE, Coyle AJ, Gearing D, Gutierrez-Ramos JC. Mouse monocyte-derived chemokine is involved in airway hyperreactivity and lung inflammation. J Immunol 1999; 163:403–411.

138. Nikolic B, Lee S, Bronson RT, Grusby MJ, Sykes M. Th1 and Th2 mediate acute graft-versus-host disease, each with distinct end-organ targets. J Clin Invest 2000; 105:1289–1298.

139. Rus V, Svetic A, Nguyen P, Gause WC, Via CS. Kinetics of Th1 and Th2 cytokine production during the early course of acute and chronic murine graft-versus-host disease. J Immunol 1995; 155:2396–2406.

140. Sasaki M, Hasegawa H, Kohno M, Inoue A, Ito MR, Fujita S. Antagonist of secondary lymphoid-tissue chemokine (CCR ligand 21) prevents the development of chronic graft-versus-host disease in mice. J Immunol 2003; 170:588–596.

141. Schneider GP, Salcedo R, Welniak LA, Howard OM, Murphy WJ. The diverse role of chemokines in tumor progression: prospects for intervention (Review). Int J Mol Med 2001; 8:235–244.

142. Salcedo R, Wasserman K, Young HA, Grimm MC, Howard OM, Anver MR, Kleinman HK, Murphy WJ, Oppenheim JJ. Vascular endothelial growth factor and basic fibroblast growth factor induce expression of CXCR4 on human endothelial cells: In vivo neovascularization induced by stromal-derived factor-1alpha. Am J Pathol 1999; 154:1125–1135.

143. Salcedo R, Martins-Green M, Gertz B, Oppenheim JJ, Murphy WJ. Combined administration of antibodies to human interleukin 8 and epidermal growth factor receptor results in increased antimetastatic effects on human breast carcinoma xenografts. Clin Cancer Res 2002; 8:2655–2665.

144. Sasaki M, Hasegawa H, Kohno M, Inoue A, Ito MR, Fujita S. Antagonist of secondary lymphoid-tissue chemokine (CCR ligand 21) prevents the development of chronic graft-versus-host disease in mice. J Immunol 2003; 170:588–596.

145. Zhang Y, McCormick LL, Desai SR, Wu C, Gilliam AC. Murine sclerodermatous graft-versus-host disease, a model for human scleroderma: cutaneous cytokines, chemokines, and immune cell activation. J Immunol 2002; 168:3088–3098.

6

Graft-vs.-Leukemia Effects

JEFFREY J. MOLLDREM

The University of Texas M. D. Anderson Cancer Center, Houston, Texas, U.S.A.

WARREN D. SHLOMCHIK

Yale University School of Medicine, New Haven, Connecticut, U.S.A.

I. INTRODUCTION

The most compelling clinical evidence that lymphocytes meditate an anti-leukemia effect comes from studies that used allogeneic donor lymphocyte infusions (DLI) to treat relapse of myeloid leukemia after allogeneic hemopoietic cell transplantation (HCT) (1–5). Lymphocyte transfusions from the original bone marrow (BM) donor induces both hematological and cytogenetic responses in approximately 70–80% of patients with chronic myelogenous leukemia (CML) in the chronic phase (CP) (4). Complete cytogenetic responses are usually obtained between 1 and 4 months after DLI (6), and approximately 80% of responders will achieve reverse transcriptase-polymerase chain reaction (RT-PCR) negativity for the *bcr-abl* translocation gene [the fusion product of the t(9;22) translocation found in CML] within 6 months (6). Acute myeloid leukemia (AML) is also susceptible to the GVL effect, with 15–40% of patients obtaining remissions with DLI alone (7). While significant GVHD occurs in approximately 50% of CML patients treated with DLI and 90% of those patients respond, 55% of patients without GVHD also have disease responses (1,2). These observations suggest that GVL may be separable from GVHD.

In this chapter we will briefly review the history of the study of tumor immunity and of transplantation biology as they pertain to the study of GVL. We will discuss murine models of GVL and subsequently examine the effector cells that potentially mediate GVL in the clinical setting.

II. HISTORICAL BACKGROUND

Harnessing the body's immune system to treat malignancy is a concept that dates back more than 100 years. The approach taken by HCT physicians is based on observations made by Barnes and colleagues in 1956 (8). They observed that an allogeneic reaction of the graft against the recipient's leukemia might contribute to the cure of leukemia. Similar anecdotal observations were made in humans. However, leukocyte (tissue) antigens, now termed HLA, were described only in 1958 (9), and HCT performed with knowledge of these antigens did not occur until 1968 (10). In 1981 peripheral blood stem cells began to supplant bone marrow as a source of hematopoietic progenitors, and in the last 15 years HLA-mismatched products and cord blood have been increasingly used.

Based upon the observation that patients with malignancies who developed severe infections would occasionally experience regression of their tumors, physicians in Europe intentionally induced bacterial infections in cancer patients (8). Dr. William B. Coley, a New York physician, documented many anecdotal cases of such treatments using bacterial extracts (Coley's toxins) instead of bacteria (9). We now know that the active component, lipopolysaccharide (LPS), binds to surface Toll-like receptors (TLR) on host antigen-presenting cells (APC) such as dendritic cells (DC), and these activated (8,9) DC stimulate antigen-specific lymphocytes.

During the 1940s it was shown in inbred mouse models that when chemically induced sarcoma cells were used to elicit immunity in one animal, the resulting sarcoma-specific T lymphocytes could be adoptively transferred to syngeneic-naïve recipient animals and would protect against secondary tumor challenges (10,11). The use of allogeneic tumor-sensitized lymphocytes in humans was first reported in 1966 (12). Irradiated tumors from one patient were subcutaneously implanted into the thigh of another patient, and 2 weeks later 500 mL of blood containing leukocytes from the recipient were transfused back into the original tumor donor. Some minor responses were reported. Eventually recombinant cytokines such as interleukin 2 (IL-2) were used to expand autologous lymphocytes that showed some antitumor activity in vitro. Such lymphokine-activated killer (LAK) cells were first described in 1980, and since then LAK cells with or without IL-2 have been used to treat patients with many different tumor types (13–15). In patients with renal cell cancer or melanoma, response rates were seen in up to 15–30% of patients (16).

Beginning in 1988, tumor-infiltrating lymphocytes (TIL), collected from human melanoma lesions and expanded ex vivo with IL-2, were used to induce both partial and complete and partial regressions (17). There was no significant relationship between response rate and the number of infused TIL, although there was a highly significant association of tumor response with the ability of TIL to lyse autologous tumor targets in vitro (18). The administration of cyclophosphamide was significantly associated with the ability of TIL to localize to tumor, and localization to tumor correlated with clinical response (19). More recently, megadoses of TIL ($>10^{12}$) were shown to contribute to remission of melanoma when the cells were infused following lympholytic chemotherapy. These investigators used a combination of peptide/MHC I tetramers and molecular sequencing of TCR derived from the TIL to demonstrate tumor specificity (20).

TIL taken either directly from the tumors or from the peripheral blood of these patients exhibit cross-reactivity with autologous and allogeneic tumors in a MHC-restricted manner. These observations led to the first successful characterization of a human tumor antigen, MAGE-1, in 1991 (21). The phenomenon of MHC-restricted tumor cell specificity has now also been observed in patients with other cancers, and many other tumor-associated antigens (TAA) have since been isolated (22,23).

III. ANIMAL MODELS OF GVL

The earliest murine transplant models suggested that the donor immunity in the allogeneic hemopoietic cell transplant (allo HCT) could be harnessed to treat leukemias (24–26). GVL research has focused on solving two key clinical problems:) Is GVL separable from GVHD? and How can we augment GVL against relatively resistant diseases? Murine models offer important advantages over studies in other species. Mice are relatively inexpensive to maintain, and well-characterized inbred strains allow experiments with large groups of nearly identical mice. Of all potential animal models, the murine immune system is the best defined, and a wide range of reagents including antibodies, cytokines, and growth factors are readily available. Finally, the rapid growth in the numbers of transgenic and gene-deficient strains has enabled a detailed examination of specific immune mechanisms.

However, murine models also have some drawbacks and limitations. Models rarely parallel human transplantation in that up-front immunosuppression is infrequently used in murine experiments, and spleen cells, as opposed to peripheral blood T cells, are most commonly infused as a source of alloreactive lymphocytes. Generalizations are often difficult to make because GVHD responses in different strain combinations are unique. Finally, the types of leukemias studied are typically derived from cell lines, which share only a subset of important biological features with de novo human leukemias.

A. Variables Examined in Murine Models

1. Donor : Recipient Strain Pair

To understand the outcomes of various murine transplant models, it is first helpful to review the various strains that have been investigated. Donor : recipient strain pairings fall into five main categories: (a) MHC identical, minor histocompatibility antigen (mHA) incompatible [e.g., B10.BR (H-2^k) $\rightarrow$ CBA (H-2^k)]; (b) MHC disparate on different background strains [e.g., B6 (H-2^b) $\rightarrow$ BALB/c (H-2^d)]; (c) MHC disparate on identical background strains (e.g., B10 (H-2^b) $\rightarrow$ B10.BR (H-2^k)]; (d) the use of strains in which single MHC I or MHC II alleles differ by only a small number of residues that mostly affect TCR recognition rather than peptide binding (e.g., B6 $\rightarrow$ B6^{bm12} or B6 $\rightarrow$ B6^{bm1})]; and (e) parent $\rightarrow$ F1 models such as B6 $\rightarrow$ (B6 $\times$ DBA/2)F1. In the latter case, model leukemias share MHC restriction with only one of the parental strains.

2. Leukemia Models

Model leukemias and lymphomas are listed in Table 1. Most of these leukemia cell lines were derived from spontaneous or mutagen-induced neoplasms. There is variability due to subcloning efficiency and the outgrowth of more dominant clones within these cell lines. The most commonly used lines are the P815 mastocytoma line, the EL4 T-cell lymphoma line, and the 32D myeloid line (see Table 1). Retrovirus-mediated insertion of oncogenes has also been used to induce leukemias, although this can complicate an understanding of the immune response against those leukemia lines (27,28). A commonly used model (considered separately below) is immunodeficient NOD/SCID mice, which are then used

Table 1 Murine Leukemia Models and Strain Combinations Studied

Model leukemia	Descriptions	Background strain	Ref.
p815	Mastocytoma cell line	DBA/2 (H-2^d)	37,39,44,220–222
32D	Myeloid different differentiation based on culture conditions subclone variation IL-3 dependent	C3H/HeJ (H-2^k)	223
32D-p210	As per 32D, p210 transduced, IL-3 independent	C3H/HeJ (H-2^k)	39,43,49,224
BCL-1	Spontaneous B-cell lymphoma	BALB/c (H-2^d)	225–228
A20	Spontaneous B-cell lymphoma	BALB/c	229
AKR Leukemia	T-cell leukemia/lymphoma	AKR	31,33,35,230,231
C1498	Spontaneous myeloid tumor	B6 (H-2^b)	66,232–234
EL4	T-cell lymphoma induced by 9,10-dimethyl-1,2-benzanthracene	B6 (H-2^b)	32,80,81,235,236
LE750, 833, 9107, 7929	Irradiation-induced leukemias	C3H/HeJ (H-2^k)	237
MMBX.X	c-myo–transformed myeloid lines with macrophage features	B6	27,41,238

to study antileukemia responses by human effector cells against human leukemias, both of which have been adoptively transferred to the mouse (29,30).

3. Transplant Protocols

Transplant protocols for murine study vary substantially. Total body irradiation (TBI) is the most commonly used conditioning regimen; chemotherapy has been used alone or in combination with TBI, and doses of both have varied significantly. Similar to human transplantation, increasing conditioning dose intensity typically worsens GVHD (31) and likely promotes alloimmune responses in general. With the advent of lower intensity conditioning regimens in humans, those conditions are also being explored in murine systems, including the intentional establishment of mixed chimerism (32). Most investigators model minimal residual disease by infusing a small number of leukemic cells after the conditioning regimens or a somewhat larger dose prior to irradiation. It is not clear which approach is closer to the human situation. Some studies have infused leukemic cells after T cells that are given either at the time of transplant or days to weeks posttransplant (32–36).

4. Source of Donor T Cells

Splenocytes are the most common source of T cells. The role of T-cell subsets in GVL has been studied using both positive (cell-selecting) and negative (cell-depleting) selection methods and by the use of antibodies to recipient cell surface markers that deplete T-cell subsets. The use of defined genetically deficient T cells has been a powerful technique to study modes of T-cell activation and effector function in both knockout and transgenic models. In particular, T cells deficient in FasL, perforin, TNF-α, and TRAIL have been studied (37–46). Results of these studies tend to support the notion that while perforin is an important mediator of CD8 CTL-mediated GVL, FasL may be more important for mediating GVHD. T cells from donors immunized to host splenocytes, leukemic cells, or to peptide antigens have also been studied as a way to understand the target antigens involved in GVL (47,48). Ex vivo cultured cells polarized to Th1 or Th2 phenotypes have also been studied, and some evidence suggests that Th1 subsets may convey more GVHD while Th2 subsets favor GVL (49).

5. Reagents Tested

As shown in Table 2, a large number of potential mediators of GVL have been tested. In many cases these reagents were found to decrease GVHD before being tested in GVL models. Such reagents include cytokines (IL-2, IL-12, IL-11, IL-18), growth factors [keratinocyte growth factor (KGF) and G-CSF], agents that block the activity of costimulatory molecules and cytokines, the LPS antagonist B975, and FTY720, which alters T-cell trafficking.

B. Summary of Findings from GVL Models

1. Target Antigens in MHC-Identical, but Multiple mHA-Disparate Allo HCT

Minor histocompatibility antigens, the principal targets of alloimmune responses in MHC-identical allo HCT, are derived from the protein products of genes that are most commonly polymorphic between donor and recipient. Splice variants and incomplete gene expression may also result in mHA. Although donor and recipient mouse pairs differ at many loci, genetic studies have suggested that, for example, between B6 (H-2^b) and BALB.B (H-2^b) mice, more than 50 potential mHA exist. Pioneering studies using mHA congenic mice generated by crossing B6 and BALB.B strains suggested that, similar to antiviral CD8 responses, alloimmune CD8 responses target only a few immunodominant epitopes among the many possible target peptides. These studies also showed a hierarchy of dominance, i.e., responses against some targets could only be detected in the absence of more dominant epitopes (50–55). These studies were pivotal in providing an overall framework for understanding alloimmune responses.

   The results of these genetic studies were later confirmed at the molecular level and served to confirm the underlying hypotheses. Bulk CTL cultures from the different MHC-matched strains, which had the potential to recognize multiple mHA, in fact only recognized a few HPLC-separated peptide fractions from the surface of the target cells (56–58), consistent with the hypothesis that immunodominance is an important feature of MHC-identical alloimmune responses. That the presence or absence of an immunodominant target peptide could influence GVL was suggested from experiments in which CTL lines raised against one dominant antigen were not able to kill MHC-identical leukemia cells that lacked the immunodominant peptide fraction (59). Until more is known about the distribution of immunodominant epitopes in different donor : recipient pairs, it is difficult to assess how frequently an absence of an immunodominant epitope in a neoplasm can account for the lack of a GVL effect.

   It is not clear whether these peptides are endogenously expressed in host APC or are cross-presented by host or donor APC. We have shown in an MHC-compatible CD8-dependent GVHD model that host APC are absolutely required for GVHD induction and that neither the engrafting nor the long-term resident donor APC are effective in priming GVHD reactions (60). If the same is true for GVL reactions, then immunodominant

Table 2 Potential Mediators and Modifiers of GVL and Various Murine Models Used to Investigate Them

Reagent/Approach	Transplant model	Model leukemia	T-cell dose(s)	Death by GVHD	Comments/Mechanism	Ref.
IL-2	A/J → B10 10.25 Gy	EL-4 500 cells/mouse	Varied	Median about 50 days	aGVHD requires CD4 cells; GVL CD8-mediated; IL-2 reduces CD4-mediated alloreactivity	80
IL-12	A/J + B10 → B10 10.25 Gy	EL-4 500 cells/mouse	$15-18 \times 10^6$ spleen cells	Varied; median 10–50 days	aGVHD requires CD4 cells; GVL CD8-mediated; IL-12 reduces CD4-mediated alloreactivity	81
IL-11	B6 → B6D2F1 B6 → B6C3F1 1500 cGy, 11 Gy	p815 2000/mouse 32D, 500 cells 5000/mouse	1×10^6	> 50% by day 5 7/40 overall	GVHD CD4 mediated; IL-11 acts on CD4 cells and less so on CD8 cells	39
IL-18	B6 → B6D2F1 13 Gy	p815, 2000/mouse	2×10^6, 1×10^6	50% by day 30	CD4 dependent GVHD model; promotes apoptosis of CD4 cells	44,82
KGF (keratinocyte growth factor)	B6 → B6D2F1 13 Gy	p815, 5000/mouse	2×10^6	50% day 5	Protection of gut epithelium	38
IL-1 antagonism	B6 → B6D2F1 CTX 100 mg/kg 900 Gy	p815, 50,000/mouse	2×10^6	50% day 15	CD4 dependent GVHD model; CTL activity preserved with anti-IL-1R antibody	37
GCSF	B6 → B6D2F1 11 Gy	p815, 5–25,000/mouse	10^7 splenocytes	w/o GCSF—100% at 12 days w/GCSF—5% at 75 days	CD4 dependent GVHD model; CTL activity preserved	83

B975 (LPS antagonism)	B6 → B6D2F1 14 Gy	p815 mastocytoma 2000/mouse	2×10^6	> 50% by D7	No effect on CTL activity?	222
FTY720	C3HD2F1 → B6D2F1 9.75 Gy	EL4 5000/animal	1–3×10^6 spleen cells	3×10^6 90% D10 1×10^6 0% D100	FTY720 traps T cells in lymphoid organs?	239
Anti-CTLA-4	B10.Br → B6 800 cGy DLI day 21	C1498 2×10^6 D28	25×10^6 D28	50% D130	Anti-CTLA-4 increased leukemia protection, but no increase in overall survival	36
Mixed chimera/DLI	B10.A → B6 B10.A + B6 → B6 10.25 Gy	EL4 cells 500/mouse	3×10^7	0%	A protection assay; DLI day 56; EL4 cells day 63; most APCs important for maximal GVL	32
Tc1/Tc2	B6 → B6C3F1 1050 cGy	32D/p210 10^4/mouse	0.5–2.5×10^7	Varied	Modest survival advantage in recipients of Tc1 > Tc2 cells; less GVHD with Tc2 > Tc1	49
DLI	B10.BR → AKR SJL → [SJL × AKR]F1 9 Gy	AKR T cell leukemia/ lymphoma 5×10^4/ mouse	3×10^7	0% with DLI on D21	A protection assay; DLI given on day 21, AKR leukemia on day 28	33–35
Antigen specificity	B10.H7^b (B6^{dom1} primed) → B10 or B10.H7^b 1000 cGy	EL4 10^5/mouse on D1	5×10^7 spleen 0.5×10^5 B6dom1	0%	B6dom1 specific T cells alone do not cause GVHD; GVL more effective in recipients not expressing B6^{dom1}	47
Immunize donors with MHC disparate 3rd party cells	CBA → AKR	AKR leukemia 10^5/animal	10^7 spleen or LN	varied	Mice immunized against 3rd party cells had increased GVL without GVHD; mechanism not known.	48

(Continued)

Table 2 Continued

Reagent/ Approach	Transplant model	Model leukemia	T-cell dose(s)	Death by GVHD	Comments/Mechanism	Ref.
FasL-deficient T cells	B6 → B6D2F1 12 Gy	p815 10^5/ mouse D-2 L1210 10^4/ mouse D-2	2×10^7 spleen cells	wt 50% D28 gld 0% PKO 0%	GVL does not require FasL; GVHD attenuated with FasL−/− T cells	40
FasL-deficient T cells	B6 → B6D2F1 B6 → B6C3F1 13 Gy	32D/p210 1– 5×10^3/ mouse p815	$1–2 \times 10^6$	wt 50% D30 PKO 50% D35 gld 70& D90	GVL does not require FasL; GVHD attenuated with FasL−/− T cells; GVHD CD4 dominated with FasL mechanism; GVL CD8 dominated with perforin-mediated killing	43
Regulatory DCs (rDC)	B6 → DBA/2 10 Gy	p815, 2×10^5 D-2	1.5×10^7	no rDC, 100% D8	rDC suppress alloimmune responses via generation of regulatory T cells; sufficient alloreactivity to mediate GVL	74
Regulatory	CD4 + CD25 + cells	B6 → BALB/c	BCL1-luciferase A20-luciferase		Overall suppression of alloreactivity; intact CD8 CTL activity	84

peptides must be endogenously expressed in host APCs, and one would expect that for leukemia cells to be sensitive to spontaneous GVL reactions, they must also express the genes encoding immunodominant epitopes expressed in APC.

2. Mechanisms of T-Cell Killing

Is GVL mediated by CD4+ T cells or CD8+ T cells alone, or are both required? In part, the answer depends upon the model, but effective GVL by either CD8 cells or CD4 cells alone has been demonstrated, while in some models maximal GVL depends on a mix of CD4 and CD8 cells. The roles of FasL and perforin in killing have been evaluated using FasL$-/-$ or perforin$-/-$ T cells (39–44). Perforin appears to be more critical than FasL-mediated killing for CD8 CTL responses. The role of TNF-α has also been shown to be important in GVL responses via experiments with anti-TNF-α antibodies, TNF-$\alpha-/-$, and TNFR1$-/-$ T cells (37,40,46). It has been difficult to directly implicate TNF-α as a direct cytolytic mediator since TNF-α also plays a role in the initiation of alloimmune responses (61). For example, in one model, anti-TNF-α antibodies decreased GVL while the target cells themselves were resistant to TNF-α in vitro (40). Another TNF-α family member expressed on T cells, TRAIL (TNF-related apoptosis-inducing ligand), has also been implicated as being important for GVL (46). The role of TRAIL was examined in MHC-disparate and MHC-identical allo HCT models against p815 and 32D-p210 cell lines. Overall, the absence of TRAIL had little effect on GVHD but significantly reduced GVL in the three model systems tested. The authors suggested that augmentation of TRAIL-mediated killing might induce more effective GVL without increasing GVHD.

We have studied GVL in an MHC-identical, multiple mHA-disparate system using a murine model of chronic phase CML (mCP-CML) induced by retrovirus expressing the human p210 cDNA (28,62–65). Because mCP-CML is induced by a retrovirus-encoding gene, we have been able to transfer it to mice that are deficient in genes that might be important mediators of GVL killing. An advantage of this approach over using gene-deficient T cells is that the T-cell response is left intact and only the posited effector mechanisms are tested. For CD8 CTL-mediated GVL in this model, mCP-CML targets deficient in Fas or doubly deficient in TNFR1 and TNFR2 were as sensitive to GVL as wild-type targets (W. Shlomchik, unpublished data). For CD4 T cell–mediated GVL, we have found that GVL is impaired, although not absent, against MHC II$-$ mCP-CML (W. Shlomchik, unpublished data), suggesting that direct cognate interactions are required for maximal CD4-mediated killing.

3. Antigen Presentation in GVL

In alloimmune responses, naïve T-cell responses are primed by so-called professional APC, including DC, B cells, and macrophages. These APC provide requisite costimulatory signals to T cells critical for their activation, proliferation, and maturation into effector and memory T cells. Antigen presentation has been the focus of numerous GVHD studies, but has been less well examined in GVL responses.

Costimulatory molecule blockade has been proposed as a method to prevent GVHD, and obviously the impact of these interventions on GVL responses would be of particular interest. A priori, one would expect that interventions that block costimulation would weaken GVL, whereas those that promote antigen-driven T-cell expansion will promote it.

To study this question, Blazar and colleagues (66) have examined antibody-mediated blockade of B7 engagement with both CD28 and CTLA-4 and blockade of B7 engagement only with CTLA-4 in an MHC-disparate DLI model. Blocking antibodies to

B7-1 and B7-2 inhibited GVL against C1498 cells as completely as depleting antibodies to both CD4 and CD8. The same study suggested that B7-1 overexpression on leukemic cell lines might promote GVL responses. This left unanswered whether the infusion of a small number of B7-modified leukemia cells could enhance protection against unmodified leukemic cells, which could be a useful clinical strategy. In contrast to B7 blockade, blocking antibodies to CTLA-4 augmented DLI-mediated GVL against C1498 cells (36). Although GVHD was not noted to be increased in recipients of anti-CTLA-4 as compared to controls, overall survival was not improved due to the number of deaths from GVHD. The same study showed that anti-CTLA-4, when given on day 0, augmented GVHD, suggesting that its use in the DLI setting would likely still carry an increased risk for GVHD. Nevertheless, these murine experiments provide important preclinical data supporting the use of CTLA-4 blockade to augment GVL, especially against relatively GVL-resistant neoplasms or in patients who do not develop GVHD after DLI given for relapsed or persistent disease.

These studies suggest that blocking B7-mediated activation of CD28 will impair alloimmunity in general, as would be expected. This effect could be T-cell dose dependent, as CD28$-/-$ T cells have been shown to cause GVHD in MHC I$-$ and MHC II$-$disparate models, although their capacity to do so at lower T-cell doses is impaired (36,67,68). These studies also highlight that the net effect of B7 blockade reflects the activity of both the CD28 and CTLA-4 pathways. It remains untested whether B7 blockade begun on day 0 or in MHC identical models would enhance GVL over GVHD.

Blazar et al. used the same MHC-disparate DLI model to examine augmentation of signaling via 4-1BB (69). 4-1BB is a TNF-receptor family member expressed on activated cytolytic and helper T cells (70–72). The 4-1BB ligand is expressed on B cells, macrophages, and DC. Infusion of an agonist antibody to 4-1BB augmented GVL mediated by only a modest dose of donor spleen cells. However, at higher DLI doses, survival was decreased due to more severe GVHD, supporting the conclusion that a dose effect of T cells might separate GVL and GVHD in the setting of modified T-cell costimulation. As with anti-CTLA4, this could be a promising approach in some high-risk clinical settings, albeit with a significant increased risk for probability of GVHD.

In the mCP-CML GVL model system described above using MHC-dentical, multiple mHA-mismatched pairings, CD8-mediated GVL was intact if donor bone marrow was MHC-I$-$ and, thus, unable to interact with donor CD8 T cells. We examined the role of antigen presentation by leukemia cells via generation of mCP-CML in B7.1/B7.2$-/-$ cells and found that GVL mediated by a mix of CD4 and CD8 cells was intact (W. Shlomchik, unpublished data). These studies are ongoing and may help shed more light on the role of costimulation in GVL.

4. Separation of GVL and GVHD

The holy grail of allo SCT has been the ability to deliver a potent antitumor effect without GVHD. Table 2 summarizes some different approaches. Separation of GVHD and GVL could be achieved in several general ways. Overall T-cell alloreactivity can be reduced such that it is sufficient for GVL but insufficient for GVHD. For example, T-cell doses can be decreased to numbers that can mediate GVL without GVHD, and this has already been demonstrated clinically (73). A novel approach for globally suppressing alloimmune responses is the infusion of regulatory DC (rDC) at the time of transplant (74). In a Pto F1 model, this approach achieved GVHD suppression with sufficient remaining alloreactivity to kill p815 mastocytoma cells. The data from this innovative study suggest that GVHD is suppressed via the generation of donor-derived CD4+/CD25+ regulatory T cells, a subject discussed elsewhere in this book.

GVL and GVHD could also be separated on the basis of T-cell subset selection. This has been studied in human allo HCT as well, with the suggestion that CD8-depleted DLI or the selective depletion of CD8 T cells from initial grafts can still mediate GVL against chronic phase CML, but with less GVHD (75,76). We have found this to be true in the mCP-CML GVL model where CD4 cells alone can mediate GVL without GVHD when performed in a strain pairing in which CD4 cells alone do not cause GVHD (28). These data suggest that there can be CD4 T-cell–mediated reactivity against malignant hematopoietic cells without clinical GVHD. However, when we tested the efficacy of CD4 cells in a strain pairing in which CD4 cells mediate GVHD, GVL was accompanied by GVHD (W. Shlomchik, unpublished data), suggesting that this might be also be true in humans if CD4 T cells did not contribute to GVHD, which does not appear likely. In a separate clinical trial of a small group of CP-CML patients, CD4 T-cell–depleted grafts that were augmented with CD8 CTL also showed less GVHD and better engraftment, without higher than expected relapse rates (77). Furthermore, graded doses of DLI have shown that GVL can be induced with less GVHD for treatment of CML (78). Taken together, this may imply that both CD4 and CD8 subsets are important mediators of both GVL and GVHD in humans, and that any method that produces a modest degree of T-cell depletion can translate into a reduction in GVHD with retention of some GVL. This is supported by a larger study from the IBMTR that shows that "narrow specificity" antibodies are associated with better preservation of the GVL effect, as measured by leukemia-free survival (79).

In some Pto F1 models, GVHD is primarily mediated by CD4 T cells, while GVL against at least some cell lines has been found to be mostly CD8 CTL-dependent. This difference has been exploited by manipulations that suppress the alloreactivity of CD4 cells greater than that of CD8 cells. For example, a number of mediator reagent-based interventions in the B6to B6D2F1 Pto F1 model are capable of suppressing CD4 T-cell–mediated GVHD while leaving CD8 CTL responses relatively intact (37,39,44,80–83).

Regulatory CD4+ CD25+ cells have also been tested for their ability to suppress GVHD while leaving GVL intact (84). In an MHC-disparate model with the BCL1 lymphoma and A20 leukemic cell lines, CD4+CD25+ cells suppressed GVHD while leaving adequate alloreactivity to mediate effective GVL. Specifically, perforin-mediated CD8+ CTL activity was shown to be intact. Another novel feature of this model was the use of leukemia cell lines that express luciferase, which allowed simultaneous in vivo imaging based on bioluminescence.

GVL and GVHD might also be separated on the basis of unique effector mechanisms. In some models, GVHD is FasL-dependent, but GVL can be mediated by perforin, TNF-α, and TRAIL, independent of FasL (40,43).

Furthermore, it may also be possible to separate GVL and GVHD via the use of T cells that recognize only a single dominant mHA, as single mHA differences have been shown to be insufficient for GVHD (51,85). In an MHC-matched model, CD8 T cells only recognizing the B6 mHA B6^{dom1} mediated GVL without inducing GVHD (47).

Finally, in another approach, T cells that recognize hematopoietically restricted antigens might also be able to mediate GVL with less GVHD (86–93). This is a very attractive approach for augmenting GVL without GVHD, although it would not solve the problem of reconstituting T cells without inducing GVHD. A novel way in which this approach might be used therapeutically would be to elicit T cells from a donor, for example, of MHC type A, against a hematopoietically restricted antigen presented by recipient cells of MHC type B (91–93). The T cells would need to retain their peptide specificity and also have the necessary MHC type B restriction. If used in the MHC-disparate allo HCT setting, recipient hematopoietic cells should be susceptible, but donor hematopoietic cells would not be as they are of a different MHC type. This approach would not be limited to mHA, but would apply to any hematopoietic-restricted peptide that sufficiently bound to two or more HLA alleles (see below).

5. NOD/SCID Mice for the Study of GVL Effects with Human T Cells and Natural Killer Cells

As introduced above, the use of CD8+ T-cell lines or clones that recognize antigens restricted to hematopoietic cells restricted antigens has been suggested as a potential strategy for inducing GVL without GVHD. In vitro studies demonstrated that such cells could kill bulk populations of leukemia blasts. However, it has been more difficult to determine whether clonogenic leukemia blasts are susceptible to such killing. The use of NOD/SCID mice has been suggested as an in vivo model reservoir of adoptively transferred patient leukemia cells, which can then be assayed to determine the spectrum of primitive hematopoietic cells, including clonogenic AML blasts (94–96). Cells that can colonize NOD/SCID mice have been termed SCID leukemia-initiating cells, or SL-IC. Using this model, human CD8+ CTL clones when cultured with AML blasts were shown to reduce the engraftment of those blasts in NOD/SCID mice (29). If T-cell clones are to be applied clinically, such a model system could be useful in predicting their in vivo efficacy in patients. Questions about toxicity or epitope spread could not be easily addressed due to potential differences in gene expression and tissue distribution of the target antigen between humans and mice and due to differences in MHC.

The NOD/SCID system has also been used to demonstrate the efficacy of alloreactive natural killer cell (NK) lines and clones to kill clonogenic AML cells (30). However, unlike human T cells, human alloreactive NK cells were shown to kill AML blasts in vivo in NOD/SCID mice after engraftment. This result was important in providing evidence that alloreactive NK cells directly kill AML blasts in humans rather than mediating an indirect effect (see below).

IV. PRECLINICAL AND CLINICAL STUDIES OF GVL EFFECTS IN HUMANS

A. Effector Cells of GVL

Because T-cell depletion of donor cells is associated with significant relapse rates after HCT, and because enrichment of T cells in either the original graft or in subsequent DLI increases the likelihood of remaining in durable remission, it is thought that $\alpha\beta$-T lymphocytes are the most significant mediators of GVL (Table 3). Although unconventional T-cell subsets such as $\gamma\delta$ T cells, NKT cells, or certain other CD1-restricted $\alpha\beta$ T cells have been studied for their GVL potential, these cells may have only limited, if any, involvement. Likewise, the humoral immune response is unlikely to play a significant role in GVL. However, recent data have emerged that NK cells may contribute to GVL very early after HCT in AML patients that are transplanted with donor cells mismatched at specific MHC class I loci. In this section, we will examine the biology of these mediators of GVL by reviewing relevant preclinical and clinical studies.

Table 3 Clinical Evidence of Lymphocyte-Mediated GVL Effects

Relapse increased in recipients of T-cell–depleted transplants (79)

Relapse decreased in recipients who develop acute/chronic GVHD (240)

Remission associated with GVHD flares (7,241)

Relapse higher in recipients of T-cell–depleted matched related donor allograft recipients who develop GVHD compared to recipients of matched related donor allografts who do not develop GVHD (242)

Remission in up to 90% of CML patients who receive DLI administered for relapse after transplant (2,243)

B. T Lymphocytes

T cells recognize peptide antigens that are presented on the cell surface in combination with major histocompatibility complex (MHC, in humans termed HLA) antigens (Fig. 1). Peptides derived from intracellular cytoplasmic proteins that are 8–11 amino acids in length bind within the groove of class I MHC molecules and are transported via the endoplasmic reticulum to the cell surface and are subsequently recognized by CD8 T cells. Larger peptides, 12–18 amino acids in length, usually derived from extracellular proteins, bind class II MHC molecules and are presented on the cell surface to CD4 T cells. Both peptide/MHC I and peptide/MHC II are recognized by the heterodimeric $\alpha\beta$ T-cell receptor (TCR-$\alpha\beta$) with very rapid off rates and k_D that are typically in the range of 10^{-4}– 10^{-5} M (97) (Fig. 2). Points of contact between the TCR and the peptide/MHC surface

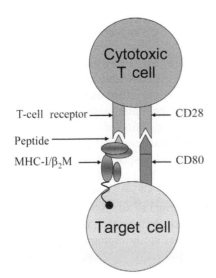

Figure 1 Antigen recognition by T lymphocytes. Peptide antigen, presented in the peptide-binding groove of an MHC molecule, is recognized and bound by the T-cell receptor (TCR), as shown for a CD8 T-lymphocyte response. The T lymphocyte also receives other co-stimulatory signals from antigen-presenting cells that modulate the antigen-specific signal. As an example, the CD28 receptor on CD8 Ty lymphocytes binds CD80 on the antigen-presenting cell, which decreases the activation threshold of the T lymphocyte.

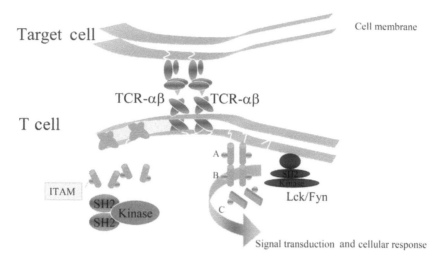

Figure 2 T-cell receptor (TCR) signaling. After binding to cognate antigen/MHC complexes on the antigen-presenting cell (APC) surface, TCRs assemble toward the center of an enlarging synapse between the T lymphocyte and the APC. Phosphorylation of the immune receptor tyrosine activation motif (ITAM) on the various CD3 subunits associated with the TCR complex then occurs mediated by tyrosine kinases such as lck/fyn. The strength of the signal that is thereby transduced is related to the degree of ITAM phosphorylation. TCE-binding affinity and avidity contribute to prolonged signaling, and the signal strength progressively increases from activation threshold to possible overstimulation with saturation of the ITAMs, which may lead to eventual cell death.

include surface amino acids contributed by the two alpha helical domains of the MHC molecule that flank the peptide antigen binding pocket as well as amino acids from the peptide itself.

Following an initial limited contact of surface TCR-$\alpha\beta$ heterodimers with their cognate peptide/MHC target antigen, a complex signaling network leads to the formation of an immune synapse (98–101). Further modulation occurs via costimulatory molecules and cell adhesion molecules (99,100,102). In this way the initial signaling event is amplified, leading to further downstream events such as upregulation of IL-2 and the IL-2 receptor. These events are essential for subsequent T-cell functions (103).

Our understanding of the nature of antigen-specific T cell responses has been greatly improved by the discovery that antigen-specific TCR can be reversibly labeled with soluble peptide/MHC tetramers (104) (Fig. 3). Up to 45% of all peripheral circulating T cells may be specific for a single dominant antigen at the height of an immune response to EBV infection (105), and similar dominance may be seen during other viral infections (106,107). Tetramers have also been used to discover and study immune responses to tumor antigens (108,109).

C. Potential GVL T-Lymphocyte Antigens

Tissue-restricted mHA that are derived from proteins expressed only in hematopoietic tissue have been shown to be the targets of alloreactive T cells. These mHA may result from polymorphic differences between donor and recipient in the coding regions of peptide antigens. Heterologous T-cell clones with alloreactivity toward mHA have been

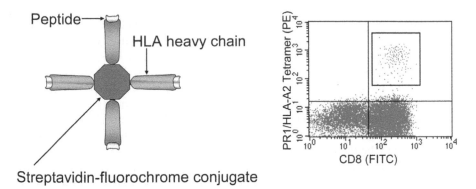

Streptavidin-fluorochrome conjugate

Figure 3 Peptide/MHC tetramers can be used to identify antigen-specific T lymphocytes. Recombinant MHC heavy chains are folded together with β_2-microglobulin and synthetic peptide antigens, and they are then attached via a biotin-streptavidin link at the C terminus of the MHC heavy chain to a fluorochrome, such as phycoerythrin (PE). The avidity of the TCR-peptide/MHC binding is increased by increasing the number of peptide/MHC monomers attached to the streptavidin up to four, with the geometry of the resulting tetramers being optimal for TCR binding.

established from patients with severe GVHD following HCT with an HLA-matched donors (110–113). Some of these mHA-specific CTL clones react only with hematopoietic-derived cells targets, suggesting tissue specificity (112), and therefore may be useful because of potentially shared antigens with leukemia cells. In one study, GVHD correlated closely with differences in the minor antigen HA-1 in HLA identical sibling transplants (114). Expression of two human mHAs, identified as HA-1 and HA-2, is confined to hematopoietic tissues, and HA-2 was identified as a peptide derived from the non–filament-forming class I myosin family by using mHA-reactive CTL clones to screen peptide fractions eluted from MHC class I molecules (115). This methodology is extremely labor intensive, and it is unclear whether CTL specific for any minor antigens identified thus far convey leukemia-specific immunity without concomitant GVHD. Adoptive cellular immunotherapy of leukemia using antigen-specific T cells that target mHA may promote GVL and reduce GVHD if appropriate mHA restricted to hematopoietic cells could be targeted. However, a practical limit of any immunotherapy approach targeting these mHAs is that only 10% of individuals would be expected to have the relevant HA-1 alternate allele, and <1% would have the HA-2 alternate allele, which makes donor availability quite limiting. An alternative immunological method, using peptides synthesized on the basis of an "educated guess" of which proteins are potential targets for a selective antileukemia CTL response, has been applied to determine whether BCR-ABL fusion region peptides could be used to elicit CML-specific T-cell responses. Since BCR-ABL is present in nearly all Philadelphia chromosome-positive CML patients, it is thought to represent a potentially unique leukemia antigen. The ABL coding sequences upstream (5') of exon II on chromosome 9 are translocated to chromosome 22 and fused in-frame with the BCR gene downstream (3') of exon III, resulting in a chimeric mRNA (b3a2) (the most common transcript), which is translated into a chimeric protein ($p210^{BCR-ABL}$). Translation of b3a2 mRNA results in the coding of a unique amino acid (lysine) within the fusion region. Some HLA-B8–restricted overlapping peptides inclusive of this lysine bind to HLA-B8 and could be used to elicit T-cell proliferative responses (116–118). However, when the b3a2 peptides were used to elicit b3a2-specific T lymphocyte lines in vitro, the resulting T cells could did not specifically lyse fresh CML cells which had not previously been pulsed with the peptide (118). This could have been due to a low affinity or lack of processing or presentation to CML cells. However, some b3a2-specific CTL have now been identified in the peripheral blood of CML patients using soluble b3a2 peptide/MHC tetramers (119). Although the tetramer-positive CTL from the patients were not tested to determine whether they killed CML targets, b3a2-specific CTL from healthy donors elicited in vitro were able to kill CML cells, suggesting that bcr-abl fusion peptides may be the targets of GVL reactions.

In tumors other than leukemia, many peptide targets for tumor-specific CTL have been identified. Nearly all tumor antigens identified as targets of tumor-specific CTL are derived from normal tissue proteins (23,120). Thus, many self-antigenic determinants have not induced self-tolerance, and these peptide determinants supply target structures for autoimmune attacks (120,121). Since these proteins are often aberrantly expressed or overexpressed in tumors, this may result in a relative tumor specificity of CTL that recognize these epitopes (122,123).

Melanomas have been studied extensively in regards to tumor immunity. MAGE-3–derived peptides, for example, are presented to CTL in the context of HLA-A1 and -A2 alleles (124–127). A phase I clinical trial using a MAGE-3 peptide showed some clinical responses (128). In addition, tyrosinase, gp100, and Melan-A-MART-1, normal self-proteins that are expressed only in the melanocyte lineage, are recognized by T cells in many melanoma patients (120,129,130).

Several patients with breast and ovarian cancer have existent have shown immune recognition of HER-2/neu, including T-cell recognition of specific HER-2/neu–derived peptides (131,132). The fact that patients have cancer despite an immune recognition is probably due to many reasons. For instance, tumors show heterogeneity in the level of expression of MHC, B7.1, and ICAM-1 on individual tumor cells (133). Cells with a low level of expression of these molecules may escape immune recognition (133). There may also be quantitative differences in antigen processing and presentation in the tumor cells (134).

Tumor cells (just like the virus-infected fibroblasts) may not process and present the tumor antigens to elicit responses against the dominant epitopes. This may be important in the search for tumor antigens among self-antigens in many tumors such as leukemia. For instance, T-cell recognition of self-proteins expressed in hematopoietic tissues might be preserved against many subdominant epitopes because the T cells that recognize them have escaped negative selection and may be tolerant. Alternatively, these T cells may exist in a state of "ignorance" toward the subdominant epitopes because they never encountered the antigen after maturation. Importantly, if there is tolerance to these self-antigens, it may be quantitative rather than absolute. In animal models vaccination with such self-antigens can activate specific T cells that are able to reject tumor cells that express high levels of the self-antigen. If we could determine what might be the subdominant epitopes selectively expressed in hematopoietic tissues, they may provide targets for leukemia-specific CTL.

With this background we studied myeloid-restricted proteins that are highly expressed in the leukemia cells relative to normal hematopoietic progenitors. Myeloid leukemias express a number of differentiation antigens associated with granule formation. An example is proteinase 3 (Pr3), a 26 kDa neutral serine protease that is stored in primary azurophil granules and is maximally expressed at the promyelocyte stage of myeloid differentiation (135–137). Pr3 and two other azurophil granule proteins, neutrophil elastase and azurocidin, are coordinately regulated, and the transcription factors PU.1 and C/EBPα, which are responsible for normal myeloid differentiation from stem cells to monocytes or granulocytes, are important in mediating their expression (138). In particular, PU.1 induces expression of the macrophage colony-stimulating factor receptor and the development of monocytes, whereas C/EBPα increases the expression of the granulocyte colony-stimulating factor receptor and leads to mature granulocytes (138,139). These transcription factors have been implicated in leukemogenesis (139), and Pr3 antisense oligonucleotides can halt cell division and induce maturation of the HL-60 promyelocytic leukemia cell line HL-60 (140).

We have also studied another the myeloid-restricted protein myeloperoxidase (MPO) (141). MPO and Pr3 are both overexpressed in a variety of myeloid leukemia cells, including 75% of CML patients, approximately 50% of acute myeloid leukemia patients, and approximately 30% of patients with myelodysplastic syndrome (142).

Pr3 is known to be the target of autoimmune attack in Wegener's granulomatosis (143), and MPO is the target antigen in small vessel vasculitis (141,144,145). There is evidence for both abnormal T cell and humoral immunity in patients with these diseases (146–148). T cells taken from affected individuals proliferate in response to crude extracts from neutrophil granules and to the purified proteins (144,149), suggesting that T-cell responses against these proteins might be relatively easy to elicit in vitro using a deductive strategy to identify HLA-restricted peptide epitopes. We identified PR1, an HLA-A2.1–restricted nonamer derived from Pr3, as a leukemia-associated antigen (109,150–152). Peptides predicted to have high-affinity binding to HLA-A2.1 were synthesized, confirmed to bind, and then used to elicit peptide-specific CTL in vitro from healthy donor lymphocytes.

PR1 can be used to elicit CTL from HLA-A2.1+ normal donors in vitro, and T-cell immunity to PR1 is present in healthy donors and in many patients with CML that are in remission. These PR1-specific CTL show preferential cytotoxicity toward allogeneic HLA-A2.1+ myeloid leukemia cells over HLA-identical normal donor marrow (150). In addition, PR1-specific CTL inhibit colony-forming unit granulocyte-macrophage (CFU-GM) from the marrow of CML patients, but not CFU-GM from normal HLA-matched donors (151), suggesting that leukemia progenitors are also targeted.

Using PR1/HLA-A2 tetramers to detect CTL specific for PR1 (PR1-CTL), we showed a significant correlation with cytogenetic remission in patients with CML after treatment with interferon-α and the presence of PR1-CTL (109). PR1-CTL were also identified in the peripheral blood of some allogeneic HCT recipients who achieved molecular remission and who had converted to 100% donor chimerism. PR1/HLA-A2 tetramer-sorted allogeneic CTL from patients in remission were able to kill CML cells but not normal bone marrow cells in 4-hour cytotoxicity assays, demonstrating that the PR1 self-antigen is also recognized by allogeneic CTL (109). These findings have recently been confirmed and extended to CML patients treated with imatinib mesylate, where PR1-CTL do not appear to be expanded. High numbers of PR1-CTL are also present in AML patients in remission after HCT.

Another HLA-A2–restricted nonomer peptide, derived from MPO, can also be used to elicit CTL from HLA-A2.1+ normal donors in vitro (153). MPO-specific CTL show preferential cytotoxicity toward allogeneic HLA-A2.1+ myeloid leukemia cells over HLA-identical normal donor marrow (153). MPO-specific CTL also inhibit CFU-GM from the marrow of CML patients, but not CFU-GM from normal HLA-matched donors. The many striking similarities between immunity to Pr3 and MPO suggest that similar methods applied to the study of immunity against MPO-derived peptides should establish these and other peptides as important leukemia-associated antigens (154).

The Wilms' tumor antigen-1 (WT1) has also emerged as a potent immunogen containing multiple unique HLA-restricted epitopes (93,155–158). Like PR1, WT1-specific CTL are also present in high numbers in myeloid leukemia patients after HCT, and WT1-CTL can inhibit the colony growth of leukemia progenitors.

Various surface molecules on leukemia cells, such as isoforms of CD45, present on all hematopoietic cells, and CD33 and CD19 on myeloid and lymphoid cells, respectively, have been studied by deductive means to uncover potentially immunogenic epitopes (159–161). While some HLA-restricted epitopes have been identified, it is unclear if any of these are leukemia-associated antigens. The method of serological screening of cDNA expression libraries with autologous serum (SEREX) (162,163) has been used to identify MAGE-1 and to confirm WT1 as potential leukemia-associated antigens (164,165).

Other potential antigens that act as target antigens for T lymphocytes that may convey GVL activity include the idiotypes associated with lymphoid malignancies, such as immunoglobulin idiotypes and the TCR-CDR3 variable regions. Furthermore, antigens such as telomerase (166) and CYP1B1 (167,168) contain epitopes that are recognized by CTL in vitro that preferentially kill leukemia cells but not normal cells. Also of interest are EBV-derived antigens (169,170). Although viral antigens are not strictly GVL antigens, they might be considered as GVL targets in the context of allogeneic donor T cells mediating anti-B cell immunity in the case of posttransplant lymphoproliferative disorder (PTLD) (169).

We have recently shown that distinct populations of PR1-CTL with either high or low TCR affinity for PR1 can be elicited from PBMC of healthy donors (171). The high-affinity PR1-CTL cause higher specific lysis of CML cells than low-affinity PR1-CTL. When high-affinity PR1-CTL were exposed to target cells that expressed high concentration of target antigen, the PR1-CTL underwent apoptosis within 18 hours. However, there was no apoptosis when the high-affinity PR1-CTL were exposed to a 2 log lower concentration of PR1 antigen. We have been unable to either detect or elicit high-affinity PR1-CTL in vitro from PBMC of untreated CML patients. Since healthy HLA-A2+ individuals have PR1-CTL with high-affinity TCR, however, this suggests that the high-affinity PR1-CTL may have been deleted during the outgrowth of the leukemia by CML cells that overexpress the PR1 tumor antigen.

These findings suggest that, in addition to HLA disparities and polymorphic mHAs, self-antigens may be the targets of alloreactive T cells. These observations form the basis for a mechanism of alloreactivity and subsequent new treatment strategies based on targeting self-antigens in the allogeneic setting. Specifically, GVL alloreactivity may in part be due to the transfer from donor to recipient of high-affinity CTL with leukemia self-antigen specificity that were not deleted from the T-cell repertoire during normal T-cell development in the donor. On this basis, GVL could be separated from GVHD if the target self-antigen expression was limited to hematopoietic tissue only. Further, specificity from aberrant expression of the target self-antigen in the leukemia compared to normal hematopoietic cells might give rise to a critical number of recognizable surface peptide epitopes that would surpass the activation threshold of high-affinity T cells, whereas the lower level of antigen expressed in the normal hematopoietic cells would not. This would result in preferential killing and elimination of leukemia cells over normal hematopoietic cells by the transplanted high-affinity donor T cells. As a consequence, residual normal recipient hematopoietic cells would be spared and could then coexist with donor hematopoietic cells after successful elimination of the leukemia, a phenomenon that occurs in some HCT recipients who achieve cytogenetic remission.

Arguing against this hypothesis is the observation that CML recipients of syngeneic stem cell grafts, which have few mHA differences but which should also contain high-affinity PR1-CTL, suffer higher relapse rates than do recipients of allogeneic grafts (172). However, because high-affinity PR1-CTL are present at a very low precursor frequency in healthy donors, major and minor histocompatibility antigenic differences may be required to provide generalized heightened immunity via indirect effects mediated by cytokine secretion, which might broadly decrease the threshold of TCR activation and drive the expansion of high-affinity self-antigen–specific T cells. This would also explain the development of GVHD, since this could lead to the uncovering of cryptic antigens and also to epitope spreading (173). More effective GVL might therefore be observed after syngeneic HCT if higher numbers of high-affinity CTL were initially transplanted. Consistent with this is the clinical observation that fewer relapses occur in syngeneic graft recipients who receive higher total nucleated cell doses during initial transplant (174), suggesting that an initially large number of high-affinity self-antigen–specific CTL might compensate for their innately low precursor frequency and the absence of significant alloreactivity in this setting.

Like CD8+ T lymphocytes, CD4+ T lymphocytes are important mediators of GVL (175), both directly because of their capacity to kill leukemia cells (110,176) and indirectly due to their capacity to provide help for expanding CD8+ T lymphocytes (177,178). In a study of adoptively transferred CD8+ T-lymphocyte clones specific for CMV antigens, long-term engraftment and immune memory of the CD8+ T lymphocytes was not observed in the absence of CMV-specific CD4+ T lymphocytes (177).

Much less is known about the nature of the potential GVL antigens targeted by CD4+ T lymphocytes, despite the clinical and laboratory evidence that CD4+ T lymphocytes are important mediators of GVL (179–181). This is due in part to the weaker interaction of TCR with the cognate peptide/MHC ligand, which makes the identification of target peptide antigens and the use of peptide/MHC II tetramers more difficult (182–184). Despite difficulties, some CD4+ T-lymphocyte target antigens with the potential to be relevant GVL antigens have been identified, such as the HLA-DQ–restricted DBY antigen (185). Since the tissue distribution of this antigen is unlikely to be restricted to hematopoietic cells, its potential as a GVL antigen is low, although it may be an important target of GVHD-producing T lymphocytes.

D. Natural Killer Cells

Natural killer cells have been studied for their potential to kill tumors, but until recently there has been little clinical benefit spin-off (186,187). NK cells are lymphocytes involved in the innate immune response, that have the ability to quickly respond to foreign antigens early during infection, frequently at barrier surfaces of the host where the immune system first encounters an invader. Unlike T cells, however, NK cells are not able to rearrange their receptor genes from the germ line configuration, which limits the repertoire of their potential antigen diversity. Nonetheless, recent studies indicate that these cells may be important mediators of GVL effects in patients with myeloid leukemia who have been transplanted from haploidentical donors with alloreactive NK cells.

The heterogeneity that has been recognized among NK-cell subsets arises due to the different expression of various inhibitory and activating receptors on the cell surface. Alloreactive NK cells are predominantly defined by the activity of inhibitory receptors, which have specificity for HLA class I determinants. The killer-cell immunoglobulin-like inhibitory receptor (KIR) family includes inhibitory receptors for certain HLA-A, -B, and -C polymorphic determinants (Table 4) (188–193). The determinants on the HLA molecules that are recognized by these receptors are called KIR epitopes. In addition to the KIR, there are lectin-like receptors that are heterodimers of CD94 with an NKG2-family member protein. These receptors have specificity for complexes of HLA-E plus peptides that are derived from most of the leader sequences of many HLA-A, HLA-B, and HLA-C heavy-chain proteins (194–196).

Every NK cell expresses one or more inhibitory receptors, which, through interactions with HLA class I molecules, prevent NK cells from killing healthy autologous cells (197). The alloreactivity of NK cells results when the HLA type of the NK cell donor includes a KIR epitope that is not part of the HLA type of the allogeneic recipient target cell. Under these circumstances there are certain donor-derived NK cells in the HCT recipient that have an inhibitory receptor specific for a donor KIR epitope that is not expressed on the recipient target cells. The subsequent ensuing lack of any inhibitory signal mediated through the KIR allows for the activation of the NK cell through other activating receptors. This has been referred to as "missing self" on the recipient target cells (198), and it is the basis of the "F1 hybrid resistance" described much earlier in murine transplant experiments (199,200).

The gene locus of the KIR is found on chromosome 19q and is organized into three conserved framework region genes (KIR3DL3, KIR2DL4, and KIR3DL2) and variable region genes (187). Similar to the nomenclature applied to the HLA locus, the cluster of KIR genes located on one chromosome is referred to as the KIR haplotype, which is further organized into a group A and group B haplotype. The group A haplotype has fewer genes, but they tend to show more polymorphisms, while the group B haplotype has more genes and also contains the activating KIR genes. The KIR genotype is therefore a sum of each of the two KIR haplotypes, which in turn are either group A or group B. The overall diversity that is contributed by the gene content and by gene polymorphisms accounts for a less than 2% probability that any given unrelated human donor-recipient pair will have the same KIR genotype (201).

Although there is substantial diversity of NK cell receptors, the most dominant pattern of alloreactivity is due to a dimorphism that results in the expression of two epitopes of HLA-C, which in turn results in a single amino acid difference at position 80

Table 4   Killer-Cell Immunoglobulin-like Receptor (KIR) Types with Specificity for HLA Class I

KIR	Ligand
KIR3DL2	HLA-A
KIR3DL1	HLA-B
KIR2DL1	HLA-C
KIR2DL2	HLA-C
KIR2DL3	HLA-C

(202). Therefore, individuals may be homozygous for either dimorphism or they may be heterozygous. Because most individuals have KIR that are specific for both HLA-C epitopes, however, the pattern of alloreactivity between two individuals can often be predicted by their HLA-C types (203). For instance, heterozygous individuals would have some NK cells that recognize and kill target cells from either homozygous individual, whereas homozygous donor-derived NK cells would not kill a heterozygous recipient since the target cells would express both dimorphisms and could therefore send an inhibitory signal to either type of homozygous donor-derived NK cell.

Alloreactive NK cells have recently been found to contribute to the GVL effect in myeloid leukemia patients that who are the recipients of haploidentical transplants with significant T-cell depletion and transplanted with large numbers of CD34+ progenitor cells (30). For such HLA-mismatched haploidentical transplants, the donor and recipient share one HLA-C allele, but the second HLA-C allele differs. After transplantation, there are three potential outcomes for NK-cell alloreactivity: (a) no alloreactivity (due to compatibility of the KIR epitopes), (b) GVL (and GVHD) alloreactivity, or (c) host-vs.-graft alloreactivity, threatening graft rejection.

In a recent study, NK cell clones with predicted GVL alloreactivity were derived from haploidentical transplant recipients that were inhibited by the HLA-C epitope present in the donor but not present in the recipient (30,204). This alloreactivity was no longer seen by 4 months after transplant (204). In the same group of patients, the event-free survival was significantly better in AML patients who that received grafts with predicted GVL alloreactive NK cells than in those with no predicted GVL alloreactive NK cells. This was not true for the ALL patients in the study, however, which may be due to from a lack of effective GVL effect due related to a lack absence of adhesion molecules such as LFA-1 on ALL cells (204). The lack of GVHD in these patients may also be due to poor LFA-1 expression on nonhematopoietic cells, although a more intriguing possibility is that the alloreactive NK cells may have killed the recipient DC in tissues that are ordinarily susceptible to GVHD (205–207). The basis for this has been substantiated in murine models (60) and suggests a future role of eliminating or reducing host APC prior to donor T-cell engraftment as a means to ameliorate GVHD.

Some, though not all, retrospective studies have confirmed the initial findings of NK-cell alloreactivity as a means to predict transplant survival outcome (Table 5) (30,208–211). Some of these studies examined the outcomes of recipients of unrelated

Table 5 Clinical Studies on the Effect of HLA-C KIR Epitope Mismatching on BMT Outcome

No. of patients	BMT type	Favorable BMT outcome based on KIR epitope mismatch	Ref.
92	Haploidentical	+	30
62	Haploidentical	−	208
122	Unrelated	−	209
175	Unrelated	−	210
130	Unrelated	+	211

transplants, while others reviewed haploidentical transplant outcomes. Although the initial study of haploidentical transplant recipients found a favorable effect of KIR epitope mismatching on AML relapse (30), a study of unrelated transplant recipients that reported a favorable effect on overall survival did not find that epitope mismatching significantly reduced the relapse rate of AML (211).

The failure to find a favorable effect on the relapse outcome based on KIR epitope mismatch may be due to differences in the conditioning regimens that were given in each of the studies or because of differences in the doses of either the hematopoietic progenitor cells or the T cells, which might compete with NK-cell expansion. Alternatively, because of the large diversity of KIR genes, simple typing of the HLA-C alleles alone between donor-recipient pairs may not be sufficient to predict relapse outcome (212–214). Complete KIR genotyping may need to be performed to learn of the full potential of NK-KIR incompatibility to add to the GVL effect. In addition, prospective studies are needed.

V. CLINICAL STRATEGIES TO ENHANCE GVL

The traditional distinction between active and passive immunity provides some context to discuss the current therapeutic approaches being explored to elicit GVL without GVHD, although there is overlap and they are not mutually exclusive. Passive immune approaches center around ex vivo manipulations of the donor cells prior to infusion into the recipient, whereas active immune approaches can be used to treat either the donor or the recipient.

A. Donor Allograft Modification and Adoptive Cellular Immunotherapy

GVHD is induced by donor T lymphocytes, and efforts to deplete these cells from the graft have gradually become more refined (Table 6). The capability exists to deplete enough total T lymphocytes to eliminate GVHD, typically after infusing less than 1×10^4 cells/ kg, but at the expense of early relapse and an increased incidence of infectious complications. Complicating matters is the fact that merely increasing the CD34+ progenitor cell dose, regardless of the number of T lymphocytes that are subsequently transferred, may also increase the incidence of GVHD.

Early attempts to select hematopoietic progenitor cells and leave behind lymphocytes were based on size selection through counterflow current elutriation.

Table 6   Methods of Lymphocyte Selection

Nonselective
  Elutriation
  CD34 selection
Semiselective
  Antithymocyte globulin OKT3 (anti-CD3)
T10B9 (anti-T-cell receptor)
  Anti-CD52 (Campath)
  Anti-CD8 depletion
  Anti-CD6 depletion
Selective
  Alloreactive depletion
  Antigen-specific selection

Progenitor cell selection based on phenotypic markers such as CD34 provides more selectivity and greater subsequent T-cell depletion, typically 2–3 log versus 1–2 log of lymphocyte depletion. Selective methods to enhance GVL over GVHD include removing the most alloreactive T cells from the graft or, conversely, enriching for antigen-specific T cells based that recognize potential leukemia-associated antigens or mHA. In the first approach, by incubating the graft ex vivo with recipient lymphocyes, the donor lymphocytes that proliferate or upregulate activation markers such as CD25 can be targeted for removal, often by monoclonal antibodies. These methods have shown promise in preclinical reports (214a,b,c).

Finally, selecting T lymphocytes that are reactive against only the malignant cells based on antigen specificity may be a logical next step after relevant antigens are identified. This strategy holds promise since proof of principle has been established by investigators who used CML-reactive donor T cells that were derived from limiting dilution and subsequently expanded prior to transfer to a patient with relapsed CML (214d). The patient experienced a cytogenetic remission but did not develop GVHD. The barriers to expanding the clinical use of these highly selective adoptive cellular approaches are both economical and technical.

B. Vaccination

Results of tumor vaccine clinical trials have generally been disappointing. However, the potential to immunize either the donor directly prior to grafting or to immunize the donor lymphocytes after transplantation offers a unique opportunity to boost a competent donor immune system selectively against the tumor.

Aside from peptides derived from the idiotypes of lymphoid malignancies, peptides derived from the bcr-abl fusion transcript have undergone the most extensive clinical testing thus far. The results of a previous phase I trial in CML patients showed that although a combination of fusion region-derived peptides was safe when administered subcutaneously and immune responses could also be measured by ELISPOT after vaccination, meaningful clinical responses were not observed (215). More recently, the same group at Memorial Sloan-Kettering Cancer Center reported on 14 patients in a phase II study who were given five injections of six peptides over 10 weeks. A decrease in the percentage of Ph+ cells was noted in four patients in previous hematological remission; three were also receiving interferon, and one was receiving imatinib mesylate (216). Transient PCR negativity was also noted in a few additional patients who had received prior allogeneic transplants and donor lymphocyte infusions.

Because heat shock protein 70 (HSP70) is associated with antigenic peptides and is involved in chaperoning these peptides in the MHC I antigen processing pathway, autologous cellular extracts containing HSP70-peptide complexes have been studied as a vaccine in chronic phase CML patients. At the University of Connecticut, HSP70-peptide complexes purified from leukapheresis products were administered to CML patients who had not yet achieved a major cytogenetic response after 6 months of imatinib mesylate treatment. Of the first five patients who completed all 8 weekly subcutaneous injections, major cytogenetic responses were noted in all five, and only mild cutaneous reactions were seen (217). Importantly, ELISPOT responses to the vaccine preparation were also noted in some of the patients.

Although results from both the HSP70 and the bcr-abl vaccine studies are important because they demonstrate that the vaccines can induce immune responses, true cause and effect has not been established since patients in both studies concomitantly received other therapies. Major cytogenetic remissions after imatinib treatment continue to be observed in more than 30% of patients beyond 6 months of therapy, and small fluctuations in the percentage of Ph+ cells may be seen throughout treatment.

The PR1 peptide has also undergone phase I/II study, and the single peptide epitope has been combined with an incomplete Freund's adjuvant and GM-CSF and administered every 3 weeks for a total of three total vaccinations. To judge whether a clinical response was due to the vaccine, eligible patients were required to have evidence of leukemia progression, relapse, or be in second or greater CR remission (for AML patients only) prior to vaccination. Immune responses, measured using PR1/HLA-A2 tetramers, were noted in eight of the patients, and clinical responses were noted in five of those patients. Notably, the TCR avidity of the vaccine-induced PR1-specific CTL was reported to be higher in the clinical responders than in the nonresponders, and durable molecular remissions were noted in two refractory AML patients who were followed for 8 months to nearly 3 years (J. Molldrem, unpublished data).

VI. THE FUTURE

Several authors have suggested that one way to improve GVL and reduce GVHD would be to adoptively transfer antigen-specific T cells from the donor to the recipient (218,219). Several transplant centers are currently conducting such clinical trials using antigen-specific T cells, and some centers are prospectively selecting donors based on KIR epitope mismatching to favor NK alloreactivity. Undoubtedly, successful GVL strategies will also depend upon the pace of the malignant cell growth and the pace and cytolytic potential of the delivered immune manipulation. While hematopoietic tissue-restricted mHA-specific adoptive T-cell transfer offers a relatively straightforward way to test whether antigen-specific T-cell therapies have the potential to produce GVL without GVHD, there are many practical limitations to eventual widespread use. These limitations are related to the relative genotype frequencies and mHA mismatching, precise HLA matching, mHA tissue distribution, technical limitations of cell expansions, and cost.

Adoptive transfer to HCT recipients of alloreactive T cells with specificity for self-peptides after an initial T-cell–depleted MHC-mismatched transplant offers several potential advantages over strategies utilizing precise HLA matching and the eventual use of mHA matching to reduce the incidence of GVHD. First, it would greatly expand the number of potential donors for allogeneic stem cell transplantation, which is the largest obstacle to extending this potentially curative treatment modality to more patients. Donor-recipient pairs that shared a common HLA supertype would be sufficient. Second, the time required to expand peptide antigen-specific CTL ex vivo for adoptive transfer to recipients to induce GVL might be eliminated or greatly reduced because of the high initial precursor frequency of the alloreactive CTL. Third, since the target peptide is a self-antigen, it would eliminate the need to find tissue-restricted mHA differences between donor and recipient if mHA-specific CTL were to be adoptively transferred to the recipient to induce GVL reactivity.

This strategy of self-peptide–directed alloreactivity might also be applied to the treatment of solid tumors, where many self-antigens have already been discovered but where effective autologous immune responses are lacking (108). It also suggests a possible future strategy for the treatment of autoimmune diseases if suitable peptide antigens could be identified and their gene expression was restricted to T cells or even to hematopoietic cells.

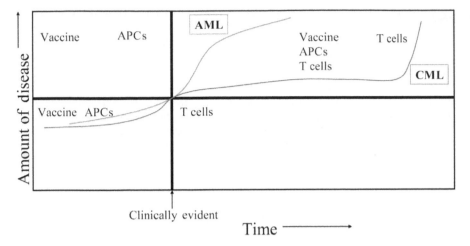

Figure 4 Timing of immunotherapy strategies. The delivery of immunotherapies such as vaccines or adoptive T-cell transfers to elicit or convey GVL will ultimately depend on the availability of the specific therapy and the state of the tumor in the host. For example, fast-growing tumors such as AML may require large numbers of specific T cells in passive transfer cellular immune therapy strategies because the kinetics of the disease may outpace the kinetics of an immune response that is elicited by active immunization strategies such as vaccination.

Many obstacles to the leukemia-associated self-antigen targeting approach remain, as well. We must (a) determine the key MHC residues that are involved in positive selection, (b) identify certain tissue-restricted self-peptides that are recognized by T cells, and (c) determine which of those peptides also bind to different alleles that are confined to a given HLA supertype. In addition, such approaches will still require choosing the appropriate antigens, the cell dose, treatment frequency, and how to maintain long-term memory cells.

In the future, allogeneic HCT is likely to evolve as a platform for delivering antigen-specific adoptive cellular therapies and for posttransplant vaccination strategies where donor CTL are elicited in the recipient. Both autologous and allogeneic transplants may reset T-cell homeostasis and allow a more complete T-cell repertoire to emerge postgrafting that could be further expanded selectively against tumor antigens by vaccination posttransplant. Alloreactive NK cells, delivered in large numbers as part of the original graft, may have the added potential to help eliminate recipient DC, which could reduce the incidence of GVHD. Elimination of donor T cells that cause GVHD, perhaps by targeting activation markers on alloreactive T cells ex vivo, could be used to treat an allograft to favor GVL. Eventual combinations of each of these strategies could be investigated, with the timing of individual therapies dependent in part upon the type and number of malignant cells (Fig. 4).

Exactly how we will move from the current clinical methods of adoptive transfer of nonspecific alloreactivity to highly specific targeted therapy remains uncertain, but it appears likely that the current approach will soon be supplanted by a next generation of antigen-specific allogeneic immunotherapies with highly specific cell subsets. More work on the fundamental biology of GVL remains, however, before this can become a reality.

REFERENCES

1. Giralt SA, Kolb HJ. Donor lymphocyte infusions. Curr Opin Oncol 1996; 8:96–102.
2. Kolb HJ, Holler E. Adoptive immunotherapy with donor lymphocyte transfusions. Curr Opin Oncol 1997; 9:139–145.
3. Kolb HJ, Schattenberg A, Goldman JM, Hertenstein B, Jacobsen N, Arcese W, Ljungman P, Ferrant A, Verdonck L, Niederwieser D, et al. Graft-versus-leukemia effect of donor lymphocyte transfusions in marrow grafted patients. European Group for Blood and Marrow Transplantation Working Party Chronic Leukemia. Blood 1995; 86:2041–2050.
4. Kolb HJ, Mittermuller J, Holler E, Thalmeier K, Bartram CR. Graft-versus-host reaction spares normal stem cells in chronic myelogenous leukemia. Bone Marrow Transplant 1996; 17:449–452.
5. Antin JH. Graft-versus-leukemia: no longer an epiphenomenon. Blood 1993; 82:2273–2277.
6. van Rhee F, Lin F, Cullis JO, Goldman J. Relapse of chronic myeloid leukemia after allogeneic bone marrow transplant: the case for giving donor lymphocyte transfusions before the onset of hematological relapse. Blood 1994; 83.
7. Collins RH, Jr., Shpilberg O, Drobyski WR, Porter DL, Giralt S, Champlin R, Goodman SA, Wolff SN, Hu W, Verfaillie C, List A, Dalton W, Ognoskie N, Chetrit A, Antin JH, Nemunaitis J. Donor leukocyte infusions in 140 patients with relapsed malignancy after allogeneic bone marrow transplantation. J Clin Oncol 1997; 15:433–444.
8. Schwarz K, Storni T, Manolova V, Didierlaurent A, Sirard JC, Rothlisberger P, Bachmann MF. Role of Toll-like receptors in costimulating cytotoxic T cell responses. Eur J Immunol 2003; 33:1465–1470.
9. Wagner H. Toll meets bacterial CpG-DNA. Immunity 2001; 14:499–502.
10. Gross L. Intradermal immunization of C3H mice against a sarcoma that originated in an animal of the same line. Cancer Res 1943; 3:326–330.
11. Foley EJ. Antigenic properties of methylcholanthrene-induced tumors in mice of the strain of origin. Cancer Res 1953; 13:835–844.
12. Nadler SH, Moore GE. Clinical immunologic study of malignant disease: Response to tumor transplants and transfer of leukocytes. Ann Surg 1966; 482–490.
13. Lotze MT, Line BR, Mathisen DJ. The in vivo distribution of autologous human and murine lymphoid cells grown in T cell growth factor (TCGF): implications for the adoptive immunotherapy of tumors. J Immunol 1980; 125:1487–1493.
14. Rosenberg SA. Immunotherapy of cancer by the systemic administration of lymphoid cells plus interleukin-2. J Biol Respir Mod 1984; 3:501–511.
15. Mazumder A, Eberlein TJ, Grimm EA. Phase I study of the adoptive immunotherapy of human cancer with lectin activated autologous mononuclear cells. Cancer 1984; 53:896–905.
16. Rosenberg SA. Cell transfer therapy: clinical applications. In: Rosenberg SA, ed. Biologic Therapy of Cancer. 2d ed. Philadelphia: Lippincott, 1995.
17. Rosenberg SA, Packard BS, Aebersold PM. Use of tumor-infiltrating lymphocytes and interleukin-2 in the immunotherapy of patients with metastatic melanoma, special report. N Engl J Med 1988; 319:1676–1680.
18. Schwartzentruber DJ, Hom SS, Dadmarz R, White DE, Yannelli JR, Steinberg SM, Rosenberg SA, Topalian SL. In vitro predictors of therapeutic response in melanoma patients receiving tumor-infiltrating lymphocytes and interleukin-2. J Clin Oncol 1994; 12:1475–1483.
19. Pockaj BA, Sherry R, Wei J, Yannelli JR, Carter CS, Leitman SF, Carrasquillo JR, White DE, Steinberg S, Rosenberg SA, Yang JD. Localization of indium-111-labelled tumor infiltrating lymphocytes to tumor in patients receiving adoptive immunotherapy: augmentation with cyclophosphamide in association with response. Cancer 1994; 73:1731–1737.
20. Dudley ME, Wunderlich JR, Robbins PF, Yang JC, Hwu P, Schwartzentruber DJ, Topalian SL, Sherry R, Restifo NP, Hubicki AM, Robinson MR, Raffeld M, Duray P, Seipp CA,

Rogers-Freezer L, Morton KE, Mavroukakis SA, White DE, Rosenberg SA. Cancer regression and autoimmunity in patients after clonal repopulation with antitumor lymphocytes. Science 2002; 298:850–854.

21. van der Bruggen P, Traversari C, Chomez P, Lurquin C, De Plaen E, Van den Eynde B, Knuth A, Boon T. A gene encoding an antigen recognized by cytolytic T lymphocytes on a human melanoma. Science 1991; 254:1643–1646.

22. Robbins PF, Kawakami Y. Human tumor antigens recognized by T cells. Curr Opin Immunol 1996; 8:628–636.

23. Boon T, Coulie PG, Van den Eynde B. Tumor antigens recognized by T cells. Immunol Today 1997; 18:267–268.

24. Barnes DW, Corp MJ, Loutit JF, Neal FE. Treatment of murine leukaemia with x rays and homologous bone marrow. Br M J 1956; 2:626–627.

25. Weiden PL, Flournoy N, Thomas ED, Prentice R, Fefer A, Buckner CD, Storb R. Antileukemic effect of graft-versus-host disease in human recipients of allogeneic-marrow grafts. N Engl J Med 1979; 300:1068–1073.

26. Thomas ED, Buckner CD, Clift RA, Fefer A, Johnson FL, Neiman PE, Sale GE, Sanders JE, Singer JW, Shulman H, Storb R, Weiden PL. Marrow transplantation for acute nonlymphoblastic leukemia in first remission. N Engl J Med 1979; 301:597–599.

27. Korngold R, Leighton C, Manser T. Graft-versus-myeloid leukemia responses following syngeneic and allogeneic bone marrow transplantation. Transplantation 1994; 58:278–287.

28. Shlomchik WD, Pear WS. Graft-vs-leukemia in a retrovirally induced murine CML model: mechanisms of leukemia recognition (abstr). Blood 2001; 98:812a.

29. Bonnet D, Warren EH, Greenberg PD, Dick JE, Riddell SR. CD8(+) minor histocompatibility antigen-specific cytotoxic T lymphocyte clones eliminate human acute myeloid leukemia stem cells. Proc Natl Acad Sci USA 1999; 96:8639–8644.

30. Ruggeri L, Capanni M, Urbani E, Perruccio K, Shlomchik WD, Tosti A, Posati S, Rogaia D, Frassoni F, Aversa F, Martelli MF, Velardi A. Effectiveness of donor natural killer cell alloreactivity in mismatched hematopoietic transplants. Science 2002; 295:2097–2100.

31. Truitt RL, Atasoylu AA. Impact of pretransplant conditioning and donor T cells on chimerism, graft-versus-host disease, graft-versus-leukemia reactivity, and tolerance after bone marrow transplantation. Blood 1991; 77:2515–2523.

32. Mapara MY, Kim YM, Wang SP, Bronson R, Sachs DH, Sykes M. Donor lymphocyte infusions mediate superior graft-versus-leukemia effects in mixed compared to fully allogeneic chimeras: a critical role for host antigen-presenting cells. Blood 2002; 100:1903–1909.

33. Johnson BD, Drobyski WR, Truitt RL. Delayed infusion of normal donor cells after MHC-matched bone marrow transplantation provides an antileukemia reaction without graft-versus-host disease. Bone Marrow Transplant 1993; 11:329–336.

34. Johnson BD, Truitt RL. Delayed infusion of immunocompetent donor cells after bone marrow transplantation breaks graft-host tolerance allows for persistent antileukemic reactivity without severe graft-versus-host disease. Blood 1995; 85:3302–3312.

35. Johnson BD, Becker EE, Truitt RL. Graft-vs.-host and graft-vs.-leukemia reactions after delayed infusions of donor T-subsets. Biol Blood Marrow Transplant 1999; 5:123–132.

36. Blazar BR, Taylor PA, Panoskaltsis-Mortari A, Sharpe AH, Vallera DA. Opposing roles of CD28:B7 and CTLA-4:B7 pathways in regulating in vivo alloresponses in murine recipients of MHC disparate T cells. J Immunol 1999; 162:6368–6377.

37. Hill GR, Teshima T, Gerbitz A, Pan L, Cooke KR, Brinson YS, Crawford JM, Ferrara JL. Differential roles of IL-1 and TNF-alpha on graft-versus-host disease and graft versus leukemia. J Clin Invest 1999; 104:459–467.

38. Krijanovski OI, Hill GR, Cooke KR, Teshima T, Crawford JM, Brinson YS, Ferrara JL. Keratinocyte growth factor separates graft-versus-leukemia effects from graft-versus-host disease. Blood 1999; 94:825–831.

39. Teshima T, Hill GR, Pan L, Brinson YS, van den Brink MR, Cooke KR, Ferrara JL. IL-11 separates graft-versus-leukemia effects from graft-versus-host disease after bone marrow transplantation. J Clin Invest 1999; 104:317–325.

40. Tsukada N, Kobata T, Aizawa Y, Yagita H, Okumura K. Graft-versus-leukemia effect and graft-versus-host disease can be differentiated by cytotoxic mechanisms in a murine model of allogeneic bone marrow transplantation. Blood 1999; 93:2738–2747.

41. Hsieh MH, Korngold R. Differential use of FasL- and perforin-mediated cytolytic mechanisms by T-cell subsets involved in graft-versus-myeloid leukemia responses. Blood 2000; 96:1047–1055.

42. Hsieh MH, Patterson AE, Korngold R. T-cell subsets mediate graft-versus-myeloid leukemia responses via different cytotoxic mechanisms. Biol Blood Marrow Transplant 2000; 6:231–240.

43. Schmaltz C, Alpdogan O, Horndasch KJ, Muriglan SJ, Kappel BJ, Teshima T, Ferrara JL, Burakoff SJ, van den Brink MR. Differential use of Fas ligand and perforin cytotoxic pathways by donor T cells in graft-versus-host disease and graft-versus-leukemia effect. Blood 2001; 97:2886–2895.

44. Reddy P, Teshima T, Hildebrandt G, Duffner U, Maeda Y, Cooke KR, Ferrara JL. Interleukin 18 preserves a perforin-dependent graft-versus-leukemia effect after allogeneic bone marrow transplantation. Blood 2002; 100:3429–3431.

45. Schmaltz C, Alpdogan O, Kappel BJ, Muriglan SJ, Rotolo JA, Ongchin J, Willis LM, Greenberg AS, Eng JM, Crawford JM, Murphy GF, Yagita H, Walczak H, Peschon JJ, van den Brink MR. T cells require TRAIL for optimal graft-versus-tumor activity. Nat Med 2002; 8:1433–1437.

46. Schmaltz C, Alpdogan O, Muriglan SJ, Kappel BJ, Rotolo JA, Ricchetti ET, Greenberg AS, Willis LM, Murphy GF, Crawford JM, van den Brink MR. Donor T cell-derived TNF is required for graft-versus-host disease and graft-versus-tumor activity after bone marrow transplantation. Blood 2003; 101:2440–2445.

47. Fontaine P, Roy-Proulx G, Knafo L, Baron C, Roy DC, Perreault C. Adoptive transfer of minor histocompatibility antigen-specific T lymphocytes eradicates leukemia cells without causing graft-versus-host disease [comment]. Nat Med 2001; 7:789–794.

48. Bortin MM, Truitt RL, Rimm AA, Bach FH. Graft-versus-leukaemia reactivity induced by alloimmunisation without augmentation of graft-versus-host reactivity. Nature 1979; 281:490–491.

49. Fowler DH, Breglio J, Nagel G, Eckhaus MA, Gress RE. Allospecific CD8+ Tc1 and Tc2 populations in graft-versus-leukemia effect and graft-versus-host disease. J Immunol 1996; 157:4811–4821.

50. Wettstein PJ, Korngold R. T cell subsets required for in vivo and in vitro responses to single and multiple minor histocompatibility antigens. Transplantation 1992; 54:296–307.

51. Korngold R, Wettstein PJ. Immunodominance in the graft-vs-host disease T cell response to minor histocompatibility antigens. J Immunol 1990; 145:4079–4088.

52. Wettstein PJ, Bailey DW. Immunodominance in the immune response to "multiple" histocompatibility antigens. Immunogenetics 1982; 16:47–58.

53. Wettstein PJ. Immunodominance in the T cell response to multiple non-H-2 histocompatibility antigens. III. Single histocompatibility antigens dominate the male antigen. J Immunol 1986; 137:2073–2079.

54. Berger M, Wettstein PJ, Korngold R. T cell subsets involved in lethal graft-versus-host disease directed to immunodominant minor histocompatibility antigens. Transplantation 1994; 57:1095–1102.

55. Berger MA, Korngold R. Immunodominant CD4+ T cell receptor Vbeta repertoires involved in graft-versus-host disease responses to minor histocompatibility antigens. J Immunol 1997; 159:77–85.

56. Yin L, Poirier G, Neth O, Hsuan JJ, Totty NF, Stauss HJ. Few peptides dominate cytotoxic T lymphocyte responses to single and multiple minor histocompatibility antigens. Int Immunol 1993; 5:1003–1009.

57. Pion S, Fontaine P, Desaulniers M, Jutras J, Filep JG, Perreault C. On the mechanisms of immunodominance in cytotoxic T lymphocyte responses to minor histocompatibility antigens. Eur J Immunol 1997; 27:421–430.

58. Perreault C, Jutras J, Roy DC, Filep JG, Brochu S. Identification of an immunodominant mouse minor histocompatibility antigen (MiHA). T cell response to a single dominant MiHA causes graft-versus-host disease. J Clin Invest 1996; 98:622–628.

59. Pion S, Fontaine P, Baron C, Gyger M, Perreault C. Immunodominant minor histocompatibility antigens expressed by mouse leukemic cells can serve as effective targets for T cell immunotherapy. J Clin Invest 1995; 95:1561–1568.

60. Shlomchik WD, Couzens MS, Tang CB, McNiff J, Robert ME, Liu J, Shlomchik MJ, Emerson SG. Prevention of graft versus host disease by inactivation of host antigen-presenting cells. Science 1999; 285:412–415.

61. Hill GR, Teshima T, Rebel VI, Krijanovski OI, Cooke KR, Brinson YS, Ferrara JL. The p55 TNF-alpha receptor plays a critical role in T cell alloreactivity. J Immunol 2000; 164:656–663.

62. Gishizky ML, Johnson-White J, Witte ON. Efficient transplantation of BCR-ABL-induced chronic myelogenous leukemia-like syndrome in mice. Proc Natl Acad Sci USA 1993; 90:3755–3759.

63. Okuda K, Golub TR, Gilliland DG, Griffin JD. p210BCR/ABL, p190BCR/ABL, and TEL/ABL activate similar signal transduction pathways in hematopoietic cell lines. Oncogene 1996; 13:1147–1152.

64. Pear WS, Miller JP, Xu L, Pui JC, Soffer B, Quackenbush RC, Pendergast AM, Bronson R, Aster JC, Scott ML, Baltimore D. Efficient and rapid induction of a chronic myelogenous leukemia-like myeloproliferative disease in mice receiving P210 bcr/abl-transduced bone marrow. Blood 1998; 92:3780–3792.

65. Li S, Ilaria RL, Jr., Million RP, Daley GQ, Van Etten RA. The P190, P210, and P230 forms of the BCR/ABL oncogene induce a similar chronic myeloid leukemia-like syndrome in mice but have different lymphoid leukemogenic activity. J Exp Med 1999; 189:1399–1412.

66. Blazar BR, Taylor PA, Boyer MW, Panoskaltsis-Mortari A, Allison JP, Vallera DA. CD28/B7 interactions are required for sustaining the graft-versus- leukemia effect of delayed post-bone marrow transplantation splenocyte infusion in murine recipients of myeloid or lymphoid leukemia cells. J Immunol 1997; 159:3460–3473.

67. Speiser DE, Bachmann MF, Shahinian A, Mak TW, Ohashi PS. Acute graft-versus-host disease without costimulation via CD28. Transplantation 1997; 63:1042–1044.

68. Yu XZ, Martin PJ, Anasetti C. Role of CD28 in acute graft-versus-host disease. Blood 1998; 92:2963–2970.

69. Blazar BR, Kwon BS, Panoskaltsis-Mortari A, Kwak KB, Peschon JJ, Taylor PA. Ligation of 4-1BB (CDw137) regulates graft-versus-host disease, graft- versus-leukemia, and graft rejection in allogeneic bone marrow transplant recipients. J Immunol 2001; 166:3174–3183.

70. Shuford WW, Klussman K, Tritchler DD, Loo DT, Chalupny J, Siadak AW, Brown TJ, Emswiler J, Raecho H, Larsen CP, Pearson TC, Ledbetter JA, Aruffo A, Mittler RS. 4-1BB costimulatory signals preferentially induce CD8+ T cell proliferation and lead to the amplification in vivo of cytotoxic T cell responses. J Exp Med 1997; 186:47–55.

71. Takahashi C, Mittler RS, Vella AT. Cutting edge: 4-1BB is a bona fide CD8 T cell survival signal. J Immunol 1999; 162:5037–5040.

72. Goodwin RG, Din WS, Davis-Smith T, Anderson DM, Gimpel SD, Sato TA, Maliszewski CR, Brannan CI, Copeland NG, Jenkins NA, et al. Molecular cloning of a ligand for the inducible T cell gene 4-1BB: a member of an emerging family of cytokines with homology to tumor necrosis factor. Eur J Immunol 1993; 23:2631–2641.

73. Mackinnon S, Papadopoulos EB, Carabasi MH, Reich L, Collins NH, Boulad F, Castro-Malaspina H, Childs BH, Gillio AP, Kernan NA, et al. Adoptive immunotherapy evaluating escalating doses of donor leukocytes for relapse of chronic myeloid leukemia after bone marrow transplantation: separation of graft-versus-leukemia responses from graft-versus-host disease. Blood 1995; 86:1261–1268.

74. Sato K, Yamashita N, Baba M, Matsuyama T. Regulatory dendritic cells protect mice from murine acute graft-versus-host disease and leukemia relapse. Immunity 2003; 18:367–379.

75. Champlin R, Giralt S, Przepiorka D, Ho W, Lee K, Gajewski J, Nimer S, Andersson B, Wallerstein R, Ippolito C, et a. Selective depletion of CD8-positive T-lymphocytes for allogeneic bone marrow transplantation: engraftment, graft-versus-host disease and graft-versus leukemia. Prog Clin Biol Res 1992; 377:385–394.

76. Giralt S, Hester J, Huh y, Hirsch-Ginsber C, Rondon G, Seong D, Lee M, Gajewski J, Van Besien K, Khouri I, Rakesha M, Przepiorka D, Korbling M, Talpaz M, Kantarjian H, Fischer H, Deisseroth A, Champlin R. CD8-depleted donor lymphocyte infusion as treatment for relapsed chronic myelogenous leukemia after allogeneic bone marrow transplantation. Blood 1995; 86:4337–4343.

77. Gallardo D, Garcia-Lopez J, Sureda A, Canals C, Ferra C, Cancelas JA, Berlanga JJ, Brunet S, Boque C, Picon M, Torrico C, Amill B, Martino R, Martinez C, Martin-Henao G, Domingo-Albos A, Granena A. Low-dose donor CD8+ cells in the CD4-depleted graft prevent allogeneic marrow graft rejection and severe graft-versus-host disease for chronic myeloid leukemia patients in first chronic phase. Bone Marrow Transplant 1997; 20:945–952.

78. Mackinnon S, Papadopoulos EB, Carabasi MH, Reich L, Collins NH, O'Reilly RJ. Adoptive immunotherapy using donor leukocytes following bone marrow transplantation for chronic myeloid leukemia: is T cell dose important in determining biological response? Bone Marrow Transplant 1995; 15:591–594.

79. Champlin RE, Passweg JR, Zhang MJ, Rowlings PA, Pelz CJ, Atkinson KA, Barrett AJ, Cahn JY, Drobyski WR, Gale RP, Goldman JM, Gratwohl A, Gordon-Smith EC, Henslee-Downey PJ, Herzig RH, Klein JP, Marmont AM, O'Reilly RJ, Ringden O, Slavin S, Sobocinski KA, Speck B, Weiner RS, Horowitz MM. T-cell depletion of bone marrow transplants for leukemia from donors other than HLA-identical siblings: advantage of T-cell antibodies with narrow specificities. Blood 2000; 95:3996–4003.

80. Sykes M, Abraham VS, Harty MW, Pearson DA. IL-2 reduces graft-versus-host disease and preserves a graft-versus-leukemia effect by selectively inhibiting CD4+ T cell activity. J Immunol 1993; 150:197–205.

81. Yang YG, Sergio JJ, Pearson DA, Szot GL, Shimizu A, Sykes M. Interleukin-12 preserves the graft-versus-leukemia effect of allogeneic CD8 T cells while inhibiting CD4-dependent graft-versus-host disease in mice. Blood 1997; 90:4651–4660.

82. Reddy P, Teshima T, Kukuruga M, Ordemann R, Liu C, Lowler K, Ferrara JL. Interleukin-18 regulates acute graft-versus-host disease by enhancing Fas-mediated donor T cell apoptosis. J Exp Med 2001; 194:1433–1440.

83. Pan L, Teshima T, Hill GR, Bungard D, Brinson YS, Reddy VS, Cooke KR, Ferrara JL. Granulocyte colony-stimulating factor-mobilized allogeneic stem cell transplantation maintains graft-versus-leukemia effects through a perforin-dependent pathway while preventing graft-versus-host disease. Blood 1999; 93:4071–4078.

84. Edinger M, Hoffmann P, Ermann J, Drago K, Beilhack A, G. FC, Strober SS, Negrin RS. Donor CD4+ CD25+ regulatory T cells suppress acute GVHD lethality without loss of GVL activity. Blood 2002; 100.

85. Blazar BR, Roopenian DC, Taylor PA, Christianson GJ, Panoskaltsis-Mortari A, Vallera DA. Lack of GVHD across classical, single minor histocompatibiliTy (miH) locus barriers in mice. Transplantation 1996; 61:619–624.

86. van Lochem E, de Gast B, Goulmy E. In vitro separation of host specific graft-versus-host and graft-versus-leukemia cytotoxic T cell activities. Bone Marrow Transplant 1992; 10:181–183.

87. De Bueger M, Bakker A, Van Rood JJ, Goulmy E. Minor histocompatibility antigens, defined by graft-vs.-host disease-derived cytotoxic T lymphocytes, show variable expression on human skin cells. Eur J Immunol 1991; 21:2839–2844.

88. Marijt WA, Veenhof WF, Goulmy E, Willemze R, van Rood JJ, Falkenburg JH. Minor histocompatibility antigens HA-1-, -2-, and -4-, and HY-specific cytotoxic T-cell clones inhibit human hematopoietic progenitor cell growth by a mechanism that is dependent on direct cell-cell contact. Blood 1993; 82:3778–3785.

89. Warren EH, Greenberg PD, Riddell SR. Cytotoxic T-lymphocyte-defined human minor histocompatibility antigens with a restricted tissue distribution. Blood 1998; 91:2197–2207.

90. Mutis T, Blokland E, Kester M, Schrama E, Goulmy E. Generation of minor histocompatibility antigen HA-1-specific cytotoxic T cells restricted by nonself HLA molecules: a potential strategy to treat relapsed leukemia after HLA-mismatched stem cell transplantation. Blood 2002; 100:547–552.

91. Sadovnikova E, Stauss HJ. Peptide-specific cytotoxic T lymphocytes restricted by nonself major histocompatibility complex class I molecules: reagents for tumor immunotherapy. Proc Natl Acad Sci USA 1996; 93:13114–13118.

92. Gao L, Yang TH, Tourdot S, Sadovnikova E, Hasserjian R, Stauss HJ. Allo-major histocompatibility complex-restricted cytotoxic T lymphocytes engraft in bone marrow transplant recipients without causing graft-versus-host disease. Blood 1999; 94:2999–3006.

93. Gao L, Bellantuono I, Elsasser A, Marley SB, Gordon MY, Goldman JM, Stauss HJ. Selective elimination of leukemic CD34(+) progenitor cells by cytotoxic T lymphocytes specific for WT1. Blood 2000; 95:2198–2203.

94. Sirard C, Lapidot T, Vormoor J, Cashman JD, Doedens M, Murdoch B, Jamal N, Messner H, Addey L, Minden M, Laraya P, Keating A, Eaves A, Lansdorp PM, Eaves CJ, Dick JE. Normal and leukemic SCID-repopulating cells (SRC) coexist in the bone marrow and peripheral blood from CML patients in chronic phase, whereas leukemic SRC are detected in blast crisis. Blood 1996; 87:1539–1548.

95. Wang JC, Lapidot T, Cashman JD, Doedens M, Addy L, Sutherland DR, Nayar R, Laraya P, Minden M, Keating A, Eaves AC, Eaves CJ, Dick JE. High level engraftment of NOD/SCID mice by primitive normal and leukemic hematopoietic cells from patients with chronic myeloid leukemia in chronic phase. Blood 1998; 91:2406–2414.

96. Larochelle A, Vormoor J, Hanenberg H, Wang JC, Bhatia M, Lapidot T, Moritz T, Murdoch B, Xiao XL, Kato I, Williams DA, Dick JE. Identification of primitive human hematopoietic cells capable of repopulating NOD/SCID mouse bone marrow: implications for gene therapy. Nat Med 1996; 2:1329–1337.

97. Alam SM, Travers PJ, Wung JL, Nasholds W, Redpath S, Jameson SC, Gascoigne NR. T-cell-receptor affinity and thymocyte positive selection. Nature 1996; 381:616–620.

98. Savage PA, Davis MM. A kinetic window constricts the t cell receptor repertoire in the thymus. Immunity 2001; 14:243–252.

99. Dustin ML, Bromley SK, Davis MM, Zhu C. Identification of self through two-dimensional chemistry and synapses. Annu Rev Cell Dev Biol 2001; 17:133–157.

100. Bromley SK, Burack WR, Johnson KG, Somersalo K, Sims TN, Sumen C, Davis MM, Shaw AS, Allen PM, Dustin ML. The immunological synapse. Annu Rev Immunol 2001; 19:375–396.

101. Savage PA, Boniface JJ, Davis MM. A kinetic basis for T cell receptor repertoire selection during an immune response. Immunity 1999; 10:485–492.

102. Krummel MF, Sjaastad MD, Wulfing C, Davis MM. Differential clustering of CD4 and CD3zeta during T cell recognition. Science 2000; 289:1349–1352.

103. Richie LI, Ebert PJ, Wu LC, Krummel MF, Owen JJ, Davis MM. Imaging synapse formation during thymocyte selection: inability of CD3zeta to form a stable central accumulation during negative selection. Immunity 2002; 16:595–606.

104. Altman JD, Moss PAH, Goulder PJR, Barouch DH, McHeyzer-Williams MG, Bell JI, McMichael AJ, Davis MM. Phenotypic analysis of antigen-specific T lymphocytes. Science 1996; 274:94–96.

105. Callan MF, Tan L, Annels N, Ogg GS, Wilson JD, O'Callaghan CA, Steven N, McMichael AJ, Rickinson AB. Direct visualization of antigen-specific CD8+ T cells during the primary immune response to Epstein-Barr virus in vivo. J Exp Med 1998; 187:1395–1402.

106. Komanduri KV, Donahoe SM, Moretto WJ, Schmidt DK, Gillespie G, Ogg GS, Roederer M, Nixon DF, McCune JM. Direct measurement of CD4+ and CD8+ T-cell responses to CMV in HIV-1-infected subjects. Virology 2001; 279:459–470.

107. Komanduri KV, Viswanathan MN, Wieder ED, Schmidt DK, Bredt BM, Jacobson MA, McCune JM. Restoration of cytomegalovirus-specific CD4+ T-lymphocyte responses after ganciclovir and highly active antiretroviral therapy in individuals infected with HIV-1. Nat Med 1998; 4:953–956.

108. Lee PP, Yee C, Savage PA, Fong L, Brockstedt D, Weber JS, Johnson D, Swetter S, Thompson J, Greenberg PD, Roederer M, Davis MM. Characterization of circulating T cells specific for tumor-associated antigens in melanoma patients. Nat Med 1999; 5:677–685.

109. Molldrem JJ, Lee PP, Wang C, Felio K, Kantarjian HM, Champlin RE, Davis MM. Evidence that specific T lymphocytes may participate in the elimination of chronic myelogenous leukemia. Nat Med 2000; 6:1018–1023.

110. Faber LM, van Luxemburg-Heijs SA, Veenhof WF, Willemze R, Falkenburg JH. Generation of CD4+ cytotoxic T-lymphocyte clones from a patient with severe graft-versus-host disease after allogeneic bone marrow transplantation: implications for graft-versus-leukemia reactivity. Blood 1995; 86:2821–2828.

111. Faber LM, van der Hoeven J, Goulmy E, Hooftman-den Otter AL, van Luxemburg-Heijs SA, Willemze R, Falkenburg JH. Recognition of clonogenic leukemic cells, remission bone marrow and HLA-identical donor bone marrow by CD8+ or CD4+ minor histocompatibility antigen-specific cytotoxic T lymphocytes. J Clin Invest 1995; 96:877–883.

112. Faber LM, van Luxemburg-Heijs SA, Rijnbeek M, Willemze R, Falkenburg JH. Minor histocompatibility antigen-specific, leukemia-reactive cytotoxic T cell clones can be generated in vitro without in vivo priming using chronic myeloid leukemia cells as stimulators in the presence of alpha-interferon. Biol Blood Marrow Transplant 1996; 2:31–36.

113. van der Harst D, Goulmy E, Falkenburg JH, Kooij-Winkelaar YM, van Luxemburg-Heijs SA, Goselink HM, Brand A. Recognition of minor histocompatibility antigens on lymphocytic and myeloid leukemic cells by cytotoxic T-cell clones. Blood 1994; 83:1060–1066.

114. Goulmy E, Schipper R, Pool J, Blokland E, Falkenburg JH, Vossen J, Grathwohl A, Vogelsang GB, van Houwelingen HC, van Rood JJ. Mismatches of minor histocompatibility antigens between HLA-identical donors and recipients and the development of graft-versus-host disease after bone marrow transplantation. N Engl J Med 1996; 334:281–285.

115. den Haan JMM, Sherman NE, Blokland E, Huczko E, Koning F, Drijfhout JW, Skipper J, Shabanowitz J, Hunt DF, Engelhard VH, Goulmy E. Identification of a graft versus host disease-associated human minor histocompatibility antigen. Science 1995; 268:1476–1480.

116. Dermime S, Molldrem J, Parker KC, Jiang YZ, Mavroudis D, Hensel N, Couriel D, Mahoney M, Coligan JE, Barrett AJ. Human CD8+ T lymphocytes recognize the fusion region of bcr/abl hybrid protein present in chronic myelogenous leukemia. Blood 1995; 86.

117. Bocchia M, Wentworth PA, Southwood S, Sidney J, McGraw K, Scheinberg DA, Sette A. Specific binding of leukemia oncogene fusion protein peptides to HLA class I molecules. Blood 1995; 85:2680–2684.

118. Bocchia M, Korontsvit T, Xu Q, Mackinnon S, Yang SY, Sette A, Scheinberg DA. Specific human cellular immunity to bcr-abl oncogene-derived peptides. Blood 1996; 87:3587–3592.

119. Clark RE, Dodi IA, Hill SC, Lill JR, Aubert G, Macintyre AR, Rojas J, Bourdon A, Bonner PL, Wang L, Christmas SE, Travers PJ, Creaser CS, Rees RC, Madrigal JA. Direct evidence that leukemic cells present HLA-associated immunogenic peptides derived from the BCR-ABL b3a2 fusion protein. Blood 2001; 98:2887–2893.

120. Nanda NK, Sercarz EE. Induction of anti-self-immunity to cure cancer. Cell 1995; 82: 13–17.

121. Rosenberg SA, White DE. Vitiligo in patients with melanoma: normal tissue antigens can be targets for cancer immunotherapy. J Immunother Emphasis Tumor Immunol 1996; 19:81–84.

122. Pardoll DM. Spinning molecular immunology into successful immunotherapy. Nat Rev Immunol 2002; 2:227–238.

123. Pardoll DM. Tumour antigens. A new look for the 1990s. Nature 1994; 369:357.

124. Gaugler B, Van den Eynde B, Van der Bruggen P, Romero P, Gaforio JJ, De Plaen E, Lethe B, Brasseur F, Boon T. Human gene MAGE-3 codes for an antigen recognized on a melanoma by autologous cytolytic T lymphocytes. J Exp Med 1994; 179:921–930.

125. Tanaka F, Fujie T, Tahara K, Mori M, Takesako K, Sette A, Celis E, Akiyoshi T. Induction of antitumor cytotoxic T lymphocytes with a MAGE-3-encoded synthetic peptide presented by human leukocytes antigen-A24. Cancer Res 1997; 57:4465–4468.

126. van der Bruggen P, Bastin J, Gajewski T, Coulie PG, Boel P, De Smet C, Traversari C, Townsend A, Boon T. A peptide encoded by human gene MAGE-3 and presented by HLA-A2 induces cytolytic T lymphocytes that recognize tumor cells expressing MAGE-3. Eur J Immunol 1994; 24:3038–3043.

127. Celis E, Tsai V, Crimi C, DeMars R, Wentworth PA, Chesnut RW, Grey HM, Sette A, Serra HM. Induction of anti-tumor cytotoxic T lymphocytes in normal humans using primary cultures and synthetic peptide epitopes. Proc Natl Acad Sci USA 1994; 91:2105–2109.

128. Marchand M, Weynants P, Rankin E, Arienti F, Belli F, Parmiani G, Cascinelli N, Bourlond A, Vanwijck R, Humblet Y, et al. Tumor regression responses in melanoma patients treated with a peptide encoded by gene MAGE-3. Int J Cancer 1995; 63:883–885.

129. Zarour H, De Smet C, Lehmann F, Marchand M, Lethe B, Romero P, Boon T, Renauld JC. The majority of autologous cytolytic T-lymphocyte clones derived from peripheral blood lymphocytes of a melanoma patient recognize an antigenic peptide derived from gene Pmel17/gp100. J Invest Dermatol 1996; 107:63–67.

130. Boon T, Coulie P, Marchand M, Weynants P, Wolfel T, Brichard V. Genes coding for tumor rejection antigens: perspectives for specific immunotherapy. Important Adv Oncol 1994; 53–69.

131. Linehan DC, Peoples GE, Hess DT, Summerhayes IC, Parikh AS, Goedegebuure PS, Eberlein TJ. In vitro stimulation of ovarian tumour-associated lymphocytes with a peptide derived from HER2/neu induces cytotoxicity against autologous tumour. Surg Oncol 1995; 4:41–49.

132. Peoples GE, Goedegebuure PS, Smith R, Linehan DC, Yoshino I, Eberlein TJ. Breast and ovarian cancer-specific cytotoxic T lymphocytes recognize the same HER2/neu-derived peptide. Proc Natl Acad Sci USA 1995; 92:432–436.

133. Dermime S, Mavroudis D, Jiang YZ, Hensel N, Molldrem J, Barrett AJ. Immune escape from a graft-versus-leukemia effect may play a role in the relapse of myeloid leukemias following allogeneic bone marrow transplantation. Bone Marrow Transplant 1997; 19:989–999.

134. Croft M, Joseph SB, Miner KT. Partial activation of naive CD4 T cells and tolerance induction in response to peptide presented by resting B cells. J Immunol 1997; 159:3257–3265.

135. Sturrock AB, Franklin KF, Rao G, Marshall BC, Rebentisch MB, Lemons RS, Hoidal JR. Structure, chromosomal assignment, and expression of the gene for proteinase 3. J Biol Chem 1992; 267:21193.

136. Chen T, Meier R, Ziemiecki A, Fey MF, Tobler A. Myeloblastin/proteinase 3 belongs to the set of negatively regulated primary response genes expressed during in vitro myeloid differentiation. Biochem Biophys Res Commun 1994; 200:1130–1135.

137. Muller-Berat N, Minowada J, Tsuji-Takayama K, Drexler H, Lanotte M, Wieslander J, Wiik A. The phylogeny of proteinase 3/myeloblastin, the autoantigen in Wegener's granulomatosis, and myeloperoxidase as shown by immunohistochemical studies on human leukemic cell lines. Clin Immunol Immunopathol 1994; 70:51–59.

138. Zhang P, Nelson E, Radomska HS, Iwasaki-Arai J, Akashi K, Friedman AD, Tenen DG. Induction of granulocytic differentiation by 2 pathways. Blood 2002; 99:4406–4412.

139. Behre G, Zhang P, Zhang DE, Tenen DG. Analysis of the modulation of transcriptional activity in myelopoiesis and leukemogenesis. Methods 1999; 17:231–237.

140. Bories D, Raynal MC, Solomon DH, Darzynkiewicz Z, Cayre YE. Down-regulation of a serine protease, myeloblastin, causes growth arrest and differentiation of promyelocytic leukemia cells. Cell 1989; 59:959.

141. Borregaard N, Cowland JB. Granules of the human neutrophilic polymorphonuclear leukocyte. Blood 1997; 89:3503–3521.

142. Dengler R, Munstermann U, al-Batran S, Hausner I, Faderl S, Nerl C, Emmerich B. Immunocytochemical and flow cytometric detection of proteinase 3 (myeloblastin) in normal and leukaemic myeloid cells. Br J Haematol 1995; 89:250–257.

143. Franssen CF, Cohen Tervaert JW, Stegeman CA, Kallenberg CG. c-ANCA as a marker of Wegener's disease. Lancet 1996; 347:116, 118.

144. Brouwer E, Stegeman CA, Huitema MG, Limburg PC, Kallenberg CG. T cell reactivity to proteinase 3 and myeloperoxidase in patients with Wegener's granulomatosis (WG). Clin Exp Immunol 1994; 98:448–453.

145. Franssen CF, Stegeman CA, Kallenberg CG, Gans RO, De Jong PE, Hoorntje SJ, Tervaert JW. Antiproteinase 3- and antimyeloperoxidase-associated vasculitis. Kidney Int 2000; 57:2195–2206.

146. Williams RC, Staud R, Malone CC, Payabyab J, Byres L, Underwood D. Epitopes on proteinase 3 recognized by antibodies from patients with Wegener's granulomatosis. J Immunol 1994; 152:4722–4732.

147. Jennette JC, Thomas DB, Falk RJ. Microscopic polyangiitis (microscopic polyarteritis). Semin Diagn Pathol 2001; 18:3–13.

148. Savige J, Gillis D, Benson E, Davies D, Esnault V, Falk RJ, Hagen EC, Jayne D, Jennette JC, Paspaliaris B, Pollock W, Pusey C, Savage CO, Silvestrini R, van der Woude F, Wieslander J, Wiik A. International consensus statement on testing and reporting of antineutrophil cytoplasmic antibodies (ANCA). Am J Clin Pathol 1999; 111:507–513.

149. Ballieux BE, van der Burg SH, Hagen EC, van der Woude FJ, Melief CJ, Daha MR. Cell-mediated autoimmunity in patients with Wegener's granulomatosis (WG). Clin Exp Immunol 1995; 100:186–193.

150. Molldrem J, Dermime S, Parker K, Jiang YZ, Mavroudis D, Hensel N, Fukushima P, Barrett AJ. Targeted T-cell therapy for human leukemia: cytotoxic T lymphocytes specific for a peptide derived from proteinase 3 preferentially lyse human myeloid leukemia cells. Blood 1996; 88:2450–2457.

151. Molldrem JJ, Clave E, Jiang YZ, Mavroudis D, Raptis A, Hensel N, Agarwala V, Barrett AJ. Cytotoxic T lymphocytes specific for a nonpolymorphic proteinase 3 peptide preferentially inhibit chronic myeloid leukemia colony-forming units. Blood 1997; 90:2529–2534.

152. Molldrem JJ, Lee PP, Wang C, Champlin RE, Davis MM. A PR1-human leukocyte antigen-A2 tetramer can be used to isolate low-frequency cytotoxic T lymphocytes from healthy donors that selectively lyse chronic myelogenous leukemia. Cancer Res 1999; 59:2675–2681.

153. Braunschweig I, Wang C, Molldrem J. Cytotoxic T lymphocytes (CTL) specific for myeloperoxidase-derived HLA-A2-restricted peptides specifically lyse AML and CML cells. Blood 2000; 96:3291.

154. Kochenderfer JN, Molldrem JJ. Leukemia vaccines. Curr Oncol Rep 2001; 3:193–200.

155. Azuma T, Makita M, Ninomiya K, Fujita S, Harada M, Yasukawa M. Identification of a novel WT1-derived peptide which induces human leucocyte antigen-A24-restricted anti-leukaemia cytotoxic T lymphocytes. Br J Haematol 2002; 116:601–603.

156. Bellantuono I, Gao L, Parry S, Marley S, Dazzi F, Apperley J, Goldman JM, Stauss HJ. Two distinct HLA-A0201-presented epitopes of the Wilms tumor antigen 1 can function as targets for leukemia-reactive CTL. Blood 2002; 100:3835–3837.

157. Scheibenbogen C, Letsch A, Thiel E, Schmittel A, Mailaender V, Baerwolf S, Nagorsen D, Keilholz U. CD8 T-cell responses to Wilms tumor gene product WT1 and proteinase 3 in patients with acute myeloid leukemia. Blood 2002; 100:2132–2137.

158. Oka Y, Elisseeva OA, Tsuboi A, Ogawa H, Tamaki H, Li H, Oji Y, Kim EH, Soma T, Asada M, Ueda K, Maruya E, Saji H, Kishimoto T, Udaka K, Sugiyama H. Human cytotoxic T-lymphocyte responses specific for peptides of the wild-type Wilms' tumor gene (WT1) product. Immunogenetics 2000; 51:99–107.

159. Chen W, Chatta K, Rubin W, Liggitt DH, Kusunoki Y, Martin P, Cheever MA. Polymporphic segments of CD45 can serve as targets for GVHD and GVL responses. Blood 1995; 86.

160. Raptis A, Clave E, Mavroudis D, Molldrem J, Van Rhee F, Barrett AJ. Polymorphism in CD33 and CD34 genes: a source of minor histocompatibility antigens on haemopoietic progenitor cells? Br J Haematol 1998; 102:1354–1358.

161. Amrolia PJ, Reid SD, Gao L, Schultheis B, Dotti G, Brenner MK, Melo JV, Goldman JM, Stauss HJ. Allo-restricted cytotoxic T cells specific for human CD45 show potent antileukemic activity. Blood 2002.

162. Tureci O, Sahin U, Pfreundschuh M. Serological analysis of human tumor antigens: molecular definition and implications. Mol Med Today 1997; 3:342–349.

163. Chen YT. Cancer vaccine: identification of human tumor antigens by SEREX. Cancer J 2000; 6 Suppl 3:S208–217.

164. Greiner J, Ringhoffer M, Simikopinko O, Szmaragowska A, Huebsch S, Maurer U, Bergmann L, Schmitt M. Simultaneous expression of different immunogenic antigens in acute myeloid leukemia. Exp Hematol 2000; 28:1413–1422.

165. Chambost H, van Baren N, Brasseur F, Olive D. MAGE-A genes are not expressed in human leukemias. Leukemia 2001; 15:1769–1771.

166. Vonderheide RH, Hahn WC, Schultze JL, Nadler LM. The telomerase catalytic subunit is a widely expressed tumor-associated antigen recognized by cytotoxic T lymphocytes. Immunity 1999; 10:673–679.

167. Xie HJ, Lundgren S, Broberg U, Finnstrom N, Rane A, Hassan M. Effect of cyclophosphamide on gene expression of cytochromes p450 and beta-actin in the HL-60 cell line. Eur J Pharmacol 2002; 449:197–205.

168. Nagai F, Hiyoshi Y, Sugimachi K, Tamura HO. Cytochrome P450 (CYP) expression in human myeloblastic and lymphoid cell lines. Biol Pharm Bull 2002; 25:383–385.

169. Rooney CM, Smith CA, Heslop HE. Control of virus-induced lymphoproliferation: Epstein-Barr virus-induced lymphoproliferation and host immunity. Mol Med Today 1997; 3:24–30.

170. Heslop HE, Ng CY, Li C, Smith CA, Loftin SK, Krance RA, Brenner MK, Rooney CM. Long-term restoration of immunity against Epstein-Barr virus infection by adoptive transfer of gene-modified virus-specific T lymphocytes. Nat Med 1996; 2:551–555.

171. Molldrem JJ, Lee PP, Kant S, Wieder E, Jiang W, Lu S, Wang C, Davis MM. Chronic myelogenous leukemia shapes host immunity by selective deletion of high-avidity leukemia-specific T cells. J Clin Invest 2003; 111:639–647.

172. Gale RP, Horowitz MM, Ash RC, Champlin RE, Goldman JM, Rimm AA, Ringden O, Stone JA, Bortin MM. Identical-twin bone marrow transplants for leukemia. Ann Intern Med 1994; 120:646–652.

173. Anderton SM, Wraith DC. Selection and fine-tuning of the autoimmune T-cell repertoire. Nat Rev Immunol 2002; 2:487–498.

174. Barrett AJ, Ringden O, Zhang MJ, Bashey A, Cahn JY, Cairo MS, Gale RP, Gratwohl A, Locatelli F, Martino R, Schultz KR, Tiberghien P. Effect of nucleated marrow cell dose on relapse and survival in identical twin bone marrow transplants for leukemia. Blood 2000; 95:3323–3327.

175. Jiang YZ, Barrett J. The allogeneic CD4+ T-cell-mediated graft-versus-leukemia effect. Leuk Lymphoma 1997; 28:33–42.

176. Jiang YZ, Couriel D, Mavroudis DA, Lewalle P, Malkovska V, Hensel NF, Dermime S, Molldrem J, Barrett AJ. Interaction of natural killer cells with MHC class II: reversal of HLA-DR1-mediated protection of K562 transfectant from natural killer cell-mediated cytolysis by brefeldin-A. Immunology 1996; 87:481–486.

177. Walter EA, Greenberg PD, Gilbert MJ, Finch RJ, Watanabe KS, Thomas ED, Riddell SR. Reconstitution of cellular immunity against cytomegalovirus in recipients of allogeneic bone marrow by transfer of T-cell clones from the donor. N Engl J Med 1995; 333:1038–1044.

178. Fearon ER, Pardoll DM, Itaya T, Golumbek P, Levitsky HI, Simons JW, Karasuyama H, Vogelstein B, Frost P. Interleukin-2 production by tumor cells bypasses T helper function in the generation of an antitumor response. Cell 1990; 60:397–403.

179. Giralt S, Hester J, Huh Y, Hirsch-Ginsberg C, Rondon G, Seong D, Lee M, Gajewski J, Van Besien K, Khouri I, et al. CD8-depleted donor lymphocyte infusion as treatment for relapsed chronic myelogenous leukemia after allogeneic bone marrow transplantation. Blood 1995; 86:4337–4343.

180. Posthuma EF, Falkenburg JH, Apperley JF, Gratwohl A, Hertenstein B, Schipper RF, Oudshoorn M, Biezen JH, Hermans J, Willemze R, Roosnek E, Niederwieser D. HLA-DR4 is associated with a diminished risk of the development of chronic myeloid leukemia (CML). Chronic Leukemia Working Party of the European Blood and Marrow Transplant Registry. Leukemia 2000; 14:859–862.

181. Dodi IA, Van Rhee F, Forde HC, Roura-Mir C, Jaraquemada D, Goldman JM, Madrigal JA. CD4(+) bias in T cells cloned from a CML patient with active graft versus leukemia effect. Cytotherapy 2002; 4:353–363.

182. Reijonen H, Kwok WW. Use of HLA class II tetramers in tracking antigen-specific T cells and mapping T-cell epitopes. Methods 2003; 29:282–288.

183. Gebe JA, Falk BA, Rock KA, Kochik SA, Heninger AK, Reijonen H, Kwok WW, Nepom GT. Low-avidity recognition by CD4+ T cells directed to self-antigens. Eur J Immunol 2003; 33:1409–1417.

184. Cohen CJ, Denkberg G, Schiffenbauer YS, Segal D, Trubniykov E, Berke G, Reiter Y. Simultaneous monitoring of binding to and activation of tumor-specific T lymphocytes by peptide-MHC. J Immunol Methods 2003; 277:39–52.

185. Vogt MH, van den Muijsenberg JW, Goulmy E, Spierings E, Kluck P, Kester MG, van Soest RA, Drijfhout JW, Willemze R, Falkenburg JH. The DBY gene codes for an HLA-DQ5-restricted human male-specific minor histocompatibility antigen involved in graft-versus-host disease. Blood 2002; 99:3027–3032.

186. Farag SS, Fehniger TA, Becknell B, Blaser BW, Caligiuri MA. New directions in natural killer cell-based immunotherapy of human cancer. Expert Opin Biol Ther 2003; 3:237–250.

187. Parham P, McQueen KL. Alloreactive killer cells: hindrance and help for haematopoietic transplants. Nat Rev Immunol 2003; 3:108–122.

188. Dohring C, Scheidegger D, Samaridis J, Cella M, Colonna M. A human killer inhibitory receptor specific for HLA-A1,2. J Immunol 1996; 156:3098–3101.

189. Litwin V, Gumperz J, Parham P, Phillips JH, Lanier LL. NKB1: a natural killer cell receptor involved in the recognition of polymorphic HLA-B molecules. J Exp Med 1994; 180:537–543.

190. Colonna M, Samaridis J. Cloning of immunoglobulin-superfamily members associated with HLA-C and HLA-B recognition by human natural killer cells. Science 1995; 268:405–408.

191. Wagtmann N, Rajagopalan S, Winter CC, Peruzzi M, Long EO. Killer cell inhibitory receptors specific for HLA-C and HLA-B identified by direct binding and by functional transfer. Immunity 1995; 3:801–809.

192. Gumperz JE, Litwin V, Phillips JH, Lanier LL, Parham P. The Bw4 public epitope of HLA-B molecules confers reactivity with natural killer cell clones that express NKB1, a putative HLA receptor. J Exp Med 1995; 181:1133–1144.

193. D'Andrea A, Chang C, Franz-Bacon K, McClanahan T, Phillips JH, Lanier LL. Molecular cloning of NKB1. A natural killer cell receptor for HLA-B allotypes. J Immunol 1995; 155:2306–2310.

194. Lee N, Llano M, Carretero M, Ishitani A, Navarro F, Lopez-Botet M, Geraghty DE. HLA-E is a major ligand for the natural killer inhibitory receptor CD94/NKG2A. Proc Natl Acad Sci USA 1998; 95:5199–5204.

195. Borrego F, Ulbrecht M, Weiss EH, Coligan JE, Brooks AG. Recognition of human histocompatibility leukocyte antigen (HLA)-E complexed with HLA class I signal sequence-derived peptides by CD94/NKG2 confers protection from natural killer cell-mediated lysis. J Exp Med 1998; 187:813–818.

196. Braud VM, Allan DS, O'Callaghan CA, Soderstrom K, D'Andrea A, Ogg GS, Lazetic S, Young NT, Bell JI, Phillips JH, Lanier LL, McMichael AJ. HLA-E binds to natural killer cell receptors CD94/NKG2A, B and C. Nature 1998; 391:795–799.

197. Valiante NM, Uhrberg M, Shilling HG, Lienert-Weidenbach K, Arnett KL, D'Andrea A, Phillips JH, Lanier LL, Parham P. Functionally and structurally distinct NK cell receptor repertoires in the peripheral blood of two human donors. Immunity 1997; 7:739–751.

198. Ljunggren HG, Karre K. In search of the 'missing self': MHC molecules and NK cell recognition. Immunol Today 1990; 11:237–244.

199. Cudkowicz G, Bennett M. Peculiar immunobiology of bone marrow allografts. II. Rejection of parental grafts by resistant F1 hybrid mice. J Exp Med 1971; 134:1513–1528.

200. Cudkowicz G, Bennett M. Peculiar immunobiology of bone marrow allografts. I. Graft rejection by irradiated responder mice. J Exp Med 1971; 134:83–102.

201. Shilling HG, Guethlein LA, Cheng NW, Gardiner CM, Rodriguez R, Tyan D, Parham P. Allelic polymorphism synergizes with variable gene content to individualize human KIR genotype. J Immunol 2002; 168:2307–2315.

202. Colonna M, Brooks EG, Falco M, Ferrara GB, Strominger JL. Generation of allospecific natural killer cells by stimulation across a polymorphism of HLA-C. Science 1993; 260:1121–1124.

203. Farag SS, Fehniger TA, Ruggeri L, Velardi A, Caligiuri MA. Natural killer cell receptors: new biology and insights into the graft-versus-leukemia effect. Blood 2002; 100:1935–1947.

204. Ruggeri L, Capanni M, Casucci M, Volpi I, Tosti A, Perruccio K, Urbani E, Negrin RS, Martelli MF, Velardi A. Role of natural killer cell alloreactivity in HLA-mismatched hematopoietic stem cell transplantation. Blood 1999; 94:333–339.

205. Piccioli D, Sbrana S, Melandri E, Valiante NM. Contact-dependent stimulation and inhibition of dendritic cells by natural killer cells. J Exp Med 2002; 195:335–341.

206. Ferlazzo G, Tsang ML, Moretta L, Melioli G, Steinman RM, Munz C. Human dendritic cells activate resting natural killer (NK) cells and are recognized via the NKp30 receptor by activated NK cells. J Exp Med 2002; 195:343–351.

207. Ruggeri L, Capanni M, Martelli MF, Velardi A. Cellular therapy: exploiting NK cell alloreactivity in transplantation. Curr Opin Hematol 2001; 8:355–359.

208. De Santis D, Witt C, Nagler A, Brautbar C, Christiansen F, Bishara A. HLA-C KIR ligands and donor recipient KIR genotypes influence outcome of haploidentical stem cell transplantation. Hum Immunol 2002; 63:17.

209. Schaffer M, Remberger M, Ringden O, Olerup O. Role of HLA-C incompatibilities in unrelated donor hematopoietic stem cell transplantation. Tissue Antigens 2002; 59:18.

210. Davies SM, Ruggieri L, DeFor T, Wagner JE, Weisdorf DJ, Miller JS, Velardi A, Blazar BR. Evaluation of KIR ligand incompatibility in mismatched unrelated donor hematopoietic transplants. Killer immunoglobulin-like receptor. Blood 2002; 100:3825–3827.

211. Giebel S, Locatelli F, Lamparelli T, Velardi A, Davies S, Frumento G, Maccario R, Bonetti F, Wojnar J, Martinetti M, Frassoni F, Giorgiani G, Bacigalupo A, Holowiecki J. Survival advantage with KIR ligand incompatibility in hematopoietic stem cell transplantation from unrelated donors. Blood 2003; 102:814–819.

212. Cook MA, Norman PJ, Curran MD, Maxwell LD, Briggs DC, Middleton D, Vaughan RW. A multi-laboratory characterization of the KIR genotypes of 10th International Histocompatibility Workshop cell lines. Hum Immunol 2003; 64:567–571.

213. Gomez-Lozano N, Vilches C. Genotyping of human killer-cell immunoglobulin-like receptor genes by polymerase chain reaction with sequence-specific primers: an update. Tissue Antigens 2002; 59:184–193.

214. Gagne K, Brizard G, Gueglio B, Milpied N, Herry P, Bonneville F, Cheneau ML, Schleinitz N, Cesbron A, Follea G, Harrousseau JL, Bignon JD. Relevance of KIR gene polymorphisms in bone marrow transplantation outcome. Hum Immunol 2002; 63:271–280.

214a. Barrett AJ, Mavroudis D, Tisdale J, et al. T cell-depleted bone marrow transplantation and delayed T cell add-back to control acute GVHD and conserve a graft-versus-leukemia effect. Bone Marrow Transplant 1998; 21:543–551.

214b. Mavroudis DA, Dermime S, Molldrem J, Jiang YZ, Raptis A, van Rhee F, Hensel N, Fellowes V, Eliopoulos G, Barrett AJ. Specific depletion of alloreactive T cells in HLA-identical siblings: a method for separating graft-versus-host and graft-versus-leukaemia reactions. Br J Haematol 1998; 101:565–570.

214c. Amrolia PJ, Muccioli-Casadei G, Yvon E, et al. Selective depletion of donor allo-reactive T-cells without loss of anti-viral or anti-leukemic responses. Blood 2003; 102:2292–2299.

214d. Falkenburg JH, Wafelman AR, Joosten P, et al. Complete remission of accelerated phase chronic myeloid leukemia by treatment with leukemia-reactive cytotoxic T lymphocytes. Blood 1999; 94:1201–1208.

215. Pinilla-Ibarz J, Cathcart K, Korontsvit T, Soignet S, Bocchia M, Caggiano J, Lai L, Jimenez J, Kolitz J, Scheinberg DA. Vaccination of patients with chronic myelogenous leukemia with bcr-abl oncogene breakpoint fusion peptides generates specific immune responses. Blood 2000; 95:1781–1787.

216. Panilla J, Cathcart K, Korontsvit T, Schwartz JD, Zakheleva E, Papadopoulos E, Scheinberg DA. A phase II trial of patients with CML using a multivalent BCR-ABL oncogene product fusion peptide vaccine. American Society of Clinical Oncology, San Francisco, 2003:674.

217. Li Z, Qiao Y, Laska E, Julko J, Bona R, Gaffney J, Hegde U, Moyo P, Srivastava P. Combination of imatinib mesylate with autologous leukocyte-derived heat shock protein 70 vaccine for chronic myelogenous leukemia. American Society of Clinical Oncology, San Francisco, 2003:664.

218. Appelbaum FR. Haematopoietic cell transplantation as immunotherapy. Nature 2001; 411:385–389.

219. Barrett J, Jiang Y-Z. Allogeneic Immunotherapy for Malignant Diseases. Basic and Clinical Oncology. Vol. 22. New York: Marcel Dekker, 2000.

220. Ralph P, Moore MA, Nilsson K. Lysozyme synthesis by established human and murine histiocytic lymphoma cell lines. J Exp Med 1976; 143:1528–1533.

221. Hill GR, Cooke KR, Teshima T, Crawford JM, Keith JC, Jr., Brinson YS, Bungard D, Ferrara JL. Interleukin-11 promotes T cell polarization and prevents acute graft-versus-host disease after allogeneic bone marrow transplantation. J Clin Invest 1998; 102:115–123.

222. Cooke KR, Gerbitz A, Crawford JM, Teshima T, Hill GR, Tesolin A, Rossignol DP, Ferrara JL. LPS antagonism reduces graft-versus-host disease and preserves graft-versus-leukemia activity after experimental bone marrow transplantation [comment]. J Clin Invest 2001; 107:1581–1589.

223. Greenberger JS, Sakakeeny MA, Humphries RK, Eaves CJ, Eckner RJ. Demonstration of permanent factor-dependent multipotential (erythroid/neutrophil/basophil) hematopoietic progenitor cell lines. Proc Natl Acad Sci USA 1983; 80:2931–2935.

224. Tauchi T, Boswell HS, Leibowitz D, Broxmeyer HE. Coupling between p210bcr-abl and Shc and Grb2 adaptor proteins in hematopoietic cells permits growth factor receptor-independent link to ras activation pathway. J Exp Med 1994; 179:167–175.

225. Knapp MR, Jones PP, Black SJ, Vitetta ES, Slavin S, Strober S. Characterization of a spontaneous murine B cell leukemia (BCL1). I. Cell surface expression of IgM, IgD, Ia, and FcR. J Immunol 1979; 123:992–999.

226. Weiss L, Morecki S, Vitetta ES, Slavin S. Suppression and elimination of BCL1 leukemia by allogeneic bone marrow transplantation. J Immunol 1983; 130:2452–2455.

227. Slavin S, Yatziv S, Weiss L, Morecki S, Abeliuk P, Fuks Z. Total lymphoid irradiation (TLI) and allogeneic marrow transplantation for enzyme replacement therapy and immunotherapy of leukemia in mice. Transplant Proc 1981; 13:439–442.

228. Slavin S, Strober S. Spontaneous murine B-cell leukaemia. Nature 1978; 272:624–626.

229. Kim KJ, Kanellopoulos-Langevin C, Merwin RM, Sachs DH, Asofsky R. Establishment and characterization of BALB/c lymphoma lines with B cell properties. J Immunol 1979; 122:549–554.

230. Bortin M, Truitt RL. AKR T-cell acute lymphoblastic leukemia: a model for human T-cell leukemia. Biomedicine 1977; 26:309–311.

231. Truitt RL, Atasoylu AA. Contribution of CD4+ and CD8+ T cells to graft-versus-host disease and graft-versus-leukemia reactivity after transplantation of MHC-compatible bone marrow. Bone Marrow Transplant 1991; 8:51–58.

232. Ralph P. Retention of lymphocyte characteristics by myelomas and theta + -lymphomas: sensitivity to cortisol and phytohemagglutinin. J Immunol 1973; 110:1470–1475.

233. Ralph P, Nakoinz I. Inhibitory effects of lectins and lymphocyte mitogens on murine lymphomas and myelomas. J Natl Cancer Inst 1973; 51:883–890.

234. Anderson LD, Jr., Savary CA, Mullen CA. Immunization of allogeneic bone marrow transplant recipients with tumor cell vaccines enhances graft-versus-tumor activity without exacerbating graft-versus-host disease.[erratum appears in Blood 2000; 96(2):783]. Blood 2000; 95:2426–2433.

235. Sykes M, Bukhari Z, Sachs DH. Graft-versus-leukemia effect using mixed allogeneic bone marrow transplantation. Bone Marrow Transplant 1989; 4:465–474.

236. Yang YG, Sykes M. The role of interleukin-12 in preserving the graft-versus-leukemia effect of allogeneic CD8 T cells independently of GVHD. Leuk Lymphoma 1999; 33:409–420.

237. Aizawa S, Kamisaku H, Sado T. An MHC-compatible allogeneic bone marrow donor with a distinct role of T cell subsets in graft-versus-leukemia effect and lethal graft-versus-host disease. Bone Marrow Transplant 1995; 16:603–609.

238. Patterson AE, Korngold R. Cross-protective murine graft-versus-leukemia responses to phenotypically distinct myeloid leukemia lines. Biol Blood Marrow Transplant 2000; 6:537–547.

239. Kim YM, Sachs T, Asavaroengchai W, Bronson R, Sykes M. Graft-versus-host disease can be separated from graft-versus-lymphoma effects by control of lymphocyte trafficking with FTY720. J Clin Invest 2003; 111:659–669.

240. Drobyski WR, Ash RC, Casper JT, McAuliffe T, Horowitz MM, Lawton C, Keever C, Baxter-Lowe LA, Camitta B, Garbrecht F, et al. Effect of T-cell depletion as graft-versus-host disease prophylaxis on engraftment, relapse, and disease-free survival in unrelated marrow transplantation for chronic myelogenous leukemia. Blood 1994; 83:1980–1987.

241. Porter DL, Roth MS, McGarigle C, Ferrara JL, Antin JH. Induction of graft-versus-host disease as immunotherapy for relapsed chronic myeloid leukemia. N Engl J Med 1994; 330:100–106.

242. Hessner MJ, Endean DJ, Casper JT, Horowitz MM, Keever-Taylor CA, Roth M, Flomenberg N, Drobyski WR. Use of unrelated marrow grafts compensates for reduced graft-versus-leukemia reactivity after T-cell-depleted allogeneic marrow transplantation for chronic myelogenous leukemia. Blood 1995; 86:3987–3996.

243. Slavin S, Naparstek E, Nagler A, Ackerstein A, Kapelushnik J, Or R. Allogeneic cell therapy for relapsed leukemia after bone marrow transplantation with donor peripheral blood lymphocytes. Exp Hematol 1995; 23:1553–1562.

7

The Immune System in Graft-vs.-Host Disease: Target and Effector Organ

CRYSTAL L. MACKALL and FRANCES T. HAKIM

National Institutes of Health, Bethesda, Maryland, U.S.A.

ANDREA VELARDI

University of Perugia, Perugia, Italy

I. INTRODUCTION

Allogeneic stem cell transplantation has emerged as the treatment of choice for a variety of lymphohematopoietic malignancies, immunodeficiencies, and marrow failure syndromes. For each of these diseases, the primary goal of allogeneic bone marrow transplantation is replacement of the recipient lymphohematopoietic system with a fully competent one from the donor. Transfer of hematopoiesis is readily accomplished with current therapies, but successful transfer of a fully functional immune system remains a substantial problem. The extent to which immune reconstitution occurs and the rate at which it occurs are heavily influenced by the presence or absence of graft-vs.-host disease (GVHD). Profound immunosuppression with infectious complications occurs commonly in patients with GVHD and is further exacerbated by the immunosuppressive therapy administered for the treatment of GVHD. Moreover, T-cell depletion of the stem cell graft to reduce the incidence of GVHD exacerbates post-transplant immunodeficiency. Therefore, since the pathophysiology, therapy, and prevention of GVHD converge at immunosuppression, resulting in the clinical complications of infection and recurrence of malignancy, GVHD and immune reconstitution are inextricably linked to one another within the biology of allogeneic stem cell transplantation (SCT). The challenge for the future is to develop new therapies that can enhance the competence of the transferred immune system against both infection and malignancy without exacerbating GVHD.

This chapter will focus on the interface between immune reconstitution and GVHD. We will summarize current data, derived from murine and clinical studies, which illustrate how the immune system functions as both the effector and target organ of GVHD. We will also discuss a variety of emerging strategies which hold promise for improving the competency of the transplanted immune system against infection and/or malignancy with an eye toward the potential impact that these may have on GVHD. Finally, because of emerging interest in the biology of natural killer (NK)-cell–mediated responses following SCT, we will discuss the dual role of NK cells as potential cofactors in the pathophysiology of T-cell–initiated GVHD as well as potential preventative agents for the GVH reaction in the setting of T-cell–depleted major histocompatibility complex (MHC)-mismatched SCT.

II. THE GVH REACTION

A. Three Critical Elements: Alloreactive T Cells, Recipient Antigen-Presenting Cells, and Inflammation

Current models hold that there are three critical elements that come together to generate the clinical syndrome of acute GVHD: donor T cells, recipient antigen presenting cells (APC), and inflammatory stimulation, usually introduced by the conditioning regimen. To briefly summarize material discussed at length in Chapter 1, donor T cells have long been known to be the key element in GVHD. Depletion of donor T cells, or even of recipient-reactive T cells, prevents GVHD. Donor CD4+ and CD8+ T cells, clonally expanding in response to host antigens, generate cytokines [primarily interleukin (IL)-2 and interferon (IFN-γ)] that support differentiation of cytotoxic T cells specific for the host as well as nonspecific effector cells, such as macrophages and NK cells. Shlomchik et al. (1) demonstrated that recipient APC were critical for activation of these donor T cells; indeed, alloantigen-expressing recipient APC are sufficient to activate donor T cells and induce GVHD in the absence of any other alloantigen-expressing cells in the host (2). Activation of recipient APC, through triggering of the innate immune system by bacterial antigens during conditioning, enhances stimulation of donor T cells and also contributes to a massive release of tumor necrosis factor (TNF)-α and other factors that contribute to tissue damage in the gut, liver, and skin. Together, these three elements interact in a self-perpetuating cycle, which has been described as a "cytokine storm" (3,4).

One of the primary characteristics of GVHD is a profound and long-lasting immune deficiency. This is an exacerbation of the predictable immune deficiency that occurs in all transplant recipients as a result of the ablation of host immunity that occurs during the preparative regimen and is reconstituted only slowly by donor-derived cells. Of the many variables analyzed posttransplant, the time elapsed after transplant and the presence of GVHD have been consistently shown to be the most critical factors affecting the degree of immune recovery. Furthermore, while acute GVHD-associated inflammation of the liver, gut, and skin is adequately treated with currently available immunosuppressive therapies, these same therapies only contribute to problems in immune recovery.

Immune reconstitution following high-intensity cytotoxic therapy is a dynamic process involving major alterations in lymphocyte and APC populations, local and systemic fluxes in cytokines and chemokines, changes in the structural organization of lymphoid organs, and marked shifts in cell trafficking. Each of these processes is exacerbated by GVHD, resulting in an immune deficiency that is complex and multifactorial in etiology. Three main factors will be discussed that are primarily responsible for limiting immune reconstitution in hosts with acute GVHD: limitations in the repertoire and function of the transferred mature T cells (including recipient-reactive T cells), nonspecific suppression of lymphocyte function, and deficient lymphopoiesis of new B- and T-cell populations from the transferred graft. Depending upon the time when the patient with GVHD is studied, the relative contribution of each of these factors may vary. In general, alterations in the repertoire and function of mature T cells and nonspecific immune suppression occur in the first weeks to months of GVHD, while deficiencies in lymphopoiesis are critical factors in the chronic immunodeficiency associated with GVHD, which can remain for months to years.

B.   GVHD Impairs Thymic-Independent Peripheral Expansion

GVHD induces dramatic abnormalities in both the alloreactive and the non-alloreactive bystander populations transferred as part of the stem cell graft. These effects substantially limit the capacity for mature T cells to contribute to effective immune reconstitution in hosts with GVHD. Following cytoreductive therapy and graft administration, mature T-cell populations residual in the recipient or contained in the donor graft are induced into a state of flux. Proliferative expansion of residual mature cells in the periphery increase lymphocyte populations; trafficking shifts and cell death reduce the circulating cells. The balance between these processes modulates T-cell numbers, and GVHD intensifies these changes. The two main factors driving mature T-cell expansion are homeostatic regulation and antigenic stimulation.

In general, homeostatic feedback loops attempt to maintain steady population levels such that when T cells are transplanted into T-replete host mice, there is little proliferative activity, whereas when T cells are transferred into lymphopenic recipients (which occurs in the context of SCT), donor T cells rapidly expand (5). Thus, a high frequency of T cells transferred within the graft in the setting of SCT are in cycle in the early weeks posttransplant (6). Data from mouse models have shown that this homeostatic process is primarily cytokine dependent since naïve CD4 and CD8 T cells transferred into lymphopenic hosts require IL-7 for survival and expansion and memory CD8+ T cells require either IL-7 or IL-15 to expand (5). Adding IL-7 posttransplant accelerates T-cell recovery in part through dramatically enhancing this process of peripheral T-cell expansion (7). Human T-cell expansion is likely also under the control of cytokine feedback loops posttransplant (8). When lymphocytes are depleted, circulating IL-7 levels rise and the higher levels of IL-7 enhance survival and stimulate proliferative expansion, allowing mature T-cell numbers to compensate for the loss. Indeed, increased serum levels of IL-7 are present in lymphopenic SCID and leukemia patients (9). Following chemotherapy or transplant, IL-7 levels increase during the period of severe lymphopenia and then decline with recovery of CD4 levels (8,9). IL-15 may also be involved in expansion and stabilization of CD8+ T-cell populations.(5) Although serum IL-15 levels are normally undetectable, conditioning regimens for transplant result in elevated serum levels for the first few weeks (10). Furthermore, elevated IL-15 levels remain detectable in the serum during grade II–IV acute GVHD (10). It remains unclear whether IL-15 acts as a homeostatic regulator in this setting, as IL-7 appears to, or whether IL15 is produced primarily as an inflammatory cytokine in conditions of early transplant and GVHD.

Regardless, it appears clear that cytokine levels play a key role in regulating T-cell expansion posttransplant and thus may have a significant impact on the immunopathology of GVHD.

The thymic-independent peripheral expansion that occurs post-SCT is comprised of cells responding to both cognate (high-affinity) antigens and intermediate or low-affinity antigens. Hazenberg et al. demonstrated that individuals with ongoing inflammatory processes—whether GVHD or infection—have higher frequencies of cycling peripheral blood T cells than patients without such complications (6). A characteristic of antigenic stimulation during peripheral lymphocyte expansion is the selective expansion of antigen-specific cells, resulting in skewing the TCR repertoire (11). In MHC-matched, *mls*-disparate murine models, in which recipient-reactive T cells could be identified by T-cell receptor $V\beta$ usage, CD4 and CD8 T cells reactive to the recipient expand to 75–90% of the T-cell population within one week (12). In humans, oligoclonal TCR repertoires are characteristic of CD4+ and especially CD8+ T cells in the first months posttransplant. This is due in part to severe reductions in T-cell numbers with resultant decreases in repertoire diversity, but is also related to antigen-driven expansion with resultant skewing in the setting of GVHD (13,14). Importantly, oligoclonal expansions of T cells arise in the setting of GVHD and are stably maintained for many months (15–17). Circulating expanded clones are matched by similar $V\beta$ usage in GVHD target tissues (18). Further, chronically stimulated T cells (phenotypically CD28-CD27-CD57+)(19) typically become the dominant CD8+ T-cell population posttransplant (20). Thus, it appears that a large proportion of the T cells that circulate in the hosts of patients with GVHD have been subjected to chronic antigen stimulation.

Peripherally expanding lymphocytes in the early posttransplant period are phenotypically memory, not naive, T cells with a high degree of expression of activation markers (21). Coincident with activation is an increase in susceptibility to activation-induced cell death (AICD) (21–24). During the early period of rapid peripheral expansion, T cells undergo apoptosis at elevated rates when cultured in vitro, with or without mitogenic stimulation (21,23,25). Apoptosis occurs more frequently in HLA-DR+ cells, and the overall frequency of apoptosis is correlated with the percentage of DR+ cells, an indicator of activation (21). AICD is increased in the setting of mismatched transplants and in severe GVHD (21–25). The key finding is that the frequency of early apoptosis is inversely correlated with later CD4+ T-cell levels (23).

Murine studies have similarly observed that rapidly expanding recipient-reactive populations subsequently undergo swift declines in number (12,26). The dramatic loss of alloreactive T cells is considered to be due in large part to AICD (27–30). Importantly, this depletion effectively diminishes the number of dangerous alloreactive T cells, but also leads to significant apoptosis of bystander, nonalloreactive populations, severely limiting the number and diversity of residual T cells available for immune reconstitution via homeostatic T-cell expansion (31) (Fig. 1). Furthermore, those donor T cells that survive following this massive expansion and contraction are abnormal, as they are anergic to stimulation with alloantigen and nonspecific stimuli (12). While responses to mitogens and third-party stimuli gradually recover, the regenerated T cells typically show prolonged anergy to recipient alloantigens, which is not corrected by addition of IL-2 and is not due to suppressor activity (32). Thus activated, peripherally expanding T cells do not give rise to stable peripheral T-cell repopulation. While early peripheral expansion in GVHD may occur rapidly, the resultant populations are limited in number and repertoire, and the efficiency of the expansion is limited by apoptotic instability. While the process of

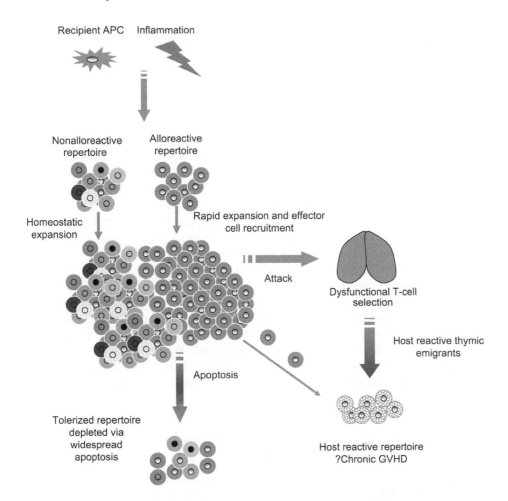

Figure 1 GVHD impedes both thymic-independent and thymic-dependent T-cell regeneration. T cells are regenerated through homeostatic expansion of mature T cells and through thymopoietic pathways. In the presence of GVHD, alloantigen-induced expansion is followed by profound activation-induced cell death. Bystander, homeostatically expanding cells are simultaneously depleted through bystander apoptosis. Simultaneously, alloreactivity directed toward thymic epithelium diminishes the number of thymic emigrants and leads to the export of recipient reactive T cells as a result of impaired thymic selection.

expansion and subsequent contraction is a general feature of immune reconstitution via peripheral expansion, it appears to be magnified in the setting of GVHD.

C. GVHD-Associated Immune Suppression

Immune deficiencies in GVHD have long been associated with experimental and phenomenological evidence for immune suppression, but many of cells or cytokines involved and the molecular mechanisms utilized are poorly defined at best. A rapid loss of host immune function is observed in vitro within the first 2 days of acute GVHD, when the donor T cells are still a minority (33). Evidence for active suppression of T- and B-cell responses has been observed as early as one week following initiation of the alloreaction (33,34). Several suppressor populations have been identified in the setting of GVHD—including CD8+ T cells, macrophages, and natural suppressor (NS) cells)—and it appears likely that multiple different regulatory cells may function through different effector mechanisms at different time points associated with the GVH reaction. CD8 suppressor cells have been detected in both murine and clinical studies (34,35), but the soluble mediators have not been characterized. Proinflammatory macrophages isolated from the spleen or liver of mice undergoing acute GVHD have also been found to inhibit T- and B-cell responses to mitogens, particularly when stimulated with lipopolysaccharide (LPS), perhaps through nitric oxide (NO) release (36–39). Macrophages from mobilized peripheral blood stem cells suppress the proliferative responses of normal T cells in coculture, perhaps by stimulating apoptosis of activated T cells (40,41). Natural suppressor cells present in the first weeks after transplant were found to inhibit both concanavalin (ConA) and LPS-stimulated proliferation in an MHC nonrestricted manner (42), yet these populations were never defined further than by their lack of T, B, or macrophage markers. Recently donor-derived CD4 + CD25+ regulatory T cells (43) have been reported to serve a role in limiting alloreactivity. Removal of these cells increases the severity of GVHD, whereas infusion of these cells reduces alloreactivity (44–47). Multiple cytokines and other factors, notably IL-10, transforming growth factor (TGF)-β and NO, have been found to be produced in GVHD and are known to be suppressive in vitro. Thus, while there is ample evidence that immunosuppression, both allospecific and nonallospecific, occurs commonly in GVHD, the mediators of such suppression and the mechanisms by which immune suppression is induced and regulated remains poorly characterized.

D.   Delayed and Deficient Lymphopoiesis in GVHD

The third and perhaps the most important element contributing to the prolonged immune deficiency associated with clinical GVHD is the dramatic reduction in lymphopoiesis that occurs as a result of the GVH reaction. Conditioning regimens produce a severe depletion of all lymphocyte populations (48,49). Even in non-myeloablative "minitransplants," lymphoid populations are specifically targeted for depletion. Restoration of peripheral lymphocytes through lymphopoiesis is a slow and variable process, which commonly requires many months following both autologous or allogeneic SCT, even in the absence of GVHD (21,50,51) (Fig. 2).

Following completion of chemotherapy or transplant conditioning regimens, NK cell numbers are the first lymphocyte subset to return to pretreatment levels, and global NK function is restored with weeks as evidenced by ex vivo assays (52). Interestingly, however, more recent studies evaluating NK subsets have revealed significant long-standing alterations post-SCT. Although traditional assays have identified NK cells solely as CD3− CD56+ or CD3− CD16+, more recent studies have suggested important distinctions between CD56^{dull}CD16+ and CD56^{bright} subsets. CD56^{dull}CD16+ cells generally express higher levels of inhibitory KIRs and are highly cytotoxic, whereas the CD56^{bright} cells express higher levels of activating CD94/NKG2A NK cell receptors and are robust cytokine producers (53). Interestingly, following allogeneic SCT, even in the absence of GVHD, there is increased expression of CD94/NKG2A, and the expression of several KIR is reduced (54). These alterations in NK receptor levels do not return to donor patterns of receptor expression for one year or longer. Similarly, the relative

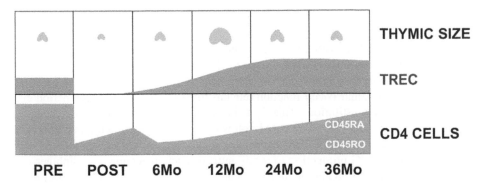

Figure 2 CD4 + T cell regeneration is protracted due to thymic insufficiency. Following T-cell–depleting therapy, regeneration of new T cells is highly dependent upon thymic-dependent pathways. Because age-associated thymic involution occurs relatively early in life, most patients sustaining T-cell depletion have involuted thymi at baseline, which undergo further damage related to cytotoxic therapy. Thymic function can be monitored by following either recovery of CD4 + CD45RA + T cells or TREC levels.

populations of CD56^{dull}CD16+ cytotoxic NK cells and CD56^{bright} cytokine–producing NK cells also are altered (53). CD56^{bright} cells, which normally comprise less than 10% of the NK repertoire, increase to become the majority of NK cells in the first weeks, and then decline by 3 months, perhaps reflecting shifts in the cytokine milieu supporting their maturation (55,56). Thus, although global NK number and function rapidly normalizes following SCT, alterations in NK subsets that may have important implications for overall NK function persist for several months. Thus, although NK cells generally rapidly recover to normal or elevated levels following SCT, in the presence or absence of GVHD, the full effects of SCT and GVHD on NK subsets and NK receptor repertoire are still unknown.

In the absence of GVHD, total B-cell numbers recover within approximately 3 months and may continue to increase to levels well above normal (57). Reconstituting B cells initially resemble cord blood B cells and subsequently follow a pattern that recapitulates ontogeny with a particularly notable increase in CD5+ B cells (57,58). Essentially all murine models of GVHD show dramatic reductions or delays in B-cell regeneration (59,60). Mechanistically, diminished B-cell lymphopoiesis is associated with significant reductions in IL-7–induced colony-forming units (CFU) from the marrow of mice with GVHD (60), consistent with a decrease in pro-B-cell numbers. The extent to which this reflects abnormalities in hematopoietic pluripotent stem cells and/or abnormalities in lymphoid progenitor cells remains unclear. In general, while the number and the self-renewal capacity of the bone marrow stem cells and erythroid and myeloid progenitors are modestly reduced in GVHD (61–63), there is a dramatic skewing of the transferred stem cell graft away from the generation of B and T cells. Part of this deficit may be related to a decrease in progenitor cells, since donor T cells express elevated levels of Fas ligand and stem cells are susceptible to Fas/Fas ligand mediated cytotoxicity (64). Secretion of IFN-γ by host-reactive donor T cells in the marrow microenvironment could also result in alterations in progenitor cell lineage commitment, since IFN-γ can directly inhibit proliferation of developing B cells or indirectly inhibit B-cell proliferation via macrophage activation and secretion of IL-1 (65). Important in this regard is the evidence that IL-1 has an overall stimulatory effect on myelopoiesis, but reduces the generation of B cells and pre-T cells from the bone marrow (66).

Clinically, GVHD is well known to dramatically alter normal B-cell reconstitution. The frequencies of both early (CD19[low]) and total B cells in bone marrow are reduced in GVHD throughout the first year (67). There are fewer CD5+ B cells in GVHD, no CD5 overshoot period (58), and B-cell function remains impaired for a prolonged period even after quantitative reconstitution. This is evidenced by impaired T-cell–independent humoral responses, such as is observed following immunization with pneumococcal polysaccharide vaccine (68). T-cell–dependent B-cell responses are impaired as well. There is diminished IgG production to recall antigens such as tetanus and diphtheria, as well as essentially absent IgG production to neoantigens such as bacteriophage ØX174 and keyhole limpet hemocyanin (68).

T-cell–dependent isotype switching is also adversely affected by GVHD. While total serum IgM and IgG levels are not dramatically altered in the setting of GVHD (51), patients with GVHD have monoclonal gammopathies or homogeneous Ig components indicative of clonal dysregulation (69–71). Further, diminished plasma IgA levels occur in GVHD (51), and there is decreased IgA secretion in saliva and reduced numbers of IgA- and IgM-bearing plasma cells in the mucosa-associated lymphoid tissues of patients with GVHD (72,73). The result of this B-cell deficiency is a prolonged susceptibility to infection, particularly with pneumococcus and other encapsulated organisms. More than any other lymphoid population, low B-cell counts at day 80 are associated with elevated infection rates throughout the first year in patients with GVHD (74).

With regard to T-cell lymphopoiesis, alterations in the marrow microenvironment or in lymphoid commitment could also diminish the generation of pre-T cells (75). However, a major contributing factor in delayed T-cell recovery is the damage to the thymic epithelium and stromal elements that occurs during the GVH reaction. Animal models have shown that the thymus plays a crucial role in CD4+ T-cell regeneration following SCT (76). While the thymus may be damaged by chemotherapy agents or radiation used in the context of SCT preparative regimens (77–79), it is a particular target organ of cytolytic attack early in acute GVHD. Donor NK and T cells invade the thymus, and the thymic structure is destroyed (80–85). The cortex shrinks, the cortical-medullary demarcation disappears, and the characteristic clusters of pale epithelial cells and Hassall's bodies are lost (86). In murine models, although new T cells begin to emerge in the periphery within 10 weeks, recovery of normal structure does not occur for approximately 6 months (86). First the thymic cortex regenerates, at about the same time that new pre-B cells appear in the bone marrow; this correlation is consistent with a common recovery of pre-B and pre-T-cell lymphopoiesis (87). Subsequently, medullary thymocytes appear and finally medullary epithelia and Hassall's bodies normalize. Recovery of thymic structure occurs coincident with normalization of mitogen-stimulated T-cell proliferation and T-dependent B-cell responses to sRBC. For comparison, mice that undergo SCT but do not develop GVHD recover normal peripheral T-cell number and function within 3 months following lethal irradiation, whereas this takes 6–9 months in mice with GVHD. Thus, the structural disruption of the thymus by GVHD significantly prolongs the time course of T-cell repopulation.

Clinical reports similarly demonstrate that GVHD effectors invade the thymus (88,89), exacerbate the damage that conditioning regimens produce in the thymus (79,90), and severely delay recovery of thymopoiesis, profoundly limiting the efficiency of immune recovery. Renewal of thymopoiesis and repopulation of naïve T-cell pools is a protracted process following cytoreductive therapy, particularly in adults, but recent evidence clearly demonstrates that thymopoiesis continues in adults. Although thymic epithelia dwindle with age, cortical and medullary tissues are detectable in the elderly (91), and cells at all thymopoietic stages reside in adult and even aged thymuses (92). Thymocytes undergo T-cell-receptor (TCR) rearrangement, as evidenced by the production of TCR rearrangement excision circles (TREC), and recent thymic emigrants (i.e., cells still bearing TREC) are evident in the periphery (93–95). Although memory phenotype CD4+ and CD8+ T cells often have skewed TCR repertoires in the elderly, naïve T cells continue to include a broad TCR repertoire (96) consistent with ongoing replenishment of naive cells. Nevertheless, thymic productivity declines sharply with age (97). When challenged by severe depletion of T-cell populations, the time course of thymic-dependent recovery in adults is slow compared to that in children. Thymic expansion ("thymic rebound") generally occurs within 3–6 months following cytotoxic therapy in children and is correlated with recovery of naive CD4+ T cells in the periphery (79). A lesser expansion requires 9–12 months in middle-aged adults (F. Hakim, in preparation). As a result, CD4+ T cells bearing a naïve phenotype (CD45RA+) and recovery of TREC-bearing cells occurs more rapidly in children than in adult recipients (14). Comparison of children and adults receiving umbilical cord stem cell transplants noted recovery of normal TREC levels and diverse TCR repertoire by 1–2 years in children, but found that recovery of even the lower "adult levels" of TREC and TCR repertoire diversity occurred only after 3 years in adults (14). TREC frequencies in peripheral blood T cells increase from the transplant nadir by 3–6 months, but the greatest numerical increases in naïve T cells and total TREC per mL of lymphocytes occur only in the second and third year posttransplant in adults (14,97). Further, in adults treated with chemotherapy or autologous transplant, the total CD4+ T-cell number after 2 years is proportional to the recovery of naïve T cells. Higher overall CD4+ T-cell numbers are strongly correlated with recovery of naïve phenotype (CD45RA+ CD62L+) CD4 T cells or with higher frequencies of TREC-bearing CD4 cells (F. Hakim, in preparation). Furthermore, while naïve T cells, whatever their frequency, recover a broad TCR repertoire within 1–2 years posttransplant (14,98), only those individuals with a high frequency of naïve T cells have diverse polyclonal repertoires among the total CD4 population (99). Indeed, protracted deficits in recovery of repertoire diversity and total CD4+ T-cell levels have been found to persist for 3 years or longer (14,100,101).

Thus, recovery of thymopoiesis is critical to the recovery of stable peripheral T-cell populations and to the recovery of a diverse TCR repertoire. Not surprisingly, then, thymic function is critical for functional immune competence as well. Recovery of vaccine responses to tetanus toxoid (TT) has been observed not only to occur earlier in pediatric transplant recipients than in adults, but also to be correlated with recovery of naïve (CD45RA+ CD45RO−) CD4+ T cells (102). Indeed, the TT-specific response in several pediatric recipients after one year was found to incorporate a different TCR Vβ repertoire usage than was present in the donor's response (103). This de novo vaccine response was identifiable for 3 consecutive years, demonstrating the stability of the reestablished T-cell repertoire. Thus, the more rapid recovery of the thymic-dependent pathway underlies the more rapid recovery of lymphocyte numbers, repertoire diversity, and functional competence in children than in adults. As discussed below, because adults are more susceptible to GVHD than children, it is not surprising that the combined thymic toxicity of the GVHD reaction added to a relatively aged thymus results in a high likelihood for chronic T-cell depletion in adults with GVHD.

While the time course required for renewed thymopoiesis may be months to years in the absence of GVHD, data derived from human studies provides evidence that GVHD delays the process of thymic recovery even more. Frequencies of phenotypically naïve (CD45RA+ CD45RO−) T cells have long been observed to be reduced in GVHD (104). When TREC frequencies have been assessed at 1–2 years posttransplant across a spectrum of patients under 25 years in age, TREC frequencies were found to be significantly lower in individuals with ongoing chronic GVHD than in those with no GVHD (79,98,105). The low frequencies of TREC are consistent with a diminished production and export of new T cells to the peripheral blood, even after 2 years. It remains possible that some component of the TREC deficit observed in patients with GVHD is due to the greater activation and expansion of GVHD T cells in the early months posttransplant (6), since cycling of peripheral T cells also reduces TREC levels. Some investigators have used calculations of total CD4+ or CD8+ T cells bearing TREC per mL of blood to counter this concern by comparing total TREC, not TREC frequency. Using this approach, there are also reductions in absolute numbers of TREC levels in GVHD as compared to non-GVHD allogeneic transplants as early as 80 days posttransplant (106). Together, the substantial animal data showing the thymus to be a target organ of GVHD and the clinical data providing evidence for diminished thymopoiesis in patients with GVHD lead to the likely conclusion that diminished thymopoiesis is likely to be a major factor contributing to the chronic immunodeficiency observed in patients with GVHD.

Thus, multiple factors contribute to the prolonged immune deficiency in GVHD. First, the early expansion of host-reactive T cells is short-lived; through processes that probably include AICD and anergy, the expanded donor T-cell population is severely reduced with an adverse impact on both the number and function of nonalloreactive populations which serve as the source for thymic-independent T-cell reconstitution. Second, there is widespread immunosuppression induced by a myriad of regulatory cells. Finally, prolonged delays in the development of new B and T cells from the hematopoietic graft occur as a result of GVH-induced damage to lymphoid progenitors and the thymic microenvironment.

III. IMMUNE DEFICIENCY AND DYSFUNCTION IN CHRONIC GVHD

The immune deficits observed initially in acute GVHD merge gradually into long-lasting deficiencies which are characteristic of chronic GVHD. In addition, however, chronic GVHD is also disorder of immune dysregulation characterized by autoantibody production, increased collagen deposition, and clinical symptoms similar to those seen in patients with autoimmune diseases (107). Whereas acute GVHD is associated with hypogammaglobulinemia, serum IgM and IgG levels are elevated in chronic GVHD, with associated monoclonal gammopathies indicative of clonal dysregulation (69). Even when the same organs are affected, the pathology is distinct, with necrosis dominating in acute GVHD and fibrosis dominating in chronic GHVD.

Murine models of chronic GVHD have demonstrated three elements that contribute to the immunopathology of chronic GVHD. The first is that the cytokine production patterns of acute and chronic GVH reactions differ markedly. Whereas the predominant cytokines produced in acute GVHD are type I cytokines, such as IL-2, IFNγ, and TNF, those in chronic GVHD are typically type II cytokines such as IL-4, IL-5, and IL-13. These cytokines are central to both the pathology and the immune dysfunctions of chronic

GVHD. IL-4 and IL-5 contribute to the eosinophilia, B-cell hyperactivity, and elevated IgG1 and IgE titers observed in chronic GVHD.

The second major distinction between acute and chronic GVHD is that the disease pathology in chronic GVHD is dependent upon the continued presence of host-reactive donor T cells, which, unlike those in acute GVHD, fail to become tolerant of the host (108). Evidence for this comes from the observation that chronic GVHD is transferable even many weeks after its initiation: the transfer of DBA/2 → B6D2F1 chronic GVHD splenic T cells can induce autoantibody production in new secondary B6D2F1 hosts, but not in DBA/2 (donor strain) hosts (108). This is distinct from acute GVHD wherein donor T cells initially expand and then undergo massive AICD followed by anergy. This Fas-Fas ligand-dependent apoptosis is dependent on IFN-γ production and is found in acute but not chronic GVHD (30).

Third, evidence suggests that the developmental pathway differs between mediators of acute and chronic GVHD. Whereas it is clear that alloreactive T cells responsible for inducing acute GVHD are mature donor T cells which are transferred as part of the graft, the origin of the dysfunctional, recipient-reactive T cells that mediate chronic GVHD has not been established. Certainly these cells may also derive from the original donor inoculum, perhaps retaining a type II rather than type I cytokine profile (Fig. 1). But a second potential source is the cells that develop in the recipient thymus following thymic damage induced by acute GVHD. Indeed, when an acute GVHD is induced in (B10xB10.BR)F1 mice by injection of a mixture of B6 (Thy1.2 +) lymph node and B6.PL (Thy 1.1+) T-depleted bone marrow, the cells involved in the initial attack on the host are entirely Thy 1.2+, that is, derived from the mature donor T-cell populations. After 9 months, however, more than 75% of the CD4 cells and 50% of the CD8 cells in the periphery expressed Thy 1.1, indicating derivation from pre-T cells in the donor marrow (12). Because the host thymus is extensively damaged in GVHD, errors in negative selection during thymic maturation could occur, which could result in the maturation and export of recipient-reactive T cells. Several groups have reported a failure of thymic clonal deletion of potentially autoreactive Vβ6 expressing T cells in mls[a] host mice (109,110), and T cells escaping negative selection in an aberrant GVHD thymus were found to be present within the recipient spleen after several weeks. These recipient-reactive cells are not tolerant or anergic and can induce GVHD in secondary irradiated mls[a] hosts (110,111). Thus, autoreactive or, more accurately, recipient-reactive cells may mature following acute GVHD and generate peripheral T cells, which are not adequately tolerized toward host antigens, leading to ongoing immune reactivity.

IV. ENHANCING RECOVERY OF IMMUNE FUNCTION

Delayed immune reconstitution results in a high risk for viral, bacterial, and fungal infections and remains a central contributor to the morbidity and mortality associated with allogeneic bone marrow transplant (BMT). Further, the success of immunotherapeutic strategies developed to augment GVL or GVT following allogeneic SCT depend in large part on the immune competence of the newly developing immune system within the recipient. Therefore, there is great interest in developing therapies which can accelerate the pace of immune restoration following allogeneic BMT without aggravating GVHD. Theoretically, ideal immunorestorative agents for use in the setting of allogeneic SCT would enhance the number of thymic-dependent progeny without accelerating the potency of alloreactive immune responses. Thymic-dependent progeny are known to have a diverse repertoire (112), and, assuming thymic selection is adequate in hosts that have not undergone damaging acute GVH reactions, thymic emigrants are predicted to be rendered tolerant to recipient minor and major histocompatibility alleles during the process of thymic selection. Importantly, however, some agents that have "thymopoietic" effects also augment peripheral T-cell responses, which could potentially augment T-cell–mediated alloreactivity with a paradoxical decrease in overall immune reconstitution. Thus, the extent to which immunorestorative agents can augment the number and function of thymic emigrants versus their effects on antigen-driven peripheral expansion are critical factors determining the overall effectiveness of immunorestoratives used in the setting of allogeneic SCT.

Several new approaches that could be used to enhance immune competence following SCT will be explored. Considerations have ranged from cytokine modulation to enhance T-cell recovery, growth factor administration to protect thymic epithelia, and adoptive cell therapy to selectively reduce alloreactive T cells or to selectively administer T cells with specificities for tumor or uniquely problematic pathogens. In the MHC mismatched setting where profoundly T-cell–depleted stem cell grafts are administered, unique approaches must be considered. In this context, recent promising strategies focusing on the use of natural killer (NK) effectors to provide antitumor effects against residual leukemia without inducing GVHD will be reviewed.

A. Cytokines

IL-7 is a T-cell active cytokine that is remarkably effective at improving the pace and extent of immune reconstitution following syngeneic SCT in murine models. Initial reports of its action emphasized its potential to increase thymopoiesis presumably through its capacity to increase proliferation of early thymic progenitors (reviewed in Refs. 113–115). More recent studies, however, have clearly shown that IL-7 also has potent effects on peripheral T cells and dramatically modulates thymic-independent immune reconstitution by increasing the magnitude of both antigen-driven expansion in response to cognate antigen and "homeostatic" peripheral expansion, which results from a proliferative response to low-affinity "self" antigens (7). Indeed, recent studies have actually begun to question whether the "thymopoietic" effects of IL-7 actually reflect enhanced thymic throughput or rather a potent capacity for IL-7 to induce cycling of a existing resting naïve T cells through low-affinity TCR-mediated reactions (116). Thus, it remains formally possible that the thymopoietic effects of IL-7 observed in murine transplant models might actually represent enhanced expansion of recent thymic emigrants following thymic selection. Such an effect would be predicted to increase the availability of diverse recent thymic emigrants, but it would not increase diversity beyond that generated via baseline thymopoiesis.

With this as a background, the question is raised as to whether IL-7 could be used clinically to enhance immune function following allogeneic SCT. An initial report by Alpdogan et al. suggested that IL-7 could improve immune reconstitution in HLA-mismatched allogeneic BMT without aggravating GVHD (117). However, in this study a high rate of GVHD lethality was already present in the mouse model used and the length of IL-7 therapy was quite limited. Thus, while IL-7 did not enhance GVHD in this report, it remained unclear whether the more prolonged course of IL-7 that would be required to "enhance immune reconstitution" might increase the frequency or severity of GVHD, and the issue of whether IL-7 would increase the incidence of GVHD when subthreshold doses of T cells were administered was not addressed. A subsequent report by Sinha et al. showed that when subthreshold doses of T cells were administered with a 4-week course of IL-7 given at doses shown to be immunorestorative in syngeneic models, the incidence and severity of GVHD was substantially increased (118). Importantly, this was not due to concomitant toxicity of the cytokine, as there is no significant morbidity seen with IL-7 in syngeneic recipients. Rather, a typical picture of GVHD occurred with inflammatory cellular infiltrates in liver, gut, and skin, which were quantitatively increased at low T-cell doses. This capacity for IL-7 to induce a more potent immune response with fewer T cells was predicted based upon previous studies which showed that the effects of IL-7 amplify antigen-specific responses, leading to improved immune competence in athymic T-cell–depleted hosts receiving syngeneic T cells (8). Importantly, however, because of the vicious cycle induced between GVHD and immune reconstitution, IL-7 therapy in the setting of T-cell–replete allogeneic BMT actually diminished immune restoration by amplifying GVHD (Fig. 3). Indeed, in this study of T-cell–replete BMT, direct evidence for increased thymic inflammation and diminished numbers of thymic emigrants was observed in animals administered both IL-7 and T-cell inocula (118). Thus, these results illustrate the basic principle that there is an intimate linkage between immune reconstitution and GVHD in the setting of allogeneic SCT, which must be addressed carefully as immunorestoratives are developed for use in this setting. Importantly, it remains possible that IL-7 might prove useful if it is carefully utilized in the setting of T-cell–depleted BMT. Here, one would expect that IL-7 may increase numbers of recent thymic emigrants, which have already been rendered tolerant through negative thymic selection and would thus not be capable of inducing GVHD. Furthermore, it is possible that delayed administration of IL-7 at a time when recipient APC are already eliminated

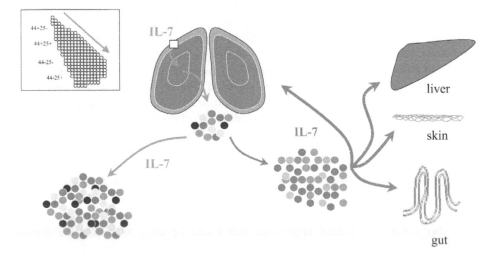

Figure 3 IL-7–induced GVHD diminishes immune reconstitution in recipients of T-cell replete allogeneic SCT. IL-7 exerts potent immunorestorative effects by enhancing proliferation of early triple negative thymocytes, enhancing homeostatic expansion of recent thymic emigrants and enhancing antigen-driven expansion. In allogeneic recipients that receive T cells plus IL-7, the increased antigen-driven expansion induced leads to worsened GVHD with increased thymic damage.

and the inflammatory milieu has resolved would potentially allow donor leukocyte infusions plus antigen-directed therapies to be administered without an overall increase in GVHD.

With regard to other T-cell active cytokines, IL-2 has been widely used as a CD4 immunorestorative in HIV-infected patients where clear increases in CD4 counts are observed (119). While most investigators have attributed this effect to enhanced peripheral expansion of CD4 cells, and we have observed low TREC levels in CD4 cells generated in IL-2–treated patients suggesting increased peripheral expansion rather than increased thymic output (C. L. Mackall, unpublished data), animal studies have shown increased numbers of thymic-derived progeny with IL-2 therapy (7). In clinical settings of allogeneic SCT, IL-2 has been administered with variable effects (120). Some investigators have shown that it is capable of inducing autologous GVHD and that it may exacerbate GVHD when administered with DLI, while others have suggested that it may be administered safely. Clearly the emerging field of exploiting NK alloreactivity as a means for eliminating recipient APC and potentially improving GVL may lead to further use of this agent since it can potently enhance NK cell number and function.

B. Protection of Thymic Epithelial Function in Hosts with GVHD with Keratinocyte Growth Factor

The observation that lymphoid progenitors are much more adversely effected by GVHD than hematopoietic progenitors has given rise to a model that holds that GVH diminishes lymphopoiesis primarily due to alterations in the microenvironment responsible for thymopoieis and B-cell lymphopoiesis rather than through direct effects on progenitor populations themselves. Direct evidence for this is most clearly shown in the thymus where the GVH reaction leads to a clear loss of stromal cell populations and alterations in the epithelial cells of both the cortex and the thymic medulla (80,81,83,84,86). On this basis, one potential approach to ameliorate the damage induced by GVHD is protection of the stromal elements within the thymus. Recent data by Rossi et al. have shown that keratinocyte growth factor (KGF) binds to receptors, which are expressed by thymic cortical and medullary epithelium but not by the thymocytes themselves. When KGF was administered to mice in a parent into an F1 model of GVHD, there was potent protection against thymic damage induced by the GVH reaction (85). Indeed, whereas control mice with GVH show a loss of all thymic subsets, diminished proliferation of triple negative thymocytes, and a dramatic disruption of thymic architecture, KGF-treated recipients were protected. It is important to note that this was not due to amelioration of the GVH response per se, since the severity of the GVHD-induced changes in the spleen was not altered. Rather, the protective effects of KGF on thymic function appear to represent provision of growth or trophic signals through the KGF receptor to the epithelial components within the thymus that provide the microenvironment milieu so critical for T-cell lymphopoiesis.

Other nonimmunological approaches that could be used to protect the thymic microenvironment or to enhance thymic function are currently under study. One potential agent is growth hormone, which appears capable of inducing modest protection against age-associated thymic involution in murine models (121). Recent studies in HIV infection have also suggested that growth hormone (GH) may enhance thymopoiesis directly (122,123). The mechanisms responsible for this are unknown, although it seems unlikely to represent a direct effect on thymocytes and GH does not have potent effects of mature T cells. Thus, it remains possible that growth hormone, or its mediator insulin-like growth factor 1, could also enhance thymic function in the setting of allogeneic BMT without exacerbating GVHD.

C. Adoptive Cell Transfer

As discussed above, it appears that three critical elements come together to generate the clinical disease entity known as acute GVHD: alloreactive donor T cells, presentation of alloantigens by recipient APC, and an inflammatory milieu which is amplified by transplant preparative regimens and environmental pathogens. Because donor T cells themselves undergo homeostatic expansion in response to low-affinity antigens and this process is known to provide an important source for immune reconstitution, it is plausible that strategic approaches could be used to allow donor leukocyte infusions (DLI) to improve immune reconstitution without augmenting GVHD (124). Indeed, investigators have long appreciated that delayed administration of DLI in the setting of myeloablative BMT is often associated with diminished GVHD, and recent studies have shown some beneficial impacts of DLI on immune reconstitution (16,124). One could also administer selected populations of T cells that have either been depleted of all CD8+ T cells (125) or have been more specifically depleted of alloreactive populations, as has been done through the use of CD25 targeted depletion (126). Here, one is attempting to prevent major or minor histocompatibility antigen–driven expansion while allowing homeostatic expansion in response to self antigens to proceed (31). One potential problem associated with CD25 depletion is the potential for depletion of regulatory T cells which also express CD25 and may paradoxically increase alloreactivity (44,46,47). Alternatively, the transfer of specific immunity to one or another of viral and malignant antigens is currently under investigation by numerous groups (127–129). Finally, it should be noted that incomplete donor engraftment, or chronic mixed chimerism appears to provide some protection against GVHD (130). This is likely due to tolerance which is established in both directions during the very slow pace of engraftment that occurs in this setting. Such hosts potentially have the advantage of recognizing antigen in the context of both donor and host MHC which could be potentially advantageous for immune competence. While this approach has had success recently in benign conditions (130), it is generally not acceptable for transplant for malignant conditions and may be associated with a relatively high rate of graft rejection as well.

D. MHC Mismatched BMT

1. Impaired Immune Reconstitution in MHC Mismatched BMT

Because a matched sibling or matched unrelated donor is not available for some patients with diseases that are only curable through SCT, attention has long been focused on the use of alternative sources of stem cells. Among these is the transplantation of stem cells from a relative with one identical HLA haplotype and variable mismatches for zero, one, two, or three HLA-A, -B, and -DR loci of the unshared haplotype. Nearly all patients have at least one HLA-haploidentical parent, child, or sibling who is immediately available as a transplant donor, but the morbidity and mortality associated with such transplants has historically been high due to problems associated with graft failure and GVHD (131). Recent progress in donor immune ablation, progenitor cell mobilization, and progenitor cell selection has allowed grafts to be engineered that combine very high doses of hematopoietic progenitors with very limited numbers of mature T cells (132–134). This has led to high rates of full donor hematopoietic engraftment, rapid hematopoietic recovery, and an incidence of Grade II–IV acute GVHD of <5%. Thus, while state-of-the-art approaches have overcome the primary barriers of hematopoietic engraftment and GVHD in MHC mismatched SCT, overall success is still limited, with <30% of patients alive and free of disease with a median follow-up of 18 months (133). Analyses of several transplant series demonstrate that survival correlates with both age and disease status at transplant in mismatched transplants as well as matched unrelated transplants (124,135). In the Perugia haploidentical transplant series (133,136) and in other reports, most patients were in advanced stage of disease at transplant (at or over 3rd complete remission or relapse) and had been heavily pretreated, thus confounding interpretation of the outcome and of the infectious mortality in full haplotype mismatched transplants. Nonetheless, mortality and morbidity in these patients often occurs as a result of infection or recurrence of malignancy. Thus, future progress in this arena likely involves the development of new strategies to improve the capacity for the transplanted immune system to provide adequate immunity toward environmental pathogens and toward the underlying malignancy.

Following the administration of profoundly T-cell–depleted haploidentical grafts, there appear to be two major factors limiting immune reconstitution. The first relates to the extent of T-cell depletion itself. It is well known that mature T cells provide a primary source for immune reconstitution in the early phase following BMT. In the setting of haploidentical SCT, however, even small numbers of residual mature T cells can result in clinically severe GVHD. Thus, current SCT protocols using haploidentical donors typically require profound T-cell depletion of the graft with a T-cell dose administered in the range of 10^4 cells/kg (133,137). This profound T-cell depletion of both the hematopoietic graft and the host results in a very limited T-cell repertoire available for homeostatic peripheral expansion in the initial months following SCT, impeding the capacity to generate immune responses to infectious agents and to tumor-associated antigens (102,112). Any new approach that could allow the subsequent transfer of mature T cells without initiating a GVH reaction could potentially result in a long-term benefit for immune reconstitution by providing a larger repertoire that would be available to undergo peripheral expansion.

The use of HLA mismatched donor/recipient pairs means that the hematopoietic progenitors that develop within the thymus will undergo positive selection in an MHC-restricted milieu, which will primarily select T cells that recognize antigen in the context of recipient HLA, as this is expressed on thymic epithelium. However, donor APC repopulate the periphery, resulting in some mismatch between thymic selection and peripheral MHC restriction in HLA mismatched SCT. While the shared haplotype allows some measure of "matching" between those cells positively selected in the thymus and the antigen-presenting haplotype in the periphery, experimental data from murine models predict that perhaps half of the maturing T cells will be positively selected to recognize antigen in the context of the nonshared haplotype, limiting the efficiency of positive selection overall (138). While the exact impact of reducing by half the productive HLA repertoire capable of presenting antigen has not been specifically measured, significant limitations in host immune competence occur in hosts with HLA homozygosity in HIV infection, suggesting that a 50% reduction in antigen-presenting capacity may adversely impact immune competence (139). Thus, the underlying limitations in thymic regenerative capacity, which are well appreciated in patients treated with allogeneic SCT, plus the inefficiency of thymic selection due to the existence of only one shared MHC haplotype makes it likely that thymic regenerative pathways will be a primary limitation in restoring immune competence following MHC-mismatched transplantation. Furthermore, even low-level T-cell–mediated alloreactivity, which may occur as a result of the small numbers of mature T cells transferred, could adversely effect thymic function and further limit the efficacy of thymic-dependent pathways in this setting.

2. NK Cells: Dual Roles as Mediators and Modulators of GVHD

Because the inoculum of T cells that can be administered is very low and the efficiency of thymic-dependent pathways is limited in the setting of HLA mismatched BMT, recent attention has focused on NK cells as potential modulators of immune competence in this setting. T cells are central to initiating GVHD, but non-T cells also play important roles in initiating and perpetuating the "cytokine storm" responsible for GVHD-associated immunopathology. A large amount of experimental data suggests that NK cells contribute to the immunopathology that accompanies T-cell–induced GHVD either through direct cell killing of susceptible targets or through production of IFN-γ or other inflammatory mediators (140,141). For example, an increase in NK activity early in nonirradiated mouse models of GVHD has correlated with the development of histopathological lesions in lymphoid and nonlymphoid organs (80), and NK cell infiltrates have been found in association with GVHD-induced tissue damage in the thymus, liver, colon, pancreas, and skin (87,142). Furthermore, when NK-deficient bg/bg mutant mice are used as the donors in nonirradiated mouse models of GVHD, the development of histopathological lesions associated with GVHD is greatly reduced (142). Despite this evidence of the contribution of NK cells to T-cell–initiated GVHD, depletion of endogenous NK cells from the donor inoculum does not block lethal GVHD in MHC-disparate mice (143). Even in irradiation-based models in which an inflammatory milieu would be expected to be induced by the preparative regimen, the isolated transfer of "alloreactive" NK cells in the absence of alloreactive T cells does not induce GVHD (144). Taken together, the data show that NK cells are neither necessary nor sufficient to induce GVHD, but in the setting wherein a GVHD response is already underway, NK cells contribute to the overall immuno-pathology.

Recent murine experiments suggest that NK-mediated cytotoxicity, in the absence of T cells, generates an alloreaction that is limited to lymphohematopoietic tissues and can potentially benefit the recipient in the clinical setting of allogeneic BMT. Unlike T cells and B cells that are activated in a clonal fashion following antigen-specific recognition, NK cell activation is largely negatively regulated by inhibitory receptors for MHC class I molecules on target cells (e.g., the missing self hypothesis)(145,146). Thus, NK cells kill some tumor or virally infected cells which express reduced levels of self-MHC class I molecules. In the setting of mismatched allogeneic BMT, NK cells can be stimulated to attack allogeneic lymphohematopoietic cells that lack self-MHC, but in the absence of T-cell help, NK cells do not kill nonhematopoietic cells lacking self-MHC. Indeed, animal models have clearly shown that F1 rodents reject parent hematopoietic grafts (which lack self-MHC) but do not reject parental skin grafts and other organ grafts (reviewed in Ref. 147). This may be due to the presence of requisite, but as yet unidentified, ligands for activating NK receptors which are uniquely expressed on hematopoietic tissues. Thus, as predicted by the emerging paradigms to explain NK cell killing of allogeneic tissues, in the absence of alloreactive T cells but in the presence of MHC disparity, "alloreactive" NK donor cells (i.e., NK cells responding to a lack of self-MHC on recipient tissues) can enhance donor chimerism in sublethally irradiated mice by depleting host stem cells, granulocytes, and T cells. NK cells that are not "alloreactive" to the host fail to enhance

212 Mackall et al.

engraftment under comparable conditions (144). Further, when a reduced conditioning regimen without alloreactive NK cells results in mixed chimerism, the subsequent administration of alloreactive NK cells 6 weeks posttransplant converts mixed chimeras to stable full-donor chimerism (144). Thus, NK cells are uniquely poised to induce lysis of allogeneic hematopoietic targets that lack self-MHC, but to spare other allogeneic tissues. Although the exact mechanisms responsible for the unique susceptibility of hematopoietic cells to NK cell killing remains unclear, this phenomenon has important implications for NK cells as modulators of GVHD. It also suggests that NK alloreactivity may also be exploited to eradicate leukemic cells, which are generally susceptible to NK-mediated killing (148–151). Indeed, when human alloreactive NK clones are infused into human AML-engrafted NOD-SCID mice, alloreactive NK cells clear the leukemia and the mice survive to 120 days, whereas all mice given nonalloreactive human NK clones die within 3 weeks (144).

3. NK Alloreactivity Provides Antileukemic Effects in MHC Mismatched BMT

One potential beneficial aspect of the use of haploidentical donor/recipient pairs in SCT is that there is the potential for NK alloreactivity, which, in the absence of GVHD, could benefit the host with regard to hematopoietic engraftment and GVL. In humans, inhibitory control of NK-cell function is exerted by two families of receptors specific for HLA class I molecules: killer-cell Ig-like receptors, or KIRs, and the CD94/NKG2A receptor. KIR 2D refers to receptor molecules with two Ig-like domains, whereas KIR 3D denotes those displaying three Ig-like domains. Receptors having long (inhibitory) cytoplasmic tails are designated as L (long), whereas those having short activating tails are termed S. KIR bind amino acid sequences which are shared by specific class I alleles at the HLA-C locus. Two distinct allelic groups of HLA-C molecules are distinguished by KIR on the basis of alternative amino acid sequence motifs at positions 77 and 80 of the α1 helix (reviewed in Ref. 152). KIR2DL1 are inhibited through recognition of HLA-C group 2 alleles (including HLA-Cw2,4,6,8), while KIR2DL2/3 are inhibited through recognition of HLA-C group 1 alleles (Table 1) reviewed in 152,153)). Thus, NK cells expressing the KIR2DL1 (P58.1) lyse targets expressing group 1 HLA-C alleles and NK cells expressing one of the two inhibitory receptors (KIR2DL2 or KIR2DL3) specific for group 1 HLA-C alleles lyse target cells expressing group 2, but not group 1 HLA-C alleles (154,155). Obviously, individual NK cells that coexpress inhibitory receptors for both HLA-C groups are not alloreactive because every individual expresses alleles from either one or both HLA-C groups. Cells expressing the Bw4-specific, KIR3DL1 receptor are also alloreactive and kill Bw4− (Bw6+) cells, but not cells expressing Bw4+ alleles. As new alleles are discovered, they are grouped according to their amino acid sequence. CD94-NKG2A expression is regulated to fill the holes in the KIR repertoire, being expressed primarily on NK cells that do not express an inhibitory KIR for self HLA class I. In humans, NK cells that solely express CD94-NKG2A are generally not alloreactive since HLA-E, the ligand for this receptor, is expressed on cells from all individuals (156,157).

Recent evidence has shown that HLA-C mismatched transplants that result in a transfer of NK cells not inhibited through KIRs can provide beneficial effects with regard to engraftment and GVL. This benefit arises because, although multiple KIR receptors may be coexpressed on the same NK cell, some NK cells express a single KIR and are therefore blocked only by a specific (self) class I molecule. For these NK cells, missing expression of the inhibitory MHC class I allele on allogeneic targets triggers alloreactivity (158–161)(Fig. 4). Thus, in any given individual, KIR-bearing NK cells make up a

Table 1 HLA Class I Allele Specificity of the Main KIR Expressed by Human NK Cells

KIR genes	Encoded protein	HLA specificity
KIR2DL1	P58.1 receptor	HLA-C group 2 (Asn77, Lys80[a])
		Cw2 (all)[b]
		Cw4 (all)
		Cw5 (all)
		Cw6 (all)
		Cw0307, C*0315
		C*0707, C*0709
		C*1205, C*12041, C*12042
		Cw15 (all except C*1507)
		C*1602
		Cw17 (all)
		Cw18 (all)
KIR 2DL2/3	P58.2 receptor	HLA-C group 1 (Ser77, Asn80)[a]
		Cw1 (all)
		Cw3: (all except C*0307, C*0310, C*0315)
		Cw7, (all except C*0707, C*0709)
		Cw8 (all)
		Cw12 (all except C*1205, C*12041, C*12042)
		Cw13 (all)
		Cw14 (all except C*1404)
		C*1507
		Cw16 (all except C*1602)
KIR 3DL1	P70/NKB1 receptor	Bw4 alleles
		B5, B13, B17, B27, B37, B38, B44, B47, B49, B51, B52, B53, B57, B59, B63, B77, B*1513, B*1516, B*1517, B*1523, B*1524
KIR 3DL2	P140 receptor	HLA-A3 and A11

[a] Note that the two groups of HLA-C alleles can be distinguished on the basis of alternative amino acid sequence motif at positions 77 and 80 of the α1 helix. Site-directed mutagenesis unequivocally demonstrated that these residues are crucial for KIR-mediated recognition.

[b] All molecular types within a serologically defined group of alleles.

Note: C*0310 (Ser77, Lys80) behaves as if it belonged to Group 1 and to Group 2 HLA-C. If a patient expresses this allele, he or she should be considered to express both allele groups. In other words, C*0310 blocks NK cells expressing any HLA-C–specific receptor, it does not block clones expressing the Bw4 receptor. C*1404 (Asn77, Asn80) is the opposite. It does not belong to Group 1 or Group 2 HLA-C. In other words, it does not block NK cells expressing HLA-C–specific receptors. So, expression of C*1404 may be ignored in a patient, because it is as if the patient did not express HLA-C alleles at all. Of course one has to consider the other allele. C*1207 Gly77, Asn80, cannot be assigned to either group based on its amino acid sequence, and still needs to be tested functionally.

discrete repertoire that is tolerant of self because it is blocked by the self class I allele groups, but it may also give rise to alloreactions when confronted with allogeneic targets failing to express its inhibiting class I alleles. The factors that regulate NK repertoire acquisition during NK cell differentiation is an active area of investigation. KIR and HLA genes are inherited independently. While the HLA genotype has some influence on which KIR genes are expressed, most individuals of European descent have a full complement of KIR genes for inhibitory receptors and thus generate a diverse NK repertoire (54,162).

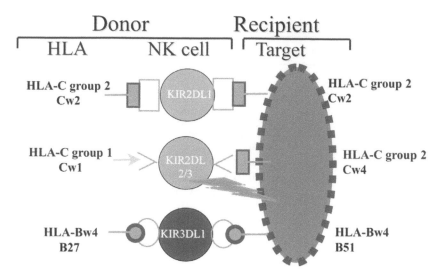

Figure 4 NK-cell–mediated attack of target cells through loss of KIR-mediated inhibition. In this example, a graft that expresses HLA-C Group 1 (Cw1) gives rise to a repertoire of NK cells bearing a variety of KIRs. While KIR2DL1 and KIR2DL2 cells are inhibited by the HLA-C group 2 allele expressed by the recipient, the cells bearing KIR2DL2 or KIR2DL3 are not inhibited due to the absence of any HLA-C Group 1 in the recipient. The NK cells thus kill the target (thunderbolt). Note that the recipient cell must also express an activating ligand to be susceptible to killing. The identity and distribution of such activating ligands have not yet been fully identified but presumably result in the specificity of this killing for hematopoietic and neoplastic tissues.

With regard to HLA, individuals may express one to three KIR reactive alleles (group 1 and group 2 HLA-C, and HLA-Bw4 alleles). Approximately 30% of the population express class I alleles belonging to all three major HLA class I groups (HLA-C group 1, HLA-C group 2, and HLA-Bw4 alleles) and therefore will not induce any KIR-mediated killing since their KIR-reactive alleles will block all known NK-cell patterns of reactivity from every donor. Thus, every donor is likely to possess NK cells with reactivity to multiple KIR ligands and, depending upon the HLA Bw/C allele expressed by the recipient, there may be a mismatch that drives NK-mediated alloreactivity.

Importantly, in addition to the absence of signaling through KIR, cytokine release and killing by NK cells also require triggering of activating NK receptors. The nature of one family of activating NK receptors has recently been identified as a heterogeneous family of NK-specific Ig-like molecules termed natural cytotoxicity receptors (including NKp30, NKp46, and NKp44). A second NK-activating receptor is NKG2D, a member of the lectin superfamily, which is expressed by both NK and cytolytic T cells (163,164). The cellular ligands for NCR still remain to be determined, while those for NKG2D have been identified as class I–like molecules MICA/B (165) and ULBP (166). The function of NK-cell–triggering receptors is normally counterbalanced by that of the HLA-specific inhibitory receptors. This balance, however, is rapidly altered as soon as the magnitude of the inhibitory signals is decreased by insufficient engagement of the HLA-specific inhibitory receptors. Thus, some tissues display no susceptibility to NK-mediated cytotoxicity even when they fail to express inhibitory HLA class I molecules. In this case the level of expression of adhesion molecules and/or ligands recognized by the triggering receptors may be insufficient to induce NK-cell activation. This may explain the selectivity of NK-mediated effects on hematopoietic tissues, the lack of NK-mediated GVHD (144) and potentially the resistance of ALL cells to alloreactive NK killing (discussed below).

Since NK cells distinguish groups of HLA class I molecules, haploidentical transplants can be classified in at least two categories: (a) NK-matched transplants in which donor-vs.-recipient NK alloreactivity does not occur because all regenerated NK cells recognize the HLA class I alleles of the host and are blocked, and (b) NK-mismatched transplants in which at least some of the regenerated NK cells do not recognize the class I alleles of the host and thus kill host targets. After transplantation of T-cell–depleted PBSC from NK-mismatched donors, Ruggeri et al. observed that the engrafted stem cells give rise to an NK-cell wave of donor origin consistent with the early recovery of NK cells following SCT (155). Alloreactive NK clones of donor origin were isolated and killed recipient lymphocytes. Killing was blocked by targets expressing the donor HLA class I allele that was missing in the recipient. Alloreactive NK clones killed all acute and chronic myeloid leukemias tested, but only a rare example of acute lymphoblastic leukemia (ALL). ALL resistance to killing was associated with the lack of expression of LFA-1, a leukocyte adhesion receptor. These data suggest that donor alloreactive NK cells could enhance the probability of cure for patients with myeloid leukemia.

Ruggeri et al. evaluated the impact of donor-vs.-recipient NK-cell alloreactivity on relapse, rejection, GVHD, and survival in 92 high-risk acute leukemia patients who had received hematopoietic transplants from HLA haplotype–mismatched relatives (144). Donor-recipient pairs were divided into two groups: those with and without KIR ligand incompatibility in the GVH direction. Donors were evaluated for NK alloreactivity by screening their NK repertoire (by analysis of NK clones). Detection of donor NK clones that killed recipient targets correlated closely with KIR ligand incompatibility in the GVH direction. Transplantation from NK alloreactive donors prevented rejection, GVHD, and relapse of AML. In AML, the probability of event-free survival after a median follow-up of 5 years (range 1–8 years) was 5% in the NK-non–alloreactive group vs. 60% in the NK-alloreactive group ($p < 0.0005$)(Fig. 5). Multivariate analysis that considered crucial variables affecting transplantation outcome, such as conditioning regimens, number of stem cells and T cells in the graft, and status of disease at transplant, showed that GVH KIR ligand incompatibility was the only independent predictor of survival in AML. Conversely, an absence of GVH KIR ligand incompatibility was the only independent factor predicting poor outcome (hazard ratio 0.33, 95% CI 0.11–0.94, $p < 0.04$). GVH KIR ligand incompatibility had no effect on ALL. Since this report was published, another 20 patients with AML have received haploidentical transplants in the Perugia transplant center. An updated analysis of the 77 transplants (follow-up range 3 months to 9.75 years) confirms the striking survival advantage of transplantation from an NK-alloreactive donor for patients with AML (probability of survival 56% vs. 5%, $p < 0.001$) (A. Velardi, unpublished observations).

Thus, in the setting of MHC-mismatched BMT, the absence of T cells that are required to initiate GVHD and the presence of MHC mismatch, which allows for the possibility of NK-mediated recognition, has given rise to new strategies for exploiting NK alloreactivity to enhance GVL. Importantly, however, such effects appear to be active only in unique settings. As alluded to above, approximately one third of the population expresses class I alleles belonging to all three major HLA class I groups (HLA-C group 1,

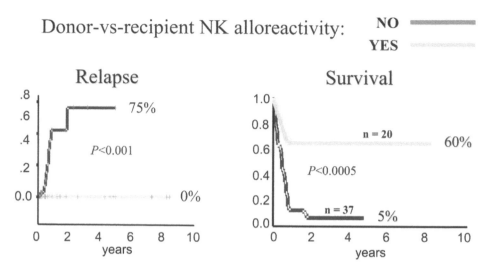

Figure 5 The presence of an MHC mismatch which leads to NK alloreactivity in the GVHD direction dramatically reduces relapse and improves survival of patients with AML following haploidentical, T-cell–depleted BMT. At the time of transplant, > 85% of patients were in 3rd or later relapse.

HLA-C group 2, and HLA-Bw4 alleles), and these recipients will block all known NK-cell patterns of reactivity. Furthermore, when analysis of the effects of MHC class C/Bw4 mismatch was evaluated in mismatched unrelated donor cell transplants, no benefit with regard to leukemic relapse of survival was observed (167). This likely relates to the fact that such transplants did not utilize T-cell depletion and used postgrafting immunosuppression that may adversely impact on the posttransplant NK-mediated function. Furthermore, T-replete allogeneic transplants result in reduced expression of KIR (and increased expression of CD94/NKG2A) for much of the first year (54). Thus, modulation of the T-cell population and/or the cytokine milieu posttransplant may alter the frequency of KIR-expressing NK cells. Nonetheless, in the appropriate clinical scenario, it appears that donor selection could be modified to include a deliberate search for the "perfect mismatch" at HLA class I to drive donor-vs.-recipient NK-cell alloreactivity with a potential for improved outcome (168).

As discussed earlier in this chapter, the recipient APC is now known to be a critical element responsible for initiating alloreactivity (1,2). Thus, the ability for NK cells to eradicate recipient APC without inducing GVHD could prove to be a critical first step for subsequent introduction of alloreactive T cells with potential long-term implications for immune reconstitution. Based upon this hypothesis, Ruggeri et al. tested whether a priori NK "conditioning" to eradicate recipient APC could allow the subsequent administration of alloreactive T cells (144). After conditioning with TBI and alloreactive or nonalloreactive NK cells, cohorts of transplanted mice were given escalating doses of allogeneic donor T cells. Even following administration of large numbers of alloreactive T cells, 100% of mice that had previously received alloreactive NK cells survived for 120 days with no signs of GVHD, whereas control mice that received no NK cells or nonalloreactive NK cells rapidly died from GVHD. In order to determine whether NK-mediated ablation of host APC was responsible for protection from GVHD, B6xBALB/c into B6 ($H - 2^{d/b} \rightarrow H - 2^b$) bone marrow chimeras were generated to replace the NK-cell–sensitive $H - 2^b$ APC with $H - 2^{d/b}$ cells that would be resistant to NK-cell killing. When these chimeras were reconditioned with TBI plus $H - 2^b$-reactive, but $H - 2^{d/b}$-nonreactive NK cells followed by alloreactive T cells, 100% of the mice died from GVHD while control $H - 2^b \rightarrow H - 2^b$ chimeras given the same NK-cell conditioning followed by alloreactive T cells survived with no signs of GVHD. This study also provided direct evidence that alloreactive NK cells accelerated the loss of bone marrow, spleen, and gut APC, as compared to mice conditioned with either TBI or TBI plus non-alloreactive NK cells. Taken together, these results indicate that alloreactive NK cells prevent GVHD via elimination of recipient APC, thus allowing the subsequent safe infusion of otherwise lethal doses of allogeneic T cells (144). Because the homeostatic peripheral expansion of mature T cells is not dependent upon recipient APC, such NK-facilitated T-cell transfer might improve immune reconstitution by allowing the introduction of a sizable T-cell inocula that could then undergo thymic-independent peripheral expansion (144).

V. SUMMARY

GVHD and immune reconstitution are inextricably linked to one another in the setting of allogeneic SCT. GVHD adversely impacts immune reconstitution by limiting both thymic-independent peripheral expansion and by damaging the microenvironments of the marrow and the thymus required for posttransplant lymphopoiesis. Paradoxically, however, standard approaches used to prevent GVHD also limit immune reconstitution and approaches that could enhance immune reconstitution may also worsen GVHD. Thus, ongoing success in the field of BMT requires that creative and careful strategies be developed, which can specifically enhance immune reconstitution without aggravating GVHD. In recent years, much progress has been made in identifying the factors critical for initiating GVHD and the factors required for optimal immune reconstitution. With this knowledge in hand, it is to be expected that new approaches to enhance immune reconstitution without aggravating GVHD will soon come to fruition.

REFERENCES

1. WD Shlomchik, MS Couzens, CB Tang, J McNiff, ME Robert, J Liu, MJ Shlomchik, SG Emerson. Prevention of graft versus host disease by inactivation of host antigen-presenting cells. Science 1999; 285:412–415.
2. T Teshima, R Ordemann, P Reddy, S Gagin, C Liu, KR Cooke, JL Ferrara. Acute graft-versus-host disease does not require alloantigen expression on host epithelium. Nat Med 2002; 8:575–581.
3. JH Antin, JL Ferrara. Cytokine dysregulation and acute graft-versus-host disease. Blood 1992; 80:2964–2968.
4. JL Ferrara. Cytokine dysregulation as a mechanism of graft versus host disease. Curr Opin Immunol 1993; 5:794–799.
5. JT Tan, B Ernst, WC Kieper, E LeRoy, J Sprent. Interleukin (IL)-15 and IL-7 jointly regulate homeostatic proliferation of memory phenotype CD8+ cells but are not required for memory phenotype CD4+ cells. J Exp Med 2002; 195:1523–1532.
6. MD Hazenberg, SA Otto, ES de Pauw, H Roelofs, WE Fibbe, D Hamann, F Miedema. T-cell receptor excision circle and T-cell dynamics after allogeneic stem cell transplantation are related to clinical events. Blood 2002; 99:3449–3453.

218

Mackall et al.

7. CL Mackall, TJ Fry, C Bare, P Morgan, A Galbraith, RE Gress. IL-7 increases both thymic-dependent and thymic-independent T-cell regeneration after bone marrow transplantation. Blood 2001; 97:1491–1497.

8. TJ Fry, BL Christensen, KL Komschlies, RE Gress, CL Mackall. Interleukin-7 restores immunity in athymic T-cell-depleted hosts. Blood 2001; 97:1525–1533.

9. E Bolotin, G Annett, R Parkman, K Weinberg. Serum levels of IL-7 in bone marrow transplant recipients: relationship to clinical characteristics and lymphocyte count. Bone Marrow Transplant 1999; 23:783–788.

10. S Kumaki, M Minegishi, H Fujie, Y Sasahara, Y Ohashi, S Tsuchiya, T Konno. Prolonged secretion of IL-15 in patients with severe forms of acute graft-versus-host disease after allogeneic bone marrow transplantation in children. Int J Hematol 1998; 67:307–312.

11. CL Mackall, CV Bare, LA Granger, SO Sharrow, JA Titus, RE Gress. Thymic-independent T cell regeneration occurs via antigen-driven expansion of peripheral T cells resulting in a repertoire that is limited in diversity and prone to skewing. J Immunol 1996; 156:4609–4616.

12. FT Hakim, S Payne, GM Shearer. Recovery of T cell populations after acute graft-vs-host reaction. J Immunol 1994; 152:58–64.

13. J Gorski, M Yassai, X Zhu, B Kissela, B Kissella, C Keever, N Flomenberg. Circulating T cell repertoire complexity in normal individuals and bone marrow recipients analyzed by CDR3 size spectratyping. Correlation with immune status. J Immunol 1994; 152:5109–5119.

14. AK Klein, DD Patel, ME Gooding, GD Sempowski, BJ Chen, CX Liu, J Kurtzberg, BF Haynes, NJ Chao. T-cell recovery in adults and children following umbilical cord blood transplantation. Biology of Blood and Marrow Transplantation 2001; 7:454–466.

15. M Hirokawa, T Matsutani, H Saitoh, Y Ichikawa, Y Kawabata, T Horiuchi, A Kitabayashi, T Yoshioka, Y Tsuruta, R Suzuki, AB Miura, K Sawada. Distinct TCRAV and TCRBV repertoire and CDR3 sequence of T lymphocytes clonally expanded in blood and GVHD lesions after human allogeneic bone marrow transplantation. Bone Marrow Transplant 2002; 30:915–923.

16. E Orsini, EP Alyea, R Schlossman, C Canning, RJ Soiffer, A Chillemi, D Neuberg, KC Anderson, J Ritz. Changes in T cell receptor repertoire associated with graft-versus-tumor effect and graft-versus-host disease in patients with relapsed multiple myeloma after donor lymphocyte infusion. Bone Marrow Transplant 2000; 25:623–632.

17. S Verfuerth, K Peggs, P Vyas, L Barnett, RJ O'Reilly, S Mackinnon. Longitudinal monitoring of immune reconstitution by CDR3 size spectratyping after T-cell-depleted allogeneic bone marrow transplant and the effect of donor lymphocyte infusions on T-cell repertoire. Blood 2000; 95:3990–3995.

18. DA Margolis, JT Casper, AD Segura, T Janczak, L McOlash, B Fisher, K Miller, J Gorski. Infiltrating T cells during liver graft-versus-host disease show a restricted T-cell repertoire. Biol Blood Marrow Transplant 2000; 6:408–415.

19. F Kern, E Khatamzas, I Surel, C Frommel, P Reinke, SL Waldrop, LJ Picker, HD Volk. Distribution of human CMV-specific memory T cells among the CD8pos. subsets defined by CD57, CD27, and CD45 isoforms. Eur J Immunol 1999; 29:2908–2915.

20. T Horiuchi, M Hirokawa, Y Kawabata, A Kitabayashi, T Matsutani, T Yoshioka, Y Tsuruta, R Suzuki, AB Miura. Identification of the T cell clones expanding within both CD8(+)CD28(+) and CD8(+)CD28(−) T cell subsets in recipients of allogeneic hematopoietic cell grafts and its implication in post-transplant skewing of T cell receptor repertoire. Bone Marrow Transplant 2001; 27:731–739.

21. FT Hakim, R Cepeda, S Kaimei, CL Mackall, N McAtee, J Zujewski, K Cowan, RE Gress. Constraints on CD4 recovery postchemotherapy in adults: thymic insufficiency and apoptotic decline of expanded peripheral CD4 cells. Blood 1997; 90:3789–3798.

22. NC Hebib, O Deas, M Rouleau, A Durrbach, B Charpentier, F Beaujean, JP Vernant, A Senik. Peripheral blood T cells generated after allogeneic bone marrow transplantation: lower levels of bcl-2 protein and enhanced sensitivity to spontaneous and CD95-mediated apoptosis in

vitro. Abrogation of the apoptotic phenotype coincides with the recovery of normal naive/primed T-cell profiles. Blood 1999; 94:1803–1813.

23. MT Lin, LH Tseng, H Frangoul, T Gooley, J Pei, A Barsoukov, Y Akatsuka, JA Hansen. Increased apoptosis of peripheral blood T cells following allogeneic hematopoietic cell transplantation. Blood 2000; 95:3832–3839.

24. D Brugnoni, P Airo, M Pennacchio, G Carella, A Malagoli, AG Ugazio, F Porta, R Cattaneo. Immune reconstitution after bone marrow transplantation for combined immunodeficiencies: down-modulation of Bcl-2 and high expression of CD95/Fas account for increased susceptibility to spontaneous and activation-induced lymphocyte cell death. Bone Marrow Transplant 1999; 23:451–457.

25. S Rutella, G Bonanno, L Pierelli, F Sora, S Sica, G Scambia, G d'Onofrio, C Rumi, G Leone. Enhanced susceptibility to apoptosis in T cells recovering after autologous peripheral blood progenitor cell transplantation: reversal by interleukin-15. Cytokines Cell Mol Ther 2000; 6:189–198.

26. J Sprent, H Kosaka, EK Gao, CD Surh, SR Webb. Intrathymic and extrathymic tolerance in bone marrow chimeras. Immunol Rev 1993; 133:151–176.

27. S Webb, C Morris, J Sprent. Extrathymic tolerance of mature T cells: clonal elimination as a consequence of immunity. Cell 1990; 63:1249–1256.

28. J Sprent, SR Webb. Intrathymic and extrathymic clonal deletion of T cells. Curr Opin Immunol 1995; 7:196–205.

29. CS Via, P Nguyen, A Shustov, J Drappa, KB Elkon. A major role for the Fas pathway in acute graft-versus-host disease. J Immunol 1996; 157:5387–5393.

30. A Shustov, P Nguyen, F Finkelman, KB Elkon, CS Via. Differential expression of Fas and Fas ligand in acute and chronic graft-versus-host disease: up-regulation of Fas and Fas ligand requires CD8+ T cell activation and IFN-gamma production. J Immunol 1998; 161:2848–2855.

31. S Brochu, B Rioux-Masse, J Roy, DC Roy, C Perreault. Massive activation-induced cell death of alloreactive T cells with apoptosis of bystander postthymic T cells prevents immune reconstitution in mice with graft-versus-host disease. Blood 1999; 94:390–400.

32. RB Levy, M Jones, C Cray. Isolated peripheral T cells from GvHR recipients exhibit defective IL-2R expression, IL-2 production, and proliferation in response to activation stimuli. J Immunol 1990; 145:3998–4005.

33. ST Pals, T Radaszkiewicz, E Gleichmann. Allosuppressor- and allohelper-T cells in acute and chronic graft-vs-host disease. IV. Activation of donor allosuppressor cells is confined to acute GVHD. J Immunol 11984; 132:1669–1678.

34. AG Rolink, E Gleichmann. Allosuppressor- and allohelper-T cells in acute and chronic graft-vs.-host (GVH) disease. III. Different Lyt subsets of donor T cells induce different pathological syndromes. J Exp Med 1983; 158:546–558.

35. B Autran, V Leblond, B Sadat-Sowti, E Lefranc, P Got, L Sutton, JL Binet, P Debre. A soluble factor released by CD8+ CD57+ lymphocytes from bone marrow transplanted patients inhibits cell-mediated cytolysis. Blood 1991; 77:2237–2241.

36. Y Ikarashi, K Kawai, H Watanabe, Y Matsumoto, S Omata, M Fujiwara. Immunosuppressive activity of macrophages in mice undergoing graft-versus-host reaction due to major histocompatibility complex class I plus II difference. Immunology 1993; 79:95–102.

37. CD Howell, TD Yoder, JM Vierling. Suppressor function of hepatic mononuclear inflammatory cells during murine chronic graft-vs-host disease. I. Macrophage-enriched cells mediate suppression in the liver. Cell Immunol 1991; 132:256–268.

38. FP Nestel, KS Price, TA Seemayer, WS Lapp. Macrophage priming and lipopolysaccharide-triggered release of tumor necrosis factor alpha during graft-versus-host disease. J Exp Med 1992; 175:405–413.

39. RA Hoffman, NC Nussler, SL Gleixner, G Zhang, HR Ford, JM Langrehr, AJ Demetris, RL Simmons. Attenuation of lethal graft-versus-host disease by inhibition of nitric oxide synthase. Transplantation 1997; 63:94–100.

40. JE Talmadge, R Singh, K Ino, A Ageitos, S Buyukberber. Mechanisms of immune dysfunction in stem cell transplantation. Int J Immunopharmacol 2000; 22:1041–1056.

41. RK Singh, ML Varney, S Buyukberber, K Ino, AG Ageitos, E Reed, S Tarantolo, JE Talmadge. Fas-FasL-mediated CD4+ T-cell apoptosis following stem cell transplantation. Cancer Res 1999; 59:3107–3111.

42. JH Holda, T Maier, HN Claman. Murine graft-versus-host disease across minor barriers: immunosuppressive aspects of natural suppressor cells. Immunol Rev 1985; 88:87–105.

43. S Sakaguchi, N Sakaguchi, M Asano, M Itoh, M Toda. Immunologic self-tolerance maintained by activated T cells expressing IL-2 receptor alpha-chains (CD25). Breakdown of a single mechanism of self-tolerance causes various autoimmune diseases. J Immunol 1995; 155:1151–1164.

44. BD Johnson, MC Konkol, RL Truitt. CD25+ immunoregulatory T-cells of donor origin suppress alloreactivity after BMT. Biol Blood Marrow Transplant 2002; 8:525–535.

45. JL Cohen, A Trenado, D Vasey, D Klatzmann, BL Salomon. CD4(+)CD25(+) immunoregulatory T cells: new therapeutics for graft-versus-host disease. J Exp Med 2002; 196:401–406.

46. P Hoffmann, J Ermann, M Edinger, CG Fathman, S Strober. Donor-type CD4(+)CD25(+) regulatory T cells suppress lethal acute graft-versus-host disease after allogeneic bone marrow transplantation. J Exp Med 2002; 196:389–399.

47. PA Taylor, CJ Lees, BR Blazar. The infusion of ex vivo activated and expanded CD4(+)CD25(+) immune regulatory cells inhibits graft-versus-host disease lethality. Blood 2002; 99:3493–3499.

48. P Schlenke, S Sheikhzadeh, K Weber, T Wagner, H Kirchner. Immune reconstitution and production of intracellular cytokines in T lymphocyte populations following autologous peripheral blood stem cell transplantation. Bone Marrow Transplant 2001; 28:251–257.

49. CL Mackall, D Stein, TA Fleisher, MR Brown, FT Hakim, CV Bare, SF Leitman, EJ Read, CS Carter, LH Wexler, RE Gress. Prolonged CD4 depletion after sequential autologous peripheral blood progenitor cell infusions in children and young adults. Blood 2000; 96:754–762.

50. MM Roberts, LB To, D Gillis, J Mundy, C Rawling, K Ng, CA Juttner. Immune reconstitution following peripheral blood stem cell transplantation, autologous bone marrow transplantation and allogeneic bone marrow transplantation. Bone Marrow Transplant 1993; 12:469–475.

51. K Kalwak, E Gorczynska, J Toporski, D Turkiewicz, M Slociak, M Ussowicz, E Latos-Grazynska, M Krol, J Boguslawska-Jaworska, A Chybicka. Immune reconstitution after haematopoietic cell transplantation in children: immunophenotype analysis with regard to factors affecting the speed of recovery. Br J Haematol 2002; 118:74–89.

52. CA Keever, J Klein, N Leong, EA Copelan, BR Avalos, N Kapoor, I Cunningham, PJ Tutschka. Effect of GVHD on the recovery of NK cell activity and LAK precursors following BMT. Bone Marrow Transplant 1993; 12:289–295.

53. MA Cooper, TA Fehniger, MA Caligiuri. The biology of human natural killer-cell subsets. Trends Immunol 2001; 22:633–640.

54. HG Shilling, N Young, LA Guethlein, NW Cheng, CM Gardiner, D Tyan, P Parham. Genetic control of human NK cell repertoire. J Immunol 2002; 169:239–247.

55. LR Gottschalk, RA Bray, H Kaizer, HM Gebel. Two populations of CD56 (Leu-19)+/CD16+ cells in bone marrow transplant recipients. Bone Marrow Transplant 1990; 5:259–264.

56. R Jacobs, M Stoll, G Stratmann, R Leo, H Link, RE Schmidt. CD16- CD56+ natural killer cells after bone marrow transplantation. Blood 1992; 79:3239–3244.

57. TN Small, CA Keever, S Weiner-Fedus, G Heller, RJ O'Reilly, N Flomenberg. B-cell differentiation following autologous, conventional, or T-cell depleted bone marrow transplantation: a recapitulation of normal B-cell ontogeny. Blood 1990; 76:1647–1656.

58. J Storek, S Ferrara, N Ku, JV Giorgi, RE Champlin, A Saxon. B cell reconstitution after human bone marrow transplantation: recapitulation of ontogeny? Bone Marrow Transplant 1993; 12:387–398.

59. A Xenocostas, WS Lapp, DG Osmond. Suppression of B lymphocyte genesis in the bone marrow by systemic graft-versus-host reactions. Transplantation 1987; 43:549–555.

60. BA Garvy, JM Elia, BL Hamilton, RL Riley. Suppression of B-cell development as a result of selective expansion of donor T cells during the minor H antigen graft-versus-host reaction. Blood 1993; 82:2758–2766.

61. PJ van Dijken, J Wimperis, JM Crawford, JL Ferrara. Effect of graft-versus-host disease on hematopoiesis after bone marrow transplantation in mice. Blood 1991; 78:2773–2779.

62. M Seddik, TA Seemayer, WS Lapp. The graft-versus-host reaction and immune function. IV. B cell functional defect associated with a depletion of splenic colony-forming units in marrow of graft-versus-host-reactive mice. Transplantation 1986; 41:242–247.

63. T Iwasaki, H Fujiwara, GM Shearer. Loss of proliferative capacity and T cell immune development potential by bone marrow from mice undergoing a graft-vs-host reaction. J Immunol 1986; 137:3100–3108.

64. K Saheki, Y Fujimori, Y Takemoto, E Kakishita. Increased expression of Fas (APO-1, CD95) on CD34+ haematopoietic progenitor cells after allogeneic bone marrow transplantation. Br J Haematol 2000; 109:447–452.

65. BA Garvy, RL Riley. IFN-gamma abrogates IL-7-dependent proliferation in pre-B cells, coinciding with onset of apoptosis. Immunology 1994; 81:381–388.

66. P Morrissey, K Charrier, L Bressler, A Alpert. The influence of IL-1 treatment on the reconstitution of the hemopoietic and immune systems after sublethal radiation. J Immunol 1988; 140:4204–4210.

67. J Storek, D Wells, MA Dawson, B Storer, DG Maloney. Factors influencing B lymphopoiesis after allogeneic hematopoietic cell transplantation. Blood 2001; 98:489–491.

68. RP Witherspoon, R Storb, HD Ochs, N Fluornoy, KJ Kopecky, KM Sullivan, JH Deeg, R Sosa, DR Noel, K Atkinson, ED Thomas. Recovery of antibody production in human allogeneic marrow graft recipients: influence of time posttransplantation, the presence or absence of chronic graft-versus-host disease, and antithymocyte globulin treatment. Blood 1981; 58:360–368.

69. AJ Mitus, R Stein, JM Rappeport, JH Antin, HJ Weinstein, CA Alper, BR Smith. Monoclonal and oligoclonal gammopathy after bone marrow transplantation. Blood 1989; 74:2764–2768.

70. E Gokmen, FM Raaphorst, DH Boldt, JM Teale. Ig heavy chain third complementarity determining regions (H CDR3s) after stem cell transplantation do not resemble the developing human fetal H CDR3s in size distribution and Ig gene utilization. Blood 1998; 92:2802–2814.

71. EJ Gerritsen, MJ van Tol, AC Lankester, CP van der Weijden-Ragas, CM Jol-van der Zijde, NJ Oudeman-Gruber, J Radl, JM Vossen. Immunoglobulin levels and monoclonal gammopathies in children after bone marrow transplantation. Blood 1993; 82:3493–3502.

72. WE Beschorner, JH Yardley, PJ Tutschka, GW Santos. Deficiency of intestinal immunity with graft-vs.-host disease in humans. J Infect Dis 1981; 144:38–46.

73. KT Izutsu, KM Sullivan, MM Schubert, EL Truelove, HM Shulman, GE Sale, TH Morton, JC Rice, RP Witherspoon, R Storb, ED Thomas. Disordered salivary immunoglobulin secretion and sodium transport in human chronic graft-versus-host disease. Transplantation 1983; 35:441–446.

74. J Storek, G Espino, MA Dawson, B Storer, ME Flowers, DG Maloney. Low B-cell and monocyte counts on day 80 are associated with high infection rates between days 100 and 365 after allogeneic marrow transplantation. Blood 2000; 96:3290–3293.

75. PL McCarthy, Jr., S Abhyankar, S Neben, G Newman, C Sieff, RC Thompson, SJ Burakoff, JL Ferrara. Inhibition of interleukin-1 by an interleukin-1 receptor antagonist prevents graft-versus-host disease. Blood 1991; 78:1915–1918.

76. CL Mackall, L Granger, MA Sheard, R Cepeda, RE Gress. T-cell regeneration after bone marrow transplantation: differential CD45 isoform expression on thymic-derived versus thymic-independent progeny. Blood 1993; 82:2585–2594.

77. B Chung, L Barbara-Burnham, L Barsky, K Weinberg. Radiosensitivity of thymic interleukin-7 production and thymopoiesis after bone marrow transplantation. Blood 2001; 98:1601–1606.

78. GA Perry, JD Jackson, JE Talmadge. Effects of a multidrug chemotherapy regimen on the thymus. Thymus 1994; 23:39–51.

79. CL Mackall, TA Fleisher, MR Brown, MP Andrich, CC Chen, IM Feuerstein, ME Horowitz, IT Magrath, AT Shad, SM Steinberg, et al. Age, thymopoiesis, and CD4+ T-lymphocyte regeneration after intensive chemotherapy. N Engl J Med 1995; 332:143–149.

80. T Ghayur, TA Seemayer, WS Lapp. Association between the degree of thymic dysplasia and the kinetics of thymic NK cell activity during the graft-versus-host reaction. Clin Immunol Immunopathol 1988; 48:19–30.

81. N Fukushi, H Arase, B Wang, K Ogasawara, T Gotohda, RA Good, K Onoe. Thymus: a direct target tissue in graft-versus-host reaction after allogeneic bone marrow transplantation that results in abrogation of induction of self-tolerance. Proc Natl Acad Sci USA 1990; 87:6301–6305.

82. C Cray, RB Levy. Evidence that donor cells are present in the thymus of recipients undergoing a P→F1 graft-versus-host reaction exacerbated by concurrent murine cytomegalovirus infection. Transplantation 1992; 53:696–699.

83. M Seddik, TA Seemayer, WS Lapp. The graft-versus-host reaction and immune function. I. T helper cell immunodeficiency associated with graft-versus-host-induced thymic epithelial cell damage. Transplantation 1984; 37:281–286.

84. M Seddik, TA Seemayer, WS Lapp. T cell functional defect associated with thymic epithelial cell injury induced by a graft-versus-host reaction. Transplantation 1980; 29:61–66.

85. S Rossi, BR Blazar, CL Farrell, DM Danilenko, DL Lacey, KI Weinberg, W Krenger, GA Hollander. Keratinocyte growth factor preserves normal thymopoiesis and thymic microenvironment during experimental graft-versus-host disease. Blood 2002; 100:682–691.

86. T Ghayur, TA Seemayer, A Xenocostas, WS Lapp. Complete sequential regeneration of graft-vs.-host-induced severely dysplastic thymuses. Implications for the pathogenesis of chronic graft-vs.-host disease. Am J Pathol 1988; 133:39–46..

87. T Ghayur, TA Seemayer, WS Lapp. Kinetics of natural killer cell cytotoxicity during the graft-versus-host reaction. Relationship between natural killer cell activity, T and B cell activity, and development of histopathological alterations. Transplantation 1987; 44:254–260.

88. WE Beschorner, GM Hutchins, GJ Elfenbein, GW Santos. The thymus in patients with allogeneic bone marrow transplants. Am J Pathol 1978; 92:173–181.

89. HK Muller-Hermelink, GE Sale, B Borisch, R Storb. Pathology of the thymus after allogeneic bone marrow transplantation in man. A histologic immunohistochemical study of 36 patients. Am J Pathol 1987; 129:242–256.

90. B Chung, L Barbara-Burnham, L Barsky, K Weinberg. Radiosensitivity of thymic interleukin-7 production and thymopoiesis after bone marrow transplantation. Blood 2001; 98:1601–1606.

91. BF Haynes, ML Markert, GD Sempowski, DD Patel, LP Hale. The role of the thymus in immune reconstitution in aging, bone marrow transplantation, and HIV-1 infection. Ann Rev Immunol 2000; 18:529–560.

92. CL Mackall, JA Punt, P Morgan, AG Farr, RE Gress. Thymic function in young/old chimeras: substantial thymic T cell regenerative capacity despite irreversible age-associated thymic involution. Eur J Immunol 1998; 28:1886–1893.

93. JF Poulin, MN Viswanathan, JM Harris, KV Komanduri, E Wieder, N Ringuette, M Jenkins, JM McCune, RP Sekaly. Direct evidence for thymic function in adult humans. J Exp Med 1999; 190:479–486.

94. BD Jamieson, DC Douek, S Killian, LE Hultin, DD Scripture-Adams, JV Giorgi, D Marelli, RA Koup, JA Zack. Generation of functional thymocytes in the human adult. Immunity 1999; 10:569–575.

95. CM Steffens, L Al-Harthi, S Shott, R Yogev, A Landay. Evaluation of thymopoiesis using T cell receptor excision circles (TRECs): differential correlation between adult and pediatric TRECs and naive phenotypes. Clin Immunol 2000; 97:95–101.

96. R Schwab, P Szabo, JS Manavalan, ME Weksler, DN Posnett, C Pannetier, P Kourilsky, J Even. Expanded CD4+ and CD8+ T cell clones in elderly humans. J Immunol 1997; 158:4493–4499.

97. DC Douek, RA Vescio, MR Betts, JM Brenchley, BJ Hill, L Zhang, JR Berenson, RH Collins, RA Koup. Assessment of thymic output in adults after haematopoietic stem-cell transplantation and prediction of T-cell reconstitution. Lancet 2000; 355:1875–1881.

98. F Dumont-Girard, E Roux, RA van Lier, G Hale, C Helg, B Chapuis, M Starobinski, E Roosnek. Reconstitution of the T-cell compartment after bone marrow transplantation: restoration of the repertoire by thymic emigrants. Blood 1998; 92:4464–4471.

99. K Talvensarri, E Clave, C Douay, C Rabian, L Garderet, M Busson, F Garnier, D Douek, E Gluckman, D Charron, A Toubert. A broad T-cell repertoire diversity and an efficient thymic function indicate a favorable long-term immune reconstitution after cord blood stem cell transplantation. Blood 2002; 99:1458–1464.

100. T Nordoy, A Kolstad, P Endresen, H Holte, S Kvaloy, G Kvalheim, A Husebekk. Persistent changes in the immune system 4-10 years after ABMT. Bone Marrow Transplant 1999; 24:873–878.

101. S Mariani, M Coscia, J Even, S Peola, M Foglietta, M Boccadoro, L Sbaiz, G Restagno, A Pileri, M Massaia. Severe and long-lasting disruption of T-cell receptor diversity in human myeloma after high-dose chemotherapy and autologous peripheral blood progenitor cell infusion. Br J Haematol 2001; 113:1051–1059.

102. E Roux, F Dumont-Girard, M Starobinski, CA Siegrist, C Helg, B Chapuis, E Roosnek. Recovery of immune reactivity after T-cell-depleted bone marrow transplantation depends on thymic activity. Blood 2000; 96:2299–2303.

103. BC Godthelp, MJD van Tol, JM Vossen, PJ van den Elsen. T-cell immune reconstitution in pediatric leukemia patients after allogeneic bone marrow transplantation with T-cell-depleted or unmanipulated grafts: evaluation of overall and antigen-specific T-cell repertoires. Blood 1999; 94:4358–4369.

104. K Weinberg, G Annett, A Kashyap, C Lenarsky, SJ Forman, R Parkman. The effect of thymic function on immunocompetence following bone marrow transplantation. Biol Blood Marrow Transplant 1995; 1:18–23.

105. K Weinberg, BR Blazar, JE Wagner, E Agura, BJ Hill, M Smogorzewska, RA Koup, MR Betts, RH Collins, DC Douek. Factors affecting thymic function after allogeneic hematopoietic stem cell transplantation. Blood 2001; 97:1458–1466.

106. J Storek, A Joseph, MA Dawson, DC Douek, B Storer, DG Maloney. Factors influencing T-lymphopoiesis after allogeneic hematopoietic cell transplantation. Transplantation 2002; 73:1154–1158.

107. Lee SJ, Vogelsang G, Flowers ME. Chronic graft-versus-host disease. Biol Blood Marrow Transplant 2003; 9:215–233.

108. L Rozendaal, ST Pals, E Gleichmann, CJ Melief. Persistence of allospecific helper T cells is required for maintaining autoantibody formation in lupus-like graft-versus-host disease. Clin Exp Immunol 1990; 82:527–532.

109. J Desbarats, WS Lapp. Thymic selection and thymic major histocompatibility complex class II expression are abnormal in mice undergoing graft-versus-host reactions. J Exp Med 1993; 178:805–814.

110. MR van den Brink, E Moore, JL Ferrara, SJ Burakoff. Graft-versus-host-disease-associated thymic damage results in the appearance of T cell clones with anti-host reactivity. Transplantation 2000; 69:446–449.

111. GA Hollander, B Widmer, SJ Burakoff. Loss of normal thymic repertoire selection and persistence of autoreactive T cells in graft vs host disease. J Immunol 1994; 152:1609–1617.

112. E Roux, C Helg, F Dumont-Girard, B Chapuis, M Jeannet, E Roosnek. Analysis of T-cell repopulation after allogeneic bone marrow transplantation: significant differences between recipients of T-cell depleted and unmanipulated grafts. Blood 1996; 87:3984–3992.

113. R Hofmeister, AR Khaled, N Benbernou, E Rajnavolgyi, K Muegge, SK Durum. Interleukin-7: physiological roles and mechanisms of action. Cytokine Growth Factor Rev 1999; 10:41–60.

114. TJ Fry, CL Mackall. Interleukin-7: from bench to clinic. Blood 2002; 99:3892–3904.

115. H Spits. Development of alphabeta T cells in the human thymus. Nat Rev Immunol 2002; 2:760–772.

116. TJ Fry, M Moniuszko, S Creekmore, SJ Donohue, DC Douek, S Giardina, TT Hecht, BJ Hill, K Komschlies, J Tomaszewski, G Franchini, CL Mackall. IL-7 therapy dramatically alters peripheral T-cell homeostasis in normal and SIV-infected non-human primates. Blood 2002.

117. O Alpdogan, C Schmaltz, SJ Muriglan, BJ Kappel, MA Perales, JA Rotolo, JA Halm, BE Rich, MR van den Brink. Administration of interleukin-7 after allogeneic bone marrow transplantation improves immune reconstitution without aggravating graft-versus-host disease. Blood 2001; 98:2256–2265.

118. ML Sinha, TJ Fry, DH Fowler, G Miller, CL Mackall. Interleukin 7 worsens graft-versus-host disease. Blood 2002; 100:2642–2649.

119. C Katlama, G Carcelain, C Duvivier, C Chouquet, R Tubiana, M De Sa, L Zagury, V Calvez, B Autran, D Costagliola. Interleukin-2 accelerates CD4 cell reconstitution in HIV-infected patients with severe immunosuppression despite highly active antiretroviral therapy: the ILSTIM study—ANRS 082. AIDS 2002; 16:2027–2034.

120. A Fefer, N Robinson, MC Benyunes, WI Bensinger, O Press, JA Thompson, C Lindgren. Interleukin-2 therapy after bone marrow or stem cell transplantation for hematologic malignancies. Cancer J Sci Am 1997; 3(suppl 1):S48–53.

121. Y Bar-Dayan, M Small. Effect of bovine growth hormone administration on the pattern of thymic involution in mice. Thymus 1994; 23:95–101.

122. LA Napolitano, JC Lo, MB Gotway, K Mulligan, JD Barbour, D Schmidt, RM Grant, RA Halvorsen, M Schambelan, JM McCune. Increased thymic mass and circulating naive CD4 T cells in HIV-1-infected adults treated with growth hormone. AIDS 2002; 16:1103–1111.

123. E Montecino-Rodriguez, R Clark, K Dorshkind. Effects of insulin-like growth factor administration and bone marrow transplantation on thymopoiesis in aged mice. Endocrinology 1998; 139:4120–4126.

124. TN Small, EB Papadopoulos, F Boulad, P Black, H Castro-Malaspina, BH Childs, N Collins, A Gillio, D George, A Jakubowski, G Heller, M Fazzari, N Kernan, S MacKinnon, P Szabolcs, JW Young, RJ O'Reilly. Comparison of immune reconstitution after unrelated and related T-cell-depleted bone marrow transplantation: effect of patient age and donor leukocyte infusions. Blood 1999; 93:467–480.

125. RJ Soiffer, EP Alyea, E Hochberg, C Wu, C Canning, B Parikh, D Zahrieh, I Webb, J Antin, J Ritz. Randomized trial of CD8+ T-cell depletion in the prevention of graft-versus-host disease associated with donor lymphocyte infusion. Biol Blood Marrow Transplant 2002; 8:625–632.

126. DA Mavroudis, YZ Jiang, N Hensel, P Lewalle, D Couriel, RJ Kreitman, I Pastan, AJ Barrett. Specific depletion of alloreactivity against haplotype mismatched related individuals by a recombinant immunotoxin: a new approach to graft-versus-host disease prophylaxis in haploidentical bone marrow transplantation. Bone Marrow Transplant 1996; 17:793–799.

127. SR Riddell, PD Greenberg. T cell therapy of human CMV and EBV infection in immunocompromised hosts. Rev Med Virol 1997; 7:181–192.

128. S Gottschalk, OL Edwards, MH Huls, T Goltsova, AR Davis, HE Heslop, CM Rooney. Generating CTL against the subdominant Epstein-Barr virus LMP1 antigen for the adoptive immunotherapy of EBV-associated malignancies. Blood 2003; 101(5):1905–1912.

129. RJ O'Reilly, TN Small, E Papadopoulos, K Lucas, J Lacerda, L Koulova. Adoptive immunotherapy for Epstein-Barr virus-associated lymphoproliferative disorders complicating marrow allografts. Springer Semin Immunopathol 1998; 20:455–491.

130. ME Horwitz, AJ Barrett, MR Brown, CS Carter, R Childs, JI Gallin, SM Holland, GF Linton, JA Miller, SF Leitman, EJ Read, HL Malech. Treatment of chronic granulomatous disease with nonmyeloablative conditioning and a T-cell-depleted hematopoietic allograft. N Engl J Med 22001; 344:881–888.

131. RJ O'Reilly, D Kirkpatrick, N Kapoor, N Collins, J Brochstein, N Kernan, N Flomenberg, M Pollack, B Dupont, C Lopez, et al. A comparative review of the results of transplants of fully allogeneic fetal liver and HLA-haplotype mismatched, T-cell depleted marrow in the treatment of severe combined immunodeficiency. Prog Clin Biol Res 1985; 193:327–342.

132. F Aversa, A Tabilio, A Terenzi, A Velardi, F Falzetti, C Giannoni, R Iacucci, T Zei, MP Martelli, C Gambelunghe, et al. Successful engraftment of T-cell-depleted haploidentical "three-loci" incompatible transplants in leukemia patients by addition of recombinant human granulocyte colony-stimulating factor-mobilized peripheral blood progenitor cells to bone marrow inoculum. Blood 1994; 84:3948–3955.

133. F Aversa, A Tabilio, A Velardi, I Cunningham, A Terenzi, F Falzetti, L Ruggeri, G Barbabietola, C Aristei, P Latini, Y Reisner, MF Martelli. Treatment of high-risk acute leukemia with T-cell-depleted stem cells from related donors with one fully mismatched HLA haplotype. N Engl J Med 1998; 339:1186–1193.

134. Y Reisner, MF Martelli. Bone marrow transplantation across HLA barriers by increasing the number of transplanted cells. Immunol Today 1995; 16:437–440.

135. J Sierra, B Storer, JA Hansen, JW Bjerke, PJ Martin, EW Petersdorf, FR Appelbaum, E Bryant, TR Chauncey, G Sale, JE Sanders, R Storb, KM Sullivan, C Anasetti. Transplantation of marrow cells from unrelated donors for treatment of high-risk acute leukemia: the effect of leukemic burden, donor HLA-matching, and marrow cell dose. Blood 1997; 89:4226–4235.

136. F Aversa, A Velardi, A Tabilio, Y Reisner, MF Martelli. Haploidentical stem cell transplantation in leukemia. Blood Rev 2001; 15:111–119.

137. R Handgretinger, M Schumm, P Lang, J Greil, A Reiter, P Bader, D Niethammer, T Klingebiel. Transplantation of megadoses of purified haploidentical stem cells. Ann NY Acad Sci 1999; 872:351–362.

138. RM Zinkernagel, A Althage, G Callahan, RM Welsh, Jr. On the immunocompetence of H-2 incompatible irradiation bone marrow chimeras. J Immunol 1980; 124:2356–2365.

139. J Tang, C Costello, IP Keet, C Rivers, S Leblanc, E Karita, S Allen, RA Kaslow. HLA class I homozygosity accelerates disease progression in human immunodeficiency virus type 1 infection. AIDS Res Hum Retroviruses 1999; 15:317–324.

140. P Garside, AK Hutton, A Severn, FY Liew, AM Mowat. Nitric oxide mediates intestinal pathology in graft-vs.-host disease. Eur J Immunol 1992; 22:2141–2145.

141. WJ Murphy, CW Reynolds, P Tiberghien, DL Longo. Natural killer cells and bone marrow transplantation. J Natl Cancer Inst 1993; 85:1475–1482.

142. T Ghayur, TA Seemayer, PA Kongshavn, JG Gartner, WS Lapp. Graft-versus-host reactions in the beige mouse. An investigation of the role of host and donor natural killer cells in the pathogenesis of graft-versus-host disease. Transplantation 1987; 44:261–267.

143. T Ghayur, A Xenocostas, TA Seemayer, WS Lapp. Induction, specificity and elimination of asialo-GM1+ graft-versus-host effector cells of donor origin. Scand J Immunol 1991; 34:497–508.

144. L Ruggeri, M Capanni, E Urbani, K Perruccio, WD Shlomchik, A Tosti, S Posati, D Rogaia, F Frassoni, F Aversa, MF Martelli, A Velardi. Effectiveness of donor natural killer cell alloreactivity in mismatched hematopoietic transplants. Science 2002; 295:2097–2100.

145. HG Ljunggren, K Karre. Host resistance directed selectively against H-2-deficient lymphoma variants. Analysis of the mechanism. J Exp Med 1985; 162:1745–1759.

146. HG Ljunggren, K Karre. In search of the 'missing self': MHC molecules and NK cell recognition. Immunol Today 1990; 11:237–244.

147. WJ Murphy, CY Koh, A Raziuddin, M Bennett, DL Longo. Immunobiology of natural killer cells and bone marrow transplantation: merging of basic and preclinical studies. Immunol Rev 20201; 181:279–289.

148. CY Koh, BR Blazar, T George, LA Welniak, CM Capitini, A Raziuddin, WJ Murphy, M Bennett. Augmentation of antitumor effects by NK cell inhibitory receptor blockade in vitro and in vivo. Blood 2001; 97:3132–3137.

149. O Asai, DL Longo, ZG Tian, RL Hornung, DD Taub, FW Ruscetti, WJ Murphy. Suppression of graft-versus-host disease and amplification of graft-versus-tumor effects by activated natural killer cells after allogeneic bone marrow transplantation. J Clin Invest 1998; 101:1835–1842.

150. B Glass, L Uharek, M Zeis, H Loeffler, W Mueller-Ruchholtz, W Gassmann. Graft-versus-leukaemia activity can be predicted by natural cytotoxicity against leukaemia cells. Br J Haematol 1996; 93:412–420.

151. M Zeis, L Uharek, B Glass, J Steinmann, P Dreger, W Gassmann, N Schmitz. Allogeneic MHC-mismatched activated natural killer cells administered after bone marrow transplantation provide a strong graft-versus-leukaemia effect in mice. Br J Haematol 1997; 96:757–761.

152. SS Farag, T Fehniger, L Ruggeri, A Velardi, MA Caligiuri. Natural killer cells: biology and application in stem-cell transplantation. Cytotherapy 2002; 4:445–446.

153. A Velardi, L Ruggeri, A Moretta, L Moretta. NK cells: a lesson from mismatched hematopoietic transplantation. Trends Immunol 2002; 23:438–444.

154. A Moretta, M Vitale, C Bottino, AM Orengo, L Morelli, R Augugliaro, M Barbaresi, E Ciccone, L Moretta. P58 molecules as putative receptors for major histocompatibility complex (MHC) class I molecules in human natural killer (NK) cells. Anti-p58 antibodies reconstitute lysis of MHC class I-protected cells in NK clones displaying different specificities. J Exp Med 1993; 178:597–604.

155. L Ruggeri, M Capanni, M Casucci, I Volpi, A Tosti, K Perruccio, E Urbani, RS Negrin, MF Martelli, A Velardi. Role of natural killer cell alloreactivity in HLA-mismatched hematopoietic stem cell transplantation. Blood 1999; 94:333–339.

156. LL Lanier. NK cell receptors. Annu Rev Immunol 1998; 16:359–393.

157. NM Valiante, M Uhrberg, HG Shilling, K Lienert-Weidenbach, KL Arnett, A D'Andrea, JH Phillips, LL Lanier, P Parham. Functionally and structurally distinct NK cell receptor repertoires in the peripheral blood of two human donors. Immunity 1997; 7:739–751.

158. E Ciccone, D Pende, O Viale, C Di Donato, G Tripodi, AM Orengo, J Guardiola, A Moretta, L Moretta. Evidence of a natural killer (NK) cell repertoire for (allo) antigen recognition: definition of five distinct NK-determined allospecificities in humans. J Exp Med 1992; 175:709–718.

159. E Ciccone, A Moretta, L Moretta. Specific functions of human NK cells. Immunol Lett 1992; 31:99–103.

160. M Colonna, EG Brooks, M Falco, GB Ferrara, JL Strominger. Generation of allospecific natural killer cells by stimulation across a polymorphism of HLA-C. Science 1993; 260:1121–1124.

161. M Colonna, G Borsellino, M Falco, GB Ferrara, JL Strominger. HLA-C is the inhibitory ligand that determines dominant resistance to lysis by NK1- and NK2-specific natural killer cells. Proc Natl Acad Sci USA 1993; 90:12000–12004.

162. M Uhrberg, NM Valiante, NT Young, LL Lanier, JH Phillips, P Parham. The repertoire of killer cell Ig-like receptor and CD94:NKG2A receptors in T cells: clones sharing identical

alpha beta TCR rearrangement express highly diverse killer cell Ig-like receptor patterns. J Immunol 2001; 166:3923–3932.

163. R Biassoni, C Cantoni, D Pende, S Sivori, S Parolini, M Vitale, C Bottino, A Moretta. Human natural killer cell receptors and co-receptors. Immunol Rev 2001; 181:203–214.

164. L Moretta, R Biassoni, C Bottino, MC Mingari, A Moretta. Human NK-cell receptors. Immunol Today 2000; 21:420–422.

165. S Bauer, V Groh, J Wu, A Steinle, JH Phillips, LL Lanier, T Spies. Activation of NK cells and T cells by NKG2D, a receptor for stress-inducible MICA. Science 1999; 285:727–729.

166. CL Sutherland, NJ Chalupny, D Cosman. The UL16-binding proteins, a novel family of MHC class I-related ligands for NKG2D, activate natural killer cell functions. Immunol Rev 2001; 181:185–192.

167. SM Davies, L Ruggieri, T DeFor, JE Wagner, DJ Weisdorf, JS Miller, A Velardi, BR Blazar. Evaluation of KIR ligand incompatibility in mismatched unrelated donor hematopoietic transplants. Killer immunoglobulin-like receptor. Blood 2002; 100:3825–3827.

168. K Karre. Immunology. A perfect mismatch. Science 2002; 295:2029–2031.

8

Pathology and Pathogenesis
of Cutaneous Graft-vs.-Host Disease

JOHN L. WAGNER

*Thomas Jefferson University, Philadelphia, Pennsylvania
and Harvard Medical School, Boston, Massachusetts, U.S.A.*

GEORGE F. MURPHY

*Thomas Jefferson University, Philadelphia, Pennsylvania,
Harvard Medical School and Brigham and Women's Hospital,
Boston, Massachusetts, U.S.A.*

I. PATHOBIOLOGY OF CUTANEOUS GRAFT-VS.-HOST DISEASE

A. Brief Overview

Understanding the cellular pathology of cutaneous graft-vs.-host disease (GVHD) requires attention to at least three issues: the gross or clinical pathology of disease, the histopathology of lesions, including the use of novel adjunctive modalities that may facilitate diagnosis, and the pathobiology that underlies the morphological alterations that produce lesions at these clinical and histological levels. This chapter has been organized accordingly. The last section deals with pathobiology and presents a conceptual model for disease initiation and progression that involves three distinctive phases, namely allostimulation, homing, and targeting. It is hoped that this approach will not only facilitate understanding of the morphological correlates of the fundamental cellular and molecular events, but also provide a framework that promotes future insights into translationally relevant research aimed at abrogating this all too often devastating disorder.

B. Changing Paradigms and Diagnostic Dilemmas

The cutaneous effects of GVHD were originally described in 1955 as a "secondary disease" (as distinct from the primary toxicity of radiation sickness) in a murine model of hematopoietic stem cell transplantation (SCT) (1). Since that time, enormous strides have been made in defining the pathology and understanding the pathogenesis of cutaneous GVHD. In spite of this, the clinical diagnosis of cutaneous GVHD has become more complicated. The term acute GVHD has traditionally been used to describe a distinctive syndrome of hepatitis, gastroenteritis, and dermatitis developing within 100 days of allogeneic hematopoietic SCT. The term chronic GVHD has indicated a syndrome involving dermatitis, often with sclerosis, and systemic manifestations suggestive of autoimmunity that develops after day 100. However, in an era of increased numbers of haploidentical, cord blood, nonmyeloablative, and unrelated transplants, "stem cell boosts," and donor lymphocyte infusions, the time frames for distinguishing between acute and chronic GVHD become potentially less relevant. For example, signs and symptoms of chronic GVHD may be observed soon after donor lymphocyte infusions, and manifestations more commonly associated with acute GVHD (such as diarrhea unrelated to bacterial overgrowth) may be encountered well beyond day 100 posttransplant. Moreover, the related histopathological alterations, as assessed by skin biopsy, need not adhere to a specific time course; the occasional patient can show contemporaneous changes of both acute and chronic GVHD.

The clinical and histopathological changes of cutaneous GVHD may occur in a variety of clinical settings in addition to traditional allogeneic SCT, including syngeneic SCT (2,3), following blood transfusions (4,5), and following solid organ transplants (6). In some patients acute cutaneous GVHD may be difficult to distinguish from certain viral exanthemas or from some toxic and allergic drug eruptions (7). Moreover, GVHD in the autologous setting may be difficult to distinguish from that in the allogeneic setting (8). Finally, the finding of suspected GVHD in one organ system need not imply that abnormalities in other potential target sites are secondary to GVHD.

Certain clinical features have conventionally been used to differentiate GVHD from other conditions that may occur in the post-SCT period. For example, involvement of the palms and soles has been considered to be suggestive of acute GVHD and potentially related to the concentration of target epithelial cells in the rete ridges of the epidermal layer at these sites (9). In our experience, however, involvement of the palms and soles may be highly variable, with only 20% of recently diagnosed patients showing this manifestation of disease.

Skin biopsies, especially when performed serially to assess disease evolution, may be useful in distinguishing GVHD from other disorders in the posttransplant period. It must be remembered, however, that the skin biopsy is neither entirely sensitive of nor specific for GVHD. Accordingly, close correlation of skin biopsy results with other pathological and clinical parameters is necessary to enhance diagnostic accuracy. When an exanthem appears early (e.g., within one week) after infusion of a cellular product (e.g., a stem cell or donor lymphocyte infusion), skin biopsies may be of limited utility in diagnosing GVHD (10). To complicate matters, agents such as intravenous contrast media and exposure to ultraviolet (UV) light, which in themselves may cause skin rashes, also have the ability to trigger or potentiate GVHD (11). Furthermore, debate exists as to whether certain infectious processes, such as cytomegalovirus, can provoke or exacerbate GVHD, as opposed to simply arising as events secondary to the immune dysregulation that typically accompanies this disease (12,13).

II. GROSS PATHOLOGY

A. Acute GVHD

Unlike most other forms of pathology, where the gross features of affected organs are evaluated ex vivo and correlated with histological changes, the gross pathology of a skin biopsy is the disease itself as it presents in the living patient. The initial manifestation

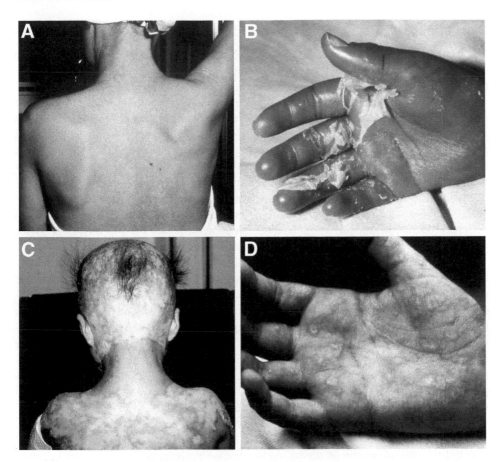

Figure 1 Clinical manifestations of acute and chronic GVHD. (A) Maculopapular exanthem of early acute GVHD; (B) diffuse epithelial sloughing of advanced and severe acute GVHD (toxic epidermal necrolysis-like variant); (C) thickened, tight skin showing poikilodermatous changes and hair loss in chronic GVHD of the dermal type; (D) multiple violaceous and hyperkeratotic papules typical of chronic GVHD of the epidermal (lichen planus-like) type.

of acute GVHD in the skin is a maculopapular rash (Fig. 1A). This rash may be punctate, correlating with early and preferential involvement of hair follicles and thus resembling folliculitis, or it may be more diffuse, resembling a sunburn. Pruritis and/or burning are often prominent components. Confluence of the exanthem may correlate with increased clinical stage of disease in certain patients. Rarely (<7% of cases) there is epidermal necrosis with sloughing and formation of bullae resembling toxic epidermal necrolysis (14) (Fig. 1B). The incidence of this severe type of cutaneous acute GVHD appears to be decreasing, possibly as the result of improved immunosuppressive regimens to prevent GVHD, alterations in conditioning regimens, improved HLA matching, or perhaps as a consequence of earlier diagnosis and more rapid intervention with immunosuppressive agents.

Recently a syndrome has been described in which patients receiving transplants, particularly from unrelated donors, exhibit a form of hyperacute GVHD manifested by generalized erythroderma with desquamation and diarrhea before there are signs of myeloid engraftment (15).

B. Chronic GVHD

The clinical manifestations of chronic cutaneous GVHD are often more protean than its acute counterpart, although the skin is the most commonly affected organ in this form of the disease. Chronic GVHD may begin at sites of trauma, UV irradiation, or localized infection, as with varicella zoster. There are two major types of cutaneous chronic GVHD: sclerodermoid and lichenoid. In the sclerodermoid form, affected individuals develop indurated, whitish plaques with hypo- and hyperpigmentation (Fig. 1C). Skin coloration often acquires a gray hue. Initially localized, the skin thickening may become progressively more diffuse. Localized sclerodermoid GVHD can develop on the legs, and at this site the skin may become adherent to underlying fascia, with associated development of ischemic and traumatically induced ulceration. Blisters may also develop, presumably as a consequence of compromised lymphatic drainage. Entrapment of nerve endings by fibrous tissue may result in peripheral axonal neuropathy (16). When sclerodermoid plaques are located over joints, fibrous entrapment of ligaments and joint contractures also may develop.

In some patients, the cutaneous manifestations of chronic GVHD are predominantly lichenoid, with no typical pattern of distribution. Individual papules and small plaques are erythematous to violaceous and exhibit a variably shiny to scaling, flat-topped surface (Fig. 1D). Hypo- and hyperpigmented areas may develop as a result of chronic injury to the basal cell layer, and over time larger plaques may arise due to coalescence of individual papules. Patients with darker skin may only have areas of cutaneous dryness or regions of hypo- or hyperpigmentation, without evidence of a rash. Poikilodermatous changes may eventuate in some patients. The lichenoid form may occur earlier after transplantation than the sclerodermoid form. Occasional patients exhibit both lichenoid and sclerodermoid features of chronic GVHD contemporaneously.

Other less common manifestations of chronic GVHD include total leukoderma (17), macroscopic mucinosis (18), and fasciitis (19). In the latter, the skin may initially present as cellulitis with subcutaneous edema. As the disease evolves, the involved area becomes progressively indurated and the lesion is visible as a depression, although the epidermis may remain normal. The fasciitis can result in significant decrease in range of motion, especially if skin overlying joints is involved. However, patients also may have fasciitis without involvement of overlying skin.

Dermal appendages are often involved in chronic GVHD. Body or scalp hair may become brittle, prematurely gray, or fall out entirely (Fig. 1C). Nails may develop deep ridges or flaking, and occasionally are lost completely. Nail changes may persist long after the cutaneous manifestations have become inactive. Sweat glands may be destroyed by inflammation, leading to increased risk of heat stroke.

Mucosal alterations are observed in both acute and chronic GVHD, although lesions tend to be more widespread in the chronic form, with involvement of the mouth, conjunctiva, and genitalia. Oral involvement is characterized by focal to diffuse mucosal atrophy and erythema, especially affecting the tongue, pallet, lips, and buccal surfaces (20). In severe oral GVHD, there may be painful ulcerative lesions with impairment of taste sensation. Ocular involvement from keratitis sicca may result in symptoms of burning, itching, pain, and photophobia (21,22). Vaginal involvement, when severe, is manifested in the formation of strictures (23), and penile lesions may eventuate in phimosis (24) or Peyronie's disease (25). It is often difficult to differentiate these lesions clinically from the mucosal toxicity that may result from the conditioning regimen, particularly when they occur soon after the infusion of a cellular product.

III. DIAGNOSTIC PATHOLOGY

A. Acute GVHD

The first histological alterations that occur in acute cutaneous GVHD involve adhesion and transvascular diapedesis of lymphocytes through postcapillary venules situated within the uppermost dermis (superficial vascular plexus) (Fig. 2A). Such changes are often observed in biopsies 2–3 weeks after transplantation or in association with the first clinical

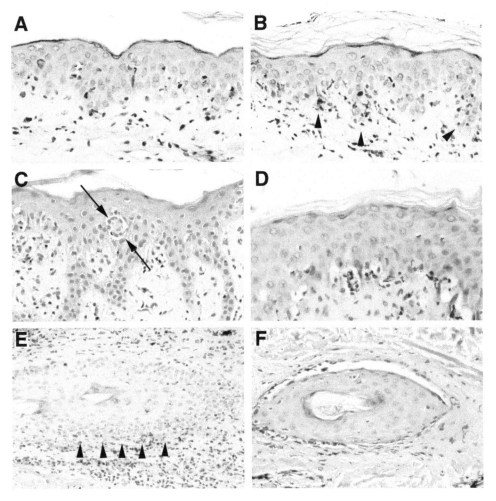

Figure 2 Histopathology of acute GVHD. (A) Early lesion showing sparse infiltrate of lymphocytes about superficial dermal vessels, with rare cells accumulating at the dermal-epidermal interface; (B) more advanced early lesion, with unequivocal accumulation of infiltrating lymphocytes along the dermal epidermal junction, particularly at the rete tips (arrowheads); (C) satellitosis, showing lymphocytes surrounding an apoptotic, centrally located keratinocyte (arrows); (D) higher grade lesion, with basal cell layer apoptosis and vacuolization resulting in incipient microscopic focus of dermal epidermal detachment; (E) follicular infiltration by lymphocytes in early lesion (arrowheads); (F) higher grade follicular injury, with follicular basal cell layer injury resulting in perifollicular cleft formation.

signs and symptoms of cutaneous involvement. Mast-cell degranulation around the affected venules appears to be related to activation of microvascular endothelial cells responsible for initial recruitment of effector cells. It is of interest, therefore, that pruritis, a common sign of mast-cell degranulation, may also accompany early clinical lesions of acute GVHD. Migration of leukocytes into the perivascular interstitutium of the superficial (papillary) dermis is the result of adhesive interaction between the effector cells and microvascular endothelial cells. Remarkably few cells seem to be involved in this phase, and their migratory fate is influenced by the secondary induction of chemokines and adhesion molecules by cells in the overlying epidermal layer.

The diagnostic histology of this endothelial phase of acute GVHD is nonspecific, and serial biopsies are often required to establish a definitive diagnosis. Maculopapular viral exanthemas are probably the most common cause of a superficial perivascular lymphocytic infiltrate, and this possibility must always be considered when the diagnosis of GVHD is entertained. Although viral exanthemas may be hemorrhagic and therefore associated with superficial perivascular extravasation of erythrocytes, altered coagulation status may also produce this finding after SCT. Drug eruptions must also be considered in the early endothelial phase of acute GVHD. Generally, drug eruptions will involve both superficial and deep dermal vessels, and the inflammatory infiltrate will include eosinophils as well as lymphocytes. However, in the setting of the immunosuppression and leukopenia that accompanies the posttransplant period, these characteristic features may be lacking. Moreover, although most lesions of acute GVHD do not harbor eosinophils, occasional lesions do. Cutaneous eruption of lymphocyte recovery, seen after chemotherapy and a period of marrow aplasia, shows an upper dermal, usually perivascular infiltrate with variable exocytosis of lymphocytes and spongiosis. Apoptotic keratinocytes are seen rarely. Thus, histological and clinical evolution over time (see below), as assessed in serial biopsies, is often the best diagnostic indicator of the presence of evolving acute GVHD.

Lymphocytes that initially accumulate about superficial dermal venules migrate from the perivascular interstitium into the overlying epidermal layer (epidermotropism). Some of these cells may seem to align along the dermal-epidermal junction (Fig. 2B), while others are present in all levels of the epidermis. The finding of lymphocytes in the epidermis is diagnostically important in early acute GVHD, for it is the harbinger of target-cell injury. Unlike other forms of dermatitis that show lymphoid epidermotropism, such as various forms of eczematous dermatitis, acute GVHD generally fails to show significant intercellular edema (spongiosis) within the epidermal layer. However, we have seen examples of true spongiotic dermatitis that, upon serial sampling, have demonstrated transition to lesions more typical of acute GVHD. Whether this represents the blending of two independent immune responses in the post-SCT period or the potential for rare examples of early GVHD to show prominent spongiosis remains unclear.

The most characteristic histological finding in acute GVHD is the finding of "satellitosis," indicating target-cell injury within the epidermis or follicular epithelium (Fig. 2C). Satellitosis consists of multiple lymphocytes intimately surrounding one or several keratinocytes that shows signs of eosinophilic degeneration and cell death. Such keratinocytes usually contain condensed, hyperchromatic, and sometimes fragmented nuclei. The cytoplasm is dark red due to increased eosin uptake (acidophilia). Recent evidence indicates that such dying target keratinocytes are actually undergoing apoptosis (26), although original reports referred to such cells as "dyskeratotic" (27,28). In general, the degree of epidermal injury in acute GVHD seems out of proportion to the sparse numbers of lymphocytes present within the superficial dermal and epidermal layers. It is important to realize that a small number of degenerating keratinocytes independent of lymphocytic apposition may be the sequelae of the pretransplant conditioning regimen alone. Accordingly, care should be taken to attribute epidermal necrosis to acute GVHD only when such changes are associated with unequivocal clustering of epidermotropic lymphocytes. A helpful feature in early acute GVHD is the preferential lymphoid infiltration around apoptosis of keratinocytes within the tips of epidermal rete ridges. With disease progression, vacuolization of contiguous basal cells may accompany satellitosis, and the former may be so pronounced in some patients as to result in diffuse epidermal sloughing in a manner akin to toxic epidermal necrolysis (Fig. 2D).

Migration by lymphocytes into the upper third of the hair follicle (follicular infundibulum) is also commonly observed in acute GVHD (Fig. 2E). This phenomenon has been termed "cytotoxic folliculitis" and is a helpful indicator of early GVHD even in biopsies that fail to show significant lymphocytic infiltration of the interfollicular epidermis. When GVHD is extensive and severe, separation of follicular epithelium from surrounding adventitia may occur as a result of contiguous apoptosis within the basal cell layer (Fig. 2F).

Acute GVHD may also involve other squamous epithelial surfaces that differ in architecture and cytology from most cutaneous regions. These include acral skin and oral mucosa. Biopsies of acral acute GVHD frequently reveal subtle alterations, consisting of superficial perivascular lymphoid infiltration and focal epidermotropism and keratinocyte apoptosis that selectively involves the often well-developed rete tip epithelium (Fig. 3A). It must be remembered that the stratum corneum is normally thick and compacted in these regions and thus should not be interpreted as a component of the pathology. Squamous mucosal acute GVHD is characterized by a band-like infiltrate of lymphocytes (and usually some plasma cells) directly beneath the epithelial layer (Fig. 3B). Infiltration of the epithelium by lymphocytes may be associated with apoptosis and satellitosis (Fig. 3B,C), although this feature is variable. Occasionally the inflammation extends to involve the epithelium of minor salivary glands, which shows prominent lymphoid infiltration and, with chronicity, periductal fibrosis (Fig. 3D).

1. Sensitivity, Specificity, and Predictive Value of Histopathology

In murine models of acute GVHD, the number of apoptotic epidermal cells (26) has been found to correlate with the number of effector T cells in the donor marrow inoculum, the presence and extent of hepatic and intestinal disease (27), and the overall severity of clinical disease (28). It therefore is reasonable to ask whether the severity of disease, as assessed histopathologically in a skin biopsy, permits similar predictions in humans. By inference, the Lerner system of histological grading (29) suggests that the extent of epidermal injury may be of biological significance in predicting clinical disease severity and outcome. Massi and coworkers have suggested that one potential drawback of this approach is its failure to take into account inflammatory infiltrate as a criterion in early (stage I and II) lesions (30). This issue has been addressed in one study where 69 cyclosporine-treated, allogeneic SCT patients were evaluated to determine early clinical, laboratory, or histopathological indicators for the development of progressive, fatal acute GVHD (31). Whereas substantial increases in total bilirubin, stool output, extent of rash, and overall clinical GVHD stage proved useful in predicting severe, potentially fatal forms of the disease, the number of lymphocytes entering into the epidermal layer and the number of dyskeratotic (apoptotic) keratinocytes did not. In other studies, skin biopsy findings correlated poorly with outcome in patients treated based on clinical severity of skin

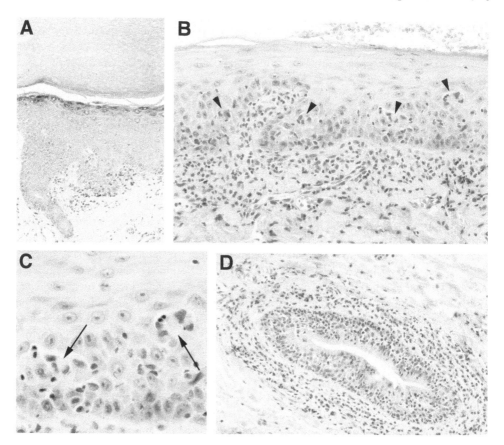

Figure 3 Acral and squamous mucosal manifestations of acute GVHD. (A) Lymphocyte infiltration favors the rete ridge (arrows) of palm skin showing normally thickened and compacted orthokeratotic scale; (B) buccal mucosal lesion, with lymphocyte migration into the squamous mucosa accompanied by focal apoptosis (arrowheads); (C) higher magnification of apoptotic cells (arrows) in buccal mucosa surrounded by lymphocytes (satellitosis); (D) minor salivary duct heavily infiltrated by lymphocytes; note developing mantle of early periductal fibrosis.

rashes suggestive of acute GVHD (10). Accordingly, although we provide qualitative descriptions for skin biopsy specimens consistent with GVHD by indicating the nature and extent of effector cell infiltration and epidermal injury, we do not provide histological grades as predictors of disease severity. It must also be emphasized that in any given patient, the skin biopsy may be of limited sensitivity for the early detection of disease, particularly with respect to other target sites (e.g., gut). In addition, because the histopathology of early acute GVHD has considerable overlap with other conditions that occur in the posttransplant period (e.g., viral exanthemas, drug eruptions, eruptions associated with immunological reconstitution), specificity is enhanced dramatically when the biopsy is correlated with other signs of disease.

2. Adjunct Studies for Diagnosis of Cutaneous Acute GVHD

While histopathology remains the mainstay of diagnosis for both acute and chronic GVHD, problems with specificity and sensitivity have resulted in the need to develop special ancillary techniques that may assist in more accurate recognition of this often protean and diagnostically elusive condition.

Histochemical Approaches. The ability to differentiate between acute GVHD and erythema multiforme, a cytotoxic hypersensitivity condition that may closely resemble GVHD, has been examined using histochemical stains to detect bile pigment (associated with hyperbilirubinemia) within the epidermal layer (32). No lesions of erythema multiforme stained for intraepidermal bile pigment ($n = 50$), whereas 6% of the acute GVHD cases showed bile pigment within the epidermal layer (3 of 50 cases evaluated). Thus it appears that in a very small minority of acute GVHD cases, intraepidermal bile pigment serves as a built-in marker for the hyperbilirubinemia of GVHD-associated liver dysfunction, and therefore may assist in distinguishing between erythema multiforme and acute GVHD. The practical significance of this observation, however, is limited by the small number of cases that actually harbor intraepidermal bile pigment, the assumptions that clinical parameters of liver dysfunction are not available to the pathologist, and are secondary to hepatic GVHD.

Immunohistochemical Approaches. Interface drug eruptions, where cytotoxic lymphocytes attack the epidermal basal cell layer, may closely mimic acute GVHD. A recent study sought to compare acute interface drug eruptions with acute GVHD using immunohistochemistry. Unfortunately, both conditions were found to have a predominance of CD8+ T cells in the infiltrate, reduction in the number of CD1a+ Langerhans cells, and increased epidermal expression of HLA-DR and ICAM-1 (33). Thus, by these parameters, both acute interface drug eruptions and acute GVHD could not be reliably distinguished. In contrast, a similar approach taken to differentiate epidermal-type chronic GVHD (lichen planus type) from true lichen planus showed more promising results (34) based on a limited numbers of patients. Whereas lichen planus was characterized by infiltration of CD4+ T cells and increased numbers of Langerhans cells, lichenoid chronic GVHD demonstrated predominantly CD8+ T cells, associated LAK cell markers CD16 and CD28, and diminished numbers of Langerhans cells.

Molecular Approaches. The unanticipated development of acute GVHD after massive blood transfusion was reportedly confirmed in one study by examining the T lymphocytes infiltrating a skin biopsy by PCR directed against a Y chromosome–specific sex-determining region Y (SRY) gene (35). The diagnosis was established by HLA-DNA typing with PCR sequence–specific oligonucleotides that revealed the presence of complex HLA-DR chimerism in the peripheral lymphocytes collected after the onset of GVHD. Thus, the use of SRY-directed PCR could promise to be a rapid technique for the early diagnosis of GVHD in female patients. However, it remains unclear as to whether mere infiltration of skin by chimeric donor cells implies effector function, since passive infiltration of donor cells at sites of inflammation due to non–GVHD-related stimuli (e.g., drug-induced and viral exanthemas) could produce similar findings.

In Vitro Assays. Recently, skin organ culture has been rediscovered for the examination of numerous histological and immunopathological changes relevant to acute GVHD, such as the induction of MHC class II molecules and related adhesion pathways (36,37). Human skin has been used in in vitro assays to predict the likelihood of acute GVHD developing in HLA-matched sibling SCT (38). This model involves sensitizing donor lymphocytes in vitro in a primary mixed lymphocyte reaction and then evaluating the secondary response in patient skin biopsies by grading the resultant GVHD-like alterations histopathologically. Sviland et al. suggested that this model permits an 82% correlation between histopathological changes in the explants and clinical outcome (39). This strategy may be refined further by using the TUNEL approach to mark apoptotic target cells in the explants (40), thereby enhancing the capacity of this assay to predict more severe grades of GVHD. These approaches remain in developmental stages; however, a potential limitation lies in the fact that nonspecific degenerative alterations that occur within the epidermal layer upon skin explantation in vitro may bear marked similarity to early evolutionary stages of acute GVHD. An exciting potential alternative to this approach has recently been discovered where viable and structurally normal human skin xenografts on genetically immunosuppressed (SCID) mice can be induced to express the phenotype of cytotoxic dermatitis with features of epidermal-type GVHD (41).

B. Chronic GVHD

Chronic GVHD has traditionally been divided into epidermal (lichen planus-like) and dermal (sclerodermoid) types. However, we have frequently reviewed biopsies where both epidermal and dermal alterations are present, and the former may represent an early manifestation of what will eventuate in the dermal sclerotic form of the disease. Accordingly, the epidermal and dermal alterations are described separately with the caveat that in certain patients, epidermal and dermal pathology will not be mutually exclusive and hybrid features may be present.

1. Epidermal Alterations

The epidermal manifestations of chronic GVHD are far less subtle than those observed in the acute disease. Satellitosis, with epidermotropic lymphocytes surrounding degenerating and necrotic keratinocytes, is common to both forms of disease, in contrast to acute GVHD. However, the inflammatory infiltrate in chronic GVHD is not sparse and angiocentric, but it may fill the papillary dermis in a bandlike manner (Fig. 4A–D). The epidermis is generally thickened, and the stratum corneum is thickened and compacted. In rare cases, foci of spongiosis may be observed, mimicking subacute eczematous dermatitis (e.g., as in a subacute spongiotic drug eruption) (Fig. 4A). However, a careful search will often reveal foci of follicular cytotoxicity (Fig. 4B). The more common form is nonspongiotic and dominated by thickening of the stratum corneum, stratum granulosum, and stratum spinosum. These features, along with a band-like infiltrate of lymphocytes in the papillary dermis that results in vacuolization, apoptosis, and squamatization of the basal cell layer, result in histopathology that bears a striking similarity to lichen planus (Fig. 4C,D). Whether dealing with spongiotic or nonspongiotic variants of epidermal-type chronic GVHD, cytotoxic injury to basal layer or follicular keratinocytes is key to establishing a correct diagnosis.

An additional feature that may facilitate the diagnosis of epidermal-type chronic GVHD is the presence of coarse, early fibrosis within the perifollicular adventitial of affected hair follicles (Fig. 4B) or in the inflamed papillary dermis (Fig. 4D). Such alterations may actually be a harbinger of the development of deeper sclerosis and a sclerodermoid picture clinically.

In addition to follicular injury and focal superficial sclerosis, the variants of epidermal-type chronic GVHD may be further identified by the composition of the inflammatory infiltrate. In general, drug-related subacute immune responses producing either spongiotic

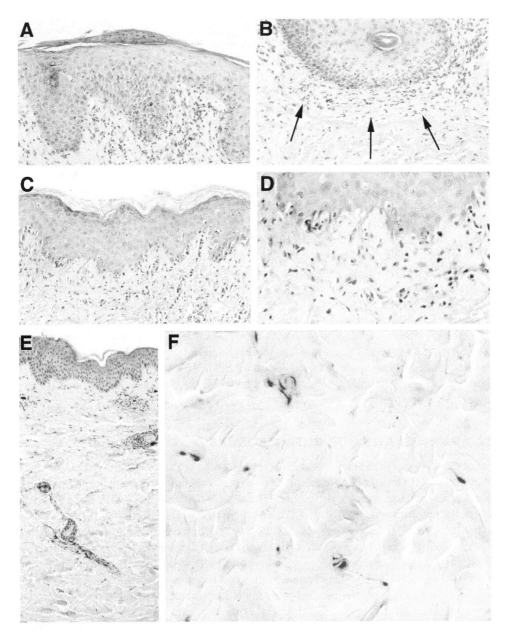

Figure 4 Cutaneous manifestation of chronic GVHD. (A) This patient's skin showed a mixture of subacute spongiotic changes as well as keratinocyte apoptosis, leading to the initial impression of a drug eruption—note the epidermal thickening and abnormal scale formation; (B) hair follicle from biopsy represented in panel A showing cytotoxic folliculitis and early perifollicular fibrosis (arrows; this patient rapidly evolved to a more classical sclerodermoid picture); (C) more classical epidermal-type chronic GVHD, showing epidermal thickening and papillary dermal infiltration by lymphocytes; (D) higher magnification of C, depicting vacuolization, apoptosis, and squamous changes within the basal cell layer as well as early fibrosis within the papillary dermis; (E) sclerodermatous chronic GVHD with progressive thickening, hyalinization, and compaction of collagen bundles within the deep dermis; (F) markedly sclerotic dermal collagen in advanced chronic GVHD of the dermal/sclerodermatous type.

or lichen planus-like epidermal alterations will generate inflammatory infiltrates that are comprised of lymphocytes with numerous admixed eosinophils. While both acute and chronic skin GVHD rarely have significant numbers of eosinophils, this feature must always be assessed in the absence of peripheral blood eosinophilia (a condition where infiltrates may be secondarily seeded with these cells). Although the absence of eosinophilic infiltrates is of some practical value, we have not found it to be consistent in view of occasional cases of evolving mixed epidermal/dermal chronic GVHD where inflammatory infiltrates contained both lymphocytes and eosinophils.

2. Dermal Alterations

The dermal alterations of chronic GVHD often follow a phase of chronic epidermal injury (discussed above) and consist of deep-seated sclerosis remarkably similar to that seen in morphea and progressive systemic sclerosis (Fig. 4E,F). These deeper alterations begin at the interface of the reticular dermis and subcutaneous fat, where thick bundles of pale, homogeneous collagen are deposited. Early changes are frequently accompanied by a deep dermal perivascular lymphoplasmacytic infiltrate. Over time, the abnormally deposited collagen replaces subcutaneous fat and extends to involve thickened interlobular septa. The overlying reticular dermis is also progressively replaced, with encasement and eventual atrophy of adnexal epithelium (Fig. 4E). When eccrine coils persist, their placement approximates the now obscured normal junction that separated the reticular dermis from underlying fat and may be helpful in determining the extent of subcutaneous replacement. The end result is a markedly thickened dermal layer composed of enlarged bundles of pale, hyalinized collagen. The adnexae are generally absent in advanced disease, and the overlying epidermis is frequently diffusely atrophic.

IV. PATHOBIOLOGY OF CUTANEOUS GVHD

Acute and chronic GVHD may appear to occur on a continuum in a single individual. However, they probably represent two different, albeit related, disease processes. Acute GVHD is a cytotoxic attack of donor lymphocytes on host tissues, most dramatically on cells associated with epithelial compartments (gut, liver, skin), which are seen as foreign. Chronic GVHD, on the other hand, involves not only cytotoxicity, but also a derangement of host immune function, stimulated by donor lymphocytes and allowing the development of autoimmunity in a permissive genetic background. In situations of GVHD where there is no tissue incompatibility (syngeneic GVHD), this immune dysfunction becomes paramount.

We have conceptually divided acute GVHD into three distinct phases: allostimulation, homing, and targeting. A fourth phase, resolution/chronicity, also exists and will be discussed separately under the pathobiology of chronic GVHD. Throughout the three phases of acute GVHD, and ostensibly driving these events to a crescendo by the point of targeting, is an ever-increasing background of cytokine dysregulation. As will be seen, circulating cytokines appear to direct and enhance events related to cell stimulation, organ-directed migration, and cytotoxicity, and thus represent an integral part of the disease process.

A. Phase I: Allostimulation and the Initiation of Cytokine Cascades

Whereas many, if not most, of the inflammatory elements detected in a skin biopsy of acute GVHD are likely to represent secondary, nonspecific responders, the fundamental cutaneous lesion involves the initial influx of specifically allostimulated T cells. The donor T cells that mediate acute cutaneous GVHD are directed against HLA or minor histocompatibility antigen (miHA) disparities expressed by host tissues (42–44). The site(s) at which alloreactive responses are generated are not fully understood, although recent experimental evidence implicates secondary lymphoid tissues, such as Peyer's patches in gut (45). Although specifically allostimulated T cells account for disease by infiltrating and damaging host tissues, broad-spectrum T-cell depletion from the donor stem cell inoculum often results in increased graft failure, leukemic relapse, and opportunistic infections (46). Accordingly, identification of the specific alloreactive T cells responsible for the induction of acute GVHD is important not only in defining the histopathology of the earliest cutaneous lesions, but also in developing approaches for their selective depletion. Such strategies would leave residual, nonalloreactive T cells to potentially support engraftment and mediate immune interactions against persistent leukemic cells as well as infectious agents.

In animal models, specific subsets of allostimulated cells that cause acute GVHD have now been defined by examining the T-cell receptor (TCR) Vβ repertoire of CD4+ T cells. Using both phenotypic analysis of CD4+ T cells coupled with CDR3-size spectratyping in a murine model of miHA-induced acute GVHD (47), expansion of specific Vβ families has been documented. Moreover, using antibodies specific for these Vβ populations, skin and squamous mucosal infiltration by these allostimulated cells can be documented. The homing patterns of these effector T-cell subpopulations are likely to provide insight into the identification of cellular targets within tissues.

It is important to remember that cytokines represent a major driving force in the events leading to the formation of cutaneous acute GVHD. Induction of cytokines occur early and is related to the effects of SCT-conditioning regimens (48) and develops further as a consequence of transplantation and allostimulation. Additional cytokines are released locally during effector phases of GVHD due in part to allostimulation and as a result of tissue injury consequent to the conditioning regimen. The release of these inflammatory cytokines in GVHD has been documented at the protein and mRNA levels, promoting the concept of GVHD as a "cytokine storm" (49). The time course of cytokine mRNA transcription suggests a hierarchy of cytokine dysregulation in this process. Cytokine dysregulation may explain pathological features of acute GVHD in which tissue damage appears to be more severe than would be attributable to direct cytotoxicity of rare infiltrating T cells (49). The consequence of systemic and local cytokine release is cellular activation, induction of cell-adhesion pathways that mediate organ-specific homing, and direct cytotoxicity.

Some of the key cytokines released during the evolution of acute GVHD include interleukin-1 (IL-1) (50–53), IL-2 (50–52), interferon-gamma (IFNγ) (54), tumor necrosis factor-alpha (TNFα) (51,55–57), and T-cell growth factor-beta (TGFβ) in the setting of chronicity (58,59). Indeed, studies have shown that either direct inhibition or receptor blockade of cytokines, such as TNFα and IL-2, may lessen the severity of experimental acute GVHD (60,61). Therapeutic agents such as cyclosporine, which inhibit cytokine production by lymphocytes, can thereby ameliorate GVHD. Krenger et al. (48) have suggested that activation of specific cytokine cascades during GVHD occurs in the context of three phases. In the first phase, the conditioning regimen in the form of irradiation and/or chemotherapy results in damage to and activation of host tissues, inducing the secretion of inflammatory cytokines TNFα and IL-1. These cytokines result in enhanced expression of MHC adhesion molecules (Fig. 5). In the second phase, donor T-cell activation results in proliferation of Th1 T cells and secretion of IL-2 and IFNγ, which

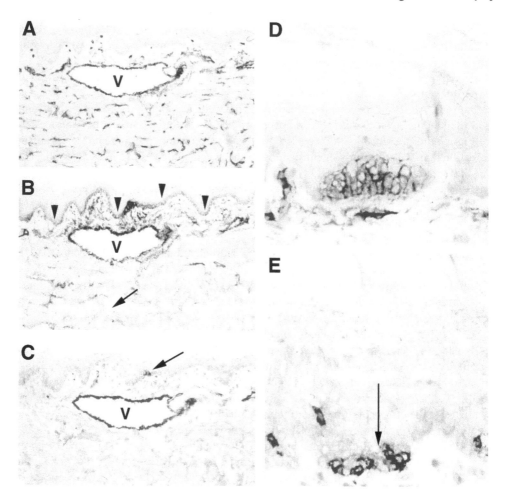

Figure 5 Immunohistochemistry of murine acute GVHD depicting effects of cytokine stimulation on lingual epithelium and endothelium. (A) CD31 staining indicating normal vascular distribution (V = vessel lumen); (B) ICAM-1 is induced in the lower layers of the squamous mucosa (arrowheads) and is upregulated on dermal vessels; (C) VCAM-1 is induced focally in the squamous mucosa (arrow) and in endothelium lining superficial submucosal vessels (A–C represent adjacent sections); (D) ICAM-1 is focally expressed at the tip of a rete ridge-like downgrowth of the dorsal mucosal; (E) CD3-positive T cells (arrow) in adjacent section, indicating that infiltration is restricted to this cytokine-simulated microdomain.

in turn induce further T-cell expansion, cytotoxic T-lymphocyte (CTL) and natural killer (NK) cell responses, and prime mononuclear phagocytes to produce additional IL-1 and TNFα. Finally in the last phase, effector functions are triggered by lipopolysaccharide (LPS), which leaks through intestinal mucosa damaged initially by the conditioning regimen, and ultimately LPS may stimulate gut-associated mononuclear cells as well as skin cells to produce additional proinflammatory cytokines. As we discuss the progression of disease from allostimulation through the homing and targeting phases, additional mention of specific cytokine pathways will be made.

B. Phase II: Homing

One of the great mysteries of acute GVHD has been why and how allostimulated effector T cells find their way to target organs, such as skin. It is now known that T cells normally percolate freely between tissue microenvironments and the systemic circulation. The expression of adhesion molecules and ligands in these tissues may tend, however, to slow their migration, resulting in their localized accumulation over time. A potentially useful and well-studied paradigm for such highly directed cellular homing is found in the cutaneous delayed-type hypersensitivity (DTH) reaction. For several decades it has been recognized that T-cell influx into sites of epicutaneous antigen challenge initially involves the postcapillary venule within the superficial dermis (62,63). This observation, left dormant for many years, is now the central theme of an enormous body of data indicating a critical role for this migratory pathway in antigen-driven cutaneous inflammation.

The microanatomy of the superficial dermis is critical to understanding the cellular and molecular interactions responsible for target-specific leukocyte homing. Exogenous and endogenous antigenic targets within the epidermal layer are separated from a complex microvascular plexus by a thin layer of type III collagen, called the papillary dermis. The microvascular plexus is composed of small anastomosing arterioles and venules, the former of which gives rise to capillary loops extending upward within conical dermal papillae that invaginated into the epidermal layer. The immediate perivascular microenvironment of postcapillary venules contains mast cells, monocyte/macrophages, and dermal dendritic cells. Ultrastructural studies show an intimate relationship between mast cells and these microvenules. During the earliest phases (minutes to hours) of cutaneous inflammation, there are prominent alterations of the postcapillary venule and the cells that surround it. The changes consist of degranulation of perivenular mast cells and associated changes in endothelium, namely prominence of endothelial cytoplasmic filaments, endothelial bulging into the venular lumen, and gap formation between adjacent endothelial cells. The endothelial alterations, initially believed to be solely the result of liberation of histamine from mast cells and termed "histamine effect," occur at timepoints that correlate with the earliest recruitment of leukocytes to affected venules.

Today it is known that this "endothelial activation" involves complicated and precisely orchestrated molecular signals that result in the efficient display of endothelial adhesion molecules that serve to promote leukocyte binding to the lumenal endothelial surface. Such molecules are expressed in a cascade. P-selectin appears within minutes, mediates the weakest binding, and brings circulating leukocytes to slow "roll" along the endothelial membrane. Display of subsequent molecules may serve either to favor adhesion of specific subpopulations of skin-homing effector cells (e.g., E-selectin) or to strengthen leukocyte-endothelial binding and promote diapedesis, e.g., vascular cell adhesion molecule-1 (VCAM-1), intercellular adhesion molecule-1 (ICAM-1), and platelet endothelial cell adhesion molecule-1 (PECAM-1, or CD31) (Fig. 5A–C). Reciprocal ligands on effector cells may be either constitutively expressed by certain subpopulations (e.g., as in lymphocyte function–associated antigen-1, or LFA-1, the ligand for ICAM) (64,65) or progressively upregulated during the binding process (66,67). Mast-cell degranulation may facilitate the display of these binding cascades, since mast cells liberate secretory substances that either induce or alter distribution of endothelial adhesion molecules (e.g., histamine for P-selectin; tumor necrosis factor for E-selectin, ICAM-1, and VCAM-1).

The nature of the stimuli that results in early mast-cell degranulation is potentially of critical importance in understanding what triggers initial effector-cell binding to microvenular endothelium. In experimental delayed-type hypersensitivity (DTH) reactions, it appears that antigen-specific antibody molecules that function like IgE may be generated during sensitization (68). Subsequent challenge with epicutaneous antigen provokes mast-cell degranulation by local cross-linking of these antibodies on mast-cell membranes, setting into motion an endothelial adhesion cascade that results in recruitment of specific memory T cells. With reference to acute GVHD, mast-cell degranulating properties have been characterized in supernatants of allostimulated T cells (69). In human GVHD, early expression of endothelial adhesion molecules (e.g., E-selectin) possibly induced in part by mast-cell cytokines, has also been documented (70). Moreover, the potential importance of mast cells to the early inflammatory phases of GVHD is emphasized by ultrastructural studies indicating that degranulation of these cells consistently precedes effector cell influx. In keeping with this observation, cutaneous GVHD lesions are delayed in onset when genetically mast-cell–deficient animals serve as transplant recipients. Disease eventually occurs only when granulated mast cells develop, either from donor stem cells or due to microenvironmental factors that are as yet unclear (61).

Based upon these and other observations, it is likely that the homing phase of acute GVHD results from the enhanced expression of adhesion molecules within microvessels of specific target organs. These adhesion cascades may be induced by the growing concentrations of proinflammatory cytokines that typify the immediate post-SCT period, as well as by cytokines produced and released locally from skin cells such as mast cells. Certain subsets of T cells express skin-homing characteristics owing to the expression of receptors and ligands that interact with adhesive proteins preferentially expressed by dermal microvessels (e.g., E-selectin). This may further enhance the organ-selective homing of effector cells to relevant target sites, such as skin. Once effector T cells have accumulated in sufficient numbers in the skin, final localization to microanatomical domains that harbor target cells and antigens may result in the cellular injury that typifies cutaneous acute GVHD.

C. Phase III: Targeting

1. Epidermotropic Localization

Once effector leukocytes have successfully infiltrated the dermis, they must then complete their journey into the epidermal layer, where putative target alloantigens are displayed. Navigation into the epidermal layer, a process referred to as "epidermotropism," is likely to involve molecular interactions that are equally or more complicated than what has already transpired within the underlying dermis. The first adhesive events between effector leukocytes and epidermal cells appear to involve the basal-cell layer and the basement membrane zone, which defines the boundary between epidermis and superficial dermis. In human and experimental GVHD, many T cells infiltrating the epidermal layer become localized in close proximity to the basement membrane zone. Such T cells, lymphokine-activated killer cells, and alloreactive cytotoxic cells, but not B cells, express the $\alpha 3 \beta 1$ membrane integrin, which is a receptor for the basement membrane ligand, epiligrin, also termed laminin 5 (71). This molecule is synthesized by basal keratinocytes and is expressed primarily in the lamina lucida of the basement membrane. Binding interactions between specific subsets of T cells and basal epidermal cells are therefore likely to influence early epidermotropic migration and adhesion in GVHD.

Binding of T lymphocytes to cells that constitute the suprabasal epidermal layers is likely to be mediated by interactions between leukocytes and keratinocytes, including well-established LFA-1/ICAM-1–mediated adhesion. Unlike endothelial cells, keratino-cytes do not constitutively express ICAM-1, and therefore expression must be induced by systemic cytokines as well as those produced by early migrant T cells. Both ICAM-1 and HLA-DR are upregulated on epidermal cells by INFγ, and both are prominently displayed during the epidermotropic phases of GVHD (Fig. 5D). By analogy to the trafficking patterns of intestinal intraepithelial T cells and malignant lymphocytes of cutaneous T-cell lymphoma, it has been suggested that leukocytes may also bind to epidermal cells via heterophilic adhesion between keratinocyte E-cadherin and the lymphocyte integ-rin αEβ7 (72,73).

A novel observation has recently been made by Kim and coworkers (74) indicating that in addition to endothelial cells, VCAM-1 is also expressed by squamous epithelium in the setting of experimental murine acute GVHD. VCAM-1 expression antecedes accumu-lation of effector T cells and coincides with rete tip–like downgrowths of dorsal lingual mucosa. This finding suggests that differential induction of adhesion molecules in specific epithelial microdomains may dictate initial injury to defined subsets of target cells. Indeed, recent evidence indicates that keratinocytes are injured by the process of apoptosis in acute GVHD (26) and that these apoptotic cells are confined to rete tips and their equivalents. Thus, it now appears that site specificity of injury in GVHD involves not only specific organs, but also precisely localized cellular domains within their epithelial components.

2. Identity of Epidermotropic Effector Cells

Effector T cells that initiate and perpetuate epidermal injury in acute GVHD after successful homing to skin include NK cells, lymphokine-activated killer (LAK) cells, and CTL. Cells bearing markers for NK cells have been identified as possible effector cells infiltrating organs of mice with acute GVHD; indeed, they have been found in close association with dead or dying epithelial cells in skin, liver, and colon (75,76). These cells are donor in origin and can mediate cytotoxicity in the absence of class I or II on target cells. Mature donor CD8+ CTL have also been shown to play an important role in acute GVHD. CTL kill via recognition of self-MHC (class I) molecules and pro-cessed foreign antigens expressed on the surface of a targeted cell, typically a virally infected cell or a tumor cell. Hess (77) showed that the presence of CD8+ cytotoxic T cells correlates with the onset of the acute phase of syngeneic GVHD in rats and that these cells recognize a public determinant of class II histocompatibility antigens. The his-tological changes in mucosa of the tongue show CD4− CD8+ lymphocytes infiltrating the mucosa, with prominent epithelial cell destruction and satellitosis.

A useful murine model for the study of various donor lymphocyte subsets in GVHD utilizes highly purified populations of these subsets to generate GVHD across minor histocompatibility loci (78,79). In multiple different mouse strain combinations, mature CD8+ T cells can mediate GVHD without help from donor CD4+ helper lymphocytes. CD4+ lymphocytes can produce GVHD alone, but only in certain strain combinations, suggesting that genetic factors play an important role in GVHD. In two strain combinations designated to evaluate the histopathology of GVHD mediated by either CD4+ or CD8+ lymphocytes, epidermal cytotoxicity is present in both, indicating that a final common pathway of cytotoxicity may exist for these T-cell subsets. Significantly, dermal fibrosis is evident only in CD8+-mediated disease in these murine modes (27). The use of this Korngold Sprent model for murine GVHD has illustrated the complexity of effector lymphocyte pathways as well as the importance of histocompatibility target antigens in initiation and progression of GVHD.

3.   Mechanisms of Apoptosis Induction in Cellular Targets

Molecular mechanisms potentially responsible for the induction of apoptosis by skin-infiltrating cytotoxic effector cells (80–82) appear to involve one or more of at least three pathways, namely Fas/Fas ligand, perforin/granzyme (83–86), and TNF/TNF receptor-TRAIL (87–90). The Fas/Fas ligand pathway is involved in an array of regulatory mechanisms potentially important to GVHD, including target cell cytolysis by CTL, regulation of inflammatory responses, peripheral deletion of autoimmune cells, costimulation of T cells, and activation-induced cell death (AICD). In studies employing Fas-deficient *lpr* mice as recipients of SCT, hepatic disease was significantly ameliorated, but injury to other tissues, including skin, was unexpectedly augmented (91). Similarly, when Fas ligand–deficient *gld* mice were used as recipients (92), disease was also exacerbated, suggesting that, on balance, expression of Fas ligand in the SCT recipient is important to the host's ability to control GVHD. However, when donor T cells deficient in Fas ligand are employed in experimental SCT, there is diminished GVHD activity (93). Interestingly, perforin-deficient donor T cells retain ability to produce disease. These data suggest that donor T cells may mediate GVHD activity primarily through the Fas ligand effector pathway. Moreover, a reciprocal effect is seen with regard to graft-vs.-leukemia (GVL) effects, with only donor T cells deficient in perforin, but not Fas ligand, resulting in diminished GVL activity. Taken together, it would appear, at least in certain experimental systems and strain combinations, that donor T cells make differential use of cytolytic pathways and that the specific blockade of these pathways may preferentially ameliorate GVHD while preserving beneficial GVL activity. However, it is important to realize that both Fas/Fas ligand and perforin/granzyme pathways have been implicated in acute GVHD, along with cytokines and other cytotoxic factors. Moreover, the dominant pathways may vary according to the nature of the effector T cells and the target antigens that are involved.

Recently, studies employing donor murine T cells deficient in TRAIL (tumor necrosis factor–related apoptosis-inducing ligand) demonstrated diminished GVL but not GVHD effects, suggesting that TRAIL is also an important mediator of the former (90). In graft-vs.-myeloid leukemia responses, differential use of Fas ligand and perforin-mediated cytolytic mechanisms by specific T-cell subsets has also been demonstrated (94). The ultimate goal of these and other studies will be to identify differences in effector T-cell cytolytic pathways that will permit development of inhibitory agents for GVHD target cell injury, while preserving GVL potency.

Although the levels of TNFα mRNA transcripts in the skin are upregulated only four- to sixfold in GVHD (51), this cytokine has been implicated as a major contributor to cytotoxicity. Circulating levels of TNFα protein are high and correlate with the severity and course of cutaneous GVHD. Piguet et al. (55,56) have shown that neutralizing antibodies against TNFα administered to mice with acute GVHD will reduce morbidity and mortality of disease. Furthermore, administration of TNFα to normal mice will reproduce some of the clinical and pathological features of GVHD. As noted earlier, mast cells degranulate in early GVHD and release TNFα locally. The effects of TNFα on keratinocytes are diverse, from upregulation of ICAM-1 expression to direct cytotoxicity. Although TNFα can produce apoptotic cell death with characteristic laddered DNA degradation in certain sensitive cells, it is not known if it causes a necrotic or an apoptotic type of cell death in skin keratinocytes. TNFα also upregulates mRNA production and protein expression of endothelial cell molecules such as ICAM-1 and E-selectin, and it may play an important role in the endothelial phase of cutaneous GVHD.

4.   Identity of Target Cells

A final question relates to precisely what cells and molecules in the skin are being targeted by the apoptotic process. Epidermal cells (keratinocytes) showing injury in acute GVHD have been termed "dyskeratotic" in recognition of their characteristically hypereosinophilic cytoplasm (28). However, it has been demonstrated that these cells actually succumb by the process of apoptosis (26). It is important to recognize that some apoptosis occurs as a result of conditioning regimen (95,96), and accordingly, the epidermal injury of acute GVHD develops upon a background of already compromised cells. Moreover, from a practical viewpoint, pathologists must be careful not to overread baseline apoptosis as early disease.

But are epithelial cells such as epidermal keratinocytes, and the molecules that they express, actually the targets in acute GVHD? One recent study examining experimental acute GVHD across class I and II MHC barriers addressed this issue by using murine bone marrow chimeras in which alloantigen was expressed only by antigen-presenting cells (APC) (97). It was discovered that in these transplant settings, acute GVHD did not require alloantigen expression on host target epithelium. Moreover, neutralization of IL-1 and TNFα prevented epithelial injury. These findings, which were most pronounced in disease mediated by CD4+ effector T cells, suggested a central role for APC and cytokines in the targeting phase of disease. While these data imply that dendritic cells may represent primary cellular targets when disease is elicited by MHC antigenic differences, this may not be the case in miHA mismatches (98).

In the epidermis and squamous mucosal epithelium of the skin, the principal dendritic cell is the epidermal Langerhans cell. This cell is depleted post-SCT, and at least some of this injury appears to be related to the effects of the conditioning regimen (99,100). Nonetheless, we have observed degenerative alterations in Langerhans cells in murine acute GVHD (101). Moreover, in murine lingual mucosa, where adhesion molecule expression, T-cell infiltration, and apoptosis occur preferentially in rete tip–like downgrowths (26,74), Langerhans cells are consistently localized to these microanatomical domains (G.F. Murphy, unpublished observation). If Langerhans cells are the primary targets of disease in certain transplantation settings, then keratinocyte apoptosis known to occur in acute GVHD could represent a nonspecific innocent bystander effect. Alternatively, histocompatibility differences displayed by target keratinocytes may require nearby dendritic cells to communicate these signals to infiltrating allostimulated T cells. If this is so, injury may be spatially restricted to microdomains, where these three cell types are most concentrated. Further exploration of these issues is required in order to clarify more precisely the target cells and molecules required for apoptotic injury in cutaneous GVHD.

The three-step model for the cellular pathogenesis of acute GVHD is summarized in Figure 6, taking into account the role of progressive background cytokine amplification as a force that drives allostimulated T cells to their effector fates involving organ-specific homing and cell-selective targeting.

4.   Mesenchymal Alterations and Transition to Chronicity

Compared to acute GVHD, relatively little is known concerning the mechanism(s) whereby sclerodermoid alterations are induced to occur in chronic cutaneous GVHD. One important clue, however, may reside in the similarities between the skin changes in GVHD and those seen in scleroderma of both the localized and systemic forms

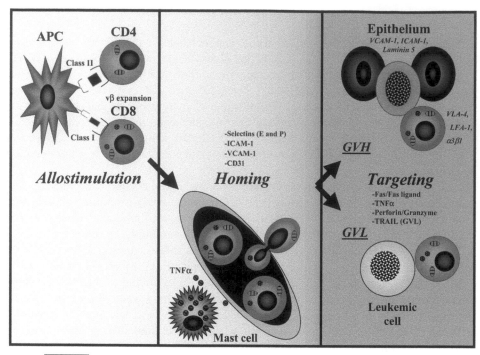

= progressive increase in proinflammatory cytokines

Figure 6 Schematic representation of the proposed three-step model for the pathogenesis of acute GVHD. Cytokine secretion begins as early as the start of SCT conditioning and increases in breadth and strength during the allostimulation, homing, and targeting phases. During the allostimulation phase, antigen-presenting cells (APC) display donor-derived alloantigens (MHC class I or II, or minor histocompatibility antigens) to specific subsets of CD4+ or CD8 + T cells. Allostimulation results in expansion of specific Vβ families, which circulate and eventually home to target tissues as a consequence of growing cytokine concentrations. Systemic along with locally released cytokines (e.g., mast cell TNFα) promote adhesive interactions between circulating effector cells and the endothelium lining microvascular complexes within the relevant target tissues. These interactions are facilitated by induction, expression, and relocalization of cell adhesion molecules (e.g., P- and E-selectin, ICAM-1, VCAM-1, and CD31) on the lumenal endothelial surface that promote the binding and localization of circulating skin-homing effector leukocyte populations. Transvascular diapedesis of effector cells is followed by subsequent epidermotropic migration potentially mediated by adhesive interactions between T-cell VLA-4, LFA-1, and $\alpha 3\beta 1$ with epidermal VCAM-1, ICAM-1, and basement membrane–associated laminin 5, respectively. This heralds the targeting phase, where effector cells come into direct apposition with squamous epithelial targets in the GVHD response (red basal keratinocyte) as well as in the GVL reaction, inducing apoptosis (signified by nuclei with interrupted patterns) via molecular pathways that appear to involve Fas/Fas ligand interactions, the perforin/granzyme pathway, cytokine-receptor binding interactions, and, in the case of GVL, the TRAIL pathway.

(morphea and progressive systemic sclerosis, respectively). In a seminal report (101), lesional skin biopsies from women with scleroderma were found to harbor fetal DNA and lymphocytes many years after the delivery of offspring, which at times occurred before onset of disease. These provocative findings raised the possibility that scleroderma itself could represent a form of chronic GVHD where fetal lymphocytes that enter the maternal circulation serve as the graft, with maternal cells within the dermis representing the host targets.

Other avenues of investigation have centered on mast cells. The involvement of mast cells in fibrosing disorders is supported by many independent reports showing increased numbers of mast cells in the following conditions: healing wounds and keloids, bleomycin fibrosis, eosinophilic fasciitis, pulmonary fibrosis, and radiation-induced fibrosis, as well as in early progressive systemic sclerosis and chronic GVHD (103–106). Often in these conditions the mast cells also are degranulated, suggesting activation. We have shown that mast-cell degranulation precedes acute GVHD target-cell injury in two different combinations of irradiated murine strains with minor histocompatibility differences, and, as described earlier, the onset of GVHD can be delayed when mast-cell–deficient B6WWv mice are used as allogeneic SCT recipients. The eventual onset of GVHD in these animals can be correlated with appearance of granulated mast cells (61). TNFα and TGFβ released as a consequence of mast-cell degranulation in mice has recently been linked to induction of collagen type I mRNA in dermal fibroblasts (58). In humans, release of mast-cell TNFα may be linked to increased numbers of dendritic stromal cells, termed dermal dendrocytes (107), during early phases of experimental murine GVHD (108). Therefore, mast cells may not only play an important role in the endothelial cell phase of acute GVHD, but may also trigger stromal alterations integral to the development of chronic GVHD.

Models for chronic cutaneous GVHD will be of paramount importance to better understand the pathogenesis of this disabling form of the disease. The laboratory of Gilliam and coworkers has made major strides in this regard. For example, Zhang et al. (109) have recently characterized the sequential inflammatory events that result in development of sclerodermatous skin changes, lung fibrosis, and upregulation of collagen mRNA expression in a relevant murine model. They found that male donor T cells (defined by PCR analysis of Y-chromosome sequences) increase at early timepoints post-transplantation in skin of female recipients. Monocyte/macrophages and T cells showed upregulation of MHC class II molecules and class A scavenger receptors consistent with active antigen presentation early in disease. Moreover, upregulated cutaneous TGFβ1 mRNA and elevated C-C chemokines preceded the development of skin and lung fibrosis. Accordingly, TGFβ1–producing donor mononuclear cells and C-C chemokines may be potential critical effectors in the development of sclerodermoid changes. In addition, antibodies to TGFβ would appear to ameliorate chronic GVHD in murine models by blocking influx of monocyte/macrophages and T cells and by blocking collagen synthesis at the level of this potentially critical cytokine.

V. CONCLUSIONS AND FUTURE DIRECTIONS

GVHD in its acute and chronic forms is all too often clinically protean, histologically deceptive, and pathogenically mysterious. As we learn more about its diagnosis and pathobiology, the complexity of this disorder seems to paradoxically increase. Yet enormous strides have been accomplished at the molecular level in an effort to tease out pathways that may themselves be targets for therapeutic intervention. For example, synthetic peptides crafted by computer modeling that bind to and block specific molecular interactions involving the T-cell receptor have shown promise in experimental systems (110). Inhibition of mast-cell activity, cytokines, and the adhesion molecules they induce are known to influence effector cell homing (111,112) and thus represent additional strategies for disease amelioration. Approaches to alter molecular interactions that result in apoptotic targeting while preserving the ability of donor T cells to kill residual leukemic cells are under active exploration, and early results are encouraging (90). All of these initiatives depend upon more sensitive and specific modalities to diagnose disease and assess its activity, particularly in major target organs such as the skin. Recognition of the three-step pathogenesis of GVHD (allostimulation, homing, and targeting) and the mechanisms responsible for these progressive phases is integral to the identification of novel strategies to interrupt the relevant disease pathways at molecular levels. Because acute and chronic GVHD are possible paradigms for a number of potentially related and more common skin diseases (e.g., erythema multiforme and Stevens-Johnson syndrome, lichen planus, scleroderma), the insight gained from the study of GVHD at the clinical and experimental levels is likely to have implications that reach far beyond the population of patients receiving allogeneic SCT.

ACKNOWLEDGMENTS

This work was supported by grants CA40538, CA77401, CA55593, and AI45009 from the National Cancer Institute of the NIH. Dr. Anita Gilliam, in serving as coauthor of the previous version of this chapter, has provided valuable input and information that will benefit this and the future versions that are yet to be written.

REFERENCES

1. Barnes DWH, Loutit JF. Spleen protection: the cellular hypothesis. In: Bacq ZM, ed. Radiobiology Symposium. Butterworth: London, 1955:134–135.
2. Gluckman E, Devergie A, Sohier J, Saurat J, Saurat JH. Graft-versus-host disease in recipients of syngeneic bone marrow. Lancet 1980; 1:253–254.
3. Tokime K, Isoda K, Yamanaka K, Mizutani H. A case of acute graft versus host disease following autologous peripheral blood stem cell transplantation. J Dermatol 2000; 27:446–449.
4. Greenbaum BH. Transfusion-associated graft-versus-host disease: historical perspectives, incidence, and current use of irradiated blood products. J Clin Oncol 1991; 9:1889–1902.
5. Hull RJ, Bray RA, Hillyer C, Swerlick RA. Transfusion-associated chronic cutaneous graft-versus-host disease. J Am Acad Dermatol 1995; 33:327–332.
6. Schmuth M, Vogel W, Weinlich G, Margreiter R, Fritsch P, Sepp N. Cutaneous lesions as the presenting sign of acute graft-versus-host disease following liver transplantation. Br J Hematol 1999; 141:779–780.
7. Takatsuka H, Takemoto Y, Yamada S, Mori A, Wada H, Fujimori Y, Okamoto T, Kanamaru A, Kakishita E. Similarity between eruptions induced by sulfhydryl drugs and acute cutaneous graft-versus-host disease after bone marrow transplantation. Hematology 2002; 7:55–57.
8. Esteban JM, Somolo G. Skin biopsy in allogeneic and autologous bone marrow transplant patients: a histologic and immunohistochemical study and review of the literature. Mod Pathol 1995; 8:59–64.
9. Sale GE, Shulman HM, Gallucci BB, Thomas ED. Young rete ridge keratinocytes are preferred targets in cutaneous graft-versus-host disease. Am J Pathol 1985; 118:278–287.
10. Zhou Y, Barnett MJ, Rivers JK. Clinical significance of skin biopsies in the diagnosis and management of graft-versus-host disease in early post allogeneic bone marrow transplantation. Arch Dermatol 2000; 136:717–721.
11. Vavricka SR, Halter J, Furrer K, Wolfensberger U, Schanz U. Contrast media triggering cutaneous graft-versus-host disease. Bone Marrow Transplant 2002; 29:899–901.

12. Boström L, Ringdén O, Sundberg B, Ljungman P, Linde A, Nilsson B. Pretransplantation herpes virus serology and chronic graft-versus-host disease. Bone Marrow Transplant 1989; 4:547–552.
13. Ljungman P, Niederwieser D, Pepe MS, Longton G, Storb R, Meyers JD. Cytomegalovirus infection after bone marrow transplantation for aplastic anemia. Bone Marrow Transplant 1990; 6:295–300.
14. Villada G, Roujeau J, Cordonnier C, Bagot M, Kuentz M, Wechsler J, Vernant JP. Toxic epidermal necrolysis after bone marrow transplantation; study of nine cases. J Am Acad Dermatol 1990; 23:870–875.
15. Sullivan KM, Deeg HJ, Sanders J, Klosterman A, Amos D, Shulman H, Sale G, Martin P, Witherspoon R, Appelbaum F, et al. Hyperacute graft-versus-host disease in patients not given immunosuppression after allogeneic marrow transplantation. Blood 1986; 67:1172–1175.
16. Aractingi S, Socié G, Devergie A, Dubertret L, Glukman E. Localized scleroderma-like lesions on the legs in bone marrow transplant recipients: association with polyneuropathy in the same distribution. Br J Dermatol 1993; 129:201–203.
17. Nagler A, Goldenhersh MA, Levi-Schaffer F, Bystryn JC, Klaus SN. Total leucoderma: a rare manifestation of cutaneous chronic graft-versus-host disease. Br J Dermatol 1996; 134:780–783.
18. Ameen M, Russell-Jones R. Macroscopic and microscopic mucinosis in chronic sclerodermoid graft-versus-host disease. Br J Dermatol 2000; 142:529–532.
19. Janin A, Socié G, Devergie A, Aractingi S, Esperou H, Verola O, Gluckman E. Fasciitis in chronic graft-versus-host disease. A clinicopathologic study of 14 cases. Ann Intern Med 1994; 120:993–998.
20. Schubert MM, Sullivan KM, Morton TH, Izutsu KT, Peterson DE, Flournoy N, Truelove EL, Sale GE, Buckner CD, Storb R, et al. Oral manifestations of chronic graft-versus-host disease. Arch Intern Med 1984; 144:1591–1595.
21. Gratwohl AA, Moutsopoulous HM, Chused TM, Akizuki M, Wolf RO, Sweet JB, Deisseroth AB. Sjögren-type syndrome after allogeneic bone marrow transplantation. Ann Intern Med 1977; 87:703–706.
22. Tichelli A, Duell T, Weiss M, Socie G, Ljungman P, Cohen A, vanLint M, Gratwohl A, Kolb HJ. Late onset keratoconjunctivitis sicca syndrome after bone marrow transplantation: incidence and risk factors. Bone Marrow Transplant 1996; 17:1105–1111.
23. Corson SL, Sullivan K, Batzer F, August C, Storb R, Thomas ED. Gynecologic manifestations of chronic graft-versus-host disease. Obstet Gynecol 1992; 60:448–492.
24. Karni M, Kanda Y, Sasaki M, Takeda N, Tanaka Y, Saito T, Ogawa S, Honda H, Ohba S, Mitani K, Hirai H, Yazaki Y. Phimosis as a manifestation of chronic graft-versus-host disease after allogeneic bone marrow transplantation. Bone Marrow Transplant 1998; 21:721–728.
25. Grigg AP, Underhill C, Russell J, Sale G. Peyronie's disease as a complication of chronic graft versus host disease. Hematology 2002; 7:165–168.
26. Gilliam A, Whitaker-Menezes, Korngold R, Murphy GF. Apoptosis is the predominant form of epithelial target cell injury in acute experimental graft-versus-host disease. J Invest Dermatol 1996; 107:377–383.
27. Murphy GF, Whitaker D, Sprent J, Korngold R. Characterization of target injury of murine acute graft-versus-host disease directed to multiple minor histocompatibility antigens elicited by either CD4+ or CD8+ effector cells. Am J Pathol 1991; 138:983–990.
28. Ferrara J, Guillen FJ, Sleckman B, Burakoff SJ, Murphy GF. Cutaneous acute graft-versus-host disease to minor histocompatibility antigens in a murine model: histologic analysis and correlation to clinical disease. J Invest Dermatol 1986; 86:371–375.
29. Lerner KG, Kao GF, Storb R, Buckner CD, Clift RA, Thomas ED. Histopathology of graft-vs.-host reaction (GvHR) in human recipients of marrow from HL-A-matched sibling donors. Transplant Proc 1974; 6:367–371.

30. Massi D, Franchi A, Pimpinelli N, Laszlo D, Bosi A, Santucci M. A reappraisal of the histopathologic criteria for the diagnosis of cutaneous allogeneic acute graft-vs-host disease. Am J Clin Pathol 1999; 112:791–800.
31. Darmstadt GL, Donnenberg AD, Vogelsang GB, Farmer ER, Horn TD. Clinical, laboratory, and histopathologic indicators of the development of progressive acute graft-versus-host disease. J Invest Dermatol 1992; 99:397–402.
32. Dilday BR, Smoller BR. Intracytoplasmic bile pigment in skin biopsy specimens for graft-versus-host disease versus erythema multiforme. Mod Pathol 1998; 11:1005–1009.
33. Osawa J, Kitamura K, Saito S, Ikezawa Z, Nakajima H. Immunohistochemical study of graft-versus-host reaction (GVHR)-type drug eruptions. J Dermatol 1994; 21:25–30.
34. Hitchins L, Fucich LF, Freeman SM, Millikan LE, Marrogi AJ. Immunophenotyping as a diagnostic tool to differentiate lichen planus from chronic graft-versus-host disease: diagnostic observations on two patients. J Invest Med 1997; 45:463–468.
35. Hayakawa S, Chishima F, Sakata H, Fujii K, Ohtani K, Kurashina K, Hayakawa J, Suzuki K, Nakabayashi H, Esumi M. A rapid molecular diagnosis of posttransfusion graft-versus-host disease by polymerase chain reaction. Transfusion 1993; 33:413–417.
36. Messadi DV, Pober JS, Fiers W, Gimbrone MA, Murphy GF. Induction of an activation antigen on post-capillary venular endothelium in human skin organ culture. J Immunol 1987; 139:1557–1562.
37. Messadi DV, Pober JS, Murphy GF. Effects of recombinant gamma-interferon on HLA-DR and DQ expression by skin cells in short-term organ culture. Lab Invest 1988; 58:61–67.
38. Sviland L, Dickinson AM. A human skin explant model for predicting graft-versus-host disease following marrow transplantation. J Clin Pathol 1999; 52:910–913.
39. Sviland L, Hromadnikova I, Sedlacek P, Cermakova M, Holler E, Eissner G, Schulz U, Kolb HJ, Jackson G, Wang XN, Dickinson AM. Histological correlation between different centers using the skin explant model to predict graft-versus-host disease following bone marrow transplantation. Human Immunol 2001; 62:1277–1281.
40. Jarvis M, Schulz U, Dickinson AM, Sviland L, Jackson G, Konur A, Wang XN, Hromadnikova I, Kolb HJ, Eissner G, Holler E. The detection of apoptosis in a human in vitro skin explant assay for graft versus host reactions. J Clin Pathol 2002; 55:127–132.
41. Christofidou-Solomidou M, Albelda SM, Bennett FC, Murphy GF. Experimental production and modulation of human cytotoxic dermatitis in human-murine chimeras. Am J Pathol 1997; 150:631–639.
42. Gale RP. Graft-versus-host disease. Immunol Rev 1985; 88:1193–1214.
43. Santos GW, Hess AD, Vogelsamg GB. Graft-versus-host reactions and disease. Immunol Rev 1985; 88:169–192.
44. Ferrara J, Deeg HJ. Graft-versus-host disease. N Engl J Med 1991; 324:667–674.
45. Murai M, Yoneyama H, Ezaki T, Suematsu M, Terashima Y, Harada A, Asakura H, Ishikawa H, Matsushima K. Peyer's patch is the essential site in initiating murine acute and lethal graft-versus-host reaction. Nature Immunol 2003; 4:154–160.
46. Kernan NA. T-cell depletion for prevention of graft-versus-host disease. In: Forman SJ, Thomas ED, eds. Bone Marrow Transplantation. Cambridge, MA: Blackwell Scientific; 1994:124–135.
47. Friedman TM, Statton D, Jones SC, Berger MA, Murphy GF, Korngold R. Vb spectratype analysis reveals heterogeneity of CD4+ T-cell responses to minor histocompatibility antigens involved in graft-versus-host disease: correlations with epithelial tissue infiltrate. Biol Blood Bone Marrow Transplant 2001; 7:2–13.
48. Krenger W, Hill GR, Ferrara JLM. Cytokine cascades in acute graft-versus-host disease. Transplantation 1997; 64:553–558.
49. Ferrara JL. Cytokine dysregulation as a mechanism of graft versus host disease. Curr Opin Immunol 1993; 5(5):794–799.

50. Jadus MR, Wepsic HT. The role of cytokines in graft-vs-host reactions and disease. Bone Marrow Transplant 1992; 10:1–14.
51. Abhyanker S, Gilliland DG, Ferrara JL. Interleukin-1 is a critical effector molecule during cytokine dysregulation in graft-vs-host disease to minor histocompatibility antigens. Transplantation 1993; 56:1518–1523.
52. Ferrara JLM, Abhyankar S, Gilliland DG. Cytokine storm of graft-vs-host disease: a critical effector role for interleukin-1. Transplant Proc 1993; 25:1216–1217.
53. McCarthy PL, Abhyankar S, Neben S, et al. Inhibition of interleukin-1 receptor antagonist prevents graft-vs-host disease. Blood 1991; 78:1915–1918.
54. Volc-Platzer B, Stingl G. Cutaneous graft-vs.-host disease. In: Burakoff SJ, Deeg HJ, Ferrara J, Atkinson K, eds. Graft-vs.-Host Disease. New York: Marcel Dekker, 1990:245–254.
55. Piguet PF, Grau GE, Allet B, Vassalli P. Tumor necrosis factor/cochectin is an effector of skin and gut lesions of the acute phase of graft-versus-host disease. J Exp Med 1987; 166:1280–1289.
56. Piguet PF. Tumor necrosis factor and graft-vs.-host disease. In: Burakoff SJ, Deeg HJ, Ferrara J, Atkinson K, eds. Graft-vs.-Host Disease. New York: Marcel Dekker, 1990:255–276.
57. Walsh LJ, Murphy GF. Role of adhesion molecules in cutaneous inflammation and neoplasia (review). J Cutan Pathol 1992; 19:161–171.
58. Gordon JR, Galli SJ. Promotion of mouse fibroblast collagen gene expression by mast cells stimulated via the FceRI: role for mast cell-derived transforming growth factor β and tumor necrosis factor α. J Exp Med 1994; 180:2027–2037.
59. Reed JA, Albino AP, McNutt NS. Human cutaneous mast cells express basic fibroblast growth factor. Lab Invest 1995; 72:215–222.
60. Ferrara J, Marion A, McIntyre JF, Murphy GF, Burakoff SJ. Amelioration of acute graft-versus-host disease to minor histocompatibility antigens by in vivo administration of anti-interleukin 2 receptor antibody. J Immunol 1986; 87:1874–1877.
61. Murphy GF, Sueki H, Teuscher C, Whitaker D, Korngold R. Role of mast cells in early epithelial target cell injury in experimental acute graft-vs-host disease. J Invest Dermatol. 1994; 102:451–461.
62. Dvorak HF, Mihm MC, Dvorak AM. Morphology of delayed-type hypersensitivity reaction in man. J Invest Dermatol 1976; 67:391–401.
63. Dvorak AM, Mihm MC, Dvorak HF. Morphology of delayed-type hypersensitivity reactions in man: II. Ultrastructural alteration affecting the microvasculature and the tissue mast cells. Lab Invest 1976; 1976:179–191.
64. Springer TA. Adhesion receptors of the immune system. Nature 1990; 346:425–434.
65. Springer TA. Traffic signals for lymphocyte recirculation and leukocyte emigration: the multistep paradigm. Cell 1994; 76:301–314.
66. Lasky LA. Selectins: Interpreters of cell-specific carbohydrate information during inflammation. Science 1992; 258:964–969.
67. Picker LJ. Control of lymphocyte homing. Curr Opin Immunol 1994; 6:349–405.
68. Askenase PW. Delayed-type hypersensitivity recruitment of T-cell subsets via antigen-specific non-IgE factors or IgE antibodies: relevance to asthma, autoimmunity and immune responses to tumors and parasites. Chem Immunol 1992; 54:166–211.
69. Levi-Schaffer F, Mekori YA, Segal V, Claman HN. Histamine release from mouse and rat mast cells cultured with supernatants from chromic murine graft-vs-host splenocytes. Cell Immunol 1990; 127:146–158.
70. Shen N, Ffrench P, Guyotat D, Ffrench M, et al. Expression of adhesion molecules in endothelial cells during allogeneic bone marrow transplantation. Eur J Haematol 1994; 52:296–301.
71. Wayner EA, Gil SG, Murphy GF, et al. Epiligrin, a component of epithelial basement membranes, is an adhesive ligand for $\alpha E\beta 7$ positive T cell lymphocytes. J Cell Biol 1993; 121:1141–1152.

72. Simonitsch I, Volc-Platzer B, Mosberger I, Radaszkicwicz T. Expression of monoclonal anti-body HML-1-defined $\alpha E\beta 7$ integrin in cutaneous T cell lymphoma. Am J Pathol 1994; 145:1148–1158.
73. Cepek KL. Adhesion between epithelial cells and T lymphocytes mediated by E-cadherin and $\alpha E\beta 7$ integrin. Nature 1994; 372:190–193.
74. Kim JC, Whitaker-Menezes D, Deguchi M, Adair BS, Korngold R, Murphy GF. Novel expression of vascular cell adhesion molecule-1 (CD106) by squamous epithelium in experimental acute graft-versus-host disease. Am J Pathol 2002; 161:763–770.
75. Guillén FJ, Ferrara J, Hancock WW, et al. Acute cutaneous graft-versus-host disease to minor histocompatibility antigens in a murine model: evidence that large granular lymphocytes are effector cells in the immune response. Lab Invest 1996; 55:35–42.
76. Ferrara JL, Guillén FJ, van Dijken PJ, et al. Evidence that large granular lymphocytes of donor origin mediate acute graft-versus-host disease. Transplantation 1989; 47:50–54.
77. Hess AD. Syngeneic graft-vs.-host disease. In: Burakoff SJ, Deeg HJ, Ferrara J, Atkinson K, eds. Graft-vs.-Host Disease. New York: Marcel Dekker, 1990:95–107.
78. Korngold R, Sprent J. Lethal graft-vs-host disease following bone marrow transplantation across minor histocompatibility barriers in mice: prevention by removing mature T cells from marrow. J Exp Med 1978; 148:1687–1698.
79. Korngold R. Biology of graft-versus-host disease. Am J Pediatr Hematol/Oncol 1993; 15:18.
80. Berke G. The binding and lysis of target cells by cytotoxic lymphocytes: molecular and cellular aspects. Annu Rev Immunol 1994; 12:735–773.
81. Squier MKT, Cohen JJ. Cell-mediated cytotoxic mechanisms. Curr Opin Immunol 1994; 6:447–452.
82. Sale GE, Anderson P, Browne M, Myerson D. Evidence of cytotoxic T-cell destruction of epidermal cells in human graft-versus-host disease: immunohistology with monoclonal antibody TIA-1. Arch Pathol Lab Med 1992; 116:622–625.
83. Sale GE, Beauchamp M, Myerson D. Immunohistologic staining of cytotoxic T and NK cells in formalin-fixed paraffin-embedded tissue using microwave TIA-1 antigen retrieval. Transplantation 1994; 57:287–289.
84. Kägi D, Vignaux F, Ledermann B, et al. Fas and perforin pathways as major mechanisms of T cell-mediated cytotoxicity. Science 1994; 265:528–530.
85. Itoh N, Yonehara S, Ishii A, et al. The polypeptide encoded by the cDNA for human cell surface antigen Fas can mediate apoptosis. Cell 1991; 66:233–243.
86. Sayama K, Yonehara S, Watanabe Y, Miki Y. Expression of Fas antigen on keratinocytes in vivo and induction of apoptosis in cultured keratinocytes. J Invest Dermatol 1994; 103:330–334.
87. Antin JH, Ferrara JLM. Cytokine dysregulation and acute graft-versus-host disease. Blood 1992; 80:2964–2968.
88. Nickoloff BJ, Naidu Y. Pertubation of epidermal barrier function correlates with initiation of cytokine cascade in human skin. J Am Acad Dermatol 1994; 30:535–546.
89. Groves RW, Sherman L, Mizutani H, et al. Detection of interleukin-1 receptors in human epidermis: induction of the type II receptor after organ culture and in psoriasis. Am J Pathol 1994; 145:1048–1056.
90. Schmaltz C, Alpdogan O, Kappel BJ, Muriglan SJ, Rotolo JA, Ongchin J, Willis LM, Greenberg AS, Eng JM, Crowford JM, Murphy GF, Yagita, Wlaczak H, Peschon JJ, van den Brink MRM. T cells require TRAIL for optimal graft-versus-host activity. Nature Med 2002; 8:1433–1437.
91. van den Brink MRM, Moore E, Horndasch KJ, Crawford JM, Hoffman J, Murphy GF, Burakoff SJ. Fas-deficient lpr mice are more susceptible to graft-versus-host disease. J Immunol 2000; 164:469–480.
92. van den Brink MRM, Moore E, Horndasch K, Crawford J, Murphy G, Burakoff S. Fas ligand-deficient gld mice are more susceptible to graft-versus-host disease. Transplantation 2000; 70:184–191.

93. Schmaltz C, Alpdogan O, Horndasch KJ, Muriglan SJ, Kappel BJ, Teschima T, Ferrara JL, Burakoff SJ. Differential use of Fas ligand and perforin cytotoxic pathways by donor T cells in graft-versus-host disease and graft-versus-leukemia effect. Blood 2001; 97:2886–2895.
94. Hsieh MH, Korngold R. Differential use of FasL- and perforin-mediated cytolytic mechanisms by T-cell subsets in graft-versus-myeloid leukemia responses. Blood 2000; 96:1047–1055.
95. Shulman HM, Sale GE. Pathology of acute and chronic cutaneous GVHD. In: Sale GE, Shulman WM, eds. The Pathology of Bone Marrow Transplantation. New York: Masson Publ., 1984:40–76.
96. LeBoit PE. Subacute radiation dermatitis: a histologic imitator of acute cutaneous graft-versus-host disease. J Am Acad Dermatol 1989; 20:236–241.
97. Teshima T, Ordmann R, Reddy P, Gagin P, Liu C, Cooke KR, Ferrara JLM. Acute graft-versus-host disease does not require alloantigen expression on host epithelium. Nature Med 2002; 8:575–581.
98. Korngold R, Sprent J. Features of T cells causing H2-restricted lethal graft-versus-host disease across minor histocompatibility barriers. J Exp Med 1982; 155:872–883.
99. Murphy GF, Merot Y, Tong AKF, Mihm Jr MC. Depletion and repopulation of epidermal dendritic cells after allogeneic bone marrow transplantation in humans. J Invest Dermatol 1985; 84:210–214.
100. Murphy GF, Messadi D, Fonferko E, Hancock WW. Phenotypic transformation of macrophages to Langerhans cells in the skin. Am J Pathol 1986; 123:401–406.
101. Sueki H, Korngold R, Whitaker-Menezes D, Murphy GF. Changes in the ultrastructure of epidermal Langerhans/indeterminate cells in experimental acute graft-versus-host disease. Showa J Med Sci 1998; 9:103–108.
102. Artlett CM, Smith JB, Jimenez SA. Identification of fetal DNA and cells in skin lesions from women with systemic sclerosis. N Engl J Med 1998; 338:1186–1191.
103. Claman HN. Mast cells, T cells and abnormal fibrosis. Immunol Today 1985; 6:192–196.
104. Claman HN. Mast cells and fibrosis: the relevance to scleroderma. Rheum Dis Clin North Am 1990; 16:141–151.
105. Choi KL, Claman HN. Mast cells in murine graft-versus-host disease: a model of immunologically induced fibrosis. Immunol Ser 1989; 46:641–651.
106. Hawkins RA, Claman HN, Clark RAF, Steigerwald JC. Increased dermal mast cell populations in progressive systemic sclerosis: a link in chronic fibrosis? Ann Intern Med 1985; 102:182–186.
107. Sueki H, Whitaker D, Buchsbaum M, Murphy GF. Novel interactions between dermal dendrocytes and mast cells in human skin. Implications for hemostasis and matrix repair (see comments). Lab Invest 1993; 69:160–172.
108. Yoo YH, Whitaker-Menezes D, Korngold R, Murphy GF. Dermal dendrocytes participate in the cellular pathology of experimental acute graft-versus-host disease. J Cutan Pathol 1998; 25:426–434.
109. Zhang Y, McCormick LL, Desai SR, Wu C, Gilliam AC. Murine sclerodermatous graft-versus-host disease, a model for human scleroderma: cutaneous cytokines, chemokines, and immune cell activation. J Immunol 2002; 168:3088–3098.
110. Townsend RM, Briggs C, Marini JC, Murphy GF, Korngold R. Inhibitory effect of a CD4-CDR3 peptide analog on graft-versus-host disease across a major histocompatibility complex-haploidentical barrier. Blood 1996; 88(8):3038–3047.
111. Korngold R, Jameson BA, McDonnell JM, Leighton C, Sutton BJ, Gould HJ, Murphy GF. Peptide analogs that inhibit IgE-Fc epsilon RI alpha interactions ameliorate the development of lethal graft-versus-host disease. Biol Blood & Marrow Transplant 1997; 3(4):187–193.
112. Yan, H-C, Juhasz I, Pilewski J, Murphy GF, Herlyn M, Albelda SM. Human/SCID mouse chimeras: an experimental in vivo model system to study the regulation of human endothelial cell-leukocyte adhesion molecules. J Clin Invest 1993; 91:986–996.

9

Graft-vs.-Host Disease of the Liver

CHEN LIU and JAMES M. CRAWFORD

University of Florida College of Medicine, Gainesville, Florida, U.S.A.

I. INTRODUCTION

Hematopoietic stem cell transplantation (SCT) subjects the liver to numerous potential insults. The types of injury fall into the broad categories of infection, toxic damage due to medication, recurrence of the primary disease, and immunologically mediated injury (1) (Table 1). Liver toxicity is commonly attributed to the cytoreductive therapy used during induction for SCT and may take the form of generalized impairment of liver function in the immediate posttransplantation period (2), such as venoocclusive disease (VOD), or nodular regenerative hyperplasia months later (3,4). Systemic infections involving the liver or infections by hepatotrophic viruses are ever-present threats. Emerging from this morass of potential problems is the clinical syndrome of graft-vs.-host disease (GVHD), featuring, to varying degrees, skin rashes, diarrhea, weight loss, and predominantly cholestatic liver dysfunction. GVHD involving the liver is a frequent complication after SCT, and this chapter will address features of this form of hepatic dysfunction.

II. CLINICAL SYNDROMES

A. Acute GVHD

The conditions necessary for the development of GVHD (the infusion of immunocompetent cells, histocompatibility difference between donor and the recipient, and the inability of the recipient to destroy donor lymphocytes) are met most frequently in the setting of allogeneic hematopoietic SCT. The likelihood of developing GVHD increases with the degree of histoincompatibility between donor and recipient (5). It needs to be mentioned that a GVHD-like reaction can also occur in autologous stem cell transplantation, although the underlying mechanisms are not clear (6). Clinical GVHD has been separated into

Table 1 Differential Diagnosis of Hepatic Dysfunction in Bone Marrow
Transplantation Patients

Timing	Common causes	Less common causes
Pretransplant	Viral hepatitis	Drug toxicity
	Malignancy	Venoocclusive disease
		Opportunistic infection
		Biliary tract disease
Day 0–25	Venoocclusive disease	Hyperacute or acute GVHD
	Drug toxicity	Opportunistic infection
		Nodular regenerative hyperplasia
		Total parenteral nutrition toxicity
		Cholestasis of sepsis
		Acalculous cholecystitis
Day 25–100	Acute GVHD	Total parenteral nutrition toxicity
	Venoocclusive disease	Nodular regenerative hyperplasia
	Opportunistic infections	
	Drug toxicity	
Day >100	Chronic GVHD	Opportunistic infections
	Viral hepatitis	Drug toxicity
	(hepatotrophic)	Epstein-Barr virus–induced
		lymphoproliferative disorder

hyperacute, acute, and chronic forms based on how long after SCT the symptoms occur (7). Hyperacute GVHD is a severe fulminant form of acute GVHD that is frequently fatal and occurs in the first few weeks after SCT (8). It is an extremely rare condition due to GVHD prophylaxis and will not be discussed further. Acute GVHD usually develops within 7–50 days after SCT, and chronic GVHD usually evolves 100 or more days after transplantation. Although rare, hepatic GVHD may also occur following blood transfusions or transplantation of organs containing abundant lymphoid tissue, particularly the small intestine, lung, or liver (9–11).

GVHD-related liver dysfunction may develop within days, but more commonly, abnormalities are encountered 2–4 weeks after SCT. Onset of liver GVHD is heralded by a gradual rise in serum levels of both direct and indirect bilirubin and in serum alkaline phosphatase and transaminases (SGOT/AST, SGPT/ALT). Elevations of bilirubin may be mild or may reach 10–20 times normal. Values for some serum enzymes (γ-glutamyl transpeptidase and alkaline phosphatase) may be elevated even when others (alanine aminotransferase, aspartate aminotransferase) remain within the normal range. In more severe cases, clinically evident jaundice and icterus develop and all serum liver enzymes are elevated. Hepatomegaly may occur and is usually without pain. The incidence of acute GVHD ranges from 10% to more than 80% of SCT recipients, depending on the degree of histoincompatibility, number of T cells in the graft, patient age (incidence increases with age), and immunoprophylactic regimen (5,12). Clinical symptomatology, attributable in part to hepatic dysfunction, includes fatigue, easy bruising, and onset of confusion.

The severity of acute GVHD is graded according to the extent of organ involvement (2,13,14). In mild GVHD (grade 1), symptoms are limited to the skin; hepatic involvement is subclinical, with serum bilirubin <3 mg/dL. In moderate GVHD (grade 2), skin rash, diarrhea, and jaundice may be evident, and serum bilirubin is in the 3–6 mg/dL range.

With severe GVHD (grade 3), generalized erythroderma and severe diarrhea predominate. Jaundice is more marked, with serum bilirubin values in excess of 6 mg/dL. With the progression of disease to life-threatening grade 4 GVHD, coagulopathy and a bleeding diathesis develop, along with other features of hepatic failure including encephalopathy. Survival is directly related to the clinical severity, and the proximate causes of death are multifactorial.

B.   Chronic GVHD

Chronic GVHD has traditionally been defined as a syndrome arising after day 100 and may arise de novo, after a disease-free interval following an episode of acute GVHD (quiescent) or as a continuous extension of acute GVHD (progressive) (5). It can significantly affect the quality of life of long-term survivors and also lead to mortality (see Chapter 20) (15). Since the syndrome may occasionally develop as early as 40–50 days after transplantation, the time frames for acute and chronic GVHD can overlap. Unlike acute GVHD, in which skin, gut, and liver symptoms predominate, chronic GVHD may involve a much wider ranges of organ systems. Chronic GVHD can include the skin (systemic sclerosis), ductal epithelia of salivary and lacrimal glands (Sjögren's syndrome), intestine and oral mucosa, and the liver, lymph nodes, lungs, and musculoskeletal system.

The incidence of chronic GVHD in allogeneic bone marrow transplant recipients ranges from 30 to 60% and correlates with the occurrence of acute GVHD. This syndrome is the most common cause of cholestatic liver disease (hyperbilirubinemia and elevated serum alkaline phosphatase) in long-term survivors of SCT and may occur in the absence of extrahepatic GVHD (16). However, since such laboratory findings are nonspecific, other causes such as cholestatic drug injury (e.g., from trimethoprim-sulfamethoxazole, azathioprine, cyclosporine), infiltrative liver disease (fungus, recurrent tumor), and extrahepatic biliary disease (stones, infection) must also be considered. Since significant immunosuppression occurs in nearly all SCT recipients, these patients are highly susceptible to bacterial, viral, fungal, and other opportunistic infections. In particular, chronic GVHD and viral hepatitis may coexist, and liver biopsy may be necessary to distinguish between the etiologies (see below).

Limited chronic GVHD consists of localized skin disease and/or mild liver dysfunction (mild hyperbilirubinemia and elevations in serum alkaline phosphatase). The designation of severe chronic GVHD is reserved for patients with generalized skin involvement or liver dysfunction with one of the following: severe chronic hepatitis (confirmed by histology; see below); ocular, salivary, or oral mucosal involvement; or disease involvement of other target organs (17).

An unusual form of hepatic GVHD has been recently reported. Patients with chronic GVHD of the liver exhibited significantly elevated transaminases and significant parenchymal damage on liver biopsy, resembling acute viral hepatitis (18–20). However, the characteristic bile duct destructive features of chronic GVHD were still present. Therefore liver biopsy plays an important role in accurate diagnosis of long-term survivors of stem cell transplantation with evidence of hepatic dysfunction.

III.   PATHOLOGY

The morphological diagnosis of GVHD in the liver is based on 1) identifying a constellation of nonspecific alterations, of which bile duct damage and portal inflammation with mononuclear cells are the most characterized features (see Table 2), and 2) excluding other causes of liver damage. It is important to note that the characteristic histological changes secondary to GVHD may not be obvious in the early stages of the disease. For example, bile duct damage is rarely identified in the first 35 days after SCT (21), whereas isolated apoptotic cells in the liver parenchyma are the main feature. In murine models of allo-geneic SCT, the most frequent findings in the first week are apoptotic hepatocytes and mild inflammatory cell infiltrates (22,23). Modifications of SCT-conditioning regimens and widespread use of prophylaxis have not only reduced the incidence and severity of clinical hepatic GVHD, but at the same time have rendered the histological diagnosis of GVHD more difficult; the number of typical lesions has decreased while the number of nonspecific, low-grade, atypical or masked lesions has increased (24).

A. Acute GVHD

The sine qua non of acute GVHD is selective epithelial damage of target organs (skin, intestine, and liver) (7,24). In the liver, the most characterized lesion is the direct attack of donor lymphocytes on bile duct epithelial cells (7,21,25) (see Fig. 1a). Small-caliber bile ducts are most frequently involved (26). Lymphocytic infiltrates are seen surrounding, invading, and disrupting the walls of interlobular bile ducts. Lymphocytic attachment is

Table 2   Key Histological Features of Hepatic GVHD

Disease condition	Key features
Acute GVHD	Bile ducts:
	Lymphocytic infiltrate
	Nuclear pleomorphism and pyknosis
	Cytoplasmic swelling and eosinophilia
	Segmental duct disruption and loss
	Portal tracts:
	Inflammation: mononuclear cells, occasional eosinophils, endotheliitis
	Parenchyma
	Hepatocyte apoptosis
	Ballooning degeneration of hepatocytes
	Centrilobular cholestasis
Chronic GVHD	Bile ducts:
	Lymphocytic infiltrate
	Nuclear pleomorphism and pyknosis
	Cytoplasmic swelling and eosinophilia
	Segmental duct disruption and loss
	Paucity of bile ducts
	Portal tracts:
	Inflammation: mononuclear cells, occasional eosinophils
	Fibrosis (advanced cases)
	Parenchyma
	Minimal hepatocyte apoptosis
	Cholestasis

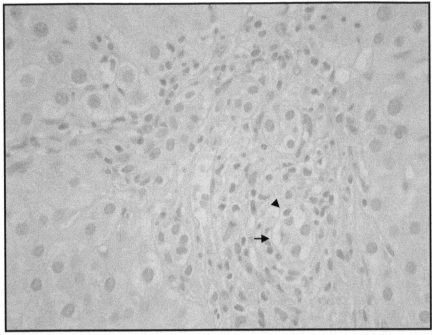

(A)

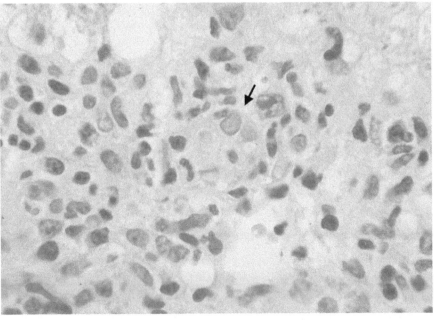

(B)

Figure 1 Acute hepatic GVHD. (A) Portal tract. A mild infiltrate is present in an expanded portal tract; the bile ducts show reactive change, epithelial vaculation is indicated by an arrow, and intraepithelial lymphocytes are present (arrowhead). (Original magnification, 400×.) (B) Interlobular bile duct. The arrow indicates a destructive bile duct. (Original magnification, 500×.)

accompanied by necrosis of bile duct epithelial cells, as evidenced by cytoplasmic vacuo-lization, nuclear pleomorphism or loss of nuclei, and sloughing of epithelial cells into the bile duct lumens (27). By electron microscopy, lymphocytes are found to be in close contact with the bile epithelial cells (28,29). Residual duct epithelial cells may become attenuated to the point of appearing squamous in character. The withered appearance of the ductal epithelium is to be distinguished from the heaped-up, reactive duct epithelial cells commonly encountered in viral hepatitis, particularly with hepatitis C virus (30). Because patients with acute GVHD are usually pancytopenic, the degree of ductal and portal tract inflammation may be quite minimal, despite obvious damage to bile ducts.

Damage to hepatocytes also occurs, giving rise to a hepatitis-like picture. The his-tological pattern of hepatocellular ballooning, intralobular lymphocytic infiltration, and hepatocyte apoptosis shown in Figure 2 may be hard to distinguish from viral infections from cytomegalovirus (CMV) and herpes virus, both of which occur in SCT patients (21). Immunostaining for peptide antigens or in situ hybridization for viral genomic material may be used to exclude the presence of viruses within tissue sections (31,32). Hepatocellular cholestasis may also be observed, particularly when intralobular bile ducts are severely damaged or lost.

An additional feature of GVHD is endotheliitis, in which portal veins and terminal hepatic veins exhibit attachment of lymphocytes and damage to the endothelium (see Fig. 3). This particular feature is a relatively specific but less sensitive marker for GVHD and is observed infrequently and generally only in more severe cases of acute

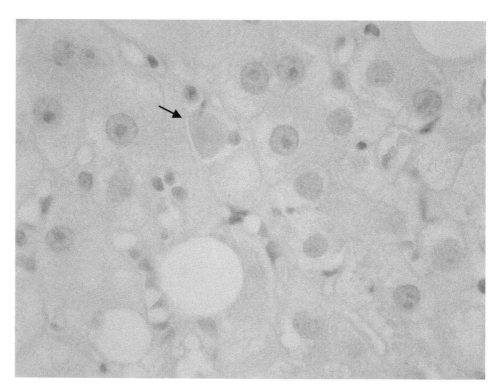

Figure 2 Acute hepatic GVHD-hepatitis–like features. A hepatocyte is undergoing apoptosis (arrow). (Original magnification, 600×.)

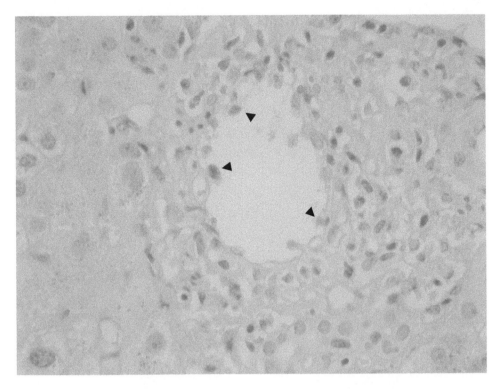

Figure 3   Acute hepatic GVHD-endotheliitis. A portal vein exhibits lumenal attachment of lymphocytes (arrowheads) and subendothelial lymphocytic infiltrates. (Original magnification, 600×.)

(and chronic) GVHD (32). Although rarely observed in other conditions, such as alcoholic and viral hepatitis, endotheliitis is a common accompaniment in solid organ liver allograft rejection. The usual vascular lesion observed during liver allograft rejection includes the subendothelial collection of lymphocytes and associated hepatocellular necrosis. By contrast, GVHD is characterized by the attachment of lymphoid cells to the luminal endothelium and the absence of hepatocellular necrosis in the immediate vicinity of venous endotheliitis.

B.   Chronic GVHD

Chronic GVHD is chiefly characterized by the portal infiltration of lymphocytes (with or without plasma cells and eosinophils) and damage to small (<45 μm in diameter), interlobular bile ducts (33). Although bile duct epithelial degeneration resembling that seen during acute GVHD may be observed, duct epithelial cells more commonly appear eosinophilic and coagulated when compared to healthy neighboring cells (see Fig. 4). As with acute GVHD, lymphocytes are seen in close point contact with bile duct epithelial cells. Loss of bile ducts tends to be a relatively late phenomenon in chronic GVHD, although it has been observed as early as 1 month after SCT (32,34). Regardless of the time frame, bile duct loss may lead to a "vanishing bile duct" syndrome or outright cirrhosis

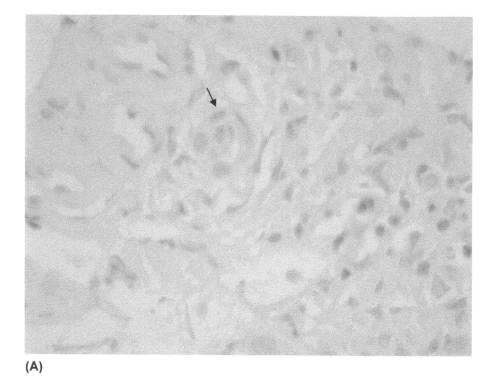

(A)

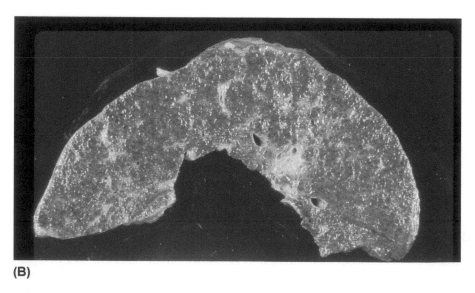

(B)

Figure 4   Chronic GVHD. (A) A portal tract is expanded, and scattered lymphocytes are present. The bile duct exhibits epithelial apoptosis (arrow) and reactive changes. (Original magnification, 400×.) (B) Gross photograph of end-stage cirrhosis due to chronic GVHD.

(35–37). Degenerative changes in the epithelium of intrahepatic periductal glands have also been described (38), but with rare exception extrahepatic biliary injury is absent (39).

Unlike acute GVHD, hepatocellular damage is minimal in most cases of chronic GVHD, except when the loss of interlobular bile ducts gives rise to progressive hepatocellular cholestasis. The entirely liver can be greenish due to severe cholestasis (Fig. 4b). In the more advanced stages of chronic GVHD, cholestasis may be so severe that it results in actual degeneration of hepatocytes, particularly along the portal tract margins. Venous endotheliitis is not a prominent feature of chronic GVHD. Noncaseating granulomata of the portal tract are encountered only rarely.

Several studies have attempted to distinguish the morphological changes of GVHD from other conditions affecting the liver after SCT. However, alterations specific to GVHD have not been consistently identified. Although extensive bile duct damage with minimal portal inflammatory changes are the most characteristic morphological findings in both acute and chronic GVHD, features of GVHD vary greatly in severity from one portal tract to another, and the damage to interlobular and septal bile ducts is segmental (7,21,40). This variability can make interpretation of liver biopsies quite difficult. The diagnosis of GVHD is reinforced by using molecular techniques to demonstrate that the inflammatory cells in the liver are of donor origin (41), although this is not part of the usual diagnostic armamentarium. Nevertheless, the biopsy diagnosis of hepatic GVHD has a sensitivity of 66%, a specificity of 91%, and a predictive value of 86% (7), and there has been little alteration in histological diagnosis of hepatic GVHD in the past 20 years.

IV. PATHOGENESIS

The liver is one of the major sites of involvement in both acute and chronic forms of GVHD (5), and hepatic disease in both humans and experimental animals is reproducibly encountered (5,42–44). Many insights into the mechanisms responsible for hepatic GVHD have been obtained primarily from the investigation of systemic disease, but the detailed molecular mechanisms of hepatic GVHD are far from completely understood. Most of the investigative efforts have focused on the function of donor T cells and allo-antigen expression on bile duct epithelial cells. Many studies have also examined the pathogenesis of bile duct lesions in chronic GVHD, as these are most characteristic of this disorder (32). The mechanisms by which hepatocytes are attacked in acute GVHD have recently been studied by a number of groups. Current concepts related to hepatic GVHD are reviewed in this section, whereas the more general immunology of GVHD is covered extensively in Chapters 1 and 2.

A.   Antigenicity of the Host Liver

Traditionally, two processes were believed to be required for immunologically mediated events: recognition of foreign antigens by immunologically competent cells and reaction to these antigens. However, very recent studies have challenged this concept. Teshima et al. (23) and Pratt et al. (45) have demonstrated that antigen-independent mechanisms can cause tissue damage in the setting of transplantation. Nevertheless, an antigen-mediated immunoreaction in the setting of GVHD still plays a central role, particularly in the induction process. One must ask, therefore, which antigens in the host liver are recognized as foreign? While the specific antigens are unknown, significant emphasis has been placed on the major histocompatibility complex (MHC) system of HLA antigens and to a lesser extent on the minor MHC antigens (46). Recently, certain adhesion molecules expressed in the liver have also been proposed to be antigens involved in hepatic GVHD (47).

In the normal liver, MHC class I antigens are constitutively expressed on the cells lining the vascular sinusoids (e.g., endothelial cells and the tissue-resident macrophages, or Kupffer cells), on bile duct epithelial cells, and to a lesser extent on hepatocytes (48). While all somatic cells express MHC class I antigens, MHC class II antigens are expressed only by Kupffer cells and by dendritic cells in the portal tracts. Under normal conditions and in SCT patients without GVHD, bile duct epithelial cells and large vessel endothelial cells express little or no detectable MHC class II antigen (49). By contrast, a consistent observation during both acute and chronic GVHD of the liver is the aberrant expression of MHC class II antigens by vascular endothelial and bile duct epithelial cells (32,50–52). Increased bile duct MHC class II antigen expression has also been noted in liver allograft rejection. In both conditions, the upregulation occurs in temporal association with the onset of immunological damage to the bile ducts and appears to be mediated by inflammatory cytokines like TNFα and IFNγ (see below). It is possible that unique biliary epithelial peptides are expressed with the MHC class II molecules, rendering bile ducts vulnerable to immunological attacks.

While class II MHC disparities are among the most potent inducers of alloimmune responses to other GVHD target organs or during graft rejection (e.g., heart and kidney) (53,54), the role of MHC class II antigens in hepatic GVHD is still controversial (53). The current data seem to suggest that alloantigen expression responsible for hepatic GVHD is multifactorial, at least in murine models. Class I MHC, class II MHC, or non–MHC-encoded antigenic differences between donor and recipient are sufficient to generate lymphocytic infiltrates in and around the walls of interlobular bile ducts (40). Frank destruction of bile ducts is most dramatic when hepatic GVHD is elicited by isolated class I MHC differences (40), although an isolated class II disparity can induce this damage in some models (55). It is possible that recognition of allogeneic MHC class I and class II antigens expressed in the liver may occur in a temporal fashion. Class I MHC antigenic differences occur ab initio, given the constitutive expression of class I molecules on the biliary epithelium. Thus, early in the course of GVHD, immunological responses may occur only to class I antigens or to non–MHC-encoded antigens. Later in the course of GVHD, enhanced class II MHC expression is encountered on bile duct epithelium and the vascular endothelium. The large number of MHC class II–restricted effector cells associated with more chronic cholangitic lesions seen in a variety of allograft models suggests that a MHC class II–restricted response to biliary and vascular antigens may be operative after hepatic GVHD has been established. Despite uncertainty about the specific hepatic antigens involved and the timing of their recognition and attack, it is likely that alloantigenic disparities contribute to the development of hepatic GVHD. However, as mentioned earlier, non–alloantigen-specific liver damage from GVHD has been demonstrated in murine models (22,23). Hence, hepatic GVHD may involve both alloantigen-dependent and independent mechanisms.

Finally, the wide variation in the incidence of GVHD and the occasional occurrence of GVHD when donor and recipient are HLA-identical have raised the issue of whether foreign antigenic influences, particularly viruses, may also contribute to a graft-vs.-host response (56,57). For example, the association between herpes infections and an increased incidence of GVHD has led to the speculation that latent viruses might act as antigenic targets for a donor immune attack (58). Alternatively, immunological imbalances produced by cytoreductive induction therapy prior to SCT may be responsible for the occurrence of GVHD in recipients of marrow from HLA-identical siblings (59).

B. Immunological Effector Cells

1. Resident Antigen-Presenting Cells

While effector lymphocytes are the most notable inflammatory cells entering the liver during GVHD, the interplay between effector cells and antigen-presenting cells (APCs) must be considered. Recent studies have shown that host APCs are necessary and sufficient to induce GVHD. Several cell types capable of antigen presentation are present in the liver. Kupffer cells are an abundant APC population in the liver, and the life span of these adherent sinusoidal cells is estimated to be between 7 days and 3 months (60). It is expected, but not proven, that the number of host Kupffer cells would be significantly reduced by SCT induction therapy. Kupffer cells are migratory cells, and repopulation of the liver by circulating monocytes is observed after allogeneic SCT (32) and in liver transplant recipients (61). This replacement can occur within one month of transplantation and is persistent (32). The role of newly acquired donor-derived Kupffer cells in the evolution of hepatic GVHD has yet to be clearly established. Experimental studies have also shown that vascular endothelial cells, which are not usually replaced after SCT, can process and display antigens (62). Expression of MHC class II antigens is also up regulated on endothelial cells after SCT, implying that these cells present host antigens to alloreactive T lymphocytes. Repopulation kinetics of portal tract dendritic cells and the role these cells play in the induction of hepatic GVHD remain unknown.

It is also possible that resident APCs are not necessary for the development of hepatic GVHD; donor T-cell populations may instead encounter host antigens and become activated at distant sites and subsequently migrate to target tissue. Recent work from Murai and colleagues supports this hypothesis and demonstrates that host Peyer's patches are critical for the generation of CTL that ultimately home to the liver and cause hepatocellular damage. Furthermore, when recruitment of donor T cells into Peyer's patches was prevented by either disruption of the gene encoding the chemokine receptor CCR5 or by blocking integrin $\alpha 4 \beta 7$: MAdCAM-1 interactions, mortality and liver enzyme elevation from GVHD was significantly reduced (63).

2. Lymphocytes

T lymphocytes dominate the inflammatory infiltrates accompanying hepatic GVHD (5,32,64) in accordance with the concept that T cells of donor origin react against recipient histocompatibility antigens (65,66). CD4+ (helper/inducer) and CD8+ (cytolytic) T cells along with natural killer (NK) cells have all been shown to contribute to GVHD of the liver (67–69). In particular, CD8+ lymphocytes are increased relative to the distribution of lymphocytes found in the livers of SCT patients without hepatic GVHD (70,71). Recent experimental data demonstrate that CCR5 expression is critical for the migration of CD8+ cells during the pathogenesis of liver injury during GVHD (72). By contrast, B lymphocytes are few in number and are present in liver GVHD only in cases where lymphoid follicular aggregates have been found.

MHC class II antigens are essential for the activation of CD4+ T cells, whereas class I antigens are required for the cytolytic activity of CD8+ cells (73). Thus, it is not surprising that in murine models, GVHD arising from class II MHC differences is mediated by CD4+ donor cells, whereas GVHD directed at class I MHC differences appears to be mediated by CD8+ donor T cells (74–76). In most instances, CD4+ donor T cells are capable of generating only inflammatory infiltrates and not bile duct destruction (66). However, in selected murine strain combinations, CD4+ helper T cells alone are sufficient to generate bile duct destruction (40,77) and do so primarily by using the Fas/FasL cytolytic pathway (78,79).

When the murine host is different at both MHC class I and class II loci, a sequence of interdependent immune reactions evolves (80,81). Injection of donor CD4+ lymphocytes alone into recipients leads to mononuclear cell infiltrates in portal tracts and bile ducts but not to destruction of bile duct epithelial cells. Injection of donor CD4+ lymphocytes followed by injection of host CD8+ lymphocytes leads to similar changes, but also precipitates destructive injury to bile ducts. Thus, alloreactive CD4+ cells can mediate initial inflammation, but progression to cytodestruction may require activation of alloreactive CD8+ cells. Cytolytic activity is then perpetuated and extended by the local release of cytokines capable of enhancing the expression of MHC class I and class II antigens on host cells (73).

Collectively, these studies suggest that hepatic GVHD is initiated by an alloresponse to host antigens. The observation that mononuclear cells isolated from the livers of mice with GVHD show increased homing to liver when these cells are injected into normal animals expressing the same MHC differences supports this hypothesis (82). In these studies homing was directed toward minor histocompatibility antigens expressed by the host biliary epithelial cells. However, the progression of injury may relate to changes in the microenvironment and activation of host cells cytodestructive mechanisms (66) rather than continued exposure to fixed antigetic differences. Furthermore, we cannot conclude that alloreactive CD4+ and CD8+ cells are the sole effector cells for bile duct damage in GVHD. On the one hand, the CD4+ and CD8+ cells used in experimental studies are not pure cell populations. Suppressor cell subsets are present in both CD4+ (ostensibly helper/inducer) and CD8 (ostensibly cytotoxic) cell preparations. On the other hand, the role of cell types such as CD22+ cells and CD45RO+ cells (which respond to recall stimulation) have yet to be explored. NK cells have no MHC restrictions, but they have been described in the cellular milieu of murine GVHD.

3. Monocytes and Macrophages

As detailed in the previous section, phenotypic analysis of leukocytes infiltrating GVHD target organs has focused on lymphocytes. However, an evolving hypothesis invokes a role for macrophages primed by gut-derived endotoxin (lipopolysaccharide) in the pathogenesis of acute GVHD (83–85). A key feature of this hypothesis is the failure of hepatic clearance of lipopolysaccharide (LPS) from splanchnic blood in the setting of intestinal injury, resulting in the spillover of LPS into the systemic circulation and generalized triggering of macrophages (84). We must ask, therefore, whether LPS-induced shock induces hepatic changes similar to those of acute GVHD and, conversely, whether cells of monocytes/macrophage lineage are found in the inflammatory infiltrates of hepatic GVHD.

Kupffer cells (of either host or donor origin) play a key role in clearing LPS released into the splanchnic circulation following gut injury. Hepatic exposure to LPS results in Kupffer cell and platelet activation, intravenous thrombosis, and neutrophil infiltration (86). Kupffer cells in turn release a whole spectrum of protein and lipid mediators, including TNFα, interleukin-1 (IL-1), IL-6, and eicosanoids (87–89). Some LPS is taken up by hepatocytes, most likely following initial clearance and modification, and usually leads to focal hepatocellular necrosis and a predominantly neutrophilic infiltration (86,88,90). The portal tracts per se are not significantly affected following acute exposure to LPS. In human liver biopsies from septic patients, the predominant features are ductular cholestasis at the margins of portal tracts and a periductal infiltrate of neutrophils (89). It would appear, therefore, that the liver in septic shock does not bear much resemblance to the liver affected by acute GVHD.

With regard to the second question, monocytes are present in hepatic GVHD. Donor lymphocytes are the predominant inflammatory cell of both acute and chronic hepatic GVHD (32,91), but cells of myeloid/histiocytic lineage also are abundant when specific immunotyping studies are performed. Interestingly, these cells are of donor origin, and murine studies indicate that such monocytes appear to home to the liver (82). Donor monocytes accumulate preferentially in hepatic portal spaces and in close proximity to interlobular bile ducts, suggesting that sensitized monocytes may contribute to bile duct destruction during GVHD. Furthermore, Cooke and coworkers have demonstrated that the responsiveness of donor cells to LPS stimulation predicts the severity of GVHD (85,92). In these studies, allogeneic SCT using LPS-resistant donors resulted in a reduction of both gut and liver GVHD. However, hepatic monocytes do not always appear to enhance local immunological function; murine livers affected by chronic GVHD contain monocytes that exhibit defective proliferation when stimulated by LPS (42). Thus, while monocytes are clearly present during both human and experimental hepatic GVHD, further studies are required to determine the specific role of these cells in this process.

4. Immunomodulation: Cytokines

Cytokines facilitate cell-to-cell communication and modulate immune responses in the local microenvironment. They promote the expression of class II MHC antigens, enhance target antigen presentation, activate neutrophils, T cells, and B cells, modulate the expression of intracellular adhesion molecules, and may also promote tissue damage by direct action. Cytokines, particularly lymphokines produced locally during the immune response, likely contribute to the immunomodulation of hepatic GVHD (47,93).

The nature and interrelationships of cytokine-mediated events have been difficult to clarify, particularly since cytokines are a continuous variable with counterbalancing actions within the microenvironment (5,94). Possible contributions of cytokines to the induction of GVHD have recently been reviewed (5,44,95) and can be summarized as follows. First, secretion of inflammatory cytokines induced by SCT conditioning regimens contributes to diffuse, nonspecific injury to host tissues immediately after transplant and also facilitates the ability of host APC to present antigen to donor T cells. Conversely, they can also stimulate natural suppressor cells that promote immunosuppression. Second, macrophages or Kupffer cells (both host or donor origin) primed by IFNγ produced by Th1 T lymphocytes can produce large amounts of cytokines that can be both cytopathic and immunosuppressive (43,49,52,96–98).

Thus there are indications that cytokines play a major role in the evolution of hepatic GVHD (5), and their influence on general immunological function is well documented. Data on the direct effect of cytokines on liver function and histology have recently been published. LPS-induced release of IL-6 from Kupffer cells can have a profound effect on hepatocellular function, as evidenced by a marked inhibition in hepatic bile salt uptake (99,100). In addition, it is likely that the liver is sensitive, at least in part, to the effects of TNFα and IL-1. TNFα released by Kupffer cells during hepatic GVHD (101,102) is also associated with cholestatic jaundice (103). Furthermore, the neutralization of TNFα and IL-1 after allogeneic SCT has been shown to significantly reduce or prevent the progression of hepatic GVHD in experimental models (23,104). In a related study, the administration of hepatocyte growth factor (HGF), a potent hepatocyte growth factor with antiapoptotic activity in a variety of epithelial cells, was found to ameliorate acute GVHD after allogeneic SCT. The protective effect of HGF was attributed in part to a reduction of IFNγ and TNFα expression in the gut and liver of allogeneic SCT recipients (105).

By contrast, using a nonirradiated allogeneic SCT model, Hattori et al. found that Fas-FasL interactions, rather than TNFα, significantly contributed to the development of liver GVHD (79). It is therefore clear that additional studies are needed before the exact mechanisms of cytokine-induced hepatic injury are elucidated.

V. DIAGNOSIS AND MANAGEMENT

A. Differential Diagnosis

The clinical abnormalities arising from GVHD of the liver are quite nonspecific. The primary conditions to be distinguished from hepatic GVHD are drug effects (including those used in cytoreductive therapy), infectious processes (viral, bacterial, and fungal), the cholestatic effects of parenteral alimentation, extrahepatic obstruction, and posttransplant lymphoproliferative disorders (Table 1).

During the first 100 days after SCT, specific clinical indicators of hepatic GVHD are largely absent. The development of ascites and hepatomegaly would favor drug toxicity or venoocclusive disease more than GVHD. Viral serologies are helpful in excluding infection by hepatotropic viruses. Hepatic infection by nonhepatotropic viruses such as herpes or cytomegalovirus or by yeast such as *Candida* may be exceedingly difficult to exclude clinically, although negative serologies and cultures are reassuring. Perhaps the most pertinent information for the diagnosis of liver GVHD is whether there are signs and symptoms of GVHD of the skin and gastrointestinal tract (7,34).

After day 100, evidence of GVHD-induced hepatic damage (e.g., persistent low grade elevation of serum bilirubin and alkaline phosphatase) may occur with or without clinically apparent GVHD in other systems (5) or may lag behind the evolution of disease in other organs (37). Cholestasis (characterized by increases in the levels of serum alkaline phosphatase, aminotransferases, and bilirubin) is a prominent feature of chronic liver GVHD and occurs in 80% of affected patients (106).

B. The Role of Liver Biopsy

In the acute situation (<100 days after transplantation), liver biopsy can play an important role in the exclusion of causes of hepatic damage, but diagnosis of hepatic GVHD itself may be quite difficult. Trans-venous biopsy via the jugular vein is the preferred approach and in experienced hands may provide satisfactory amounts of hepatic tissue. Unfortunately, biopsies from the earliest stages of hepatic GVHD (<35 days after transplantation) show hepatocyte apoptosis and portal tract inflammatory infiltrates, which are quite nonspecific. In addition, hemodynamic instability and coexisting coagulopathy in more severely affected patients often precludes the ability to obtain a liver biopsy. Thus, for these various reasons, liver biopsies in the early weeks after transplantation are not widely obtained for the diagnosis of hepatic GVHD, but may play a role if other conditions are suspected, particularly since improvement in hepatic clinical indices may lag behind those of skin and gut during treatment of acute GVHD.

In contrast, liver biopsies are an important diagnostic test in establishing a diagnosis of chronic GVHD following allogeneic SCT and the key features of hepatic GVHD described earlier serve as important discriminators (7,21). Specifically, the findings of extensive bile duct damage involving >50% of bile ducts with minimal inflammatory changes or evidence of bile duct paucity (<80% of portal tracts containing bile ducts) (107) is highly suggestive of GVHD. Although observed infrequently, the presence of endotheliitis of portal or terminal veins is even more predictive of GVHD. Parenchymal inflammation and hepatocyte necrosis, cholestasis, and secondary bile ductular proliferation may be observed, but they are not satisfactory discriminators between GVHD and other etiologies (such as drug toxicity, hepatotropic and nonhepatotropic viral infection, and bile duct obstruction). Moreover, GVHD may be accompanied by viral hepatitis or drug toxicity, producing overlapping histological features. Confident exclusion of viral causes may require in situ hybridization techniques using specific antiviral probes that are not routinely used.

Avoidance of false-positive diagnosis requires both careful correlation with clinical data and appropriate caution in invoking GVHD as the solitary diagnosis. Given the common occurrence of bile duct damage or loss in hepatic GVHD, false-negative diagnoses are less problematic than false positivity. However, the patchy distribution of the bile duct lesion may lead to their absence in biopsy specimens from patients with milder forms of the disease (108). Finally, pretransplant biopsies on all patients with evidence of preexisting liver disease will help to reduce the likelihood of misinterpreting prior liver disease as newly evolving GVHD.

C. Clinical Management

The overall prognosis of patients with acute GVHD correlates directly with the severity of the clinical disease. Severe hepatic compromise plays a major role in multisystem failure that can be seen after allogeneic SCT, and the management of deficiencies in hepatic function (e.g., in hepatic synthesis of clotting factors) is supportive in nature (109). In the case of chronic GVHD, hepatic dysfunction from progressive chronic hepatitis or cirrhosis may eventuate in hepatic failure, with ensuing demise. Since hepatic GVHD in the acute and chronic setting is secondary to systemic immune dysregulation, oral/ parenteral immunosuppressive agents would presumably have a favorable impact on hepatic function and are the mainstay of therapy.

At the present time, only one treatment modality may have specific relevance to the liver. Given that bile duct injury and ultimately destruction is a prominent feature of hepatic GVHD, attention has recently given to the maintenance of adequate hepatic bile flow (106). The exogenous bile salt ursodeoxycholate acid (also called ursodiol, UDCA) is more hydrophilic than the predominant bile salts (cholate and chenodeoxycholate) normally present in the human enterohepatic circulation. When taken orally, this supplemental bile salt promotes secretion and bile flow in individual a with cholestatic syndromes (110). This reasoning prompted Fried and coworkers to treat patients with chronic GVHD unresponsive to immunosuppressive therapy for 6 weeks with 10–15 mg/kg per day ursodiol (111). Administration of UDCA resulted in transient reductions in serum levels of alkaline phosphatase, aminotransferases, and bilirubin during therapy, but pruritus secondary to cholestasis did not improve during treatment. Importantly, no adverse effects were encountered. The ability of UDCA to prevent hepatic complications early after allogeneic SCT was recently studied in a prospective randomized trial (112). Although a smaller proportion of patients receiving UDCA developed significant elevations in serum bilirubin levels compared to controls, there was no observable difference in VOD. However, the incidence of VOD was quite low in both treatment arms and ranged from 2% to 4%. The administration of UDCA was, however, associated with a significant reduction in grades III–IV acute GVHD. Of particular note, treatment with ursodiol was well tolerated and was associated with significantly improved survival at one year and lower nonrelapse mortality.

Although liver transplantation is an important therapy for treatment of many end-stage cholestatic liver disorders, there is as yet no consensus that chronic hepatic GVHD is an indication for liver transplantation (113). This approach has been utilized only in isolated instances (114).

D. Long-Term Sequelae

Acute GVHD is a potentially reversible, or at least controllable, systemic illness, provided that prompt therapy is instituted upon its detection (115). In addition to generalized hepatic dysfunction, extensive bile duct destruction can generate a so-called "vanishing bile duct syndrome," which is the most severe form of acute liver GVHD. Evolution from acute to chronic GVHD is a worrisome problem. Although the debilitation caused by chronic GVHD can result from multiorgan involvement, the most ominous long-term hepatic condition is progressive fibrosis culminating in end-stage cirrhosis (Fig. 4b). The life-threatening problems with esophageal bleeding and hepatic encephalopathy are much like those encountered with cirrhosis from other causes.

VI. CONCLUSION

Hepatic GVHD has a major clinical impact in both the acute and chronic settings. Severe acute liver GVHD contributes to multiorgan decompensation and exceedingly high mortality rates. Chronic hepatic GVHD may lead to a progressive cholestatic syndrome with associated morbidity and potential mortality from end-stage liver disease. In both settings, exclusion of other potential causes of liver disease on clinical grounds may be exceedingly difficult. Liver biopsy, particularly in the chronically affected patient, is an important diagnostic tool. Immunosuppressive therapy can lead to improvement in hepatic function in some patients with liver GVHD. Oral bile salt therapy has been advocated as an adjunct for the treatment of cholestasis and may be efficacious in reducing acute GVHD and transplant-related mortality after allogeneic SCT. Although significant progress with respect to the diagnosis and treatment of GVHD has been made over the past decade, the detailed molecular mechanisms responsible for hepatic damage from GVHD are only partially mapped out. Further investigation of the roles of donor-derived T cells, Fas/FasL-mediated apoptosis, and cytokines secreted by immune and nonimmune cells in the liver may facilitate the design of more effective therapeutic interventions for hepatic GVHD in the future.

REFERENCES

1. Crawford JM, Ferrell L. The liver in transplantation. In: Rustgi VK, Van Thiel DH, eds. The Liver in Systemic Diseases. New York: Raven Press; 1993:337–364.
2. McDonald GB, Shulman HM, Wolford JL, Spencer GD. Liver disease after human marrow transplantation. Semin Liver Dis 1987; 7:210–229.
3. Shulman HM, Fisher LB, Schoch HG, Henne KW, McDonald GB. Veno-occlusive disease of the liver after marrow transplantation: histological correlates of clinical signs and symptoms. Hepatology 1994; 19:1171–1181.
4. Snover DC, Weisdorf S, Bloomer J, McGlave P, Weisdorf D. Nodular regenerative hyperplasia of the liver following bone marrow transplantation. Hepatology 1989; 9:443–448.
5. Ferrara JL. Pathogenesis of acute graft-versus-host disease: cytokines and cellular effectors. J Hematother Stem Cell Res 2000; 9:299–306.
6. Saunders MD, Shulman HM, Murakami CS, Chauncey TR, Bensinger WI, McDonald GB. Bile duct apoptosis and cholestasis resembling acute graft-versus-host disease after autologous hematopoietic cell transplantation. Am J Surg Pathol 2000; 24:1004–1008.
7. Snover DC, Weisdorf SA, Ramsay NK, McGlave P, Kersey JH. Hepatic graft versus host disease: a study of the predictive value of liver biopsy in diagnosis. Hepatology 1984; 4:123–130.
8. Sullivan KM, Deeg HJ, Sanders J, Klosterman A, Amos D, Shulman H, Sale G, Martin P, Witherspoon R, Appelbaum F, et al. Hyperacute graft-v-host disease in patients not given immunosuppression after allogeneic marrow transplantation. Blood 1986; 67:1172–1175.
9. Watanabe K, Yagi T, Iwagaki H, Kimura Y, Mitsuoka N, Inagaki M, Tanaka S, Tanaka N. Graft-versus-host reaction in small-bowel transplantation and possibilities for its circumvention. J Int Med Res 2001; 29:222–228.
10. Randhawa P, Yousem SA. The pathology of lung transplantation. Pathol Annu 1992; 27:247–279.
11. Demetris AJ. Immune cholangitis: liver allograft rejection and graft-versus-host disease. Mayo Clin Proc 1998; 73:367–379.
12. Ferrara JL, Deeg HJ. Graft-versus-host disease. N Engl J Med 1991; 324:667–674.
13. Ferrara J, ed. Graft-vs-Host Disease. 2nd ed. New York: Marcel Dekker, 1997.
14. Wick MR, Moore SB, Gastineau DA, Hoagland HC. Immunologic, clinical, and pathologic aspects of human graft-versus-host disease. Mayo Clin Proc 1983; 58:603–612.
15. Socie G, Stone JV, Wingard JR, Weisdorf D, Henslee-Downey PJ, Bredeson C, Cahn JY, Passweg JR, Rowlings PA, Schouten HC, Kolb HJ, Klein JP. Long-term survival and late deaths after allogeneic bone marrow transplantation. Late Effects Working Committee of the International Bone Marrow Transplant Registry. N Engl J Med 1999; 341:14–21.
16. Gholson CF, Yau JC, LeMaistre CF, Cleary KR. Steroid-responsive chronic hepatic graft-versus-host disease without extrahepatic graft-versus-host disease. Am J Gastroenterol 1989; 84:1306–1309.
17. Shulman HM, Sullivan KM, Weiden PL, McDonald GB, Striker GE, Sale GE, Hackman R, Tsoi MS, Storb R, Thomas ED. Chronic graft-versus-host syndrome in man. A long-term clinicopathologic study of 20 Seattle patients. Am J Med 1980; 69:204–217.
18. Strasser SI, Shulman HM, Flowers ME, Reddy R, Margolis DA, Prumbaum M, Seropian SE, McDonald GB. Chronic graft-versus-host disease of the liver: presentation as an acute hepatitis. Hepatology 2000; 32:1265–1271.
19. Fujii N, Takenaka K, Shinagawa K, Ikeda K, Maeda Y, Sunami K, Hiramatsu Y, Matsuo K, Ishimaru F, Niiya K, Yoshino T, Hirabayashi N, Harada M. Hepatic graft-versus-host disease presenting as an acute hepatitis after allogeneic peripheral blood stem cell transplantation. Bone Marrow Transplant 2001; 27:1007–1010.
20. Akpek G, Boitnott JK, Lee LA, Hallick JP, Torbenson M, Jacobsohn DA, Arai S, Anders V, Vogelsang GB. Hepatitic variant of graft-versus-host disease after donor lymphocyte infusion. Blood 2002; 100:3903–3907.

21. Shulman HM, Sharma P, Amos D, Fenster LF, McDonald GB. A coded histologic study of hepatic graft-versus-host disease after human bone marrow transplantation. Hepatology 1988; 8:463–470.

22. Blatter DD, Crawford JM, Ferrara JL. Nuclear magnetic resonance of hepatic graft-versus-host disease in mice. Transplantation 1990; 50:1011–1018.

23. Teshima T, Ordemann R, Reddy P, Gagin S, Liu C, Cooke KR, Ferrara JL. Acute graft-versus-host disease does not require alloantigen expression on host epithelium. Nat Med 2002; 8:575–581.

24. Hyemer B. Clinical and Diagnostic Pathology of Graft-Versus-Host Disease. New York: Springer, 2002:1–2.

25. Shulman HM, Gooley T, Dudley MD, Kofler T, Feldman R, Dwyer D, McDonald GB. Utility of transvenous liver biopsies and wedged hepatic venous pressure measurements in sixty marrow transplant recipients. Transplantation 1995; 59:1015–1022.

26. Tanaka M, Umihara J, Shimmoto K, Cui SJ, Sata H, Ishikawa T, Ishikawa E. The pathogenesis of graft-versus-host reaction in the intrahepatic bile duct. An immunohistochemical study. Acta Pathol Jpn 1989; 39:648–655.

27. Desmet VJ. Vanishing bile duct disorders. Prog Liver Dis 1992; 10:89–121.

28. Nonomura A, Kono N, Yoshida K, Nakanuma Y, Ohta G. Histological changes of bile duct in experimental graft-versus-host disease across minor histocompatibility barriers. II. Electron microscopic observations. Liver 1988; 8:32–41.

29. Bernuau D, Gisselbrecht C, Devergie A, Feldmann G, Gluckman E, Marty M, Boiron M. Histological and ultrastructural appearance of the liver during graft-versus-host disease complicating bone marrow transplantation. Transplantation 1980; 29:236–244.

30. Bach N, Thung SN, Schaffner F. The histological features of chronic hepatitis C and autoimmune chronic hepatitis: a comparative analysis. Hepatology 1992; 15:572–577.

31. Brainard JA, Greenson JK, Vesy CJ, Tesi RJ, Papp AC, Snyder PJ, Western L, Prior TW. Detection of cytomegalovirus in liver transplant biopsies. A comparison of light microscopy, immunohistochemistry, duplex PCR and nested PCR. Transplantation 1994; 57:1753–1757.

32. Andersen CB, Horn T, Sehested M, Junge J, Jacobsen N. Graft-versus-host disease: liver morphology and pheno/genotypes of inflammatory cells and target cells in sex-mismatched allogeneic bone marrow transplant patients. Transplant Proc 1993; 25:1250–1254.

33. Vierling JM. Immune disorders of the liver and bile duct. Gastroenterol Clin North Am 1992; 21:427–449.

34. Yeh KH, Hsieh HC, Tang JL, Lin MT, Yang CH, Chen YC. Severe isolated acute hepatic graft-versus-host disease with vanishing bile duct syndrome. Bone Marrow Transplant 1994; 14:319–321.

35. Alpini G, McGill JM, Larusso NF. The pathobiology of biliary epithelia. Hepatology 2002; 35:1256–1268.

36. Yau JC, Zander AR, Srigley JR, Verm RA, Stroehlein JR, Korinek JK, Vellekoop L, Dicke KA. Chronic graft-versus-host disease complicated by micronodular cirrhosis and esophageal varices. Transplantation 1986; 41:129–130.

37. Knapp AB, Crawford JM, Rappeport JM, Gollan JL. Cirrhosis as a consequence of graft-versus-host disease. Gastroenterology 1987; 92:513–519.

38. Nakanuma Y, Terada T, Ohtake S, Govindarajan S. Intrahepatic periductal glands in graft-versus-host disease. Acta Pathol Jpn 1988; 38:281–289.

39. Geubel AP, Cnudde A, Ferrant A, Latinne D, Rahier J. Diffuse biliary tract involvement mimicking primary sclerosing cholangitis after bone marrow transplantation. J Hepatol 1990; 10:23–28.

40. Williams FH, Thiele DL. The role of major histocompatibility complex and non-major histocompatibility complex encoded antigens in generation of bile duct lesions during hepatic graft-vs.-host responses mediated by helper or cytotoxic T cells. Hepatology 1994; 19:980–988.

41. Anderson JE, Appelbaum FR, Schoch G, Barnett T, Chauncey TR, Flowers ME, Storb R. Relapse after allogeneic bone marrow transplantation for refractory anemia is increased by shielding lungs and liver during total body irradiation. Biol Blood Marrow Transplant 2001; 7:163–170.

42. Howell CD, Yoder TY, Vierling JM. Suppressor function of liver mononuclear cells isolated during murine chronic graft-vs-host disease. II. Role of prostaglandins and interferon-gamma. Cell Immunol 1992; 140:54–66.

43. Howell CD, Yoder TD, Vierling JM. Suppressor function of hepatic mononuclear inflammatory cells during murine chronic graft-vs-host disease. I. Macrophage-enriched cells mediate suppression in the liver. Cell Immunol 1991; 132:256–268.

44. Goker H, Haznedaroglu IC, Chao NJ. Acute graft-vs-host disease: pathobiology and management. Exp Hematol 2001; 29:259–277.

45. Pratt JR, Basheer SA, Sacks SH. Local synthesis of complement component C3 regulates acute renal transplant rejection. Nat Med 2002; 8:582–587.

46. Margolis DA, Casper JT, Segura AD, Janczak T, McOlash L, Fisher B, Miller K, Gorski J. Infiltrating T cells during liver graft-versus-host disease show a restricted T-cell repertoire. Biol Blood Marrow Transplant 2000; 6:408–415.

47. Itoh S, Matsuzaki Y, Kimura T, Unno R, Ikegami T, Shoda J, Doy M, Fujiwara M, Tanaka N. Suppression of hepatic lesions in a murine graft-versus-host reaction by antibodies against adhesion molecules. J Hepatol 2000; 32:587–595.

48. Vierling JM, Hu K. Immunologic mechanisms of hepatobiliary injury. In: Kaplowwitz N, ed. Liver and Biliary Diseases. Baltimore: Williams & Wilkins, 1992:48–69.

49. Suitters AJ, Lampert IA. Class II antigen induction in the liver of rats with graft-versus-host disease. Transplantation 1984; 38:194–196.

50. Siegert W, Stemerowicz R, Hopf U. Antimitochondrial antibodies in patients with chronic graft-versus-host disease. Bone Marrow Transplant 1992; 10:221–227.

51. Nonomura A, Yoshida K, Kono N, Nakanuma Y, Ohta G. Histological changes of bile duct in experimental graft-versus-disease across minor histocompatibility barriers. III. Immunoelectron microscopic observations. Acta Pathol Jpn 1988; 38:269–280.

52. Stet RJ, Thomas C, Koudstaal J, Hardonk MJ, Hulstaert CE, Nieuwenhuis P. Graft-versus-host disease in the rat: cellular changes and major histocompatibility complex antigen expression in the liver. Scand J Immunol 1986; 23:81–89.

53. Donaldson P, Underhill J, Doherty D, Hayllar K, Calne R, Tan KC, O'Grady J, Wight D, Portmann B, Williams R. Influence of human leukocyte antigen matching on liver allograft survival and rejection: "the dualistic effect." Hepatology 1993; 17:1008–1015.

54. Calne RY, White HJ, Yoffa DE, Binns RM, Maginn RR, Herbertson RM, Millard PR, Molina VP, Davis DR. Prolonged survival of liver transplants in the pig. Br Med J 1967; 4:645–648.

55. Itoh S, Matsuzaki Y, Kimura T, Ikegami T, Shoda J, Fujiwara M, Tanaka N. Cytokine profile of liver-infiltrating CD4+ T cells separated from murine primary biliary cirrhosis-like hepatic lesions induced by graft-versus-host reaction. J Gastroenterol Hepatol 2000; 15:443–451.

56. Chen YC, Lin KH, Huang WS, Tang JL. Bone marrow transplantation in Taiwan: an overview. Bone Marrow Transplant 1994; 13:705–708.

57. Fujii Y, Kaku K, Tanaka M, Kaneko T, Matumoto N, Shinohara K. Hepatitis C virus infection and liver disease after allogeneic bone marrow transplantation. Bone Marrow Transplant 1994; 13:523–526.

58. Appleton AL, Sviland L, Peiris JS, Taylor CE, Wilkes J, Green MA, Pearson AD, Kelly PJ, Malcolm AJ, Proctor SJ, et al. Human herpes virus-6 infection in marrow graft recipients: role in pathogenesis of graft-versus-host disease. Newcastle upon Tyne Bone Marrow Transport Group. Bone Marrow Transplant 1995; 16:777–782.

59. Snover DC. Acute and chronic graft versus host disease: histopathological evidence for two distinct pathogenetic mechanisms. Hum Pathol 1984; 15:202–205.

60. Kuiper J, Brouwer A, Knook D. Kupffer and sinusoidal endothelial cells. In: Aries IM, et al., eds. The Liver: Biology and Pathobiology. Vol. 3. New York: Raven Press, 1994; pp 791–818.

61. Demetris AJ, Murase N, Fujisaki S, Fung JJ, Rao AS, Starzl TE. Hematolymphoid cell trafficking, microchimerism, and GVH reactions after liver, bone marrow, and heart transplantation. Transplant Proc 1993; 25:3337–3344.

62. Rubinstein D, Roska AK, Lipsky PE. Antigen presentation by liver sinusoidal lining cells after antigen exposure in vivo. J Immunol 1987; 138:1377–1382.

63. Murai M, Yoneyama H, Ezaki T, Suematsu M, Terashima Y, Harada A, Hamada H, Asakura H, Ishikawa H, Matsushima K. Peyer's patch is the essential site in initiating murine acute and lethal graft-versus-host reaction. Nat Immunol 2003; 4:154–160.

64. Zhang Y, Shlomchik WD, Joe G, Louboutin JP, Zhu J, Rivera A, Giannola D, Emerson SG. APCs in the liver and spleen recruit activated allogeneic CD8(+) T cells to elicit hepatic graft-versus-host disease. J Immunol 2002; 169:7111–7118.

65. Hirokawa M, Matsutani T, Saitoh H, Ichikawa Y, Kawabata Y, Horiuchi T, Kitabayashi A, Yoshioka T, Tsuruta Y, Suzuki R, Miura AB, Sawada K. Distinct TCRAV and TCRBV repertoire and CDR3 sequence of T lymphocytes clonally expanded in blood and GVHD lesions after human allogeneic bone marrow transplantation. Bone Marrow Transplant 2002; 30:915–923.

66. Saitoh T, Fujiwara M, Asakura H. L3T4+ T cells induce hepatic lesions resembling primary biliary cirrhosis in mice with graft-versus-host reactions due to major histocompatibility complex class II disparity. Clin Immunol Immunopathol 1991; 59:449–461.

67. Jansen J, Hanks S, Akard LP, Thompson JM, Burns S, Chang Q, English D, Garrett P. Immunomagnetic CD4+ and CD8+ cell depletion for patients at high risk for severe acute GVHD. Bone Marrow Transplant 1996; 17:377–382.

68. Cray C, Levy RB. CD8+ and CD4+ T cells contribute to the exacerbation of class I MHC disparate graft-vs-host reaction by concurrent murine cytomegalovirus infection. Clin Immunol Immunopathol 1993; 67:84–90.

69. Arai S, Lee LA, Vogelsang GB. A systematic approach to hepatic complications in hematopoietic stem cell transplantation. J Hematother Stem Cell Res 2002; 11:215–229.

70. Kataoka Y, Iwasaki T, Kuroiwa T, Seto Y, Iwata N, Hashimoto N, Ogata A, Hamano T, Kakishita E. The role of donor T cells for target organ injuries in acute and chronic graft-versus-host disease. Immunology 2001; 103:310–318.

71. Dilly SA, Sloane JP. An immunohistological study of human hepatic graft-versus-host disease. Clin Exp Immunol 1985; 62:545–553.

72. Murai M, Yoneyama H, Harada A, Yi Z, Vestergaard C, Guo B, Suzuki K, Asakura H, Matsushima K. Active participation of CCR5(+)CD8(+) T lymphocytes in the pathogenesis of liver injury in graft-versus-host disease. J Clin Invest 1999; 104:49–57.

73. Czaja AJ. Chronic graft-versus-host disease and primary biliary cirrhosis: sorting the puzzle pieces. Lab Invest 1994; 70:589–592.

74. Korngold R, Sprent J. Surface markers of T cells causing lethal graft-vs-host disease to class I vs class II H-2 differences. J Immunol 1985; 135:3004–3010.

75. Sprent J, Korngold R. T cell subsets controlling graft-v-host disease in mice. Transplant Proc 1987; 19:41–47.

76. Korngold R, Sprent J. Graft-versus-host disease in experimental allogeneic bone marrow transplantation. Proc Soc Exp Biol Med 1991; 197:12–18.

77. Miconnet I, de La Selle V, Bruley-Rosset M. Relative importance of CD4+ and CD8+ T cell repertoires in the development of acute graft-versus-host disease in a murine model of bone marrow transplantation. Bone Marrow Transplant 1998; 21:583–590.

78. Via CS, Nguyen P, Shustov A, Drappa J, Elkon KB. A major role for the Fas pathway in acute graft-versus-host disease. J Immunol 1996; 157:5387–5393.

79. Hattori K, Hirano T, Miyajima H, Yamakawa N, Tateno M, Oshimi K, Kayagaki N, Yagita H, Okumura K. Differential effects of anti-Fas ligand and anti-tumor necrosis factor alpha antibodies on acute graft-versus-host disease pathologies. Blood 1998; 91:4051–4055.

80. Suzuki K, Narita T, Yui R, Asakura H, Fujiwara M. Mechanism of the induction of auto-immune disease by graft-versus-host reaction. Role of CD8+ cells in the development of hepatic and ductal lesions induced by CD4+ cells in MHC class I plus II-different host. Lab Invest 1994; 70:609–619.

81. Hayashi A, Suzuki K, Narita T, Yui R, Inada S, Kimura T, Aizawa Y, Zeniya M, Toda G, Fujiwara M. Induction of autoimmune-like hepatic and ductal lesions by administration of lipopolysaccharide in mice undergoing graft-versus-host reaction across MHC class I difference. Immunol Lett 1997; 59:159–170.

82. Howell CD, Yoder T, Claman HN, Vierling JM. Hepatic homing of mononuclear inflammatory cells isolated during murine chronic graft-vs-host disease. J Immunol 1989; 143:476–483.

83. Nestel FP, Price KS, Seemayer TA, Lapp WS. Macrophage priming and lipopolysaccharide-triggered release of tumor necrosis factor alpha during graft-versus-host disease. J Exp Med 1992; 175:405–413.

84. Hill GR, Ferrara JL. The primacy of the gastrointestinal tract as a target organ of acute graft-versus-host disease: rationale for the use of cytokine shields in allogeneic bone marrow transplantation. Blood 2000; 95:2754–2759.

85. Cooke KR, Gerbitz A, Crawford JM, Teshima T, Hill GR, Tesolin A, Rossignol DP, Ferrara JL. LPS antagonism reduces graft-versus-host disease and preserves graft-versus-leukemia activity after experimental bone marrow transplantation. J Clin Invest 2001; 107:1581–1589.

86. Fox ES, Thomas P, Broitman SA. Clearance of gut-derived endotoxins by the liver. Release and modification of 3H, 14C-lipopolysaccharide by isolated rat Kupffer cells. Gastroenterology 1989; 96:456–461.

87. Crawford AR, Smith AJ, Hatch VC, Oude Elferink RP, Borst P, Crawford JM. Hepatic secretion of phospholipid vesicles in the mouse critically depends on mdr2 or MDR3 P-glycoprotein expression. Visualization by electron microscopy. J Clin Invest 1997; 100:2562–2567.

88. Spitzer JA, Zhang P, Mayer AM. Functional characterization of peripheral circulating and liver recruited neutrophils in endotoxic rats. J Leukoc Biol 1994; 56:166–173.

89. Crawford JM, Boyer JL. Clinicopathology conferences: inflammation-induced cholestasis. Hepatology 1998; 28:253–260.

90. Fox ES, Broitman SA, Thomas P. Bacterial endotoxins and the liver. Lab Invest 1990; 63:733–741.

91. Leskinen R, Volin L, Taskinen E, Ruutu T, Renkonen R, Hayry P. Monitoring of bone marrow transplant recipient liver by fine-needle aspiration biopsy. Transplantation 1989; 48:969–974.

92. Cooke KR, Hill GR, Crawford JM, Bungard D, Brinson YS, Delmonte J, Jr., Ferrara JL. Tumor necrosis factor-alpha production to lipopolysaccharide stimulation by donor cells predicts the severity of experimental acute graft-versus-host disease. J Clin Invest 1998; 102:1882–1891.

93. De Bueger M, Bakker A, Van Rood JJ, Goulmy E. Minor histocompatibility antigens, defined by graft-vs.-host disease-derived cytotoxic T lymphocytes, show variable expression on human skin cells. Eur J Immunol 1991; 21:2839–2844.

94. Nikolic B, Lee S, Bronson RT, Grusby MJ, Sykes M. Th1 and Th2 mediate acute graft-versus-host disease, each with distinct end-organ targets. J Clin Invest 2000; 105:1289–1298.

95. Deeg HJ. Cytokines in graft-versus-host disease and the graft-versus-leukemia reaction. Int J Hematol 2001; 74:26–32.

96. Greve JW, Gouma DJ, Buurman WA. Bile acids inhibit endotoxin-induced release of tumor necrosis factor by monocytes: an in vitro study. Hepatology 1989; 10:454–458.

97. Howell CD, Li J, Chen W. Role of intercellular adhesion molecule-1 and lymphocyte function-associated antigen-1 during nonsuppurative destructive cholangitis in a mouse graft-versus-host disease model. Hepatology 1999; 29:766–776.

98. Hreha G, Jefferson DM, Yu CH, Grubman SA, Alsabeh R, Geller SA, Vierling JM. Immortalized intrahepatic mouse biliary epithelial cells: immunologic characterization and immunogenicity. Hepatology 1999; 30:358–371.

99. Sonne O, Davidsen O, Moller BK, Munck Petersen C. Cellular targets and receptors for interleukin-6. I. In vivo and in vitro uptake of IL-6 in liver and hepatocytes. Eur J Clin Invest 1990; 20:366–376.

100. Green RM, Whiting JF, Rosenbluth AB, Beier D, Gollan JL. Interleukin-6 inhibits hepatocyte taurocholate uptake and sodium- potassium-adenosinetriphosphatase activity. Am J Physiol 1994; 267:G1094–G1100.

101. Remberger M, Ringden O, Markling L. TNF alpha levels are increased during bone marrow transplantation conditioning in patients who develop acute GVHD. Bone Marrow Transplant 1995; 15:99–104.

102. Remberger M, Svahn BM, Hentschke P, Lofgren C, Ringden O. Effect on cytokine release and graft-versus-host disease of different anti-T cell antibodies during conditioning for unrelated haematopoietic stem cell transplantation. Bone Marrow Transplant 1999; 24:823–830.

103. Jones A, Selby PJ, Viner C, Hobbs S, Gore ME, McElwain TJ. Tumour necrosis factor, cholestatic jaundice, and chronic liver disease. Gut 1990; 31:938–939.

104. Cooke KR, Hill GR, Gerbitz A, Kobzik L, Martin TR, Crawford JM, Brewer JP, Ferrara JL. Tumor necrosis factor-alpha neutralization reduces lung injury after experimental allogeneic bone marrow transplantation. Transplantation 2000; 70:272–279.

105. Kuroiwa T, Kakishita E, Hamano T, Kataoka Y, Seto Y, Iwata N, Kaneda Y, Matsumoto K, Nakamura T, Ueki T, Fujimoto J, Iwasaki T. Hepatocyte growth factor ameliorates acute graft-versus-host disease and promotes hematopoietic function. J Clin Invest 2001; 107:1365–1373.

106. Rubin RA, Kowalski TE, Khandelwal M, Malet PF. Ursodiol for hepatobiliary disorders. Ann Intern Med 1994; 121:207–218.

107. Crawford AR, Lin XZ, Crawford JM. The normal adult human liver biopsy: a quantitative reference standard. Hepatology 1998; 28:323–331.

108. Sloane JP, Farthing MJ, Powles RL. Histopathological changes in the liver after allogeneic bone marrow transplantation. J Clin Pathol 1980; 33:344–350.

109. Sherlock S. Fulminant hepatic failure. Adv Intern Med 1993; 38:245–267.

110. Jazrawi RP, de Caestecker JS, Goggin PM, Britten AJ, Joseph AE, Maxwell JD, Northfield TC. Kinetics of hepatic bile acid handling in cholestatic liver disease: effect of ursodeoxycholic acid. Gastroenterology 1994; 106:134–142.

111. Fried RH, Murakami CS, Fisher LD, Willson RA, Sullivan KM, McDonald GB. Ursodeoxycholic acid treatment of refractory chronic graft-versus-host disease of the liver. Ann Intern Med 1992; 116:624–629.

112. Ruutu T, Eriksson B, Remes K, et al. Ursodeoxycholic acid for the prevention of hepatic complications in allogeneic stem cell transplantation. Blood 2002; 100:1977–1983.

113. Bismuth H. Consensus statement on indications for liver transplantation. Hepatology 1994; 20:63S–68S.

114. Rhodes DF, Lee WM, Wingard JR, Pavy MD, Santos GW, Shaw BW, Wood RP, Sorrell MF, Markin RS. Orthotopic liver transplantation for graft-versus-host disease following bone marrow transplantation. Gastroenterology 1990; 99:536–538.

115. Ramsay NK, Kersey JH, Robison LL, McGlave PB, Woods WG, Krivit W, Kim TH, Goldman AI, Nesbit ME, Jr. A randomized study of the prevention of acute graft-versus-host disease. N Engl J Med 1982; 306:392–397.

10

Intestinal Graft-vs.-Host Disease

ALLAN MOWAT

University of Glasgow, Glasgow, Scotland

GERARD SOCIÉ

Hospital St. Louis, Paris, France

I. INTRODUCTION

Early studies of graft-vs.-host reaction (GVHR) quickly identified intestinal damage as an important component of host disease (1). Most animals with severe GVHR developed diarrhea, and this feature remains one of the characteristic signs of graft-vs.-host disease (GVHD) both in humans and in experimental animals. Nevertheless, the mechanisms responsible for intestinal damage have not been clearly identified. Partly this reflects a failure to discriminate between intestinal alterations that are true consequences of GVHR and those that are artefacts of irradiation or infection. Furthermore, the mucosal features vary markedly with time, even within a single experimental model, and many studies have failed to appreciate that the intestinal changes present in moribund patients or animals may not necessarily be relevant to the condition as a whole. Finally, the intestine is a distinct component of the host immune response, and therefore measurements of systemic immune responsiveness in animals with GVHR may not reflect events within the intestine. This chapter will review the intestinal pathology that characterizes GVHD in experimental animals and under clinical conditions and discuss the possible mechanisms involved.

II. THE INTESTINE AND ITS IMMUNE SYSTEM

A. Epithelial Pathophysiology

The gut-associated lymphoid tissues (GALT) are the largest immune compartment in the body and contain populations of lymphoid cells whose origin and function are distinct from those in other tissues (for reviews see Refs. 2–5). Furthermore, this enormous population is in intimate contact with a specialized epithelial layer whose function is essential for the survival of the animal (Fig. 1). Both the epithelial and lymphoid cells in the gut are constantly changing and local immune responses can produce rapid and profound changes

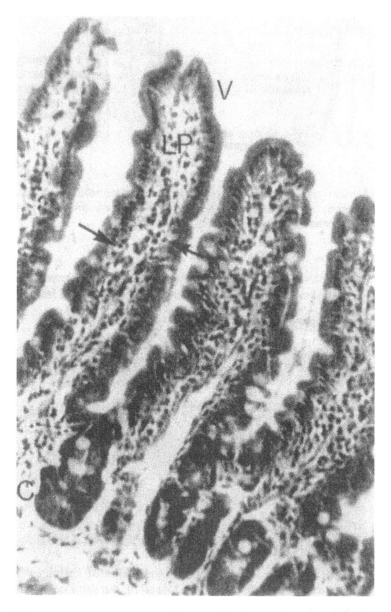

Figure 1 The appearance of the normal small intestine. The villus (V) is clothed by a layer of columnar epithelial cells, which arise from dividing cells in the crypts (C). The lamina propria (LP) is separated from the epithelium by a basement membrane and contains a wide variety of lymphoid cells. Intraepithelial lymphocytes (arrows) are found between the epithelial cells. (H&E ×500.)

in intestinal structure and function (Fig. 2). An appreciation of these aspects of intestinal immunology and physiology are essential for understanding enteropathy in GVHR.

The principal function of the small intestine is the digestion and absorption of foods. These activities are performed by enzymes found on the microvilli present on the luminal surface of columnar enterocytes. Any form of insult that compromises the production and function of these cells will inevitably have profound consequences for the well-being of the host. The functional unit of the small intestine is the villus (Figs. 1, 2), which comprises a cylinder consisting of sheets of enterocytes, and these finger-like processes greatly increase the surface area of epithelial cells available for digestive functions. Atrophy or disruption of the villus architecture causes intestinal failure, and GVHD is one of the most potent means of producing this type of intestinal pathology.

The enterocytes that cover the surface of the villus move upwards in continuous sheets from their origin in the crypts of Lieberkühn, where a self-renewing population of stem cells normally balances loss of effete enterocytes from the villus tip (Figs. 1, 2). In the steady state, around 10 new cells are produced in each crypt per hour, and the migration of enterocytes from the crypt to the villus tip takes 2–3 days. However, when there is epithelial cell damage or increased cell loss, both the production of new cells by the crypts and their subsequent migration increase in an attempt to repair the damage. However, certain stimuli can have direct effects on crypt cell turnover, one of which is the immune response in intestinal GVHD. Increased epithelial cell turnover can itself interfere with intestinal function, as when enterocytes leave the crypts. They are immature with no microvilli and poorly developed enzymes; they acquire the ability to digest and absorb foods only after they enter the villus compartment. Conditions that enhance crypt cell turnover or enterocyte migration result in the appearance of a large number of recently produced, immature cells on the part of the villus normally covered by mature cells. As a result there is an effective decrease in absorptive surface area.

Pathogenic insults can therefore alter intestinal function either by direct damage to villus enterocytes or by interfering with the dynamic balance between epithelial cell renewal and differentiation. Another potential cause of intestinal damage is disruption of the tissues that underlie the epithelium. The three-dimensional structure of the villus is central to maintaining the functional surface area of the gut. In turn, this is dependent on the integrity of the epithelial basement membrane and the extracellular matrix of the

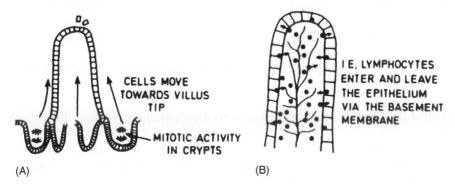

(A)   (B)

Figure 2 The villus/crypt unit as a dynamic structure. Enterocyte loss from the villus tip is normally balanced by continual upward movement of new cells produced in the crypts. Lymphocytes move constantly in and out of the epithelium.

underlying lamina propria, structures that are formed by myofibroblasts and related mesenchymal cells. As these cells also produce important factors that regulate enterocyte turnover and differentiation, damage to them is likely to have profound effects on epithelial behavior. Finally, the epithelium is invested closely by a complex network of blood vessels, as well as autonomic and peptidergic nerves. Their function is also essential for intestinal integrity and function.

B. Mucosal Lymphoid Cells

The most cursory microscopic examination reveals that the lamina propria which underlies the intestinal epithelium contains a wide variety of lymphoid and myeloid cells (Fig. 1). These include dendritic cells (DC), macrophages, eosinophils, mast cells, and basophils, as well as B lymphocytes, T lymphocytes, and plasma cells. Many of these cells are quite distinct from their peripheral counterparts, as is typified by the predominance of IgA-producing B cells in the intestine, where up to 90% of plasma cells are committed to IgA synthesis. In humans these are all derived from precursors that are primed by antigen in the Peyer's patch (PP) and then migrate back to the mucosa via the draining mesenteric lymph node (MLN), thoracic duct, and bloodstream. This migration process is determined by the selective upregulation of the $\alpha_4\beta_7$ integrin only on lymphocytes that have been primed in the GALT $\alpha_4\beta_7$ integrin binds to MADCAM-1 expressed specifically by blood vessels in mucosal surfaces; this means that only mucosally derived lymphocytes can migrate into tissues such as the gut wall. In addition, mucosally primed lymphocytes express the CCR9 chemokine receptor whose ligand is produced selectively by small bowel enterocytes. Together, these factors account for the anatomical separation of the intestine from the rest of the immune system (4,6).

IgA-producing plasma cells reside in the lamina propria, mainly in the crypt area, whereas mucosal T cells are distributed in a number of different locations throughout the villus-crypt unit. CD8+ T cells migrate preferentially to the epithelium, whereas T cells in the lamina propria have a CD4+ : CD8 + ratio of 2 : 1, similar to that in peripheral lymphoid organs. Epithelial and lamina propria T cells are distinct from each other and from T cells in other tissues. Their exact functions are still largely uncertain, but cells with a "memory" phenotype predominate in both sites, suggesting that they have been exposed to antigen.

The intestinal lamina propria is a complex and rather unique immunological niche, and the T cells there may be of particular relevance to the effector mechanisms of intestinal GVHD. As noted above, the majority of lamina propia (LP) CD4+ T cells in normal animals have a "memory" phenotype, and although they are generally unresponsive to TcR-mediated proliferative signals, they can be induced to proliferate when CD2 is used as an accessory molecule. In addition, they produce large amounts of cytokines, especially interferon-gamma (IFNγ), but also interleukin-4 (IL-4) and IL-10 even under physiological conditions (7–11). In conditions such as inflammatory bowel disease, LP CD4+ T cells are believed to be responsible for much of the IFNγ production that is critical for the local pathology (12). Thirty to 40% of LP T cells are CD8+, and these are also capable of potent effector functions, including cytotoxic T-lymphocyte (CTL) activity and IFNγ production in response to, for example, virus infection (13).

Fifteen to 20% of cells in the intestinal epithelium are also lymphocytes, making this one of the largest single populations in the immune system. Virtually all intraepithelial lymphocytes (IEL) are CD3+ T cells, 80–90% of which are CD8 + , with the remainder comprising small populations of CD4+CD8+, CD4+CD8− and CD4−CD8− cells. There are no B cells, plasma cells, or macrophages within the epithelium, underlining how different this population is from that of the adjacent lamina propria (2,5,13). All IEL express a unique integrin molecule (αEβ7) whose ligand is E cadherin on epithelial cells. In humans, the vast majority of IEL normally expresses the $\alpha\beta$ T-cell receptor (TcR), but in some species a substantial proportion may be $\gamma\delta$ T cells (5,14). The number of $\gamma\delta$ TcR+ IEL is also expanded in humans with celiac disease (15). In all species, CD8+IEL have many unusual properties, with a low expression of markers found on all other peripheral CD8 + T cells, including CD2, CD5, CD28, and Thy1. Of particular note, a variable, occasionally large proportion of CD8+ IEL (up to 60%) express a homodimeric CD8$\alpha\alpha$ molecule, in contrast to the CD8$\alpha\beta$ heterodimer found on other T cells (5,16). The expression of the CD8$\alpha\alpha$ molecule may be indicative of extrathymic development, and studies in rodents show that many IEL may be derived from local T-cell differentiation in the intestine itself, perhaps in the structures referred to as "cryptopatches" (17,18).

Increased numbers of IEL are found in immunologically based disorders such as celiac disease and GVHR. They lie between epithelial cells on the basement membrane (Fig. 3) and are therefore likely to be in contact with luminal antigen. In addition, most IEL appear to represent the progeny of oligoclonal expansion, which occurs in response to local antigen. Together these findings suggest that IEL could contribute to the pathogenesis of epithelial damage in GVHD, but the functions of these unusual T cells are still unclear. Many IEL may recognize self antigen or nonpeptide antigens presented by nonclassical MHC molecules, such as Tl in mice or MIC-A/MIC-B in humans (19,20), and although most IEL show marked nonspecific cytolytic activity when their T-cell receptor (TcR) is cross-linked in vitro, much of this is due to spontaneous lytic activity. Classical antigen-specific CTL activity is limited to a small subset of CD8$\alpha\beta^+$ $\alpha\beta$TcR$^+$ IEL

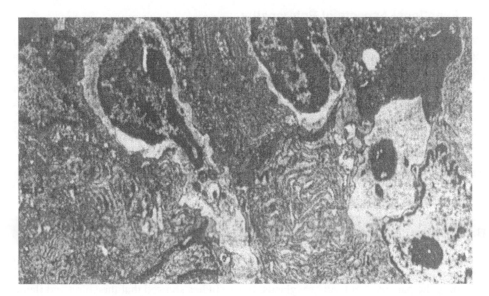

Figure 3 Electron microscopic appearance of two intraepithelial lymphocytes, one of which is crossing into the epithelium through the basement membrane ($\times$ 16,000) Ep, epithelial cell nucleus).

(5,21,22). They can also secrete lymphokines such as IL-5 and IFNγ in vitro, but show little or no proliferative activity to antigen or T-cell mitogens (5,13). Therefore, the contribution of IEL to local immune responses remains uncertain.

Mucosal mast cells (MMC) are a further population of intestinal effector cells, which differ from the equivalent cells in the periphery and may be important in enteropathies such as GVHD. MMC occur predominantly in the lamina propria and differ from classical connective tissue mast cells in staining pattern, chemical content, and response to mast cell activators (23,24). They contain little or no histamine and secrete a serine protease mast cell protease II (MMCP), which is antigenically different from the related proteases found in peripheral mast cells. MMCP has a number of potentially harmful effects in the mucosa, including increasing epithelial permeability, direct destruction of basement membrane type IV collagen, and the activation of tissue metalloproteinases (24). In addition, other MMC-derived mediators may increase epithelial permeability and ion secretion (23), indicating that MMC could play an important pathogenic role in intestinal GVHD. The differentiation and function of MMC are highly dependent on T lymphocytes, and MMC hyperplasia is a characteristic feature of cell-mediated responses to intestinal parasite infections and allergic reactions in the intestine, where their mediators can influence epithelial secretion and permeability, among other effects (24).

III. INTESTINAL GVHR IN EXPERIMENTAL ANIMALS

The runting disease found in the earliest studies of tolerance to allogeneic cells in neonatal mice was accompanied by diarrhea (1,25). Subsequent studies of "graft-vs.-host" disease also noted the presence of diarrhea (26), and since then, this sign has provided one of the most important indicators of both clinical and experimental GVHD.

A. Functional Aspects of Enteropathy

Much of the morbidity and mortality of GVHD reflects the malabsorption, fluid loss, and increased intestinal permeability that occur as a result of damage to the epithelium. To a great extent, this reflects the loss of total surface area and damage to individual enterocytes that leads to deficiency of the epithelial cell enzymes required for absorption and digestion of nutrients (27,28). Colonic damage in GVHR could also potentially interfere with normal water-absorption mechanisms. The damaged epithelium also becomes hyperpermeable to serum and tissue proteins, with concomitant water loss into the lumen (29–31). In parallel, there is increased inward permeability of the epithelium to luminal materials, the most important of which are endotoxins and related products of local bacteria (32,33). We shall discuss how this increased uptake of endotoxins may contribute significantly to the evolution of acute GVHD.

B. Distribution of Intestinal Pathology

Acute GVHD in humans can affect the entire gastrointestinal tract, sparing few sites from the mouth to the rectum and causing lesions in several of the associated exocrine glands, including the pancreas and salivary glands. Early studies showed that the colon and ileum are the worst affected areas of the bowel in human GVHD (34) and suggested that the ileum was the most seriously damaged site in neonatal mice with acute GVHR (35). However, as we shall discuss, the upper small intestine is in fact a major site of involvement, and this probably accounts for much of the metabolic effects of the disorder. Colonic disease also occurs in mice with GVHR (29), and it may even occur before pathology in other parts of the intestine (36). Acute GVHD occurring in rats after small bowel transplantation damages both the small intestine and colon, with colonic disease being more severe in the distal region (37).

Scleroderma-like lesions have been found in the esophagus and tongue of rats undergoing a chronic form of GVHR across minor histocompatibility differences (38). It should be noted, however, that intestinal pathology is entirely absent in models of chronic GVHD in mice (39,40).

IV. NATURE OF THE INTESTINAL PATHOLOGY

A. Epithelial Damage

1. Evolution of Enteropathy

Severe intestinal inflammation, with macroscopic ulceration of the ileum and colon and focal degeneration of the crypts, was found in the earliest studies of GVHR in mice (25,41). Later, more detailed studies found intestinal dilatation and bloody exudates accompanied by severe villus atrophy, crypt necrosis, and increased extrusion of necrotic cells from the villus tip (29,35,42). This destructive pattern of pathology has also been emphasized in most studies of human GVHD and is often believed to represent the entire spectrum of the disease. However, this is a misinterpretation, and intestinal damage of this severity is in fact the end stage of a complex enteropathy that evolves through distinct phases, each of which seems to reflect the effects of distinct immune mechanisms (Table 1). These phases are:

1. Proliferative: characterized by increased epithelial cell turnover, crypt hypertrophy, and infiltration of the mucosa by lymphoid cells in the absence of villus atrophy or damage to mature enterocytes (Fig. 4A). This comprises the initial phase of damage in severe acute GVHD and may be the only evidence of gut disease in less severe models.
2. Destructive: depending on the model system, a second phase of enteropathy may ensue, in which continuing and intense crypt hyperplasia is accompanied by the rapid onset of villus damage. Shortly thereafter there is a sudden cessation in crypt cell proliferation, associated with apoptosis of stem cells, and the mucosa begins to show evidence of the necrosis familiar from clinical studies. If this persists, it will lead to complete intestinal destruction unless sufficient crypts survive to allow regeneration. These destructive changes are accompanied by the loss of lymphoid infiltrates and the appearance of the inflammatory cells more typical of necrosis (Fig. 4B).
3. Atrophic: this lesion is characterized by thinning and shortening of both villi and crypts, as well as a complete absence of lymphoid cells. It may occur as an end-stage event after destructive enteropathy has resolved, or, under some circumstances, it may be the only manifestation of intestinal GVHR.

2. Crypt Cell Pathology

Crypt epithelial cells are the principal target of small intestinal GVHR, irrespective of the type of enteropathy. Apoptosis of stem cells, together with focal necrosis and degeneration

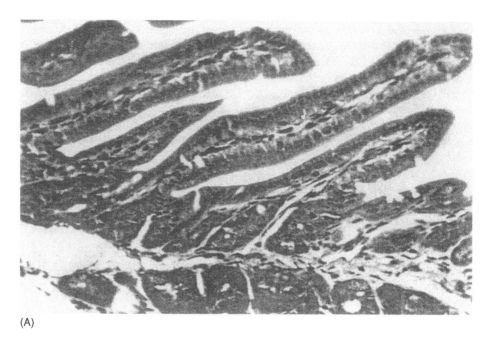

(A)

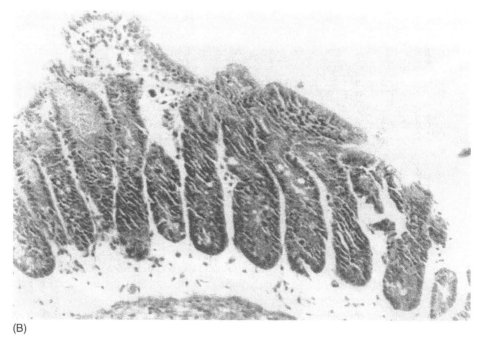

(B)

Figure 4 Enteropathy in murine graft-vs.-host reaction. (A) In the proliferative form, there is crypt lengthening and increased numbers of mucosal lymphoid cells, but no villus atrophy or enterocyte damage. (H&E ×320.) (B) In the destructive form, many crypts remain long and hyperplastic, but there is also necrosis of individual enterocytes and severe villus atrophy. The mucosa is devoid of lymphoid cells. (H&E×320.) (C) Crypt cell apoptosis also occurs in late destructive disease.

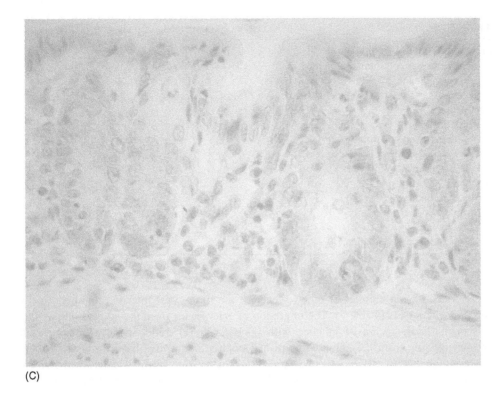

(C)

Figure 4 *Continued.*

of individual crypts, is the cardinal feature of the terminal stages of intestinal GVHD. However, early studies showed that these destructive changes were often accompanied by histological evidence of crypt lengthening and increased mitotic activity (29,35). As this hyperplasia was always accompanied by marked villus atrophy, it was concluded that the increased crypt cell mitotic activity was an attempt to repair the loss of mature enterocytes. However, subsequent studies showed that an increase in crypt cell production rate (CCPR) in the jejunum occurred during the first few days of GVHR in mice and this preceded any evidence of villus atrophy (43,44). Similar findings were made in a later study of a GVHD model in which villus atrophy never occurred (45). Identical findings have also been reported in rats with GVHR (46), supporting the idea that stimulation of dividing crypt stem cells is the primary consequence of GVHR.

Subsequent alterations in crypt cell behavior depend on the model under study. In mild forms of disease, the enhanced mitotic activity returns to normal and the intestine shows no other evidence of damage (45). Destructive forms of GVHR are associated with prolonged crypt hyperplasia, which may continue for some time after resolution of other aspects of intestinal pathology (39). In the most severe cases of intestinal GVHR, there is a sudden cessation of crypt cell proliferative activity, associated with apoptosis of basal crypt enterocytes (29,35,42,47–50). This highly characteristic feature (Fig. 4C) is now frequently used as an index of intestinal GVHD, but it is important to note that this is the last effect of the local immune response on crypt cells and so is not an appropriate index of all aspects of the condition.

Table 1 Pathological Stages of Intestinal GVHD in Experimental Animals

Early proliferative
   Increased crypt cell mitotic activity
   Crypt lengthening ($\pm$ villus lengthening)
   Increased density of intraepithelial lymphocytes, MMC
Destructive
   Villus atrophy
   Continued crypt hyperplasia + crypt cell turnover
   Crypt stem cell apoptosis + necrosis
   Loss of mucosal lymphoid cells
Atrophic
   Mucosal thinning
   Normal/short villi
   Crypt hypoplasia
   Absence of local lymphoid cells

GVHD has a number of other effects on the biology of intestinal epithelial cells and their precursors (Table 2). The migration of enterocytes from the crypts up the villus is also markedly increased in mice with GVHR (28,51), reflecting a greater upward pressure arising from the enlarged crypt cell population. As we have discussed above, one consequence of the more rapid appearance of recently formed enterocytes on the villus is that the proportion of cells with mature enzyme function will be decreased. This has been confirmed in GVHR, where jejunal lactase and aminopeptidase activities do not develop until much higher up the villus than normal (28). Interestingly, however, the increased production of immature cells is balanced partly by a concomitant enhancement of the rate of differentiation of new enterocytes, with more rapid acquisition of mature enzyme activity than normal (27,28). Enhanced expression of class II MHC molecules by the epithelium is a further effect of GVHR on enterocyte differentiation. Class II MHC molecules are expressed in the cytoplasm and on the surface of small bowel villus enterocytes in most species. In normal animals, this is usually at a low level and is restricted to mature epithelial cells, with none being found on crypt cells (2). However, in acute GVHR, villus enterocytes have markedly increased levels of MHC expression, and this phenomenon now involves the entire epithelium, including the crypts. In addition, the intestinal epithelium of GVHR animals begins to express class II MHC products not normally found on enterocytes (52,53). Intestinal class II MHC expression in murine GVHR appears within the first few days of inducing GVHR and peaks before villus atrophy is detected (50,53). However, the appearance of class II MHC molecules on crypt cells is not directly related to the alterations in mitotic activity,

Table 2 Effects of GVHR on the Behavior of Intestinal Crypt Cells

Increased proliferation rate
Enhanced migration on to villus
More rapid differentiation of enzymes
Induction of expression of class II MHC molecules
Ultimately, suppression of proliferation + necrosis

as class II MHC expression does not continue to increase as the CCPR rises later in GVHR (50). There is also no clear evidence of a gradient of class II MHC expression along the villus-crypt axis (53). These findings suggest that immune mediators such as IFNγ may influence MHC gene expression by both mature and immature epithelial cells.

3. Evolution of Villus Damage

The findings discussed above indicate that the primary effects of a GVHR on the intestine are to modify the behavior of crypt cells. Nevertheless, villus atrophy remains the best recognized feature of intestinal GVHR, and in many cases there can be complete loss of the normal villus architecture (Fig. 4). Villus atrophy occurs in severe forms of GVHR, such as those found in neonatal or irradiated hosts or in certain unirradiated adults. Even in advanced GVHR, there is little evidence of direct damage to mature villus enterocytes (51). Minor changes such as the cytoplasmic vacuolization reported by some workers (29,35,54) are unlikely to account for the major structural abnormalities found in villus atrophy and may simply reflect the alterations in differentiation and migration described above. Villus atrophy is preceded by intense crypt hyperplasia, which normally reaches its peak shortly before villus atrophy can be demonstrated. The villus atrophy may develop because very intense crypt hyperplasia creates a hyper-dynamic, unstable mucosa, which cannot maintain the usual column of mature entero-cytes. An additional factor is that the stem cell apoptosis described above may lead to a failure to repopulate the villus. This latter possibility was suggested by studies of GVHR in irradiated (CBA $\times$ BALB/c)F$_1$ mice in which significant crypt hyperplasia occurred within 1–2 days of inducing the GVHR, rising to very high levels by 3–4 days (49). Villus atrophy appeared only on day 5 and was accompanied by a sudden ces-sation in crypt cell mitotic activity, rather than the further rise in CCPR that would be anticipated if crypt cell turnover was merely responding to epithelial cell damage. There-after, progressive mucosal destruction occurred, with evidence of crypt necrosis and ulceration.

In summary, the intestinal epithelium is an important target for the pathogenic effects of GVHR, and most evidence seems to favor the idea that crypt cells are the principal focus of this attack. Initially, the immune stimulus produces a proliferative enteropathy characterized by increased crypt cell proliferation, migration, and differen-tiation, but with few effects on mature enterocytes (Table 2). In severe cases, this early phase intensifies rapidly and progresses to a destructive disorder associated with cessation of crypt cell mitotic activity and crypt necrosis. Only at this stage does villus atrophy and damage to mature enterocytes appear, and we propose that these events are secondary to the alterations in crypt cell turnover and function.

B. Pathology of NonEpithelial Structures in Intestinal GVHR

Direct damage to the functioning epithelial tissues of the gut has obvious and important consequences for the host, but as we have noted, the extracellular matrix (ECM) is also involved in maintaining the integrity of the intestine. Thickening of the epithelial base-ment membrane occurs early in GVHR, but later, the basement membrane and underlying ECM appear to disintegrate as villus atrophy develops (unpublished observations). This is supported by decreased levels of the ECM protein tenascin found in the intestine of animals with acute GVHD, and, interestingly, prevention of the enteropathy with an OX40L-Ig protein leads to a concomitant increase in tenascin expression (55). Destruction of the ECM by local tissue MMP is an important late component of the Th1-mediated immune response in clinical and experimental models of inflammatory bowel diseases (56,57), and both the systemic and intestinal features of destructive acute GVHD in mice can be prevented by treatment with an MMP inhibitor (58).

The vascular system is also involved in intestinal GVHD. Swelling of the intestinal vascular endothelium has been noted in irradiated mice with severe GVHR (48), and hemorrhagic exudates and segmental ischemia are present during the terminal stages of intestinal GVHR (35,54). Notably, all these features can be reproduced by administering tumor necrosis factor-alpha (TNFα) to mice (59,60). Immune-mediated destruction or occlusion of the local blood supply may contribute significantly to the failure of intestinal function in GVHR.

C. Effects of GVHR on Intestinal Lymphoid Cells

1. General

Initial studies on intestinal GVHR emphasized that atrophy of Peyer's patches and depletion of mucosal lymphoid cells accompanied the destructive changes in mucosal architecture (25,26,35,61). These findings are again biased by studying late stages of severe disease using nonquantitative methods. Some groups reported that early, acute GVHR in mice was associated with infiltration of the mucosa by lymphoblasts (29,54). Subsequent work showed marked infiltration of the lamina propria by T lymphocytes, which correlated with the severity of mucosal damage in different models of murine GVHR (47,62). Interestingly, the majority of infiltrating T cells is found near the crypts, the major targets of the GVHR. Both donor and host T cells can be found in the infiltrate, but infiltration of the mucosa by donor CD4+ and CD8+ T cells occurs early in GVHD and is preceded by their expansion in the subepithelial region of Peyer's patch (MLN) (63,64). Interestingly, this area is particularly rich in DC that are exposed to luminal antigens (65). The donor T cells activated in PP express the $\alpha_4\beta_7$ integrin and the CCR5 chemokine receptor, and the epithelial damage and infiltration of the lamina propria and epithelium by donor T cells can be prevented by local irradiation of the PP, or by ablation of PP in utero (62,64). Therefore, the mucosal infiltrating cells appear to be derived from stimulation by host antigens in intestinal, rather than peripheral lymphoid tissues.

The organized tissues of the GALT are also involved in the intestinal phase of GVHR and show a similar biphasic pattern of damage. Depletion and atrophy of Peyer's patches is a characteristic feature of late, acute GVHR, and, of course, this may contribute to depletion of mucosal lymphocytes. However, the presence of a proliferative GVHR accelerates the development of PP in isografts of fetal small intestine implanted under the kidney capsule of mice (66), indicating that the depletion of PP may be preceded by initial lymphoid hyperplasia. The crypts supplying the dome epithelium of PP share the biphasic pattern of crypt hyperplasia and atrophy found elsewhere during intestinal GVHR (67).

2. Intraepithelial Lymphocytes

A characteristic component of the lymphocytic infiltration of the gut in GVHR is an increased proportion and mitotic activity of intraepithelial lymphocytes. An increased IEL count is one of the earliest detectable signs of intestinal GVHR, occurring within

24 hours of inducing GVHR in neonatal or irradiated mice and continuing to rise in parallel with the other proliferative features of GVHR, such as crypt hyperplasia and splenomegaly (45,49). Although this increase in IEL involves both crypt and villus epithelium, the enhanced number of IEL in crypt epithelium precedes that in the villus compartment (50). This finding is reminiscent of the pattern of IEL hyperplasia that occurs during the evolution of the mucosal lesion in human celiac disease, where a relative increase in the number of crypt IEL is the earliest feature of the local immune response to gluten antigen (68,69). The subsequent behavior of IEL depends on the type of intestinal GVHR (Fig. 5). Whereas the IEL count falls to normal levels after the peak of the GVHR in mice undergoing an entirely proliferative enteropathy, a GVHR that causes villus atrophy and mucosal destruction is associated with almost complete loss of IEL (Fig. 5) (45,66).

Given their location and increased number, it is tempting to speculate that IEL could play an important role in the mucosal pathology. As noted above, the vast majority of normal IEL are CD8+ T cells, and this remains the case during GVHR (47,50). These cells retain the low Thy 1 expression characteristic of murine IEL (47), but as the GVHR evolves, the proportion of conventional $\alpha\beta$ TcR+ CD8+ T cells bearing the $\alpha\beta$ form of the CD8 molecule increases (16,50) (Table 1). Initially, the vast majority of IEL is of host origin, but in the destructive phase of disease, most IEL are of donor origin, and the number of host-derived $\gamma\delta$ TcR+ IEL decreases (50,64,70). As we have noted, the donor IEL that appear in GVHR appear to derive via the thoracic duct and bloodstream from lymphoblast precursors that were first activated in the Peyer's patches (16,47,62,64,71). The replacement of host IEL by donor-derived T cells parallels the appearance of fas ligand–mediated cytolytic activity against host cells by IEL (70,72,73) and the onset of crypt cell apoptosis. Thus, the elimination of host IEL and destruction of crypt stem cells may both be consequences of the donor antihost response in severe disease.

The reasons for the early infiltration by host-derived IEL are unknown, but it has been suggested that they may be potentially autoreactive CD8+ T cells that recognize self antigens expressed at abnormally high levels on the damaged epithelium (5). It is equally possible that the infiltration by host IEL is part of a generalized, nonspecific recruitment of inflammatory cells which occurs in the mucosa during GVHR.

3. Other Lymphoid Cells

The biphasic increases and decreases in IEL and lamina propria T lymphoblasts are accompanied by parallel changes in other mucosal lymphoid cells. Increased numbers of class II MHC-expressing accessory cells are found in the lamina propria early in GVHR (53), and the density of MHC expression is higher. Subsequently, there is marked depletion of class II MHC+ macrophages and dendritic cells in established GVHR (47). Similar effects on IgA-producing plasma cells in the lamina propria have been observed, with substantial loss of these cells occurring in severe murine GVHR (74), preceded by a phase of enhanced IgA production and hyperplasia of IgA plasma cells. It is important to note that the depletion of both these cell types late in GVHR could compromise local defense mechanisms and hence contribute to the evolution of intestinal damage.

Hyperplasia of mucosal mast cells is a further indicator of the proliferative consequences of intestinal GVHR. Several studies have reported an increase in MMC in rodent GVHR (45,62). In parallel, there is an increase in serum levels of IL-3 (75), while the intestine and serum show increased levels of the mucosal mast cell specific protease (46,76). The time course of MMC hyperplasia and release of protease parallels other

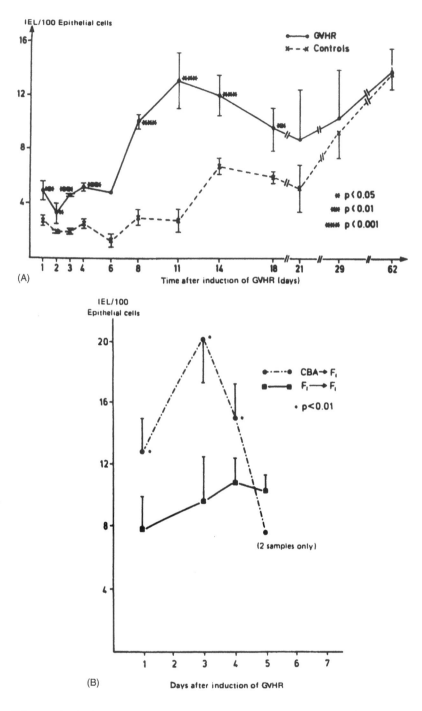

Figure 5 Behavior of intraepithelial lymphocyte populations in different forms of intestinal GVHR. IEL counts increase rapidly in both proliferative (A) and destructive (B) enteropathy. However, the IEL counts remain increased for some time in the proliferative GVHR in unirradiated (CBA × BALB/c)F_1 mice, while IEL disappear rapidly as GVHR progresses in irradiated F_1 hosts given CBA donor cells (B).

proliferative changes of GVHR but does not seem to reduce to the same extent as other indices of host inflammation during the destructive phase of GVHR (76).

In conclusion, the pattern of damage to intestinal lymphoid components parallels that found in the associated epithelium. As in other peripheral lymphoid organs, there is an early period of infiltration by donor T lymphoblasts and an associated proliferation of many host-derived immune cells. In mild forms of GVHR this proliferation may be the only abnormality, but in acute, destructive models of GVHR there is progression to the lymphoid depletion often thought to be the principal feature of GVHR.

IV. MECHANISMS OF INTESTINAL GVHD

Intestinal GVHD shows the same requirement for T cells as GVHR in other sites, being inhibited by elimination of mature T cells from the donor inoculum (36) and by administration of cyclosporin A (77). Although there are also many similarities between the mechanisms responsible for systemic and intestinal GVHD, there are several important differences. In this review, we will first address the cellular and genetic factors that determine the induction of intestinal GVHR before discussing local and systemic effector mechanisms.

A. Cellular and Genetic Basis of Intestinal GVHR

Most work on intestinal GVHR across MHC incompatibilities has emphasized the importance of CD4+ T cells to the disease. In our own experience, both CD4+ and CD8+ T cells were required to induce fully developed enteropathy in either proliferative or destructive models of fully allogeneic GVHR in mice. However, CD8-depleted T cells were fully capable of inducing hyperplasia of IEL in adult, unirradiated mice with proliferative GVHR, as well as significant villus atrophy and crypt hyperplasia in either adult or neonatal hosts. In contrast, purified CD8+ T cells only produced a small degree of villus atrophy and crypt hyperplasia in destructive GVHR and were incapable alone of inducing hyperplasia of IEL or crypts in adult hosts (78). In analogous studies of three different models of destructive GVHR in (C3H × DBA/2)F$_1$ mice, Guy-Grand and Vassalli (47) also found that both CD4+ and CD8+ T cells could produce some degree of intestinal pathology. However, CD4+ T cells were much more efficient than CD8+ T cells at inducing crypt hyperplasia, class II MHC expression by crypts, and mucosal infiltration by donor lymphoblasts in irradiated hosts. Interestingly though, only CD8+ T cells induced significant enteropathy in unirradiated adults and were more efficient than CD4+ T cells in newborn hosts (47). Colonic GVHR can also be induced in BDF1 hosts using either CD4+ or CD8+ T cells of DBA/2 origin, but again, CD4+ cells are much more effective (36).

The genetic requirements for intestinal GVHR in experimental mice underline the predominant role of CD4 + T cells, as a number of groups have shown that a class II MHC incompatibility alone is sufficient for the induction of both proliferative and destructive enteropathy (31,47,78,79). The ability of isolated class I MHC disparities to induce intestinal GVHR is less certain. Some studies have reported that no enteropathy occurs in congenic mice differing only at the class I MHC locus, even if very sensitive techniques are used to measure intestinal damage and in models that produce significant systemic disease (31,78). However, if sufficient donor T cells are transferred into class I MHC disparate congenic recipients, or if a sufficiently potent mutant class I alloantigen is used as the stimulus, intestinal GVHR can be produced in irradiated hosts (47,79). Interestingly, class I MHC-disparate recipients that undergo acute intestinal GVHR after transfer of CD8+ T cells may also go on to develop the unusual atrophic form of enteropathy described above (79).

Few studies have examined intestinal GVHR induced by minor histocompatibility differences in experimental animals. Mild crypt hyperplasia and villus edema has been reported in irradiated, minor antigen-incompatible $(DBA/2 \times B10.D2)F_1$ mice with GVHR induced by unseparated donor lymphocytes (54). Although systemic GVHR can be induced across minor histoincompatibility antigens by both CD4+ and CD8+ T cells (80,81), only CD4+ T cells have been found to produce enteropathy across minor histocompatibility differences (81).

Together, these studies show that although both major subsets of T lymphocyte can induce intestinal GVHR, class II MHC−restricted CD4+ T cells are much more potent than their class I MHC−restricted counterparts. Nevertheless, activation of both CD4+ and CD8+ T cells may usually be required to generate the full scope of enteropathy in GVHR. In addition, the two subsets may each be responsible for individual aspects of the pathology, with CD4+ T cells appearing to be of particular importance in recruiting local inflammatory cells such as IEL.

B. Effector Mechanisms in Intestinal GVHR

1. Nature of the Local Cell-Mediated Immune Response

Much of the initial interest in the mechanisms of intestinal GVHR focused on the possible role of cytotoxic T cells in the epithelial pathology. As we have discussed, class I MHC−restricted CD8+ T cells may be required to induce full-blown intestinal GVHR. Furthermore, the most severe forms of intestinal pathology tend to occur in experimental models of GVHR in which class I MHC−restricted antihost CTL are generated (49). A possible role for CTL is supported further by the finding that CD8 + T cells dominate the population of donor T lymphoblasts found in the PP, thoracic duct, and intestinal lamina propria of mice with acute GVHR directed at full MHC differences (47). In addition, the increased population of intraepithelial T cells in GVHR contains a large proportion of $\alpha\beta$ TcR+ CD8+ T cells with the cytoplasmic granules and potent spontaneous lytic functions characteristic of activated CTL (16,21,47,50). IEL of this type express high levels of fas ligand (fasL) and are capable of fasL-mediated lytic activity against enterocytes (82).

Several pieces of evidence argue against an essential role for CTL in the pathogenesis of intestinal GVHR. First, there is no consistent correlation between CTL activity and intestinal damage in experimental models of GVHR (83), while crypt hyperplasia and increased IEL counts occur in adult, unirradiated F_1 hosts in the absence of antihost CTL in the gut or other lymphoid tissues (84). Furthermore, the full scope of proliferative enteropathy develops in parental strain mice made chimeric for class II MHC−disparate BM cells of F_1 origin, despite the fact that the intestinal epithelium of these animals remains syngeneic to the parental donor T cells. Conversely, F_1 mice made chimeric for donor BM do not develop intestinal GVHR (85). Thus, the enteropathy is not due to a direct attack by donor CTL on the intestinal tissue itself, but rather it is secondary to recognition of recirculating, class II MHC+ "passenger leukocytes" of BM origin. The best evidence of this "bystander effect" of GVHR comes from experiments in which pieces of fetal small intestine of parental type are implanted under the kidney capsule of adult F_1 hybrid mice. After some weeks, grafts of this kind develop relatively normal intestinal architecture of donor type, but are infiltrated by recirculating BM-derived cells of host origin. As shown in Figure 6, when a GVHR is induced in the F_1 hosts by injection of parental lymphocytes, the donor-type grafts show increases in IEL count, CCPR, and crypt length similar to those found in the host jejunum (44). T-cell infiltration, villus atrophy, crypt hyperplasia, and crypt cell apoptosis/necrosis can all also occur as bystander phenomena in fetal intestine of donor type implanted in mice with destructive GVHR (Fig. 6) (42,62). Together these experiments show that the gut itself does not need to present an allogeneic stimulus to the alloreactive donor cells and suggest that the alterations such as crypt hyperplasia are due to nonspecific mechanisms originally induced by BM-derived cells.

Colonic GVHD is also not dependent on CTL, as it is not affected by the elimination of actively cytotoxic donor cells using the lysosomotropic agent L-leucyl-leucine-O-methyl ester, even under conditions in which systemic disease is inhibited (36).

2. Role of Cytokines

Cytokines have been the most widely studied of nonspecific effector mechanisms of this kind.

Production of Cytokines During GVHD. Several groups have found that acute GVHD in mice GVHR is accompanied by increased levels of a wide range of different cytokines in peripheral lymphoid organs and in circulation. These include IL-1, IL-2, IL-3, IL-4, IL-5, IL-10, IL-12, IFNγ, and TNFα, although the most prominent are usually those associated with Th1-dependent immune responses, particularly IFNγ and TNFα (63,70,86–92). Interestingly one of the most recent of these studies showed that the production of IFNγ in the MLN draining the gut was higher and earlier than in peripheral lymphoid tissues, indicating that much of the stimulus to the production of this cytokine occurred in the intestine (63). Studies of cytokine production in the intestine itself have also emphasized the predominance of Th1-dependent mediators in acute GVHD, as increased levels of IFNγ and TNFα have been found in both lamina propria and IEL T cells, many of which are donor derived (47,63,70,72,92,93). In parallel, local production of Th2-dependent cytokines such as IL-4, IL-5, and IL-10 may be downregulated (63).

In most reports, cytokine production has been examined at the peak of intestinal disease, but in a time course study, we found that the different phases of GVHD are characterized by different patterns of systemic cytokine production. Thus, the hyperplastic features of early GVHD are always accompanied by increasing levels of IFNγ, and these peak at the time of maximal crypt cell proliferation (Fig. 7) (90,94). IFNγ production then falls rapidly, even in models in which the enteropathy continues to progress to villus atrophy. Conversely, enhanced TNFα production is not always found in acute GVHD, but when it occurs, it is associated with the late, destructive phase of disease (94) (Fig. 7). The levels of TNFα vary considerably, even within the same disease model, probably reflecting the requirement for several independent factors to trigger the release of this cytokine (see below).

Role of Cytokines in Pathogenesis of Intestinal GVHD. Our early studies showed that treatment of mice with monoclonal anti-IFNγ antibody prevented all aspects of enteropathy, despite having much less effect on the systemic components of GVHR such as splenomegaly, weight loss, and antihost CTL activity (95). Donor T cells from IFNγ knockout

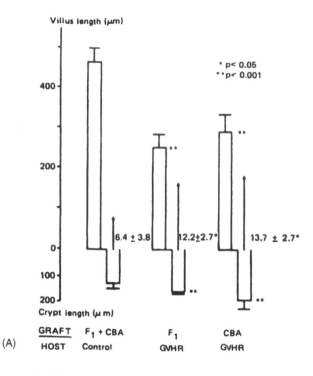

(A)

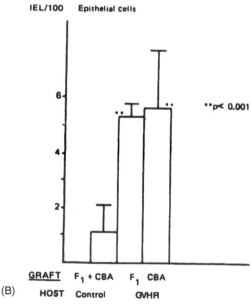

(B)

Figure 6 Intestinal GVHR occurs as a "bystander phenomenon." Mucosal architecture (A) and IEL counts (B) in grafts of fetal (CBA × BALB/c)F_1 or CBA small intestine implanted in irradiated (CBA × BALB/c)F_1 mice given CBA donor cells. Villus atrophy, as well as increases in CCPR, crypt length, and IEL count occur, irrespective of whether the gut grafts are syngeneic to the donor.

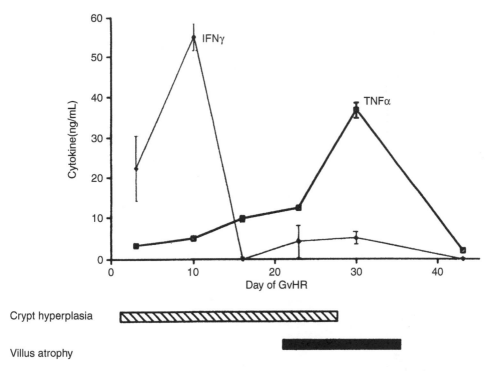

Crypt hyperplasia

Villus atrophy

Figure 7 Correlation between IFNγ and TNFα production and intestinal pathology in acute GVHR. During the early proliferation period, there is a rapid rise in splenic IFNγ production, which parallels the development of crypt hyperplasia. At this time, there is no TNFα production, but this appears as villus atrophy and mucosal destruction progresses.

(KO) mice also cannot induce crypt hyperplasia and apoptosis in GVHD (40,96), while T cells from mice lacking Stat4, the transcription factor responsible for the differentiation of IFNγ-producing Th1 cells, also have a reduced capacity to induce intestinal GVHD (97). Although one further report has suggested that intestinal GVHD occurs normally after neutralising IFNγ or IL-12 or in recipients of IFNγ KO T cells (98), the balance of evidence therefore indicates a central role for IFNγ in intestinal GVHD.

In support of this idea, parenteral administration of nontoxic doses of recombinant IFNγ induces enteropathy in mouse small intestine (59,99). Significant crypt hypertrophy and hyperplasia are found after a single dose of intraperitoneal IFNγ, and these become more marked if the cytokine is given continuously over a period of days by osmotic pump (Fig. 8) or if it is derived from a growing tumour mass in vivo (100). IFNγ alone is unable to induce villus atrophy in normal animals, but it will act in synergy to cause significant villus damage when given with TNFα (Fig. 8A). The effects of IFNγ can be reproduced by administration of IL-12 (99), and acute GVHD in mice can be prevented by anti-IL-12 antibodies (89,90). For these reasons, we believe that an IFNγ-dependent Th1 response is the critical event in the initial, proliferative stages of acute GVHD. As a consequence, this process is also the essential precursor to the later stages of the disease.

The other mediator that has been studied intensively in intestinal GVHD is TNFα. Indeed, it is now often assumed that TNFα is the principal pathogenic mechanism in the disorder. However, the evidence for this is rather equivocal. As noted above, a marked

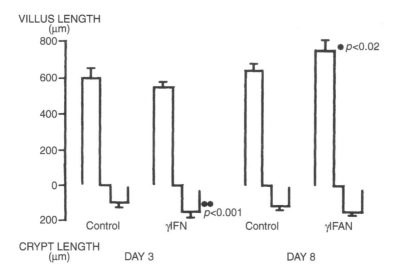

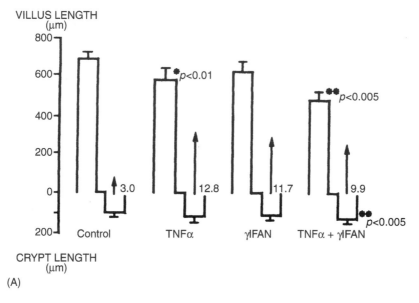

(A)

Figure 8 (A) Induction of intestinal pathology by systemic administration of IFNγ or TNFα. Continuous intraperitoneal administration of IFNγ by osmotic minipump produces significant crypt hyperplasia in the jejunum, which becomes less marked with time. Villus atrophy is not found, and indeed chronic treatment with IFNγ stimulates villus lengthening (top). A single injection of IFNγ or TNFα produces mild crypt hypertrophy 24 hours later, but not significant villus damage. However, the two cytokines together produce synergistic changes in crypt and villus lengths (bottom). (B) Administration of TNFα also rapidly induces release of mucosal mast cell protease (MMCP) in the serum of normal mice.

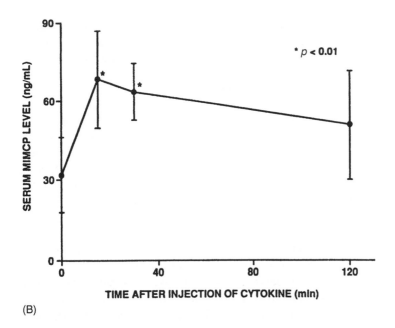

(B)

Figure 8   *Continued.*

increase in intestinal and systemic TNFα production has been reported in the established phase of several models of acute GVHD. However, this is not a consistent finding, and TNFα production appears to be determined by the amount of bacterial endotoxin that gains access to the circulation through an already damaged intestine and can interact with macrophages that have been primed by the initial release of IFNγ (see below). Early work showing that all the consequences of destructive intestinal GVHR in irradiated mice could be prevented by administration of a polyclonal anti-TNFα antibody (48) has been supported by similar findings using monoclonal anti-TNFα antibodies (93,101), DNA encoding a soluble inhibitory form of the type 2 TNF receptor (TNFR) (102), or by the TNFα inhibitor pentoxifylline (101). Recent studies indicate that the source of TNFα in these systems is donor-derived, as TNFα KO T cells have a defective ability to induce severe intestinal and systemic disease (103). Interestingly, the enterocyte apoptosis found in the small intestine of mice given anti-CD3 antibody in vivo is partially dependent on TNFα (104). In contrast to these findings, we have been completely unable to influence any aspect of intestinal GVHR by administering a number of different polyclonal or monoclonal anti-TNFα antibodies, or by treatment with soluble TNFR2 (unpublished observations). In addition, pentoxifylline has been shown to influence epithelial cell behavior via mechanisms that are independent of TNFα (105), while others have found that crypt cell apoptosis does not necessarily correlate with TNFα production in acute GVHD (96). Administration of TNFα to normal animals causes enterocyte damage and apoptosis, villus shortening, mucosal necrosis and vascular lesions within 1 hour. Although crypt hyperplasia also occurs, it appears to be a secondary event (59,60) and may be dependent on early release of IFNγ (Fig. 8A). Overall, these features are reminiscent of the terminal stages of late stage intestinal GVHD, and together they suggest that TNFα is not an essential initiating factor in intestinal GVHD.

Consistent with the evidence discussed above that Th1-dependent immune responses may be critical for intestinal GVHD, a number of reports have implicated macrophage products such as IL-1 and type 1 IFN in the disorder. Treatment of mice with polyclonal anti-IL1α antibody inhibits the development of crypt hyperplasia and increased IEL counts in GVHR, but has little effect on the systemic manifestations of disease (106). In support of this finding, administration of IL-1α induces severe enteropathy in normal mice, with intense crypt hyperplasia, villus atrophy, focal necrosis, and increased IEL counts (106). Administration of the type I IFN inducer polyinosinic:polycytydylic acid (polyI:C) exacerbates the intestinal and systemic consequences of murine GVHD and induces crypt hyperplasia and villus atrophy in normal animals (107). Purified type I IFN has similar effects in normal animals, stimulating crypt hyperplasia very rapidly (107). Interestingly, type I IFN also provokes villus atrophy and crypt hyperplasia in explants of human intestine in vitro (108), and increased levels of the cytokine have been found in the mucosa of patients with celiac disease (109), an enteropathy with many similar architectural and immunological features to intestinal GVHD. Both these cytokines may therefore play accessory roles in the early and late stages of intestinal GVHD.

Rather surprisingly, IL-4 also appears to be involved in the enteropathy of GVHR, as administration of either anti-IL-4 antibody or a soluble form of the IL-4 receptor, and prevents crypt hyperplasia, crypt hypertrophy, and IEL hyperplasia in a dose-dependent fashion (110). Depletion of IL-4 had no effect on the progress of destructive enteropathy and had only a minor effect on the systemic manifestations of GVHR, including CTL activity. Although these findings would appear to conflict with the idea that intestinal GVHD is a Th1-mediated disorder, more recent work shows that donor T cells from mice lacking Stat 6, the transcription factor that controls the action of IL-4, have some impairment in their ability to induce enteropathy in irradiated recipients (97). Interestingly, IL-4 has also been found to play a role in other forms of immune-mediated enteropathies that are normally associated more with Th1-cell activity, including chronic inflammatory bowel disease and helminth infections. In theses cases, IL-4 appears to play a similar role to IFNγ, inducing a similar final common pathway of macrophage activation, TNFα production, and nitric oxide (NO) release (12,111). Both IL-4 and IL-13 can also directly influence enterocyte function (112), and therefore Th2 cytokines of this kind may help initiate intestinal GVHD under some circumstances.

Transforming growth factor-beta (TGFβ) is an important autocrine and paracrine mediator of epithelial cell proliferation. It is produced by normal enterocytes and, as a product of activated T lymphocytes and macrophages, also has many immunoregulatory properties (110). TGFβ therefore offers a potential link between immune activation and epithelial pathology in disorders like GVHR. TGFβ is expressed constitutively by villus epithelial cells in mouse small intestine, but during the proliferative phase of intestinal GVHR, enterocyte TGFβ expression falls dramatically (113). Thereafter, as the epithelial pathology and crypt hyperplasia resolve, TGFβ expression returns to normal or above normal levels. Thus, production of this cytokine may normally play a homeostatic role in regulating the epithelial manifestations of GVHR. This is supported by the finding that neutralization of TGFβ in vivo with anti-TGFβ antibody enhances many of the intestinal and systemic features of GVHD, including crypt hyperplasia, increased IEL counts, and NK cell activation (113). In parallel, administration of TGFβ inhibits the proliferative manifestations of GVHR both in the intestine and elsewhere (113). This is not only due to downregulation of the immune response in GVHR, as TGFβ also inhibits crypt cell turnover in normal mice. Again, these results support the concept that TGFβ is an endogenous regulatory mediator which is part of the host response to epithelial insult in conditions like GVHR.

Taken together, these studies emphasize the importance of an IL-12-dependent, IFNγ-mediated Th1 response in the development of acute intestinal GVHD. IFNγ production is the initial event that produces enteropathy, and it appears to be responsible for much of the proliferative pathology in epithelial cells. In addition, it induces the production of additional potentially pathogenic mediators, including TNFα and type I IFN. However, the initiating role can be taken by other cytokines, including IL-4.

3. Mechanisms of Cytokine-Induced Intestinal Pathology

Cytokines may produce intestinal pathology either by direct effects on enterocytes or via indirect actions on nonspecific effector cells.

Direct Interactions Between Cytokines and Intestinal Epithelial Cells. Enterocytes possess receptors for many cytokines, and several epithelial cell functions can be influenced directly by cytokines. In addition, enterocytes are themselves capable of producing a range of cytokines with the potential both to modify the immune response and to influence epithelial function, including IL-1, IL-6, IL-8, IL-15, TNFα, and TGFβ (114–122). Thus, direct interactions between cytokines and epithelial cells offer the potential for both paracrine and autocrine regulation of local immunopathology.

IFNγ upregulates the expression of a number of surface proteins on purified enterocytes in vitro, including class I and II MHC molecules, adhesion molecules, and the polymeric immunoglobulin receptor (Fig. 9A) (123–126). IFNγ also decreases the ability of enterocyte monolayers to secrete Cl⁻ anions and to maintain an intact barrier, properties that translate in vivo to increased permeability to luminal contents (127–129). Abnormalities of these functions in vivo could produce many of the characteristic features of intestinal GVHR, including diarrhea, malabsorption, and increased epithelial permeability. In contrast to its proposed role in enteropathy and to its predominantly hyperplastic effects in vivo, IFNγ is usually profoundly cytostatic to enterocytes in vitro (Fig. 9B). Similar findings have been made in the skin, where the proliferation of isolated keratinocytes is inhibited by IFNγ, but local injection of the cytokine induces epidermal hyperplasia in vivo (130). These results confirm the potential for IFNγ to interact directly with enterocytes, but also underline that its overall effect in intestinal GVHD in vivo is likely to involve a number of different cell types.

IL-1 stimulates mitosis of crypt stem cells in vitro (106), as can TNFα, although the effects of TNFα are dependent on the stage of the cell cycle at which the epithelial cell is studied (our unpublished observations). In addition, TNFα causes apoptosis of enterocytes and enhanced expression of secretory component, adhesion molecules, and MHC molecules in vitro, as well as altering the barrier and secretion functions of epithelial monolayers (Fig. 9A) (126,131,132). It also induces the production of enterocyte-derived cytokines, such as IL-6 and IL-8 (114,116). Many of the effects of TNFα are enhanced by IFNγ (Fig. 8A) or if the epithelial cells have been subjected to other insults. These findings are compatible with the in vivo evidence that TNFα is involved late in intestinal GVHR, requiring the presence of other mediators both for its production and functional effects.

IL-1 and IL-6 also have a number of direct effects on enterocytes, including stimulating the release of inflammatory cytokines from enterocytes in vitro (114). IL-4 and

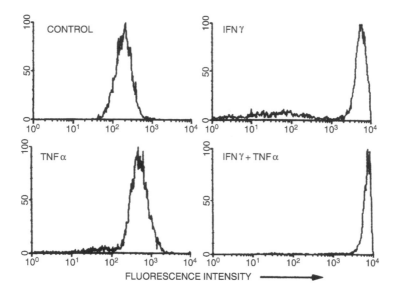

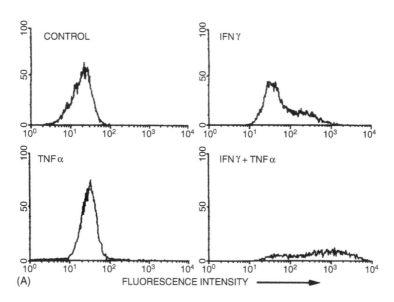

Figure 9   Effects of cytokines on enterocytes in vitro. (A) Induction of MHC expression on crypt stem cells by treatment with IFNγ and/or TNFα in vitro. Both cytokines alone produce increased levels of class I MHC antigens by RIE cells after 48 hours of culture and produce maximal expression when added together (top). Although RIE cells do not normally express class II MHC antigens, treatment with IFNγ alone produces some increase in expression, and addition of both cytokines together induces the appearance of class II MHC on most cells (bottom). (B) IFNγ is directly cytostatic to crypt stem cells in vitro. The RIE epithelial cell line shows a dose-dependent inhibition of growth in the presence of recombinant IFNγ.

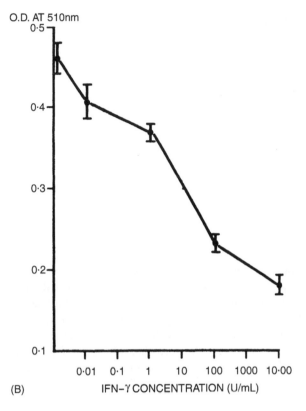

O.D. AT 510nm

IFN-γ CONCENTRATION (U/mL)

(B)

Figure 9 *Continued.*

IL-13 can also enhance epithelial expression of MHC and adhesion molecules in vitro, as well as interfering with ion secretion and transepithelial migration of neutrophils (112,133,134). Thus, a number of the cytokines implicated in intestinal GVHD have the capacity to alter epithelial function by interacting directly with enterocytes.

Indirect Effects of Cytokines in Intestinal GVHR. A major role of cytokines in enteropathy is to recruit and activate a number of inflammatory and/or mesenchymal cells.

MACROPHAGES. Release of cytokines and other inflammatory mediators by IFNγ-activated macrophages appears to be central to many aspects of intestinal GVHD. Activation of macrophages is an important feature of systemic GVHD and depletion of macrophages in vivo by administration of silica or liposomes containing the lysosomal toxin CL1,2 MDP reduces the intestinal consequences of GVHR in mice (Table 3). As we have discussed, GVHR in mice is associated with increased levels of macrophage-derived cytokines. There is also enhanced production of NO in the small intestine, which is entirely dependent on donor cell production of IFNγ and is enhanced by bacterial lipopolysaccharide (LPS) (96). Inhibition of macrophage-dependent NO production by treatment with analogues of L-arginine prevents crypt hyperplasia, enterocyte apoptosis, and increased IEL counts in murine GVHD (96,135). Macrophage products such as NO, IL-1, TNFα, and IL-6 may have direct effects on epithelial cells as discussed above, or they may alter the activities of other cell types in the gut. In particular, NO

Table 3   Effects of Macrophage Depletion on Intestinal
GVHR

Group	C1,2 MDP lips	Crypt length (μm)
Control	—	103.6 ± 4.1
Control	+	98.1 ± 7.9
GVHR	—	125.6 ± 10.8*
GVHR	+	106.0 ± 10.8+

(CBA × BALB/c)F$_1$ mice were depleted of macrophages 1 day
before induction of GVHR by intravenous injection of liposomes
containing the lysosomotropic agent C1,2 MDP. On day 8 of
GVHR, these mice had significantly less crypt lengthening in the
jejunum compared with untreated GVHR mice. * $p < 0.02$ vs. control; +$p < 0.02$ vs. GVHR.

can interact with blood vessels, epithelial cells, and neural cells of the gut, producing
apoptosis, inflammation, fluid secretion, increased motility, and other pathological effects
(136,137). IL-1 and TNFα can activate mesenchymal cells such as myofibroblasts to
release keratinocyte growth factor that regulates epithelial growth, while TNFα stimulates
the production of matrix metalloproteinases, which destroy the extracellular matrix of the
mucosa (57). Again, this latter property supports the idea that TNFα is of particular
importance in the terminal stages of intestinal GVHD, when mucosal necrosis occurs.
Macrophages themselves may release other proteolytic enzymes that are likely to contribute to the inflammation.

NATURAL KILLER CELLS.   Enhanced NK cell activity by peripheral lymphocytes is
a feature of the early proliferative phase of experimental GVHD (49,84,138,139). It parallels splenomegaly and IFNγ production, precedes the development of villus atrophy and
other destructive features of GVHD, and is dependent on the production of IL-12 during
the initiation of disease (90). Depletion of NK cells from the host or of NK1.1 + cells
from the donor inoculum also prevents systemic disease in destructive forms of GVHD
(140–142).

The ways in which NK cells could influence intestinal pathology are unknown. The
systemic NK cell activation in acute GVHD is accompanied by enhanced NK cell function
by small intestinal IEL (84) and the ability of cytokines such as IFNγ and IL-12 to produce
enteropathy correlates with the presence of IEL with natural cytolytic activity (99).
In addition, mice treated with anti-AsGM1 antibody have somewhat reduced IEL counts,
as well as being protected from enteropathy (143). Thus, mucosal NK cells may be of central importance in intestinal GVHD, perhaps by exerting cytotoxic activity on epithelial
cells or, more likely, by producing enteropathic cytokines such as IFNγ or TNFα (144).
Alternatively, it has been suggested that NK1.1 + cells may play a secondary role in intestinal damage in GVHD by virtue of the fact that their production of cytokines is important
for the differentiation of pathogenic Th1 (142).

MUCOSAL MAST CELLS.   As we have discussed, hyperplasia of mucosal mast cells is
a histological feature of many experimental models of GVHR and probably reflects
recruitment by IL-3. Administration of TNFα to normal animals also activates MMC
(Fig. 8B), and TGFβ has a potent ability to promote the recruitment and differentiation
of MMC (145). The hyperplasia of MMC in rodent GVHR is accompanied by increased

levels of MMC-specific protease in the serum and intestinal mucosa (46,76). MMCP has a number of potentially harmful effects in the mucosa, including increasing epithelial permeability, direct destruction of basement membrane type IV collagen, and the activation of tissue metalloproteinases (24). In addition, other MMC-derived mediators may increase epithelial permeability and ion secretion (23), indicating that MMC could play an important pathogenic role in intestinal GVHD. However, the peak of hyperplasia of MMC is much delayed compared with crypt hyperplasia in unirradiated hosts (45) and is not a significant feature of GVHR in irradiated hosts, despite the more severe enteropathy which occurs under these circumstances (46). More importantly, intestinal GVHD is more severe in W/W^v mice that lack all mast cells, including MMC (76). Thus, MMC may play a protective rather than a harmful role in intestinal GVHD, perhaps via their ability to promote tissue remodeling (24).

4. Other Mechanisms of Intestinal GVHD

An additional way in which T cells could cause enteropathy without the need for specific recognition of tissue cells or the production of soluble mediators is via non–antigen-specific membrane molecules. Of these, the most obvious candidate is fas ligand, which can induce apoptosis in target cells by cross-linking to fas. As we have noted, there is upregulation of fasL by mucosal T cells of donor origin in acute GVHD. IEL shows concomitant increases in expression of fasL and IFNγ (70,72,73,146). These lymphocytes can then induce cell death in epithelial cells in vitro, and the crypt cell apoptosis and villus destruction found in the enteropathy induced by administration of anti-CD3 antibody is partly dependent on fasL, although perforin and TNFR-mediated cytotoxicity also play important roles (104). It is less clear if the fas-fasL pathway is necessary for intestinal pathology in acute GVHD. Cellular damage in liver GVHD is dependent on fas (147), and the appearance of fasL + donor T cells in the gut correlates with the ability of different parental cells to induce intestinal GVHD in F$_1$ mice (70). It has also been reported that the depletion of host lymphocytes from the gut mucosa does not occur in GVHD if the donor T cells derive from gld mice that lack fasL (70). However, treatment with anti-fasL antibody does not affect the development of crypt hyperplasia, crypt cell apoptosis, or villus atrophy in acute GVHD (101). In addition, lpr recipient mice that lack fas expression undergo more severe intestinal pathology and infiltration by IFNγ–producing donor T cells than wild-type recipients (147). FasL KO (gld) recipients also develop more severe tissue damage in acute GVHD (148), indicating that this pathway may actually have a protective role in GVHD. Clearly more work is required on this potentially important issue.

C. Host Factors in Intestinal GVHR

Several host factors other than the capacity of tissue antigens to activate donor T cells influence the development of intestinal GVHR in experimental animals.

1. Intestinal Microflora

Bacteria.   The beneficial effect of bowel decontamination on survival after clinical BMT is well documented (149,150), and this clearly reflects a role for bacterial products on the outcome of systemic disease, probably via their ability to enhance the production of pathogenic cytokines (151). Early studies showed that removal of aerobic gut flora prevented much of the liver and gut damage normally associated with severe GVHD. If the animals are subsequently returned to conventional conditions or associated with gram-negative aerobes, mortality and tissue damage reappear (152,153). Administration of *Escherichia coli* or purified LPS exacerbates systemic GVHD in irradiated mice, while passive immunization with antibody to *E. coli* has a moderately beneficial effect (154,155). Together, these findings suggest that gram-negative aerobes in the gut flora are critical for the pathogenesis of systemic GVHD, although the beneficial effects of the germ-free state are frequently transient, with final mortality rates and pathology ultimately being similar to those in conventional hosts (33,152,153).

The harmful effects of intestinal bacteria probably reflect the increased amounts of endotoxin that can be found in serum and liver during the disease (33,91,156,157). Presumably other bacterially derived immunomodulators may also contribute. The increased uptake of endotoxin reflects the increased permeability that occurs early in GVHD due to the initial T-lymphocyte response (32). As we have discussed, this also primes macrophages, making them hyperreactive to the increased levels of endotoxin. Together, these effects lead to the release of macrophage-derived mediators such as TNFα and NO, which may then be responsible for the severe systemic manifestations and death (91,96,156,157). Although the most likely candidate for causing both the early intestinal pathology and priming of macrophages is IFNγ (see above), IFNγ KO donor T cells can also prime endotoxin sensitivity and TNFα production by macrophages in GVHD (40). Thus, additional mediators may also be involved in macrophage priming.

As discussed above, there is conflicting evidence on the role of TNFα in GVHD, and recent work indicates that NO may play a much more central role in both the systemic and intestinal effects (96). Not only does inhibition of NO production prevent intestinal GVHD (96,135), but the effects of endotoxin in GVHD correlate better with the induction of NO synthesis than that of TNFα (96). Together, these findings suggest that while endotoxin-induced NO may be an essential component of systemic GVHD, TNFα may be more important in end-stage disease, with its production requiring particularly high levels of circulating endotoxin or the presence of different bacterial immunomodulators. The amount and nature of the products present in circulation may be influenced by the species present in the intestinal flora, as well as by nonimmune factors that can add to the initial intestinal damage. Of these, the most important are likely to be components of the conditioning regime such as radiation and cytotoxic drugs. Intestinal damage in GVHD is much more severe and develops more rapidly in irradiated recipients, while it has been shown that even relatively modest increases in the dose of irradiation can greatly increase the severity of intestinal and systemic GVHD in a TNFα-dependent manner (158). Similar findings have been made in human bone marrow transplantation (see below). Given these conditions, TNFα may exacerbate the lesions of terminal GVHR, including bone marrow aplasia, cachexia, and destruction of epithelia via stem cell apoptosis. In contrast, the production of NO (and perhaps other mediators such as IL-1 or type I IFN) by primed macrophages may be less dependent on intense stimulation by endotoxaemia and so may play a more critical role in the induction of GVHD.

Despite the clear influence of bacterial products absorbed through a damaged intestine on the systemic consequences of GVHD, it is important to emphasize that the induction of intestinal pathology itself is not dependent on the presence of local bacteria. Although the terminal stages of intestinal GVHD may involve secondary infection causing local abscess formation and necrosis (153), crypt hyperplasia, villus atrophy, and lymphocytic infiltration can all occur in sterile, antigen-free grafts of small intestine implanted under the kidney capsule of mice with GVHD (44,49,66). As in the intact gut, the terminal stages of this may require the presence of luminal bacteria in the host intestine, presumably reflecting a role for circulating endotoxin (42). However, secondary bacterial infection of the mucosa may undoubtedly exacerbate the intestinal lesion, and systemic sepsis can also induce epithelial hyperplasia in the gut (159). Focal necrosis and abscesses are also particularly characteristic of severe GVHD in the colon.

Viral Infection. Virus infection is an important differential diagnosis of intestinal GVHD. BMT patients are already at risk of immunosuppression and this is likely to be exacerbated by the consequences and treatment of acute GVHD. For these reasons, GVHD patients are particularly susceptible to intestinal virus infection. There are no studies on the interactions between local viruses and intestinal GVHD in experimental animals, but the fact that CMV infection can exacerbate lung disease in mice with GVHD (160) indicates how local virus infection may synergize with immune-mediated damage to the intestine.

2. Endogenous Host Factors

The influence of host factors on intestinal GVHD is illustrated by the varying spectrum of disease seen in different types of host using the same donor-host strain combination. As we have noted, intestinal pathology is much more severe when the hosts used are irradiated (158,161). Irradiation and other conditioning agents have profound effects on the integrity and renewal of the intestinal epithelium, many of which overlap with those induced by the immune response in GVHD. These include apoptosis of crypt stem cells, loss of barrier function, and secondary effects on epithelial cell turnover and villus architecture. Thus, synergistic effects of GVHD and irradiation on intestinal damage can readily be imagined. Similar exacerbation of enteropathy is found in athymic or immature hosts (49,83). This may partly reflect an absence of the host T cells and other lymphocytes thought to be capable of resisting the proliferation of alloreactive donor T cells (162). In addition, the intestine of immature hosts may be unusually susceptible to the effects of GVHR, as major physiological alterations occur in mucosal architecture during the neonatal period.

V. TREATMENT OF INTESTINAL GVHD IN ANIMALS

Therapy for the intestinal symptoms of acute GVHD normally relies on the use of conventional immunosuppressive agents (see below). As we have noted, CsA can inhibit experimental intestinal GVHD (77), but as many generalized immunomodulatory agents can themselves damage the gut, it would be preferable to have more targeted therapies. The evidence that individual mediators such as TNFα, IFNγ, and NO may be important has led to clinical trials based on their depletion in vivo, and, as we discuss below, some success has been achieved. Analogous strategies have recently proved useful in the treatment of inflammatory bowel diseases. In addition to appropriate monoclonal antibodies and soluble, antagonistic forms of cytokine receptors, such approaches may also include the use of agents such as pentoxifylline or thalidomide, which inhibit the production and activity of TNFα (101,163), as well as recently described small molecule inhibitors of Th1 differentiation (164). Studies using an equivalent reagent to antagonize the activity of endotoxin in vivo have shown that by blocking the environmental trigger to the production of TNFα and other mediators, this can inhibit systemic and intestinal

GVHD in mice, indicating that this may also be feasible in humans (165). However, as we have discussed, this form of treatment may only be useful in the later stages of disease. A similar proviso applies to the use of inhibitors of other effector molecules such as MMPs, which can inhibit lethal GVHD, either by preventing the shedding of TNFα family molecules or the tissue-destroying enzymes themselves (58). Thus, it would be preferable to intervene at an earlier stage.

One way of doing this may be to inhibit the migration and accumulation of activated effector T cells in the mucosa by blocking the relevant adhesion molecules and/or chemokines. As $\alpha_4\beta_7+$ cells predominate among the cytokine-producing mucosal effector cells (63) and their precursors acquire $\alpha_4\beta_7$ in the PP (64), this would seem an obvious target molecule. Recent work has confirmed this idea by showing that blocking $\alpha_4\beta_7$ ligation in vivo using an anti-MADCAM-1 antibody abolishes the influx of donor effector CD8+ T cells into the epithelium (64). Importantly, this study also showed that ablation of PP or blocking the subsequent migration of PP-derived effector T cells also prevented the hepatic and lethal consequences of acute GVHD (64). Together these studies indicate that inhibiting the intestinal phase of GVHD might also have significant beneficial effects on the wider manifestations of the disease. Nevertheless, it should be noted that the severe pathology found in conditions such as intestinal GVHD may disrupt the anatomical pathways that normally regulate the distribution of lymphocytes. Indeed, blocking these tissue-specific molecules has less effect than would be expected in other forms of T-cell–mediated immunopathology in the intestine, including allograft rejection and IBD (166–169). Here, blocking other, more widely expressed adhesion molecules has much more effect under these conditions, suggesting that a more systemic approach may be necessary (166). A related group of molecules that may offer a way of intervening in intestinal T-cell dissemination are the chemokine receptors. Although not yet studied in detail, it has been reported that disruption of CCR5 ligation on donor T cells prevents systemic GVHD, because it may prevent the accumulation and activation of these cells in the PP (64).

The ideal way of preventing tissue pathology in GVHD is to block the activation of alloreactive T lymphocytes during the induction phase of disease. A variety of such strategies have been described in other situations, where interfering with accessory molecules and growth factors such as CD4, CD2, CD28, and IL-2 has proved useful in preventing clinical and experimental graft rejection and other inflammatory conditions. There are few direct studies of this kind in intestinal GVHD, and although the desired outcome is specific tolerance to host tissues, these strategies carry the potential risk of inducing generalized immunosuppression. A more selective approach would be to interfere with those accessory molecules that play a primary role in the induction of Th1-dependent immune responses. We have noted how neutralizing IL-12 can prevent acute GVHD in mice (89,90); this can also prevent and treat experimental models of IBD (170). Other approaches that have been reported to have had some success in preventing intestinal GVHD by preventing Th1 cell activation include blockade of the TNFR2 receptor (171), of CD40-CD40L, and of OX40-OX40L (55). Again, many of these molecules are under study in other forms of inflammatory disease. However, it is important to remember that blocking Th1 activity alone may not be entirely effective, or even desirable. Th1 cells are important in protection against many of the organisms that patients with GVHD are most susceptible to, such as viruses and other intracellular pathogens. Furthermore, although several studies have shown that inhibition of Th1 cells does inhibit acute GVHD, this may simply allow a Th2-biased disease to develop, with autoantibody formation and other forms of tissue pathology (89,97,172). In addition, we have alluded to the possibility that some "Th2" mediators such as IL-4 or IL-13 may be involved in intestinal GVHD, meaning that Th1-targeted therapy may not always be useful.

In addition to these immunologically based therapies, it may also be feasible to design treatment regimens that specifically target the intestine's own repair mechanisms. One report has shown that systemic injection of KGF can reduce intestinal pathology in irradiated mice with acute GVHD, presumably reflecting its ability to stimulate epithelial cell renewal and hence preventing the crypt cell failure that is normally the terminal event in enteropathy. As a consequence, the uptake of endotoxin into serum, the production of TNFα, and the systemic consequences of the disease are reduced (173). Similar results have been reported using the transfection of DNA encoding hepatocyte growth factor (HGF), which shares the mitogenic effects of KGF on crypt cells (92). KGF and epidermal growth factor (EGF) both have protective effects on intestinal architecture in other models of local inflammation and radiation-induced damage (174–176), indicating the potential for using such growth factors as local therapy in GVHD. One final strategy might be to use analogous approaches to help maintain the structure and function of the mesenchymal network of the villus-crypt unit. As we have noted, maintenance of the ECM protein tenascin in the stroma correlates with protection against intestinal GVHD (55) and co-culture with intestinal myofibroblasts reduces the ability of T cells to cause barrier abnormalities of enterocytes in vitro (177). If appropriate mediators could be found to stimulate the production of such factors, they would be valuable therapeutic tools.

VI. CLINICAL INTESTINAL GVHD

As discussed above, there is now a considerable amount of information on the mechanisms of intestinal GVHD in experimental animals. In most cases these studies have employed highly defined model systems using mice with limited genetic disparities and have been performed under specific pathogen-free conditions. Although this tight control helps to maximize the clarity of experimental results, it may not directly reflect the more variable clinical reality of human bone marrow transplantation. It is unlikely that the mechanisms of murine and human GVHD differ completely, but the relative contribution of a given effector pathway to specific organ damage may well differ between humans and mice. In the following sections we will review the phenomenon of clinical intestinal GVHD and indicate how it may compare with what has been described under experimental systems.

A. Occurrence and Clinical Features of Acute Intestinal GVHD

Acute intestinal GVHD is reported to occur in 30–50% of allogeneic stem cell transplant recipients. Although acute GVHD may occur simultaneously in all three classical target organs (skin, intestine, and liver), intestinal involvement may occur in isolation. In a recent prospective study at the Hospital Saint Louis in Paris, GI biopsies confirmed histopathological changes in 37% of 150 patients with suspected intestinal GVHD after allogeneic stem cell transplantation (G. Socie, unpublished data). The incidence of skin and liver involvement in these patients was 43% and 20%, respectively. The GI tract alone was by far the most frequent location of the first symptoms (Fig. 10). An earlier study also reported that a large proportion (14/24) of patients with biopsy proven acute GVHD of the intestine did not have histopathological changes in skin biopsies performed at the same time (178).

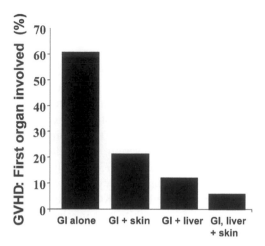

Figure 10   Target organ involvement at the time of initial diagnosis of GVHD. Acute intestinal GVHD occurs in 30–50% of allogeneic SCT recipients. Although acute GVHD may occur simultaneously in all three target organs, isolated intestinal disease represents the most frequent site of initial involvement.

The lower small intestine and colon are the parts of the intestine that are most frequently associated with symptomatic complications, producing diarrhea, intestinal bleeding, crampy abdominal pain, and ileus. The incidence of severe GI bleeding has declined significantly in recent years, now occurring in 2% or fewer of patients at risk (179). Even with cessation of oral intake, voluminous secretory diarrhea may persist, and stool volumes represent an important parameter of the grading systems of the severity of the disease. The commonly used Seattle system distinguishes four stages of intestinal GVHD based mainly on the volume of diarrhea: Stage 1, <500 mL; Stage 2, 500–1000 mL; Stage 3, >1500 mL; Stage 4, severe abdominal pain with or without ileus. The diarrhea that is frequently seen within a week after bone marrow transplant is usually secondary to the BMT preparative regimen and resolves within a few weeks; it is not considered as part of GVHD. Intestinal infection is much more difficult to distinguish from acute GVHD (180,181). Superinfection in patients with GVHD is common, and CMV infection can trigger the development of acute GVHD. In a Seattle study evaluating the etiology and outcome of diarrhea in 296 bone marrow transplant recipients, 150 acute diarrheal episodes were reported in 126 patients (182). Intestinal infection was documented in 20 of these 150 episodes and was associated with viruses (astrovirus, adenovirus, CMV, and rotavirus) in 12 patients, *Clostridium difficile* in 7 patients, and mixed infection in 1 patient. Acute GVHD was documented in only 72 of the 150 episodes; it was notable that the clinical signs and symptoms of infection and GVHD were very similar.

An upper gastrointestinal form of acute GVHD has been described that presents with anorexia, dyspepsia, food intolerance, and vomiting (183,184). In that study the diagnosis of GVHD was confirmed histologically for this syndrome in 62/469 (13%) of patients undergoing allogeneic stem cell transplantation (183). The nonspecific nature of the symptoms require histological and microbiological studies to confirm the diagnosis of upper gastrointestinal GVHD. It appears to be more common in older patients and often responds well to immunosuppressive therapy.

B. Endoscopic and Histological Evaluation of Intestinal GVHD

Endoscopic biopsy is a valuable tool in the diagnosis of intestinal GVHD, where the findings range from a normal or mildly erythematous mucosa to extensive edema and ulceration. The best site for biopsy remains controversial, although one study using simultaneous upper and recto-sigmoid endoscopic evaluation showed that 15/24 (63%) patients had both gastroduodenal and colonic GVHD; 9 patients had GVHD restricted to the upper GI tract, and none had colonic GVHD alone (178). In another study evaluating 77 patients with simultaneous upper and lower GI tract biopsies, upper GI GVHD was found in 44% of patients, of whom 59% had also positive lower GI tract biopsy (182). Upper GI biopsy is now therefore considered to be a more sensitive means of diagnosing GVHD in the intestine than sigmoid biopsy and is preferred by many groups.

The original histological criteria for intestinal GVHD were established by Sale, who proposed four grades (185). Subsequently, Epstein added criteria which recognized that early GVHD could cause crypt cell degeneration, even without crypt dilatation and crypt abscesses (186). Washington showed that crypt cell apoptosis or single cell necrosis with carryorhectic debris was the most useful marker of acute intestinal GVHD (187). Therefore, the current histological grading is as follows:

Grade I: crypt cell degeneration or epithelial cell apoptosis, without crypt loss.
Grade II: loss of up to three contiguous crypts.
Grade III: loss of four or more crypts without sloughing.
Grade IV: total sloughing.

It is important to note that the histological grade often does not correlate with the clinical grade described above, which is based on the volume of diarrhea. These two measures of severity should not be confused; the histological changes are most useful in confirming the presence of GVHD, not in quantitating its severity.

C. Pathogenesis of Intestinal GVHD in Humans

Experimental BMT data suggest that damage to the GI tract during acute GVHD plays a major pathophysiological role in the amplification of systemic disease. As noted above, endotoxin or LPS is a constituent of normal bowel flora. In the clinical setting, gram-negative gut decontamination has also been shown to reduce GVHD. Furthermore, the intensity of this decontamination has recently been demonstrated to be an important predictor of GVHD severity (149,150). Additional evidence for the importance of GI tract integrity during GVHD comes from studies of the effect of pretransplant conditioning on GVHD severity after allogeneic BMT. Clinical studies first suggested a correlation between GVHD severity and radiation dose (<12 vs. >12 Gy) (188,189) and more severe GVHD after conditioning regimens that included radiation therapy than those that included only chemotherapy (190,191). The increased incidence of conditioning-related toxicity has also been associated with GVHD. However, these studies demonstrated an inverse correlation between conditioning intensity and compliance with immunosuppression prophylaxis, which might partially account for the increase in GVHD. Indeed, only one of these studies identified increased radiation intensity as an independent risk factor for GVHD, and there was no demonstrable association with severe disease (189). By contrast, the association of increased GVHD with dose reductions in cyclosporine was maintained throughout all GVHD grades. Using clinical data alone, it has thus been difficult to separate the influence of conditioning intensity and suppression of T-cell function on subsequent GVHD severity.

Perhaps the best evidence of the role of conditioning regimen in triggering GVHD comes from data on the use of nonmyeloablative conditioning before transplantation of allo-geneic peripheral blood stem cells. After such conditioning GVHD still occurs in a signifi-cant proportion of patients, but they are generally older than those receiving myeloablative conditioning, and most have been heavily pre-treated. The Seattle group has recently pub-lished a study showing decreased incidence rates of GVHD following reduced intensity con-ditioning (192). The cumulative incidences of both grades II–IV and III–IV acute GVHD were lower in nonablative transplant recipients (64% vs. 85%, $p = 0.001$; 14% vs. 27%, $p = 0.08$). Nonablative transplantation was associated with a 2-month delay in the initiation of steroid treatment for GVHD, with a predominance of disease in the skin and GI tract within the first year after BMT. Stigmata of acute GVHD were frequently observed after day 100 in the nonablative group. Thus, nonablative HSCT is associated with a syndrome of acute GVHD occurring beyond day 100 in a considerable proportion of patients and is perhaps best considered as "late-onset acute" GVHD rather than "chronic" GVHD.

As mentioned above, the role of TNFα in the genesis of GVHD has been extensively studied in rodent models (48,193–198). In human beings, the role of TNFα release in GVHD is suggested by two lines of evidence. Hervé and coworkers reported data on 19 patients with severe acute GVHD refractory to conventional therapy who were treated by in vivo infusion of a monoclonal anti-TNFα (199). In responding patients, gut lesions showed the most improvement. However, GVHD recurred in the majority of patients when treatment was discontinued. Although this study showed that a monoclonal anti-TNFα antibody may benefit some patients with severe refractory GVHD, mediators other than TNFα might also be important. Holler et al. (200) performed a phase I/II trial using a monoclonal antibody to neutralize TNFα during pretransplant conditioning as additional prophylaxis in high-risk patients (200–202). TNFα serum levels and clinical courses in 21 patients receiving anti-TNFα prophylaxis were compared to 22 historical controls. In that study, prophylactic application of monoclonal anti-TNFα seemed to postpone onset of acute GVHD.

Recently, the group from Hospital Saint Louis in Paris analyzed GI biopsies from 95 patients after allogeneic BMT. This analysis included characterization and quantification of the cellular infiltrate, TNF, TNF receptors, and Fas expression in in situ expression and quantitation of apoptotic cells (203). Both TNFα and Fas expression correlated with GVHD histopathological changes, implicating these molecules in the disease process. TNFα was expressed in all (100%) biopsies of patients with acute GVHD. Quantitative assessment showed that TNF expression in more than 10 cells per high-power fluid was specific of acute GVHD (203). The number of lymphocytes and of inflammatory cells within the lamina propria in gut biopsies was also assessed. Cell counts were based on an individually defined mucosal tissue unit and the intensity of edema was assessed. Lymphocyte number (>20 per field) and edema intensity appeared to be both sensitive and specific of GVHD (203). Interestingly, increased early transplant-related mortality was associated with the number of neutrophils in the cellular infiltrate. Furthermore, this same group recently observed that activated eosinophils are associated with pathologi-cally aggressive GI GVHD (204). Both studies suggest a role for effector cells of the innate immune system in human GVHD. Since these cells are attracted to damaged tissues by soluble factors including chemokines, it would be of interest to examine the in situ expression of these molecules and/or of genetic polymorphisms associated with increased chemokine production in human GVHD. IL-5, the major mediator that recruits, activates, and prolongs eosinophils survival, is expressed in human gut GVHD by mononuclear cells infiltrating the lamina propina, suggesting an autocrine mechanism (203).

D. Treatment of Intestinal GVHD

Glucocorticosteroids are the treatment of choice as first line treatment of acute GVHD (reviewed in Chapter 16). Although 2 mg/kg is the usual starting dose, if steroids have been included within the prophylaxis regimen, some centers begin treatment with 5 mg/kg. There is no definitive proof, however, of a dose-effect of steroids in the treatment of acute GVHD. There is also no general consensus regarding the length of time for such treatment.

Topical active steroids may also be used in the management of intestinal disease (205,206). A placebo-controlled study in patients with anorexia and poor oral intake GVHD (grade I disease) showed a better response after oral beclamethasone diproprionate (207). Somatostatin analogues may aid in the management of unremitting diarrhea, but randomized trials have not yet been performed and the treatment is costly (208). Finally, supportive care is of obvious major importance in the practical management of patients with acute GVHD. Gut rest, hyperalimentation, pain control, and antibiotic prophylaxis are routine elements of such supportive care.

VII. CONCLUSIONS AND WIDER IMPLICATIONS

A hypothetical basis for the immunopathogenesis of intestinal GVHD is illustrated in Figure 11. We believe that dividing stem cells are the principal target of the immune response in GVHR, with the initial effect being stimulation of proliferation. This is followed either by resolution and a return to normal levels, or by stem cell death via apoptosis. In parallel, there is crypt hypertrophy and hyperplasia, followed by a period in which villus atrophy accompanies persistent crypt hypertrophy. Finally, crypt loss, villus ablation, and mucosal necrosis occur. These pathological features are accompanied by distinctive immunological events. The early, proliferative enteropathy is preceded by infiltration of the epithelium by T lymphocytes and is associated with the production of large amounts of IFNγ. This phase is triggered by recognition of IL-12–producing host APC in the gut or its draining lymphoid tissues by donor CD4+ T cells and does not require intestinal bacteria or their products. IL-12–activated NK cells may also provide an important source of IFNγ during this early stage. IFNγ primes nonspecific effector cells such as macrophages and is itself responsible for the initial features of intestinal pathology, including the crypt cell hyperplasia, enhanced MHC expression, and alterations in epithelial barrier and digestive functions. The resulting enhanced uptake of bacterial products such as endotoxin allows further activation of IFNγ-primed macrophages and the release of inflammatory cytokines such as NO, IL-1, type I IFN, and TNFα. These macrophage-derived mediators may contribute to the evolving enteropathy in two ways. First, they can exacerbate the crypt cell pathology, either by their effects on proliferation or by causing stem cell apoptosis. In addition, they can act on the mesenchymal components of the mucosa, including myofibroblasts and vascular endothelial cells, leading to increased vascular permeability, thrombosis, influx of further inflammatory cells, and destruction of the extracellular matrix of the villus/crypt unit via the effects of matrix metalloproteinases. Villus atrophy is the main consequence of these effects on mucosal infrastructure

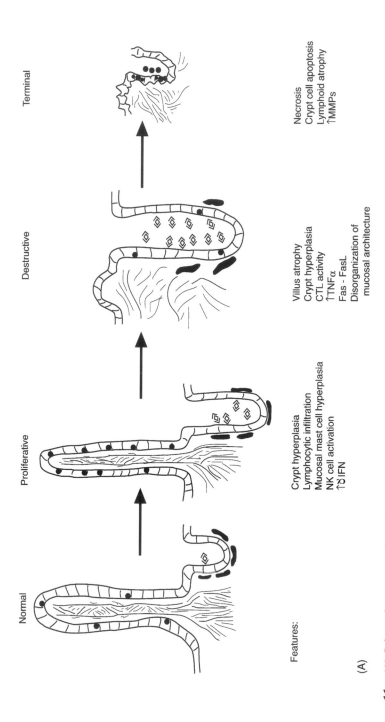

Figure 11 (A) Schematic representation of evolving intestinal GVHR. Early proliferative GVHR is characterized by crypt hyperplasia, IFNγ production, recruitment of IEL, and nonspecific activation of host cells, as indicated by NK cell activation and splenomegaly. Subsequently, villus atrophy develops due to a combination of continued dysregulation of epithelial cell turnover and damage to the intestinal stroma. This destructive phase may be accompanied by the appearance of antihost CTL and the production of toxic cytokines such as TNFα. In some cases, a final phase ensues, in which the antihost immune response destroys crypt stem cells and ablates intestinal repair. (B) Mechanisms of intestinal immunopathology mediated by CD4+ T lymphocytes in GVHR. Donor CD4+ T cells initiate the response by production of IFNγ. Together with its direct effects on crypt stem cells, IFNγ activates nonspecific effector cells such as macrophages, whose soluble products continue the evolving stem cell damage (see text for details).

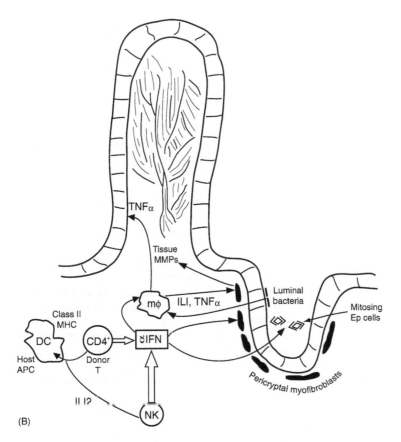

Figure 11 *Continued.*

and, ultimately, mucosal necrosis and autolysis may ensue if there is also a failure of epithelial repair due to overwhelming apoptotic loss of crypt stem cells. TNFα is commonly regarded as the most important mediator of these events, but its production may require high levels of circulating endotoxin, and it may only be responsible for the terminal features of the pathology such as mucosal necrosis. In contrast, NO may be more important, requiring less endotoxin for its production and having a wide range of properties that allow it to modulate all components of the intestinal mucosa, including the epithelium, its blood and nervous supply, and the function of mesenchymal cells. The destructive phase of intestinal GVHD may also involve the action of terminally differentiated, fasL-expressing donor T cells in the epithelium and lamina propria which contribute to the apoptosis of crypt stem cells and may also kill mature villus enterocytes. Understanding how these individual mechanisms may be associated with distinct pathological features may help in the development of better therapeutic and preventative strategies.

REFERENCES

1. Billingham RE, Brent L, Medawar PB. Acquired tolerance of skin homografts. Ann NY Acad Sci 1955; 59:409–498.

2. Mowat AM, Viney JL. The anatomical basis of mucosal immune responses. Immunol Rev 1997; 156:145–166.
3. McGhee JR, Lamm ME, Strober W. Mucosal immune responses: an overview. In: Ogra PL, Mestecky J, Lamm ME, Strober W, McGhee JR, Bienenstock J, eds. Mucosal Immunology. 2d ed. San Diego: Academic Press, 1999; pp 485–506.
4. Butcher EC. Lymphocyte homing and intestinal immunity. In: Ogra PL, Mestecky J, Lamm ME, Strober W, McGhee JR, Bienenstock J, eds. Mucosal Immunology. 2d ed. San Diego: Academic Press, 1999; pp 507–540.
5. Hayday A, Theodoridis E, Ramsburg E, Shires J. Intraepithelial lymphocytes: exploring the Third Way in immunology. Nat Immunol 2001; 2:997–1003.
6. Kunkel EJ, Butcher EC. Chemokines and the tissue-specific migration of lymphocytes. Immunity 2002; 16:1–4.
7. MacDonald TT, Pender SLF. Lamina propria T cells. Chem Immunol 1998; 71:103–117.
8. James SP, Kiyono H. Gastrointestinal lamina propria T cells. In: Ogra PL, Mestecky J, Lamm ME, Strober W, McGhee JR, Bienenstock J, eds. Mucosal Immunology. 2d ed. San Diego: Academic Press, 1999; pp 381–396.
9. Braunstein J, Qiao L, Autschbach F, Schurmann G, Meuer S. T cells of the human intestinal lamina propria are high producers of interleukin-10. Gut 1997; 41:215–220.
10. Carol M, Lambrechts A, Van Gossum A, Libin M, Goldman M, Mascart-Lemone F. Spontaneous secretion of interferon γ and interleukin 4 by human intraepithelial and lamina propria gut lymphocytes. Gut 1998; 42.
11. Hurst SD, Cooper CJ, Sitterding SM, Cho JH, Jump RL, Levine AD, Barrett TA. The differentiated state of intestinal lamina propria CD4+ T cells results in altered cytokine production, activation threshold, and costimulatory requirements. J Immunol 1999; 163:5937–5945.
12. Strober W, Fuss IJ, Blumberg RS. The immunology of mucosal models of inflammation. Annu Rev Immunol 2002; 20:495–549.
13. Beagley KW, Husband AJ. Intraepithelial lymphocytes: origins, distribution, and function. Crit Rev Immunol 1998; 18:237–254.
14. Poussier P, Julius M. Intestinal intraepithelial lymphocytes: the plot thickens. J Exp Med 1994; 180:1185–1189.
15. Halstensen T, Scott H, Brandtzaeg P. Intraepithelial T cells of the TcR g/d+ CD8− and Vd1/Jd1+ phenotypes are increased in celiac disease. Scand J Immunol 1989; 30:665–672.
16. Guy-Grand D, Cerf-Bensussan N, Malissen B, Malassis-Seris M, Briottet C, Vassalli P. Two gut intraepithelial CD8 + lymphocyte populations with different T cell receptors: a role for the gut epithelium in T cell differentiation. J Exp Med 1991; 173:471–478.
17. Suzuki K, Oida T, Hamada H, Hitotsumatsu O, Watanabe M, Hibi T, Yamamoto H, Kubota E, Kaminogawa S, Ishikawa H. Gut cryptopatches: direct evidence of extrathymic anatomical sites for intestinal T lymphopoiesis. Immunity 2000; 13:691–702.
18. Guy-Grand D, Vassalli P. Gut intraepithelial lymphocyte development. Curr Opin Immunol 2002; 14:255–259.
19. Groh V, Steinle A, Bauer S, Spies T. Recognition of stress-induced MHC molecules by intestinal epithelial $\gamma\delta$ T cells. Science 1998; 279:1737–1740.
20. Leishman AJ, Naidenko OV, Attinger A, Koning F, Lena CJ, Xiong Y, Chang HC, Reinherz E, Kronenberg M, Cheroutre H. T cell responses modulated through interaction between CD8alphaalpha and the nonclassical MHC class I molecule, TL. Science 2001; 294:1936–1939.
21. Guy-Grand D, Malassis-Seris M, Briottet C, Vassalli P. Cytotoxic differentiation of mouse gut thymodependent and independent intraepithelial T lymphocytes is induced locally. Correlation between functional assays, presence of perforin and granzyme transcripts, and cytoplasmic granules. J Exp Med 1991; 173:1549–1552.
22. Guy-Grand D, Cuenod-Jabri, B, Malassis-Seris, M, Selz F, Vassalli, P. Complexity of the mouse gut T cell immune system: identification of two distinct natural killer T cell intraepithelial lineages. Eur J Immunol 1996; 26: 2248–2256.

23. Yu LC, Perdue MH. Role of mast cells in intestinal mucosal function: studies in models of hypersensitivity and stress. Immunol Rev 2001; 179:61–73.

24. Miller HRP, Pemberton AD. Tissue-specific expression of mast cell granule serine proteinases and their role in inflammation in the lung and gut. Immunology 2002; 105:375–390.

25. Billingham RE. The biology of graft-versus-host reactions. Harvey Lectures 1967; 62:21–79.

26. Simonsen M. Graft versus host reactions. Their natural history, and applicability as tools of research. Prog Allergy 1962; 6:349–367.

27. Hedberg CA, Reiser S, Reilly RW. Intestinal phase of the runting syndrome in mice. II. Observations on nutrient absorption and certain disaccharidase abnormalities. Transplantation 1968; 6:104–110.

28. Lund EK, Bruce MG, Smith MW, Ferguson A. Selective effects of graft-versus-host reaction on disaccharidase expression by mouse jejunal enterocytes. Clin Sci 1968; 71:189–198.

29. Cornelius EA. Protein-losing enteropathy in the graft-versus-host reaction. Transplantation 1970; 9:247–252.

30. Weisdorf SA, Salati LM, Longsdorf LA, Ramsay NKC, Sharp HL. Graft-versus-host disease of the intestine: a protein losing enteropathy characterised by fecal α1-antitrypsin. Gastroenterology 1983; 85:1076–1081.

31. Piguet P-F. GvHR elicited by products of class I or class II loci of the MHC: analysis of the response of mouse T lymphocytes to products of class I and class II loci of the MHC in correlation with GvHR-induced mortality, medullary aplasia and enteropathy. J Immunol 1985; 135:1637–1643.

32. Koltun WA, Bloomer MM, Colony P, Kauffman GL. Increased intestinal permeability in rats with graft versus host disease. Gut 1996; 39:291–298.

33. Walker RI. The contribution of intestinal endotoxin to mortality in hosts with compromised resistance: a review. Exp Haematol 1978; 6:172–184.

34. Slavin RE, Woodruff JM. The pathology of bone-marrow transplantation. In: Sommers SC, ed. Pathology Annual. New York: Appleton-Century-Crofts, 1974; pp 291–344.

35. Reilly RW, Kirsner JB. Runt intestinal disease. Lab Invest 1965; 14:102–107.

36. Thiele DL, Eigenbrodt ML, Bryde SE, Eigenbrodt EH, Lipsky PE. Intestinal graft-versus-host disease is initiated by donor T cells distinct from classic cytotoxic T lymphocytes. J Clin Invest 1989; 84:1947–1956.

37. Koltun WA, Bloomer MM, Colony P, Ruggiero FM, Kauffman GL. Graft-versus-host disease after small bowel transplantation is associated with host colonic injury. Dig Dis Sci 1995; 40:1925–1933.

38. Beschorner WE, Tutschka PJ, Santos GW. Chronic graft-versus-host disease in the rat radiation chimera. I. Clinical features, haematology, histology and immunopathology in long-term chimeras. Transplantation 1982; 33:393–399.

39. Mowat AM, Felstein MV. Experimental studies of immunologically mediated enteropathy. V. Destructive enteropathy during an acute graft-versus-host reaction in adult BDF1 mice. Clin Exp Immunol 1990; 79:279–284.

40. Ellison C, Fischer JM, HayGlass KT, Gartner J. Murine graft-versus-host disease in an F1-hybrid model using IFN-γ gene knockout donors. J Immunol 1998; 161:631–640.

41. Gorer PA, Boyse ED. Pathological changes in F_1 hybrid mice following transplantation of spleen cells from donors of the parental strains. Immunology 1959; 2:182–193.

42. van Bekkum DW, Knaan S. Role of bacterial microflora in development of intestinal lesions from GvHR. J Natl Cancer Inst 1977; 58:787–790.

43. MacDonald TT, Ferguson A. Hypersensitivity reactions in the small intestine. III. The effects of allograft rejection and of GvHD on epithelial cell kinetics. Cell Tiss Kinet 1977; 10:301–312.

44. Elson CO, Reilly RW, Rosenberg IH. Small intestinal injury in the GvHR: an innocent bystander phenomenon. Gastroenterology 1977; 72:886–889.

45. Mowat AM, Ferguson A. Intraepithelial lymphocyte count and crypt hyperplasia measure the mucosal component of the graft-versus-host reaction in mouse small intestine. Gastroenterology 1982; 83:417–423.
46. Cummins AG, Munro GH, Huntley JF, Miller HR, Ferguson A. Separate effects of irradiation and of graft-versus-host reaction on rat mucosal mast cells. Gut 1989; 30:355–360.
47. Guy-Grand D, Vassalli P. Gut injury in mouse graft-versus-host reaction. Study of its occurrence and mechanisms. J Clin Invest 1986; 77:1584–1595h.
48. Piguet P-F, Grau GE, Allet B, Vassalli P. Tumor necrosis factor/cachectin is an effector of skin and gut lesions of the acute phase of graft-vs-host disease. J Exp Med 1987; 166:1280–1289.
49. Mowat AM, Felstein MV, Borland A, Parrott DMV. Experimental studies of immunologically mediated enteropathy. Delayed type hypersensitivity is responsible for the proliferative and destructive enteropathy in irradiated mice with graft-versus-host reaction. Gut 1988; 29:949–956.
50. Tsuzuki T, Yoshikai Y, Ito M, Mori N, Ohbayashi M, Asai J. Kinetics of intestinal intraepithelial lymphocytes during acute graft-versus-host disease in mice. Eur J Immunol 1994; 24:709–715.
51. Wall AJ, Rosenberg JL, Reilly RW. Small intestinal injury in the immunologically runted mouse. Morphologic and autoradiographic studies. J Lab Clin Med 1971; 78:833–834A.
52. Barclay AN, Mason DW. Induction of Ia antigen in rat epidermal cells and gut epithelium by immunological stimuli. J Exp Med 1982; 156:1665–1676.
53. Bland PW, Whiting CV. Induction of MHC class II gene products in rat intestinal epithelium during graft-versus-host disease and effects on the immune function of the epithelium. Immunology 1992; 75:366–367.
54. Rappaport H, Khalil A, Halle-Pannenko O, Pritchard L, Dantchev D, Mathe G. Histopathologic sequence of events in adult mice undergoing lethal graft-versus-host reaction developed across H-2 and/or non-H-2 histocompatibility barriers. Am J Pathol 1979; 96:121–142.
55. Stuber E, Von Freier A, Marinescu D, Folsch UR. Involvement of OX40-OX40L interactions in the intestinal manifestations of the murine acute graft-versus-host disease. Gastroenterology 1998; 115:1205–1215.
56. Pender S, Lionetti P, Murch SH, Wathan N, MacDonald TT. Proteolytic degradation of intestinal mucosal extracellular matrix after lamina propria T cell activation. Gut 1996; 39:284–290.
57. MacDonald TT, Bajaj-Elliott M, Pender SLF. T cells orchestrate intestinal mucosal shape and integrity. Immunology Today 1999; 20:505–510.
58. Hattori K, Hirano T, Ushiyama C, Miyajima H, Yamakawa N, Ebata T, Wada Y, Ikeda S, Yoshino K, Tateno M, Oshimi K, Kayagaki N, Yagita H, Okumura K. A metalloproteinase inhibitor prevents lethal acute graft-versus-host disease in mice. Blood 1997; 90:542–548.
59. Garside P, Bunce C, Tomlinson RC, Nichols BL, Mowat AM. Analysis of enteropathy induced by tumour necrosis factor alpha. Cytokine 1993; 24–30.
60. Piguet PF, Vesin C, Guo J, Donati J, Donati J, Barrazone C. TNF-induced enterocyte apoptosis in micc is mediated by the TNF receptor 1 and does not require p53. Eur J Immunol 1998; 28:3499–3505.
61. Nowell PC, Cole LJ. Lymphoid pathology in homologous disease of mice. Transplant Bull 1959; 6:4–35.
62. Guy-Grand D, Griscelli CG, Vassalli P. The mouse gut T-lymphocyte, a novel type of T-cell: nature, origin and traffic in mice in normal and graft-versus-host conditions. J Exp Med 1978; 148:1661–1677.
63. Snider D, Liang H. Early intestinal Th1 inflammation and mucosal T cell recruitment during acute graft-versus-host reaction. J Immunol 2001; 166:5991–5999.
64. Murai M, Yoneyama H, Ezaki T, Suematsu M, Terashima Y, Harada A, Hamada H, Asakura H, Matsushima K. Peyer's patch is the essential site in initiating murine acute and lethal graft-versus-host reaction. Nat Immunol 2003; 4:154–160.

65. Kelsall B, Strober W. Distinct populations of dendritic cells are present in the subepithelial dome and T cell regions of the murine Peyer's patch. J Exp Med 1996; 183:237–247.

66. Mowat AM, Ferguson A. Hypersensitivity reactions in the small intestine. 6. Pathogenesis of the graft-versus-host reaction in the small intestinal mucosa of the mouse. Transplantation 1981; 32:328–343.

67. Klein RM, Clancy J, Sheridan K. Acute lethal graft-versus-host disease stimulates cellular proliferation in Peyer's patches and follicle associated ileal epithelium of adult rats. Virch Arch (B) 1984; 47:303–311.

68. Marsh M. Grains of truth: evolutionary changes in small intestinal mucosa in response to environmental antigen challenge. Gut 1990; 31:111–114.

69. Marsh MN. Correlative aspects of mucosal pathology across the spectrum of gluten sensitivity. In O'Farrelly CFaC, ed. Gastrointestinal Immunology and Gluten-Sensitive Disease. Dublin: Oak Tree Press, 1994; pp 145–157.

70. Kataoka Y, Iwasaki T, Kuroiwa T, Seto Y, Iwata N, Hashimoto N, Ogata A, Hamano T, Kakishita E. The role of donor T cells for target organ injuries in acute and chronic graft-versus-host disease. Immunology 2001; 103:310–318.

71. Sprent J. Fate of H2-activated T lymphocytes in syngeneic hosts. I. Fate in lymphoid tissues and intestines traced with 3H-thymidine, 125I-deoxyuridine and 51chromium. Cell Immunol 1976; 21.

72. Sakai T, Kimura Y, Inagaki-Ohara K, Kusugami K, Lynch DH, Yoshikai Y. Fas-mediated cytotoxicity by intestinal intraepithelial lymphocytes during acute graft-versus-host disease in mice. Gastroenterology 1997; 113:168–174.

73. Lin T, Brunner T, Tietz B, Madsen J, Bonfoco E, Reaves M, Huflejt M, Green DR. Fas ligand-mediated killing by intestinal intraepithelial lymphocytes. Participation in intestinal graft-versus-host disease. J Clin Invest 1998; 101:570–577.

74. Gold JA, Kosek J, Wanek N, Baur S. Duodenal immunoglobulin deficiency in graft-versus-host disease (GvHD) mice. J Immunol 1976; 117:471–476.

75. Crapper RM, Schrader JW. Evidence for the in vivo production and release into the serum of a T-cell lymphokine, persisting-cell stimulating factor (PSF), during graft-versus-host reactions. Immunology 1986; 57:533–538.

76. Newlands GF, Mowat AM, Felstein MV, Miller HRP. Role of mucosal mast cells in intestinal graft-versus-host reaction in the mouse. Int Arch Allergy Appl Immunol 1990; 93:308–313.

77. Cummins AG, Munro GH, Miller HRP, Ferguson A. Effect of cyclosporin A treatment on the enteropathy of graft-versus-host reaction in the rat: a quantitative study of intestinal morphology, epithelial cell kinetics and mucosal immune activity. Immunol Cell Biol 1989; 67:153–160.

78. Mowat AM, Borland A, DMVP. Hypersensitivity reactions in the small intestine. VII. Induction of the intestinal phase of murine graft-versus-host-reaction by Lyt 2-T cells activated by I-A alloantigens. Transplantation 1986; 41:192–198.

79. Mowat AM, Sprent J. Induction of intestinal graft-versus-host reactions across mutant major histocompatiblity antigens by T lymphocyte subsets in mice. Transplantation 1989; 47:857–863.

80. Korngold R, Sprent J. Variable capacity of L3T4+ T cells to cause lethal graft-versus-host disease across minor histocompatibility barriers in mice. J Exp Med 1987; 165:1552–1564.

81. Murphy GF, Whitaker D, Sprent J, Korngold R. Characterization of target injury of murine acute graft-versus-host disease directed to multiple minor histocompatiblity antigens elicited by either CD4 + or CD8 + effector cells. Am J Pathol 1991; 138:983–990.

82. Chardes T, Buzoni-Gatel D, Lepage A, Bernard F, Bout D. *Toxoplasma gondii* oral infection induces specific cytotoxic CDa/b + Thy1 + intraepithelial lymphocytes, lytic for parasite-infected enterocytes. J Immunol 1994; 153:4596–4603.

83. Felstein MV, Mowat AM. Experimental studies of immunologically mediated enteropathy. IV. Correlation between immune effector mechanisms and type of enteropathy during a graft-versus-host reaction in neonatal mice of different ages. Clin Exp Immunol 1988; 72:108.

84. Borland A, Mowat AM, Parrott DMV. Augmentation of intestinal and peripheral natural killer cell activity during the graft-versus-host reaction in mice. Transplantation 1983; 36:513–519.

85. Mowat A. Evidence that Ia + bone-marrow-derived cells are the stimulus for the intestinal phase of the murine graft-versus-host reaction. Transplantation 1986; 42:141–144.

86. Cleveland MG, Annable CR, Klimpel GR. In vivo and in vitro production of IFNβ and IFNγ during graft versus host disease. J Immunol 1988; 141:3349–3356.

87. Clancy J, Goral J, Kovacs EJ. Expression of cytokine genes (TNF-α, TGF-β and IFN-γ) in acute lethal graft versus host disease. Progr Leuk Biol 1990; 10B:165–170.

88. Kelso A. Frequency analysis of lymphokine-secreting CD4+ and CD8+ T cells activated in a graft-versus-host reaction. J Immunol 1990; 145:2167–2176.

89. Williamson E, Garside P, Bradley JA, Mowat AM. Neutralising IL12 during induction of murine acute GvHD polarises the cytokine profile towards a TH2-type alloimmune response and confers long-term protection from the disease. J Immunol 1997; 159:1208–1215.

90. Williamson E, Garside P, Bradley JA, Mowat AM. Interleukin-12 is a central mediator of acute graft-versus-host disease in mice. J Immunol 1996; 157:689–699.

91. Nestel FP, Price KS, Seemayer TA, Lapp WS. Macrophage priming and lipopolysaccharide-triggered release of tumour necrosis factor α during graft-versus-host disease. J Exp Med 1992; 175:405–413.

92. Kuroiwa T, Kakishita E, Hamano T, Kataoka Y, Seto Y, Iwata N, Kaneda Y, Matsumoto K, Nakamura T, Ueki T, Fujimoto J, Iwasaki T. Hepatocyte growth factor ameliorates acute graft-versus-host disease and promotes hematopoietic function. J Clin Invest 2001; 107:1365–1373.

93. Hattori K, Hirano T, Miyajima H, Yamakawa N, Tateno M, Oshimi K, Kayagaki N, Yagita H, Okumura K. Differential effects of anti-Fas ligand and anti-tumor necrosis factor alpha antibodies on acute graft-versus-host disease pathologies. Blood 1998; 91:4051–4055.

94. Garside P, Reid S, Steel M, Mowat AM. Differential cytokine production associated with distinct phases of murine graft-versus-host reaction. Immunology 1994; 82:211–214.

95. Mowat AM. Antibodies to γ interferon prevent immunologically mediated intestinal damage in murine graft-versus-host reaction. Immunology 1989; 68:18–23.

96. Ellison CA, Natuik SA, McIntosh AR, Scully SA, Danilenko DM, Gartner JG. The role of IFN-γ, nitric oxide and LPS in intestinal graft-versus-host disease developing in F1 hybrid mice. Immunology 2003; 109:440–449.

97. Nikolic B, Lee S, Bronson RT, Grusby MJ, Sykes M. Th1 and Th2 mediate acute graft-versus-host disease, each with distinct end-organ targets. J Clin Invest 2000; 105:1289–1298.

98. Stuber E, Schlenger P, Von Freier A, Arendt T, Folsch UR. Interferon-gamma is not involved in the intestinal manifestations of the acute murine semiallogenic graft-versus-host disease. Int J Colorectal Dis 2001; 16:346–351.

99. Guy-Grand D, DiSanto JP, Hencoz P, Malassis-Seris M, Vassalli P. Small bowel enteropathy: role of intraepithelial lymphocytes and of cytokines (IL-12, IFN-γ, TNF) in the induction of epithelial cell death and renewal. Eur J Immunol 1998; 28:730–744.

100. Lollini PL, D'Errico A, De Giovanni C, Landuzzi L, Frabetti F, Nicoletti G, Cavallo F, Giovarelli M, Grigioni WF, Nanni P. Systemic effects of cytokines released by gene-transduced tumour cells. Marked hyperplasia induced in glands of small bowel by γ-interferon transfectants through host's lymphocytes. Int J Cancer 1995; 61:425–430.

101. Stuber E, Buschenfeld A, von Freier A, Arendt T, Folsch UR. Intestinal crypt cell apoptosis in murine acute graft versus host disease is mediated by tumour necrosis factor alpha and not by the FasL-Fas interaction: effect of pentoxifylline on the development of mucosal atrophy. Gut 1999; 45:229–235.

102. Brown GR, Lindberg G, Meddings J, Silva M, Beutler B, Thiele D. Tumor necrosis factor inhibitor ameliorates murine intestinal graft-versus-host disease. Gastroenterology 1999; 116:593–601.

103. Schmaltz C, Alpdogan O, Muriglan SJ, Kappel BJ, Rotolo JA, Ricchetti ET, Greenberg AS, Murphy GF, Crawford JM, Van Den Brink MR. Donor T cell-derived TNF is required for graft-versus-host disease and graft-versus-tumor activity after bone marrow transplantation. Blood 2003; 101:2440–2445.

104. Merger M, Viney JL, Borojevic R, Steele-Norwood D, Zhou P, Clark DA, Riddell R, Maric R, Podack ER, Croitoru K. Defining the roles of perforin, Fas/FasL, and tumour necrosis factor alpha in T cell induced mucosal damage in the mouse intestine. Gut 2002; 51:155–163.

105. Diab-Assef M, Reimund JM, Ezenfis J, Duclos B, Kedinger M, Foltzer-Jourdainne C. The phosphodiesterase inhibitor, pentoxifylline, alters rat intestinal epithelial cell proliferation via changes in the expression of transforming growth factors. Scand J Gastroenterol 2002; 37:206–214.

106. Mowat AMI, Hutton AK, Garside P, Steel M. A role for interleukin-1α in immunologically mediated intestinal pathology. Immunology 1993; 80:110–115.

107. Garside P, Felstein MV, Green EA, Mowat AM. The role of interferon α/β in the induction of intestinal pathology in mice. Immunology 1991; 74:279–283.

108. Monteleone G, Pender SL, Wathen NC, MacDonald TT. Interferon-α drives T cell-mediated immunopathology in the intestine. Eur J Immunol 2001; 31:2247–2255.

109. Monteleone G, Pender SLF, Alstead E, Hauer AC, Lionetti P, MacDonald TT. Role of interferon α in promoting T helper cell type 1 responses in the small intestine in coeliac disease. Gut 2001; 48:425–429.

110. Mowat AM, Widmer MB. A role for IL-4 in immunologically mediated enteropathy. Clin Exp Immunol 1995; 99:65–69.

111. Lawrence CE, Paterson JC, Higgins LM, MacDonald TT, Kennedy MW, Garside P. IL-4-regulated enteropathy in an intestinal nematode infection. Eur J Immunol 1998; 28:2672–2684.

112. Zund G, Madara JL, Dzus AL, Awtrey CS, Colgan SP. Interleukin-4 and interleukin-13 differentially regulate epithelial chloride secretion. J Biol Chem 1996; 271:7460–7464.

113. Mowat AM, Garside P, Fitton LA, Higley HR, Carlino JA. Regulatory activity of endogenous and exogenous transforming growth factor β in experimental intestinal immunopathology. Growth Factors 1996; 13:75–85.

114. McGee DW. Inflammation and mucosal cytokine production. In: Ogra PL, Mestecky J, Lamm ME, Strober W, McGhee JR, Bienenstock J, eds. Mucosal Immunology, 2d ed. San Diego: Academic Press, 1999: pp 559–574.

115. Eckmann L, Jung HC, Schurer-Maly C, Panja A, Morzycka-Wroblewska E, Kagnoff MF. Differential cytokine expression by human intestinal epithelial cell lines: regulated expression of interleukin 8. Gastroenterology 1993; 105:1689–1697.

116. Schuerer-Maly C, Eckmann L, Kagnoff MF, Falco T, Maly FE. Colonic epithelial cell lines as a source of interleukin-8: stimulation by inflammatory cytokines and bacterial lipopolysaccharide. Immunology 1994; 81:85–91.

117. Panja A, Siden E, Mayer L. Synthesis and regulation of accessory/proinflammatory cytokines by intestinal epithelial cells. Clin Exp Immunol 1995; 100:298–305.

118. Ziambaras T, Rubin DC, Perlmutter DH. Regulation of sucrase-isomaltase gene expression in human intestinal epithelial cells by inflammatory cytokines. J Biol Chem 1996; 271:1237–1242.

119. Shibahara T, Wilcox JN, Couse T, Madara JL. Characterization of epithelial chemoattractants for human intestinal intraepithelial lymphocytes. Gastroenterology 2001; 120:60–70.

120. Panja A, Goldberg S, Eckmann L, Krishen P, Mayer L. The regulation and functional consequence of proinflammatory cytokine binding on human intestinal epithelial cells. J Immunol 1998; 161:3675–3684.

121. Reinecker HC, MacDermot tRP, Mirau S, Dignass A, Podolsky DK. Intestinal epithelial cells both express and respond to interleukin 15. Gastroenterology 1996; 111:1706–1713.

122. Shirota K, LeDuy L, Yuan SY, Jothy S. Interleukin-6 and its receptor are expressed in human intestinal epithelial cells. Virchows Arch B Cell Pathol Incl Mol Pathol 1990; 58:303–308.

123. Kaiserlian D, Rigal D, Abello J, Revillard JP. Expression, function and regulation of the intercellular adhesion molecule-1 (ICAM-1) on human intestinal epithelial cell lines. Eur J Immunol 1991; 21:2415–2421.

124. Ackermann LW, Wollenweber LA, Denning GM. IL-4 and IFN-γ increase steady state levels of polymeric Ig receptor mRNA in human airway and intestinal epithelial cells. J Immunol 1999; 162:5112–5118.

125. Hayashi M, Takenouchi N, Asano M, Kato M, Tsurumachi T, Saito T, Moro I. The polymeric immunoglobulin receptor (secretory component) in a human intestinal epithelial cell line is up-regulated by interleukin-1. Immunology 1997; 92:220–225.

126. Nilsen EM, Johansen FE, Kvale D, Krajci P. Different regulatory pathways employed in cytokine-enhanced expression of secretory component and epithelial HLA class I genes. Eur J Immunol 1999; 29:168–179.

127. Madara J, Stafford J. Interferon-gamma directly affects barrier function of cultured intestinal epithelial monolayers. J Clin Invest 1989; 83:724–727.

128. Planchon S, Martins CA, Guerrant RL, Roche JK. Regulation of intestinal epithelial barrier function by TGF-β 1. Evidence for its role in abrogating the effect of a T cell cytokine. J Immunol 1994; 153:5730–5739.

129. Adams RB, Planchon SM, Roche JK. IFN-γ modulation of epithelial barrier function. Time course, reversibility, and site of cytokine binding. J Immunol 1993; 150:2356–2363.

130. Prinz JC, Gross B, Vollmer S, Trommler P, Strobel I, Meure M, Plewig G. T cell clones from psoriasis skin lesions can promote keratinocyte proliferation in vitro via secreted products. Eur J Immunol 1994; 24:593–598.

131. Kvale D, Brandtzaeg P, Lovhaug D. Up-regulation of the expression of secretory component and HLA molecules in a human colonic cell line by tumour necrosis factor-α and γ interferon. Scand J Immunol 1988; 28:351–357.

132. Schmitz H, Fromm M, Bentzel CJ, Scholz P, Detjen K, Mankertz J, Bode H, Epple HJ, Riecken EO, Schulzke JD. Tumor necrosis factor-α (TNF α) regulates the epithelial barrier in the human intestinal cell line HT-29/B6. J Cell Sci 1999; 112:137–146.

133. Colgan SP, Resnick MB, Parkos CA, Delp-Archer C, McGurk D, Bacarra AE, Weiler PF, Madara JL. IL-4 directly modulates function of a model human intestinal epithelium. J Immunol 1994; 153:2122–2129.

134. Madden KB, Whitman L, Sullivan C, Gause WC, Urban JFJ, Katona IM, Finkelman FD, Shea-Donohue T. Role of STAT6 and mast cells in IL-4- and IL-13-induced alterations in murine intestinal epithelial cell function. J Immunol 2002; 169:4417–4422.

135. Garside P, Hutton AK, Severn A, Liew FY, Mowat A. Nitric oxide mediates intestinal pathology in graft-vs.-host disease. Eur J Immunol 1992; 22:2141–2145.

136. Wallace JL, Miller MJ. Nitric oxide in mucosal defense: a little goes a long way. Gastroenterology 2000; 119:512–520.

137. Xu DZ, Lu Q, Deitch EA. Nitric oxide directly impairs intestinal barrier function. Shock 2002; 17:139–145.

138. Roy C, Ghayur T, Kongshavn PA, Lapp WS. Natural killer activity by spleen, lymph node, and thymus cells during the graft-versus-host reaction. Transplantation 1982; 34:144–146.

139. Kubota E, Ishikawa H, Saito K. Modulation of F1 cytotoxic potentials by GvHR. Host- and donor-derived cytotoxic lymphocytes arise in the unirradiated F1 host spleens under the condition of GvHR-associated immunosuppression. J Immunol 1983; 131:1142–1148.

140. Charley MR, Anwar M, Bennett M, Gilliam JN, Sontheimer RD. Prevention of lethal, minor-determinate graft-host disease in mice by the In vivo administration of anti-asialo GM1. J Immunol 1983; 131:2101–2103.

141. Varkila K. Depletion of asialo-GM1 + cells from the F1 recipient mice prior to irradiation and transfusion of parental spleen cells prevents mortality to acute graft-versus-host disease and induction of anti-host specific cytotoxic T cells. Clin Exp Immunol 1987; 69:652–659.

142. Ellison C, HayGlass KT, Fischer JM, Rector ES, MacDonald GC, Gartner J. Depletion of natural killer cells from the graft reduces interferon-γ levels and lipopolysaccharide-induced tumor necrosis factor-α release in F1 hybrid mice with acute graft-versus-host disease. Transplantation 1998; 66:284–294.

143. Mowat AM, MVF. Experimental studies of immunologically mediated enteropathy. II. Role of natural killer cells in the intestinal phase of murine graft-versus-host reaction. Immunology 1987; 61:179–183.

144. Biron CA, Brossay L. NK cells and NKT cells in innate defense against viral infections. Curr Opin Immunol 2001; 13:458–464.

145. Wright SH, Brown J, Knight PA, Thornton EM, Kilshaw PJ, Miller HRP. Transforming growth factor-β1 mediates coexpression of the integrin subunit alphaE and the chymase mouse mast cell protease-1 during the early differentiation of bone marrow-derived mucosal mast cell homologues. Clin Exp Allergy 2002; 32:315–324.

146. Wasem C, Frutschi C, Arnold D, Vallan C, Lin T, Green DR, Mueller C, Brunner T. Accumulation and activation-induced release of preformed Fas (CD95) ligand during the pathogenesis of experimental graft-versus-host disease. J Immunol 2001; 167:2936–2941.

147. van Den Brink MR, Moore E, Horndasch KJ, Crawford JM, Hoffman J, Murphy GF, Burakoff SJ. Fas-deficient lpr mice are more susceptible to graft-versus-host disease. J Immunol 2000; 164:469–480.

148. van den Brink MR, Moore E, Horndasch KJ, Crawford JM, Murphy GF, Burakoff SJ 2000 Fas ligand-deficient gld mice are more susceptible to graft-versus-host-disease. Transplantation 70:184–191.

149. Beelen DW, Haralambie E, Brandt H, Linzenmeier G, Muller KD, Quabeck K, Sayer HG, Graeven U, Mahmoud HK, Schaefer UW. Evidence that sustained growth suppression of intestinal anaerobic bacteria reduces the risk of acute graft-versus-host disease after sibling marrow transplantation. Blood 1992; 80:2668–2676.

150. Beelen DW, Elmaagacli A, Muller KD, Hirche H, Schaefer UW. Influence of intestinal bacterial decontamination using metronidazole and ciprofloxacin or ciprofloxacin alone on the development of acute graft-versus-host disease after marrow transplantation in patients with hematologic malignancies: final results and long-term follow-up of an open-label prospective randomized trial. Blood 1999; 93:3267–3275.

151. Krenger W, Hill GR, Ferrara JLM. Cytokine cascades in acute graft-versus-host disease. Transplantation 1997; 64:553–558.

152. Jones JM, Wilson R, Bealmear PM. Mortality and gross pathology of secondary disease in germfree mouse radiation chimeras. Rad Res 1971; 45:577–588.

153. van Bekkum DW, Roodenburg J, Heidt PJ, van der Waaij D. Mitigation of secondary disease of allogeneic mouse radiation chimeras by modification of the intestinal microflora. J Natl Cancer Inst 1974; 52:401–404.

154. Moore RH, Lampert IA, Chia Y, Aber VR, Cohen J. Influence of endotoxin on graft-versus-host disease after bone marrow transplantation across major histocompatibility barriers in mice. Transplantation 1987; 43:731–736.

155. Moore RH, Lampert IA, Chia Y, Aber VR, Cohen J. Effect of immunization with *Escherichia coli* J5 on graft-versus-host disease induced by minor histocompatibility antigens in mice. Transplantation 1987; 44:249–253.

156. Price KS, Nestel FP, Lapp WS. Progressive accumulation of bacterial lipopolysaccharide in vivo during acute murine graft-versus-host disease. Scand J Immunol 1997; 45:294–300.

157. Ellison CA, Amadeo RJ, Gartner JG. GVHD-associated enteropathy and endotoxemia in F1-hybrid recipients of NK1.1-depleted grafts. Scand J Immunol 2001; 54:375–382.

158. Hill GR, Crawford JM, Cooke KR, Brinson YS, Pan L, Ferrara JL. Total body irradiation and acute graft-versus-host disease: the role of gastrointestinal damage and inflammatory cytokines. Blood 1997; 90:3204–3213.

159. Rafferty JF, Noguchi Y, Fischer JE, Hasselgren P. Sepsis in rats stimulates cellular proliferation in the mucosa of the small intestine. Gastroenterology 1994; 107:121–127.

160. Grundy JE, Shanley JD, Shearer GM. Augmentation of graft-versus-host reaction by cytomegalovirus infection resulting in interstitial pneumonitis. Transplantation 1985; 39:548–553.

161. Mowat AM, Felstein MV, Baca ME. Experimental studies of immunologically mediated enteropathy. III. Severe and progressive enteropathy during a graft-versus-host reaction in athymic mice. Immunology 1987; 61:185–188.

162. Bellgrau D, Wilson DB. Immunological studies of T-cell receptors. I. Specifically induced resistance to graft-versus-host disease in rats mediated by host T-cell immunity to alloreactive parental T cells. J Exp Med 1978; 148:103–114.

163. Eigler A, Sinha B, Hartmann G, Endres S. Taming TNF: strategies to restrain this proinflammatory cytokine. Immunol Today 1997; 18:487–492.

164. Lu Y, Sakamaki S, Kuroda H, Kusakabe T, Konuma Y, Akiyama T, Fujimi A, Takemoto N, Nishiie K, Matsunaga T, Hirayama Y, Kato J, Kon S, Kogawa K, Niitsu Y. Prevention of lethal acute graft-versus-host disease in mice by oral administration of T helper 1 inhibitor, TAK-603. Blood 2001; 97:1123–1130.

165. Cooke KR, Gerbitz A, Crawford JM, Teshima T, Hill GR, Tesolin A, Rossignol DP, Ferrara JL. LPS antagonism reduces graft-versus-host disease and preserves graft-versus-leukemia activity after experimental bone marrow transplantation. J Clin Invest 2001; 107:1581–1589.

166. Sarnacki S, Auber F, Cretolle C, Camby C, Cavazzana-Calvo M, Muller W, Wagner N, Brousse N, Revillon Y, Fischer A, Cerf-Bensussan N. Blockade of the integrin $\alpha L\beta 2$ but not of integrins $\alpha 4$ and/or $\beta 7$ significantly prolongs intestinal allograft survival in mice. Gut 2000; 47:97–104.

167. Kellersmann R, Lazarovits A, Grant D, Garcia B, Chan B, Kellersmann A, Wang H, Jevnikar A, Wagner N, Muller W, Ulrichs K, Thiede A, Zhong R. Monoclonal antibody against $\beta 7$ integrins, but not $\beta 7$ deficiency, attenuates intestinal allograft rejection in mice. Transplantation 2002; 74:1317–1324.

168. Picarella D, Hurlbu tP, Rottman J, Shi X, Butcher E, Ringler DJ. Monoclonal antibodies specific for $\beta 7$ integrin and mucosal addressin cell adhesion molecule-1 (MAdCAM-1) reduce inflammation in the colon of scid mice reconstituted with CD45RBhigh CD4+ T cells. J Immunol 1997; 158:2099–2106.

169. Sydora BC, Wagner N, Lohler J, Yakoub G, Kronenberg M, Muller W, Aranda R. $\beta 7$ Integrin expression is not required for the localization of T cells to the intestine and colitis pathogenesis. Clin Exp Immunol 2002; 129:35–42.

170. Neurath MF, Fuss I, Kelsall BL, Stuber E, Strober W. Antibodies to IL-12 abrogate established experimental colitis in mice. J Exp Med 1995; 182:1281–1290.

171. Brown GR, Lee E, Thiele DL. TNF-TNFR2 interactions are critical for the development of intestinal graft-versus-host disease in MHC class II-disparate (C57BL/6J → C57BL/6J × bm12)F1 mice. J Immunol 2002; 168:3065–3071.

172. Ellison CA, Bradley DS, Fischer JM, Hayglass KT, Gartner JG. Murine graft-versus-host disease induced using interferon-gamma-deficient grafts features antibodies to double-stranded DNA, T helper 2-type cytokines and hypereosinophilia. Immunology 2002; 105:63–72.

173. Krijanovski OI, Hill GR, Cooke KR, Teshima T, Crawford JM, Brinson YS, Ferrara JL. Keratinocyte growth factor separates graft-versus-leukemia effects from graft-versus-host disease. Blood 1999; 94:825–831.

174. Zeeh JM, Procaccino F, Hoffmann P, Aukerman SL, McRoberts JA, Soltani S, Pierce GF, Lakshmanan J, Lacey D, Eysselein VE. Keratinocyte growth factor ameliorates mucosal injury in an experimental model of colitis in rats. Gastroenterology 1996; 110:1077–1083.

175. Riegler M, Sedivy R, Sogukoglu T, Cosentini E, Bischof G, Teleky B, Feil W, Schiessel R, Hamilton G, Wenzl E. Epidermal growth factor promotes rapid response to epithelial injury in rabbit duodenum in vitro. Gastroenterology 1996; 111:28–36.

176. Huang FS, Kemp CJ, Williams JL, Erwin CR, Warner BW. Role of epidermal growth factor and its receptor in chemotherapy-induced intestinal injury. Am J Physiol 2002; 282:G432–442.

177. Willemsen LE, Schreurs CC, Kroes H, Spillenaar Bilgen EJ, Van Deventer SJ, Van Tol EA. A coculture model mimicking the intestinal mucosa reveals a regulatory role for myofibroblasts in immune-mediated barrier disruption. Dig Dis Sci 2002; 47:2316–2324.

178. Roy J, Snover D, Weisdorf S, Mulvahill A, Filipovich A, Weisdorf D. Simultaneous upper and lower endoscopic biopsy in the diagnosis of intestinal graft-versus-host disease. Transplantation 1991; 51:642–646.

179. Schwartz JM, Wolford JL, Thornquist MD, Hockenbery DM, Murakami CS, Drennan F, Hinds M, Strasser SI, Lopez-Cubero SO, Brar HS, Ko CW, Saunders MD, Okolo CN, McDonald GB. Severe gastrointestinal bleeding after hematopoietic cell transplantation, 1987–1997: incidence, causes, and outcome. Am J Gastroenterol 2001; 96:385–393.

180. Chakrabarti S, Lees A, Jones SG, Milligan DW. *Clostridium difficile* infection in allogeneic stem cell transplant recipients is associated with severe graft-versus-host disease and non-relapse mortality. Bone Marrow Transplant 2000; 26:871–876.

181. Einsele H, Ehninger G, Hebart H, Weber P, Dette S, Link H, Horny HP, Meuter V, Wagner S, Waller HD, et al. Incidence of local CMV infection and acute intestinal GVHD in marrow transplant recipients with severe diarrhoea. Bone Marrow Transplant 1994; 14:955–963.

182. Cox GJ, Matsui SM, Lo RS, Hinds M, Bowden RA, Hackman RC, Meyer WG, Mori M, Tarr PI, Oshiro LS, et al. Etiology and outcome of diarrhea after marrow transplantation: a prospective study. Gastroenterology 1994; 107:1398–1407.

183. Weisdorf DJ, Snover DC, Haake R, Miller WJ, McGlave PB, Blazar B, Ramsay NK, Kersey JH, Filipovich A. Acute upper gastrointestinal graft-versus-host disease: clinical significance and response to immunosuppressive therapy. Blood 1990; 76:624–629.

184. Wu D, Hockenberry DM, Brentnall TA, Baehr PH, Ponec RJ, Kuver R, Tzung SP, Todaro JL, McDonald GB. Persistent nausea and anorexia after marrow transplantation: a prospective study of 78 patients. Transplantation 1998; 66:1319–1324.

185. Sale GE, Shulman HM, McDonald GB, Thomas ED. Gastrointestinal graft-versus-host disease in man. A clinicopathologic study of the rectal biopsy. Am J Surg Pathol 1979; 3:291–299.

186. Epstein RJ, McDonald GB, Sale GE, Shulman HM, Thomas ED. The diagnostic accuracy of the rectal biopsy in acute graft-versus-host disease: a prospective study of thirteen patients. Gastroenterology 1980; 78:764–771.

187. Washington K, Bentley RC, Green A, Olson J, Treem WR, Krigman HR. Gastric graft-versus-host disease: a blinded histologic study. Am J Surg Pathol 1997; 21:1037–1046.

188. Clift RA, Buckner CD, Appelbaum FR, Bearman SI, Petersen FB, Fisher LD, Anasetti C, Beatty P, Bensinger WI, Doney K, et al. Allogeneic marrow transplantation in patients with acute myeloid leukemia in first remission: a randomized trial of two irradiation regimens. Blood 1990; 76:1867–1871.

189. Nash RA, Pepe MS, Storb R, Longton G, Pettinger M, Anasetti C, Appelbaum FR, Bowden RA, Deeg HJ, Doney K, et al. Acute graft-versus-host disease: analysis of risk factors after allogeneic marrow transplantation and prophylaxis with cyclosporine and methotrexate. Blood 1992; 80:1838–1845.

190. Clift RA, Buckner CD, Thomas ED, Bensinger WI, Bowden R, Bryant E, Deeg HJ, Doney KC, Fisher LD, Hansen JA, et al. Marrow transplantation for chronic myeloid leukemia: a randomized study comparing cyclophosphamide and total body irradiation with busulfan and cyclophosphamide. Blood 1994; 84:2036–2043.

191. Socie G, Clift RA, Blaise D, Devergie A, Ringden O, Martin PJ, Remberger M, Deeg HJ, Ruutu T, Michallet M, Sullivan KM, Chevret S. Busulfan plus cyclophosphamide compared with total-body irradiation plus cyclophosphamide before marrow transplantation for myeloid leukemia: long-term follow-up of 4 randomized studies. Blood 2001; 98:3569–3574.

192. Mielcarek M, Martin PJ, Leisenring W, Flowers ME, Maloney DG, Sandmaier BM, Maris MB, Storb R. Graft-versus-host disease after nonmyeloablative versus conventional hematopoietic stem cell transplantation. Blood 2003; 102:756–762.

193. Cheng J, Turksen K, Yu QC, Schreiber H, Teng M, Fuchs E. Cachexia and graft-vs.-host-disease-type skin changes in keratin promoter-driven TNF alpha transgenic mice. Genes Dev 1992; 6:1444–1456.

194. Cooke KR, Hill GR, Crawford JM, Bungard D, Brinson YS, Delmonte J, Ferrara JL., Jr. Tumor necrosis factor-α production to lipopolysaccharide stimulation by donor cells predicts the severity of experimental acute graft-versus-host disease. J Clin Invest 1998; 102:1882–1891.

195. Hill GR, Cooke KR, Brinson YS, Bungard D, Ferrara JL. Pretransplant chemotherapy reduces inflammatory cytokine production and acute graft-versus-host disease after allogeneic bone marrow transplantation. Transplantation 1999; 67:1478–1480.

196. Hill GR, Teshima T, Gerbitz A, Pan L, Cooke KR, Brinson YS, Crawford JM, Ferrara JL. Differential roles of IL-1 and TNF-alpha on graft-versus-host disease and graft versus leukemia. J Clin Invest 1999; 104:459–467.

197. Hill GR, Teshima T, Rebel VI, Krijanovski OI, Cooke KR, Brinson YS, Ferrara JL. The p55 TNF-alpha receptor plays a critical role in T cell alloreactivity. J Immunol 2000; 164:656–663.

198. Speiser DE, Bachmann MF, Frick TW, McKall-Faienza K, Griffiths E, Pfeffer K, Mak TW, Ohashi PS. TNF receptor p55 controls early acute graft-versus-host disease. J Immunol 1997; 158:5185–5190.

199. Herve P, Flesch M, Tiberghien P, Wijdenes J, Racadot E, Bordigoni P, Plouvier E, Stephan JL, Bourdeau H, Holler E, et al. Phase I-II trial of a monoclonal anti-tumor necrosis factor alpha antibody for the treatment of refractory severe acute graft-versus-host disease. Blood 1992; 79:3362–3368.

200. Holler E, Kolb HJ, Mittermuller J, Kaul M, Ledderose G, Duell T, Seeber B, Schleuning M, Hintermeier-Knabe R, Ertl B, et al. Modulation of acute graft-versus-host-disease after allogeneic bone marrow transplantation by tumor necrosis factor alpha (TNF alpha) release in the course of pretransplant conditioning: role of conditioning regimens and prophylactic application of a monoclonal antibody neutralizing human TNF alpha (MAK 195F). Blood 1995 86:890–899.

201. Holler E, Ertl B, Hintermeier-Knabe R, Roncarolo MG, Eissner G, Mayer F, Fraunberger P, Behrends U, Pfannes W, Kolb HJ, Wilmanns W. Inflammatory reactions induced by pretransplant conditioning—an alternative target for modulation of acute GvHD and complications following allogeneic bone marrow transplantation? Leuk Lymphoma 1997; 25:217–224.

202. Holler E, Kolb HJ, Hintermeier-Knabe R, Mittermuller J, Thierfelder S, Kaul M, Wilmanns W. Role of tumor necrosis factor alpha in acute graft-versus-host disease and complications following allogeneic bone marrow transplantation. Transplant Proc 1993; 25:1234–1236.

203. Socie G, Mary J, Lemann M, Daneshpouy M, Guardiola P, Meignin V, Ades L, Esperou H, Ribaud P, Devergie A, Gluckman E, Ameisen J, Janin A. Graft-versus-host disease of the gastro-intestinal tract in humans: TNF and Fas expression; prognostic value of apoptotic cells and infiltrating neutrophils. Blood 2003; 103:50–57.

204. Daneshpouy M, Socie G, Lemann M, Rivet J, Gluckman E, Janin A. Activated eosinophils in upper gastrointestinal tract of patients with graft-versus-host disease. Blood 2002; 99:3033–3040.

205. Baehr PH, Levine DS, Bouvier ME, Hockenbery DM, Gooley TA, Stern JG, Martin PJ, McDonald GB. Oral beclomethasone dipropionate for treatment of human intestinal graft-versus-host disease. Transplantation 1995; 60:1231–1238.

206. Bertz H, Afting M, Kreisel W, Duffner U, Greinwald R, Finke J. Feasibility and response to budesonide as topical corticosteroid therapy for acute intestinal GVHD. Bone Marrow Transplant 1999; 24:1185–1189.

207. McDonald GB, Bouvier M, Hockenbery DM, Stern JM, Gooley T, Farrand A, Murakami C, Levine DS. Oral beclomethasone dipropionate for treatment of intestinal graft-versus-host disease: a randomized, controlled trial. Gastroenterology 1998; 115:28–35.

208. Ippoliti C, Champlin R, Bugazia N, Przepiorka D, Neumann J, Giralt S, Khouri I, Gajewski J. Use of octreotide in the symptomatic management of diarrhea induced by graft-versus-host disease in patients with hematologic malignancies. J Clin Oncol 1997; 15:3350–3354.

11

The Pathophysiology of Lung Injury After Hematopoietic Stem Cell Transplantation

KENNETH R. COOKE and JAMES L. M. FERRARA

University of Michigan Comprehensive Cancer Center, Ann Arbor, Michigan, U.S.A.

I. INTRODUCTION

Over the last several decades, allogeneic hematopoietic stem cell transplantation (SCT) has emerged as an important therapeutic option for a number of malignant and nonmalignant conditions. Unfortunately, this treatment strategy is limited by several side effects including pulmonary toxicity. Diffuse lung injury is a major complication of SCT that occurs in 25–55% of SCT recipients and can account for approximately 50% of transplant-related mortality (1–6). Noninfectious lung injury can be either acute (termed idiopathic pneumonia syndrome, or IPS) or chronic, depending on the time of onset after SCT and the tempo of disease progression. Historically, approximately 50% of all pneumonias seen after SCT have been secondary to infection, but the judicious use of broad-spectrum antimicrobial prophylaxis in recent years has tipped the balance of pulmonary complications from infectious to noninfectious causes (7). Chronic lung injury (by definition occurring in patients over 100 days posttransplant) is further subdivided into two types: obstructive and restrictive (8–16). Each form of noninfectious lung injury is associated with significant morbidity and mortality and responds poorly to standard therapeutic approaches. A significant body of experimental literature demonstrates that both acute and chronic noninfectious lung injuries after SCT are immunologically mediated and share similar pathogenetic mechanisms with graft-vs.-host disease (GVHD). This chapter will review the definitions, risk factors, and pathogeneses of noninfectious lung injury occurring both early and late after allogeneic SCT.

329

II. ACUTE LUNG INJURY: IDIOPATHIC PNEUMONIA SYNDROME

A. Definition and Clinical Course

In 1993 an NIH panel defined IPS as widespread alveolar injury following SCT that occurs in the absence of an active lower respiratory tract infection and cardiogenic causes (17). This entity is considered a clinical syndrome, with variable histopathological correlates and several potential etiologies (17). Diagnostic criteria of IPS include signs and symptoms of pneumonia, nonlobar radiographic infiltrates, abnormal pulmonary function, and the absence of infectious organisms as determined by bronchoalveolar lavage (BAL) or lung biopsy (2,17). Histopathological findings associated with IPS include diffuse alveolar damage with hyaline membranes, lymphocytic bronchitis, and bronchiolitis obliterans organizing pneumonia (BOOP) (18). The most frequently reported pattern, however, is interstitial pneumonitis, a term historically used interchangeably with IPS (3,19). Interstitial pneumonitis is seen in association with diffuse alveolar damage and hemorrhage early after SCT and is accompanied by bronchiolar inflammation and epithelial damage at later time points (18).

The median time of onset for IPS was initially reported to be 6–7 weeks (range 14–90 days) after the infusion of donor stem cells (17), and mortality rates range from 50 to 80% overall, and greater than 95% for patients requiring mechanical ventilation (1,3,5–7,17,20). A retrospective study from Seattle showed a lower incidence and earlier onset of IPS than previously reported, but the typical clinical course involving the rapid onset of respiratory failure leading to death remained unchanged (6). A recent review from the University of Michigan Medical Center demonstrated that the frequency of IPS after allogeneic SCT ranged from 5 to 25%, depending upon donor source and the degree of antigenic mismatch between donor and recipient (21). The median time for development of IPS at Michigan was 14 days after transplant, and the overall day 100 mortality was 80%. Of note, the median time to death from diagnosis of IPS was 13 days despite aggressive treatment with high-dose steroids and broad-spectrum antimicrobial therapy (21).

IPS also encompasses other forms of pulmonary toxicity. In one small subset of patients with IPS, acute pulmonary hemorrhage or hemorrhagic alveolitis occurs. Diffuse alveolar hemorrhage (DAH) generally develops in the immediate post-SCT period and is characterized by progressive shortness of breath, cough, and hypoxemia with or without fever (7,22–24). Progressively bloodier aliquots of BAL fluid have traditionally diagnosed DAH, but frank hemoptysis is rare (22). Sloan and colleagues identified acute hemorrhagic pulmonary edema (the histological correlate of DAH) in a subset of SCT recipients at autopsy, 80% of whom had received a non–HLA-identical SCT and had previous acute GVHD (25). Similarly, a Hopkins series reported that death from pulmonary hemorrhage was associated with grade II or greater GVHD (26). Mortality from DAH is as high as 75% despite aggressive treatment with high-dose (2 mg/kg to 1 g/m^2) steroids, and death usually occurs within 3 weeks of diagnosis (23).

Peri-engraftment respiratory distress syndrome (PERDS) and delayed pulmonary toxicity syndrome (DPTS) are also included within the definition of IPS (7). PERDS and DPTS typically occur after autologous SCT (7), and both are characterized by fever, dyspnea, and hypoxemia (27–29). By definition, PERDS occurs within 5 days of engraftment, whereas the onset of DPTS may be delayed for months and commonly occurs following conditioning regimens that contain cyclophosphamide, cisplatin, and bischloroethylinitrosurea (BCNU) as used in SCT for breast cancer (29). Although PERDS after autologous SCT appears similar to IPS after allogeneic SCT with respect to clinical presentation and time of onset, the two entities differ sharply with respect to overall outcome; injury from PERDS after autologous SCT, even when requiring mechanical support, responds promptly to corticosteroids and is associated with a favorable prognosis (27), whereas IPS occurring in an allogeneic environment responds poorly to standard therapy and results rapid respiratory failure and death in the majority of patients (6,–21).

B. Risk Factors of IPS

Potential risk factors for IPS include conditioning with total body irradiation (TBI), acute GVHD, older recipient age, initial diagnosis of malignancy other than leukemia, and the use of methotrexate (MTX) for GVHD prophylaxis (5,19,30,31). The likelihood of developing IPS increases with the number of identified risk factors (3). Although recipient age and the use of MTX are not always risk factors, the use of TBI and the development of acute GVHD have been identified as factors in multiple reports (2,5,6,31–33). A recent report from Seattle found that despite greater patient age and a similar incidence of acute GVHD, recipients of allogeneic SCT using nonmyeloablative conditioning have a reduced risk of IPS compared to patients receiving myeloablative conditioning (34). Once established, pulmonary toxicity was severe in each group and resulted in respiratory failure in the majority of patients. These findings suggest that the intensity of SCT conditioning plays an important role in the development of IPS, and they are consistent with data generated from two mouse SCT models showing that the lung is sensitive to the combined effects of radiation and alloreactive T cells (35,36).

The potential etiologies for IPS include direct toxic effects of SCT conditioning regimens, occult pulmonary infections, and the release of inflammatory cytokines that have been implicated in other forms of pulmonary injury (37–41). Immunological factors may also be important as suggested by the association of IPS and severe GVHD in several large series (2,3,5–7,20). Acute GVHD often precedes IPS, suggesting a possible causal relationship between the two disorders (5,19,42,43). Although IPS can also occur when signs and symptoms of GVHD are limited or absent (44–47), the consistent association between lung injury and GVHD after experimental SCT also supports such an etiology (2,3,5,6,48–52).

The role of GVHD and specifically alloreactive donor T lymphocytes in the pathogenesis of IPS remains a topic of considerable debate. Epithelial apoptosis is usually attributed to T-cell–mediated injury and is considered pathognomonic for acute GVHD. Although observed in the lungs of some patients with IPS (18), epithelial apoptosis has not been consistently identified in allogeneic SCT recipients with pulmonary dysfunction (25,43,53,54). Lymphocytic bronchitis was, however, reported as a potential histopathological correlate of GVHD of the lung (43). This pattern was initially observed in allogeneic SCT recipients with GVHD but not in patients receiving autologous SCT or in untransplanted controls, but this association was not confirmed in subsequent reports (25,53,54). More recently, Yousem described the histological spectrum of pulmonary GVHD in 17 allogeneic SCT recipients. Findings ranged from diffuse alveolar injury early after SCT to cicatrical bronchiolitis obliterans, which represented a late and irreversible form of lung injury (18). In this report, bronchitis/bronchiolitis with interstitial pneumonitis (BIP) was the most common finding and included a lymphocytic infiltration around bronchial structures along with a mononuclear inflammation in the perivascular zones and alveolar septa. The heterogeneity of pulmonary histopathology after allogeneic

SCT is complicated further by the nonspecific changes that occur after mechanical ventilation and by the limited quality and quantity of lung biopsy tissue. Yet despite the lack of
classic acute GVHD histopathology, several lines of evidence suggest that the lung is a
target of immunologically mediated damage after allogeneic SCT.

C. Murine Models of IPS

Several laboratories have explored the relationship between alloreactivity and IPS
in rodent SCT models and have consistently shown that animals with systemic
GVHD develop lung injury, whereas those receiving syngeneic SCT do not (Fig. 1)
(48,51,55,56). Even under tightly controlled experimental conditions, several patterns
of lung injury have emerged, including acute hemorrhagic alveolitis, late onset interstitial
pneumonitis, and lymphocytic bronchiolitis (48). In several models where the GVH

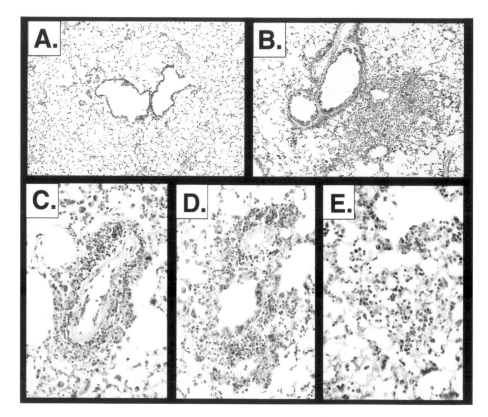

Figure 1 IPS pathology. Following lethal irradiation, mice received hematopoietic SCT from
either allogeneic (MHC-matched) or syngeneic donors. Lungs were harvested and prepared for
microscopic analysis. At 6 weeks, lungs of mice receiving syngeneic SCT maintain virtually
normal histology (A), whereas allogeneic SCT recipients develop significant lung histopathology
(B–E). Two major abnormalities are apparent after allogeneic SCT. First, dense mononuclear
cell infiltrates are observed around both pulmonary vessels (C) and bronchioles (D). Second,
an acute pneumonitis is present involving both the interstitial and alveolar spaces (E). The
alveolar infiltrate is composed of macrophages, lymphocytes, epithelial cells, and scattered
polymorphonuclear cells within a fibrin matrix. Original magnification: 200× (A, B); 400× (C–E).

reaction is induced to 1) minor H antigens, 2) class I or class II MHC antigens only, or 3) both major and minor H antigens, two major abnormalities are apparent after allogeneic SCT: a dense mononuclear cell infiltrate around both pulmonary vessels (Fig. 1B) and bronchioles (Fig. 1C) and an acute pneumonitis involving the interstitium and alveolar spaces (Fig. 1D) (51,57,58). The alveolar infiltrate is composed of macrophages, lymphocytes, epithelial cells, and scattered polymorphonuclear cells within a fibrin matrix. Both of these histopathological patterns closely resemble those of the nonspecific, diffuse interstitial pneumonias seen in allogeneic SCT recipients (17,18,25,43). However, evidence for diffuse alveolar injury including alveolar hemorrhage, edema, and hyaline membranes has not been demonstrated in these models.

In those studies where it has been measured, pulmonary function is significantly decreased in animals with IPS after SCT, demonstrating that the observed lung pathology was physiologically relevant (52,56). In one report, mice with IPS showed significant reductions in both dynamic compliance and airway conductance compared with syngeneic controls, consistent with changes expected from both the interstitial and peribronchial infiltrates (52). Lung injury correlated with the presence but not the severity of GVHD in that study, consistent with clinical reports of IPS in allogeneic SCT recipients whose signs and symptoms of GVHD were mild or absent (8,9,21,46,59,60) (see Sec. II.D).

D. The Pathogenesis of IPS

1. The Inflammatory Effectors TNFα and LPS

The mixed inflammatory alveolar infiltrates found in mice with IPS are accompanied by significant increases in the number of total number of cells, lymphocytes, macrophages, and neutrophils in the BAL fluid (51). These infiltrates are also associated with increased TNFα in both lung tissue and BAL fluid (49–51,61,62). Increases in neutrophils and TNFα in the absence of infection suggested that endogenous endotoxin (LPS) might play an important role in IPS pathophysiology. LPS is a component of the innate immune response and is a potent enhancer of inflammatory cytokine release. In non-SCT experimental models, intratracheal administration of LPS elicits a severe, acute inflammatory response in the lungs of animals (63–65). Recent work has also demonstrated that LPS is an important effector molecule in the development of acute GVHD; translocation of LPS across a gut mucosa damaged early in the posttransplant period provides access to the systemic circulation where it stimulates leukocytes to release inflammatory mediators that subsequently contribute to GVHD target organ damage and dysfunction (66–72) (see Chapter 1). LPS levels are elevated in the BAL fluid of mice with IPS, and LPS stimulates the release of inflammatory cytokines that directly contribute to lung damage: intravenous LPS injection 6 weeks after allogeneic SCT significantly amplifies lung injury (51). This amplification is only seen in mice with advanced GVHD and is associated with large increases in BAL fluid levels of TNFα and LPS and the development of alveolar hemorrhage (51,62). Furthermore, direct antagonism of LPS early in the time course of SCT reduces systemic and BAL fluid levels of TNFα and significantly decreases the severity of IPS compared to control treated animals (68) (K. R. Cooke, unpublished observation).

A causal role for TNFα in the development of IPS has been established by neutralizing this cytokine in experimental SCT models (61,62,73). Administration of a soluble, dimeric, TNF-binding protein (rhTNFR : Fc; Immunex Corp., Seattle, WA) at the time of LPS challenge effectively prevents increases in pathology, BAL fluid cellularity, and LPS levels, confirming the linkage between LPS and TNFα in this setting (62). Neutralization of TNFα from week 4 to week 6 after SCT reduces the development of IPS in the absence of LPS challenge (62). Recent data also demonstrate that signaling through the p75 TNF receptor (TNFR) is critical for the development of IPS; when used as allogeneic SCT recipients, p75 TNFR-deficient mice develop significantly less pulmonary toxicity compared to wild-type controls and animals deficient in the p55 receptor (74). The incomplete protection provided by TNFα neutralization after SCT is consistent with reports from many groups (48,61,71,72,75–77) and suggests that other inflammatory and cellular mechanisms such as the Fas-FasL pathway that mediate acute GVHD may also contribute to the development of IPS (75,78,79). For example, IL-1β, TGFβ, and nitrating species including nitric oxide and peroxynitrite have also been implicated in the development of IPS, particularly when cyclophosphamide is included in the conditioning regimen (56,80,81).

TNFα likely contributes to the development of IPS through both direct and indirect mechanisms. In addition to being directly cytotoxic, TNFα increases expression of inflammatory chemokines and MHC antigens, modulates leukocyte migration, and facilitates cell-mediated cytotoxicity (61,82). TNFα may also contribute to lung injury by increasing the severity of GVHD in other target organs such as the gut and liver, promoting the release of other inflammatory mediators and their ultimate passage to the pulmonary vascular bed. The ability of TNFα neutralization to reduce BAL fluid LPS levels after the systemic administration of endotoxin strongly suggests that rhTNFR : Fc alters the systemic inflammatory response to LPS "upstream" from the lung in addition to directly neutralizing TNFα in the alveolar space (63). Because damage to the GI tract precedes lung injury in these allogeneic SCT models, we hypothesize that inflammatory mediators (i.e., LPS and TNFα) released in response to GI GVHD later contribute to the development of IPS. From this perspective, the structural and functional integrity of the liver is critical. The liver is pivotally located between the intestinal reservoir of gram-negative bacteria and their toxic byproducts and the rich capillary network in the lung. Kupffer cells in the liver detoxify and subsequently clear endotoxin from the systemic circulation (83) and protect the lung in experimental models of sepsis and ARDS (84,85). Inflammation engendered during the normal clearance of endotoxin remains contained within the reticulo-endothelial system of the liver (83). If the capacity of the liver to clear an endotoxin challenge is exceeded, however, both inflammatory cytokines and unprocessed LPS can enter into the systemic circulation and damage other organs. Several experimental studies have shown that preexisting injury to the liver decreases its ability to neutralize endotoxin effectively (86–89). In the setting of acute GVHD, an endotoxin surge into the systemic bloodstream can arise from increased leakage of LPS across damaged intestinal mucosa. In this scenario, underlying damage to the liver could decrease its capacity for LPS uptake and clearance. Animals with mild or no GVHD can effectively detoxify endotoxin and protect their lungs from further damage, whereas mice with severe GVHD are unable to do so and develop severe extensive lung injury including alveolar hemorrhage (51). Systemic neutralization of TNFα after allogeneic SCT prevents damage to the liver caused by endotoxin, which may also help protect the lung from injury (62).

Collectively, these data demonstrate that the inflammatory mediators TNFα and LPS both contribute to experimental IPS. Moreover, they support the hypothesis of a "gut-liver-lung" axis of inflammation in IPS pathophysiology (Fig. 2). Any process that ultimately results in large amounts of endotoxin and/or TNFα in the pulmonary circulation may contribute to the development of lung injury in this setting. This hypothesis is consistent with the observation that serum TNFα levels are increased in patients

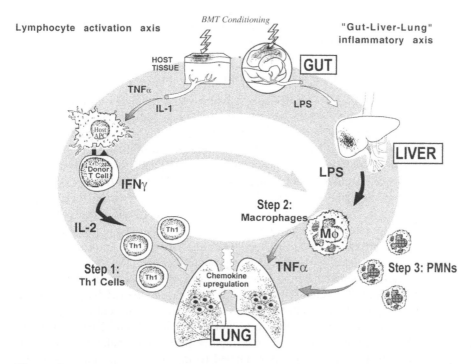

Figure 2   Pathophysiology of IPS after allogeneic SCT. Data generated using murine SCT models have been incorporated into a working hypothesis of IPS physiology. This schema postulates that the lung is susceptible to two distinct but interrelated pathways of immune-mediated injury that occur along a T-lymphocyte activation axis and a "gut-liver-lung" axis of inflammation. The lymphocyte activation axis fundamentally depends upon interactions between donor T cells and host antigen-presenting cells. Chemo-radiotherapy of SCT conditioning causes TNFα and IL-1 release that enhance the ability of host APC to present alloantigens to mature donor T cells and upregulate chemokine expression in the lung. Once engaged, donor T cells become activated and secrete IFNγ and IL-2. IFNγ primes donor macrophages (Mφ) and monocytes, whereas IL-2 facilitates T-cell activation and the generation of Th1-lymphocyte effectors that migrate to the lung early after SCT in response to inflammatory chemokine gradients (step 1) and contribute to pulmonary toxicity via Fas-FasL–mediated cell killing. The inflammatory axis focuses on the relationship between the cellular activating effects of LPS and the downstream production of TNFα as it occurs along a gut-liver-lung axis of inflammation. LPS enters the systemic circulation through gaps in the intestinal mucosa. The ability of systemic endotoxin to reach the alveolar space is related to the consequences of GVHD in other target organs, particularly the liver, which is pivotally located immediately downstream (via the splanchnic circulation) of the intestinal reservoir of gram-negative bacteria and their toxic byproducts. Underlying liver damage from hepatic GVHD decreases the liver's capacity for LPS uptake and clearance and allows passage of LPS into the pulmonary circulation. Donor macrophages primed by IFNγ are recruited to the lung (step 2), where they are triggered by LPS to secrete inflammatory cytokines like TNFα, resulting in enhanced chemokine expression, the recruitment of neutrophils to the lung (step 3), and increased tissue damage.

with IPS (90). A clinical linkage of hepatic dysfunction to lung injury after SCT is also suggested by associations between VOD and IPS and between hepatic failure and death from IPS (2,21). Furthermore, evidence for cytokine activation and LPS amplification observed in the BAL fluid of ARDS patients (91) has been demonstrated in patients with IPS after allogeneic SCT; increased pulmonary vascular permeability and increases in BAL fluid levels of IL-1, IL-12, IL-6, TNFα LPS-binding protein (LBP), and soluble CD14 were also observed in these patients (1).

2. Cellular Effectors and the Development of IPS

The Role of Donor-Derived T-Cell Effectors.   Although the induction of GVHD fundamentally depends upon interactions between donor T cells and host antigen-presenting cells (APCs) (92), the role of alloreactive donor T cells in the pathogenesis of IPS has been a topic of considerable debate. Pulmonary endothelial and epithelial cells can express MHC class I, MHC class II, and minor histocompatibility (H) antigens, and the expression of these molecules on vascular endothelium is enhanced by TNFα and IFNγ (93). It is conceivable, therefore, that pulmonary parenchymal cells can serve as targets for direct cell-mediated damage. The recovery of donor specific, alloreactive T cells in the BAL fluid of heart-lung transplant recipients heralds the onset of acute rejection and provides support for cell-mediated lung injury (94). The importance of lymphocytes to lung injury after experimental SCT has been shown by several groups (49,56,95,96). Donor T cells are critical to the early proinflammatory events associated with lung injury that develops within the first week of SCT across MHC antigens, whereas in minor H antigen mismatch systems, donor lymphocytes continue to respond to host antigens and contribute to physiologically significant lung injury at later time points (52,56). Donor T-cell clones that recognize CD45 polymorphisms result in a rapidly progressive pulmonary vasculitis within 3 days of their injection into nonirradiated recipients (49,96). The speed of this injury directed at a single minor H antigen is probably accounted for by the clonal nature of the effector population. The origin and functional capacity of T cells infiltrating the lung have been examined by using differences in the T-cell Vβ repertoire between donor and recipient (52). Flow cytometry demonstrated that the TCR$\alpha\beta$ + T cells found in the lung 6 weeks after allogeneic SCT were of donor origin. When these donor derived T cells were recultured with irradiated host APCs, they proliferated vigorously and produced significant amounts of IFNγ (52). Similar results have been obtained using a P $\rightarrow$ F1 mouse model and congenic SCT donors expressing allelic differences of CD45 on all leukocytes. Greater than 95% of CD4+ and CD8+ lymphocytes in the bronchoalveolar space were of donor origin by the first week, and turnover was complete by week 2 after SCT. A significant proportion of these donor T cells secreted IFNγ (K. Cooke, unpublished observations). Comparable findings were observed for lymphocytes obtained from whole lung digests. These experimental data support the hypothesis that the alveolar lymphocytosis associated with IPS after clinical SCT represents a pulmonary manifestation of GVHD (97).

Both cytotoxic T lymphocytes (CTLs) and natural killer (NK) cells may play a role in IPS. Gartner and colleagues showed that pulmonary NK-cell activity remained increased over an extended period of time during GVHD in contrast to the transient and mild increase in NK-cell activity that occurred in the spleen during the same interval (98). Donor CTL effectors can contribute to lung injury via two primary cytolytic mechanisms: the perforin-granzyme pathway and the Fas-Fas ligand (FasL) pathway (99–102). During GVHD, CD4+ T cells use primarily the Fas pathway (103), whereas perforin CD8+ CTLs can kill using both perforin and Fas pathways (78,104). Each cytolytic pathway can play a role in the development of lung injury in non-SCT models (105–108). Cytolytic T cells expressing granzyme B are present in the lungs of mice after a fully mismatched allogeneic SCT, and they colocalize with macrophages expressing the costimulatory molecules B7.1 (DC80) and B7.2 (CD86). Pretreatment of allogeneic SCT recipients with keratinocyte growth factor (KGF) has been shown to decrease B7 and granzyme B expression and hasten repair in the lungs of mice with IPS (109). Alloantigen-specific killing by donor T cells using both perforin and Fas/FasL pathways has also been identified in the lung using a P → F1 allogeneic SCT model. CTL activity is present as early as week 2 after transplant and persists over time, but in this system only the Fas pathway contributes to the development of IPS (57).

Despite these compelling data supporting a role for alloreactive donor lymphocytes in the development of noninfectious lung injury after SCT, IPS has been reported in patients in whom systemic GVHD is mild or absent, making a causal relationship between the two entities difficult to establish (8,9,18,46,59,60). The relationship between lung injury and GVHD severity has been examined in a SCT model across minor H antigens. T-cell depletion (TCD) at the time of allogeneic SCT reduced the number of T cells by more than 99% and eliminated evidence of clinical or histological GVHD. Nevertheless, significant lung injury was noted after allogeneic TCD SCT and donor lymphocytes reactive to host antigens were present in the BAL fluid, but not the spleens, of these animals (52). This intriguing result suggested that the lung may be particularly sensitive to the effects of small numbers of host-reactive donor T cells even when systemic tolerance has been established. Consistent with these findings, BAL fluid lymphocytosis has been described after TCD SCT in association with pneumonitis that resulted from a local immune response; pulmonary T cells appeared to be activated despite systemic immune suppression (44). Furthermore, pulmonary toxicity has been reported after nonconditioned allogeneic SCT for severe combined immunodeficiency (SCID) where donor lymphocytes were noted in the lung during a period of rapid engraftment without evidence of systemic GVHD. Suppression of cellular immunity with high-dose methylprednisolone resulted in complete resolution of lung disease (110).

Taken together, these data suggest that donor-derived, IFNγ-secreting T cells home to the lungs early after SCT, persistently respond to host antigens, and can cause clinically and histologically significant tissue injury even when systemic GVHD is limited or absent. However, the precise mechanisms by which these cells interact with host antigens and cause injury remain unresolved. This process is likely to be complex and to involve interactions with pulmonary APCs (111,112). The pulmonary dendritic cell (DC) is significantly more efficient than the alveolar macrophage (AM) in antigen presentation and functions as the dominant APC in the lung (113–115). Pulmonary DCs are located in the pulmonary interstitium and in the bronchial epithelium and submucosa, where DC tissue density diminishes with decreasing airway diameter (116). During steady-state conditions, pulmonary DCs constitute the sole source of MHC class II expression within the epithelial lining of the airway (117). Lung DCs serve as sentinels at the epithelial surface of the airways. DCs can efficiently internalize and process antigen at this location, but paradoxically, their capacity to present antigen and to stimulate T cells is limited. DCs must migrate to regional lymph nodes where they become potent APCs, but at this point, their capacity to process antigen diminishes. This maturation process is associated with upregulation of costimulatory, adhesion, and MHC class II antigens (114). The antigen-presenting capacity of pulmonary DCs is regulated by AMs, which exist in close proximity to DCs in both the airway and lung parenchyma, and this process likely involves the secretion of soluble factors like nitric oxide; addition of AMs to in vitro DC cultures enhances this regulatory effect, whereas depletion of AMs in vivo enhances the APC function of freshly isolated DCs (117).

Pulmonary dendritic cells play a critical role in the initiation and regulation of immune responses in the lung, and recent data suggest that they are important to both acute and chronic rejection of lung allografts (115,118–120). The necessity of host APCs for the generation of acute GVHD has been demonstrated in a CD8+ T-cell–driven GVHD model (92). These results were recently extended by Teshima and colleagues, who showed that alloantigen expression on host APCs alone is both necessary and sufficient to induce a graft-vs.-host reaction and that GVHD target organ damage can be mediated by inflammatory cytokines (121). It is possible that radioresistant host DCs persist longer in the lung than in other organs and allow for sustained presentation of host antigens in that organ. In experiments using congenic rats, host DC populations in tracheal epithelium were depleted by 80% 3 days after 1000 cGy of TBI and were completely eliminated 14 days after syngeneic SCT. By contrast, lung parenchymal DCs were only reduced by 50% at day 3 and 60% by day 6 and declined at a rate that was intermediate between airway and epidermal DC populations (122). Activated donor T cells that can cause progressive lung injury might therefore remain within the pulmonary microvascular circulation because persistent host DCs function as a continuing site of alloantigen presentation. This scenario could account for the apparent "sanctuary" status of the lung with respect to alloreactive donor T cells and may have important implications with regard to the evaluation and treatment of IPS after allogeneic SCT even when clinical GVHD is absent.

It is also possible that donor T cells responsible for IPS initially encounter host APCs residing in more distant secondary lymphoid tissues and are later specifically recruited to the lung. Recent experimental data demonstrate that the subepithelial dome of intestinal Peyer's patches (PPs) is required for the generations of antihost CTL and the resultant induction of acute GVHD (123). Interrupting donor T-cell–host APC interactions at this site by using CCR5-deficient SCT donors, monoclonal antibodies to MAdCAM-1 or PP-deficient mice as SCT recipients prevented lethal GVHD resulting from marrow aplasia. However, GVHD target organ histopathology was not examined. These findings suggest that PPs are essential for initiating acute GVHD, but whether they are critical for the generation of donor effectors that contribute to damage in target organs, including the lung, must still be evaluated.

The Role of Donor Accessory Cells in the Development of IPS.   A significant body of experimental data suggests that synergistic interactions between cells from the lymphoid and myeloid lineage are critical to the development of GVHD (67,68,72). Specifically, the production of IFNγ from activated donor T cells primes mononuclear cells and macrophages to secrete cytopathic amounts of TNFα when stimulated with LPS (66). The contribution of donor accessory cells (monocytes/macrophages) to IPS has been investigated using several models. Kinetic studies of macrophage recruitment to the lung after allogeneic SCT show that the percentage of donor macrophages in the BAL fluid increases from approximately 40% at week 1 to >90% by week 4. Additional experiments showed that these donor derived macrophages are major sources of TNFα after SCT (K. Cooke, unpublished observations).

The role of accessory cell populations in the pathophysiology of IPS was further examined using SCT donors that differ in their response to LPS (124). A genetic mutation in the Toll-like receptor 4 (Tlr 4) gene makes C3H/Hej mice resistant to LPS (LPS-r) (124–127). SCT from LPS-r donors results in a significant decrease in lung injury when compared to SCT using wild-type, LPS-sensitive (LPS-s) donors even though T-cell responses to host antigens are identical between the two donor strains (72). Recipients of LPS-r SCT also develop significantly less GVHD. Furthermore, BAL cells collected from LPS-r recipients produce 30-fold less TNFα when restimulated with LPS compared to cells collected after LPS-s SCT, reproducing the phenotype of naïve LPS-r and LPS-s donor cells (73). Lung injury is also reduced when animals deficient in CD14, a cell surface receptor critical to the innate immune response and an important receptor for LPS, are used as donors (128). These results are consistent with the report that monocytes recruited to an inflamed lung upregulate CD14 expression and show enhanced sensitivity to LPS stimulation (129) and with the clinical observation that components of the LPS-activating system are elevated in the BAL fluid of SCT patients with IPS (1). Collectively, these data demonstrate that donor macrophages/monocytes cells are recruited to the lungs of allogeneic SCT recipients, and their secretion of TNFα in response to LPS stimulation directly correlates with IPS severity. Strategies that disrupt the innate immune response by targeting interactions between CD14/Tlr4 and LPS may, therefore, reduce the severity of IPS or prevent its development.

The Role of Neutrophils/Polymorphonuclear (PMN) Cells. Neutrophils are a major component of the inflammatory infiltrates seen in animals with IPS (51). Neutrophilia is a prominent finding in acute respiratory distress syndrome (ARDS) and in bronchiolitis obliterans syndrome (BOS) characteristic of lung allograft rejection (130–135). PMN products such as elastase, myeloperoxidase, metalloproteinases, and oxidants are abundant in the BAL fluid of patients with ARDS and are believed to contribute to the endothelial and epithelial damage that occurs in this setting (130,135). Increases in PMN activation markers may also be early indicators of BOS after lung transplant (132). Neutrophils are likely to play a role in lung injury after SCT as well; their appearance in the bloodstream is often temporarily associated with lung injury; more than 60% of patients diagnosed with IPS at the University of Michigan developed signs and symptoms of pulmonary dysfunction within seven days of neutrophil engraftment (21). In mouse IPS models, the influx of neutrophils into BAL fluid is prominent between weeks 4 and 6 after SCT and is associated with increases in BAL fluid levels of TNFα and LPS (51,62). Neutralization of TNFα with rhTNFR:Fc during this time interval prevents the influx of neutrophils and reduces the progression of lung injury and dysfunction (62). Administration of rhTNFR:Fc following LPS challenge completely abrogates the influx of PMNs into the lungs and prevents further damage (including hemorrhage) underscoring the relationship between neutrophils, TNFα, and LPS in this setting. These data support a role for neutrophils in the injury incurred during IPS and suggest that aspects of the innate immune response contribute to this process.

3. Mechanisms of Leukocyte Recruitment to the Lung After Allogeneic SCT Overview

Cellular effectors play a significant role in development of IPS, but the molecular mechanisms by which white blood cells (WBCs) traffic to the lung and cause inflammation have yet to be determined. WBC migration to sites of inflammation is a complex process involving interactions between leukocytes and endothelial cells that are mediated by adhesion molecules, chemokines, and their receptors (136,137). The recruitment of leukocytes from the vascular space and into target tissue can be divided into four steps: 1) week adhesion of WBCs to the vascular endothelium, 2) firm adhesion of WBCs to endothelial cells, 3) transmigration of leukocytes through the vascular wall, and 4) migration of cells through the extracellular matrix along a chemotactic gradient.

Adhesion Molecules and IPS.   Selectins and integrins are families of adhesion molecules that are critical to steps one and two, respectively, and the expression of each is enhanced by pro-inflammatory cytokines like TNFα. Selectins function to slow the passage of WBCs in the main flow of blood. Selectin interactions do not firmly anchor leukocytes but facilitate their rolling along the endothelial surface (137), whereas firm adhesion of WBCs is dependent on the interaction between intercellular adhesion molecule-1 (ICAM-1) and leukocyte function antigen-1 (LFA-1). The role of adhesion molecules in the development of IPS has been examined using mouse models (58,138,139), and mRNA expression of ICAM, VCAM, and E-selectin is increased in the lungs of mice with IPS after allogeneic SCT compared to syngeneic controls (139). Furthermore, the severity of IPS is dramatically reduced when ICAM deficient (ICAM $-/-$) mice are used as SCT recipients of either MHC-matched or mismatched allogeneic donor cells (58,138). Surprisingly, in each scenario, ICAM deficiency selectively protects the lung from injury even though ICAM expression is elevated in the liver, colon, and spleen of animals with acute GVHD (140).

Chemokines and the Pathogenesis of IPS.   As noted above, leukocyte migration to sites of inflammation can be conceptualized as a four-step process involving interactions between leukocytes and endothelial cells. A subset of chemoattractant molecules called chemokines contribute to steps 2, 3, and 4 of this process. Chemokines secreted at the site of tissue injury are retained within the extracellular matrix and on the surface of the overlying endothelial cells (141). Leukocyte rolling is facilitated by selectin molecules and brings WBCs into contact with chemokines present on the endothelial surface. Chemokine signaling activates leukocyte integrin molecules resulting in arrest and extravasation. Once through the vascular wall, the WBC enters the tissue space, where it is exposed to an existing chemokine concentration gradient surrounding the inflammatory stimulus.

Chemokines are classified into four main groups according to the configuration of cysteine residues near the NH_2 terminus (see Chapter 5), and their effects are mediated through a family of seven-transmembrane-spanning, G-protein–coupled receptors. Chemokines and their receptors can be classified functionally into two broad categories: "inflammatory" and "homeostatic". Inflammatory chemokines orchestrate the recruitment of leukocytes to sites of inflammation during an immunological challenge, whereas homeostatic chemokines contribute to the development of secondary lymphoid organs during organogenesis and are responsible for leukocyte migration during routine immune surveillance. Inflammatory chemokines are produced by a variety of hematopoietic and nonhematopoietic cells, and their expression is augmented by molecules such as LPS, IL-1, and TNFα (136). Receptors for inflammatory chemokines tend to bind in a more promiscuous or redundant fashion than homeostatic receptors and are generally expressed on cells with an effector rather than resting phenotype (142).

Chemokines facilitate the recruitment of leukocytes to the lung in a variety of inflammatory states including asthma, ARDS, infectious pneumonia, pulmonary fibrosis, and lung allograft rejection (142,143), but investigators have just recently begun to explore their role in IPS. The specific composition of a pulmonary leukocytic infiltrate is determined by the pattern of chemokine expression in the inflamed lung. The mixed pulmonary infiltrate observed after experimental allogeneic SCT therefore suggests that those chemokines responsible for the recruitment of lymphocytes, monocytes, and neutrophils will be up-regulated during the development of IPS.

The pulmonary expression of four inflammatory chemokine receptors of T-cell effectors (CCR5 and CXCR3), monocytes and macrophages (CCR2), and neutrophils (CXCR2) and their respective ligands have been analyzed using an irradiated P → F1 (C57BL/6 → B6D2F1) SCT model wherein IPS develops in response to both minor and major HC antigens. Lung injury in this model is present at week 2 after allogeneic SCT and progresses steadily through week 6 (data not shown). Whole lung mRNA expression was determined at weeks 1, 2, 4, and 6 after SCT using RNAse protection assays (RPA). As shown in Figure 3, mRNA expression of each chemokine receptor and ligand is increased in allogeneic SCT recipients compared to syngeneic controls at every time point. Elevations in CCR5 and CXCR3 expression peaked early after allogeneic SCT, whereas expression of CCR2 and CXCR2 continued to rise over time. Importantly, the kinetics of chemokine ligand expression correlated with the corresponding receptors; increases in RANTES, MIP-1α (CCR5), and IP-10 (CXCR3) peaked at week 1 after allogeneic SCT and then tapered off, whereas increases in MCP-1 (CCR2) and MIP-2 (CXCR2) peaked at weeks 2 and 4, respectively. These data are consistent with the findings of Panoskaltsis-Mortari and coworkers, who reported that enhanced expression of monocyte and T cell attracting chemokines in the lungs correlated with lung injury that developed within the first 2 weeks after SCT (144) and with prominent increases in the expression of IFNγ-inducible chemokines observed in a model of lung injury induced by alloreactive Th1 cells (145).

Significant increases in chemokine ligand expression in the lung therefore precede the development of IPS and herald the influx of leukocyte subsets bearing the corresponding chemokine receptors. Inflammatory chemokine expression is induced by a variety of mediators of the immune response, including cytokines and LPS, which are also critical to the induction of acute GVHD. We have previously shown that serum levels of IFNγ,

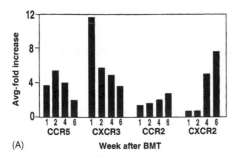
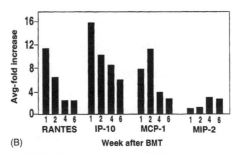

(A)   (B)

Figure 3 Chemokine expression in the lung after allogeneic SCT. B6D2F1 mice were lethally irradiated and received SCT from syngeneic or allogeneic (B6) donors. Lungs were harvested on weeks 1, 2, 4, and 6 after SCT and evaluated from chemokine receptor and ligand mRNA expression. RNA was prepared and hybridized to multiprobe templates and analyzed using RNase protection assays. The intensity of the mRNA signals was measured and standardized to the L32 signal for each sample in order to generate mean intensity values from 3 to 6 mice per group. The averagefold increase in RNA expression after allogeneic SCT (compared to syngeneic SCT) was then calculated for chemokine receptors (A) and ligands (B).

TNFα, IL-1, and LPS are significantly increased within the first week after SCT. Thus, upregulation of pulmonary chemokine expression early after SCT occurs in the setting of systemic inflammation.

We hypothesize that enhanced chemokine expression and leukocyte infiltration that occurs during the development of IPS can be conceptualized in three distinct steps, as described in Figure 4. These steps describe the kinetics of chemokine receptor expression on activated donor derived, cellular effectors and are identical to the three steps depicted in Figure 2. Activation of donor T cells by host alloantigens after hematopoietic SCT creates a systemic proinflammatory environment that enhances pulmonary chemokine expression and results in the sequential recruitment of donor derived Th1 T cells, followed by macrophages and finally neutrophils to the lung during the development of IPS. Each cell type modifies the local chemokine milieu and directly contributes to the recruitment of the next. In step 1 of the process, SCT conditioning and the initial allogeneic donor T-cell response result in systemic inflammation within 7 days of transplant. This proinflammatory environment is characterized by the release of IFNγ, TNFα, and LPS and causes increased chemokine expression in the lung. Increased production of RANTES, MIP-1α, and IP-10 recruit donor-derived, Th1 lymphocyte effectors (CCR5+/CXCR3+) from day 7 to day 14 after SCT. In step 2, these T cells proliferate, cause local tissue injury, and

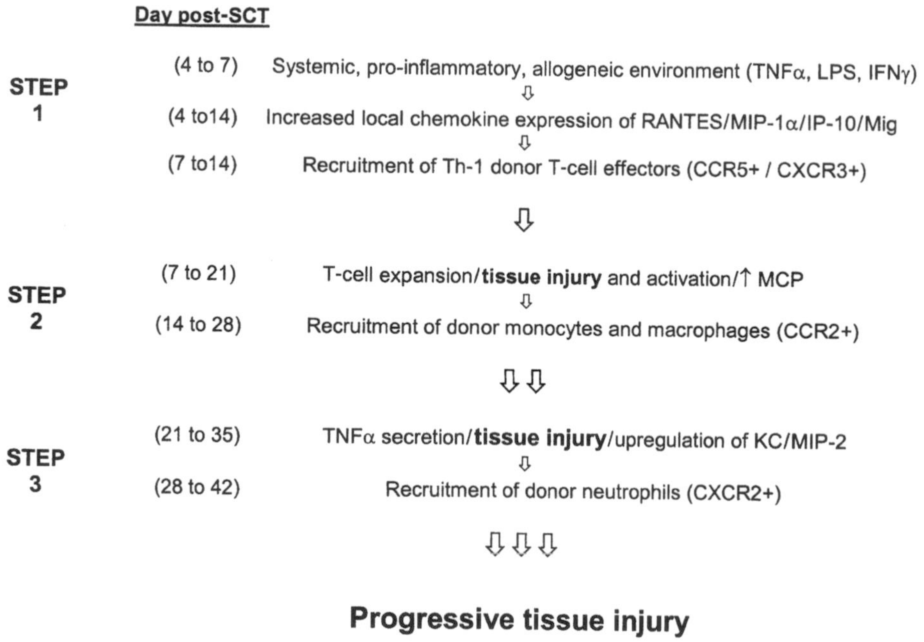

Day post-SCT

STEP 1	(4 to 7)	Systemic, pro-inflammatory, allogeneic environment (TNFα, LPS, IFNγ)
		⇩
	(4 to 14)	Increased local chemokine expression of RANTES/MIP-1α/IP-10/Mig
		⇩
	(7 to 14)	Recruitment of Th-1 donor T-cell effectors (CCR5+ / CXCR3+)

⇩

STEP 2	(7 to 21)	T-cell expansion/**tissue injury** and activation/↑ MCP
		⇩
	(14 to 28)	Recruitment of donor monocytes and macrophages (CCR2+)

⇩ ⇩

STEP 3	(21 to 35)	TNFα secretion/**tissue injury**/upregulation of KC/MIP-2
		⇩
	(28 to 42)	Recruitment of donor neutrophils (CXCR2+)

⇩ ⇩ ⇩

Progressive tissue injury

Figure 4   Chemokine dysregulation during the development of IPS. SCT conditioning and the initial allogeneic donor T-cell response result in systemic inflammation within 7 days of transplant. This pro-inflammatory environment directly enhances pulmonary chemokine expression and results in the sequential recruitment of donor derived Th1 T cells (step 1), followed by macrophages (step 2) and finally neutrophils (step 3) to the lung during the development of IPS. Each cell type modifies the local chemokine milieu and directly contributes to the recruitment of the next, culminating in tissue injury and acute pulmonary dysfunction that characterize IPS.

activate endothelial and epithelial cells to secrete additional chemokines, including MCP-1. Enhanced expression of MCP-1 in turn recruits CCR2+ donor monocytes, macrophages, and additional T cells. In step 3, recruited macrophages secrete TNFα in response to LPS stimulation, which results in additional tissue injury, the upregulation of KC and MIP-2, and the recruitment of donor neutrophils. These neutrophils amplify progressive lung injury and dysfunction. This hypothesis stipulates that the migration of each leukocyte subset controls the recruitment of the next wave of effectors. Thus the recruitment of Th1 effectors initiates the cascade, and interruption of this first step will have the most profound effect on the development of IPS. Prevention of steps 2 or 3 will result in significant, but less complete, amelioration of disease.

Data in support of this hypothesis have recently been generated by using CCR2-deficient mice as donors in the B6 → B6D2F1 system described above (146). CCR2−/− SCT recipients developed significantly less severe IPS compared to mice receiving allogeneic SCT from wild-type donors. Mild lung injury was identified in all animals at 3 weeks after SCT, consistent with a normal step 1 in both groups. However, the absence of CCR2 on engrafting donor leukocytes completely prevented the increase in lung pathology seen by week 6 in the wild-type controls. The reduction in histopathology after CCR2−/− SCT was associated with decreased macrophages, CD8+ lymphocytes, and TNFα levels in the BAL fluid. Similar findings were observed when recipients of wild-type SCT were treated with polyclonal antibodies to MCP-1 from days 10 to 28 after transplant. Thus, interruption of CCR2 : MCP-1 receptor : ligand interactions significantly impaired the recruitment of cellular effectors to the lung, reduced TNF secretion in the bronchoalveolar space, and abrogated the progression pulmonary toxicity after allogeneic SCT.

E. Treatment Strategies for IPS After Allogeneic SCT

Current standard treatment regimens for IPS include supportive care measures in conjunction with broad-spectrum antimicrobial agents with or without intravenous corticosteroids (6,21). Although anecdotal reports of responses to standard therapy are available, such responses are limited, and the mortality of patients diagnosed with IPS remains unacceptably high (7). Prospective studies addressing the treatment of IPS, including the specific use of steroids, are lacking in the literature. A recent study from Michigan reported the use of etanercept (Enbrel; Immunex Corp., Seattle, WA) in three pediatric patients with IPS (21). In all three patients, BAL fluid was negative for infection, and pulmonary edema from fluid overload or cardiogenic factors was also ruled out before the administration of etanercept. Each patient received empiric broad-spectrum antimicrobial therapy and methylprednisolone (2 mg/kg d) prior to and during etanercept therapy. The administration of etanercept was well tolerated, and in combination with standard immunosuppressive therapy it was associated with significant improvements in pulmonary function within the first week of therapy (21). Clinical trials using etanercept for the treatment of IPS are now ongoing.

F. Summary

IPS remains a frequently fatal complication of allogeneic SCT despite significant advances in critical care medicine. Extensive preclinical and clinical data suggest that both inflammatory and cellular effectors participate in the development of IPS after allogeneic SCT. TNFα and LPS are significant, albeit not exclusive, contributors to IPS, and cells of both lymphoid and myeloid origin play a direct role in lung injury that occurs in this setting. In particular, the contribution of donor, nonlymphoid, accessory cells may be linked to the cellular activation by LPS and the ultimate secretion of TNFα within a "gut-liver lung" axis of inflammation, whereas donor T-cell effectors can home to and damage the lung even when systemic GVHD is mild or absent. These findings have led to the hypothesis that the lung is susceptible to two distinct but interrelated pathways of injury after SCT involving aspects of both the adaptive and the innate immune response (Fig. 2). In step 1, interactions between host APC and donor T cells result in the generation of Th1/Tc1 CTLs that express CCR5 and CXCR3. This effector pathway is augmented by two related steps wherein the expression of CCR2 and CXCR2 contribute to the sequential recruitment of donor-derived monocytes/macrophages followed by neutrophils, respectively, during the development of IPS. These findings support a shift away from the current paradigm of acute lung injury after SCT as an idiopathic clinical syndrome to a process in which the lung is the target of an alloantigen-specific, immune-mediated attack. Mechanistic insights from these experimental models should form the basis for translational clinical research protocols with the goal of treating or preventing IPS after SCT.

III. CHRONIC PULMONARY DYSFUNCTION AFTER SCT: OBSTRUCTIVE LUNG DISEASE AND RESTRICTIVE LUNG DISEASE

A. Definition, Risk Factors, and Clinical Course

Two forms of chronic pulmonary dysfunction are common in patients surviving greater than 100 days posttransplant: obstructive lung disease (OLD) and restrictive lung disease (RLD) (8,9,14,60,147,148). The incidence of both patterns of lung toxicity ranges from 20 to 50%, depending upon donor source and the time interval after SCT (8–15,46,147). In each scenario, collagen deposition and the development of fibrosis either in the interstitial (RLD) or peribronchiolar space (OLD) are believed to contribute to the patterns of lung dysfunction displayed on pulmonary function testing.

RLD is defined by reductions in forced vital capacity (FVC), total lung capacity (TLC), and diffusion capacity of the lung for carbon monoxide (DLCO) as measured by standard pulmonary function tests (PFTs). In restrictive disease, the ratio of the forced expiratory volume in one second (FEV_1) to FVC (FEV_1/FVC) is maintained near 100% (7,10,14,60,147). RLD is common after SCT; significant decreases in FVC or TLC have been reported in as many as 25–45% of allogeneic SCT recipients at day 100 and occur with greater frequency than obstructive abnormalities at this time (10,14,15,147). An increase in nonrelapse mortality has been associated with a decline in TLC or FVC at 100 days and one year after SCT compared to pretransplant values, even if the absolute values for each measurement remained within the normal range (10,14). TBI containing conditioning regimens and the presence of acute GVHD have been associated with RLD and higher mortality rates (10,14,15,149–151). By contrast, the impact of age on the development of RLD is less clear. Early reports suggested that the incidence of RLD is lower in children compared to adults and that the incidence increases with advancing recipient age (15), but more recent studies have revealed significant RLD in children receiving SCT (147,152). In contrast to OLD (discussed below), RLD after SCT has not been associated with the presence of chronic GVHD.

Histological features of RLD after SCT are rarely described in the clinical literature, although varying degrees of interstitial and alveolar inflammation and fibrosis as seen in patients with other forms of interstitial lung disease such as idiopathic pulmonary fibrosis (IPF) would be expected. One exception, which merits specific mention, is bronchiolitis obliterans organizing pneumonia. Although reported in less than 2% of SCT recipients, BOOP is associated with restrictive (rather than obstructive) changes on PFTs (7). Presenting symptoms of dry cough, shortness of breath, and fever are accompanied by radiographic findings of diffuse, peripheral, fluffy infiltrates consistent with airspace consolidation (153). The diagnosis of BOOP requires histological evidence on lung biopsy of several signature features: patchy fibrosis, granulation tissue within alveolar spaces, alveolar ducts and respiratory bronchioles, and the absence of infectious organisms (153). The term BOOP should not be used interchangeably with bronchiolitis obliterans (BrOb) or bronchiolitis obliterans syndrome (BOS) to describe a patient with chronic lung dysfunction after SCT, although such usage is unfortunately widespread. The two disorders differ with respect to histopathology, pulmonary function characteristics, and, most importantly, response to therapy; BOOP after SCT is quite responsive to corticosteroids and in other settings may resolve spontaneously, whereas, as discussed later in this chapter, BrOb and BOS are not (7,153).

OLD involves enhanced resistance to airflow on expiration and reflects conditions in the smaller airways and bronchioles. Obstructive defects are demonstrated by decreases in FEV_1 and in FEV_1/FVC (147,154). OLD was first recognized as a complication of allogeneic SCT in the mid-1980s. Of the first 35 patients described, 75% had evidence of extensive, chronic GVHD and presented with cough, wheezing, or shortness of breath. Despite aggressive therapy with immunosuppressive agents and bronchodilators, only 3 patients showed improvement in lung function, and the case-fatality rate was 50% (154). OLD is now a well-documented cause of morbidity after allogeneic SCT (8,60,148,154–156), and obstructive defects as defined by a FEV_1/FVC of <70% have been observed in approximately 15–25% of allogeneic SCT recipients by day 100 and can persist for years (10,46,60,147).

OLD results from extensive narrowing and/or destruction of small airways. Lung biopsies from patients with OLD have shown histological patterns of lymphocytic bronchitis, acute and chronic interstitial pneumonitis, and bronchiolar inflammation, including BrOb (8,46,155,157,158). This variation in histopathology is complicated further by the methods used to procure lung tissue. Specifically, transbronchial biopsies rarely include an adequate sampling of distal bronchial structures, and therefore such specimens can reveal cellular infiltrates involving larger airways and the interstitium but may not detect bronchiolar inflammation.

Despite these limitations, BrOb remains the most common form of histopathology associated with OLD and has been used historically to describe "chronic GVHD of the lung" (8,46,155,157,158). As the name implies, BrOb depicts small airway inflammation with fibrinous obliteration of the bronchiolar lumen that is classically associated with a fixed obstructive defect on PFT (8,9,12,46,159). Airflow obstruction may, however, occasionally exist without BrOb and vice versa (160). Moreover, in the vast majority of cases, OLD is diagnosed by PFT findings without histopathological confirmation, and in this context, two phrases that identify affected patients are found in the literature. "Obstructive bronchiolitis" describes functional airflow obstruction in patients with signs and symptoms of bronchial inflammation (148), and "bronchiolitis obliterans syndrome" describes the deterioration of graft function that accompanies chronic lung allograft rejection (161). BOS is defined as an irreversible decline in FEV_1 of at least 20% from baseline and is graded using the international heart and lung transplantation criteria: BOS stage 0 = FEV_1 of = 80% baseline; stage 1 ≥ FEV_1 of 66–79%; stage 2 = FEV_1 of 51–65%; stage 3 = FEV_1 of ≤50% of baseline value (161). This system requires the establishment of a posttransplant baseline value of FEV_1 and is commonly reported in clinical studies of lung allograft rejection.

The lack of consistent terminology for OLD, along with the variability in diagnostic criteria, have contributed to the wide variation in the reported incidence of this form of lung injury after SCT. Afessa and colleagues found that OLD was reported in 8.3% of over 2000 allogeneic SCT patients in nine studies and was identified in 6–20% of long-term survivors with chronic GVHD (7). The onset of OLD occurs later than IPS (3–18 months after SCT) and is more insidious. A review of 35 allogeneic SCT recipients with OLD from a single institution demonstrated that approximately 40% of cases developed between 50 and 150 days after transplantation, whereas the remainder occurred between 150 and 500 days (154). Respiratory symptoms may include cough, dyspnea, and wheezing, but many patients remain asymptomatic despite showing signs of moderate to severe airway obstruction on PFTs (8,60). Chest radiographs may show patchy, diffuse infiltrates but are more often normal except for signs of hyperinflation (8,46,59). Likewise, chest CT findings range from normal early in the course of disease to extensive peribronchial inflammation, bronchiectasis, significant air trapping, and diffuse parenchymal hypoattenuation at later time points (9,162,163).

The clinical course of OLD also varies from mild with slow deterioration to severe with necrotizing bronchiolitis, a rapid decline in FEV_1 and a mortality rate of 25–50%. Unfortunately, clear predictors of outcome have not been identified (8,9,11–13,59,154). Response to bronchodilator therapy is usually marginal since airflow obstruction tends to be fixed rather than reversible. Responses to immunosuppressive therapy (including various combinations of steroids cyclosporine and azathioprine) are limited and typically result in preservation of remaining lung function rather than in significant improvement. Since enhanced immunosuppression significantly increases the risk of infection, the utility of such therapy is questionable when a clinical response is not seen within the first months of treatment or when pulmonary dysfunction is longstanding. The partial response to immunosuppressive therapy suggests that early detection of disease may be important (8,9,13,154). In this light, two reports have suggested that a decrease of maximum mid-expiratory flow rates (MMFR) may be an earlier indicator of OLD than changes in FEV_1 (13,59). Additional studies are required to determine whether such a parameter can serve as an early diagnostic tool and improve efforts to prevent the development of significant, irreversible dysfunction.

As with IPS, risk factors for OLD are several and include the effects of pretransplant conditioning regimens, concomitant infections, chronic aspiration, and GVHD. OLD has been reported in association with older donor age, the use of methotrexate for GVHD prophylaxis, the presence of esophageal dysfunction (with aspiration), the use of mismatched donors, and the use of busulfan (rather than TBI) in SCT conditioning regimens (8,9,13,60,148,154,164). From an infectious disease perspective, the CMV status of neither donor nor recipient prior to SCT correlates with the development of OLD. However, previous RSV and adenoviral infections are possible risk factors for the higher incidence of OLD in the pediatric population (9). The development of OLD is strongly associated with chronic GVHD, particularly in patients with low serum IgG levels (8,154) and with chronic hepatic GVHD (9). Furthermore, recipients of HLA-mismatched related donor or matched unrelated donor grafts have a much higher incidence of OLD than patients receiving 6/6-HLA-matched related donor transplants (40% vs. 13%) (9). Thus, OLD and chronic GVHD may share immunopathogenic mechanisms.

B. Pathogenesis of Chronic Pulmonary Toxicity

The pathophysiology of chronic lung injury after SCT is less well defined than for IPS. This limitation stems from the lack of correlative data obtained from afflicted SCT recipients and the paucity of suitable SCT animal models for either the restrictive or the obstructive form of chronic lung injury. The development of chronic pulmonary toxicity likely involves an initial insult to lung parenchyma followed by an ongoing inflammatory process involving the interplay between recruited immune effector cells and the resident cells of the pulmonary vascular endothelium and interstitium. Duration of the inciting stimulus determines the ultimate outcome of the ensuing inflammatory response: a static, limited insult results in wound healing with resolution and repair, whereas a persistent stimulus could lead to an over-exuberant reparative response and greater destruction with permanent scarring and fibrosis. Normal repair mechanisms depend upon the proper balance between pro-inflammatory and anti-inflammatory mediators, and changes in this balance significantly influence the ultimate outcome of the immune response. Most of what is known about the pathogenesis of OLD is based upon observations made in lung allograft recipients and from data generated in murine heterotopic tracheal transplant models. The absence of an initial inflammatory response from SCT conditioning regimens and the presence of a "host-vs.-graft" rather than a "graft-vs.-host" reaction are just two of the issues that limit the extrapolation of such data to OLD after hematopoietic SCT. Similarly, our understanding of the mechanisms responsible for RLD is inferred from patients with various forms of interstitial fibrosis and from animal models of these diseases. Despite these limitations, lung allograft rejection and pulmonary fibrosis are characterized by epithelial cell injury in the terminal bronchioles or alveoli, respectively, and by a profound defect in reepithelialization and normal repair. Each response also involves T-cell activation, leukocyte recruitment, and enhanced expression of inflammatory mediators, all of which are likely operative in chronic lung injury after SCT.

1. Pathogenesis of OLD

Mechanisms of OLD are derived primarily from lung allograft rejection, which is classified as acute or chronic histologically. Acute rejection is driven primarily by T-helper lymphocytes that recognize donor MHC epitopes, secrete cytokines, and facilitate the generation of CTL effectors. The factors responsible for the progression from acute to chronic rejection, which is characterized by fibrous obliteration of epithelialized bronchial structures, remain to be determined. The direct correlation between the intensity and duration of acute rejection episodes and the subsequent development of chronic rejection suggests, however, that the obstructive lesions characteristic of chronic rejection and BOS progress through a cascade of events involving persistent and antigen-dependent injury of endothelium and epithelium followed by the induction of repair mechanisms. Although direct cytotoxicity by cellular or cytokine effectors may be responsible for damage and loss of airway epithelium in the transplanted lung, the inability to regenerate and heal injured epithelium is believed to be an equally important factor to the development of bronchiolitis obliterans and BOS (165). In this context, interactions between activated epithelial cells and lung fibroblasts rather than inflammatory cells may be critical (166,167).

Data generated from both humans and mice support the hypothesis that the development of OLD during chronic lung allograft rejection involves the secretion of inflammatory cytokines and chemokines and interactions between APCs and activated lymphocytes. Analysis of BAL fluid and biopsy specimens obtained from lung allograft recipients with BOS has revealed elevations in IL-1ra, TGFβ, IL-8, and MCP-1, all of which have been implicated in other fibro-proliferative processes (132,168–170). Alveolar macrophages from patients with BOS also produce significant amounts of TNFα and RANTES after stimulation with IFNγ (171). Since IL-8 is a potent chemoattractant for neutrophils, BAL fluid elevations of this chemokine in patients with BOS are consistent with the observed influx of neutrophils into the bronchial walls and bronchoalveolar space (21,135,172).

Murine models of lung allograft rejection have confirmed many of the associations seen clinically and have begun to elucidate the mechanisms that contribute to leukocyte migration and rejection of allograft epithelium. Boehler and colleagues found that rat heterotopic lung allografts undergoing rejection showed a strong Th1 immune response even after fibrosis and airway obliteration was complete (173). This response was characterized by enhanced production of IL-2 and IFNγ and was associated with upregulation of MCP-1 and RANTES. Work by this same group demonstrated that the administration of IL-10 either in the recombinant form or by gene transfer using an adenoviral vector inhibited the development of fibrous airway obstruction (174). Subsequent studies by Belperio and others showed enhanced expression of TNFα and TGFβ during allograft rejection and revealed critical roles for both RANTES and MCP-1 in the development of experimental BOS (168,175,176).

The lung is a rich source of MHC antigens and APCs (93,177,178), and both clinical and experimental data suggest that interactions between pulmonary APCs and donor lymphocytes contribute to the development of OLD. Donor-specific, alloreactive lymphocytes have been identified in the BAL fluid and lung biopsy specimens from patients with acute and chronic rejection (165,179,180). In particular, the clonal expansion of T cells responding to a limited number of immunodominant epitopes has been identified in the peripheral blood and BAL fluid of patients with BOS, and the oligoclonal expansion of circulating CD4+ T cells recognizing alloantigen determinants had 100% specificity and 80% specificity for the presence of or imminent development of allograft rejection (180). Dendritic cells expressing the co-stimulatory molecules CD80 and CD86 have also been identified in the lungs of patients with BOS (181,182), and experimental studies have shown that CD28-B7 interactions contribute to the alloreactive response since the use of CTLA4Ig abrogates the development of OLD (183). Furthermore, rodent heterotropic tracheal allograft models have demonstrated that the development of BOS requires APCs from the transplanted trachea and can be initiated against either MHC class I or class II antigens on donor tissue. These findings suggest that direct allorecognition by either CD8+ or CD4+ cells is critical to the development of this form of airway injury (184).

2. The Pathogenesis of RLD

The mechanisms responsible for RLD after SCT are also poorly characterized, but factors that regulate the development of lung damage in other forms of interstitial fibrosis likely contribute. As with OLD, such factors include underlying injury to lung epithelial cells, immune cell activation, and the secretion of inflammatory chemokines and cytokines (185). The prevailing hypothesis holds that most forms of interstitial fibrosis are initiated by an acute inflammatory event that injures the lung and subsequently modulates pulmonary fibrogenesis (186). The etiology of the initial cellular insult may involve direct toxicity from drugs, toxins, or ionizing irradiation. Alternatively, the insult may represent a dysregulated immune response to an environmental antigen, (e.g., hypersensitivity pneumonitis) or to an aberrantly expressed self-antigen, as occurs when interstitial fibrosis accompanies autoimmune disorders (187).

The role of T cells in the development of interstitial fibrosis is variable and depends upon the inciting stimulus. T cells significantly contribute to hypersensitivity pneumonitis and pulmonary fibrosis that complicates collagen vascular diseases, whereas they are less critical for interstitial fibrosis secondary to radiation and other toxins (187–189). Significant increases in eosinophils and lymphocytes accompany the airway remodeling and peribronchial fibrosis that characterize the chronic, allergic, airway disease that results from the inhalation of *Aspergillus fumigatus* (190). Furthermore, macrophages and T lymphocytes contribute to pulmonary fibrosis induced by the instillation of bleomycin or silica, but fibrosis caused by the intratracheal administration of FITC can occur in the absence of T cells (189).

By contrast, the etiology of the inciting injurious event and the potential role for antigen specific T-cell responses in the development of lung fibrosis in patients with idiopathic pulmonary fibrosis are matters of considerable debate (186,191,192). The lungs of patients with IPF show increases in lymphocytes, macrophages, and neutrophils in interstitial and intra-alveolar spaces, and T-cell responses are believed by some to occur early in the time course of IPF; T cells harvested from the lungs of patients with IPF are activated and may contribute both to direct epithelial injury and the modulation of disease progression (187). Activated lymphocytes and alveolar macrophages can secrete inflammatory mediators that propagate epithelial cell injury and result in the destruction of the basal lamina and the deposition of fibrin rich exudates in the intra-alveolar space. If these exudates are not successfully cleared, fibroblasts migrate to the inflamed area and release matrix proteins that contribute to scar formation (187). Recent data suggest, however, that acute inflammation may not be a critical pathogenic event in IPF; epithelial injury without ongoing inflammation may be sufficient to stimulate the development of fibrosis (186,193). In this alternative hypothesis, injured alveolar epithelium stimulate parenchymal fibroblasts (rather than leukocytes) to produce an exuberant reparative response characterized by proliferation, differentiation to myofibroblasts, and excess matrix deposition (186,193). The function of lung fibroblasts has traditionally been limited to normal structural maintenance and the latter stages of tissue repair. However, recent data demonstrate that fibroblasts can both respond to and secrete a variety of inflammatory mediators including CC and CXC chemokines, which allow these cells to migrate to sites of ongoing inflammation and subsequently recruit activated immune cells (194,195). In this context, pulmonary fibroblasts may represent an important link in the development of both RLD and OLD after allogeneic SCT.

Several proteins that are known to have pro-fibrotic activity, including TNFα, IL-1, IL-6, TGFβ, IL-8, MCP-1, and MIP-1α have been identified in the BAL fluid of patients with IPF and in animal models of interstitial fibrosis. A growing body of scientific evidence suggests that the cytokine profile present during an evolving immune response determines its pathological outcome. In this context, a Th1/Th2 paradigm has emerged to help predict

whether a specific pulmonary response will ultimately resolve or progress toward end-stage
fibrosis. Much of the scientific evidence supporting this concept is derived from studies
showing that the interferons, and specifically IFNγ, have profound regulatory activity on
collagen synthesis and possess potent antifibrotic effects, whereas Th2 cytokines like IL-
4 and IL-13 activate fibroblasts and stimulate the production of extracellular matrix proteins. Recent data also demonstrate that a variety of cell types contribute to pulmonary
fibrosis, including epithelial cells, macrophages, eosinophils, and fibroblasts. Since these
cells can synthesize type 2 cytokines, it may be more appropriate to consider certain diseases in terms of their predominant cytokine profile rather than by T-helper cell subsets
involved (185). The Th2 dominant paradigm appears to be particularly useful for pulmonary inflammation engendered by antigens to either the parasite *Schistosoma mansoni* or the
fungus *A. fumigatus* (190,196), whereas its relevance in other models of fibrosis is less clear
(197,198). For example, fibrosis induced by bleomycin or silica is attenuated in IFN$\gamma-/-$
and IL-12p40$-/-$ mice (favoring Th2) (197,199), and a recent study found that fibrosis
from bleomycin was increased in IL-4–deficient mice (favoring Th1) and significantly
reduced in IL-4–overexpressing transgeneic animals (200).

The role of TNFα in interstitial fibrosis has also been underscored in several
experimental studies and clinical reports. TNFα may stimulate fibroblast proliferation and
collagen gene upregulation through a TGFβ- or platelet-derived growth factor pathway
(201). Human alveolar macrophages and type II epithelial cells from patients with IPF
express increased amounts of TNFα (202,203), and recent data suggest an association
between polymorphisms in the promoter region of the TNFα gene and an increased risk
of developing IPF (204). Furthermore, TNFα gene expression increases after administration
of agents that cause pulmonary fibrosis (205–208). Abrogation of TNFα signaling either by
antibody neutralization or by using mutant mice deficient in both TNF receptors (p55$-/-$
and p75$-/-$ mice) significantly reduces lung fibrosis in murine models (205,206,209).
When TNFα is specifically overexpressed in the lungs of rodents, animals develop a lymphocytic infiltration followed by progressive alveolar and interstitial fibrosis that can be
accompanied by the enhanced expression of TGFβ (210–212). TNFα is also upregulated
in models where Th2 cytokines like IL-4 and IL-13 are operative, suggesting that it may
have a significant role in fibrogenesis even in a Th2 skewed cytokine environment (208).

3. The Evolution of Chronic Lung Injury After SCT

We propose a triphasic model of non-infectious lung injury after SCT in which alloantigen
recognition is the inciting stimulus of the immune response (Fig. 5). The first phase of disease is characterized by a mixed leukocytic infiltrate and acute interstitial and peri-bronchial inflammation typically observed in IPS (Fig. 5A). This injury is initiated early after
allogeneic SCT by a systemic pro-inflammatory environment that leads to chemokine
upregulation in the lung, the promotion of leukocyte recruitment and the secretion of
inflammatory cytokines (see Sec. II.D). Donor T cells recruited to the lungs of within
the first 2 weeks of allogeneic SCT are followed by the influx of donor monocytes,
macrophages, and neutrophils, all of which contribute to the secretion of TNFα and the
propagation of tissue damage as described in Figure 2.

In phase II, the persistent expression of MHC antigens on pulmonary epithelial and
vascular endothelial cells coupled with the sequestration of alloreactive T-cell effectors in
the pulmonary microcirculation result in ongoing epithelial activation and injury.
Persistence of an inflammatory signal alters the normal reparative capacity of the lung

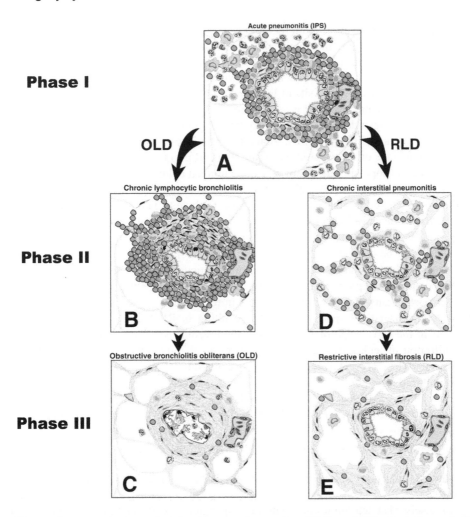

Figure 5   A triphasic model of pulmonary dysfunction (OLD or RLD) after allogeneic SCT. Immune-mediated injury to the lung after allogeneic SCT can be conceptualized in three phases. In phase I, the acute pneumonitis that characterizes idiopathic pneumonia syndrome develops as a consequence of an allogeneic immune response and results in the sequential influx of lymphocytes, macrophages, and neutrophils into an inflamed pulmonary parenchyma (A). In phase II, persistence of an inflammatory signal in the setting of dysregulated repair mechanisms promotes the transition from acute to chronic injury. If the inciting injurious stimuli predominantly involve bronchiolar epithelial cells, phase II is associated with the concentric infiltration of lymphocytes and collagen deposition in the peri-bronchiolar areas resulting in the development of chronic bronchiolitis (B). Activated lymphocytes then migrate into the airway mucosa and contribute to epithelial injury. As chronic inflammation proceeds to phase III, lung fibroblasts increase dramatically in number and contribute to the enhanced deposition of collagen and granulation tissue in and around bronchial structures, ultimately resulting in complete obliteration of small airways and fixed OLD (C). If, by contrast, the principal target of early damage is the alveolar epithelium, leukocyte recruitment and matrix deposition during phase II are confined primarily to the interstitial space (D). Fibroblast proliferation and intraseptal collagen deposition during phase III ultimately results in interstitial thickening, septal fibrosis, significant volume reduction, and severe RLD (E).

and promotes the transition from acute to chronic lung injury. This transition is accompanied by a change in the character of the leukocytic infiltrate (to one that is predominantly lymphocytic in nature) along with a shift to a pro-fibrotic environment and a proactive role of the lung fibroblast. The histological changes that occur during phase II are dependent upon the primary site of lung injury. When inflammation to the bronchiolar epithelium predominates, phase II is associated with a progressive, concentric lymphocytic infiltration, collagen deposition, and early fibrosis in the peri-bronchial areas, resulting in a chronic bronchiolitis (Fig. 5B). Activated lymphocytes then migrate through the basement membrane of the respiratory epithelium and into the airway mucosa and result in epithelial cell apoptosis and necrosis (18). Continued epithelial injury leads to areas of denudation and ulceration. As chronic inflammation proceeds into phase III, lung fibroblasts increase dramatically in number and contribute to 1) the proliferation of endothelial cells, 2) enhanced collagen deposition, and 3) the development of intraluminal granulation tissue and dense, concentric, periluminal fibrous bands (Fig. 5C) (18,166). Ultimately, this process results in complete obliteration of small airways (cicatricial bronchiolitis obliterans) and significant airflow obstruction.

By contrast, if epithelial cells in the alveolar septae are the principal targets of injury, persistent antigenic stimulation results in recruitment of lymphocytes and monocytes into the interstitial space, eventually resulting in RLD. Alveolar architecture is preserved in the early stage of phase II, but the alveolar walls are expanded by edema and infiltration of leukocytes (Fig. 5D). The resultant inflammation is associated with apoptosis and loss of septal epithelial cells, exudation of proteinacious material, the recruitment and proliferation of fibroblasts, and the deposition of intraseptal granulation tissue (18,166,213). If this extracellular matrix is not resorbed, chronic inflammation progresses to phase III, wherein collagen is deposited within the alveolar septae and the chronic leukocytic infiltrates are less evident. This results in interstitial thickening, septal fibrosis, and loss of alveolar architecture leading to dilated cystic air spaces or "honeycombing" (Fig. 5E). Such end-stage histopathology is associated with significant volume reduction and severely impaired gas exchange that is characteristic of severe RLD.

Precisely what determines the anatomical specificity (peribronchiolar vs. interstitial) of chronic lung injury remains unclear, and the development of either pattern of chronic lung injury (OLD or RLD) does not necessarily exclude the other; each pattern may develop simultaneously in an individual patient as suggested in a recent report from Trisolini and colleagues (213). Furthermore, the extremely poor survival seen in patients with IPS has precluded our ability to follow the natural history of lung injury after allogeneic SCT. Recently, PFTs completed on patients with IPS who were treated with etanercept have revealed persistent restrictive changes months after the initial episode of acute lung injury (K. R. Cooke, unpublished observation). It should be noted, however, that the role of acute inflammation and specifically of alloreactive effector cells in the initial damage to the alveolar or bronchiolar epithelium and the subsequent progression to chronic pulmonary injury are not well established. Some have suggested that an early, robust inflammatory phase may not be a prerequisite for subsequent fibrosis; persistent epithelial damage and subsequent "cross-talk" between epithelial cells and fibroblasts may be sufficient for the development of fibrotic lung disease (214). This mechanism could explain why some patients with chronic lung dysfunction do not have a clear antecedent history of acute lung inflammation; in the setting of imbalanced immune regulation, a subclinical injury, such as an allogeneic response to lung epithelial cells, could initiate a dysregulated reparative response resulting in scarring of either the terminal air-ways (OLD) or the interstitial space (RLD).

As noted above, clinical and experimental data suggest that the progression to a chronic, pro-fibrotic, and more irreversible form of pulmonary toxicity involves the secretion of cytokines and chemokines that are known to stimulate the proliferation of myofibroblasts, promote collagen synthesis, and enhance leukocyte recruitment to inflamed tissue (36,166,210). In this context, TNFα may be a central factor in the triphasic model proposed above. TNFα is an important mediator of both acute and chronic lung injury after SCT (1,21,50,51,62) and directly contributes to the development of RLD and interstitial fibrosis in several non-SCT models (166,210–212). Strong evidence for a role of TNFα in the tran-sition from acute to chronic lung injury comes from a study using transgenic mice with tar-geted over-expression of TNFα in the lungs (211). Early lung histopathology included a lymphocytic infiltrate and was similar to that seen in experimental IPS models (48,51), whereas the histological changes associated with more prolonged exposure to TNFα closely resembled those seen at later time points after SCT (18,36). Similar observations were made in other studies wherein TNFα was overexpressed in normal pulmonary tissue of adult rats. An acute inflammatory response was followed weeks later by interstitial fibrosis that was associated with the upregulation of TGFβ and the activation of fibroblasts (210). Finally, TNFα-producing cells have been associated with both acute and chronic rejection of rat lung allografts and were specifically identified in close proximity to MHC class II–positive epithelial cells at later time points of the immune response (215).

The linkage between TNFα and OLD after SCT is more indirect, but increased levels of TNFα are also known to increase the expression of several proteins that may con-tribute to this process. For example, neutralization of TNFα produced in a human MLR downregulates the production of MCP-1 that occurs during this response (216). Increased levels of TNFα are also associated with enhanced MCP-1 expression in a murine lung allograft rejection model and correlate with upregulation of CCR2 and the recruitment of mononuclear phagocytes into the allograft (168). Interruption of MCP-1/CCR2 signal-ing using CCR2-deficient recipients results in a reduction of macrophage infiltration and less rejection (168). Signaling via CCR2 is also critical to the induction of profibrotic cyto-kine cascades following the intratracheal administration of FITC and bleomycin (208). Finally, clinical studies have shown that enhanced MCP-1 is associated with the pro-gression from acute to chronic allograft rejection and with the evolution of IPF (168,217–219). Studies from our laboratory have demonstrated significant roles for both TNFα and CCR2/MCP-1 in the development of IPS (62,74,146), and experiments are ongoing to determine whether these interactions are operative in the transition from acute to chronic lung injury after SCT.

C. Treatment of Chronic Lung Injury After SCT

The clear association of OLD and chronic GVHD has resulted in a general consensus that this form of lung damage is immunologically mediated, even though the etiology of airflow obstruction after SCT is likely to be multifactorial. Thus, "standard" therapy of OLD com-bines enhanced immunosuppression in conjunction with supportive care, including sup-plemental oxygen therapy and broad-spectrum antimicrobial prophylaxis. Unfortunately, the response to multiple agents including steroids, cyclosporine, tacrolimus, and azathiopr-ine is limited and tends to occur only early in the course of treatment (8,13,46,59,154). Patients with more severe disease at the start of treatment have poor prognoses and high mortality rates, suggesting that early recognition of OLD may be important (13,59,154). The poor response to standard therapy and the unacceptable morbidity and mortality associated with chronic lung injury after SCT are underscored by the need for lung transplant in some SCT recipients with severe OLD (18,220).

The published literature contains a paucity of therapeutic trials for chronic lung injury after SCT, and most retrospective reports focus on patients treated for OLD rather than RLD. Although no agent or combination of agents has proven efficacy with respect to treating OLD, a study by Payne and colleagues showed that the use of cyclosporine and methotrexate as GVHD prophylaxis prevented the development of OLD when compared to historical controls receiving prednisone and methotrexate (221). Unfortunately, results of prospective, randomized trials studying the impact of GVHD prophylaxis regimens on the incidence and severity of OLD have not been reported. A recent clinical trial using inhaled steroids in addition to standard systemic immunosuppression to prevent BOS after lung allografting was recently completed, but no benefit was observed compared to placebo controls (222).

The potential role for TNFα in the pathogenesis of both OLD and RLD suggests that agents that neutralize this protein may have promise as novel therapeutic agents for these disorders. Etanercept (Enbrel®, rhTNFR:Fc) was recently evaluated in an open-label pilot study in 9 patients with IPF (223). All patients had worsening disease that was refractory to conventional therapy. Five of 9 patients had objective improvement in oxygen requirement, DLCO, and A-a gradient after an average follow-up of 11 months. Etanercept has also been used to treat steroid refractory chronic GVHD in a series of 10 patients, and 3 of 4 patients with lung disease were reported to have objective response (increased DLCO) as well as subjective improvement (224). A phase I–II clinical trial using etanercept specifically for patients with either OLD or RLD has recently been completed at the University of Michigan. Preliminary results demonstrate that etanercept can be safely administered in this patient population, and 6 of 15 patients showed at least a 10% improvement from baseline in either FEV_1, FVC, or DLCO within the first 2 months of finishing therapy (K. R. Cooke, unpublished observation). Additional prospective trials are needed to enhance our understanding of the immunological mechanisms responsible for this complication, to identify diagnostic and prognostic predictive factors, and to test new agents or treatment strategies in this clinical setting.

IV. CONCLUSION

Noninfectious lung injury remains a significant problem following allogeneic SCT both in the immediate posttransplant period and in the months to years that follow. Although such lung injury occasionally occurs following autologous transplants, the allogeneic setting significantly exacerbates toxicity in both the acute and chronic settings. Historically, much of this injury was assumed to be due to occult and unidentifiable infections, but animal models have clearly shown immunological mechanisms to be operative. Is the lung a target of GVHD? The weight of conceptual and experimental evidence seems to us to favor rather than disfavor this possibility.

As detailed above, a large preponderance of experimental data now demonstrate that IPS, the acute form of lung injury after allogeneic SCT, has a major immunological component. The lung, like the gut and skin, is one of the interfaces between the sterile body sanctuary and the outside environment, and the pulmonary defense system is designed to handle this particulate and antigen load. As such, the lung is a rich source of histocompatibility antigens and professional APCs and is the site of complex immunological networks involving cytokine production and lymphocyte activation. Inflammatory mediators such as TNFα and LPS along with donor-derived Th1 effector cells, which are known to play a role in acute GVHD, also directly contribute to acute lung injury in animal SCT models and have been identified in the BAL fluid of patients with IPS. Clinically, evidence supporting the concept that the lung is a target organ of acute GVHD is limited, and the major obstacle has been the lack of apoptotic epithelial injury. As already noted, however, other GVHD target organs such as the thymus do not express this particular form of injury, and recent experimental data demonstrate that direct recognition of alloantigen on host epithelium by cytotoxic effectors is not required for GVHD induction or target organ injury. The unique aspects of epithelial anatomy in the lung may also be important factors in this discrepancy. Since there is no stratification or layering of pulmonary epithelial cells as in the skin or intestine, the histopathological repertoire of pulmonary damage is very limited, making a potential diagnosis of acute GVHD in the lung by histological criteria difficult.

In the chronic setting, it is widely accepted that the lung is a target of GVHD. The striking similarities between the histopathological features of bronchiolitis obliterans seen in association with OLD after allogeneic SCT and those observed during lung allograft rejection, along with reports of improvement in lung function with immunosuppressive agents, strongly support an immunological mechanism. The case for immunological mechanisms contributing to RLD is more tenuous, and the data from experimental allogeneic models are still scant. Nonetheless, TNFα may be viewed as a common thread between acute IPS and chronic lung disease of either the obstructive or restrictive type. As animal models of lung injury after SCT yield further insights, our understanding of these disease processes should improve and ultimately lead to successful therapeutic strategies to diagnose, treat, and prevent pulmonary toxicity in recipients of allogeneic SCT.

REFERENCES

1. Clark J, Madtes D, Martin T, Hackman R, Farrand A, Crawford S. Idiopathic pneumonia after bone marrow transplantation: cytokine activation and lipopolysaccharide amplification in the bronchoalveolar compartment. Crit Care Med 1999; 27:1800.
2. Crawford S, Hackman R. Clinical course of idiopathic pneumonia after bone marrow transplantation. Am Rev Respir Dis 1993; 147:1393.
3. Weiner RS, Mortimer MB, Gale RP, Gluckman E, Kay HEM, Kolb JJ, Hartz AJ, Rimm AA. Interstitial pneumonitis after bone marrow transplantation. Ann Intern Med 1986; 104:168–175.
4. Quabeck K. The lung as a critical organ in marrow transplantation. Bone Marrow Transplant 1994; 14:S19–S28.
5. Crawford S, Longton G, Storb R. Acute graft versus host disease and the risks for idiopathic pneumonia after marrow transplantation for severe aplastic anemia. Bone Marrow Transplant 1993; 12:225.
6. Kantrow SP, Hackman RC, Boeckh M, Myerson D, Crawford SW. Idiopathic pneumonia syndrome: changing spectrum of lung injury after marrow transplantation. Transplantation 1997; 63:1079–1086.
7. Afessa B, Litzow MR, Tefferi A. Bronchiolitis obliterans and other late onset non-infectious pulmonary complications in hematopoietic stem cell transplantation. Bone Marrow Transplant 2001; 28:425–434.

8. Holland HK, Wingard JR, Beschorner WE, Saral R, Santos GW. Bronchiolitis obliterans in bone marrow transplantation and its relationship to chronic graft-versus-host disease and low serum IgG. Blood 1988; 72:621–627.

9. Schultz KR, Green GJ, Wensley D, Sargent MA, Magee JF, Spinelli JJ, Pritchard S, Davis JH, Rogers PCJ, Chan KW, Phillips GL. Obstructive lung disease in children after allogeneic bone marrow transplantation. Blood 1994; 84:3212–3220.

10. Crawford SW, Pepe M, Lin D, Benedetti F, Deeg HJ. Abnormalities of pulmonary function tests after marrow transplantation predict nonrelapse mortality. Am J Respir Crit Care Med 1995; 152:690–695.

11. Sullivan K, Mori M, Sanders J, et al. Late complications of allogeneic and autologous bone marrow transplantation. Bone Marrow Transplant 1992; 10:127–134.

12. Wiesendanger P, Archimbaud E, Mornex J, Brune J, Cordier J. Post transplant obstructive lung disease ("bronchiolitis obliterans"). Eur Respir J 1995; 8:551–558.

13. Sanchez J, Torres A, Serrano J, Romain J, Martin C, Perula L, Martinez F, Ganey P. Long term follow up of immunosuppressive treatment for obstructive airway disease after allogeneic bone marrow transplantation. Bone Marrow Transplant 1997; 20:403–408.

14. Badier M, Guillot C, Delpierre S, Vanuxem P, Blaise D, Maraninchi D. Pulmonary function changes 100 days and one year after bone marrow transplantation. Bone Marrow Transplant 1993; 12:457–461.

15. Quigley P, Yeager A, Loughlin G. The effects of bone marrow transplantation on pulmonary function in children. Pediatr Pulmon 1994; 18:361–367.

16. Abhyankar S, Gilliland DG, Ferrara JLM. Interleukin 1 is a critical effector molecule during cytokine dysregulation in graft-versus-host disease to minor histocompatibility antigens. Transplantation 1993; 56:1518–1523.

17. Clark J, Hansen J, Hertz M, Parkman R, Jensen L, Peavy H. Idiopathic pneumonia syndrome after bone marrow transplantation. Am Rev Respir Dis 1993; 147:1601–1606.

18. Yousem SA. The histological spectrum of pulmonary graft-versus-host disease in bone marrow transplant recipients. Hum Pathol 1995; 26:668–675.

19. Wingard JR, Mellits ED, Sostrin MB, et al. Interstitial pneumonitis after allogeneic bone marrow transplantation. Nine-year experience at a single institution. Medicine 1988; 67:175–186.

20. Neiman P, Wasserman PB, Wentworth BB, et al. Interstitial pneumonia and cytomegalovirus infection as complications of human marrow transplantation. Transplantation 1973; 15:478–485.

21. Yanik G, Hellerstedt B, Custer J, Hutchinson R, Kwon D, Ferrara JL, Uberti J, Cooke KR. Etanercept (Enbrel) administration for idiopathic pneumonia syndrome after allogeneic hematopoietic stem cell transplantation. Biol Blood Marrow Transplant 2002; 8:395–400.

22. Robbins RA, Linder J, Stahl MG, et al. Diffuse alveolar hemorrhage in autologous bone marrow transplant recipients. Am J Med 1989; 87:511–518.

23. Lewis ID, DeFor T, Weisdorf DJ. Increasing incidence of diffuse alveolar hemorrhage following allogeneic bone marrow transplantation: cryptic etiology and uncertain therapy. Bone Marrow Transplant 2000; 26:539–543.

24. Metcalf JP, Rennard SI, Reed EC, Haire WD, Sisson JH, Walter T, Robbins RA. Corticosteroids as adjunctive therapy for diffuse alveolar hemorrhage associated with bone marrow transplantation. University of Nebraska Medical Center Bone Marrow Transplant Group. Am J Med 1994; 96:327–334.

25. Sloane J, Depledge M, Powles R, Morgenstern G, Trickey B, Dady P. Histopathology of the lung after bone marrow transplantation. J Clin Pathol 1983; 36:546–554.

26. Wojno KJ, Vogelsang GB, Beschorner WE, Santos GW. Pulmonary hemorrhage as a cause of death in allogeneic bone marrow recipients with severe acute graft-versus-host disease. Transplantation 1994; 57:88–92.

27. Capizzi SA, Kumar S, Huneke NE, Gertz MA, Inwards DJ, Litzow MR, Lacy MQ, Gastineau DA, Prakash UB, Tefferi A. Peri-engraftment respiratory distress syndrome during autologous hematopoietic stem cell transplantation. Bone Marrow Transplant 2001; 27:1299–1303.

28. Wilczynski SW, Erasmus JJ, Petros WP, Vredenburgh JJ, Folz RJ. Delayed pulmonary toxicity syndrome following high-dose chemotherapy and bone marrow transplantation for breast cancer. Am J Respir Crit Care Med 1998; 157:565–573.

29. Bhalla KS, Wilczynski SW, Abushamaa AM, Petros WP, McDonald CS, Loftis JS, Chao NJ, Vredenburgh JJ, Folz RJ. Pulmonary toxicity of induction chemotherapy prior to standard or high-dose chemotherapy with autologous hematopoietic support. Am J Respir Crit Care Med 2000; 161:17–25.

30. Weiner RS, Horowitz MM, Gale RP, Dicke KA, van Bekkum DW, Masaoka T, Ramsay NKC, Rimm AA, Rozman C, Bortin MM. Risk factors for interstitial pneumonitis following bone marrow transplantation for severe aplastic anemia. Br J Haematol 1989; 71:535.

31. Meyers JD, Flournoy N, Thomas ED. Nonbacterial pneumonia after allogeneic marrow transplantation: a review of ten years' experience. Rev Infect Dis 1982; 4:1119–1132.

32. Atkinson K, Turner J, Biggs JC, Dodds A, Concannon A. An acute pulmonary syndrome possibly representing acute graft-versus-host disease involving the lung interstitium. Bone Marrow Transplant 1991; 8:231.

33. Della Volpe A, Ferreri AJ, Annaloro C, Mangili P, Rosso A, Calandrino R, Villa E, Lamber-tenghi-Deliliers G, Fiorino C. Lethal pulmonary complications significantly correlate with individually assessed mean lung dose in patients with hematologic malignancies treated with total body irradiation. Int J Radiat Oncol Biol Phys 2002; 52:483–488.

34. Fukuda T, Hackman R, Guthrie KA, Carter RA, Sandmaier BM, Davis C, Martin PJ, Storb RF, Madtes DK. Risks and outcomes of idiopathic pneumonia syndrome after allogeneic hematopoietic stem cell transplantation: the intensity of the conditioning regimen outweighs the effect of acute graft-versus-host disease. Biol Blood Marrow Transplant 2003; 9:65.

35. Down JD, Mauch P, Warhol M, Neben S, Ferrara JLM. The effect of donor T lymphocytes and total-body irradiation on hemopoietic engraftment and pulmonary toxicity following experimental allogeneic bone marrow transplantation. Transplantation 1992; 54:802–808.

36. Shankar G, Cohen DA. Idiopathic pneumonia syndrome after bone marrow transplantation: the role of pre-transplant radiation conditioning and local cytokine dysregulation in promoting lung inflammation and fibrosis. Int J Exp Pathol 2001; 82:101–113.

37. Kelley J. Cytokines of the lung. Am Rev Respir Dis 1990; 141:765–788.

38. Piguet P, Collart M, Grau G, Sappino A, Vassalli P. Requirement of tumour necrosis factor for development of silica-induced pulmonary fibrosis. Nature 1990; 344:245–247.

39. Schmidt J, Pliver CN, Lepe-Zuniga JL, Green I, Gery I. Silica-stimulated monocytes release fibroblast proliferation factors identical to interleukin-1. A potential role for interleukin-1 in the pathogenesis of silicosis. J Clin Invest 1984; 73:1462–1472.

40. Suter P, Suter S, Girardin E, Roux-Lombard P, Grau G, Dayer J. High bronchoalveolar levels of tumor necrosis factor and its inhibitors, interleukin-1, interferon, and elastase, in patients with adult respiratory distress syndrome after trauma, shock or sepsis. Am Rev Respir Dis 1992; 145:1016.

41. Hyers T, Tricomi S, Dettenmier P, Fowler A. Tumor necrosis factor levels in serum and bronchoalveolar lavage fluid of patients with the adult respiratory distress syndrome. Am Rev Respir Dis 1991; 144:268.

42. Bortin M, Ringden O, Horowitz M, Rozman C, Weiner R, Rimm A. Temporal relationships between the major complications of bone marrow transplantation for leukemia. Bone Marrow Transplant 1989; 4:339.

43. Beschorner W, Saral R, Hutchins G, Tutschka P, Santos G. Lymphocytic bronchitis associated with graft versus host disease in recipients of bone marrow transplants. N Engl J Med 1978; 299:1030–1036.

44. Milburn HJ, Poulter LW, Prentice HG, Du Bois RM. Pulmonary cell populations in recipients of bone marrow transplants with interstitial pneumonitis. Thorax 1989; 44:570.
45. Milburn HJ, Du Bois RM, Prentice HG, Poulter LW. Pneumonitis in bone marrow transplant recipients results from a local immune response. Clin Exp Immunol 1990; 81:232.
46. Schwarer AP, Hughes JMB, Trotman-Dickenson B, Krausz T, Goldman JM. A chronic pulmonary syndrome associated with graft-versus-host disease after allogeneic marrow transplantation. Transplantation 1992; 54:1002–1008.
47. Sutedja TG, Apperley JF, Hughes JMB, et al. Pulmonary function after bone marrow transplantation for chronic myeloid leukemia. Thorax 1988; 43:163–169.
48. Piguet PF, Grau GE, Collart MA, Vassalli P, Kapanci Y. Pneumopathies of the graft-versus-host reaction. Alveolitis associated with an increased level of tumor necrosis factor MRNA and chronic interstitial pneumonitis. Lab Invest 1989; 61:37–45.
49. Clark JG, Madtes DK, Hackman RC, Chen W, Cheever MA, Martin PJ. Lung injury induced by alloreactive Th1 cells is characterized by host-derived mononuclear cell inflammation and activation of alveolar macrophages. J Immunol 1998; 161:1913–1920.
50. Shankar G, Bryson J, Jennings C, Morris P, Cohen D. Idiopathic pneumonia syndrome in mice after allogeneic bone marrow transplantation. Am J Respir Cell Mol Biol 1998; 18:235–242.
51. Cooke KR, Kobzik L, Martin TR, Brewer J, Delmonte J, Crawford JM, Ferrara JLM. An experimental model of idiopathic pneumonia syndrome after bone marrow transplantation. I. The roles of minor H antigens and endotoxin. Blood 1996; 8:3230–3239.
52. Cooke KR, Krenger W, Hill GR, Martin T, Kobzik L, Brewer J, Simmons R, Crawford JM, van den Brink MRM, Ferrara JLM. Host reactive donor T cells are associated with lung injury after experimental allogeneic bone marrow transplantation. Blood 1998; 92:2571–2580.
53. Hackman RC, Sale GE. Large airway inflammation as a possible manifestation of a pulmonary graft-versus-host reaction in bone marrow allograft recipients. Lab Invest 1981; 44:26A.
54. Connor R, Ramsay N, McGlave P, Snover D, Kersey J, Burke B. Pulmonary pathology in bone marrow transplant recipients. Lab Invest 1982; 46:3.
55. Workman D, Clancy JJ. Interstitial pneumonitis and lymphocytic bronchiolitis/bronchitis as a direct result of acute lethal graft-versus-host disease duplicate the histopathology of lung allograft rejection. Transplant 1994; 58:207.
56. Panoskaltsis-Mortari A, Taylor PA, Yaegar TM, Wangensteen OD, Bitterman PB, Ingbar DH, Vallera DA, Blazar BR. The critical early proinflammatory events associated with idiopathic pneumonia syndrome in irradiated murine allogenic recipients are due to donor T cell infusion and potentiated by cyclophosphamide. J Clin Invest 1997; 100:1015–1027.
57. Cooke K, Kobzik L, Teshima T, Lowler K, Clouthier S, Ferrara J. A role for Fas-Fas ligand but not perforin mediated cytolysis in the development of experimental idiopathic pneumonia syndrome. Blood 2000; 96:768a.
58. Gerbitz A, Wilke A, Eissner G, Holler E, Andreesen R, Ferrara J, Cooke K. Critical role for CD54 (ICAM-1) in the development of experimental idiopathic pneumonia syndrome. Blood 2000; 96:768a.
59. Curtis DJ, Smale A, THien F, Schwarer AP, Szer J. Chronic airflow obstruction in long-term survivors of allogeneic bone marrow transplantation. Bone Marrow Transplant 1995; 16:169–173.
60. Clark JG, Schwartz DA, Flournoy N, Sullivan KM, Crawford SW, Thomas ED. Risk factors for air-flow obstruction in recipients of bone marrow transplants. Ann Intern Med 1987; 107:648–656.
61. Piguet PF, Grau GE, Allet B, Vassalli PJ. Tumor necrosis factor/cachectin is an effector of skin and gut lesions of the acute phase of graft-versus-host disease. J Exp Med 1987; 166:1280–1289.
62. Cooke KR, Hill GR, Gerbitz A, Kobzik L, Martin TR, Crawford JM, Brewer JP, Ferrara JL. Tumor necrosis factor-alpha neutralization reduces lung injury after experimental allogeneic bone marrow transplantation. Transplantation 2000; 70:272–279.

63. Smith S, Skerrett S, Chi E, Jonas M, Mohler K, Wilson C. The locus of tumor necrosis factor-α action in lung inflammation. Am J Respir Cell Mol Biol 1998; 19:881.

64. Nelson S, Bagby G, Gainton B, Wilson L, Thompson J, Summer W. Compartmentalization of intraalveolar and systemic lipopolysaccharide-induced tumor necrosis factor and the pulmonary inflammatory response. J Infect Dis 1989; 159:189.

65. Ulich TR, Watson LR, Yin SM, Guo KZ, Wang P, Thang H, del Castillo J. The intratracheal administration of endotoxin and cytokines. I. Characterization of LPS-induced IL-1 and TNF mRNA expression and the LPS-, IL-1-, and TNF-induced inflammatory infiltrate. Am J Pathol 1991; 138:1485–1496.

66. Nestel FP, Price KS, Seemayer TA, Lapp WS. Macrophage priming and lipopolysaccharide-triggered release of tumor necrosis factor alpha during graft-versus-host disease. J Exp Med 1992; 175:405–413.

67. Hill G, Ferrara J. The primacy of the gastrointestinal tract as a target organ of acute graft-versus-host disease: rationale for the use of cytokine shields in allogeneic bone marrow transplantation. Blood 2000; 95:2754–2759.

68. Cooke K, Gerbitz A, Hill G, Crawford J, Teshima T, JLM F. LPS Antagonism reduces graft-versus-host disease and preserves graft-versus-leukemia activity after experimental bone marrow transplantation. J Clin Invest 2001; 7:1581–1589.

69. Fegan C, Poynton CH, Whittaker JA. The gut mucosal barrier in bone marrow transplantation. Bone Marrow Transplant 1990; 5:373–377.

70. Jackson SK, Parton J, Barnes RA, Poynton CH, Fegan C. Effect of IgM-enriched intravenous immunoglobulin (Pentaglobulin) on endotoxaemia and anti-endotoxin antibodies in bone marrow transplantation. Eur J Clin Invest 1993; 23:540–545.

71. Hill GR, Crawford JM, Cooke KJ, Brinson YS, Pan L, Ferrara JLM. Total body irradiation and acute graft versus host disease. The role of gastrointestinal damage and inflammatory cytokines. Blood 1997; 90:3204–3213.

72. Cooke K, Hill G, Crawford J, Bungard D, Brinson Y, Delmonte J. Jr, Ferrara J. Tumor necrosis factor-α production to lipopolysaccharide stimulation by donor cells predicts the severity of experimental acute graft versus host disease. J Clin Invest 1998; 102:1882–1891.

73. Cooke K, Hill G, Gerbitz A, Kobzik L, Martin T, Crawford J, Brewer J, Ferrara J. Hyporesponsiveness of donor cells to LPS stimulation reduces the severity of experimental idiopathic pneumonia syndrome: potential role for a gut-lung axis of inflammation. J Immunol 2000; 165:6612–6619.

74. Cooke KR, Olkiewicz K, Erickson N, Hildebrandt G, Liu C, Ferrara J. A role for the p75 but not the p55 TNFa receptor in the development of idiopathic pneumonia syndrome after allogeneic stem cell transplantation. Biol Blood Marrow Transplant 2003; 9:97.

75. Hattori K, Hirano T, Miyajima H, Yamakawa N, Tateno M, Oshimi K, Kayagaki N, Yagita H, Okumura K. Differential effects of anti-Fas ligand and anti-tumor necrosis factor-α antibodies on acute graft-versus-host disease pathologies. Blood 1998; 91:4051–4055.

76. Vallera DA, Taylor PA, Vannice JL, Panoskaltsis-Mortari A, Blazar BR. Interleukin-1 or tumor necrosis factor-alpha antagonists do not inhibit graft-versus-host disease induced across the major histocompatibility barrier in mice. Transplantation 1995; 60:1371–1374.

77. Clark JG, Mandac JB, Dixon AE, Martin PJ, Hackman RC, Madtes DK. Neutralization of tumor necrosis factor-alpha action delays but does not prevent lung injury induced by alloreactive T helper 1 cells. Transplantation 2000; 70:39–43.

78. Baker MB, Altman NH, Podack ER, Levy RB. The role of cell-mediated cytotoxicity in acute GVHD after MHC-matched allogeneic bone marrow transplantation in mice. J Exp Med 1996; 183:2645–2656.

79. Braun YM, Lowin B, French L, Acha-Orbea H, Tschopp J. Cytotoxic T cells deficient in both functional Fas ligand and perforin show residual cytolytic activity yet lose their capacity to induce lethal acute graft-versus-host disease. J Exp Med 1996; 183:657–661.

80. Haddad I, Ingbar D, Panoskaltsis-Mortari A, Blazar B. Activated alveolar macrophage-derived nitric oxide predicts the development of lung damage after marrow transplantation in mice. Chest 1999; 116:37S.

81. Haddad I, Panoskaltsis-Mortari A, Ingbar D, Yang S, Milla C, Blazar B. High levels of peroxynitrite are generated in the lungs of irradiated mice given cyclophosphamide and allogeneic T cells: a potential mechanism of injury after marrow transplantation. Am J Respir Cell Mol Biol 1999; 20:1125.

82. Jasinski M, Wieckiewicz J, Ruggiero I, Pituch-Noworlska A, Zembala M. Isotype-specific regulation of MHC class II gene expression in human monocytes by exogenous and endogenous tumor necrosis factor. J Clin Immunol 1995; 15:185.

83. Crawford J. Cellular and molecular biology of the inflamed liver. Curr Opin Gastroenterol 1997; 13:175.

84. Matuschak G, Pinksy M, Klein E, Van Thiel D, Rinaldo J. Effects of D-galactosamine induced acute liver injury on mortality and pulmonary responses to *Escherichia coli* lipopolysaccharide. Am Rev Respir Dis 1990; 141:1296.

85. Matuschak GM, Mattingly ME, Tredway TL, Lechner AJ. Liver-lung interactions during *E. coli* endotoxemia. Am J Respir Crit Care Med 1994; 149:41–49.

86. Nakao A, Taki S, Yasui M, Kimura Y, Nonami T, Harada A, Takagi H. The fate of intravenously injected endotoxin in normal rats and in rats with liver failure. Hepatology 1994; 19:1251.

87. Lehmann V, Freudenberg M, Galanos C. Lethal toxicity of lipopolysaccharide and tumor necrosis factor in normal and D-galactosamine treated mice. J Exp Med 1987; 165:657.

88. Galanos C, Freudenber M, Reutter W. Galactosamine induced sensitization to the lethal effects of endotoxin. Proc Natl Acad Sci USA 1987; 76:5939.

89. Katz M, Grosfeld J, Gross K. Impaired bacterial clearance and trapping in obstructive jaundice. Am J Surg 1984; 199.

90. Holler E, Kolb HJ, Moller A, Kempeni J, Lisenfeld S, Pechumer H, Lehmacher W, Ruckdeschel G, Gleixner B, Riedner C, Ledderose G, Brehm G, Mittermuller J, Wilmanns W. Increased serum levels of tumor necrosis factor alpha precede major complications of bone marrow transplantation. Blood 1990; 75:1011–1016.

91. Martin T, Rubenfeld G, Ruzinski J. Relationship between soluble CD14, lipopolysaccharide binding protein, and the alveolar inflammatory response in patients with acute respiratory distress syndrome. Am J Respir Crit Care Med 1997; 155:937–944.

92. Shlomchik WD, Couzens MS, Tang CB, McNiff J, Robert ME, Liu J, Shlomchik MJ, Emerson SG. Prevention of graft versus host disease by inactivation of host antigen-presenting cells. Science 1999; 285:412–415.

93. Madtes DK, Crawford SW. Lung injuries associated with graft-versus-host reactions. In: Ferrara JLM, Deeg HJ, Burakoff SJ, eds. Graft-vs.-Host Disease. New York, NY: Marcel Dekker, 1997; p 425.

94. Rabinowich H, Zeevi A, Paradis IL, Yousem SA, Dauber JH, Kormos R, Hardesty RL, Griffith BP, Duquesnoy RJ. Proliferative responses of bronchoalveolar lavage lymphocytes from heart-lung transplant patients. Transplant 1990; 49:115.

95. Watanabe T, Kawamura T, Kawamura H, Haga M, Shirai K, Watanabe H, Eguchi S, Abo T. Intermediate TCR cells in mouse lung. Their effector function to induce Pneumonitis in mice with autoimmune-like graft-versus-host disease. J Immunol 1997; 158:5805.

96. Chen W, Chatta K, Rubin W, Liggit DH, Kusunoki Y, Martin P, Cheever MA. Polymorphic segments of CD45 can serve as targets for GVHD and GVL responses. Blood 1995; 86(suppl):158a.

97. Leblond V, Zouabi H, Sutton L, Guillon JM, Mayaud CM, Similowski T, Beigelman C, Autran B. Late CD8+ lymphocytic alveolitis after allogeneic bone marrow transplantation and chronic graft-versus-host disease. Am J Crit Care Med 1994; 150:1056.

98. Gartner JG, Merry AC, Smith CI. An analysis of pulmonary natural killer cell activity in F1-hybrid mice with acute graft-versus-host reactions. Transplant 1988; 46:879–886.

99. Trauth BC, Klas C, Peters AM, Matzku S, Moller P, Falk W, Debatin KM, Krammer PH. Monoclonal antibody-mediated tumor regression by induction of apoptosis. Science 1989; 245:301–305.

100. Itoh N, Yonehara S, Ishii A, Yonehara M, Mizushima SI, Sameshima M, Hase A, Seto Y, Nagata S. The polypeptide encoded by the cDNA for human cell surface antigen Fas can mediate apoptosis. Cell 1991; 66:233–243.

101. Lowin B, Hahne M, Mattmann C, Tschopp J. Cytolytic T-cell cytotoxicity is mediated through perforin and Fas lytic pathways. Nature (London) 1994; 370:650–652.

102. Lee RK, Spielman J, Zhao DY. Perforin fas ligand and tumor necrosis factor are the major cytotoxic molecules used by lymphokine-activated killer cells. J Immunol 1996; 157:1919–1925.

103. Teshima T, Hill G, Pan L, Brinson Y, van den Brink MR, Cooke K, Ferrara J. IL-11 separates graft-versus-leukemia effects from graft-versus-host disease after bone marrow transplantation. J Clin Invest 1999; 104:317–325.

104. Blazar BR, Taylor PA, Vallera DA. CD4+ and CD8+ T cells each can utilize a perforin-dependent pathway to mediate lethal graft-versus-host disease in major histocompatibility complex-disparate recipients. Transplantation 1997; 64:571–576.

105. Rafi AQ, Zeytun A, Bradley M, Sponenberg D, Grayson R, Nagarkatti M, PSN. Evidence for the involvement of Fas ligand and perforin in the induction of vascular leak syndrome. J Immunol 1998; 161:3077–3086.

106. Matute-Bello G, Liles WC, Steinberg KP, Kiener PA, Mongovin S, Chi EY, Jonas M, Martin TR. Soluble Fas ligand induces epithelial cell apoptosis in humans with acute lung injury (ARDS). J Immunol 1999; 163:2217–2225.

107. Hiroyasu S, Shiraishi M, Koji T, Mamadi T, Sugawa H, Tomori H, Muto Y. Analysis of Fas system in pulmonary injury of graft-versus-host disease after rat intestinal transplantation. Transplantation 1999; 68:933–938.

108. Hashimoto S, Kobayashi A, Kooguchi K, Kitamura Y, Onodera H, Nakajima H. Upregulation of two death pathways of perforin/granzyme and FasL/Fas in septic acute respiratory distress syndrome. Am J Respir Crit Care Med 2000; 161:237–243.

109. Panoskaltsis-Mortari A, Ingbar DH, Jung P, Haddad IY, Bitterman PB, Wangensteen OD, Farrell CL, Lacey DL, Blazar BR. KGF pretreatment decreases B7 and granzyme B expression and hastens repair in lungs of mice after allogeneic BMT. Am J Physiol Lung Cell Mol Physiol 2000; 278:L988–999.

110. Stein R, Hummel D, Bohn D, Levison H, Roifman CM. Lymphocytic pneumonitis following bone marrow transplantation in severe combined immunodeficiency. Am Rev Respir Dis 1991; 143:1406–1408.

111. Massard G, Tongiio MW, Wihlm JM, Morand G. The dendritic cell lineage: an ubiquitous antigen-presenting organization. Ann Thorac Surg 1996; 61:252.

112. Armstrong LR, Christensen PJ, Paine R, Chen GH, McDonald RA, Lim TK, Toews GB. Regulation of the immunostimulatory activity of rat pulmonary interstitial dendritic cells by cell–cell interactions and cytokines. Am J Respir Cell Mol Biol 1994; 11:682.

113. Pollard AM, Lipscomb MF. Characterization of murine lung dendritic cells: similarities to Langerhans cells and thymic dendritic cells. J Exp Med 1990; 172:159–167.

114. Masten BJ, Yates JL, Pollard Koga AM, Lipscomb MF. Characterization of accessory molecules in murine lung dendritic cell function: roles for CD80, CD86, CD54, and CD40L. Am J Respir Cell Mol Biol 1997; 16:335–342.

115. Christensen PJ, Armstrong LR, Fak JJ, Chen GH, McDonald RA, Toews GB, Paine R. Regulation of rat pulmonary dendritic cell immunostimulatory activity by alveolar epithelial cell-derived granulocyte macrophage colony-stimulating factor. Am J Respir Cell Mol Biol 1995; 13:426.

116. van Haarst JM, de Wit HJ, Drexhage HA, Hoogsteden HC. Distribution and immunophenotype of mononuclear phagocytes and dendritic cells in the human lung. Am J Respir Cell Mol Biol 1994; 10:487–492.

117. Holt PG, Oliver J, Bilyk N, McMenamin C, McMenamin PG, Kraal G, Thepen T. Downregulation of the antigen presenting cell function(s) of pulmonary dendritic cells in vivo by resident alveolar macrophages. J Exp Med 1993; 177:397–407.

118. Dupuis M, McDonald DM. Dendritic-cell regulation of lung immunity. Am J Respir Cell Mol Biol 1997; 17:284.

119. van Haarst JM, de Wit HJ, Drexhage HA, Hoogsteden HC. Distribution and immunophenotype of mononuclear and dendritic cells in the human lung. Am J Respir Cell Mol Biol 1994; 10:487.

120. Yousem SA, Ray L, Paradis IL, Dauber JA, Griffith BP. Potential role of dendritic cells in bronchiolitis obliterans in heart-lung transplantation. Ann Thorac Surg 1990; 49:424.

121. Teshima T, Ordemann R, Reddy P, Gagin S, Liu C, Cooke KR, Ferrara JL. Acute graft-versus-host disease does not require alloantigen expression on host epithelium. Nat Med 2002; 8:575–581.

122. Holt PG, Haining S, Nelson DJ, Sedgwick JD. Origin and steady-state turnover of class II MHC-bearing dendritic cells in the epithelium of the conducting airways. J Immunol 1994; 153:256–261.

123. Murai M, Yoneyama H, Ezaki T, Suematsu M, Terashim Y, Harada A, Hamada H, Asakura H, Ishikawa H, Matsushima K. Peyer's patch is the essential site in initiating murine acute and lethal graft-versus-host reaction. Nat Immunol 2003; 4:154–160.

124. Glode LM, Rosenstreich DL. Genetic control of B cell activation by bacterial lipopolysaccaride is mediated by multiple distinct genes or alleles. J Immunol 1976; 117:2061–2066.

125. Poltorak A, Ziaolong H, Smirnova I, Liu M-Y, Van Huffel C, Du X, Birdwell D, Alejos E, Silva M, Galanos C, Freudenberg M, Ricciardi-Castagnoli P, Layton B, Beutler B. Defective LPS signaling in C3H/HeJ and C57BL/20ScCr mice: mutations in Tlr4 gene. Science 1998; 282:2085–2088.

126. Watson J, Kelly K, Largen M, Taylor BA. The genetic mapping of a defective LPS response gene in C3H/Hej mice. J Immunol 1978; 120:422–424.

127. Sultzer BM, Castagna R, Bandeakar J, Wong P. Lipopolysaccharide nonresponder cells: the C3H/HeJ defect. Immunobiology 1993; 187:257–271.

128. Cooke K, Olkiewicz K, Clouthier S, Liu C, Ferrara J. Critical role for CD14 and the innate immune response in the induction of experimental acute graft-versus-host disease. Blood 2001; 98:776a.

129. Maus U, Herold S, Muth H, Maus R, Ermert L, Ermert M, Weissmann N, Rosseau S, Seeger W, Grimminger F, Lohmeyer J. Monocytes recruited into the alveolar air space of mice show a monocytic phenotype but upregulate CD14. Am J Physiol Lung Cell Mol Physiol 2001; 280:L58–68.

130. Martin T, Goodman R. The role of chemokines in the pathophysiology of the acute respiratory distress syndrome (ARDS). In Hebert C, ed Chemokines in Disease. Totowa, NJ: Humana Press, 1999; pp 81–110.

131. DiGiovine B, Lynch J, Martinez F, Flint A, Whyte R, Iannettoni M, Arenberg D, Burdick M, Glass M, Wilke C, Morris S, Kunkel S, Strieter R. Bronchoalveolar lavage neutrophilia is associated with obliterative bronchiolitis after lung transplantation: role of IL-8. J Immunol 1996; 157:4194–5202.

132. Riise GC, Andersson BA, Kjellstrom C, Martensson G, Nilsson FN, Ryd W, Schersten H. Persistent high BAL fluid granulocyte activation marker levels as early indicators of bronchiolitis obliterans after lung transplant. Eur Respir J 1999; 14:1123–1130.

133. Zheng L, Walters EH, Ward C, Wang N, Orsida B, Whitford H, Williams TJ, Kotsimbos T, Snell GI. Airway neutrophilia in stable and bronchiolitis obliterans syndrome patients following lung transplantation. Thorax 2000; 55:53–59.

134. Reynaud-Gaubert M, Thomas P, Badier M, Cau P, Giudicelli R, Fuentes P. Early detection of airway involvement in obliterative bronchiolitis after lung transplantation. Functional and bronchoalveolar lavage cell findings. Am J Respir Crit Care Med 2000; 161:1924–1929.

135. Elssner A, Vogelmeier C. The role of neutrophils in the pathogenesis of obliterative bronchiolitis after lung transplantation. Transpl Infect Dis 2001; 3:168–176.

136. Mackay CR. Chemokines: immunology's high impact factors. Nat Immunol 2001; 2:95–101.

137. Kishimoto TK, Walcheck B, Rothlein R. Leukocyte adhesion, trafficking, and migration. In: Ferrara JLM, Deeg HJ, Burakoff SJ, eds. Graft-vs.-Host Disease. New York: Marcel Dekker, 1997; pp 151–178.

138. Panoskaltsis-Mortari A, Hermanson JR, Haddad IY, Wangensteen OD, Blazar BR. Intercellular adhesion molecule-I (ICAM-I, CD54) deficiency segregates the unique pathophysiological requirements for generating idiopathic pneumonia syndrome (IPS) versus graft-versus-host disease following allogeneic murine bone marrow transplantation. Biol Blood Marrow Transplant 2001; 7:368–377.

139. Gerbitz A, Olkiewitz K, Erickson N, Williams D, Kobzik L, Eissner G, Holler E, Cooke KR. A role for TNF-alpha mediated endothelial apoptosis in the development of experimental idiopathic pneumonia syndrome. Transplantation. In press.

140. Blazar BR, Taylor PA, Panoskaltis-Mortari A, Gray GS, D.A. V. Co-blockade of the LFA1:ICAM and CD28/CTLA4:B7 pathways is a highly effective means of preventing acute lethal graft-versus-host disease induced by fully major histocompatibility complex-disparate donor grafts. Blood 1995; 85:2607–2618.

141. Luster AD. Chemokines—chemotactic cytokines that mediate inflammation. N Engl J Med 1998; 338:436–445.

142. Gerard C, Rollins BJ. Chemokines and disease. Nat Immunol 2001; 2:108–115.

143. Luster AD. The role of chemokines in linking innate and adaptive immunity. Curr Opin Immunol 2002; 14:129–135.

144. Panoskaltsis-Mortari A, Strieter RM, Hermanson JR, Fegeding KV, Murphy WJ, Farrell CL, Lacey DL, Blazar BR. Induction of monocyte- and T-cell-attracting chemokines in the lung during the generation of idiopathic pneumonia syndrome following allogeneic murine bone marrow transplantation. Blood 2000; 96:834–839.

145. Dixon AE, Mandac JB, Madtes DK, Martin PJ, Clark JG. Chemokine expression in Th1 cell-induced lung injury: prominence of IFN-gamma-inducible chemokines. Am J Physiol Lung Cell Mol Physiol 2000; 279:L592–599.

146. Hildebrandt G, Duffner U, Olkiewicz K, Willmarth N, Corrion L, Williams D, Reddy P, Moore BB, Liu C, Cooke KR. A critical role of CCR2 in the development of idiopathic pneumonia syndrome after allogeneic bone marrow transplantation. Blood 2004; 103:2417–2426.

147. Cerveri I, Fulgoni P, Giorgiani G, Zoia MC, Beccaria M, Tinelli C, Locatelli F. Lung function abnormalities after bone marrow transplantation in children: has the trend recently changed? Chest 2001; 120:1900–1906.

148. Ringden O, Remberger M, Ruutu T, Nikoskelainen J, Volin L, Vindelov L, Parkkali T, Lenhoff S, Sallerfors B, Mellander L, Ljungman P, Jacobsen N. Increased risk of chronic graft-versus-host disease, obstructive bronchiolitis, and alopecia with busulfan versus total body irradiation: long-term results of a randomized trial in allogeneic marrow recipients with leukemia. Blood 1999; 93:2196–2201.

149. Depledge MH, Barrett A, Powles RL. Lung function after bone marrow grafting. Int J Radiat Oncol Biol Phys 1983; 9:145–151.

150. Gore EM, Lawton CA, Ash RC, Lipchik RJ. Pulmonary function changes in long-term survivors of bone marrow transplantation. Int J Radiat Oncol Biol Phys 1996; 36:67–75.

151. Tait RC, Burnett AK, Robertson AG, McNee S, Riyami BM, Carter R, Stevenson RD. Subclinical pulmonary function defects following autologous and allogeneic bone marrow transplantation: relationship to total body irradiation and graft-versus-host disease. Int J Radiat Oncol Biol Phys 1991; 20:1219–1227.

152. Cerveri I, Zoia MC, Fulgoni P, Corsico A, Casali L, Tinelli C, Zecca M, Giorgiani G, Locatelli F. Late pulmonary sequelae after childhood bone marrow transplantation. Thorax 1999; 54:131–135.

153. d'Alessandro MP, Kozakewich HP, Cooke KR, Taylor GA. Radiologic-pathologic conference of Children's Hospital Boston: new pulmonary nodules in a child undergoing treatment for a solid malignancy. Pediatr Radiol 1996; 26:19–21.

154. Clark JG, Crawford SW, Madtes DK, Sullivan KM. Obstructive lung disease after allogeneic marrow transplantation. Clinical presentation and course. Ann Intern Med 1989; 111:368–376.

155. Ralph DD, Springmeyer SC, Sullivan KM, Hackman RC, Storb R, Thomas ED. Rapidly progressive air-flow obstruction in marrow transplant recipients. Possible association between obliterative bronchiolitis and chronic graft-versus-host disease. Am Rev Respir Dis 1984; 129:641–644.

156. Sullivan KM, Agura E, Anasetti C, Appelbaum F, Badger C, Bearman S, Erickson K, Flowers M, Hansen J, Loughran T, et al. Chronic graft-versus-host disease and other late complications of bone marrow transplantation. Semin Hematol 1991; 28:250–259.

157. Wyatt SE, Nunn P, Hows JM, Yin J, Hayes M, Catovsky D, Gordon-Smith EC, Hughes JMB, Goldman JM, Galton DAG. Airways obstruction associated with graft-versus-host disease after bone marrow transplantation. Thorax 1984; 39:887.

158. Urbanski SJ, Kossakowska AE, Curtis J, Chan CK, Hutcheon MA, Hyland RH, Messner H, Minden M, Sculier JP. Idiopathic small airways pathology in patients with graft-versus-host disease following allogeneic bone marrow transplantation. Am J Surg Pathol 1987; 11:965.

159. King TE, Jr. Overview of bronchiolitis. Clin Chest Med 1993; 14:607–610.

160. Crawford SW, Clark JG. Bronchiolitis associated with bone marrow transplantation. Clin Chest Med 1993; 14:741–749.

161. Cooper JD, Billingham M, Egan T, Hertz MI, Higenbottam T, Lynch J, Mauer J, Paradis I, Patterson GA, Smith C, et al. A working formulation for the standardization of nomenclature and for clinical staging of chronic dysfunction in lung allografts. International Society for Heart and Lung Transplantation. J Heart Lung Transplant 1993; 12:713–716.

162. Ooi GC, Peh WC, Ip M. High-resolution computed tomography of bronchiolitis obliterans syndrome after bone marrow transplantation. Respiration 1998; 65:187–191.

163. Bankier AA, Van Muylem A, Knoop C, Estenne M, Gevenois PA. Bronchiolitis obliterans syndrome in heart-lung transplant recipients: diagnosis with expiratory CT. Radiology 2001; 218:533–539.

164. Beinert T, Dull T, Wolf K, Holler E, Vogelmeier C, Behr J, Kolb H. Late pulmonary impairment following allogeneic bone marrow transplantation. Eur J Med Res 1996; 1:343–348.

165. Boehler A, Kesten S, Weder W, Speich R. Bronchiolitis obliterans after lung transplantation: a review. Chest 1998; 114:1411–1426.

166. Coker R, Laurent G. Pulmonary fibrosis: cytokines in the balance. Eur Respir J 1998; 11:1218–1221.

167. Hogaboam CM, Smith RE, Kunkel SL. Dynamic interactions between lung fibroblasts and leukocytes: implications for fibrotic lung disease. Proc Assoc Am Phys 1998; 110:313–320.

168. Belperio JA, Keane MP, Burdick MD, Lynch JP, 3rd, Xue YY, Berlin A, Ross DJ, Kunkel SL, Charo IF, Strieter RM. Critical role for the chemokine MCP-1/CCR2 in the pathogenesis of bronchiolitis obliterans syndrome. J Clin Invest 2001; 108:547–556.

169. Belperio JA, DiGiovine B, Keane MP, Burdick MD, Ying Xue Y, Ross DJ, Lynch JP, 3rd, Kunkel SL, Strieter RM. Interleukin-1 receptor antagonist as a biomarker for bronchiolitis obliterans syndrome in lung transplant recipients. Transplantation 2002; 73:591–599.

170. Elssner A, Jaumann F, Dobmann S, Behr J, Schwaiblmair M, Reichenspurner H, Furst H, Briegel J, Vogelmeier C. Elevated levels of interleukin-8 and transforming growth factor-beta in bronchoalveolar lavage fluid from patients with bronchiolitis obliterans syndrome: proinflammatory role of bronchial epithelial cells. Munich Lung Transplant Group. Transplantation 2000; 70:362–367.

171. Fattal-German M, Le Roy Ladurie F, Cerrina J, Lecerf F, Berrih-Aknin S. Expression and modulation of ICAM-1, TNF-alpha and RANTES in human alveolar macrophages from lung-transplant recipients in vitro. Transplant Immunol 1998; 6:183–192.

172. Reynaud-Gaubert M, Thomas P, Gregoire R, Badier M, Cau P, Sampol J, Giudicelli R, Fuentes P. Clinical utility of bronchoalveolar lavage cell phenotype analyses in the postoperative monitoring of lung transplant recipients. Eur J Cardiothorac Surg 2002;. 21:60–66.

173. Boehler A, Bai XH, Liu M, Cassivi S, Chamberlain D, Slutsky AS, Keshavjee S. Upregulation of T-helper 1 cytokines and chemokine expression in post-transplant airway obliteration. Am J Respir Crit Care Med 1999; 159:1910–1917.

174. Boehler A, Chamberlain D, Xing Z, Slutsky AS, Jordana M, Gauldie J, Liu M, Keshavjee S. Adenovirus-mediated interleukin-10 gene transfer inhibits post-transplant fibrous airway obliteration in an animal model of bronchiolitis obliterans. Hum Gene Ther 1998; 9:541–551.

175. Belperio JA, Burdick MD, Keane MP, Xue YY, Lynch JP, 3rd, Daugherty BL, Kunkel SL, Strieter RM. The role of the CC chemokine, RANTES, in acute lung allograft rejection. J Immunol 2000; 165:461–472.

176. El-Gamel A, Sim E, Hasleton P, Hutchinson J, Yonan N, Egan J, Campbell C, Rahman A, Sheldon S, Deiraniya A, Hutchinson IV. Transforming growth factor beta (TGF-beta) and obliterative bronchiolitis following pulmonary transplantation. J Heart Lung Transplant 1999; 18:828–837.

177. Glanville AR, Tazelaar HD, Theodore J, Imoto E, Rouse RV, Baldwin JC, Robin ED. The distribution of MHC class I and II antigens on bronchial epithelium. Am Rev Respir Dis 1989; 139:330–334.

178. Beaumont F, Schilizzi BM, Kallenberg CG, DeLey L. Expression of class II-MHC antigens on alveolar and bronchiolar epithelial cells in fibrosing alveolitis. Chest 1986; 89:136.

179. Duncan SR, Valentine V, Roglic M, Elias DJ, Pekny KW, Theodore J, Kono DH, Theofilopoulos AN. T cell receptor biases and clonal proliferations among lung transplant recipients with obliterative bronchiolitis. J Clin Invest 1996; 97:2642–2650.

180. Duncan SR, Leonard C, Theodore J, Lega M, Girgis RE, Rosen GD, Theofilopoulos AN. Oligoclonal CD4(+) T cell expansions in lung transplant recipients with obliterative bronchiolitis. Am J Respir Crit Care Mcd 2002; 165:1439–1444.

181. Leonard CT, Soccal PM, Singer L, Berry GJ, Theodore J, Holt PG, Doyle RL, Rosen GD. Dendritic cells and macrophages in lung allografts: a role in chronic rejection? Am J Respir Crit Care Med 2000; 161:1349–1354.

182. Ward C, Whitford H, Snell G, Bao H, Zheng L, Reid D, Williams TJ, Walters EH. Bronchoalveolar lavage macrophage and lymphocyte phenotypes in lung transplant recipients. J Heart Lung Transplant 2001; 20:1064–1074.

183. Yamada A, Konishi K, Cruz GL, Takehara M, Morikawa M, Nakagawa I, Murakami M, Abe T, Todo S, Uede T. Blocking the CD28-B7 T-cell costimulatory pathway abrogates the development of obliterative bronchiolitis in a murine heterotopic airway model. Transplantation 2000; 69:743–749.

184. Szeto WY, Krasinskas AM, Kreisel D, Popma SH, Rosengard BR. Donor antigen-presenting cells are important in the development of obliterative airway disease. J Thorac Cardiovasc Surg 2000; 120:1070–1077.

185. Lukacs NW, Hogaboam C, Chensue SW, Blease K, Kunkel SL. Type 1/type 2 cytokine paradigm and the progression of pulmonary fibrosis. Chest 2001; 120:5S–8S.

186. Selman M, King TE, Pardo A. Idiopathic pulmonary fibrosis: prevailing and evolving hypotheses about its pathogenesis and implications for therapy. Ann Intern Med 2001; 134:136–151.

187. Lynch III JP, Toews G. Idiopathic pulmonary fibrosis. In: Fishman AP, Elias JA, Fishman JA, Grippi MA, Kaiser LR, Senior RB, eds. Pulmonary Diseases and Disorders. New York: McGraw-Hill, 1998; pp 1069–1084.

188. Takizawa H, Ohta K, Horiuchi T, Suzuki N, Ueda T, Yamaguchi M, Yamashita N, Ishii A, Suko M, Okudaira H, et al. Hypersensitivity pneumonitis in athymic nude mice. Additional evidence of T cell dependency. Am Rev Respir Dis 1992; 146:479–484.

189. Christensen PJ, Goodman RE, Pastoriza L, Moore B, Toews GB. Induction of lung fibrosis in the mouse by intratracheal instillation of fluorescein isothiocyanate is not T-cell-dependent. Am J Pathol 1999; 155:1773–1779.

190. Hogaboam CM, Blease K, Mehrad B, Steinhauser ML, Standiford TJ, Kunkel SL, Lukacs NW. Chronic airway hyperreactivity, goblet cell hyperplasia, and peribronchial fibrosis during allergic airway disease induced by *Aspergillus fumigatus*. Am J Pathol 2000; 156:723–732.

191. Selman M. Idiopathic pulmonary fibrosis challenges for the future. Chest 2001; 120:8–10.

192. Crystal RG, Bitterman PB, Mossman B, Schwarz MI, Sheppard D, Almasy L, Chapman HA, Friedman SL, King TE, Jr., Leinwand LA, Liotta L, Martin GR, Schwartz DA, Schultz GS, Wagner CR, Musson RA. Future research directions in idiopathic pulmonary fibrosis: summary of a National Heart, Lung, and Blood Institute working group. Am J Respir Crit Care Med 2002; 166:236–246.

193. Pardo A, Selman M. Idiopathic pulmonary fibrosis: new insights in its pathogenesis. Int J Biochem Cell Biol 2002; 34:1534–1538.

194. Zhang K, Rekhter MD, Gordon D, Phan SH. Myofibroblasts and their role in lung collagen gene expression during pulmonary fibrosis. A combined immunohistochemical and in situ hybridization study. Am J Pathol 1994; 145:114–125.

195. Lukacs NW, Kunkel SL, Allen R, Evanoff HL, Shaklee CL, Sherman JS, Burdick MD, Strieter RM. Stimulus and cell-specific expression of C-X-C and C-C chemokines by pulmonary stromal cell populations. Am J Physiol 1995; 268:L856–861.

196. Chensue SW, Warmington K, Ruth J, Lincoln P, Kuo MC, Kunkel SL. Cytokine responses during mycobacterial and schistosomal antigen-induced pulmonary granuloma formation. Production of Th1 and Th2 cytokines and relative contribution of tumor necrosis factor. Am J Pathol 1994; 145:1105–1113.

197. Chen ES, Greenlee BS, Wills-Karp M, Moller DR. Bleomycin-induced pulmonary fibrosis is attenuated in interferon-gamma knockout mice. Chest 2001; 120(suppl):8S.

198. Keane MP, Belperio JA, Burdick MD, Strieter RM. Interleukin-12 attenuates pulmonary fibrosis via induction of interferon-gamma. Chest 2001; 120(suppl):8S.

199. Huaux F, Liu T, McGarry B, Ullenbruch M, Phan SH. Dual roles of IL-4 in lung injury and fibrosis. J Immunol 2003; 170:2083–2092.

200. Izbicki G, Or R, Christensen TG, Segel MJ, Fine A, Goldstein RH, Breuer R. Bleomycin-induced lung fibrosis in IL-4-overexpressing and knockout mice. Am J Physiol Lung Cell Mol Physiol 2002; 283:L1110–1116.

201. Kapanci Y, Desmouliere A, Pache JC, Redard M, Gabbiani G. Cytoskeletal protein modulation in pulmonary alveolar myofibroblasts during idiopathic pulmonary fibrosis. Possible role of transforming growth factor beta and tumor necrosis factor alpha. Am J Respir Crit Care Med 1995; 152:2163–2169.

202. Zhang Y, Lee TC, Guillemin B, Yu MC, Rom WN. Enhanced IL-1 beta and tumor necrosis factor-alpha release and messenger RNA expression in macrophages from idiopathic pulmonary fibrosis or after asbestos exposure. J Immunol 1993; 150:4188–4196.

203. Piguet PF, Ribaux C, Karpuz V, Grau GE, Kapanci Y. Expression and localization of tumor necrosis factor-alpha and its mRNA in idiopathic pulmonary fibrosis. Am J Pathol 1993; 143:651–655.

204. Whyte M, Hubbard R, Meliconi R, Whidborne M, Eaton V, Bingle C, Timms J, Duff G, Facchini A, Pacilli A, Fabbri M, Hall I, Britton J, Johnston I, Di Giovine F. Increased risk of fibrosing alveolitis associated with interleukin-1 receptor antagonist and tumor necrosis factor-alpha gene polymorphisms. Am J Respir Crit Care Med 2000; 162:755–758.

205. Piguet P, Collart M, Grau G, Kapanci Y, Vassalli P. Tumor necrosis factor/cachectin plays a key role in bleomycin-induced pneumopathy and fibrosis. J Exp Med 1989; 170:655–663.

206. Ortiz L, Lasky J, Lungarella G, Cavarra E, Martorana P, Banks W, Peschon J, Schmidts H-L, Brody A, Friedman M. Upregulation of the p75 but not the p55 TNFa receptor mRNA after silica and bleomycin exposure and protectin from lung injury in double receptor knockout mice. Am J Respir Cell Mol Biol 1999; 20:825–833.

207. Smith RE, Strieter RM, Phan SH, Lukacs N, Kunkel SL. TNF and IL-6 mediate MIP-1alpha expression in bleomycin-induced lung injury. J Leukoc Biol 1998; 64:528–536.

208. Moore BB, Paine R, 3rd, Christensen PJ, Moore TA, Sitterding S, Ngan R, Wilke CA, Kuziel WA, Toews GB. Protection from pulmonary fibrosis in the absence of CCR2 signaling. J Immunol 2001; 167:4368–4377.
209. Piguet P, Vesin C. Treatment by human recombinant soluble TNF receptor of pulmonary fibrosis induced by bleomycin or silica in mice. Eur Respir J 1994; 7:515–518.
210. Sime P, Marr R, Gauldie D, Xing Z, Hewlett B, Graham F, Gauldie J. Transfer of tumor necrosis factor-α to rat lung induces severe pulmonary inflammation and patchy interstitial fibrogenesis with induction of transforming growth factor-β1 and myofibroblasts. Am J Pathol 1998; 153:825–832.
211. Miyazaki Y, Araki K, Vesin C, Garcia I, Kapanci Y, Whitsett J, Piguet P-F, Vassalli P. Expression of a tumor necrosis factor-α transgene in murine lung causes lymphocytic and fibrosing alveolitis. J Clin Invest 1995; 96:250–259.
212. Nakama K, Miyazaki Y, Nasu M. Immunophenotyping of lymphocytes in the lung interstitium and expression of osteopontin and interleukin-2 mRNAs in two different murine models of pulmonary fibrosis. Exp Lung Res 1998; 24:57–70.
213. Trisolini R, Bandini G, Stanzani M, Chilosi M, Cancellieri A, Boaron M, Poletti V. Morphologic changes leading to bronchiolitis obliterans in a patient with delayed non-infectious lung disease after allogeneic bone marrow transplantation. Bone Marrow Transplant 2001; 28:1167–1170.
214. Selman M, Pardo A. Idiopathic pulmonary fibrosis: an epithelial/fibroblastic cross-talk disorder. Respir Res 2002; 3:3.
215. Sumitomo M, Sakiyama S, Tanida N, Fukumoto T, Monden Y, Uyama T. Difference in cytokine production in acute and chronic rejection of rat lung allografts. Transplant Int 1996; 9:S223–225.
216. Christensen PJ, Rolfe MW, Standiford TJ, Burdick MD, Toews GB, Streiter RM. Characterization of the production of monocyte chemoattractant protein-1 and IL-8 in allogeneic immune response. J Immunol 1993; 151:1205–1213.
217. Antoniades HN, Neville-Golden J, Galanopoulos T, Kradin RL, Valente AJ, Graves DT. Expression of monocyte chemoattractant protein 1 mRNA in human idiopathic pulmonary fibrosis. Proc Natl Acad Sci USA 1992; 89:5371–5375.
218. Iyonaga K, Takeya M, Saita N, Sakamoto O, Yoshimura T, Ando M, Takahashi K. Monocyte chemoattractant protein-1 in idiopathic pulmonary fibrosis and other interstitial lung diseases. Hum Pathol 1994; 25:455–463.
219. Standiford TJ, Rolfe MR, Kunkel SL, Lynch JP, 3rd, Becker FS, Orringer MB, Phan S, Strieter RM. Altered production and regulation of monocyte chemoattractant protein-1 from pulmonary fibroblasts isolated from patients with idiopathic pulmonary fibrosis. Chest 1993; 103:121S.
220. Rabitsch W, Deviatko E, Keil F, Herold C, Dekan G, Greinix HT, Lechner K, Klepetko W, Kalhs P. Successful lung transplantation for bronchiolitis obliterans after allogeneic marrow transplantation. Transplantation 2001; 71:1341–1343.
221. Payne L, Chan CK, Fyles G, Hyland RH, Bafundi P, Yeung M, Messner H. Cyclosporine as possible prophylaxis for obstructive airways disease after allogeneic bone marrow transplantation. Chest 1993; 104:114–118.
222. Whitford H, Walters EH, Levvey B, Kotsimbos T, Orsida B, Ward C, Pais M, Reid S, Williams T, Snell G. Addition of inhaled corticosteroids to systemic immunosuppression after lung transplantation: a double-blind, placebo-controlled trial. Transplantation 2002; 73:1793–1799.
223. Niden A, Koss MN, Boylen CT, Azizi N, Chan K. An open label pilot study to determine the potential efficacy of TNFR:Fc (Enbrel, etanercept) in the treatment of usual interstitial pneumonitis. Am J Respir Crit Care Med 2002; 165:A728.
224. Chiang KY, Abhyankar S, Bridges K, Godder K, Henslee-Downey JP. Recombinant human tumor necrosis factor receptor fusion protein as complementary treatment for chronic graft-versus-host disease. Transplantation 2002; 73:665–667.

12

Clinical Spectrum of Acute Graft-vs.-Host Disease

JOSEPH H. ANTIN

Harvard Medical School and Dana-Farber Cancer Institute, Boston, Massachusetts, U.S.A.

H. JOACHIM DEEG

Fred Hutchinson Cancer Research Center and University of Washington, Seattle, Washington, U.S.A.

I. INTRODUCTION

Pioneering studies in mice in the 1950s showed that animals irradiated with otherwise lethal doses of total body irradiation (TBI) would survive if the spleen was shielded from irradiation (1,2) or if bone marrow was infused following TBI (3). Subsequent studies showed that the infused bone marrow cells reestablished lymphohematopoiesis in the irradiated mice, but the animals generally still died, albeit later than would have been expected from marrow failure. The syndrome leading to delayed mortality was termed "secondary disease" (4,5) and clinically resembled strongly what was described by Billingham and Brent (6) as "runt disease." These investigators described diarrhea, weight loss, skin breakdown, sparse fur, odd gait, and retarded growth in unirradiated, neonatal mice transplanted with cells from genetically different donors. Both syndromes were shown to be caused by immunocompetent cells from the donor, hence the current term graft-vs.-host reaction (GvHR) and the clinical manifestations, graft-vs.-host disease (GVHD) (7–10). The first observation of GVHD in humans by George Mathé in 1960 was made after marrow cells were used to treat survivors of a nuclear accident in Belgrade, Yugoslavia (11).

The form of GVHD occurring early after transplantation is referred to as acute GVHD, while a later form with different clinical characteristics has been termed chronic

GVHD. For purposes of clinical investigation, the two forms were distinguished by time of onset—less than 100 days after transplantation was considered acute, and more than 100 days chronic (12). However, a clear distinction between acute and chronic forms of GVHD as described originally may no longer be tenable. Observations in patients transplanted with reduced intensity regimens or in patients receiving donor lymphocyte infusions at various time intervals after transplantation indicate that patients may have manifestations of acute GVHD several months after transplantation and GVHD with chronic clinical and histological characteristics can occur as early as 50 or 60 days after transplantation. It will be necessary to incorporate these insights into new grading schemes, which will, presumably, also consider a time component.

II. DESCRIPTION AND DIAGNOSIS

GVHD is characterized by a clinicopathological syndrome involving the skin, liver, or gastrointestinal tract, and possibly other organs. Any organ can be affected alone or in combination with other organs. GVHD is a clinical diagnosis—there are no laboratory tests that will confirm or refute its presence. Rather, the diagnosis of GVHD requires an interpretation of clinical and laboratory findings, recognizing that in some patients the differential diagnosis may be impossible to resolve. For instance, an elevated direct bilirubin is a relatively nonspecific abnormality, yet it is the principal criterion for the diagnosis of hepatic GVHD. In the absence of a biopsy the likelihood of mistakenly ascribing this finding to either GVHD or to other transplant-related toxicities is high. As it is often difficult to obtain an adequate tissue biopsy after transplantation, the physician or investigator is left to make a clinical judgment. Diarrhea may be due to infections, related to conditioning, drug toxicity, or GVHD. Similarly, particularly with mild or limited rashes, it can be very difficult to distinguish GVHD from a drug eruption, even on histology.

A recent multicenter phase III trial used an independent committee to assess the presence and severity of GVHD. The incidence of GVHD as determined by investigators was substantially higher than the review committee could confirm (13). Similarly, Martin and colleagues found substantial interobserver variability in assigning GVHD severity grades (14). Nevertheless, for an experienced clinician a combination of physical and laboratory findings in the appropriate context provides a working diagnosis of GVHD that is satisfactory to produce a meaningful prognostic scale (15).

III. TIME OF ONSET OF GVHD

Timing of the onset of symptoms is important. As noted above, acute GVHD generally occurs within 14–35 days of stem cell infusion. The time of onset may depend upon the degree of histocompatibility, the number of donor T cells infused, and the prophylactic regimen for GVHD. A hyperacute form of GVHD may occur in patients with severe HLA mismatches or in patients who do not receive GVHD prophylaxis (16). Hyperacute GVHD is manifested by fever, generalized erythroderma and desquamation, often edema, and may be rapidly fatal. The median time of onset is about one week after stem cell infusion. In patients receiving more conventional GVHD prophylaxis such as a combination of cyclosporine and methotrexate, the median onset of GVHD is typically 21–25 days after transplantation; however, after in vitro T-cell depletion of the graft the onset may be much later (17). Thus, findings of rash and diarrhea by one week would be likely manifestations of hyperacute GVHD if minimal or ineffective prophylaxis were administered; the same kinetics would be very unlikely with calcineurin inhibitors or in vitro T-cell depletion.

IV. SKIN MANIFESTATIONS

The most common manifestation of GVHD is a maculopapular, erythematous exanthema often involving palms and soles. Involvement of the palms is a particularly useful clinical hint, since drug eruptions are less likely to appear on the palms. However, a painful, blistering acral erythema can be related to conditioning therapy (e.g., TBI) and must be distinguished from acute GVHD. Acral erythema due to conditioning usually occurs in the second week and resembles a second-degree burn (18). GVHD may be asymptomatic, pruritic, or painful. It typically starts on the upper body—shoulders, face, arms, behind the ears—most commonly in sun-exposed areas. A skin biopsy may be helpful in substantiating the clinical diagnosis, but it cannot in and of itself prove the presence of GVHD. In its mildest manifestation, GVHD may involve less than one fourth of the body surface, but in its most severe form it can progress to whole-body erythema, gross bullae formation, and sloughing of the skin. Mild GVHD often responds to modest doses of corticosteroids (1–2 mg/kg/day) or other immunosuppressants. In its severe forms GVHD can be difficult to distinguish from Stevens-Johnson syndrome or toxic epidermal necrolysis. The loss of integrity of the integument leads to a markedly increased risk of infection with normal skin flora such as *Staphylococcus aureus* and *Staphylococcus epidermidis* as well as with gram-negative rods and fungi. In severe GVHD pain control, fluid and electrolyte replacement, metabolic support, and infection control are quite similar to the management of patients with severe burns.

Mucositis was not part of the classic description of acute GVHD. However, if infection is excluded with appropriate cultures, mucosal lesions that fail to heal with hematological recovery may well signify mucosal GVHD.

V. LIVER INVOLVEMENT

Hepatic GVHD is graded on the basis of the total bilirubin level. In addition, alkaline phosphatase is usually elevated, and there are less consistent abnormalities of transaminases. There are data to suggest that acute GVHD occurring after donor lymphocyte infusions, i.e., with some delay after transplantation, may be more likely to take the form of "hepatitic" GVHD (19). However, none of the routine serological tests of liver injury is definitive, and only the total bilirubin level is considered in GVHD grading. Mild GVHD may result only in a three- to fourfold rise in bilirubin with or without transaminase elevations, while the most severely affected patients may have serum bilirubin levels higher than 10 mg/dL and in extreme cases show a loss of liver synthetic function. The lack of a truly diagnostic test means that the diagnosis of hepatic GVHD on clinical grounds only may be quite tenuous. Drug toxicity, parenteral nutrition, hepatic veno-occlusive disease, infection, cholangitis lenta, cholelithiasis, acalculous cholecystitis, and other unrelated conditions can either coexist with or be confused with hepatic GVHD. In contrast to veno-occlusive disease, hepatic GVHD only rarely leads to weight gain, capsular pain, or ascites. Many infections can results in elevations of bilirubin. Infections with gram-negative organisms may increase bilirubin in the absence of hepatic infection per se. The presence of cytomegalovirus (CMV) may be particularly confusing, since CMV infection often occurs concomitantly with GVHD. Drugs such as cyclosporine and estrogens are some of the notorious hepatotoxins after stem cell transplantation.

Hepatic GVHD is more difficult to diagnose than cutaneous involvement. Percutaneous liver biopsies are associated with potentially prohibitive risks. Transvenous biopsies have been associated with a reasonable low morbidity and, if results are unequivocal, can result in alterations of the clinical diagnosis in almost 50% of patients (20,21). However, the small specimen size may still cause diagnostic uncertainty.

VI. INTESTINAL INVOLVEMENT

Involvement of the gut may be manifested by nausea, anorexia, pain, and watery, secretory diarrhea. In severe cases there may be failure of intestinal function resulting in protein-losing enteropathy, with hypoalbuminemia, bloody diarrhea, or frank ileus. The combination of major fluid losses through damaged skin and decreased hepatic synthetic function with massive diarrhea renders management extremely difficult. Frequent evaluation of blood, urine, and stool electrolytes and careful input and output measurements are a necessity. Infection, conditioning-related toxicity, lactose intolerance, and non-specific mucosal damage may either mimic gut GVHD or be present concurrently with GVHD, thus substantially complicating patient management. In contrast to skin histopathology, the histology of rectal and gastric mucosal biopsies is more specific or even pathognomonic such that therapeutic approaches can be targeted more narrowly (22–24).

Isolated gastric GVHD is rather common after stem cell transplantation. It must be distinguished from herpesvirus infection, candidiasis, and nonspecific gastritis (22,25,26). Gastric or upper gastrointestinal GVHD can occur alone or in conjunction with other organ involvement. When it occurs alone, it is commonly the cause of otherwise unexplained nausea and vomiting. Esophagoduodenogastroscopy and mucosal biopsies will usually lead to the correct diagnosis. GVHD of the upper intestinal tract tends to be relatively sensitive to corticosteroid therapy.

Radiographic findings of intestinal GVHD are nonspecific but include increased bowel wall thickness and increased vascularity and fluid-filled loops of bowel. An MRI may show generalized increased bowel wall thickness associated with bowel wall enhancement after administration of gadolinium (27,28).

VII. OTHER ORGANS

Whether GVHD affects organs other than the classic triad of skin, liver, and gut has remained controversial. However, numerous reports suggest additional organ manifestations. The most likely candidate is the lung. Lung toxicity including interstitial pneumonitis and diffuse alveolar hemorrhage may occur in 20–60% of allogeneic transplant recipients but in fewer autologous transplant recipients. Causes of pulmonary damage other than GVHD include "engraftment syndrome," infection, radiation pneumonitis, and chemotherapy toxicity (including methotrexate). At least one retrospective analysis failed to link severe pulmonary complications to clinical acute GVHD per se (29). The mortality of pneumonia increases with the severity of GVHD, but this association does not necessarily imply that the GVHD, as opposed to the concomitant immunosuppression and treatment, is causative. A particular histopathological syndrome of lymphocytic bronchitis has been attributed directly to GVHD (30), although this has not been confirmed by others. Nevertheless, the lungs are likely targets of GVHD because of their extensive reticuloendothelial system and direct exposure to the environment. Mouse transplant models do support the hypothesis that the lungs are a GVHD target (see Chapter 11). In addition, other chronic post-HSCT pulmonary syndromes, especially bronchiolitis obliterans, may represent manifestations of chronic GVHD (see Chapter 20).

Although renal and urinary tract symptoms commonly occur after transplantation, they are generally attributable to the conditioning regimen, the use of immunosuppressive agents, or infection. There is no convincing evidence for a role of GVHD. Similarly, neurological complications are common after transplantation but most can be attributed to drug toxicity, infection, or vascular insults. Nevertheless, data on vasculitis of the central nervous system (CNS), possibly associated with GVHD have been presented (30a,b).

VIII. HISTOPATHOLOGY

Histological manifestations of acute GVHD typically involve apoptosis of cells in the tissue layer responsible for proliferation and regeneration. In the skin the dermal-epidermal junction is most severely affected, while in the intestinal tract the main targets are the bases of the crypts. Skin involvement is reflected in epidermal and basal cell vacuolar degeneration, disorganization of epidermal cell maturation, eosinophilic body formation, and melanocyte incontinence (31–34). Hepatic small bile ducts may show segmental disruption, injury to the periductular epithelium bile duct atypia, and cellular degeneration. Cholestasis may be present (35,36). Mucosal ulcerations and crypt destruction are present in the intestinal tract. The colon is more frequently involved than the ileum and shows crypt cell apoptosis and dropout with flattening of the villous architecture (23,35,36). Mucosal ulcerations and crypt destruction are present in the intestinal tract. The colon is more frequently involved than the ileum and shows crypt cell apoptosis and dropout with flattening of the villous architecture (23). Typically, mononuclear cell infiltrates are subtle, often surprisingly mild compared with the degree of clinical illness.

IX. ENGRAFTMENT SYNDROME

A clinical entity worth noting is a constellation of findings including fever, erythematous skin rash, and low-pressure pulmonary edema that may occur during neutrophil recovery but may reflect the dysregulated production of inflammatory cytokines and the cellular response to these molecules. These clinical problems have been termed engraftment syndrome or capillary leak syndrome, and they are recognized most clearly after autologous transplantation (37–39). In allogeneic transplant recipients distinction from acute GVHD is difficult. Although this syndrome is thought to reflect cellular and cytokine activity during early recovery of blood cell counts, precise delineation of the offending cells and cytokines has not been accomplished. Engraftment syndromes may be associated with increased mortality, primarily from pulmonary failure but also from associated multi-organ dysfunction. Corticosteroid therapy may be effective particularly for the treatment of pulmonary manifestations (40).

X. DIFFERENTIAL DIAGNOSIS

The differential diagnosis of rashes, diarrhea, and liver function abnormalities can be difficult to resolve. Skin rashes may reflect delayed reactions to the conditioning regimen, reactions to antibiotics, infections, or allergic reactions. Histopathological skin changes consistent with mild to moderate acute GVHD are mimicked by the effects of the chemo-radiotherapy and drug reactions (41). Some diarrhea is expected after TBI. Viral infection, especially with CMV and other herpesviruses, parasites, *C. difficile*, nonspecific gastritis, and drug reactions, can mimic GVHD of the gut. Liver dysfunction can be due to parenteral nutrition, veno-occlusive disease, viral hepatitis, and drug-induced hepatitis (including cyclosporine, estrogens, and antifungal agents). Finally, it may be impossible to discriminate between multiple possible causes since concomitant infection and GVHD is the rule rather than the exception (42–44).

XI. RISK FACTORS FOR THE DEVELOPMENT OF ACUTE GVHD

While in vitro predictive tests for GVHD have been described (45–47), they have not been widely adopted because the results have been difficult to reproduce (48,49). Efforts to assign risk based on donor or recipient polymorphisms of the CD31, CD54, interleukin (IL)-1 receptor antagonist, IL-10, IL-6, or tumor necrosis factor (TNF) genes (or their promoter regions) have not resulted in reliable, reproducible models (50–54).

The principal risk factor for the development of GVHD in humans is histoincompatibility. Functionally, histoincompatibility is most important when crossing MHC (major histocompatibility) barriers. Presumably the risk of GVHD in fully HLA-identical recipients of either family member or unrelated donor stem cells is due to differences in minor histocompatibility antigens. At present we are severely limited in our ability to assess these antigens. Male recipients express unique antigens encoded on the Y chromosome termed H-Y antigens. These H-Y antigens can be recognized as foreign by female donor cells in the context of HLA compatibility and trigger GVHD. The effect is most profound if the female donor has been allosensitized, generally by a prior pregnancy (55–57). Other minor antigens include HA-1 and probably a host of MHC restricted antigens that have not yet been identified (58–60).

Additional risk factors for the development of acute GVHD include older age of recipient, older age of donor, prior donor transfusions, disease stage, and conditioning regimen (57,61–66). More controversial risk factors include certain HLA types (64,67), splenectomy (61,68), exposure to herpesviruses (44), CD34 cell dose (62), and ABO incompatibility (69).

XII. STAGING AND GRADING OF ACUTE GVHD

Involvement of each organ is staged independently, and the composite score of liver, gut, and skin involvement is considered the GVHD grade. Pathologists have developed histological grading systems to provide a semiquantitative estimate of severity. The histological grade must not be confused with the clinical grade of GVHD. The original grading system was proposed by the Seattle group in 1974 (12); it was modified subsequently into a "consensus" system (Table 1) (70) and complemented by the International Bone Marrow Transplant Registry (IBMTR) GVHD severity index (Table 2) (15). This IBMTR system has been validated in a retrospective analysis, and severity as determined by this system is reflected in the incidence of transplant-related mortality. IBMTR levels A, B, C, and D roughly correspond to Glucksberg grades I, II, III, and IV, respectively (14).

Table 1 Consensus Grading of Acute GVHD

	Organ/extent of involvement		
	Skin	Liver	Intestinal tract
Stage			
1	Rash on <25% of skin[a]	Bilirubin 2–3 mg/dL[b]	Diarrhea >500 mL/day[c] or persistent nausea[d]
2	Rash on 25–50% of skin	Bilirubin 3–6 mg/dL	Diarrhea >1000 mL/day
3	Rash on >50% of skin	Bilirubin 6–15 mg/dL	Diarrhea >1500 mL/day
4	Generalized erythroderma with bulla formation	Bilirubin >15 mg/dL	Severe abdominal pain with or without ileus
Grade			
0	None	None	None
I	Stage 1–2	None	None
II	Stage 3	or Stage 1	or Stage 1
III	—	Stage 2–3	or Stage 2–4
IV[e]	Stage 4	or Stage 4	—

[a]Use the "rule of nines" to determine body surface area involvement.
[b]Range given as total bilirubin. Downgrade one stage if an additional cause of elevated bilirubin has been documented.
[c]Volume of diarrhea applies to adults. For pediatric patients, the volume of diarrhea should be based on body surface area.
[d]Persistent nausea with histological evidence of GVHD in the stomach or duodenum.
[e]Grade IV may also include lesser organ involvement but with extreme decrease in performance status.
Source: Ref. 70.

GVHD grading is important for the conduct of clinical trials and for its prognostic information. Mild to moderate GVHD [grades I or II (A or B)] is associated with little morbidity, but is a significant risk factor for the development of chronic GVHD (71). Grades III and IV (C and D) GVHD carry a grave prognosis. In patients with grade IV GVHD (severity index D), mortality is 90–100%.

Table 2 IBMTR Severity Index for Acute GVHD

Index	Skin stage		Gut stage		Liver stage
0	0		0		0
A	1	and	0	and	0
B	≤2		≤1	and/or	≤1[a]
	2	and	0	and	0
	≤2	and	≤2	and/or	≤2[b]
C	3	and	≤1	and	≤1
	≤3	and/or	≤3	and/or	≤3[c]
D	≤4	and/or	≤4	and/or	≤4[d]

[a]Either gut or liver = 1 but neither >1.
[b]Any organ = 2 but none >2.
[c]Any organ = 3 but none >3.
[d]Any organ = 4.
Source: Ref. 15.

XIII. SYNGENEIC AND AUTOLOGOUS GVHD

Occasionally, patients undergoing autologous or syngeneic transplants will develop a clinical picture similar to GVHD. It is primarily manifest as a rash that usually responds promptly to corticosteroid therapy, although a recent report suggests there may also be hepatic involvement (72). The development of such a syndrome in the absence of an allogeneic barrier may be interpreted as evidence of a loss of tolerance to "self" that develops in the disrupted immune system. Hess and colleagues have proposed that infused T cells recognize MHC class II antigens in association with a peptide from the invariant chain (CLIP) (73,74). It is also possible that some cases of syngeneic GVHD reflected a mistaken assumption that the donor was syngeneic without extensive molecular confirmation. An additional hypothesis was proposed recently by Nelson and colleagues (74a). These investigators showed that maternal cells transmitted to the fetus remain present in some individuals throughout adult life. This suggests the possibility that in some instances small numbers of HLA-incompatible cells may be transmitted even with HLA-identical transplants. Maternal cells may also play a role in the development of neonatal GVHD (74b,c).

XIV. TRANSFUSION-ASSOCIATED GVHD

Most blood products administered to immunocompromised patients are now irradiated or at least leukocyte depleted to avoid the transfusion of viable alloreactive T cells. In most homologous blood products, the MHC incompatibility between donor and recipient results in rapid clearance of transfused T cells. However, occasionally transfusions from donors homozygous for one of the recipient MHC haplotypes cannot be recognized as foreign by the recipient. These cells survive and may mount an immunological attack against the unshared haplotype, resulting in transfusion-associated GVHD (75,76). This syndrome of transfusion-associated GVHD differs from GVHD occurring after hematopoietic stem cell transplantation (HSCT) in regard to its kinetics but also in regard to its manifestations in so far as the recipient marrow is a major target. This syndrome is usually fatal. Death frequently results from refractory pancytopenia in addition to other organ involvement.

XV. SUMMARY AND CONCLUSION

Acute GVHD is a complex clinical syndrome that occurs in a setting where the diagnosis may be difficult to establish. However, it is extremely important to recognize the disease, since the survival of patients may well depend on the accuracy of the clinical diagnosis and prompt institution of therapy. It is not unusual for a patient with an elevated bilirubin to be treated aggressively with corticosteroids and to die of an opportunistic infection, only to discover at postmortem examination that liver dysfunction was due to other causes. There are no simple laboratory crutches that facilitate the task. The diagnosis is left to clinical acumen supported by tissue biopsies where possible.

REFERENCES

1. Jacobsen LO, Simmons EL, Marks EL, et al. The role of the spleen in radiation injury and recovery. J Lab Clin Med 1950; 35:746.

2. Barnes DWH, Loutit JF. Spleen protection: the cellular hypothesis. In: Bacq ZM, Alexander P, eds. Radiobiology Symposium 1954. New York: Academic Press; 1955. p. 134.

3. Lorenz E, Uphoff D, Reid TR, et al. Modification of irradiation injury in mice and guinea pigs by bone marrow injections. J Natl Cancer Inst 1951; 12:197.

4. Barnes DWH, Loutit JF. Immunological and histological response following spleen treatment in irradiated mice. In: Mitchel JS, Holmes BE, and SCL, eds. Progress in Radiobiology. Edinburgh: Oliver and Boyd; 1956. p. 291.

5. Santos GW. The history of bone marrow transplantation. Clin Haematol 1983; 12:611–639.

6. Billingham RE, Brent LA. A simple method for inducing tolerance of skin homografts in mice. Transplant Bull 1957; 4:67.

7. Elkins WL. Cellular immunology and pathogenesis of graft-versus-host reaction. Prog Allergy 1971; 15:78–187.

8. Simonsen M. Graft versus host reactions. Their natural history and applicability as tools of research. Prog Allergy 1971; 6:349.

9. Van Bekkum D, De Vries M. Radiation Chimeras. New York: Academic Press; 1967.

10. Billingham RE. The biology of graft-versus-host reactions. Harvey Lecture Series 1966–1967; 62:21.

11. Mathe G, Jammet H, Pendic B, Schwartzenberg L, Duplan J-F, Maupin B, et al. Transfusions et greffes de moelle osseuse homologue chez des humans irradies a haute dose accidentelle- ment. Rev Franc Etudes Clin Biol 1959; IV:226.

12. Glucksberg H, Storb R, Fefer A, Buckner CD, Neiman PE, Clift RA, et al. Clinical manifes- tations of graft-versus-host disease in recipients of marrow from HLA-matched sibling donors. Transplantation 1974; 18:295–304.

13. Nash R, Antin J, Karanes C, Fay J, Avalos B, Yeager A, et al. A phase III study comparing methotrexate and tacrolimus with methotrexate and cyclosporine for prophylaxis of acute graft-versus-host disease after marrow transplantation from unrelated donors. Blood 2000; 96:2062–2068.

14. Martin P, Nash R, Sanders J, Leisenring W, Anasetti C, Deeg HJ, et al. Reproducibility in retro- spective grading of acute graft-versus-host disease after allogeneic marrow transplantation. Bone Marrow Transplant 1998; 21:273–279.

15. Rowlings P, Przepiorka D, Klein J, Gale R, Passweig J, Henslee-Downey P, et al. IBMTR severity index for grading acute graft-versus-host disease: retrospective comparison with Glucksberg grade. Br J Haematol 1997; 97:855–864.

16. Sullivan KM, Deeg HJ, Sanders J, et al. Hyperacute graft versus host disease in patients not given immunosuppression after allogeneic marrow transplantation. Blood 1986; 67:1172–1175.

17. Antin JH, Bierer BE, Smith BR, Ferrara J, Guinan EC, Sieff C, et al. Selective depletion of bone marrow T lymphocytes with anti-CD5 monoclonal antibodies: effective prophylaxis for graft-versus-host disease in patients with hematologic malignancies. Blood 1991; 78:2139–2149.

18. Crider M, Jansen J, Norins A, MS M. Chemotherapy-induced acral erythema in patients receiv- ing bone marrow transplantation. Arch Dermatol 1986; 122:1023–1027.

19. Akpek G, Boitnott JK, Lee LA, Hallick JP, Torbenson M, Jacobsohn DA, et al. Hepatitic variant of graft-versus-host disease after donor lymphocyte infusion. Blood 2002; 100:3903–3907.

20. Shulman HM, Gooley T, Dudley MD, Kofler T, Feldman R, Dwyer D, et al. Utility of trans- venous liver biopsies and wedged hepatic venous pressure measurements in sixty marrow transplant recipients. Transplantation 1995; 59:1015–1022.

21. Carreras E, Granena A, Navasa M, Bruguera M, Marco V, Sierra J, et al. Transjugular liver biopsy in BMT. Bone Marrow Transplant 1993; 11:21–26.

22. Weisdorf DJ, Snover DC, Haake R, Miller WJ, McGlave PB, Blazar B, et al. Acute upper gastrointestinal graft-versus-host disease: clinical significance and response to immuno- suppressive therapy. Blood 1990; 76:624–629.

23. Sale GE, Shulman HM, McDonald GB, Thomas ED. Gastrointestinal graft-versus-host disease in man. A clinicopathologic study of the rectal biopsy. Am J Surg Pathol 1979; 3:291–299.

24. Kraus MD, Feran-Doza M, Garcia-Moliner ML, Antin J, Odze RD. Cytomegalovirus infection in the colon of bone marrow transplantation patients. Mod Pathol 1998; 11:29–36.

25. Spencer GD, Hackman RC, McDonald GB, Amos DE, Cunningham BA, Meyers JD, et al. A prospective study of unexplained nausea and vomiting after marrow transplantation. Transplantation 1986; 42:602–607.

26. Wu D, Hockenberry DM, Brentnall TA, Baehr PH, Ponec RJ, Kuver R, et al. Persistent nausea and anorexia after marrow transplantation: a prospective study of 78 patients. Transplantation 1998; 66:1319–1324.

27. Klein SA, Martin H, Schreiber-Dietrich D, Hermann S, Caspary WF, Hoelzer D, et al. A new approach to evaluating intestinal acute graft-versus-host disease by transabdominal sonography and colour Doppler imaging. Br J Haematol 2001; 115:929–934.

28. Mentzel HJ, Kentouche K, Kosmehl H, Gruhn B, Vogt S, Sauerbrey A, et al. US and MRI of gastrointestinal graft-versus-host disease. Pediatr Radiol 2002; 32:195–198.

29. Ho VT, Weller E, Lee SJ, Alyea EP, Antin JH, Soiffer RJ. Prognostic factors for early severe pulmonary complications after hematopoietic stem cell transplantation. Biol Blood Marrow Transplant 2001; 7:223–229.

30. Beschorner WE, Saral R, Hutchins GM, et al. Lymphocytic bronchitis associated with graft versus host disease in recipients of bone marrow transplants. N Engl J Med 1978; 299:1030–1036.

30a. Padovan CS, Bise K, Hahn J, Sostak P, Holler E, Kolb HJ, Straube A. Angiitis of the central nervous system after allogeneic bone marrow transplantation? Stroke 1999; 30:1651–1656.

30b. Takatsuka H, Okamoto T, Yamada S, Fujimori Y, Tamura S, Wada H, Okada M, Takemoto Y, Nishimura H, Tachibana H, Kanamaru A, Kakishita E. New imaging findings in a patient with central nervous system dysfunction after bone marrow transplantation. Acta Haematol 2000; 103: 203–205.

31. Lerner KG, Kao GF, Storb R, Buckner CD, Clift RA, Thomas ED. Histopathology of graft-vs.-host reaction (GvHR) in human recipients of marrow from HL-A-matched sibling donors. Transplant Proc 1974; 6:367–371.

32. Kohler S, Hendrickson MR, Chao NJ, Smoller BR. Value of skin biopsies in assessing prognosis and progression of acute graft-versus-host disease. Am J Surg Pathol 1997; 21:988–996.

33. Zhou Y, Barnett MJ, Rivers JK. Clinical significance of skin biopsies in the diagnosis and management of graft-vs-host disease in early postallogeneic bone marrow transplantation. Arch Dermatol 2000; 136:717–721.

34. Massi D, Franchi A, Pimpinelli N, Laszlo D, Bosi A, Santucci M. A reappraisal of the histopathologic criteria for the diagnosis of cutaneous allogeneic acute graft-vs-host disease. Am J Clin Pathol 1999; 112:791–800.

35. Snover DC, Weisdorf SA, Ramsay NK, McGlave P, Kersey JH. Hepatic graft versus host disease: a study of the predictive value of liver biopsy in diagnosis. Hepatology 1984; 4:123–130.

36. Shulman HM, Sharma P, Amos D, Fenster LF, McDonald GB. A coded histologic study of hepatic graft-versus-host disease after bone marrow transplantation. Hepatology 1988; 8:463–470.

37. Lee C, Gingrich R, Hohl R, Ajram K. Engraftment syndrome in autologous bone marrow and peripheral stem cell transplantation. Bone Marrow Transplant 1995; 16:175–182.

38. Ravoet C, Feremans W, Husson B, Majois F, Kentos A, Lambermont M, et al. Clinical evidence for an engraftment syndrome associated with early and steep neutrophil recovery after autologous blood stem cell transplantation. Bone Marrow Transplant 1996; 18:943–947.

39. Cahill R, Spitzer T, Mazumder A. Marrow engraftment and clinical manifestations of capillary leak syndrome. Bone Marrow Transplant 1996; 18:177–184.

40. Spitzer TR. Engraftment syndrome following hematopoietic stem cell transplantation. Bone Marrow Transplant 2001; 27:893–898.

41. Sviland L, Pearson AD, Eastham EJ, Hamilton PJ, Proctor SJ, Malcolm AJ. Histological features of skin and rectal biopsy specimens after autologous and allogeneic bone marrow transplantation. J Clin Pathol 1988; 41:148–154.

42. Gleichmann E, Gleichmann H. Essential similarity between graft versus host disease and viral infections. Transplantation 1976; 22:399–401.

43. Gratama JW, Zwaan FE, Stijnen T, Weijers TF, Weiland HT, J DA, et al. Herpes-virus immunity and acute graft-versus-host disease. Lancet 1987; 1:471–474.

44. Gratama JW, Sinnige LG, Weijers TF, Zwaan FE, van Heugten JG, Stijnen T, et al. Marrow donor immunity to herpes simplex virus: association with acute graft-versus-host disease. Exp Hematol 1987; 15:735–740.

45. Sviland L, Dickinson AM. A human skin explant model for predicting graft-versus-host disease following bone marrow transplantation. J Clin Pathol 1999; 52:910–913.

46. Vogelsang GB, Hess AD, Berkman AW, Tutschka PJ, Farmer ER, Converse PJ, et al. An in vitro predictive test for graft versus host disease in patients with genotypic HLA-identical bone marrow transplants. N Engl J Med 1985; 313:645–650.

47. Theobald M, Nierle T, Bunjes D, Arnold R, Hempel H. Host-specific interleukin-2-secreting donor T-cell precursors as predictors of acute graft-versus-host disease in bone marrow transplantation between HLA-identical siblings. N Engl J Med 1992; 327:1613–1617.

48. Dickinson AM, Sviland L, Wang XN, Jackson G, Taylor PR, Dunn A, et al. Predicting graft-versus-host disease in HLA-identical bone marrow transplant: a comparison of T-cell frequency analysis and a human skin explant model. Transplantation 1998; 66:857–863.

49. Wang XN, Taylor PR, Skinner R, Jackson GH, Proctor SJ, Hedley D, et al. T-cell frequency analysis does not predict the incidence of graft-versus-host disease in HLA-matched sibling bone marrow transplantation. Transplantation 2000; 70:488–493.

50. Nichols WC, Antin JH, Lunetta KL, Terry VH, Hertel CE, Wheatley MA, et al. Polymorphism of adhesion molecule CD31 is not a significant risk factor for graft-versus-host disease. Blood 1996; 88:4429–4434.

51. Dickinson AM, Cavet J, Cullup H, Wang XN, Sviland L, Middleton PG. GvHD risk assessment in hematopoietic stem cell transplantation: role of cytokine gene polymorphisms and an in vitro human skin explant model. Hum Immunol 2001; 62:1266–1276.

52. Rocha V, Franco RF, Porcher R, Bittencourt H, Silva-Jr WA, Latouche A, et al. Host defense and inflammatory gene polymorphisms are associated with outcomes after HLA-identical sibling bone marrow transplant. Blood 2002; 100:3908–3918.

53. Cullup H, Dickinson AM, Jackson GH, Taylor PR, Cavet J, Middleton PG. Donor interleukin 1 receptor antagonist genotype associated with acute graft-versus-host disease in human leucocyte antigen-matched sibling allogeneic transplants. Br J Haematol 2001; 113:807–813.

54. Takahashi H, Furukawa T, Hashimoto S, Suzuki N, Kuroha T, Yamazaki F, et al. Contribution of TNF-alpha and IL-10 gene polymorphisms to graft-versus-host disease following allo-hematopoietic stem cell transplantation. Bone Marrow Transplant 2000; 26: 1317–1323.

55. Rufer N, Wolpert E, Helg C, Tiercy JM, Gratwohl A, Chapuis B, et al. HA-1 and the SMCY-derived peptide FIDSYICQV (H-Y) are immunodominant minor histocompatibility antigens after bone marrow transplantation. Transplantation 1998; 66:910–916.

56. Goulmy E, Schipper R, Pool J, Blokland E, Falkenburg JH, Vossen J, et al. Mismatches of minor histocompatibility antigens between HLA-identical donors and recipients and the development of graft-versus-host disease after bone marrow transplantation N Engl J Med 1996; 334:281–285.

57. Kollman C, Howe CW, Anasetti C, Antin JH, Davies SM, Filipovich AH, et al. Donor characteristics as risk factors in recipients after transplantation of bone marrow from unrelated donors: the effect of donor age. Blood 2001; 98:2043–2051.

58. Goulmy E, Schipper R, Pool J, Blokland E, Falkenburg JH, Vossen J, et al. Mismatches of minor histocompatibility antigens between HLA-identical donors and recipients and the development of graft-versus-host disease after bone marrow transplantation. N Engl J Med 1996; 334:281–285.

59. Tseng LH, Lin MT, Hansen JA, Gooley T, Pei J, Smith AG, et al. Correlation between disparity for the minor histocompatibility antigen HA-1 and the development of acute graft-versus-host disease after allogeneic marrow transplantation. Blood 1999; 94:2911–2914.

60. Martin PJ. Increased disparity for minor histocompatibility antigens as a potential cause of increased GVHD risk in marrow transplantation from unrelated donors compared with related donors. Bone Marrow Transplant 1991; 8:217–223.

61. Hagglund H, Bostrom L, Remberger M, Ljungman P, Nilsson B, Ringden O. Risk factors for acute graft-versus-host disease in 291 consecutive HLA-identical bone marrow transplant recipients. Bone Marrow Transplant 1995; 16:747–753.

62. Przepiorka D, Smith TL, Folloder J, Khouri I, Ueno NT, Mehra R, et al. Risk factors for acute graft-versus-host disease after allogeneic blood stem cell transplantation. Blood 1999; 94:1465–1470.

63. Nash RA, Pepe MS, Storb R, Longton G, Pettinger M, Anasetti C, et al. Acute graft-versus-host disease: analysis of risk factors after allogeneic marrow transplantation and prophylaxis with cyclosporine and methotrexate. Blood 1992; 80:1838–1845.

64. Bross DS, Tutschka PJ, Farmer ER, Beschorner WE, Braine HG, Mellits ED, et al. Predictive factors for acute graft versus host disease in patients transplanted with HLA-identical bone marrow. Blood 1984; 63:1265–1270.

65. Gale RP, Bortin MM, van Bekkum DW, Biggs JC, Dicke KA, Gluckman E, et al. Risk factors for acute graft-versus-host disease. Br J Haematol 1987; 67:397–406.

66. Weisdorf D, Hakke R, Blazar B, Miller W, McGlave P, Ramsay N, et al. Risk factors for acute graft-versus-host disease in histocompatible donor bone marrow transplantation. Transplantation 1991; 51:1197–1203.

67. Storb R, Hansen JA, Prentice RL, Thomas ED. Association between HLA-B antigens and acute graft versus host disease. Lancet 1983; 2:816–819.

68. Baughan AS, Worsley M, McCarthy DM, Hows JM, Catovsky D, Gordon-Smith EC, et al. Hematological reconstitution and severity of graft-versus-host disease after bone marrow transplantation for chronic granulocytic leukemia: the influence of previous splenectomy. Br J Haematol 1984; 56:445–454.

69. Bacigalupo A, van Lint NT, Occhini D, et al. ABO compatibility and acute graft versus-host-disease following allogeneic bone marrow transplantation. Transplantation 1988; 45:1091–1094.

70. Przepiorka D, Weisdorf D, Martin P, Klingemann HG, Beatty P, Hows J, et al. 1994 Consensus Conference on Acute GVHD Grading. Bone Marrow Transplant 1995; 15:825–828.

71. Anasetti C, Doney KC, Storb R, Meyers JD, Farewell VT, Buckner CD, et al. Marrow transplantation for severe aplastic anemia. Long term outcome in fifty "untransfused" patients. Ann Intern Med 1986; 104:461–466.

72. Saunders MD, Shulman HM, Murakami CS, Chauncey TR, Bensinger WI, McDonald GB. Bile duct apoptosis and cholestasis resembling acute graft-versus-host disease after autologous hematopoietic cell transplantation. Am J Surg Pathol 2000; 24:1004–1008.

73. Hess AD, Bright EC, Thoburn C, Vogelsang GB, Jones RJ, Kennedy MJ. Specificity of effector T lymphocytes in autologous graft-versus-host disease: role of the major histocompatibility complex class II invariant chain peptide. Blood 1997; 89:2203–2209.

74. Hess AH, Horwitz L, Beschorner WE, Santos GW. Development of graft versus host disease like syndrome in cyclosporine treated rats after syngeneic bone marrow transplantation. J Exp Med 1985; 161:718–730.

74a. Nelson JL. Microchimerisms: incidental byproduct of pregnancy or active participant in human health? Trends Mol Med 2002; 8:109–113.

74b. Murakami T, Seguchi M, Nakazawa M, Momma K. OKT3 therapy for transfusion-associated graft-versus-host disease in a neonate. Acta Paediatr Jpn 1997; 39:462–465.

74c. Ohto H, Anderson KC. Posttransfusion graft-versus-host disease in Japanese newborns (review). Transfusion 1996; 36:117–123.

75. Greenbaum BH. Transfusion-associated graft-versus-host disease: historical perspectives, incidence, and current use of irradiated blood products. J Clin Oncol 1991; 9:1889–1902.

76. Anderson KC, Weinstein HJ. Transfusion-associated graft-versus-host disease. N Engl J Med 1990; 323:315–321.

13

Role of Minor Histocompatibility Antigens in the Development of Graft-vs.-Host Disease and Graft-vs.-Leukemia Reactivity

ANNA BARBUI

Ospedali Riuniti de Bergamo, Bergamo, Italy

LISETTE VAN DE CORPUT

University Medical Center Utrecht and Wilhelmina Children's Hospital, Utrecht, The Netherlands

FREDERIK J. H. FALKENBURG

Leiden University Medical Center, Leiden, The Netherlands

I. GRAFT-VS.-HOST DISEASE AND GRAFT-VS.-LEUKEMIA REACTIVITY

Allogeneic hematopoietic stem cell transplantation (HSCT) has become the treatment of choice for many hematopoietic malignant disorders and also for certain solid tumors (1). The clinical outcome and success of allogeneic HSCT rely on the extensive knowledge of the HLA system and its accurate definition by serological and molecular typing. The application of DNA typing methods has allowed a better definition of the diversity of HLA class I and class II genes (2–5). Better HLA matching between donor and recipient may result in a lower rate of graft failure and graft rejection as well as graft-vs.-host disease (GVHD) (6). However, despite the use of immunosuppressive drugs for GVHD prophylaxis, in 20–30% of the patients clinically significant grades II–IV GVHD invariably occurs even when fully HLA-matched transplants are performed (7). These clinically significant alloreactive immune responses have been hypothesized to be due to mismatching for polymorphic genes outside the major HLA complex. Some of these genes defined as minor histocompatibility antigens (mHags) have been characterized and have been shown to act as targets for specific allo recognition by donor T cells (8–10). Such an immune activity of donor T cells is responsible not only for the detrimental GVHD but also for the therapeutic graft-vs.-leukemia (GVL) effect observed after allogeneic HSCT. The antileukemic effect of alloreactivity has been indicated by the observation that patients developing acute and/ or chronic GVHD had a significantly lower probability of leukemia relapse (11,12). Moreover, when comparing allogeneic HSCT with unmodified grafts versus T-cell–depleted allogeneic or syngeneic HSCT, the decreased risk of acute or chronic GVHD coincided with a higher rate of leukemic relapse (13,14). On the basis of these observations the crucial antineoplastic role played by immunocompetent T cells against leukemia became evident. Further conclusive evidence for the GVL effect of donor T cells after allogeneic HSCT came from the success of donor lymphocyte infusion (DLI) used as a sole procedure to reinduce a complete remission (CR) in relapsed patients (15,16). The potent capacity of donor T cells to fully eradicate massive tumor loads has prompted several investigators to challenge this dramatic therapeutic activity of the donor immune system by performing allogeneic HSCT with reduced intensity conditioning regimens (17,18).

This strategy is based on the assumption that the alloreactive immune response and not chemotherapy or irradiation is the most dominant therapeutic effect of allogeneic HSCT. These reduced intensity conditioning regimens are now currently explored for their feasibility in the treatment of acute and chronic leukemia, myeloma, lymphoma, renal cell carcinoma, and other solid tumors in patients otherwise ineligible for myeloablative allogeneic HSCT because of age or concomitant diseases (16,19). After allogeneic HSCT sustained hematological engraftment can be demonstrated with full donor chimerism of the hematopoietic system or with the coexistence of patient- and donor-derived hematopoietic and immune cells (mixed chimeric status). In both conditions donor T lymphocytes can be reinfused without the risk of being rejected, because the immunological system from the recipient is now primed to tolerate donor cells. The reinfused donor T cells are able to recognize patient-derived cells including the malignant cells but will not affect the donor-derived hematopoietic cells, and therefore the normal hematopoietic tissue after allogeneic HSCT is not under attack. Chronic myeloid leukemia (CML) in chronic phase has been shown to be the disease most susceptible to DLI, showing a durable CR in 50–80% of cases (14,15,20,21). This peculiar responsiveness to DLI could be related to the immunogenic properties of certain subpopulations of CML cells like malignant dendritic cells (DC). The ability of CML precursor cells to differentiate into DC-like cells has been demonstrated in several studies (22–25). Other malignancies, especially acute lymphoblastic leukemia (ALL) or acute myeloid leukemia (AML), do not seem to respond to DLI in many cases. Possible explanations for this differential susceptibility to DLI could be the lack of antigen expression on tumor cells, inadequate expression of adhesion or costimulatory molecules that are essential for appropriate T-cell activation, or the rapid expansion rate of the malignancy (26). Undoubtedly, however, under certain circumstances a GVL effect can be separated from clinically significant GVHD (27). One plausible explanation for this differential alloreactive effect relies on a specific immune recognition of hematopoietic restricted antigens. Although in the current clinical setting no standardized approaches have been shown to reproducibly enhance antitumor T-cell response without causing a clinical relevant GVHD, several laboratory observations have indicated an immunological basis for the separation of GVL effects from GVHD. In this chapter we will focus on the experimental background supporting the assumption that differences in expression of minor histocompatibility antigens between donor and recipient can be used to target GVL responses. Furthermore, selective differences in HLA molecules between donor and recipient can also be used to target specific antileukemic T-cell reactivity.

II. MINOR HISTOCOMPATIBILITY ANTIGENS

Minor histocompatibility antigens (mHag) can be defined as peptides derived from poly-morphic intracellular proteins that can be recognized as alloantigens by allogeneic T cells from HLA-matched individuals (28). Polymorphic genes present on Y or autosomal chromosomes have been found to code for immunogenic intracellular proteins that are pro-cessed and presented on the cell membrane in the context of HLA molecules, either HLA class I or class II (8,29,30). If the specific peptide presented in HLA class I or II molecules can be recognized by T cells derived from an HLA-identical individual and is not recog-nized as a self antigen by that same donor, this antigenic complex is considered a mHag.

To serve as a mHag, polymorphic proteins have to undergo several degradation steps to allow presentation of the polymorphic part of the protein in HLA molecules. The protein is first cleaved by intracellular proteases into smaller polypeptides in different compart-ments of the cell. For mHag that can be presented in the context of HLA class I molecules, these peptides have to be transported into the endoplasmatic reticulum, where they are bound into the groove of HLA class I molecules. This peptide/HLA complex is trans-ported to the cell membrane, where it can be presented to T cells. Several critical steps play a role in the binding and presentation of peptides in the context of class I molecules on the cell membrane. First, the intracellular proteases, and more specifically the protea-some, have to cleave the protein into appropriate fragments of 8–11 amino acids that can be transported by TAP into the endoplasmatic reticulum (31) (Fig. 1). In particular,

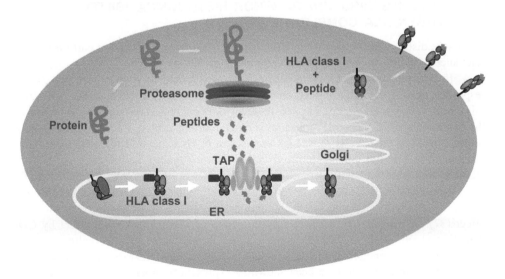

Figure 1 Proteins in the cytosol or nucleus are degraded by the proteasome into smaller peptide fragments. A peptide pump called TAP translocates the peptides over the membrane of the endoplasmatic reticulum (ER). HLA class I molecules are retained in the ER lumen until successful peptide binding occurs. These molecules are subsequently transported to the plasma membrane.

the C-terminal cleavage appears to be critical for the formation of the right immunogenic peptide. The proteases necessary for the cleavage of peptides have relative specificity for amino acids. Therefore, polymorphisms in the proteins can lead to differential formation of peptides to be processed and presented to HLA molecules. In addition, certain amino acids are critical for high-affinity binding to HLA class I molecules. Therefore, polymorphisms in these amino acids may lead to inability of the peptide to bind to HLA class I molecules, and therefore no stable HLA/peptide complex will be presented on the cell membrane. From the knowledge of the processing of peptides, several cellular mechanisms can be hypothesized by which mHag can arise. First, single or multiple amino acid substitutions in the peptide that is processed and bound to the groove of the HLA molecule may be recognized as "foreign" by allogeneic T-cell receptors (TCR) from the donor. Male specific HY antigens, several of which have been characterized recently, are the most common examples of such mHag in humans (32–34). In addition, polymorphisms in the part of the peptide that does not make direct contact with the TCR but is essential for binding to the HLA class I molecule on the target cell may lead to differential expression of the peptide/HLA complex on the cell membrane. Alternatively, polymorphisms in a protein may give rise to differential proteasome-mediated cleavage resulting in different peptides and differential formation of the specific HLA-binding peptide. Therefore, amino acid substitutions not only directly in the HLA-binding part of the peptide but also immediately adjacent to the peptide influencing the cellular processing of the peptide may result in the formation of mHag. If the specific peptide can only be presented in cells from the patient but not in donor cells, donor T cells will not be tolerant to these antigens and a T-cell response to the epitopes may occur. Several of the characterized autosomal mHag like HA-2 and HA-8 appear to be members of this family of mHag (30,35).

III. TISSUE DISTRIBUTION OF MINOR HISTOCOMPATIBILITY ANTIGEN/HLA COMPLEX

The tissue distribution of the mHag/HLA complex determines at least in part the clinical relevance of T-cell responses against these antigens (Table 1).

If a certain type of HLA molecule is not expressed in a specific tissue, T-cell responses against the HLA/mHag complex will not directly recognize the cells from this tissue. Whereas HLA class I molecules are widely expressed throughout the organism, the expression of HLA class II molecules is much more restricted. Cells of hematopoietic origin as well as other cells show high expression of HLA class II molecules during an inflammatory reaction, and therefore T-cell responses against an antigen expressed in HLA class II molecules will recognize malignant cells or normal cells depending on the expression of HLA-DR, DQ, or DP (36). It has been reported that selective depletion of CD8+ T cells from DLI may result in a reduced GVHD, with preservation of the GVL effect (37). A requisite for a successful separation of GVHD and GVL effect by CD8 depletion is obviously high expression of class II molecules on the malignant cells, especially on the clonogeneic precursor cells. CML precursor cells exhibit high expression of class II molecules and have been shown to express a number of class II–associated mHag, and therefore CML may be a good target for elective CD4-mediated GVL.

Certain mHag, including most male specific mHag, HA-3, and HA-8, have been shown to be broadly expressed in all or most tissues (8,38). Since these antigens are recognized in the context of HLA class I molecules, T-cell responses against these mHags will

Table 1   Current Status of Minor Histocompatibility Antigens

Common name	HLA restriction	Gene	Chromosome	Distribution	Ref.
HA-1	HLA-A0201	KIAA0223	19p13.3 autosome	Hematopoietic restricted	29
HA-2	HLA-A0201	Myosin-related gene	6p21.3 autosome	Hematopoietic restricted	97
HA-8	HLA-A*0201	KIAA0020	9 autosome	Ubiquitous	30
HB-1	HLA-B44	HB1	5q32 autosome	B-ALL	39,98
HY-A1	HLA-A1	DFFRY	Y	Ubiquitous	99,100
HY-A2	HLA-A2	SMCY	Y	Ubiquitous	101
HY-B7	HLA-B7	SMCY	Y	Ubiquitous	32
HY-B8	HLA-B8	UTY	Y	Ubiquitous	33
HY-B60	HLA-B60	UTY	Y	Ubiquitous	102
HY-DQ5	HLA-DQ5	DBY	Y	Ubiquitous	103

affect many tissues. In contrast, the mHag, HA-1, and HA-2 are restricted to cells from hematopoietic origin (10). Although the function of the proteins encoding these mHag have not been characterized thus far, the proteins appear to play a relevant role in hematopoiesis and lymphopoiesis since almost all normal and malignant hematopoietic cells show a highly conserved expression of these proteins. Other mHag like HB-1 have been shown to be even more restricted to subpopulations of hematopoietic cells. Both malignant and normal precursor B-cells show high expression of this antigen (39).

Tissue specificity of the polymorphic peptides in the context of HLA molecules may also be caused by a differential processing of the antigen. At least two mechanisms may be responsible for specific processing of HLA/peptide complexes. Depending on the tissue specificity and activation state of the cells, different types of proteasomes can be preferentially expressed. Most cells express regular proteasomes, whereas certain antigen presenting cells or cells stimulated with interferon IFN-γ preferentially express immunoproteasomes (40,41). It has been demonstrated that preferential processing of peptides in HLA complexes may be due to differential cleavage by the different proteasomes (31). In addition, tissue-specific mRNA splice variants may result in differential expression of mHag, even when the specific gene is expressed in most tissues. Preliminary results indicate that the male specific UTY-protein may be differentially recognized in hematopoietic and nonhematopoietic tissues.

IV. mHag AS TARGETS FOR GVHD

T-cell responses against mHag that are broadly expressed by both hematopoietic and nonhematopoietic tissues are likely to result in GVHD (42,43). For example, male patients treated with allogeneic HSCT from female donors have a high relative risk of developing GVHD (44). The likelihood that T cells recognizing specific antigens were involved in the GVHD was supported by the demonstration of high frequencies of T cells expressing a TCR specific for HY antigens as measured by flow cytometry using tetrameric HLA-peptide complexes. More broadly expressed mHag encoded by autosomal chromosomes like HA-8 may also lead to a high risk of GVHD (45).

T-cell responses against antigens mainly expressed on nonhematopoietic cells like CD31 polymorphic peptides may result in a detrimental allo reactivity as illustrated by a correlation between the occurrence of GVHD and polymorphisms in CD31 between donor and recipient (46–48).

Initially it was anticipated that disparity between donor and recipients for mHag that were specifically expressed on cells of hematopoietic origin were not likely to be associated with an increased risk of GVHD. However, several reports have indicated that disparity for mHag restricted to hematopoietic cells like HA-1 and HA-2 correlated with an increased risk of GVHD after transplantation, although not all studies could confirm this correlation (8,49–52). In addition, a high frequency of T cells recognizing hematopoiesis-specific mHag has been found in patients suffering from severe GVHD after allogeneic HSCT (45). It has recently been demonstrated in a murine transplantation model that dendritic cells endogenously expressing recipient specific antigens are likely to be essential for the induction of GVHD (53). Immune responses induced by dendritic cell–associated mHag may evoke a cascade of inflammatory responses resulting in the clinical features of GVHD. The possible explanation for the association between disparity for HA-1 and/or HA-2 and GVHD may be the very high expression of these antigens in professional antigen-presenting cells (APC) like dendritic cells or Langerhans cells. Since shortly after transplantation the APC will still be of recipient origin, HA-1–specific donor T cells recognizing the antigens may be triggered in tissues containing such professional APC. Late after allogeneic HSCT, the APC are gradually replaced by donor-derived APC (54). This may be an explanation for the observation that following donor lymphocyte infusion for the treatment of relapsed leukemia many months after allogeneic HSCT may result in the emergence of HA-1– and HA-2–specific T cells in patients without the development of severe GVHD. This hypothesis was further supported by the study of Dickinson et al., who investigated the ability of HA-1–specific T cells to induce GVHD in a skin explanted model (55). In contrast to T cells recognizing antigens with broad tissue specificity, HA-1–specific T cells induced only minor tissue damage, indicating that T cells recognizing hematopoiesis-associated mHag may not directly attack target tissues of GVHD. HA-1–specific T cells may only indirectly cause tissue damage by inducing local inflammation, which may be followed by an amplification of T-cell responses against other mHag.

V.   RELEVANCE OF MINOR HISTOCOMPATIBILITY ANTIGENS IN GVL REACTIVITY

Although there is evidence that self antigens like proteinase-3 may play a role in controlling the malignancy after allogeneic HSCT (56), the finding that allogeneic T cells but not syngeneic T cells in HLA-identical transplantation appear to be essential for GVL reactivity makes it likely that polymorphic differences between donors and recipients play a significant role in the GVL effect (27).

In vitro mHag-specific T cells have been shown to be capable of cell-mediated lysis of leukemic target cells (57,58). Both the broadly expressed male specific HY mHag as well as several autosomal mHag have been shown to be recognized in the context of the restricting HLA molecules on many hematological malignancies. However, many hematological malignancies consist of heterogeneous cell populations comprising both more differentiated malignant cells as well as clonogenic precursor cells. Since it has been demonstrated that the response to DLI is associated with the emergence of T cells reactive with clonogenic precursor cells, a prerequisite for relevant T-cell responses against mHag is the recognition of the antigens on these precursor cells. Both the broadly expressed male specific and autosomal mHag and the hematopoiesis restricted mHag described could be recognized on the clonogenic precursor cells of the malignancies tested (59). Several mHag-specific T-cell clones have been tested for their ability to recognize leukemic precursor cells capable of engrafting into immunodeficient NOD/SCID mice and have been shown to be capable of preventing the outgrowth of leukemia in these animals (58). In vitro experiments indicated that many of the mHag described, including all male specific antigens and the minor antigens HA-1 to 5, HA-8, and HB-1, may be appropriate target structures for a GVL effect.

Recent experiments also indicate that mHag-specific T cells play a role in the clinical GVL effect after DLI. In donor-patient pairs that are disparate for certain mHag that have been molecularly characterized, the appearance of T cells specific for these antigens can be monitored in vivo using fluorescent tetrameric HLA/peptide complexes. In patients positive for the mHag HA-1 or HA-2 who received DLI for relapse of their malignancy following allogeneic HSCT from their HA-1– or HA-2– negative donors, the kinetics of HA-1– and HA-2–specific T cells were monitored during the clinical response. The eradication of the malignancy coincided with a brisk emergence of HA-1– or HA-2–specific T cells. In a male patient treated with DLI from his female donor, concurrent emergence of HY-specific T cells was also found, which was associated with the occurrence of GVHD. Using the fluorescent tetrameric complexes specific for the mHag, the HA-1–, HA-2–, or HY-B7–specific T cells were isolated, expanded, and tested for their ability to recognize the clonogenic progenitor cells from the malignancy. These studies confirmed studies showing that mHag-specific T cells were capable of antigen-specific growth inhibition of the clonogenic progenitor cells (59). These results indicate that both the broadly expressed mHag as well as the hematopoiesis-associated mHag may be target structures in GVL reactivity. In accordance with the expression of the hematopoiesis-restricted mHag on both malignant and normal hematopoietic cells, all responding patients converted to 100% donor chimerism. Since the donor-derived hematopoietic cells after allogeneic HSCT are not affected by the T-cell responses against these mHag, hematopoiesis-restricted mHag can serve as malignancy-specific target structures.

Although extensive studies on tissue expression of the hematopoiesis-restricted mHag HA-1 have indicated that this antigen is solely expressed in hematopoietic cells under normal conditions, recent experiments indicated that aberrant expression of these proteins can occur. Abnormal HA-1 expression has been found in tumor cells of epithelial origin, indicating that mHag may also be target structures for graft-vs.-tumor reactivity in solid tumors (60). These findings can explain a possible graft-vs.-tumor effect that has been observed following allogeneic HSCT with reduced-intensity conditioning regimens in metastatic renal cell carcinoma (61).

VI. ADOPTIVE IMMUNOTHERAPY WITH IN VITRO SELECTED AND EXPANDED mHag-SPECIFIC T CELLS

Although it has become evident that following DLI for relapsed leukemia after allogeneic HSCT, mHag-specific T cells can arise leading to eradication of the malignancy, the response may be not sufficient to eliminate the disease in the majority of acute leukemias, non-Hodgkin's lymphomas or multiple myeloma (14,62–65). One way to amplify the specific T-cell responses may be vaccination of the patient following HSCT using mHag-specific peptides in the presence or absence of professional APC (43). Alternatively, donors could be vaccinated prior to donating T cells for immunotherapy (43,66). Although these approaches may improve the antitumor reactivity following allogeneic HSCT, the vaccination approach is likely to be successful only in the state of minimal residual disease of the patient. In addition, certain tumors, including AML and ALL, may be capable of inducing anergy in vivo by the production of suppressive cytokines or the lack or impaired expression of costimulatory or adhesion molecules (67,68). An alternative approach to bypass these problems and amplify the immune response may be the generation of mHag-specific T cells in vitro from donor peripheral blood, to expand these T cells, and to infuse high numbers of mHag-specific T cells into the patient. The feasibility of this approach has been demonstrated by the successful administration of viral antigen-specific T cells to treat or prevent viral infections following allogeneic HSCT. Both cytomegalovirus (CMV) infections and Epstein-Barr virus (EBV)–associated lymphoma have been successfully treated with in vitro isolated and expanded virus specific T-cell clones or lines (69–71).

In murine models it has been illustrated that selection of T cells specific for mHag can elicit GVL reactivity without concurrent induction of GVHD (72). Although the successful treatment of patients with resistant leukemia after allogeneic HSCT with in vitro selected and expanded T cells has been demonstrated, the logistics of generating large numbers of tumor-specific T cells in vitro against mHag or tumor-associated antigens from primary T-cell responses have been shown to be complex (43). Several approaches have been tested to efficiently induce mHag-specific T-cell responses in vitro, including the stimulation of donor T cells with professional APC loaded with synthetic peptides (57) or transduction of these APC with retroviral vectors encoding the mHag-specific genes (73). Since the in vitro expansion of mHag-specific T cells appears to be successful only in a limited number of cases, alternative approaches are being explored to isolate high numbers of mHag-specific T cells from donor peripheral blood. One approach comprises the isolation of mHag-specific T cells using tetrameric complexes, although it has been reported that this procedure may lead to anergy of a significant number of T cells (74). Recently, an isolation method has been developed that allows dissociation of the complex after isolation that may prevent the undesired incomplete activation of the T cells (75). An alternative method of isolation of T cells reactive with specific mHag is the cytokine capture assay (76,77). In this assay using bi-specific antibodies recognizing CD45 on the T cells and a specific cytokine produced by the T cells like IFN-γ, the cytokine is coupled to the cells after stimulation of a T-cell population with a specific antigen. Using antibodies directed against the captured cytokine, antigen-responding T cells can be isolated using immunomagnetic beads or cell sorting. The feasibility of isolating large numbers of antigen-specific T cells has been demonstrated for the treatment of CMV- or EBV-associated diseases (78,79).

For the large-scale application of in vitro isolated mHag-specific T cells, the number of relevant target antigens has to be significantly increased. The applicability of T-cell responses against mHag is determined by the tissue distribution of the mHag-specific protein and the relevant restriction HLA molecule necessary for presenting the antigen. By the molecular characterization of target structures recognized by T cells that can be isolated from patients that respond to DLI in the absence of GVHD, the number of relevant mHag peptides may be increased. Alternatively, by searching for nucleotide polymorphisms in genes that are solely expressed in hematopoietic cells, new target antigens may be selected from the databases. However, these proteins have to be tested first for correct processing by the target cells to estimate whether they may be appropriate targets for GVL reactivity.

VII. HEMATOPOIESIS SPECIFIC ANTIGENS AS TARGETS FOR GVL REACTIVITY AFTER HLA-MISMATCHED HSCT

This successful transplantation of hematopoietic stem cells over HLA barriers using megadoses of CD34-positive stem cells and extensive T-cell depletion of the graft allow a new application of hematopoiesis specific T cell responses for the treatment of hematological malignancies (80,81). In this situation the HLA mismatch between donor and recipient is not a disadvantage, but a prerequisite for the application of hematopoiesis-specific alloimmunotherapy (82–84). Similar to the approach using hematopoiesis-specific mHag in the context of HLA-matched transplantation, the establishment of donor chimerism is essential for the application of this form of cellular (allo)immunotherapy. This approach is based on the finding that at least a proportion of allo-HLA–recognizing T cells are specific for a single peptide recognized in the context of the mismatched HLA restriction molecule (43). The T-cell receptor from these T cells is specific for the combination of the single peptide and the polymorphic part of the HLA restriction molecule. By selecting as target antigens peptides derived from hematopoietic (sub)lineage specific proteins that can be presented in the context of mismatched HLA molecules, donor T-cell responses may be generated that specifically recognize patient hematopoietic cells, including the malignant cell population. The basics of this approach are illustrated in Figure 2.

In the example shown, the patient is HLA-A2 positive, whereas the donor is HLA-A2 negative. Donor-derived T cells that are specific for a peptide derived from a hematopoiesis-specific protein that can only be presented in the context of HLA-A2 will recognize only hematopoietic cells from the patient since donor-derived hematopoietic cells do not express the HLA restriction molecule. Patient-derived non-hematopoietic cells do not express the protein coding the peptide and will therefore not be recognized. Several hematopoiesis-associated proteins have been proposed to serve as tumor specific antigens in the context of HLA mismatched allogeneic HSCT. Recently, WT-1, CD45, as well as the mHag HA-1 and HA-2 have been shown to be plausible hematopoiesis-associated peptides that can be recognized on leukemic cells in the context of mismatched HLA-A2 molecules by HLA-A2–negative individuals (43,85–88).

The logistic challenge of this new approach is the purification of T cells that are only specific for the mismatched HLA/peptide complex without concurrent recognition of more broadly expressed peptides presented by these HLA molecules, since T cells reactive with these antigens will probable induce GVHD. Enrichment for these mismatched HLA/peptide complexes can be obtained by stimulation of donor T cells with "artificial" APC that only present these specific peptide in the groove of the HLA molecule, and no other peptides (89). By repeated stimulation of various APC specifically loaded with the antigenic peptide it has been possible to induce specific T-cell responses, which were further enriched by cell sorting using synthetic HLA/peptide tetrameric complexes (74). This strategy provides the possible targeting of hematopoiesis-specific antigens for immunotherapy of hematological malignancies after partially mismatched HSCT with limited risk of inducing GVHD.

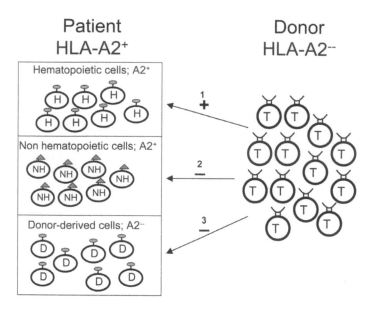

Figure 2   Donor-derived T cells that are HLA-A2⁻ specifically recognize an antigenic peptide that is only expressed by hematopoietic cells including malignant cells of the patient and presented in HLA-A2 (1), but these antigen-specific T cells are not able to recognize peptides expressed by nonhematopoietic cells of the patient and presented in HLA-A2 (2). Donor-derived T cells do not recognize other donor-derived hematopoietic cells negative for the HLA-A2 restriction molecule (3).

VIII.   TARGETING OF GVL REACTIVITY BY REDIRECTION OF ANTIGEN-SPECIFIC T-CELL REACTIVITY

For both the application of mHag-specific T cells in the context of HLA-matched transplantation and of hematopoiesis-specific T cells recognizing antigens in the context of HLA-mismatched HSCT, the generation of relatively large numbers of antigen-specific T cells is essential. Since the specificity of the T cells is determined by the TCRα and TCRβ genes, transfer of genes coding for TCR recognizing the desired antigen into immune-competent cells from the donor or from the patient after transplantation may be an alternative strategy to circumvent the logistical problems of isolation and purification of specific T cells. From a T-cell clone expressing high-affinity TCR for the antigen of choice, TCRα and TCRβ cDNA can be synthesized and cloned into retroviral vectors. Several authors have demonstrated the feasibility of redirection of the specific T-cell reactivity by gene transfer of the TCRα and TCRβ genes into other immune effector cells. By transferring the TCR specific for class I–associated antigens into CD8-positive T cells or the transfer of TCR of HLA class II–restricted specificities into CD4-positive T cells, large numbers of antigen-specific T cells could be generated (90–92). Although these experiments show the feasibility of this approach, several potential problems may occur. Since the host T cells also express endogenous TCR chains, the introduction of exogenous TCRα and TCRβ genes into these T cells may result in undesired pairing of exogenous and endogenous TCR chains leading to unpredictable specificities. The risk of the formation of undesired specificity leading to GVHD or autoimmune diseases may be minimized by limiting the variation of target T cells into which the TCR are introduced. In addition, the specificity of a TCR may not be as unidirected as thought. It has been demonstrated that single TCR cannot only recognize different peptides in the context of the same HLA class I molecule, but may also recognize different peptides in the context of HLA class I and class II molecules (93). This may result in unexpected reactivity with unrelated HLA/peptide complexes. Despite these possible pitfalls, redirection of TCR to control tumor growth has been shown to be feasible and effective in murine studies (94). Since the introduced TCRα and TCRβ chains must compete with the endogenous α and β chains for the other constituents of the CD3 complex and the signaling pathways necessary for the effector functions of the T cell, not all successfully introduced TCR may be as effective as the original T cells from which the genes have been isolated. Careful defining of T cells with the desired specificity will greatly enhance the possible application of T-cell therapy for the treatment of the malignancies.

Since retroviral gene transfer has recently been associated with possible risks of undesired proliferation of these T cells or undesired specificity, it may be necessary to introduce a safety gene into the transferred T cells. Several approaches have been explored to introduce a safety gene; the herpesvirus thymidine kinase (TK) gene has been used in clinical studies most extensively and was shown to be effective in reversing GVHD caused by T cells in the context of DLI (95). An alternative approach to introduce a safety gene into redirected T cells is the transfer of the human CD20 gene into these T cells. Effective introduction of CD20 has been shown to be feasible into CD3-positive T cells, which can subsequently be completely removed in case of a clinical emergency by exposure of the cells to the clinically available anti-CD20 monoclonal antibody rituximab (96).

IX. CONCLUSION

Minor histocompatibility antigens as well as major histocompatibility antigens play a major role in both the induction of detrimental GVHD after allogeneic HSCT and the development of the beneficial GVL effect. The tissue distribution of the HLA molecules and the proteins encoding the mHag determine at least in part the clinical outcome of T-cell responses against these antigens. T-cell responses against hematopoiesis-specific mHag may act as tumor-specific T cells following allogeneic HLA-identical HSCT by eliminating all hematopoietic cells from the recipient, including the malignant cells, while preserving normal donor hematopoiesis after transplantation. Specific T-cell responses against these antigens will eradicate the disease and induce complete donor chimerism. GVHD not only may be initiated by T-cell responses against antigens that are highly expressed in the target organs of GVHD, but may also be caused by the induction of inflammatory responses due to the presence of local T-cell reactivity against cells from hematopoietic origin like dendritic cells. An alternative approach to inducing GVL effect without severe GVHD in the context of mismatched HLA transplantation may be the targeting of T-cell responses against hematopoiesis-specific peptides presented in the context of the HLA-mismatched molecules. Several strategies including vaccination of patients after transplantation using mHag-specific peptides, ex vivo production of peptide-specific T-cell responses, and the redirection of T-cell specificity using gene transfer of T-cell receptors may be explored to specifically eradicate the malignant cells after allogeneic HSCT without concurrent induction of GVHD.

REFERENCES

1. Little MT, Storb R. History of haematopoietic stem-cell transplantation. Nat Rev Cancer 2002; 2:231–238.
2. Petersdorf EW, Hansen JA, Martin PJ, Woolfrey A, Malkki M, Gooley T, Storer B, Mickelson E, Smith A, Anasetti C. Major-histocompatibility-complex class I alleles and antigens in hematopoietic-cell transplantation. N Engl J Med 2001; 345:1794–1800.
3. Petersdorf EW, Kollman C, Hurley CK, Dupont B, Nademanee A, Begovich AB, Weisdorf D, McGlave P. Effect of HLA class II gene disparity on clinical outcome in unrelated donor hematopoietic cell transplantation for chronic myeloid leukemia: the US National Marrow Donor Program Experience. Blood 2001; 98:2922–2929.
4. Scott I, O'Shea J, Bunce M, Tiercy JM, Arguello JR, Firman H, Goldman J, Prentice HG, Little AM, Madrigal JA. Molecular typing shows a high level of HLA class I incompatibility in serologically well matched donor/patient pairs: implications for unrelated bone marrow donor selection. Blood 1998; 92:4864–4871.
5. Morishima Y, Sasazuki T, Inoko H, Juji T, Akaza T, Yamamoto K, Ishikawa Y, Kato S, Sao H, Sakamaki H, Kawa K, Hamajima N, Asano S, Kodera Y. The clinical significance of human leukocyte antigen (HLA) allele compatibility in patients receiving a marrow transplant from serologically HLA-A, HLA-B, and HLA-DR matched unrelated donors. Blood 2002; 99:4200–4206.
6. Cooper DL. HLA matching for hematopoietic stem-cell transplants. N Engl J Med 2002; 346:1251–1252.
7. Gratwohl A, Brand R, Apperley J, Biezen Av A, Bandini G, Devergie A, Schattenberg A, Frassoni F, Guglielmi C, Iacobelli S, Michallet M, Kolb HJ, Ruutu T, Niederwieser D. Graft-versus-host disease and outcome in HLA-identical sibling transplantations for chronic myeloid leukemia. Blood 2002; 100:3877–3886.
8. Goulmy E, Schipper R, Pool J, Blokland E, Falkenburg JH, Vossen J, Grathwohl A, Vogelsang GB, van Houwelingen HC, van Rood JJ. Mismatches of minor histocompatibility antigens between HLA-identical donors and recipients and the development of graft-versus-host disease after bone marrow transplantation. N Engl J Med 1996; 334:281–285.
9. Warren EH, Greenberg PD, Riddell SR. Cytotoxic T-lymphocyte-defined human minor histocompatibility antigens with a restricted tissue distribution. Blood 1998; 91:2197–2207.
10. de Bueger M, Bakker A, Van Rood JJ, Van der Woude F, Goulmy E. Tissue distribution of human minor histocompatibility antigens. Ubiquitous versus restricted tissue distribution indicates heterogeneity among human cytotoxic T lymphocyte-defined non-MHC antigens. J Immunol 1992; 149:1788–1794.
11. Weiden PL, Sullivan KM, Flournoy N, Storb R, Thomas ED. Antileukemic effect of chronic graft-versus-host disease: contribution to improved survival after allogeneic marrow transplantation. N Engl J Med 1981; 304:1529–1533.
12. Weiden PL, Flournoy N, Sanders JE, Sullivan KM, Thomas ED. Antileukemic effect of graft-versus-host disease contributes to improved survival after allogeneic marrow transplantation. Transplant Proc 1981; 13:248–251.
13. Fefer A, Sullivan KM, Weiden P, Buckner CD, Schoch G, Storb R, Thomas ED. Graft versus leukemia effect in man: the relapse rate of acute leukemia is lower after allogeneic than after syngeneic marrow transplantation. Prog Clin Biol Res 1987; 244:401–408.
14. Collins RH Jr, Shpilberg O, Drobyski WR, Porter DL, Giralt S, Champlin R, Goodman SA, Wolff SN, Hu W, Verfaillie C, List A, Dalton W, Ognoskie N, Chetrit A, Antin JH, Nemunaitis J. Donor leukocyte infusions in 140 patients with relapsed malignancy after allogeneic bone marrow transplantation. J Clin Oncol 1997; 15:433–444.
15. Kolb HJ, Mittermuller J, Clemm C, Holler E, Ledderose G, Brehm G, Heim M, Wilmanns W. Donor leukocyte transfusions for treatment of recurrent chronic myelogenous leukemia in marrow transplant patients. Blood 1990; 76:2462–2465.

16. McSweeney PA, Niederwieser D, Shizuru JA, Sandmaier BM, Molina AJ, Maloney DG, Chauncey TR, Gooley TA, Hegenbart U, Nash RA, Radich J, Wagner JL, Minor S, Appelbaum FR, Bensinger WI, Bryant E, Flowers ME, Georges GE, Grumet FC, Kiem HP, Torok-Storb B, Yu C, Blume KG, Storb RF. Hematopoietic cell transplantation in older patients with hematologic malignancies: replacing high-dose cytotoxic therapy with graft-versus-tumor effects. Blood 2001; 97:3390–3400.

17. Slavin S. Non-myeloablative stem cell transplantation for induction of host-versus-graft tolerance for adoptive immunotherapy of malignant and nonmalignant diseases and towards transplantation of organ allografts. Transplant Proc 2002; 34:3371–3373.

18. Giralt S, Estey E, Albitar M, van Besien K, Rondon G, Anderlini P, O'Brien S, Khouri I, Gajewski J, Mehra R, Claxton D, Andersson B, Beran M, Przepiorka D, Koller C, Kornblau S, Korbling M, Keating M, Kantarjian H, Champlin R. Engraftment of allogeneic hematopoietic progenitor cells with purine analog-containing chemotherapy: harnessing graft-versus-leukemia without myeloablative therapy. Blood 1997; 89:4531–4536.

19. Khouri IF, Keating M, Korbling M, Przepiorka D, Anderlini P, O'Brien S, Giralt S, Ippoliti C, von Wolff B, Gajewski J, Donato M, Claxton D, Ueno N, Andersson B, Gee A, Champlin R. Transplant-lite: induction of graft-versus-malignancy using fludarabine-based nonablative chemotherapy and allogeneic blood progenitor-cell transplantation as treatment for lymphoid malignancies. J Clin Oncol 1998; 16:2817–2824.

20. Dazzi F, Szydlo RM, Cross NC, Craddock C, Kaeda J, Kanfer E, Cwynarski K, Olavarria E, Yong A, Apperley JF, Goldman JM. Durability of responses following donor lymphocyte infusions for patients who relapse after allogeneic stem cell transplantation for chronic myeloid leukemia. Blood 2000; 96:2712–2716.

21. Mackinnon S, Papadopoulos EB, Carabasi MH, Reich L, Collins NH, Boulad F, Castro-Malaspina H, Childs BH, Gillio AP, Kernan NA, et al. Adoptive immunotherapy evaluating escalating doses of donor leukocytes for relapse of chronic myeloid leukemia after bone marrow transplantation: separation of graft-versus-leukemia responses from graft-versus-host disease. Blood 1995; 86:1261–1268.

22. Smit WM, Rijnbeek M, van Bergen CA, Willemze R, Falkenburg JH. Generation of leukemia-reactive cytotoxic T lymphocytes from HLA-identical donors of patients with chronic myeloid leukemia using modifications of a limiting dilution assay. Bone Marrow Transplant 1998; 21:553–560.

23. Yasukawa M, Ohminami H, Kojima K, Hato T, Hasegawa A, Takahashi T, Hirai H, Fujita S. HLA class II-restricted antigen presentation of endogenous bcr-abl fusion protein by chronic myelogenous leukemia-derived dendritic cells to CD4(+) T lymphocytes. Blood 2001; 98:1498–1505.

24. Westermann J, Kopp J, Korner I, Richter G, Qin Z, Blankenstein T, Dorken B, Pezzutto A. Bcr/abl+ autologous dendritic cells for vaccination in chronic myeloid leukemia. Bone Marrow Transplant 2000; 25:S46–S49.

25. Choudhury A, Gajewski JL, Liang JC, Popat U, Claxton DF, Kliche KO, Andreeff M, Champlin RE. Use of leukemic dendritic cells for the generation of antileukemic cellular cytotoxicity against Philadelphia chromosome-positive chronic myelogenous leukemia. Blood 1997; 89:1133–1142.

26. Riddell SR, Murata M, Bryant S, Warren EH. T-cell therapy of leukemia. Cancer Control 2002; 9:114–122.

27. Horowitz MM, Gale RP, Sondel PM, Goldman JM, Kersey J, Kolb HJ, Rimm AA, Ringden O, Rozman C, Speck B, et al. Graft-versus-leukemia reactions after bone marrow transplantation. Blood 1990; 75:555–562.

28. Simpson E, Scott D, James E, Lombardi G, Cwynarski K, Dazzi F, Millrain M, Dyson PJ. Minor H antigens: genes and peptides. Transplant Immunol 2002; 10:115–123.

29. den Haan JM, Meadows LM, Wang W, Pool J, Blokland E, Bishop TL, Reinhardus C, Shabanowitz J, Offringa R, Hunt DF, Engelhard VH, Goulmy E. The minor histocompatibility antigen HA-1: a diallelic gene with a single amino acid polymorphism. Science 1998; 279:1054–1057.

30. Brickner AG, Warren EH, Caldwell JA, Akatsuka Y, Golovina TN, Zarling AL, Shabanowitz J, Eisenlohr LC, Hunt DF, Engelhard VH, Riddell SR. The immunogenicity of a new human minor histocompatibility antigen results from differential antigen processing. J Exp Med 2001; 193:195–206.

31. Schultz ES, Chapiro J, Lurquin C, Claverol S, Burlet-Schiltz O, Warnier G, Russo V, Morel S, Levy F, Boon T, Van den Eynde BJ, van der Bruggen P. The production of a new MAGE-3 peptide presented to cytolytic T lymphocytes by HLA-B40 requires the immunoproteasome. J Exp Med 2002; 195:391–399.

32. Wang W, Meadows LR, den Haan JM, Sherman NE, Chen Y, Blokland E, Shabanowitz J, Agulnik AI, Hendrickson RC, Bishop CE, et al. Human H-Y: a male-specific histocompatibility antigen derived from the SMCY protein. Science 1995; 269:1588–1590.

33. Warren EH, Gavin MA, Simpson E, Chandler P, Page DC, Disteche C, Stankey KA, Greenberg PD, Riddell SR. The human UTY gene encodes a novel HLA-B8-restricted H-Y antigen. J Immunol 2000; 164:2807–2814.

34. Lahn BT, Page DC. Functional coherence of the human Y chromosome. Science 1997; 278:675–680.

35. Pierce RA, Field ED, Mutis T, Golovina TN, Von Kap-Herr C, Wilke M, Pool J, Shabanowitz J, Pettenati MJ, Eisenlohr LC, Hunt DF, Goulmy E, Engelhard VH. The HA-2 minor histocompatibility antigen is derived from a diallelic gene encoding a novel human class I myosin protein. J Immunol 2001; 167:3223–3230.

36. Faber LM, van Luxemburg-Heijs SA, Veenhof WF, Willemze R, Falkenburg JH. Generation of CD4+ cytotoxic T-lymphocyte clones from a patient with severe graft-versus-host disease after allogeneic bone marrow transplantation: implications for graft-versus-leukemia reactivity. Blood 1995; 86:2821–2828.

37. Soiffer RJ, Alyea EP, Hochberg E, Wu C, Canning C, Parikh B, Zahrieh D, Webb I, Antin J, Ritz J. Randomized trial of CD8+ T-cell depletion in the prevention of graft-versus-host disease associated with donor lymphocyte infusion. Biol Blood Marrow Transplant 2002; 8:625–632.

38. Goulmy E. Human minor histocompatibility antigens: new concepts for marrow transplantation and adoptive immunotherapy. Immunol Rev 1997; 157:125–140.

39. Dolstra H, Fredrix H, Maas F, Coulie PG, Brasseur F, Mensink E, Adema GJ, de Witte TM, Figdor CG, van de Wiel-van Kemenade E. A human minor histocompatibility antigen specific for B cell acute lymphoblastic leukemia. J Exp Med 1999; 189:301–308.

40. Morel S, Levy F, Burlet-Schiltz O, Brasseur F, Probst-Kepper M, Peitrequin AL, Monsarrat B, Van Velthoven R, Cerottini JC, Boon T, Gairin JE, Van den Eynde BJ. Processing of some antigens by the standard proteasome but not by the immunoproteasome results in poor presentation by dendritic cells. Immunity 2000; 12:107–117.

41. Rock KL, Goldberg AL. Degradation of cell proteins and the generation of MHC class I-presented peptides. Annu Rev Immunol 1999; 17:739–779.

42. Falkenburg JH, Smit WM, Willemze R. Cytotoxic T-lymphocyte (CTL) responses against acute or chronic myeloid leukemia. Immunol Rev 1997; 157:223–230.

43. Mutis T, Goulmy E. Hematopoietic system-specific antigens as targets for cellular immunotherapy of hematological malignancies. Semin Hematol 2002; 39:23–31.

44. Gratwohl A, Hermans J, Niederwieser D, van Biezen A, van Houwelingen HC, Apperley J. Female donors influence transplant-related mortality and relapse incidence in male recipients of sibling blood and marrow transplants. Hematol J 2001; 2:363–370.

45. Mutis T, Gillespie G, Schrama E, Falkenburg JH, Moss P, Goulmy E. Tetrameric HLA class I-minor histocompatibility antigen peptide complexes demonstrate minor histocompatibility antigen-specific cytotoxic T lymphocytes in patients with graft-versus-host disease. Nat Med 1999; 5:839–842.

46. Behar E, Chao NJ, Hiraki DD, Krishnaswamy S, Brown BW, Zehnder JL, Grumet FC. Polymorphism of adhesion molecule CD31 and its role in acute graft-versus-host disease. N Engl J Med 1996; 334:286–291.

47. Grumet FC, Hiraki DD, Brown BWM, Zehnder JL, Zacks ES, Draksharapu A, Parnes J, Negrin RS. CD31 mismatching affects marrow transplantation outcome. Biol Blood Marrow Transplant 2001; 7:503–512.

48. Balduini CL, Frassoni F, Noris P, Klersy C, Iannone AM, Bacigalupo A, Giorgiani G, Di Pumpo M, Locatelli F. Donor-recipient incompatibility at CD31-codon 563 is a major risk factor for acute graft-versus-host disease after allogeneic bone marrow transplantation from a human leucocyte antigen-matched donor. Br J Haematol 2001; 114:951–953.

49. Murata M, Emi N, Hirabayashi N, Hamaguchi M, Goto S, Wakita A, Tanimoto M, Saito H, Kodera Y, Morishita Y. No significant association between HA-1 incompatibility and incidence of acute graft-versus-host disease after HLA-identical sibling bone marrow transplantation in Japanese patients. Int J Hematol 2000; 72:371–375.

50. Gallardo D, Arostegui JI, Balas A, Torres A, Caballero D, Carreras E, Brunet S, Jimenez A, Mataix R, Serrano D, Vallejo C, Sanz G, Solano C, Rodriguez-Luaces M, Marin J, Baro J, Sanz C, Roman J, Gonzalez M, Martorell J, Sierra J, Martin C, de la Camara R, Granena A. Disparity for the minor histocompatibility antigen HA-1 is associated with an increased risk of acute graft-versus-host disease (GVHD) but it does not affect chronic GVHD incidence, disease-free survival or overall survival after allogeneic human leucocyte antigen-identical sibling donor transplantation. Br J Haematol 2001; 114:931–936.

51. Tseng LH, Lin MT, Hansen JA, Gooley T, Pei J, Smith AG, Martin EG, Petersdorf EW, Martin PJ. Correlation between disparity for the minor histocompatibility antigen HA-1 and the development of acute graft-versus-host disease after allogeneic marrow transplantation. Blood 1999; 94:2911–2914.

52. Lin MT, Gooley T, Hansen JA, Tseng LH, Martin EG, Singleton K, Smith AG, Mickelson E, Petersdorf EW, Martin PJ. Absence of statistically significant correlation between disparity for the minor histocompatibility antigen-HA-1 and outcome after allogeneic hematopoietic cell transplantation. Blood 2001; 98:3172–3173.

53. Shlomchik WD, Couzens MS, Tang CB, McNiff J, Robert ME, Liu J, Shlomchik MJ, Emerson SG. Prevention of graft versus host disease by inactivation of host antigen-presenting cells. Science 1999; 285:412–415.

54. Teshima T, Ordemann R, Reddy P, Gagin S, Liu C, Cooke KR, Ferrara JL. Acute graft-versus-host disease does not require alloantigen expression on host epithelium. Nat Med 2002; 8:575–581.

55. Dickinson AM, Wang XN, Sviland L, Vyth-Dreese FA, Jackson GH, Schumacher TN, Haanen JB, Mutis T, Goulmy E. In situ dissection of the graft-versus-host activities of cytotoxic T cells specific for minor histocompatibility antigens. Nat Med 2002; 8:410–414.

56. Molldrem JJ, Komanduri K, Wieder E. Overexpressed differentiation antigens as targets of graft-versus-leukemia reactions. Curr Opin Hematol 2002; 9:503–508.

57. Mutis T, Verdijk R, Schrama E, Esendam B, Brand A, Goulmy E. Feasibility of immunotherapy of relapsed leukemia with ex vivo-generated cytotoxic T lymphocytes specific for hematopoietic system-restricted minor histocompatibility antigens. Blood 1999; 93:2336–2341.

58. Bonnet D, Warren EH, Greenberg PD, Dick JE, Riddell SR. CD8(+) minor histocompatibility antigen-specific cytotoxic T lymphocyte clones eliminate human acute myeloid leukemia stem cells. Proc Natl Acad Sci USA 1999; 96:8639–8644.

59. Falkenburg JH, Goselink HM, van der Harst D, van Luxemburg-Heijs SA, Kooy-Winkelaar YM, Faber LM, de Kroon J, Brand A, Fibbe WE, Willemze R, et al. Growth inhibition of clonogenic leukemic precursor cells by minor histocompatibility antigen-specific cytotoxic T lymphocytes. J Exp Med 1991; 174:27–33.

60. Fujii N, Hiraki A, Ikeda K, Ohmura Y, Nozaki I, Shinagawa K, Ishimaru F, Kiura K, Shimizu N, Tanimoto M, Harada M. Expression of minor histocompatibility antigen, HA-1, in solid tumor cells. Transplantation 2002; 73:1137–1141.

61. Childs R, Chernoff A, Contentin N, Bahceci E, Schrump D, Leitman S, Read EJ, Tisdale J, Dunbar C, Linehan WM, Young NS, Barrett AJ. Regression of metastatic renal-cell carcinoma after nonmyeloablative allogeneic peripheral-blood stem-cell transplantation. N Engl J Med 2000; 343:750–758.

62. Collins RH Jr, Goldstein S, Giralt S, Levine J, Porter D, Drobyski W, Barrett J, Johnson M, Kirk A, Horowitz M, Parker P. Donor leukocyte infusions in acute lymphocytic leukemia. Bone Marrow Transplant 2000; 26:511–516.

63. Slavin S, Morecki S, Weiss L, Or R. Donor lymphocyte infusion: the use of alloreactive and tumor-reactive lymphocytes for immunotherapy of malignant and nonmalignant diseases in conjunction with allogeneic stem cell transplantation. J Hematother Stem Cell Res 2002; 11:265–276.

64. Marks DI, Lush R, Cavenagh J, Milligan DW, Schey S, Parker A, Clark FJ, Hunt L, Yin J, Fuller S, Vandenberghe E, Marsh J, Littlewood T, Smith GM, Culligan D, Hunter A, Chopra R, Davies A, Towlson K, Williams CD. The toxicity and efficacy of donor lymphocyte infusions given after reduced-intensity conditioning allogeneic stem cell transplantation. Blood 2002; 100:3108–3114.

65. Bellucci R, Alyea EP, Weller E, Chillemi A, Hochberg E, Wu CJ, Canning C, Schlossman R, Soiffer RJ, Anderson KC, Ritz J. Immunologic effects of prophylactic donor lymphocyte infusion after allogeneic marrow transplantation for multiple myeloma. Blood 2002; 99:4610–4617.

66. Anderson LD Jr, Mori S, Mann S, Savary CA, Mullen CA. Pretransplant tumor antigen-specific immunization of allogeneic bone marrow transplant donors enhances graft-versus-tumor activity without exacerbation of graft-versus-host disease. Cancer Res 2000; 60:5797–5802.

67. Narita M, Takahashi M, Liu A, Nikkuni K, Furukawa T, Toba K, Koyama S, Takai K, Sanada M, Aizawa Y. Leukemia blast-induced T-cell anergy demonstrated by leukemia-derived dendritic cells in acute myelogenous leukemia. Exp Hematol 2001; 29:709–719.

68. Appleman LJ, Tzachanis D, Grader-Beck T, Van Puijenbroek AA, Boussiotis VA. Induction of immunologic tolerance for allogeneic hematopoietic cell transplantation. Leuk Lymphoma 2002; 43:1159–1167.

69. Riddell SR, Watanabe KS, Goodrich JM, Li CR, Agha ME, Greenberg PD. Restoration of viral immunity in immunodeficient humans by the adoptive transfer of T cell clones. Science 1992; 257:238–241.

70. Heslop HE, Ng CY, Li C, Smith CA, Loftin SK, Krance RA, Brenner MK, Rooney CM. Long-term restoration of immunity against Epstein-Barr virus infection by adoptive transfer of gene-modified virus-specific T lymphocytes. Nat Med 1996; 2:551–555.

71. Savoldo B, Huls MH, Liu Z, Okamura T, Volk HD, Reinke P, Sabat R, Babel N, Jones JF, Webster-Cyriaque J, Gee AP, Brenner MK, Heslop HE, Rooney CM. Autologous Epstein-Barr virus (EBV)-specific cytotoxic T cells for the treatment of persistent active EBV infection. Blood 2002; 100:4059–4066.

72. Fontaine P, Roy-Proulx G, Knafo L, Baron C, Roy DC, Perreault C. Adoptive transfer of minor histocompatibility antigen-specific T lymphocytes eradicates leukemia cells without causing graft-versus-host disease. Nat Med 2001; 7:789–794.

73. Mutis T, Ghoreschi K, Schrama E, Kamp J, Heemskerk M, Falkenburg JH, Wilke M, Goulmy E. Efficient induction of minor histocompatibility antigen HA-1-specific cytotoxic T-cells using dendritic cells retrovirally transduced with HA-1-coding cDNA. Biol Blood Marrow Transplant 2002; 8:412–419.

74. Gillespie G, Mutis T, Schrama E, Kamp J, Esendam B, Falkenburg JF, Goulmy E, Moss P. HLA class I-minor histocompatibility antigen tetramers select cytotoxic T cells with high avidity to the natural ligand. Hematol J 2000; 1:403–410.

75. Knabel M, Franz TJ, Schiemann M, Wulf A, Villmow B, Schmidt B, Bernhard H, Wagner H, Busch DH. Reversible MHC multimer staining for functional isolation of T-cell populations and effective adoptive transfer. Nat Med 2002; 8:631–637.

76. Manz R, Assenmacher M, Pfluger E, Miltenyi S, Radbruch A. Analysis and sorting of live cells according to secreted molecules, relocated to a cell-surface affinity matrix. Proc Natl Acad Sci USA 1995; 92:1921–1925.

77. Brosterhus H, Brings S, Leyendeckers H, Manz RA, Miltenyi S, Radbruch A, Assenmacher M, Schmitz J. Enrichment and detection of live antigen-specific CD4(+) and CD8(+) T cells based on cytokine secretion. Eur J Immunol 1999; 29:4053–4059.

78. John Campbell. Rapid Clinical Scale Isolation and Expansion of CMV-Specific T cells using Interferon-Gamma Secretion. Barcelona: International Society for Cellular Therapy, 2002 (oral presentation).

79. Bickham K, Munz C, Tsang ML, Larsson M, Fonteneau JF, Bhardwaj N, Steinman R. EBNA1-specific CD4+ T cells in healthy carriers of Epstein-Barr virus are primarily Th1 in function. J Clin Invest 2001; 107:121–130.

80. Aversa F, Tabilio A, Velardi A, Cunningham I, Terenzi A, Falzetti F, Ruggeri L, Barbabietola G, Aristei C, Latini P, Reisner Y, Martelli MF. Treatment of high-risk acute leukemia with T-cell-depleted stem cells from related donors with one fully mismatched HLA haplotype. N Engl J Med 1998; 339:1186–1193.

81. Martelli MF, Aversa F, Bachar-Lustig E, Velardi A, Reich-Zelicher S, Tabilio A, Gur H, Reisner Y. Transplants across human leukocyte antigen barriers. Semin Hematol 2002; 39:48–56.

82. Ruggeri L, Capanni M, Urbani E, Perruccio K, Shlomchik WD, Tosti A, Posati S, Rogaia D, Frassoni F, Aversa F, Martelli MF, Velardi A. Effectiveness of donor natural killer cell alloreactivity in mismatched hematopoietic transplants. Science 2002; 295:2097–2100.

83. Ruggeri L, Capanni M, Casucci M, Volpi I, Tosti A, Perruccio K, Urbani E, Negrin RS, Martelli MF, Velardi A. Role of natural killer cell alloreactivity in HLA-mismatched hematopoietic stem cell transplantation. Blood 1999; 94:333–339.

84. Farag SS, Fehniger TA, Ruggeri L, Velardi A, Caligiuri MA. Natural killer cell receptors: new biology and insights into the graft-versus-leukemia effect. Blood 2002; 100:1935–1947.

85. Bellantuono I, Gao L, Parry S, Marley S, Dazzi F, Apperley J, Goldman JM, Stauss HJ. Two distinct HLA-A0201-presented epitopes of the Wilms tumor antigen 1 can function as targets for leukemia-reactive CTL. Blood 2002; 100:3835–3837.

86. Gao L, Bellantuono I, Elsasser A, Marley SB, Gordon MY, Goldman JM, Stauss HJ. Selective elimination of leukemic CD34(+) progenitor cells by cytotoxic T lymphocytes specific for WT1. Blood 2000; 95:2198–2203.

87. Mutis T, Blokland E, Kester M, Schrama E, Goulmy E. Generation of minor histocompatibility antigen HA-1-specific cytotoxic T cells restricted by nonself HLA molecules: a potential strategy to treat relapsed leukemia after HLA-mismatched stem cell transplantation. Blood 2002; 100:547–552.

88. den Haan JM, Mutis T, Blokland E, AP IJ, Goulmy E. General T-cell receptor antagonists to immunomodulate HLA-A2-restricted minor histocompatibility antigen HA-1-specific T-cell responses. Blood 2002; 99:985–992.

89. Sadovnikova E, Jopling LA, Soo KS, Stauss HJ. Generation of human tumor-reactive cytotoxic T cells against peptides presented by non-self HLA class I molecules. Eur J Immunol 1998; 28:193–200.

90. Clay TM, Custer MC, Sachs J, Hwu P, Rosenberg SA, Nishimura MI. Efficient transfer of a tumor antigen-reactive TCR to human peripheral blood lymphocytes confers anti-tumor reactivity. J Immunol 1999; 163:507–513.

91. Cooper LJ, Kalos M, Lewinsohn DA, Riddell SR, Greenberg PD. Transfer of specificity for human immunodeficiency virus type 1 into primary human T lymphocytes by introduction of T-cell receptor genes. J Virol 2000; 74:8207–8212.

92. Stanislawski T, Voss RH, Lotz C, Sadovnikova E, Willemsen RA, Kuball J, Ruppert T, Bolhuis RL, Melief CJ, Huber C, Stauss HJ, Theobald M. Circumventing tolerance to a human MDM2-derived tumor antigen by TCR gene transfer. Nat Immunol 2001; 2:962–970.

93. Heemskerk MH, de Paus RA, Lurvink EG, Koning F, Mulder A, Willemze R, van Rood JJ, Falkenburg JH. Dual HLA class I and class II restricted recognition of alloreactive T lymphocytes mediated by a single T cell receptor complex. Proc Natl Acad Sci USA 2001; 98:6806–6811.

94. Kessels HW, Wolkers MC, van den Boom MD, van der Valk MA, Schumacher TN. Immunotherapy through TCR gene transfer. Nat Immunol 2001; 2:957–961.

95. Bonini C, Ferrari G, Verzeletti S, Servida P, Zappone E, Ruggieri L, Ponzoni M, Rossini S, Mavilio F, Traversari C, Bordignon C. HSV-TK gene transfer into donor lymphocytes for control of allogeneic graft-versus-leukemia. Science 1997; 276:1719–1724.

96. Introna M, Barbui AM, Bambacioni F, Casati C, Gaipa G, Borleri G, Bernasconi S, Barbui T, Golay J, Biondi A, Rambaldi A. Genetic modification of human T cells with CD20: a strategy to purify and lyse transduced cells with anti-CD20 antibodies. Hum Gene Ther 2000; 11:611–620.

97. den Haan JM, Sherman NE, Blokland E, Huczko E, Koning F, Drijfhout JW, Skipper J, Shabanowitz J, Hunt DF, Engelhard VH, et al. Identification of a graft versus host disease-associated human minor histocompatibility antigen. Science 1995; 268:1476–1480.

98. Dolstra H, de Rijke B, Fredrix H, Maas F, Scherpen F, Avilo MJ, Vicario JL, Beekman NJ, Ossendorp F, de Witte TM, van de Wiel-van Kemenade E. Bi-directional allelic recognition of the human minor histocompatibility antigen HB-1 by cytotoxic T lymphocytes. Eur J Immunol 2002; 32:2748–2758.

99. Vogt MH, de Paus RA, Voogt PJ, Willemze R, Falkenburg JH. DFFRY codes for a new human male-specific minor transplantation antigen involved in bone marrow graft rejection. Blood 2000; 95:1100–1105.

100. Pierce RA, Field ED, den Haan JM, Caldwell JA, White FM, Marto JA, Wang W, Frost LM, Blokland E, Reinhardus C, Shabanowitz J, Hunt DF, Goulmy E, Engelhard VH. Cutting edge: the HLA-A*0101-restricted HY minor histocompatibility antigen originates from DFFRY and contains a cysteinylated cysteine residue as identified by a novel mass spectrometric technique. J Immunol 1999; 163:6360–6364.

101. Meadows L, Wang W, den Haan JM, Blokland E, Reinhardus C, Drijfhout JW, Shabanowitz J, Pierce R, Agulnik AI, Bishop CE, Hunt DF, Goulmy E, Engelhard VH. The HLA-A*0201-restricted H-Y antigen contains a posttranslationally modified cysteine that significantly affects T cell recognition. Immunity 1997; 6:273–281.

102. Vogt MH, Goulmy E, Kloosterboer FM, Blokland E, de Paus RA, Willemze R, Falkenburg JH. UTY gene codes for an HLA-B60-restricted human male-specific minor histocompatibility antigen involved in stem cell graft rejection: characterization of the critical polymorphic amino acid residues for T-cell recognition. Blood 2000; 96:3126–3132.

103. Vogt MH, van den Muijsenberg JW, Goulmy E, Spierings E, Kluck P, Kester MG, van Soest RA, Drijfhout JW, Willemze R, Falkenburg JH. The DBY gene codes for an HLA-DQ5-restricted human male-specific minor histocompatibility antigen involved in graft-versus-host disease. Blood 2002; 99:3027–3032.

14

Advances in Tissue Typing and Their Potential Impact on GVHD Incidence and Severity

EFFIE W. PETERSDORF

University of Washington and Fred Hutchinson Cancer Research Center, Seattle, Washington, U.S.A.

TAKEHIKO SASAZUKI

Research Institute, International Medical Center of Japan, Tokyo, Japan

I. INTRODUCTION

The HLA genetic region encodes histocompatibility molecules that play a central role in the immune response. A key feature of the HLA system is its extensive polymorphism. Availability of DNA-based typing methods for precise discrimination of HLA allelic variants has contributed to a more complete understanding of the immunogenetic barriers that lead to graft-vs.-host disease (GVHD). Data demonstrate that the overall results of unrelated hematopoietic cell transplantation (HCT) can be optimized through comprehensive and precise donor matching for HLA class I and II alleles. Furthermore, the permissibility of an HLA mismatch is shaped by a complex interaction of qualitative and quantitative differences in the HLA sequences between the donor and recipient. With the ability to type and match donors with precision, clinical experience now demonstrates that the overall outcome of unrelated HCT can approach that of sibling transplantation, especially for good risk patients. Furthermore, it is possible to achieve excellent clinical results with a less than perfectly matched donor, thereby increasing the accessibility to donors for patients in need of a transplant.

II. THE MAJOR HISTOCOMPATIBILITY COMPLEX

The HLA region spans approximately 4000 kilobases of DNA, equivalent to 0.1% of the human genome, and is comprised of three distinct regions designated class I, class II, and class III (Fig. 1). The human MHC was first recognized in the early 1950s following observations that sera from patients with febrile transfusion reactions could cause the agglutination of leukocytes from their transfusion donors (1). Subsequent studies showed that leukocyte antibodies could also be found in the sera of multiparous women. The acronym HLA is derived from the former designation human-1 (HU-1) and leukocyte antigen (LA) introduced by Dausset and Payne, respectively (1–5).

HLA alloantigens serve as the cornerstone of the immune response. T cells recognize foreign antigens presented by HLA molecules. A constellation of different peptide antigens can be processed and presented to T cells, including those derived from bacteria, viruses, and toxins, as well as peptides from autologous tissue and cellular products. Definition of the peptide-binding motifs that characterize HLA molecules provides important information on the role of the HLA system in peptide presentation, immune responsiveness, and disease susceptibility (6–8). The extensive polymorphism of the MHC assures that a vast array of foreign peptides can be presented to the immune system (9). HLA molecules represent a transplantation barrier due to the fundamental role they play in T-cell activation and initiation of an alloresponse.

Genes within the class I and class II regions are considered to be part of the immunoglobulin gene superfamily (10). The differential structural properties of HLA class I and class II molecules account for their respective roles in activating different populations of T lymphocytes. Cytotoxic (T_C) T lymphocytes recognize antigenic peptides presented by HLA class I molecules, while helper (T_H) T lymphocytes recognize antigenic peptides presented by HLA class II molecules. HLA class I and class II molecules are characterized by distinctive α and β polypeptide subunits that combine to form $\alpha\beta$ heterodimers characteristic of the mature molecule. Class I molecules were originally defined by typing with

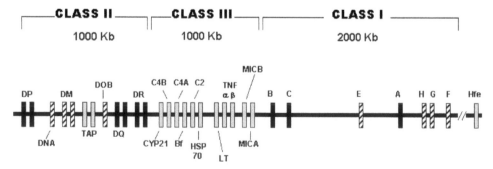

Figure 1 The human major histocompatibility complex (MHC). The class II HLA-DR, DQ, DP genes and the class I HLA-A, B, C genes are shown in black. HLA region–associated genes include transporter of antigenic peptides (TAP), 21-hydroxylase (CYP21; also termed 21-OH or P450-C21B), complement component C4, properidin factor B of the alternate complement pathway (Bf), complement component C2, heat-shock protein (HSP 70), tumor necrosis factor (TNF) complex with TNFα, TNFβ, and lymphotoxin-A (LTA), MICB, MICA, and the hemachromatosis gene (Hfe).

alloantisera and class II molecules defined by testing in functional assays such as the mixed lymphocyte culture (MLC) reaction (11,12).

A. Class I Genes

The HLA class I region encodes at least 17 resident loci. Three of these loci, termed class Ia, encode HLA-A, -B, and -C alloantigens that constitute the major class I determinants important for matching in tissue transplantation. HLA-A, -B, and -C genes show a striking degree of sequence and structural homology with one another, and all are highly polymorphic (9). Three additional class I genes, HLA-E, -F, and -G, have been defined as class Ib genes and encode cell-surface molecules that have different patterns of expression (13–15). HLA-G molecules are expressed only on the placental trophoblast, HLA-F molecules are found in the trophoblast, while HLA-E molecules are ubiquitously expressed. The function of class 1b gene products is not fully known, but recent data demonstrate that they serve as ligands for natural killer (NK) cell receptors and thus may regulate NK function (16,17).

HLA-A, -B, and -C genes are each comprised of eight exons. Exon 1 is a leader sequence; exons 2, 3, and 4 encode the $\alpha1$, $\alpha2$, and $\alpha3$ domains, respectively; exon 5 encodes the trans-membrane portion of the molecule; and exons 6, 7, and 8 encode the cytoplasmic tail. HLA class I molecules consist of a single polymorphic α (heavy) chain of approximately 338–341 residues in length, which is noncovalently bound at the cell surface to a β_2-microglobulin light chain. The gene for β_2-microglobulin is encoded on chromosome 15. Structurally, class I molecules are comprised of two α-helical regions overlying an eight-strand antiparallel β-pleated sheet that forms the groove for peptide binding (6). Nucleotide substitutions within exons 2 and 3 of class I genes are not distributed randomly, but are concentrated in discrete hypervariable regions. Polymorphic sites within the $\alpha1$ and $\alpha2$ domains facilitate the binding of peptide fragments for presentation to the T-cell receptor (18). These polymorphic sites also determine the allospecificity of the molecule and form the basis for their classification as HLA alloantigens (9).

B. Class II Genes

Class II genes have been collectively referred to as HLA-D region genes since they were initially described in the mid-1970s after the description of HLA-A, -B, and -C. Five families of class II genes are recognized and designated HLA-DR, -DQ, -DO, -DN, and -DP. Class II molecules consist of a single polymorphic (HLA-DQ and -DP) or nonpolymorphic (HLA-DR) α chain noncovalently bound to a polymorphic β chain (7). The β chains of HLA-DR, -DQ, and -DP antigens are encoded by the HLA-DRB, -DQB, and -DPB genes, respectively. Polymorphic HLA-DR β chains are encoded by four distinct HLA-DRB genes termed DRB1, DRB3, DRB4, and DRB5. The number and combination of HLA-DRB genes are inherited as a haplotype as follows: DR2 haplotypes include DRB5 and DRB1; DR3, 5, 6 haplotypes include DRB3 and DRB1; DR4, 7 haplotypes include DRB4 and DRB1. As with class I genes, HLA-DR, -DQ, and -DP genes are highly polymorphic (9). Further polymorphism of class II molecules can be generated as a result of *trans* pairing of a polymorphic HLA-DQ α chain encoded by one parental chromosome with a polymorphic DQ β chain encoded by the other parental chromosome.

Polymorphic epitopes within class II molecules are localized in specific regions of the $\alpha 1$ and $\beta 1$ domains of the α and β chains, respectively, to enable binding of a large array of peptides (18,19). The class II α and β domains also determine the allospecificity of the class II molecule and are potent stimulators of immune reactions in HCT.

C. Class III Genes

The HLA class III region maps between the class I and II regions and is comprised of at least 62 genes that span approximately one megabase of DNA. Although class III genes are located within the MHC complex, they are notably different from class I and II genes. Class III genes encode a diverse group of proteins that include complement components, tumor necrosis factor, transport proteins, and heat shock proteins; cytokine polymorphisms encoded in the class III region have relevance in GVHD after allogeneic transplantation (20).

III. HLA TYPING METHODOLOGY

Since 1964 a series of 13 international histocompatibility workshops has facilitated the development of standardized tissue typing reagents and nomenclature for HLA genes and gene products. In the early phase of these workshops, serological reagents were extensively evaluated and characterized and served as the gold standard for HLA typing until the advent of PCR in the mid-1980s.

A. Serology

The importance of matching for HLA antigens was initially demonstrated in experimental models (21,22) and applied clinically in 1968 with the first successful human allogeneic marrow transplants (23,24). At that time the HLA system was poorly defined and genes encoding HLA antigens had not been identified. Typing was performed with serological methods using a complement-dependent microcytotoxicity assay with alloantisera containing HLA antibodies capable of detecting polymorphic specificities (25). Initially two clusters of antigens were identified and named HLA-A and -B. A third group was identified in 1970 and named the HLA-C locus (5).

Antisera were highly selected for HLA specificity and usually obtained from multiparous women immunized to HLA alloantigens through pregnancy. HLA alloantigens characteristically express multiple specificities or epitopes. A public specificity describes an epitope shared by more than one distinct HLA antigen. A private specificity refers to epitopes unique to a single antigen. Such private specificities are also termed splits of the public antigen. Clusters of serologically crossreactive HLA-A and -B antigens can be classified as belonging to cross-reactive groups (CREGs). Antigens within a class I CREG are presumed to share one or more public epitopes in addition to their individual and unique private epitope(s). Although CREGs were not originally defined for class II specificities, similar relationships exist between parent antigens and split antigens (9). An increasing number of class I and class II alleles are definable by DNA-based typing methods but not by serological methods. To bridge the transition in nomenclature from serological to DNA-based typing methods, serologically equivalent designations have been defined (26).

B. Cellular Typing and Functional Assays

1. The MLC and HCT

A new family of alloantigens expressed on B cells and monocytes was identified using alloantisera that had been absorbed with platelets to remove antibodies to the class I HLA-A, -B, and -C antigens. A correlation was found between these "Ia-like" specificities and the T-cell–defined "Dw" allotypes determined by MLC typing (27,28). Eventually the human Ia antigens were shown to be encoded by three distinct loci named HLA-DR, -DQ, and -DP (29,30). The most commonly used cellular assay for the class II regions is the MLC reaction, a test in which disparity for HLA-D region antigens leads to lymphocyte activation and proliferation (11,12). Cells that proliferate in an MLC reaction belong to the helper T lymphocyte (T_H) subset. Although the strength of the proliferation measured in an MLC test correlates roughly with the degree of HLA-D region incompatibility (31), the standard one-way MLC assay has proven to be poorly predictive of GVHD in both haploidentical related and phenotypically matched unrelated donor transplants (32–34). In a study of 435 unrelated donor transplants, including 208 matched for HLA-A, -B, and -DRB1 and 191 incompatible for one HLA-A, -B, or -DR antigen mismatch, donor-vs.-recipient MLC responses were broadly reactive ranging from negative to strongly positive, and the overlap in MLC responses between cases matched and mismatched for DRB1 alleles was extensive (33). Using optimally defined cut-offs of 4% and 16% relative response, there was no correlation with the risk of acute GVHD ($p = 0.6$ and 0.5, respectively). A modified MLC assay known as the homozygous typing cell (HTC) assay was developed and was capable of detecting polymorphism (HLA-Dw) among HLA-DR-DQ alloantigens (28,35). After more complete sequence information for class II genes became available in the late 1980s, correlation of certain HLA-Dw specificities to unique HLA-DRB alleles could be defined (9).

2. CTLp and HTLp Assays

Several in vitro approaches to testing donor immune responses to host alloantigen have utility in predicting the risk of GVHD and mortality prior to transplantation. These techniques use the limiting dilution assay (LDA) to determine the frequency of donor antihost cytotoxic T-lymphocyte precursors (CTLp) and helper T-lymphocyte precursors (HTLp). The CTLp and HTLp may provide a means to select a suitable unrelated donor when more than one equally matched donor is available (36–45). High CTLp frequencies have been observed with class I donor-recipient mismatching; HTLp has been shown to detect class II disparity (37,38,42). LDAs have the potential advantage of detecting minor histocompatibility antigens; high precursor frequencies might identify alloimmunized donors whose T cells could have an increased ability to cause GVHD. Although the presence of class I mismatching correlates with high CTLp frequencies, exceptions can be found (45). In particular, disparity at residues 97, 99, 113, 114, and 116 of the HLA-C molecule has been associated with high CTLp frequencies (45), indicating that the CTLp assay is capable of identifying donor-recipient disparity for residues that influence peptide binding.

An association between the donor-vs.-recipient CTLp frequency and risk of acute GVHD after unrelated donor HCT has been observed in the setting of ex vivo or in vivo T-cell depletion (TCD) for GVHD prophylaxis (36,39,41,43,44). In T-replete transplantation, significant associations between CTLp frequency and acute GVHD could not be identified (46–48). These findings support the hypothesis that the risk of GVHD is related to the total number of transplanted donor T cells that recognize recipient alloantigens. The number of host-reactive T cells in an unmodified graft might often be sufficient to initiate GVHD regardless of the donor antirecipient CTLp frequency, while the number of specific T cells remaining in a T-cell–depleted graft might not be sufficient to initiate GVHD when the CTLp frequency is low. Alternatively, lack of association between CTLp and GVHD risk may be a consequence of inappropriate tissue distribution in vivo, low TCR affinity (which might be sufficient to generate a response in vitro but not in vivo) (49), or an inadequate helper T-cell response in vivo (50). Antigens that generate HTL responses might not evoke GVHD in the absence of a CTL response (51). Finally, the development of GVHD in the apparent absence of a CTL response could reflect the lack of appropriate peptide expression by target cells used for the in vitro assay.

C. DNA Typing Methods

The availability of DNA-based methods for HLA typing has had a dramatic impact on the clinical practice of unrelated HCT and has greatly accelerated understanding of the HLA genetic barrier. The transition from serological phenotyping to DNA-based genotyping has introduced a need for refined HLA nomenclature and the development of dictionaries of HLA alleles and antigen equivalents (26,52). Guidelines for histocompatiblity testing of volunteer donors using DNA-based methods are available (53–55), and informatics networks have been developed to effectively interpret and use molecular typing data for donor search and selection (56,57).

Most typing methods currently in use in clinical and research laboratories are based on the amplification of specific, HLA genes from genomic DNA using the polymerase chain reaction (PCR). PCR amplification of an HLA gene involves the use of locus-specific, group-specific, or allele-specific primers. Locus-specific primers amplify all alleles encoded at a given locus but not alleles encoded by other loci. Group-specific primers amplify families of alleles that share a common polymorphism(s). Allele-specific primers are used to amplify a single allele and can differentiate between two sequences that differ by only a single base change. Strategies for HLA typing can include combinations of locus-specific primers to amplify and analyze both alleles in a heterozygous sample, followed by group-specific or allele-specific amplification to isolate one of the two alleles for further characterization.

PCR-based typing methods provide either direct determination of the entire coding region sequence of an allele [e.g., sequencing-based typing (SBT)] or partial sequence information allowing inference of the HLA allele [e.g., sequence-specific oligonucleotide probe hybridization (SSOPH) or sequence-specific primer (SSP)]. As a consequence, DNA-based typing methods vary according to the level of discrimination they provide in defining the nucleotide sequence of an HLA allele. When the DNA typing method allows identification of a serologically defined antigen-equivalent (e.g., HLA-A2 or B27), the method is termed low resolution. For example, SSOPH methods that employ a restricted number of probes descriptive for key polymorphic regions of the exon provide limited sequence information about a particular HLA allele, equivalent to that achievable by serology. Typing methods that provide information beyond the serological level but short of the allele level are termed intermediate resolution and include SSOPH methods that employ a wider array of probes. Typing methods that generate nucleotide sequence information allowing complete information of an exon(s) are termed high resolution. High-resolution typing results may be achieved by direct automated SBT of an HLA gene or by the use of comprehensive panels of oligonucleotide probes that are descriptive of all known regions of variability within a gene. It follows, then, that a patient and donor who are "matched" for HLA-A and -B antigens by low-resolution typing methods may be mismatched for HLA-A or -B alleles (or both).

1. Sequence-Specific Primers

The SSP method employs a panel of amplification primers that are descriptive for known polymorphisms encoded by an HLA locus or group of alleles (58–63). After initial PCR amplification, the PCR products are electropheresed on a gel. Amplification of a PCR product of appropriate size indicates that the target DNA encoded the complementary sequence to the PCR primer. Assignment of an HLA type is made by examining the composite pattern of positive and negative PCR reactions. The SSP method is a cost-effective and simple method best suited for low- or intermediate-resolution typing. High-resolution definition of unique alleles requires large numbers of PCR primers that are descriptive for the unique polymorphisms that characterize that allele.

2. Sequence-Specific Oligonucleotide Probe Hybridization

Resolution of HLA alleles at low, intermediate, or high levels can be achieved with SSOPH methods (64–77). In forward blot SSOPH methods, the PCR-amplified product is immobilized to a solid phase support, and non–radioactive-labeled oligonucleotide probes are allowed to hybridize to the support. Probes with sequences complementary to the membrane-bound DNA will hybridize, whereas those with as little as a single nucleotide mismatch will fail to hybridize. In the reverse blot format, the probes are immobilized to the solid phase support, and the PCR-amplified target DNA is then applied and allowed to hybridize. For both approaches, the pattern of positive and negative hybridization is used to deduce the HLA type of the target DNA. SSOPH methods are informative for polymorphisms that are described by the probe panel. New sequences that differ in the regions that are probed are signaled by novel hybridization patterns. The SSOPH method is well suited to high-volume HLA typing.

3. Sequencing

Sequencing methods provide the highest resolution typing of HLA alleles, can be applied to large-scale typing of populations, and are particularly well suited for the definitive characterization of newly defined alleles (78–83). Several approaches have been used to sequence HLA genes, including the use of cloned templates (cDNA) and PCR-amplified genomic DNA. One method that has gained wide use in HLA typing is automated fluorescent sequencing. Cycle sequencing of the PCR product uses either primers labeled with a fluorescent label (dye primer, usually $5'$ primer) or dideoxynucleotides ddATP, ddTTP, ddGTP, ddCTP labeled with fluorescent tag (dye terminator). In dye primer sequencing, the label is incorporated into the $5'$ end of the HLA sequence, whereas in dye terminator sequencing the addition of a labeled dideoxynucleotide at the $3'$ end terminates the sequencing reaction. In both approaches the sequencing reaction is electropheresed on a polyacrylamide gel using an automated sequencer. The fluorescent signals are captured and interpreted as a sequence of DNA bases by a computer program. Assignment of the HLA allele(s) is performed by comparing the derived sequence to a reference sequence for a given gene.

4. Reference Strand–Mediated Conformation Analysis

Reference strand–mediated conformation analysis (RSCA) is a novel approach for high-resolution DNA typing and donor matching (84,85). This technique uses a fluorescein-labeled reference DNA that has been PCR-amplified from the HLA gene of interest. The reference DNA is allowed to hybridize to locus-specific PCR products from the test samples. Duplex formation occurs when there is complementarity between the reference and test nucleotide sequences. Each antisense nucleotide strand is uniquely different, and, thus, the mobility of the duplex on gel electropheresis can be used for discrimination. This method allows the detection of single nucleotide substitutions within a given sequence and the rapid assessment of donor-recipient identity.

5. Oligonucleotide Arrays

Oligonucleotide array technology combines nucleic acid hybridization approaches with high-density DNA array technology. Initially developed to improve sequencing efforts in the Human Genome Project, the oligonucleotide array technology has been successfully applied to many fields of molecular biology, including large-scale gene discovery, monitoring the expression of thousands of genes, mutation and polymorphism detection, as well as mapping of genomic clones.

Oligonucleotide array technology for HLA typing has high sensitivity and specificity for the detection of complex polymorphisms in heterozygous individuals (86). Multiple regions of polymorphisms in many HLA genes can be simultaneously assessed. Oligonucleotide probes can be designed to all known substitutions or to all four potential nucleotides and thereby enable detection of new sequence polymorphisms. Redundancy of probe sequences allows combinations of alleles to be distinguished in heterozygous individuals. Arrays are well suited to the analysis of very large populations for multiple polymorphic genes.

IV. IMPORTANCE OF HLA DIVERSITY AND HAPLOTYPES IN DONOR HLA MATCHING

The definition of an HLA-matched donor has been a fluid concept, made complex by the ever-increasing number of novel HLA alleles being discovered in diverse human populations. To date, over 211 HLA-A, 432 HLA- B, 110 HLA-C, 360 HLA-DRB1, and 47 HLA-DQB1 alleles have been defined (9). With the availability of DNA-based methods, it is feasible to detect single nucleotide differences that distinguish these alleles as unique. Many of the unrelated donor-patient transplant pairs initially matched for HLA-A, -B, and -DR by serology and MLC are now known to be mismatched for HLA-A, -C, -B, -DR, -DQ and -DP alleles (87–107). In one large retrospective analysis of phenotypically matched transplant pairs, molecular methods were used to define the HLA-DRB1, -DRB3, -DRB5,- DQA1, -DQB1, -DPA1, and -DPB1 alleles (106). Only 9.4% of this study population was allele-matched for all 7 loci. Loci other than HLA-A, B, and DR may contribute to additional donor-recipient disparity. In a study by Scott et al., a high percentage (35%) of mismatching at the HLA-C locus was detected using DNA-based methods among pairs who were originally selected at the time of transplantation using serological methods for HLA-A and -B (103). This study demonstrates that HLA-A/B matching does not predict HLA-C matching; furthermore, molecular methods are required for accurate typing of this locus. These studies highlight the importance of molecular typing tools for complete and precise characterization of potential unrelated donors and recipients.

The frequencies of HLA alleles, antigens, and haplotypes reflect the ethnicity and race of the transplant recipient and donor (108–117), and, as a consequence, the probability of identifying a suitable donor and the frequency of allele mismatching is a reflection of the ethnic background of the recipient and the donor. In Caucasian transplant populations, donor-recipient allele disparity is frequent for common phenotypes including A2, B27, B35, B39, and DR4 (102,104). In Asian populations, the frequency of mismatches for HLA alleles can differ dramatically from that of Caucasian patients and donors (116).

Such differences in mismatch frequencies reflect both diversity of HLA sequences and also diversity in HLA haplotypes. In general, the likelihood of identifying a donor is increased if the donor and patient share the same ethnic or racial background and when the patient has two common extended HLA haplotypes (118). HLA alleles are found in association with each other at an observed frequency that exceeds their expected frequency, a phenomenon known as linkage disequilibrium (LD) (119,120). For example, the observed association of HLA-B and -C alleles at a frequency higher than expected indicates strong positive LD and thereby increases the probability that an HLA-A, -B, or -DR matched donor will also be matched for HLA-C. Similarly, a strong degree of LD between HLA-DR and HLA-DQ increases the probability that an HLA-A, -B, or -DR matched donor will be HLA-DQ matched with the recipient (121,122). Overall, the number of common haplotypes is relatively limited. Among North American Caucasians only 7 haplotypes occur with frequencies exceeding 1% (110). Using the example of the HLA-A1, -B8, -DR3 and HLA-A3, -B7, -DR2 haplotypes in Caucasians, the chances of identifying a matched donor for a patient with these two haplotypes is exceedingly high (110). With increased use of DNA-based methods for donor registry typing, data on the probability of identifying suitable donors and estimates of optimal registry size and composition have recently become available (54,108–115,121–124).

V. SIGNIFICANCE OF HLA MATCHING AND RISK OF ACUTE GVHD AFTER UNRELATED HCT

The importance of the HLA barrier in GVH reactions was demonstrated in the early unrelated transplant experience, which uniformly reported a relatively high incidence of acute GVHD compared to that observed in HLA-identical sibling transplantation (118,125–133). The likelihood of undetected HLA allele disparity among these early serologically matched cases gave impetus to the hypothesis that the safety and efficacy of unrelated HCT could be improved through the development and application of DNA-based HLA typing methods and through a better understanding of the biological significance of allelic variation.

The long-term goal of donor HLA matching criteria is to maximize safety and efficacy of the transplant procedure and to increase availability of unrelated donor HCT for patients who have no other therapeutic option. Current criteria include the identification and prioritization of matched donors over mismatched donors using DNA-based typing methods because more complete and accurate matching is associated with lower risks of GVHD and improved survival. Furthermore, when a matched donor is not available, data demonstrate that avoidance of donors mismatched for multiple alleles is critical because multilocus disparity is associated with increased risks of GVHD and mortality. The minimal requirements for HLA matching, however, can vary depending on the clinical situation, including the conditioning regimen [T-cell depleted vs. T-replete; total body irradiation (TBI) vs. no TBI], the stem cell source, and the immunosuppressive regimen (134). For example, retrospective studies show significant differences in the number and kind of HLA mismatches (serologically detectable mismatch vs. allele mismatch in serologically matched donor) between some T-cell–depleted transplant populations compared to populations receiving unmanipulated marrow. Therefore, interpretation of retrospective studies should keep in mind the fact that permissible HLA mismatches may differ according to the specific donor-recipient allele or antigen mismatches, the transplant procedure (conditioning and immunosuppressive regimen), and other non-HLA variables.

Another important concept to aid the reader in the interpretation of retrospective studies of HLA matching and outcome pertains to the definitions used to group donor-recipient pairs for comparison. In general, published studies have used one of two different methods. One approach is to define a matched group and a mismatched group for each HLA locus (135–137). In this way, donor-recipient pairs may be variably mismatched for the other HLA loci, the presence of which is adjusted in multivariate analysis. This method assumes that the association of mismatching at the locus in question is approximately the same across all other loci. The major advantage of this method is that the effect of mismatching at a particular locus can be examined among the entire study population. The second approach is to define nonoverlapping groups of donor-recipient pairs based on match/mismatch at every HLA locus (102,138). In this model, mutually exclusive comparison groups are defined on the basis of matching information at all loci simultaneously. The major advantage to this approach is that any potential for confounding effects from other loci to the locus under examination is eliminated. Because groups are mutually exclusive, a limitation of this method may be smaller numbers of observations in each group.

Substantial data on the importance of complete and precise donor matching on clinical outcome have emerged over the last decade (98,102,117,130–159). These data support a new model for optimal donor HLA matching that considers quantitative (the total number of mismatched alleles) and qualitative (alleles vs. antigens) measures of donor-recipient disparity (Table 1). Three variables define the acceptability of an HLA mismatch: 1) the HLA genetic locus (or loci) that is (are) mismatched; 2) the number of HLA allele mismatches and 3) the specific nucleotide sequence of the mismatch. The following studies provide a basis for the current selection for unrelated donors. Identification of permissible mismatches will improve safety and efficacy of unrelated donor HCT and at the same time increase the number of patients with suitable donors.

A. Genetic Loci Involved in GVHD

1. HLA Class II Genes

Historical observations in haploidentical related transplantation demonstrated that HLA mismatching increases the incidence and severity of acute GVHD (160), the effect of which is higher with class II than with class I mismatching (161). Investigation of the

Table 1 Summary of New Donor Matching Data

Mismatching for a single locus at HLA-C affects the risks of graft failure, GVHD, and death.
The risk of death is enhanced by mismatching for a single allele at HLA-A, B, C or DRB1.
The risks of graft failure, GVHD, and death are higher with mismatching for one antigen compared to one allele.
Mismatching for multiple alleles compounds the risks of graft failure, GVHD, and death.

role of HLA allele matching and clinical outcome after unrelated HCT initially focused on the HLA-DRB1 alleles because of the availability of DNA typing technology for this gene. In early studies of HLA-A, -B, -DR serologically matched unrelated donor transplants, the risks of severe acute GVHD and mortality were significantly increased in the presence of HLA-DRB1 allele mismatching (149). This study did not take into account HLA-DQ (due to the lack of sufficient numbers of pairs with an isolated HLA-DQ mismatch). Subsequent studies uncovered a synergistic effect of two-locus HLA-DR/DQ mismatching on acute GVHD risk (96). Among 449 HLA-A, -B, -DR serologically matched pairs, allele typing for HLA-DRB1 and -DQB1 alleles revealed that 335 (75%) were HLA-DRB1 and -DQB1 matched, 41 (9%) were HLA-DRB1 matched but -DQB1 mismatched, 48 (11%) were HLA-DRB1 mismatched but -DQB1 matched, and 25 (6%) were mismatched at both HLA-DRB1 and -DQB1. The conditional probabilities of grade III–IV acute GVHD were 0.42, 0.61, 0.55, and 0.71, respectively. In multivariate analysis, HLA-DQB1 mismatching conferred a significantly increased relative risk (RR 1.8; $p = 0.01$) for grade II–IV acute GVHD demonstrating that HLA-DQ gene products function as transplantation determinants.

Recently, several large studies of unrelated transplants confirm and extend the findings of HLA-DR and -DQ disparity and risk of clinically significant acute GVHD (135,136,150,152,156). The effects of HLA-DRB1 allele disparity on acute GVHD risk were noteworthy in a good-risk subset of patients transplanted during the first chronic phase of CML from class I serologically matched unrelated donors (136). A recent NMDP analysis of a larger clinical population of patients demonstrated that HLA-DRB1 mismatching conferred a relative risk (RR) of 1.26 on GVHD [95% confidence interval (CI) 1.0–1.6; $p = 0.05$] (135). Synergistic effects of 2-locus HLA-DRB1, -DQB1 mismatching can profoundly increase the risk of grade III–IV acute GVHD (22% matched; 43% single locus; 64% two-locus mismatches) (152), and matching for both HLA-DRB1 and -DQB1 can reduce the rate of GVHD from 73% (any mismatch) to 38% (matched for both genes; $p = 0.02$) (150).

HLA-DP has recently also been shown to behave as a classical transplantation alloantigen (87,135,138,139,143,145,153,158). In most transplant populations studied to date, in which the donor was originally selected according to compatibility at HLA-A, -B, and -DR, less than 20% of HLA-A, -B, -DRB1, -DQB1 matched pairs have been found to be matched for HLA-DP. The low match rate at HLA-DP is due to the weak degree of LD between HLA-DP and the remainder of the MHC. As a consequence, retrospective examination of HLA-DP has required very large transplant populations in order that sufficient numbers of HLA-DP matched pairs can be analyzed.

Early reports failed to demonstrate significant effects of HLA-DP disparity on GVHD or mortality risk and were limited by the statistical power of too few HLA-DP–matched transplants (145). More recently, analysis of HLA-A, -C, -B, -DRB1, and -DQB1, allele matched CML transplants provided a highly homogeneous transplant population in which to evaluate the significance of isolated HLA-DP disparity on risk of clinically significant acute GVHD (138). Parallel observations have been made and indicate an increased risk of grade III–IV acute GVHD conferred independently by HLA-DPB1 disparity compared to the matched situation (153,158). However, in contrast to the data from Caucasian populations, two large studies by the Japan Marrow Donor Program (JMDP) have not confirmed a role for HLA-DP as a transplantation determinant (117,137). Taken together, these data indicate that prospective typing and matching for HLA-DP may be most useful when the search process identifies several potential

HLA-A, -C, -B, -DR, -DQ matched donors and when the patient's clinical course affords sufficient time to evaluate donor compatibility for this gene.

2.   HLA Class I Genes: HLA-A, -C, and -B

The recent availability of molecular methods for the class I region genes has enabled investigators to evaluate the potential role of class I disparity on transplant complications (95,102,117,135,137,142,151,154,155,157,159). Evidence for a role for class I in GVHD was provided in an early study in which donor-derived CTL were isolated and shown to exclusively recognize HLA-B allele sequence differences between a patient and donor (147), suggesting that class I allele differences may evoke donor-antihost responses, which may correlate with the development of acute GVHD. The first large study describing the effect of class I on GVHD risk was reported by the JMDP (117). HLA-A and HLA-C allele disparity were each independent risk factors for severe acute GVHD; interestingly, no contribution from class II was found. The JMDP experience has recently been updated and demonstrates that HLA-A, -C, -B, and -DRB1 are each independent risk factors for grade III–IV acute GVHD [(RR 1.58; 1.2–2.1; $p = 0.001$); (RR 1.58; 1.4–2.4; $p<0.001$); (RR 1.43; 1.0–2.0; $p = 0.04$) and (RR 1.42; 1.1–1.9; $p = 0.02$), respectively] (137). An NMDP analysis has likewise identified HLA-A mismatching to be a risk factor of severe GVHD (RR 1.33; 1.0–1.7; $p = 0.04$); however, HLA-B and HLA-C allele mismatches did not appear to contribute (135). These studies may have come to different conclusions regarding the relative contributions of class I and class II mismatching because of different allele and antigen mismatches between Caucasian and Japanese patients and donors.

B.   The Effect of Multiple HLA Mismatches on GVHD Risk

Early clinical experience in mismatched related transplantation uncovered the importance of the total number of HLA mismatches in determining GVHD risk. In one clinical study, grade II–IV GVHD was observed in 75% of single-locus, 78% of two-locus, and 80% of three-locus mismatches (146).

   Additive effects of multiple class I, multiple class II, or simultaneous class I and II mismatching on GVHD risk can be measured (102,117,135,137,138,140,152). The risk of clinically significant acute GVHD is increased in the presence of multiple class II mismatches (102,140,152), and additive effects of multilocus class I mismatching on GVHD risk are significant (137). In particular, HLA-C disparity in the presence of mismatching at any other HLA locus (class I or class II) is associated with significantly increased incidence of grade II–IV GVHD (60.9%, 55.7%, and 64.3% for HLA-C plus -A/B, HLA-C plus -DR/DQ, and HLA-C plus -A/B and -DR/DQ, respectively) compared to matched (34.5%), HLA-A/B mismatched (54.9%), HLA-C mismatched (42.7%), or HLA-DR/DQ mismatched (34.4%) (137).

   The cumulative effect of multiple HLA disparities on GVHD risk has been evaluated in a single center study (Table 2). When the data are stratified by the number of mismatched HLA-DPB1 alleles (0, 1, or 2), the relative associations of class I and class II disparities with GVHD appear to be unaffected. In a logistic regression model that adjusted for the presence of 0, 1, or 2 HLA-DPB1 allele mismatches, patients who were matched at HLA-DRB1 and -DQB1 tolerated a single class I HLA-A or -B or -C mismatch (OR 0.8; 0.5–1.4; $p = 0.47$). Among patients who were matched at class I, the presence of multiple class II mismatches was associated with increased risk of GVHD (OR 4.7;

Table 2   Incidence of Grades III–IV Acute GVHD According to Number of Mismatched
Class I and Class II Alleles

	0 Class I	1 Class I	≥2 Class I	Total
0 Class II	77/237 (32%)	28/94 (30%)	21/59 (36%)	126/390 (32%)
1 Class II	13/29 (45%)	4/14 (29%)	11/20 (55%)	28/63 (44%)
≥2 Class II	6/9 (67%)	2/3 (67%)	6/7 (86%)	14/19 (74%)
Total	96/275 (34%)	34/111 (31%)	38/86 (44%)	168/472 (36%)

Data for 472 patients who underwent myeloablative conditioning and unrelated bone marrow transplantation for the treatment of CML and had acute GVHD grading information available at the Fred Hutchinson Cancer Research Center, Seattle. The effect of increasing numbers of class I alleles on GVHD incidence can be viewed within a fixed number of class II mismatches. Similarly, the effect of increasing numbers of class I mismatches can be compared to a fixed number of class I mismatches.

1.1–19.6; $p = 0.03$), as were single class II mismatches (OR 1.8; 0.8–4.0; $p = 0.15$). Multiple class I mismatches were well tolerated provided there was no HLA-DRB1 or -DQB1 mismatch (OR 1.2; 0.7–2.2; $p = 0.57$). However, the combination of class I disparities with class II disparities was associated with significantly increased GVHD risk (OR 11.6; 1.4–99.5; $p = 0.03$). These data suggest that single disparities for class I are in general better tolerated than those for class II with respect to GVHD. Identification of two-locus mismatches that do not increase GVHD risk may provide a means to allow patients who lack a matched donor the option for a transplant.

C.   The Importance of Mismatching for Sequence-Specific Epitopes on GVHD Risk

As the studies described above illustrate, the relative risk conferred by specific HLA loci to GVHD differs from population to population. Examination of qualitative differences between the specific HLA sequences that are mismatched in these transplant populations may provide clues to the seemingly disparate conclusions. Although Japanese and Caucasian donor-recipient pairs encoded a similar degree of disparity for HLA-A, -B, and -DRB1 alleles (102,117,137), they differed in the specific combinations of allele mismatches (116). There was little overlap in the HLA-A, -B, -C, -DRB1, and -DQB1 allele mismatches in these two populations. Whether the nature of the specific mismatched residues played a role in defining risk to GVHD remains to be tested in larger ethnically diverse transplant populations.

The importance of the nature of the mismatched class I residue has recently be found to correlate with clinical outcome (157). Among 60 unrelated donor-recipient pairs who were mismatched for one or more class I alleles, mismatches at residue 116 were associated with a significantly increased risk of GVHD and transplant-related mortality (TRM) compared to patients without mismatches at residue 116 (58% vs. 28%; $p = 0.001$). This is the first study to implicate the importance of the HLA sequence disparity and its position within the class I heavy chain. Involvement of residue 116 is predicted to participate in peptide binding (residue P9 of the peptide) (Fig. 2). These results provide a basis for the hypothesis that the nature of amino acid substitutions at critical positions in the class I molecule may define peptide binding or involve interaction with the TCR to define alloreactivity.

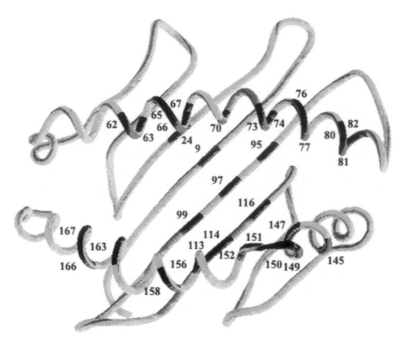

Figure 2   Ribbon diagram of the HLA class I molecule showing α-carbon backbone of the α1 and α2 domains and the β-pleated sheet. Residues implicated in peptide binding are: 5,7,9,24,25,34,45,63,67,70,73,74,77,80,81,84,95,97,99,113,114,116,123,143,147,152,156,160,   and 171. Residues implicated in TCR contact are: 58,62,65,68,69,72,76,82,145,149,150,151,154,158, 166, and 170. Residues involved in both peptide and TCR contact are: 59,66,146,155,159,162,163, and 167.

The nature of the sequence disparity distinguishing alleles from antigens influences GVHD risk has been explored in a large retrospective study by the NMDP (135). The RR of grade III–IV acute GVHD between patients with an antigen mismatch at HLA-A, -B, and -DR was significantly different from that conferred by allele mismatches at these loci (135). Furthermore, mismatching at any class I locus was associated with a significantly higher incidence of grade III–IV acute GVHD and mortality compared to matching for HLA-A, -C, and -B. Among HLA-A, -B antigen matched, -DRB1 allele matched recipients, 5-year survival was significantly inferior if additional allele disparities at HLA-A, -C, or -B were detected.

GVHD risk associated with serologically detected antigens within class I CREGs was evaluated in a single-center study of 196 patients transplanted for CML in chronic phase with unmodified marrow following conditioning with cyclophosphamide and TBI and CSP and methotrexate (MTX) as GVHD prophylaxis (162). Acute GVHD was significantly higher after HCT across an HLA-DR serological mismatch, and there was a trend for a higher incidence of grade II–IV acute GVHD following HCT across an HLA-A or -B CREG antigen mismatch. The cumulative incidence of clinically extensive chronic GVHD was 67% among patients surviving disease-free more than 100 days; there was no significant difference in the risk of clinically extensive chronic GVHD between HLA-matched and HLA-mismatched cases.

VI. ROLE OF HLA CLASS I LIGANDS AND NK-KIR RECEPTORS IN GVHD REACTIONS

Recent delineation of the genetic organization, polymorphism, and function of the NK-KIR genetic family has opened an exciting approach for the use of HLA class I–mismatched donors for transplantation by leveraging natural killer (NK) cell–mediated recognition of host cells to eliminate posttransplant relapse and GVHD.

In contrast to the HLA restriction of T-cell allorecognition, NK cells interact with HLA class I molecules through inhibitory receptors termed killer cell Ig-like receptors (KIR) and CD94/NKG2. Lack of expression of the correct inhibitory HLA class I ligands by the recipient can trigger donor NK cell alloreactivity and thereby lead to killing of recipient cells, including leukemic cells. Destruction of recipient antigen-presenting cells (APC) removes the target of GVHD; destruction of host tumor cells leads to decreased potential for posttransplant relapse. Residues 77 and 80 of HLA-C and the Bw4 epitope of HLA-B can predict the pattern of donor KIR receptor recognition. Knowledge of the donor-recipient HLA-B/C genotype can therefore be used to predict whether potential unrelated donors might be KIR mismatched. Selection of KIR mismatched donors may be desired because donor NK cells would recognize and eliminate recipient target cells that mediate GVHD and also eliminate recipient leukemic cells.

The concept of donor NK-mediated killing of recipient APC was evaluated in 92 patients who underwent haploidentical mismatched transplantation for high-risk acute myeloid or lymphoblastic leukemia (163). These patients received T-cell–depleted grafts, a high CD34+ cell dose, and no postgrafting immunosuppression, a regimen that promotes rapid NK recovery (164). KIR mismatching was associated with no acute GVHD and a 0% 5-year probability of relapse. In contrast, KIR matching was an independent risk factor for poor transplant outcome (13.7% incidence of acute GVHD and 75% 5-year probability of relapse). Patients carrying the diagnosis of acute lymphoblastic leukemia were not protected against relapse with the use of KIR-mismatched donors (90% in KIR-matched vs. 85% in KIR mismatched at 5 years).

The use of KIR-mismatched unrelated donors to leverage the effects of donor NK killing and thereby decrease the risks of acute GVHD and relapse for patients with high-risk myeloid malignancies is an intriguing approach. In a retrospective study of 175 patients who received either T-replete or T-cell–depleted unrelated grafts from class I allele mismatched donors after conditioning with TBI or busulfan/cyclophosphamide, no difference in acute GVHD or relapse was observed (165). Survival of KIR-matched recipients was superior to that of the KIR-mismatched recipients (38% vs. 13%, $p < 0.01$). The major difference in the transplant regimens between the two studies was the use of extensive T-cell depletion, high CD34+ cell dose, and no posttransplant immunosuppression in the haploidentical transplants. Whether the use of either unmanipulated or T-cell–depleted grafts with posttransplant immunosuppression for the unrelated transplants promoted higher numbers of alloreactive T cells, thereby obscuring any NK effect, still remains to be examined in a larger transplant experience.

VII. SUMMARY

There is worldwide consensus that allele typing and matching of donors is associated with superior clinical outcome after HCT. At the same time, given the extreme polymorphism of the HLA system, it is not likely that allele matching can be achieved for most patients.

If donor selection criteria are set too stringently so as to require allele identity, then the number of patients eligible for transplantation will be limited. Exhaustive efforts to find the best match may theoretically increase the success of transplantation, but a prolonged donor search may introduce delays in transplantation and increase costs without necessarily increasing the benefit to the patient. Optimal matching for individual patients may require disease-specific criteria that appropriately reflect patient diagnosis, patient age, clinical urgency, and the potential benefit of GVHD.

Currently, data demonstrate that in certain situations, single allele mismatches may be tolerated. Molecular typing tools should be used to identify and avoid donors who have multilocus hidden mismatches, as the negative impact of cumulative HLA mismatches on engraftment, GVHD, and mortality is significant.

REFERENCES

1. Dausset J. Leuco-agglutinins. IV. Leuco-agglutinins and blood transfusion. Vox Sang 1954; 4:190.
2. van Rood JJ, van Leeuwen A. Leucocyte grouping. A method and its application. J Clin Invest 1963; 42:1382–1390.
3. Payne R, Tripp M, Weigle J, Bodmer W, Bodmer J. A new leukocyte isoantigenic system in man. Cold Spring Harbor Sym Quant Biol 1964; 29:285.
4. Amos DB. Nomenclature for factors of the HL-A system. Science 1968; 160:659–660.
5. Bodmer WF. HLA:what's in a name? A commentary on HLA nomenclature development over the years. Tiss Antigens 1997; 46:293–296.
6. Bjorkman PJ, Saper MA, Samraoui B, Bennett WS, Strominger JL, Wiley DC. Structure of the human class I histocompatibility antigen, HLA-A2. Nature 1987; 329:506–512.
7. Brown JH, Jardetzky TS, Gorga JC, Stern LJ, Urban RG, Strominger JL, Wiley DC. Three-dimensional structure of the human class II histocompatibility antigen HLA-DR1. Nature 1993; 364:33–39.
8. Horn GT, Bugawan TL, Long CM, Erlich HA. Allelic sequence variation of the HLA-DQ loci: relationship to serology and to insulin-dependent diabetes susceptibility. Proc Natl Acad Sci USA 1988; 85:6012–6016.
9. Marsh SG, Bodmer JG, Albert ED, Bodmer WF, Bontrop RE, Dupont B, Erlich HA, Hansen JA, Mach B, Mayr WR, Parham P, Petersdorf EW, Sasazuki T, Schreuder GM, Strominger JL, Svejgaard A, Terasaki PI. Nomenclature for factors of the HLA system, 2000. Tiss Antigens 2001; 57:236–283.
10. Rhodes DA, Trowsdale J. Genetics and molecular genetics of the MHC. Rev Immunogenetics 1999; 1:21–31.
11. Bain B, Vas MR, Lowenstein L. The development of large immature cells in mixed leukocyte cultures. Blood 1964; 23:108–116.
12. Bach FH, Hirschhorn K. Lymphocyte interaction: a potential histocompatibility test in vitro. Science 1964; 143:813–814.
13. Geraghty DE, Wei X, Orr HT. HLA-F: an expressed HLA gene composed of a class I coding sequence linked to a novel transcribed repetitive element. J Exp Med 1990; 171:1–19.
14. Geraghty DE, Koller BH, Orr HT. A human major histocompatibility complex class I gene that encodes a protein with a shortened cytoplasmic segment. Proc Natl Acad Sci USA 1987; 84:9145–9149.
15. Koller BH, Geraghty DE, Shimizu Y, DeMars R, Orr HT. A novel HLA class I gene expressed in resting T lymphocytes. J Immunol 1988; 141:897–904.
16. Mandelboim O, Pazmany L, Davis DM, Vales-Gomez M, Reyburn HT, Rybalov B. Multiple receptors for HLA-G on human natural killer cells. Proc Natl Acad Sci USA 1997; 94:14666–14670.

17. Lee N, Llano M, Carretero M, Ishitani A, Navarro F, Lopez-Botet M, Geraghty DE. HLA-E is a major ligand for the natural killer inhibitory receptor CD94/NKG2A. Proc Natl Acad Sci USA 1998; 95:5199–5204.

18. Rammensee H-G. Chemistry of peptides associated with MHC class I and class II molecules. Curr Opin Immunol 1995; 7:85–96.

19. Marshall KW, Liu AF, Canales J, Perahia B, Jorgensen B, Gantzos RD, Aguilar B, Devaux B, Rothbard JB. Role of the polymorphic residues in HLA-DR molecules in allele-specific binding of peptide ligands. J Immunol 1994; 152:4946–4957.

20. Socie G, Loiseau P, Tamouza R, Janin A, Busson M, Gluckman E, Charron D. Both genetic and clinical factors predict the development of graft-versus-host disease after allogeneic hematopoietic stem cell transplantation. Transplantation 2001; 72:699–706.

21. Uphoff DE, Law LW. Genetic factors influencing irradiation protection by bone marrow. II. The histocompatibility-2 (H-2) locus. J Natl Cancer Inst 1958; 20:617–624.

22. Epstein RB, Bryant J, Thomas ED. Cytogenetic demonstration of permanent tolerance in adult outbred dogs. Transplantation 1967; 5:267–272.

23. Gatti RA, Meuwissen HJ, Allen HD, Hong R, Good RA. Immunological reconstitution of sex-linked lymphopenic immunological deficiency. Lancet 1968; 2:1366–1369.

24. Thomas ED, Storb R, Fefer A, Slichter SJ, Bryant JI, Buckner CD, Neiman PE, Clift RA, Funk DD, Lerner KE. A plastic anemia treated by marrow transplantation. Lancet 1972; 1(745):284–289.

25. National Institutes of Health. NIH lymphocyte microcytotoxicity technique. NIAID manual of tissue typing techniques. Publication No. NIH 80-545. Department of Health, Education, and Welfare, Atlanta, 1979.

26. Schreuder GM, Hurley CK, Marsh SG, Lau M, Maiers M, Kollman C, Noreen HJ. The HLA dictionary 2001: a summary of HLA-A, -B, -C, -DRB1/3/4/5 and -DQB1 alleles and their association with serologically defined HLA-A, -B, -C, -DR and -DQ antigens. Eur J Immunogenet 2001; 6:565–596.

27. Dupont B, Hansen JA, Yunis EJ. Human mixed-lymphocyte culture reaction: genetics, specificity, and biological implications. Adv Immunol 1976; 23:107–202.

28. Dupont B, Braun DW, Yunis EJ, Carpenter CB. Joint report: HLA-D by cellular typing. In: Terasaki PI, ed. Histocompatibility Testing. Los Angeles: Univ. California, 1980:229–267.

29. Bodmer WF. HLA: a super supergene. In: The Harvey Lectures 72. New York: Academic Press, 1978:91–138.

30. Terasaki P, Park MS, Bernoco D, Opelz G, Mickey MR. Overview of the 1980 International Histocompatibility Workshop. In: Terasaki PI, ed. Histocompatibility Testing. Los Angeles, CA: UCLA Tissue Typing Laboratory, 1980:1–17.

31. Termijtelen A, Erlich HA, Braun LA, Verduyn W, Drabbels JJ, Schroeijers WE, van Rood JJ, deKoster HS, Giphart MJ. Oligonucleotide typing is a perfect tool to identify antigens stimulatory in the mixed lymphocyte culture. Human Immunol 1991; 31:241–245.

32. Mickelson EM, Guthrie LA, Etzioni R, Anasetti C, Martin PJ, Hansen JA. Role of the mixed lymphocyte culture (MLC) reaction in marrow donor selection: matching for transplants from related haploidentical donors. Tiss Antigens 1994; 44:83–92.

33. Mickelson EM, Longton G, Anasetti C, Petersdorf EW, Martin PJ, Guthrie LA, Hansen JA. Evaluation of the mixed lymphocyte culture (MLC) assay as a method for selecting unrelated donors for marrow transplantation. Tiss Antigens 1996; 47:27–36.

34. Segall M, Noreen H, Edwins L, Haake R, Shu XO, Kersey J. Lack of correlation of MLC reactivity with acute graft-versus-host disease and mortality in unrelated donor bone marrow transplantation. Human Immunol 1996; 49:49–55.

35. Hansen JA, Mickelson EM, Choo SY, Petersdorf EW, Anasetti C, Martin PJ, Thomas ED. Clinical bone marrow transplantation: donor selection and recipient monitoring. In: Rose NR, DeMacario EC, Fahey JL, Friedman H, Penn GM, eds. Manual of Clinical Laboratory Immunology. 4th ed. American Society for Microbiology, 1992:850–866.

36. Kaminski E, Hows J, Man S, Brookes P, Mackinnan S, Hughes T, Avakian O, Goldman JM, Batchelor JR. Prediction of graft versus host disease by frequency analysis of cytotoxic T cells after unrelated donor bone marrow transplantation. Transplantation 1989; 48:608–613.

37. Zhang L, Rinke de Wit TF, Li SG, van Rood JJ, Claas FH. Subtypes of HLA-A1 defined on the basis of CTL precursor frequencies. Human Immunol 1990; 27:80–89.

38. Kaminski ER, Hows JM, Bridge J, Davey NJ, Brookes PA, Green JE, Goldman JM, Batchelor JR. Cytotoxic T lymphocyte precursor (CTLp) frequency analysis in unrelated donor bone marrow transplantation: two case studies. Bone Marrow Transplant 1991; 8:47–50.

39. Roosnek E, Hogendijk S, Zawadynski S, Speiser D, Tiercy JM, Helg C, Chapuis B, Gratwohl A, Gmur J, Seger R. The frequency of pretransplant donor cytotoxic T cell precursors with anti-host specificity predicts survival of patients transplanted with bone marrow from donors other than HLA-identical siblings. Transplantation 1993; 56:691–696.

40. Arguello R, Scott I, O'Shea J, Brookes PA, Tiercy JM, Bunce M, Goldman JM, Batchelor JR, Madrigal A. Cytotoxic T lymphocyte precursor frequency (CTLpf) analysis highlights the need for better matching in the selection of unrelated bone marrow donors (abstr). Bone Marrow Transplant 1995; 15:248:S57.

41. Spencer A, Brookes PA, Kaminski E, Hows JM, Szydlo RM, van Rhee F, Goldman JM, Batchelor JR. Cytotoxic T lymphocyte precursor frequency analyses in bone marrow transplantation with volunteer unrelated donors. Value in donor selection. Transplantation 1995; 59:1302–1308.

42. O'Shea J, Madrigal A, Davey N, Brookes P, Scott I, Firman H, Lechler R, Goldman J, Batchelor R. Measurement of cytotoxic T lymphocyte precursor frequencies reveals cryptic HLA class I mismatches in the context of unrelated donor bone marrow transplantation. Transplantation 1997; 64:1353–1356.

43. Kassar NE, Legouvello S, Joseph CM, Salesses P, Rieux C, Cordonnier C, Vernant JP, Farcet JP, Bierling P, Kuentz M. High resolution HLA class I and II typing and CTLp frequency in unrelated donor transplantation: a single-institution retrospective study of 69 BMTs. Bone Marrow Transplant 2001; 27:35–43.

44. Dolezalova L, Vrana M, Dobrovolna M, Loudova M, Cukrova V, Vitek A, Sajdova J, Stary J, Sedlacek P. Cytotoxic T lymphocyte precursor frequency analysis in the selection of HLA matched unrelated donors for hematopoietic stem cell transplantation: the correlation of CTLp frequency with HLA class I genotyping and aGVHD development. Neoplasma 2002; 49:26–32.

45. Oudshoorn M, Doxiadis IIN, van den Berg-Loonen PM, cem Voorter, Verduyn W, Claas FHJ. Functional versus structural matching: can the CTLp test be replaced by HLA allele typing? Human Immunol 2002; 63:176–184.

46. Fussell ST, Donnellan M, Cooley MA, Farrell C. Cytotoxic T lymphocyte precursor frequency does not correlate with either the incidence or severity of graft-versus-host disease after matched unrelated donor bone marrow transplantation. Transplantation 1994; 57:673–676.

47. Schwarer AP, Jiang YZ, Deacock S, Brookes PA, Barrett AJ, Goldman JM, Batchelor JR, Lechler RI. Comparison of helper and cytotoxic anti-recipient T cell frequencies in unrelated bone marrow transplantation. Transplantation 1994; 58:1198–1203.

48. Pei J, Martin PJ, Longton G, Masewicz S, Mickelson E, Petersdorf E, Anasetti C, Hansen J. Evaluation of pretransplant donor anti-recipient cytotoxic and helper T lymphocyte responses as correlates of acute graft-versus-host disease and survival after unrelated marrow transplantation. Biol Blood Marrow Transplant 1997; 3:142–149.

49. Rosenberg AS, Singer A. Cellular basis of skin allograft rejection: an in vivo model of immune-mediated tissue destruction. Ann Rev Immunol 1992; 10:333–358.

50. Sprent J, Hurd M, Schaefer M, Heath W. Split tolerance in spleen chimeras. J Immunol 1995; 154:1198–1206.

51. Braun MY, Lowin B, French Acha-Orbea L, H, Tschopp J. Cytotoxic T cells deficient in both functional Fas ligand and perforin show residual cytolytic activity yet lose their capacity to induce lethal acute graft-versus-host disease. J Exp Med 1996; 183:657–661.

52. Hurley CK, Schreuder GMT, Marsh SGE, Lau M, Middleton D, Noreen H. The search for HLA-matched donors: a summary of HLA-A*, -B*, -DRB1/3/4/5* alleles and their association with serologically defined HLA-A, -B, DR antigens. Tiss Antigens 1997; 50:401–418.

53. Hurley CK, Wade JA, Oudshoorn M, Middleton D, Kukuruga D, Navarrete C, Christiansen F, Hegland J, Ren EC, Andersen I, Cleaver SA, Brautbar C, Raffoux C. Histocompatibility testing guidelines for hematopoietic stem cell transplantation using volunteer donors: report from The World Marrow Donor Association. Quality Assurance and Donor Registries Working Groups of the World Marrow Donor Association. Bone Marrow Transplant 1999; 24:119–121.

54. O'Shea J, Cleaver S, Little A-M, Madrigal A. Searching for an unrelated haemopoietic stem cell donor—a United Kingdom perspective. In: Cecka MM, Terasaki P, eds. Clinical Transplants 1999. UCLA Immunogenetics, 2000:129–137.

55. Ottinger HD, Muller CR, Goldmann SF, Albert E, Arnold R, Beelen DW, Blasczyk R, Bunjes D, Casper J, Ebell W, Ehninger G, Eiermann T, Einsele H, Fauser A, Ferencik S, Finke J, Hertenstein B, Heyll A, Klingebiel T, Knipper A, Kremens B, Kolb HJ, Kolbe K, Lenartz E, Lindermann M, Muller CA, Mytilineos J, Niederwieser D, Runde V, Sayer H, Schaefer UW, Schmitz N, Schroder S, Schulze-Rath R, Schwerdtfeger R, Wiegert W, Thiele B, Zander AR, Grosse-Wilde H. Second German consensus on immunogenetics donor search for allotransplantation of hematopoietic stem cells. Ann Hematol 2001; 80:706–714.

56. Maiers M, Hurley CK, Capp K, Winden T, Hegland J, Ng J, Shepherd D, Hartzman RJ. A system for periodic reinterpretation of intermediate resolution DNA-based HLA types in a bone marrow registry (abstr). Human Immunol 1998; 59(S1):98.

57. Helmberg W, Hegland J, Hurley CK, Maiers M, Marsh SGE, Muller C, Rozemuller EH. Going back to the roots: effective utilization of HLA typing information for bone marrow registries requires full knowledge of the DNA sequences of the oligonucleotide reagents used in the testing. Tiss Antigens 2000; 56:99–102.

58. Browning MJ, Krausa P, Rowan A, Bicknell DC, Bodmer JG, Bodmer WF. Tissue typing the HLA-A locus from genomic DNA by sequence-specific PCR: comparison of HLA genotype and surface expression on colorectal tumor cell lines. Proc Natl Acad Sci USA 1993; 90:2842–2845.

59. Krausa P, Bodmer JG, Browning M. Defining the common subtypes of HLA-A9, A10, A28 and A19 by use of ARMS/PCR. Tiss Antigens 1993; 42:91–99.

60. Bunce M, Welsh KI. Rapid DNA typing for HLA-C using sequence-specific primers (PCR-SSP): identification of serological and nonserologically defined HLA-C alleles including several new alleles. Tiss Antigens 1994; 43:7–17.

61. Sadler AM, Petronzelli F, Krausa P, Marsh SG, Guttridge MG, Browning MJ, Bodmer JG. Low-resolution DNA typing for HLA-B using sequence-specific primers in allele or group specific ARMS/PCR. Tiss Antigens 1994; 44:148–154.

62. Guttridge MG, Burr C, Klouda PT. Identification of HLA-B35, B53, B18, B5, B78 and B17 alleles by the polymerase chain reaction using sequence-specific primers (PCR-SSP). Tiss Antigens 1994; 44:43–46.

63. Hein J, Bottcher K, Grundmann R, Kirchner H, Bein G. Low resolution DNA typing of the HLA-B5 cross-reactive group by nested PCR-SSP. Tiss Antigens 1995; 45:27–35.

64. Bugawan TL, Begovich AB, Erlich HA. Rapid HLA DPB typing using enzymatically amplified DNA and nonradioactive sequence-specific oliogonucleotide probes. Immunogenetics 1990; 32:231–241.

65. Petersdorf EW, Smith AG, Haase AM, Martin PJ, Hansen JA. Polymorphism of HLA-DRw52-associated DRB1 genes as defined by sequence-specific oligonucleotide probe hybridization and sequencing. Tiss Antigens 1991; 38:169–177.

66. Dominguez O, Coto E, Martinez-Naves E, Choo SY, Lopez-Larrea C. Molecular typing of HLA-B27 alleles. Immunogenetics 1992; 36:277–282.

67. Yoshida M, Kimura A, Numano F, Sasazuki T. Polymerase chain reaction-based analysis of polymorphism in the HLA-B gene. Human Immunol 1992; 34:257–266.

68. Rufer N, Breur-Vriesendorp BS, Tiercy J-M, Slavcev AS, Lardy NM, Francis P, Kressig R, Speiser DE, Helg C, Chapuis B. High-resolution histocompatibility testing of a group of sixteen B44-positive, ABDR serologically matched unrelated donor-recipient pairs: analysis of serologically undisclosed incompatibilities by cellular techniques, isoelectric focusing, and HLA oligotyping. Human Immunol 1993; 38:235–239.

69. Molkentin J, Gorski J, Baxter-Lowe LA. Detection of 14 HLA-DQB1 alleles by oligotyping. Human Immunol 1991; 31:114–122.

70. Allen M, Liu L, Gyllensten U. A comprehensive polymerase chain reaction-oligonucleotide typing system for the HLA-class I A locus. Human Immunol 1994; 40:25–32.

71. Gao XJ, Jakobsen IB, Serjeanson SW. Characterization of HLA-A polymorphism by locus-specific polymerase chain reaction amplification and oligonucleotide hybridization. Human Immunol 1994; 41:267–279.

72. Levine JE, Yang SY. SSOP typing of the Tenth International Histocompatibility Workshop reference cell lines for HLA-C alleles. Tiss Antigens 1994; 44:174–183.

73. Fernandez-Vina MA, Lazaro AM, Sun Y, Miller S, Forero L, Stastny P. Population diversity of B-locus alleles observed by high resolution DNA typing. Tiss Antigens 1995; 45:153–168.

74. Hurley CK, Baxter-Lowe LA, Begovich AB, Fernandez-Vina M, Noreen H, Schmeckpeper B, Awdeh Z, Chopek M, Salazar M, Williams TM, Yunis EJ, Kitajima D, Shipp K, Splett J, Winden T, Kollman C, Johnson D, Ng J, Hartzman RJ, Hegland J. The extent of HLA class II allele level disparity in unrelated bone marrow transplantation: analysis of 1259 National Marrow Donor Program donor-recipient pairs. Bone Marrow Transplant 2000; 25:385–393.

75. Erlich HA, Bugawan T, Begovich A, Scharf S, Griffith R, Saiki R, Higuchi R, Walsh PS. HLA-DR, DQ & DP typing using PCR amplification and immobilized probes. Eur J Immunogen 1991; 18:33–35.

76. Scharf SJ, Griffith RL, Erlich HA. Rapid typing of DNA sequence polymorphism at the HLA-DRB1 locus using the polymerase chain reaction and non-radioactive oligonucleotide probes. Human Immunol 1991; 30:190–201.

77. Bugawan TL, Apple R, Erlich HA. A method for typing polymorphism at the HLA-A locus using PCR amplification and immobilized oligonuclotide probes. Tiss Antigens 1994; 44:137–147.

78. Santamaria P, Lindstrom AL, Boyce-Jacino MT, Myster SH, Barbosa JJ, Faras AJ, Rich SS. HLA class I sequence-based typing. Human Immunol 1993; 37:39–50.

79. Versluis LF, Rozemuller E, Tonks S, Marsh SG, Bouwens AG, Bodmer JG, Tilanus MG. High-resolution HLA-DPB typing based upon computerized analysis of data obtained by fluorescent sequencing of the amplified polymorphic exon 2. Human Immunol 1993; 38:277–283.

80. Domena JD, Little A-M, Arnett KL, Adams EJ, Marsh SG, Parham P. A small test of a sequence-based typing method: definition of the B**1520 allele. Tiss Antigens 1994; 44:217–224.

81. Petersdorf EW, Hansen JA. A comprehensive approach for typing the alleles of the HLA-B locus by automated sequencing. Tiss Antigens 1995; 46:73–85.

82. Yao Z, Keller E, Scholz S, McNicholas A, Volgger A, Albert ED. Identification of two major HLA-B44 subtypes and a novel B44 sequence: oligotyping and solid phase sequencing of PCR products. Human Immunol 1995; 42:54–60.

83. Kotsch K, Wehling J, Blasczyk R. Sequencing of HLA class II genes based on the conserved diversity of the non-coding regions: sequencing based typing of HLA-DRB genes. Tiss Antigens 1999; 53:486–497.

84. Arguello R, Avakian H, Goldman JM, Madrigal JA. A novel method for simultaneous high resolution identification of HLA-A, HLA-B and HLA-Cw alleles. Proc Natl Acad Sci USA 1996; 93:10961–10965.

85. Madrigal JA, Arguello R, Gallardo D. High resolution HLA class I and II typing for unrelated bone marrow donors (abstr). Eur J Immunogenet 1997; 24:70.

86. Guo Z, Gatterman MS, Hood L, Hansen JA, Petersdorf EW. Oligonucleotide arrays for high-throughput SNPs detection in the MHC class I genes: HLA-B as a model system. Genome Res 2002; 12:447–457.

87. Al-Daccak R, Loiseau P, Rabian C, Devergie A, Bourdeau H, Raffoux C, Gluckman E, Colombani J. HLA-DR, DQ, and/or DP genotypic mismatches between recipient-donor pairs in unrelated bone marrow transplantation and transplant clinical outcome. Transplantation 1990; 50:960–964.

88. Baxter-Lowe LA, Eckels DD, Ash R, Casper J, Hunter JB, Gorski J. Future directions in selection of donors for bone marrow transplantation: role of oligonucleotide genotyping. Transplant Proc 1991; 23:1699–1700.

89. Petersdorf EW, Smith AG, Mickelson EM, Martin PJ, Hansen JA. Ten HLA-DR4 alleles defined by sequence polymorphisms within the DRB1 first domain. Immunogenetics 1991; 33:267–275.

90. Tiercy JM, Morel C, Freidel AC, Swahlen F, Beguhrer L, Betuel H, Jeannet M, Mach B. Selection of unrelated donors for bone marrow transplantation is improved by HLA class II genotyping with oligonucleotide hybridization. Proc Natl Acad Sci USA 1991; 88:7121–7125.

91. Santamaria P, Reinsmoen NL, Lindstrom AL, Boyce-Jacino MT, Barbosa JJ, Faras AJ, McGlave PB, Rich SS. Frequent HLA class I and sequence DP mismatches in serologically (HLA-A, HLA-B, HLA-DR) and molecularly (HLA-DRB1, HLA-DQA1, HLA-DQB1) HLA-identical unrelated bone marrow transplant pairs. Blood 1994; 83:280–287.

92. Fernández-Viña MA, Lazaro AM, Sun Y, Miller S, Forero L, Stastny P. Population diversity of B-locus alleles observed by high-resolution DNA typing. Tiss Antigens 1995; 45:153–168.

93. Nademanee A, Schmidt GM, Parker P, Dagis AC, Stein A, Snyder DS, O'Donnell M, Smith EP, Stepan DE, Molina A. The outcome of matched unrelated donor bone marrow transplantation in patients with hematological malignancies using molecular typing for donor selection and graft-versus-host disease prophylaxis regimen of cyclosporine, methotrexate, and prednisone. Blood 1995; 86:1228–1234.

94. Martinelli G, Farabegoli P, Buzzi M, Panzica G, Zaccaria A, Bandini G, Calori E, Testoni N, Rosti G, Conte R, Remiddi C, Salvucci M, DeVivo A, Tura S. Fingerprinting of HLA class I genes for improved selection of unrelated bone marrow donors. Eur J Immunogenet 1996; 23:55–65.

95. Nagler A, Brautbar C, Slavin S, Bishara A. Bone marrow transplantation using unrelated and family related donors: the impact of HLA-C disparity. Bone Marrow Transplant 1996; 18:891–897.

96. Petersdorf EW, Longton GM, Anasetti C, Mickelson EM, Smith AG, Martin PJ, Hansen JA. Definition of HLA-DQ as a transplantation antigen. Proc Natl Acad Sci USA 1996; 93:15358–15363.

97. Pursall MC, Clay TM, Bidwell JL. Combined PCR-heteroduplex and PCR-SSCP analysis for matching of HLA-A, B and C allotypes in marrow transplantation. Eur J Immunogenet 1996; 23:41–53.

98. Speiser DE, Tiercy JM, Rufer N, Grundschober C, Gratwohl A, Chapuis B, Helg C, Loliger CC, Siren MK, Roosnek E, Jeannet M. High resolution HLA matching associated with decreased mortality after unrelated bone marrow transplantation. Blood 1996; 87:4455–4462.

99. Grundschober C, Rufer N, Sanchez-Mazas A, Madrigal A, Jeannet M, Roosnek E, Tiercy J-M. Molecular characterization of HLA-C incompatibilities in HLA-ABDR-matched unrelated bone marrow donor-recipient pairs. Sequence of two new Cw alleles (Cw*02023 and Cw*0707) and recognition by cytotoxic lymphocytes. Tiss Antigens 1997; 6:612–623.

100. Szmania S, Keever-Taylor CA, Baxter-Lowe LA. Automated nucleotide sequencing reveals substantial disparity between the HLA-A2 genes of bone marrow transplant recipients and donors. Human Immunol 1997; 56:77–83.

101. Arguello R, Avakian H, Goldman JM, Madrigal JA. A novel method for simultaneous high-resolution identification of HLA-A, HLA-B and HLA-Cw alleles. Nature Genet 1998; 18:192–194.

102. Petersdorf EW, Gooley TA, Anasetti C, Martin PJ, Smith AG, Mickelson EM, Woolfrey AE, Hansen JA. Optimizing outcome after unrelated marrow transplantation by comprehensive matching of HLA class I and II alleles in the donor and recipient. Blood 1998; 92:3515–3520.

103. Scott I, O'Shea J, Bunce M, Tiercy J-M, Arguello JR, Firman H, Goldman J, Prentice HG, Little A-M, Madrigal JA. Molecular typing shows a high level of HLA class I incompatibility in serologically well matched donor/patient pairs: implications for unrelated bone marrow donor selection. Blood 1998; 12:4864–4871.

104. Prasad VK, Kernan NA, Heller G, O'Reilly RJ, Yang SY. DNA typing for HLA-A and HLA-B identifies disparities between patients and unrelated donors matched by HLA-A and HLA-B serology and HLA-DRB1. Blood 1999; 93:399–409.

105. Zanone-Ramseier R, Gratwohl A, Gmur J, Roosnek E, Tiercy J-M. Sequencing of two HLA-A blank alleles: implications in unrelated bone marrow donor matching. Transplantation 1999; 67:1336–1341.

106. Hurley CK, Baxter-Lowe LA, Begovich AB, Fernandez-Vina M, Noreen H, Schmeckpeper B, Awdeh Z, Chopek M, Salazar M, Williams TM, Yunis EJ, Kitajima D, Shipp K, Splett J, Winden T, Kollman C, Johnson D, Ng J, Hartzman RJ, Hegland J. The extent of HLA class II allele level disparity in unrelated bone marrow transplantation: analysis of 1259 National Marrow Donor Program donor-recipient pairs. Bone Marrow Transplant 2000; 25:385–393.

107. Sayer D, Whidborne R, Brestovac B, Trimboli F, Witt C, Christiansen F. HLA-DRB1 DNA sequencing based typing: an approach suitable for high throughput typing including unrelated bone marrow registry donors. Tiss Antigens 2002; 57:46–54.

108. Beatty PG, Mori M, Milford E. Impact of racial genetic polymorphism on the probability of finding an HLA-matched donor. Transplantation 1995; 60:778–783.

109. Lonjou C, Clayton J, Cambon-Thomsen A, Raffoux C. HLA-A, -B, -DR haplotype frequencies in France. Implications for recruitment of potential bone marrow donors. Transplantation 1995; 60:375–383.

110. Mori M, Beatty PG, Graves M, Boucher KM, Milford EL. HLA gene and haplotype frequencies in the North American population: The National Marrow Donor Program Donor Registry. Transplantation 1997; 64:1017–1027.

111. Oudshoorn M, Cornelissen JJ, Fibbe WE, de Graeff-Meeder ER, Lie JL, Schreuder GM, Sintnicolaas K, Willemze R, Vossen JM, van Rood JJ. Problems and possible solutions in finding an unrelated bone marrow donor. Results of consecutive searches for 240 Dutch patients. Bone Marrow Transplant 1997; 20:1011–1017.

112. Schipper RF, D'Amaro J, Bakker JT, Van Rood JJ, Oudshoorn M. HLA gene and haplotype frequencies in bone marrow donors worldwide registries. Human Immunol 1997; 52:54–71.

113. Oh HB, Kim SI, Park MH, Akaza T, Juji T. Probability of finding HLA-matched unrelated marrow donors for Koreans and Japanese from the Korean and Japan Marrow Donor Programs. Tiss Antigens 1999; 53:347–349.

114. Velickovic ZM, Carter JM. Feasibility of finding an unrelated bone marrow donor on international registries for New Zealand patients. Bone Marrow Transplant 1999; 23:291–294.

115. Brown J, Poles A, Brown CJ, Contreras M, Vavarrete CV. HLA-A, -B and -DR antigen frequencies of the London Cord Blood Bank units differ from those found in established bone marrow donor registries. Bone Marrow Transplant 2000; 25:475–481.

116. Hansen JA, Yamamoto K, Petersdorf E, Sasazuki T. The role of HLA matching in hematopoietic cell transplantation. Rev Immunogen 1999; 1:359–373.

117. Sasazuki T, Juji T, Morishima Y, Kinukawa N, Kashiwabara H, Inoko H, Yoshida T, Kimura A, Akaza T, Kamikawaji N, Kodera Y, Takaku F for the JMDP. Effect of matching of class I HLA alleles on clinical outcome after transplantation of hematopoietic stem cells from an unrelated donor. N Engl J Med 1998; 339:1177–1185.

118. Hansen JA, Clift RA, Thomas ED, Buckner CD, Storb R, Giblett ER. Transplantation of marrow from an unrelated donor to a patient with acute leukemia. N Engl J Med 1980; 303:565–567.

119. Piazza A. Haplotype and linkage disequilibrium from the three-locus phenotypes. In: Kissmeyer-Nielsen F, ed. Histocompatibility Testing. Copenhagen: Munksgaard, 1975: 923–927.

120. Begovich AB, McClure GR, Suraj VC, Helmuth RC, Fildes N, Bugawan TL, Erlich HA, Klitz W. Polymorphism, recombination, and linkage disequilibrium within the HLA class II region. J Immunol 1992; 148:249–258.

121. Beatty PG, Boucher KM, Mori M, Milford EL. Probability of finding HLA-mismatched related or unrelated marrow or cord blood donors. Human Immunol 2000; 61:834–840.

122. Tiercy J-M, Bujan-Lose M, Chapuis B, Gratwohl A, Gmur J, Seger R, Kern M, Morell A, Roosnek E. Bone marrow transplantation with unrelated donors: what is the probability of identifying an HLA-A/B/Cw/DRB1/B3/B5/DQB1-matched donor? Bone Marrow Transplant 2000; 26:437–441.

123. Takahashi K, Juji T, Miyazaki H. Determination of an appropriate size of unrelated donor pool to be registered for HLA-matched bone marrow transplantation. Transfusion 1989; 29:311–313.

124. Schipper RF, D'Amaro J, Oudshoorn M. The probability of finding a suitable related donor for bone marrow transplantation in extended families. Blood 1996; 87:800–804.

125. Speck B, Zwaan FE, van Rood JJ, Eernisse JG. Allogeneic bone marrow transplantation in a patient with aplastic anemia using a phenotypically HLA-identical unrelated donor. Transplantation 1973; 16:24–28.

126. Lohrmann H-P, Dietrich M, Goldmann SF, Kristensen T, Fliedner TM, Abt C, Pflieger H, Flad HD, Kubanek B, Heimpel H. Bone marrow transplantation for aplastic anemia from a HL-A and MLC-identical unrelated donor. Blut 1975; 31:347–354.

127. Horowitz SD, Bach FH, Groshong T, Hong R, Yunis EJ. Treatment of severe combined immunodeficiency with bone marrow from an unrelated, mixed-leukocyte culture nonreactive donor. Lancet 1975; 2:431–433.

128. L'Esperance P, Hansen JA, Jersild C, et al. Bone-marrow donor selection among unrelated four-locus identical individuals. Transplant Proc 1975; S(1):823–831.

129. O'Reilly R, Dupont B, Pahwa S, Grimes E, Smithwick EM, Pahwa R, Schwartz S, Hansen JA, Siegal FP, Sorell M, Svejgaard A, Jersild C, Thomsen M, Platz P, L'Esperance P, Good RA. Successful hematologic and immunologic reconstitution of severe combined immunodeficiency and secondary aplasia by transplantation of bone marrow from an unrelated HLA-D compatible donor. N Engl J Med 1977; 297:1311–1318.

130. Ash RC, Casper JT, Chitambar CR, Hansen R, Bunin N, Truitt RL, Lawton C, Murray K, Hunter J, Baxter-Lowe LA. Successful allogeneic transplantation of T-cell-depleted bone marrow from closely HLA-matched unrelated donors. N Engl J Med 1990; 322:485–494.

131. Gajewski JL, Ho WG, Feig SA, Hunt L, Kaufman N, Champlin RE. Bone marrow transplantation using unrelated donors for patients with advanced leukemia or bone marrow failure. Transplantation 1990; 50:244–249.

132. Beatty PG, Hansen JA, Longton GM, Thomas ED, Sanders JE, Martin PJ, Bearman SI, Anasetti C, Petersdorf EW, Mickelson EM. Marrow transplantation from HLA-matched unrelated donors for treatment of hematologic malignancies. Transplantation 1991; 51:443–447.

133. Kernan NA, Bartsch G, Ash RC, Beatty PG, Champlin R, Filipovich A, Gajewski J, Hansen JA, Henslee-Downey J, McCullough J. Analysis of 462 transplantations from unrelated donors facilitated by the National Marrow Donor Program. N Engl J Med 1993; 328:593–602.

134. Madrigal JA, Scott I, Arguello R, Szydlo R, Little AM, Goldmann JM. Factors influencing the outcome of bone marrow transplants using unrelated donors. Immunol Rev 1997; 157:153–166.

135. Flomenberg N, Baxter-Lowe LA, Confer D, Fernandez-Vina M, Filipovich A, Horowitz M, Hurley C, Kollman C, Noreen H, Weisdorf D. Impact of HLA-class I and class II high resolution matching on outcomes of unrelated donor BMT (abstr). Blood 2001; 98:813a.

136. Petersdorf EW, Kollman C, Hurley CK, Dupont B, Nademanee A, Begovich AB, Weisdorf D, McGlave P. Effect of HLA class II gene disparity on clinical outcome in unrelated donor hematopoietic cell transplantation for chronic myeloid leukemia: the US National Marrow Donor Program experience. Blood 2001; 98:2922–2929.

137. Morishima Y, Sasazuki T, Inoko H, Juji T, Akaza T, Yamamoto K, Ishikawa Y, Kato S, Sao H, Sakamaki H, Kawa K, Hamajima N, Asano S, Kodera Y for the NMDP. The clinical significance of human leukocyte antigen (HLA) allele compatibility in patients receiving a marrow transplant from serologically HLA-A, HLA-B and HLA-Dr matched unrelated donors. Blood 2002; 99:4200–4206.

138. Petersdorf EW, Gooley T, Malkki M, Anasetti C, Martin P, Woolfrey A, Smith A, Mickelson E, Hansen JA. The biological significance of HLA-DP gene variation in haematopoietic cell transplantation. Br J Haematology 2001; 112:988–994.

139. Pawlec G, Ehninger G, Schmidt H, Wernet P. HLA-DP matching and graft-versus-host disease in allogeneic bone marrow transplantation. Transplantation 1986; 42:558–560.

140. Keever-Taylor CA, Bredeson C, Loberiza FR, Casper JT, Lawton C, Rizzo D, Burns WH, Margolis DA, Vesole DH, Horowitz M, Zhang J-J, Juckett M, Drobyski WR. Analysis of risk factors for the development of GVHD after T cell-depleted allogeneic BMT: effect of HLA disparity, ABO incompatibility, and method of T-cell depletion. Biol Blood Marrow Transplant 2001; 7:620–630.

141. Anasetti C, Amos D, Beatty PG, Appelbaum FR, Bensinger W, Buckner CD, Clift R, Doney K, Martin PJ, Mickelson E. Effect of HLA compatibility on engraftment of bone marrow transplants in patients with leukemia or lymphoma. N Engl J Med 1989; 320:197–204.

142. Fleischhauer K, Kernan NA, O'Reilly RJ, Dupont B, Yang SY. Bone marrow-allograft rejection by T lymphocytes recognizing a single amino acid difference in HLA-B44. N Engl J Med 1990; 323:1818–1822.

143. Kato Y, Mitsuishi Y, Cecka M, Hopfield J, Hunt L, Champlin R, Terasaki PI, Gajewski JL. HLA-DP incompatibilities and severe graft-versus-host disease in unrelated bone marrow transplants. Transplantation 1991; 52:374–376.

144. Marks DI, Cullis JO, Ward KN, Lacey S, Syzdlo R, Hughes TP, Schwarer AP, Lutz E, Barrett AJ, Hows JM. Allogeneic bone marrow transplantation for chronic myelogenous leukemia using sibling and volunteer unrelated donors: a comparison of complications in the first 2 years. Ann Intern Med 1993; 119:207–212.

145. Petersdorf EW, Smith AG, Mickelson EM, Longton G, Anasetti C, Choo SY, Martin PJ, Hansen JA. The role of HLA-DPB1 disparity in the development of acute graft-versus-host disease following unrelated donor marrow transplantation. Blood 1993; 81:1923–1932.

146. Anasetti C, Hansen JA. Effect of HLA incompatibility in marrow transplantation from unrelated and HLA-mismatched related donors. Transfus Sci 1994; 15:221–230.

147. Keever CA, Leong N, Cunningham I, Copelan EA, Avalos BR, Klein J, Kapoor N, Adams PW, Orosz CG, Tutschka PJ. HLA-B44-directed cytotoxic T cells associated with acute graft-versus-host disease following unrelated bone marrow transplantation. Bone Marrow Transplant 1994; 14:137–145.

148. Davies SM, Shu XO, Blazar BR, Filipovich AH, Kersey JH, Krivit W, McCullough J, Miller WJ, Ramsay NK, Segall M. Unrelated donor bone marrow transplantation: influence of HLA-A and -B incompatibility on outcome. Blood 1995; 86:1636–1642.

149. Petersdorf EW, Longton GM, Anasetti C, Martin PJ, Mickelson EM, Smith AG, Hansen JA. The significance of HLA-DRB1 matching on clinical outcome after HLA-A, B, DR identical unrelated donor marrow transplantation. Blood 1995; 86:1606–1613.

150. Gajewski J, Gjertson D, Cecka M, Tonai R, Przepiorka D, Hunt L, Giralt S, Chan KW, Feig S, Territo M, Anderson B, van Besien K, Khouri I, Fischer H, Babbitt L, Ippolitti C, Schiller G, Lill M, Warkentin D, Joyce Neumann, Petz L, Terasaki P, Champlin R. The impact of T-cell depletion on the effects of HLA-DRB1 and DQB allele matching in HLA serologically identical unrelated donor bone marrow transplantation. Biol Blood Marrow Transplant 1997; 3:76–82.

151. Petersdorf EW, Longton GM, Anasetti C, Mickelson EM, McKinney SK, Smith AG, Martin PJ, Hansen JA. Association of HLA-C disparity with graft failure after marrow transplantation from unrelated donors. Blood 1997; 89:1818–1823.

152. Przepiorka D, Petropoulos D, Mullen C, Danielson M, Mattewada V, Chan KW. Tacrolimus for prevention of graft-versus-host disease after mismatched unrelated donor cord blood transplantation. Bone Marrow Transplant 1999; 23:1291–1295.

153. Varney MD, Lester S, McCluskey J, Gao X, Tait BD. Matching for HLA DPA1 and DPB1 alleles in unrelated bone marrow transplantation. Human Immunol 1999; 60:532–538.

154. Davies SM, Kollman C, Anasetti C, Antin JH, Gajewski J, Casper JT, Nadermanee A, Noreen H, King R, Confer D, Kernan NA. Engraftment and survival after unrelated-donor bone marrow transplantation: a report from the National Marrow Donor Program. Blood 2000; 96:4096–4102.

155. McGlave PB, Shu XO, Wen W, Anasetti C, Nadermanee A, Champlin R, Antin JH, Kernan NA, King R, Weisdorf DJ. Unrelated donor marrow transplantation for chronic myelogenous leukemia: 9 years' experience of the National Marrow Donor Program. Blood 2000; 95:2219–2225.

156. Prezpiorka D, Saliba R, Cleary K, Fischer H, Tonai R, Fritsche H, Khouri IF, Folloder J, Ueno NT, Mehra R, Ippoliti C, Giralt S, Gajewski S, Donato M, Claxton D, Braunschweig I, van Beisien K, Anderlini P, Andersson BS, Champlin R. Tacrolimus does not abrogate the increased risk of acute graft-versus-host disease after unrelated-donor marrow transplantation with allelic mismatching at HLA-DRB1 and HLA-DQB1. Biol Blood Marrow Transplant 2000; 6:190–197.

157. Ferrara GB, Bacigalupo A, Lamparelli T, Lanino E, Delfino L, Morabito A, Parodi AM, Pera C, Pozzi S, Sormani MP, Bruzzi P, Bordo D, Bolognesi M, Bandini G, Bontadini A, Barbanti M, Frumento G. Bone marrow transplantation from unrelated donors: the impact of mismatches with substitutions at position 116 of the human leukocyte antigen class I heavy chain. Blood 2001; 98:3150–3155.

158. Loiseau P, Esperou H, Busson M, Sghiri R, Tamouza R, Hilarius M, Raffoux C, Devergie A, Ribaud P, Socie G, Gluckman E, Charron D. DPB1 disparities contribute to severe GVHD and reduced patient survival after unrelated donor bone marrow transplantation (abstr). Blood 2001; 7:660a.

159. Petersdorf EW, Hansen JA, Martin PJ, Woolfrey A, Malkki M, Gooley T, Storer B, Mickelson E, Smith A, Anasetti C. Major histocompatibility complex class I alleles and antigens in hematopoietic cell transplantation. N Engl J Med 2001; 345:1794–1800.

160. Beatty PG, Clift RA, Mickelson EM, Nisperos BB, Flournoy N, Martin PJ, Sanders JE, Stewart P, Buckner CD, Storb R. Marrow transplantation from related donors other than HLA-identical siblings. N Engl J Med 1985; 313:765–771.

161. Servida P, Gooley T, Hansen JA, Bjerke J, Martin PJ, Petersdorf EW, Anasetti C. Improved survival of haploidentical related donor marrow transplants mismatched for HLA-A or B versus HLA-DR. Blood 1996; 88(1):484a.

162. Hansen JA, Gooley T, Martin PJ, Appelbaum F, Chauncey TR, Clift RA, Petersdorf EW, Radich J, Sanders JE, Storb RF, Sullivan KM, Anasetti C. Bone marrow transplants from unrelated donors for patients with chronic myeloid leukemia. N Engl J Med 1998; 338:962–968.

163. Ruggeri L, Capanni M, Urbani E, Perruccio K, Shlomchik WD, Tosti A, Posati S, Rogaia D, Frassoni F, Aversa F, Martelli MF, Velardi A. Effectiveness of donor natural killer cell allo-reactivity in mismatched hematopoietic transplants. Science 2002; 2097–2100.
164. Aversa F, Tabilio A, Velardi A, Falzetti F, Giannoni C, Iacucci R, Zei T, Martelli MP, Gambelunghe C. Successful engraftment of T-cell depleted haploidentical "three-loci" incompatible transplants in leukemia patients by addition of recombinant human granulocyte colony-stimulating factor-mobilized peripheral blood progenitor cells to bone marrow inoculum. Blood 1994; 84:3948–3955.
165. Davies SM, Ruggieri L, DeFor T, Wagner JE, Weisdorf DJ, Miller JS, Velardi A, Blazar BR. Evaluation of KIR ligand incompatibility in mismatched unrelated donor hematopoietic transplants. Blood 2002; 100:3825–3827.

15

Immunosuppression and Immunophilin Ligands: Cyclosporin, Tacrolimus, and Sirolimus

BARBARA E. BIERER

Harvard Medical School and Brigham and Women's Hospital, Boston, Massachusetts, U.S.A.

I. OVERVIEW

Advances in cellular and molecular immunology have heralded the application of novel modalities in clinical and experimental transplantation. The successful outcome of bone marrow and solid organ transplantation has been greatly enhanced in the last 40 years not only by improvements in surgical techniques, but by progressive understanding of HLA histocompatibility and typing, by the understanding of transplantation immunobiology, and by the development of effective immunosuppressive drugs. Activation of both T and B lymphocytes is essential for the generation of an antigen-specific immune response, as is the participation of dendritic and other cells. The inappropriate or undesired activation of these cells can lead to autoimmunity or, in the setting of allograft transplantation, graft rejection or graft-vs.-host disease (GVHD). T-lymphocyte function is central to the maintenance and regulation of the immune response and of tolerance; T cells not only mediate cytotoxicity and immune suppression, but through the production and secretion of cytokines, T cells also control the proliferation of B cells as well as their differentiation to antibody-secreting cells. Furthermore, a specific subset of regulatory T cells appears to be critical for the maintenance of immune homeostasis and tolerance. Therefore, regulation of the T-cell arm of the immune response is essential for the maintenance of immune homeostasis and for the prevention of graft rejection and GVHD.

Many immunosuppressive regimens use combinations of immunosuppressive drugs. Ideally, these agents have nonoverlapping toxicity and complementary mechanisms of action. Whereas a complete description of the pathways of T-lymphocyte antigen recognition and activation is beyond the scope of this chapter, understanding the mechanism(s) of action of these agents involves an appreciation of the normal pathways of T-cell activation and proliferation and thereby of the site of actions of specific inhibitors.

Resting, G_0 peripheral T cells express on their cell surface a heterodimeric antigen-specific T-cell receptor (TcR) complexed to an array of at least five nonpolymorphic peptides termed CD3 (Fig. 1). The TcR-CD3 complex recognizes processed peptide antigen presented in the groove of molecules of the major histocompatibility complex (MHC), which, in humans, is defined by products of the histocompatibility locus HLA, located

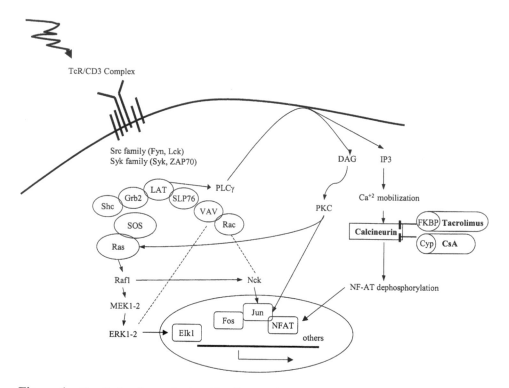

Figure 1 T-cell signal transduction. T cells are stimulated upon binding of the T-cell receptor (TcR)–CD3 complex to antigens embedded in the groove of MHC class I or class II molecules expressed on antigen-presenting cells. The signaling networks initiated upon T-cell stimulation are complex and involve recruitment of a number of intracellular intermediates to a signalosome. The src-related kinases Lck and Fyn and the Syk kinase ZAP-70 are both critical for appropriate signal transduction. These in turn phosphorylate the adaptor complex LAT that recruits the adapters Grb-2, SLP-76, and Nck, the guanine nucleotide exchange factor SOS, and other molecules to activate Ras-Raf-MEK-MAP kinase and ERK activity. Alternatively, LAT serves as the platform for the enzyme phospholipase C (PLCγ), which in turn results in the activation of diacylglycerol (DAG) and inositol trisphosphate (IP3). IP3 results in the mobilization of calcium (Ca^{2+}) stores from the endoplasmic reticulum, and calcium; calcium, along with calmodulin, are necessary cofactors for the activation of the serine/threonine phosphatase calcineurin. Calcineurin is the enzyme that is responsible for the dephosphorylation of nuclear factor of activated T cells (NFAT), a transcription factor that is essential for the transcriptional activation of cytokine genes. Calcineurin is inhibited by the complex of FKBP/tacrolimus and of cyclophilin/CsA.

on chromosome 6. Upon recognition of a specific antigen/MHC complex in concert with appropriate costimulatory signals, the TcR-CD3 complex transduces activating signals from the surface to the cytoplasm of the cell. The earliest biochemical signals that can be delineated following TcR-CD3 ligation involve the generation of protein tyrosine kinase activity and of phosphotidylinositol hydrolysis. These pathways are interdependent, but both ultimately result in the induction of gene transcription involving immediate early and late activation genes, which results, eventually, in proliferation of T cells and differentiation towards effector function. Costimulation can be provided by cytokines and by a number of T-cell coreceptor molecules, including but not limited to CD4 (or CD8), CD28, CD2, and CD40L. In the absence of costimulation, engagement of the TcR-CD3 complex alone can lead to a T-cell hypo- or unresponsiveness and the development of T-cell anergy.

Immunosuppressive agents can be generally categorized by their site of action in T-cell activation pathways. Although any categorization suffers from oversimplification (Fig. 2), few agents are thought to directly interface with antigen processing. Although the precise mechanism of action is poorly understood, 15-deoxyspergualin

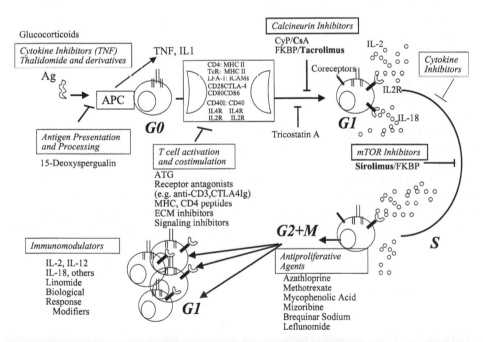

Figure 2 Mechanisms of immunosuppression. The immune response is a multistep process that is initiated by antigen processing and presentation, binding of antigen to MHC molecules, and the interaction of T cells with antigen/MHC to result in T-cell activation, a process that involves costimulation. After activation, T cells produce cytokines and express on their cell surface cytokine receptors. Cytokines, acting in a paracrine and autocrine fashion, are necessary growth factors for T-cell growth, division, and proliferation and for the acquisition of effector functions (cytotoxicity, provision of T-cell help). At each of these steps, and others, immunosuppressive and immunomodulatory agents are able to inhibit the appropriate propogation of the immune response.

(DSG), MW496 (1), a potent synthetic derivative of spergualin isolated from *Bacillus laterosporus*, is thought to inhibit antigenic processing and MHC presentation of antigen. It has been shown to associate and interact with members of the heat-shock protein (hsp) family (2) and to inhibit their ATPase activity. DSG has been shown to inhibit growth of tumor and other cell lines both in vivo and in vitro (3) and to block cell cycle progression in the G_1 phase (4). DSG has also been shown to inhibit the activation of the serine threonine kinase Akt (also termed protein kinase B), but this effect does not appear to be direct (5). Furthermore, DSG inhibits the nuclear translocation of the transcription factor NFκB (6), a transcription factor involved in determining the fate in life or death of the cell (7) as well as other processes. While DSG showed promise in preclinical animal models of both transplant rejections and GVHD, its use was limited by toxicity (8). A new immunosuppressive analog of DSG, LF 15-0195, has shown efficacy in preventing GVHD in mouse models (9). While the mechanism of action is not clear, it may relate to the ability of the drug to sensitize T cells to activation-induced cell death (apoptosis) (10).

Upon TcR-CD3 engagement of antigen successfully presented by antigen-presenting cells (APCs), the APC is stimulated to produce cytokines, which, in turn, propagate the immune response (Fig. 2). Cytokine inhibitors and neutralizing monoclonal antibodies (mAbs) directly antagonize cytokines by binding to the cytokine itself or its receptor and competing for ligand binding. Cytokine dysregulation has been implicated in and is important for the pathophysiology of both acute and chronic GVHD. A number of cytokine antagonists are now available; in fact, many cytokine receptors have naturally occurring forms that act in vitro, and possibly in vivo, as antagonists. Cytokine inhibitors may modulate the clinical manifestations of rejection or GVHD and ameliorate the tissue destruction associated with preparative conditioning and with GVHD; whether they reduce underlying T-cell alloreactivity remains to be shown.

The TNF/TNF-receptor(R)–related superfamily, important in costimulation, inflammation, cell movement, and cell survival, has been the subject of extensive investigations. TNF-α binding to the p55 TNFR1 is important in inflammation and in the induction of apoptosis in early GVHD (11). A chimeric murine anti-human IgG1 monoclonal antibody (mAb), infliximab, directed against TNF-α, and etanercept, a dimeric p75 TNFR2 receptor Fc-fusion protein both act by neutralizing the actions of TNF-α. They are both well tolerated with few serious side effects and are both approved by the U.S. Food and Drug Administration (FDA) for use in rheumatoid arthritis. When tested in early clinical trials for the treatment of GVHD, each appeared promising (12–16). The time to respond (>10 d) appeared long, and these agents have not been subject to prospective randomized clinical trials. The preliminary results, however, suggest that additional studies are warranted to define dosing, timing, and optimal combinations of these potentially effective agents.

Other members of the TNF/TNFR superfamily are also currently being investigated for use. The CD40L (CD154; TNFRSF5) on the surface of activated T cells binds to CD40 (TNFRSF5) (17) and appears to be important for costimulation and sustained, largely Th1, function (18). Blockade of the CD40L/CD40 costimulatory pathway results in tolerance induction in preclinical models (19–23). While the results using murine models of alloreactivity are encouraging, the use of anti-CD40L and of anti-CD40 mAb in humans may be constrained by toxicity associated with their use.

In addition to agents directed against the TNF/TNFR superfamily, T-cell activation and costimulation may be blocked by a number of inhibitors of signal transduction or by agents that interact with or interfere with the cell surface receptors important for stimulation. Leflunomide (previously termed HWA 486) has been shown to inhibit tyrosyl phosphorylation of a number of proteins, including the residues catalyzed by the src-related tyrosine kinases p561ck and p59fyn, and the autophosphorylation of the epidermal growth factor (EGF) receptor (for review, see Ref. 24). T-cell surface receptor antagonists, including OKT3, a mAb directed at the CD3ε chain of the TcR-CD3, and CTLA4Ig, a recombinant protein that inhibits ligand binding to CD28 (and its closely associated family member CTLA4) are examples of agents that have been approved for clinical use in other indications or are in phase II clinical trials. Ligation of the TCR-CD3 complex of newly activated cells is able to induce cell death. A humanized anti-CD3, non-FcR–binding monoclonal antibody, visilizumab, has been tested in a single arm study of patients with glucocorticoid-refractory acute GVHD (25). The treatment induced responses, but the therapy was complicated by posttransplant lymphoproliferative disease (PTLD). The addition of the anti-CD20 B-cell–specific mAb rituximab appeared to resolve the problem of PTLD, and further studies are warranted. These and other agents are directed towards the interruption of appropriate T-cell:APC interactions, thereby inhibiting activating signals to the cell.

Other immunosuppressive agents target different intermediates in lymphocyte function and proliferation. The antimetabolites act to inhibit cellular proliferation by depleting the cell of essential metabolic intermediates required for DNA synthesis; both purine (Fig. 3) and pyrimidine inhibitors have been extensively explored. Lymphocytes depend on these salvage pathways more than other cells, and these agents are clinically useful despite of their lack of specificity. In combination with other agents, antimetabolites have a role in the armamentarium of immunosuppressive drugs.

A number of inhibitors of transcriptional activation of early genes have been developed and are in clinical use. Because of their specificity, both cyclosporin A (CsA, Sandimmune®, Neoral®) and tacrolimus (FK506, Prograf®) (Fig. 4) have been widely used in solid organ and stem cell transplantation. Discovered by Borel in 1976, CsA was purified from the fungus *Tolypoladium inflatum* based on its ability to inhibit mixed lymphocyte reactions (MLR) (26). CsA, a cyclic undecapeptide of MW 1203 (Fig. 4), is synthesized by a single enzyme, CsA synthetase (27). Tacrolimus (Fig. 4) was isolated from soil samples containing *Streptomyces tsukubaensis* in 1987 by Fujisawa Pharmaceutical Co. (28,29). It, too, was purified to homogeneity based on its ability to inhibit an MLR and was shown to be a member of the macrolide antibiotic family. The chemical structure of tacrolimus revealed the drug to be homologous to another macrolide compound, sirolimus (Rapamycin, Rapamune®). Sirolimus (Fig. 4) was isolated from *Streptomyces hygroscopicus* in 1975 by Wyeth-Ayerst Pharmaceuticals and had been shown to have antifungal, antitumor, and antiproliferative activity (30,31). It was later found to have immunosuppressive activity as well. Sirolimus is now approved for use in the prevention and treatment of rejection in solid organ transplantation.

CsA and tacrolimus both share the ability to inhibit T-cell activation–dependent induction of early gene transcription, specifically the genes encoding cytokines such as IL-2. Early signal transduction events, including tyrosine kinase activation and phosphotidylinositol hydrolysis, are not perturbed by CsA or tacrolimus. It is now appreciated that both CsA and tacrolimus diffuse freely into the cell and bind to specific intracellular receptors termed immunophilins (see below). CsA binds to a family of receptors termed cyclophilins, while tacrolimus and its structural homolog sirolimus both bind to a family of proteins termed FKBPs [FK506 (tacrolimus)–binding proteins]. Both cyclophilins and

432

Bierer

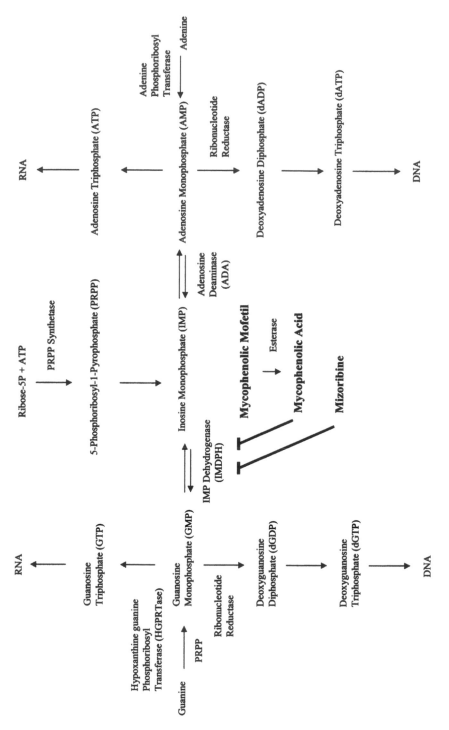

Figure 3 Pathways of purine biosynthesis and site of action of several antimetabolite agents. Synthesis of the purine nucleotides adenylic acid (AMP), inosinic acid (IMP), and guanylic acid (GMP) occurs via one of two pathways: either directly from the purine bases guanine, hypoxanthine, and adenine or de novo from nonpurine precursors such as ribose-5-phosphate. IMP is a common intermediate in both routes of synthesis. The conversion of IMP to GMP by IMP dehydrogenase (IMPDH) is inhibited by mycophenolic mofetil, mycophenolic acid, and mizoribine. By depleting the cell of essential intermediates required for DNA synthesis, these agents inhibit cellular proliferation.

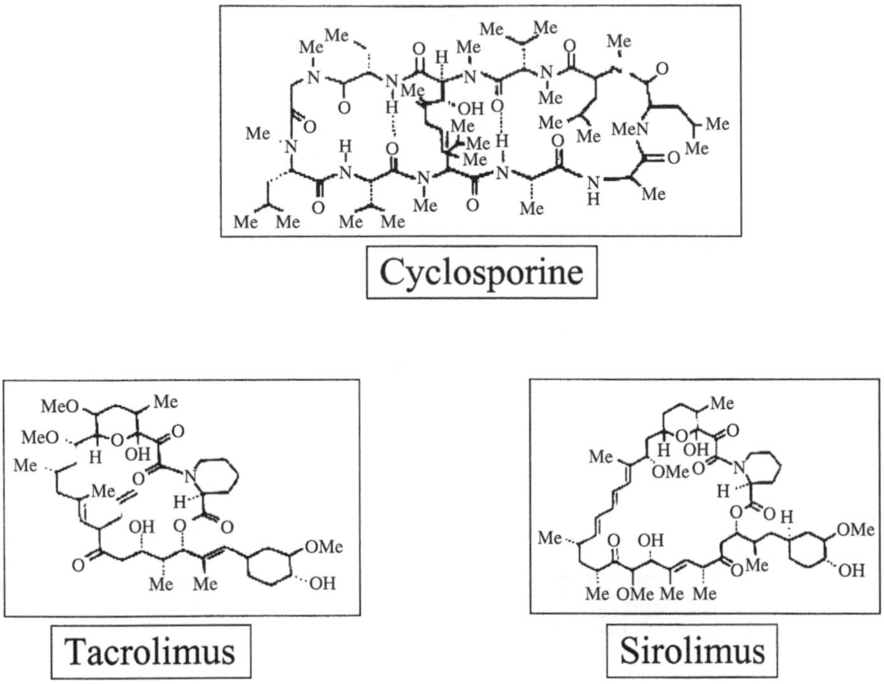

Cyclosporine

Tacrolimus

Sirolimus

Figure 4　Structure of cyclosporine (CsA), tacrolimus (FK506), and sirolimus (rapamycin). The structures of cyclosporine, a cyclic undecapeptide, and the macrolide antibiotics tacrolimus and sirolimus are shown.

FKBPs function as *cis-trans* peptidyl prolyl isomerase (PPIase or rotamase) enzymes able to catalyze the refolding of proteins in vitro (32–34). CsA inhibits rotamase activity of cyclophilins, while tacrolimus and sirolimus inhibit the rotamase activity of FKBPs (Fig. 5). However, inhibition of rotamase activity does not explain immunosuppression. Binding of drug to the receptor results in the formation of an active moiety able to bind to and inhibit specific molecular targets within the cell. CsA-cyclophilin and tacrolimus-FKBP complexes targeted the serine/threonine phosphatase calcineurin, while sirolimus-FKBP targeted a protein termed mTOR [mammalian target of rapamycin (sirolimus)] protein (reviewed below). Thus, calcineurin, inhibited by CsA and tacrolimus, is required for transcriptional activation of cytokine genes, while mTOR, inhibited by sirolimus, is required for growth factor–dependent proliferation. Sirolimus inhibits T cells at the late G_1/S interface. This chapter will review our current understanding of the molecular mechanisms of action of CsA, tacrolimus, and sirolimus.

II.　IMMUNOPHILINS: INTRACELLULAR RECEPTORS FOR CsA, TACROLIMUS, AND SIROLIMUS

A.　Cyclophilins

Cyclosporin binds to a family of intracellular receptors termed cyclophilins (CyP). A number of cyclophilin isoforms have been cloned and studied. Indeed, the number of potential

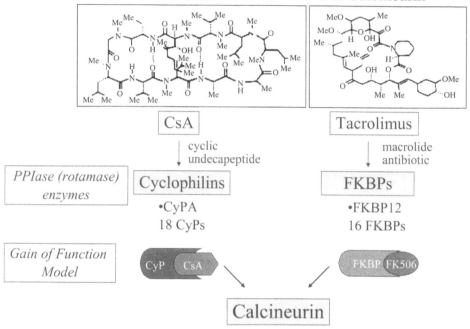

Cyclosporine (CsA) binds Cyclophilins
while FK506 binds FKBPs: both bind Calcineurin

Figure 5 Cyclosporine (CsA) binds cyclophilins while tacrolimus binds FKBPs: both bind calcineurin. CsA binds to the peptidyl proline isomerase (rotamase) enzyme cycophilin, a member of a family of cyclophilins, of which 18 have been identified in the human genome. Tacrolimus binds to another rotamase enzyme FK506-binding protein (FKBP), a member of a family of 16 human FKBPs. Both drugs inhibit the rotamase activity of the enzymes, but the rotamase activity itself is unrelated to the mechanism of drug action. Drug binding to the intracellular protein results in a gain of function and the drug/receptor complex inhibit the serine/threonine phosphatase calcineurin.

cyclophilin homologues increased substantially following the sequencing of the human genome. CyPA is by far the most abundant isoform in mammalian cells and is localized mainly to the cytoplasm (35,36). It was purified based on its high affinity for CsA and functions as a peptidyl-prolyl *cis-trans* isomerase (PPIase or rotamase) (32). Like all immunophilins, the rotamase activity of CyPA is inhibited by binding of CsA ($K_i = 6$ nM) (32). Further, the complex of CyPA bound to CsA binds to and inhibits the phosphatase activity of calcineurin (Fig. 5).

Other cyclophilins have somewhat differing properties. A 21 kDa protein, CyPB, is localized to the endoplasmic reticulum (ER), the Golgi apparatus, and plasma membrane (37–39) CyPB is less abundant than CyPA in most cells. The isomerase activity of CyPB is also inhibited by binding to CsA, but with a slightly lower K_i (9 nM). Like CyPA, the complex of CyPB bound by CsA results in the inhibition of calcineurin phosphatase activity. CyPB itself is associated with an ER resident protein termed CAML, a protein that regulates calcium release into the cytoplasm (40). Calcium signaling is a central aspect of regulation by calcineurin and, in turn, by cyclosporin and tacrolimus.

Overexpression of the CAML protein in Jurkat T cells resulted in enhancement of lymphokine gene transcription via a calcineurin-dependent mechanism (40).

Other cyclophilins have been identified, but less is known about their role. Also localized to the ER, CyPC is expressed primarily in the kidney and spleen (41,42), leading to the speculation that it may mediate nephrotoxicity; CyPC interacts with a 77 kDa protein with homology to the scavenger receptor, an association that is disrupted by CsA (42). CyPD is localized to the mitochondria and expressed ubiquitously (43). CyP40, homologous to FKBP52, is a component of the steroid receptor complex (44). The 150 kDa molecule NK-TR, expressed on the surface of natural killer cells, may be involved in tumor recognition (45). A number of cyclophilins in addition to NK-TR are thought to be expressed on the cell surface of hematopoietic and other cells.

B. Tacrolimus-Binding Proteins (FKBPs)

Like the cyclophilins, a number of FKBP isoforms have been characterized that differ in both their subcellular localization and affinity for drug. All proteins that contain a tacrolimus-binding site and a rotamase active site are capable of binding both tacrolimus and sirolimus, although the affinities for the two agents often differ. The predominant FKBP isoform in mammalian cells is the cytoplasmic 12 kDa FKBP12. In the absence of drug, FKBP12 associates with the calcium-release channel, the ryanodine receptor, in the skeletal sarcoplasmic reticulum (SR) and helps to regulate calcium flux. A homologous isoform of FKBP12, FKBP12.6, is localized to the cardiac ryanodine receptor. There, FK12.6 and the ryanodine receptors play a role in cardiomyopathy and conduction disturbances. The cardiac toxicity observed with tacrolimus may relate to this physiology (46–48).

Other FKBPs have been studied. FKBP13 is localized to the ER (49). Binding studies have shown that human FKBP13 ($K_d = 55$ nM) binds tacrolimus with lower affinity than does FKBP12 ($K_d = 0.4$ nM) (41). Nuclear in localization, FKBP25 uniquely demonstrates higher affinity for sirolimus ($K_i = 0.2$ nM) than tacrolimus; the structural basis for this wide discrepancy in drug binding remains to be shown. FKBP25 forms a nuclear complex with casein kinase II and nucleolin (50). FKBP51, also an enzymatically active rotamase, is able to bind calcineurin both in the presence of and in the absence of tacrolimus and sirolimus (51). FKBP52 is a component of the steroid receptor complex in the cytosol that contains the glucocorticoid receptor, hsp90, and hsp70 (52).

C. Endogenous Cellular Function of Immunophilins

The cellular abundance, broad tissue distribution, and evolutionary conservation of immunophilins suggest that their function is essential for cell survival. However, experimental data in lower eukaryotes fail to support the concept that these proteins are necessary. In yeast, disruption of the genes for major cyclophilins and FKBPs results in resistance to drug but has no effect on cellular viability. Thus, either cyclophilin or FKBP genes are not essential for viability or other homologous proteins subserve overlapping functions.

It is possible, of course, that immunophilins may be critical for cell survival only under specific conditions such as heat shock or cellular stress, conditions in which the rate of refolding of proteins is important. Disruption of either of the yeast cyclophilin genes, CPR1 or CPR2, confers sensitivity to heat shock. FKBP52 was first identified as a heat shock protein, complexed with hsp70 and hsp90 in the steroid receptor complex. Cyclophilins have been shown to protect cells from the destructive effects of heat shock

(53). Under conditions of cellular stress, immunophilin function appears to be critical to ensure cellular integrity.

The cellular functions of immunophilins, in addition to protein refolding and protein transport, appear to relate to regulation of associated proteins. In the absence of tacrolimus, FKBP12 associates with the ryanodine receptor of skeletal muscles and with the 1,4,5-triphosphate receptor (IP_3R). Tacrolimus regulates calcium (Ca^{+2}) release by dissociating FKBP12 from the ryanodine and IP_3 receptors, altering Ca^{+2} flux as mentioned above. Regulation by FKBP12 is not due to its isomerase activity (54) but, at least in the case of the IP_3R, to association of calcineurin and regulation of the phosphorylation state of the receptor (55). Calcineurin phosphatase activity affects the activity of voltage-gated Ca^{+2} channels and, thereby, regulates functions such as neuronal transmitter release. These findings may have direct relevance to drug-induced neurotoxicity. The cytoplasmic domain of TGFβ interacts with FKBP12, perhaps affecting the inflammatory environment and cytokine levels (56–58). CyPA and CyPB bind to HIV gag protein and modify infectivity (59,60). The molecular mechanisms of immunophilin regulation are a continuing area of investigation.

D. Immunophilins Relevant for Immunosuppressive Effects

Although all immunophilins have been shown to bind drug, it is likely that specific isoforms mediate the majority of immunosuppressive effects induced by CsA, tacrolimus, and sirolimus. In mammalian cells, CyPA and CyPB appear to mediate the effects of CsA (41). CyPC/CsA complexes have also been shown to inhibit calcineurin activity in vitro, but this has not been substantiated in vivo, perhaps secondary to sequestration of CyPC in the ER lumen (41,61). One relevant intracellular receptor for tacrolimus is FKBP12 (41,62,63). Overexpression of FKBP12, but not FKBP13 or FKBP25, in T cells resulted in increased sensitivity to tacrolimus (41). It is likely that FKBP12.6 is also able to mediate the effects of tacrolimus. At a minimum, FKBP12 is able to mediate the effects of sirolimus. The role of a number of other FKBPs (e.g., FKBP52, FKBP51) has not been rigorously examined.

III. CALCINEURIN AS A TARGET OF DRUG-IMMUNOPHILIN COMPLEXES

Several observations challenged the hypothesis that inhibition of immunophilin rotamase activity was responsible for the observed immunosuppressive properties of CsA, tacrolimus, and sirolimus. First, immunophilins are abundant intracellularly, and the concentration of drug required to fully saturate all respective receptors would be much greater than the nanomolar concentrations capable of inhibiting T-cell activation (33,64). In addition, despite potent inhibition of FKBP rotamase activity by both tacrolimus and sirolimus, their observed biological actions differ (65,66). Furthermore, the two drugs inhibited and reversed the biological actions of each other, suggesting that they competed for binding to FKBPs (65,67). Finally, analogs of tacrolimus (68) and CsA (69) were developed which lacked immunosuppressive properties, but which still bound to and inhibited the rotamase action of immunophilins. Thus, inhibition of rotamase activity alone was insufficient to explain the observed biological properties of the drug(s). The action of these agents was dependent on binding of drug to immunophilin resulting in the formation of an active drug-immunophilin complex capable of inhibiting specific steps in T-cell signal transduction pathways (64,68,70). Drug or immunophilin alone was inactive in the unbound form, but together formed a complex capable of binding to a molecular target within the cell, a gain-of-function model. Based on their identical biological activities, CsA/Cyp and tacrolimus/FKBP complexes were found to share the same intracellular target; the molecular target of sirolimus/FKBP complexes was distinct.

Both CsA and tacrolimus inhibit calcium-dependent signaling pathways in T cells (71–74). In 1991, three polypeptides from extracts of calf brain and thymus were identified as A and B subunits of the cellular phosphatase calcineurin and calmodulin, a cofactor required for calcineurin activity (42,61). Binding of these specific drug-immunophilin complexes inhibited the phosphatase activity of calcineurin in vitro, while drugs alone, immunophilins alone, or the complex sirolimus/FKBP12 had no effect (61). Subsequent studies indicated that complexes of CsA/CyPB, tacrolimus/FKBP12.6, and tacrolimus/ FKBP51 also inhibited calcineurin activity, while tacrolimus/FKBP13, tacrolimus/ FKBP25, and tacrolimus/FKBP52 did not. Inhibition of calcineurin phosphatase activity correlated with inhibition of IL-2 production (75), inhibition of activation-dependent induction of apoptosis (76), and inhibition of degranulation of CTL (77). Inhibition was specific for calcineurin, as the activity of other cellular phosphatases was unaffected in the presence of nanomolar concentrations of either CsA or tacrolimus in vivo (75,78). Similarly, in vivo treatment of cells with sirolimus at nanomolar concentrations failed to inhibit calcineurin activity, but did reverse the inhibition mediated by tacrolimus (61). Based on these observations, calcineurin was identified as the molecular target of both CsA and tacrolimus and shown to be critical in T-cell signal transduction (Fig. 5).

Calcineurin, also known as serine/threonine phosphatase 2B (or PP2B), is a heterodimeric protein that is dependent on binding of calcium and calmodulin for enzymatic activity (79,80). The two subunits calcineurin A (CnA) and calcineurin B (CnB) are noncovalently but stably and constitutively associated (79,80). The larger 59 kDa calcineurin A is composed of an aminoterminal catalytic domain, a B-subunit binding domain, a calmodulin (CaM)-binding domain, and a carboxy-terminal autoinhibitory domain. The smaller 19 kDa regulatory subunit calcineurin B contains four EF-hand sequence motifs, each of which binds a single calcium ion. Three isoforms of CnA have been cloned (CnA α, β, and γ, or PP2Bα 1, 2, and 3) (81). All are similar in structure, sharing 75–80% amino acid sequence homology, and multiple alternatively spliced forms of each isoform exist (79,81). Calmodulin must bind to CnA in the presence of Ca^{2+} for calcineurin to be enzymatically active; activity is further regulated by the carboxy-terminal portion of CnA, which contains the CaM-binding site and a putative autoinhibitory domain (82) and by reactive oxygen species (83,84). That calcineurin is the cellular target of both CsA and tacrolimus has been confirmed by a number of observations and is consistent with the apparent selectivity of both drugs for calcium-sensitive signal transduction pathways. Treatment of T cells with either CsA or tacrolimus, but not with sirolimus, resulted in inhibition of calcineurin activity and correlated with inhibition of cytokine production (75). Overexpression of one or both chains of calcineurin in T cells resulted in decreased sensitivity to CsA and tacrolimus (85). Transient transfection of a mutated, calmodulin-independent form of calcineurin demonstrated that it regulated production not only of IL-2, but also of IL-4, GM-CSF, and TNFα. Synthetic analogues of CsA and tacrolimus were used to confirm that agents possessing immunosuppressive capability effectively and selectively inhibited calcineurin activity, whereas those lacking immunosuppressive qualities, while still able to bind to immunophilins, had no effect on calcineurin activity (61,86). X-ray crystallographic structures of calcineurin/tacrolimus/FKBP12 (87) and calcineurin/calmodulin/tacrolimus/FKBP12 (88) demonstrated that tacrolimus-FKBP12 bound to calcineurin at a site 10 Å away from the phosphatase-active site. Thus, binding of drug to its immunophilin receptor was required for immunosuppression, and the target of these drug-immunophilin complexes was calcineurin.

IV. PHYSIOLOGICAL TARGETS OF CALCINEURIN

The identification of the downstream substrates of calcineurin (Fig. 6) has been an area of active study not only in an effort to understand the physiology of immunosuppression but also to understand the nuclear factor of activated T cells (NFAT) family of related transcription factors known to be involved in regulation of a number of lymphokine genes including IL-2, IL-4, GM-CSF, and TNFα (89,90). Following T-cell activation, NFAT is translocated from the cytoplasm to the nucleus where, in a complex with AP-1, it binds the IL-2 promoter (Fig. 1). Dephosphorylation of NFAT, mediated by calcineurin, is required for translocation of NFAT to the nucleus. However, none of the NFAT family members are expressed exclusively in the immune system (91), and, thus, the relative T-cell/immune cell specificity of these drugs cannot be explained by expression of NFAT isoforms.

Multiple roles for calcineurin

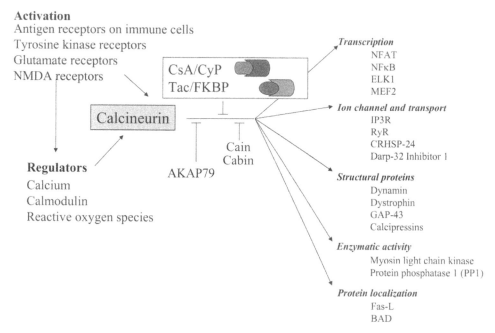

Figure 6   Multiple roles for calcineurin. Calcineurin inhibits the activation of the transcription factor NFAT, as discussed above, as well as other transcription factors. A number of other calcineurin substrates, many regulating diverse cellular processes, have been identified. In addition, calcineurin activity itself is regulated by the cofactors calcium, calmodulin, and reactive oxygen species and by the intracellular regulators AKAP79 and Cain (also termed Cabin). Calcineurin is activated not only by ligation of the TcR-CD3 complex but also by activation of a number of other receptors, depicted here.

Other transcription factors are also sensitive to tacrolimus and CsA. NFκB and rel belong to a family of transcription factors that are sequestered in an inactive state by binding of a third family of proteins termed IκBs (92,93). Phosphorylation of IκB members results in release of NFκB and rel, permitting translocation to the nucleus following T-cell activation. Calcineurin may function as an upstream regulator of IκB activity (94,95). Furthermore, calcineurin has been shown to regulate basal NFκB activity in the central nervous system, a regulation that may be important in understanding neurological side effects of drugs (96). The activity of transcription factor Elk1 regulating Map kinase (Elk1/2) activity is in turn regulated by calcineurin (97).

Substrates other than transcription factors have also been identified as targets of calcineurin. Many targets of calcineurin, in addition to transcription factors are active in brain: the molecule DARPP-32 (dopamine and cAMP-regulated phosphoprotein of Mr 32 kDa), regulated by calcium and calcineurin, is important in dopaminergic signal transduction (98). Nitric oxide synthase is a substrate of calcineurin. This regulation may be important in the mechanism by which the immunophilin ligands mediate neuronal and cardiac toxicity (99–101) cAMP-dependent protein kinase A (PKA) and one isoform of phosphodiesterase are dephosphorylated by calcineurin (102). An adenylyl cyclase has been shown to contain an FKBP12-like domain and to be regulated by calcineurin (103). Calcineurin-inhibited adenylyl cyclase is important for learning and memory (104), and specific isoforms of adenylyl cyclase may also be important in that regard (105). It is now appreciated that PKA, protein kinase C (PKC), and calcineurin form a trimolecular complex in which the calcineurin-anchoring protein AKAP79 serves as the scaffolding protein (106). Binding of calcineurin to AKAP79 results in inhibition of phosphatase activity at a site distinct from that of the immunophilin-immunosuppressant binding site (107,108). Targeting protein kinases and phosphatases by coordinating their cellular location via scaffolding proteins provides another effective mechanism of substrate selectivity and target localization within the cell.

Candidate protein sensitivity to calcineurin action in vitro, followed by functional correlation of activity, is an approach that has now been supplanted by unbiased methodologies. Molecular biological techniques (e.g., cDNA microarrays) have been used to identify genes regulated by T-cell activation and sensitive to drug. The specific genes identified depend upon the approach, cell type, and culture conditions used, and the timing and sensitivity of the assays (109,110). DNA microarray analysis has been applied to models of cardiac hypertrophy, including one mediated by calcineurin. In that analysis, no single gene or gene array emerged to explain the phenotype (111). It appears unlikely that a single critical substrate of calcineurin, one that is both necessary and sufficient, will emerge to explain biological activity or toxicity.

V. CALCINEURIN INHIBITORS IN SOLID ORGAN TRANSPLANTATION

The utilization of CsA and tacrolimus has improved the success of both solid organ and stem cell transplantation over the last quarter century. Prior to the introduction of CsA to the clinical arena, glucocorticoids and azathioprine were the main agents available to physicians for the prevention and treatment of allograft rejection. While these agents were effective, they induced significant morbidity with both long-term and short-term administration. Furthermore, once steroid therapy had been initiated, it was often difficult to taper dose without reinducing rejection. Although equally efficacious in preventing and treating graft rejection, CsA also has a spectrum of undesirable side effects that often accompany its administration. The drug can be both nephrotoxic and neurotoxic, findings consistent with the ubiquitous expression of calcineurin. Other side effects which limit its usefulness for prolonged therapy include hirsutism, hyperglycemia, and hypertension. Furthermore, maintenance of an immunosuppressed state for an extended period of time increases the risk of infectious complications, some of which may be life-threatening. Nevertheless, the availability of CsA allowed physicians to use combination immunosuppressive therapy, thereby permitting administration of lower doses of steroids for shorter periods of time.

Because they share a common intracellular target, the toxicity profiles of CsA and tacrolimus are very similar (Table 1). Common side effects encountered with the administration of either agent include nephrotoxicity (insomnia, tremor, headache), gastrointestinal disturbances, hyperglycemia, hyperkalemia, and glucose intolerance (112). While hypertension is more commonly seen with CsA, headache and other neurological side effects are more often associated with administration of tacrolimus. Hirsutism and gingival

Table 1 Comparison of Toxicities Between CsA and Tacrolimus

	U.S. study (%)		European study (%)	
	Tacrolimus ($n = 250$)	CsA ($n = 250$)	Tacrolimus ($n = 262$)	CsA ($n = 261$)
Nervous system				
Headache	64	60	31	20
Tremor	56	46	44	30
Insomnia	64	68	29	21
Paresthesia	40	30	29	21
Gastrointestinal				
Diarrhea	72	47	32	23
Nausea	46	37	30	22
Constipation	24	27	19	20
LFT abnormalities	36	30	5	2
Anorexia	34	24	6	4
Vomiting	27	15	12	9
Hypertension	47	56	31	35
Urogenital				
Kidney function	40	27	33	18
Oliguria	18	15	16	8
Metabolic				
Hyperkalemia	45	26	10	7
Hypokalemia	29	34	11	14
Hyperglycemia	47	38	29	16
Hypomagnesemia	48	45	15	8
Hematological				
Anemia	47	38	4	1
Leukocytosis	32	26	8	7
Thrombocytopenia	24	20	10	14
Pain	63	57	19	14
Rash	24	19	8	3

hypertrophy are unique to CsA. In contrast, hair loss has been reported as a side effect of tacrolimus. Both medications have parenteral and oral formulations, and both are metabolized by the liver. Drugs that inhibit activity of cytochrome P450, such as ketoconazole and erythromycin, may cause an increase in drug levels and associated toxicity (see Table 2). The incidence of posttransplant lymphoproliferative disorders occurring during treatment with either drug appears to be similar at approximately 1.5% (113). Of note, young children treated with tacrolimus following liver transplantation were reported to have a higher incidence of EBV-associated lymphoproliferative disorder (114). Whether this was related to the increased immunosuppression of patients on tacrolimus is unclear (115).

A number of trials have been conducted that directly compared CsA and tacrolimus. The large phase III, randomized registration trials that resulted in approval for tacrolimus utilized dosages and levels of tacrolimus that are higher than those used today, and thus the comparative toxicities must be interpreted with caution (Table 1). Furthermore, the availability of microemulsion preconcentrate formulations of CsA (Neoral®) has changed the bioavailability and efficacy of the drug. Now that tacrolimus is approved for use, however, direct comparisons using optimal dosages, formulations, and drug regimens are unlikely to be performed.

Although initially isolated in 1984, tacrolimus was not approved by FDA for use in orthotopic liver transplantation until 1994 (116,117). Early trials investigating the efficacy of tacrolimus often administered the drug to patients who had failed conventional therapies for rejection. The first phase II trial to be reported compared the combination of tacrolimus and prednisone to a historical control group receiving a CsA-based regimen for prevention of hepatic allograft rejection (118). Patients receiving tacrolimus were more often rejection-free at one month following transplantation and experienced fewer episodes of steroid-refractory rejection. Patients receiving tacrolimus had less hypertension and fewer infectious complications overall, probably secondary to the much lower doses of corticosteroids required to control or prevent rejection. Two prospective, randomized trials comparing prophylaxis with tacrolimus to traditional CsA-based regimens have been published (116,117). More than 500 patients were enrolled in both trials, and similar conclusions were drawn from the two studies. In the United States, the U.S. Multicenter FK506 Liver Study Group randomized patients undergoing ABO-matched orthotopic liver transplantation to receive corticosteroids and either a CsA- or tacrolimus-based regimen as prophylaxis for graft rejection (116). Patients were monitored for clinical evidence of graft rejection. In addition, liver biopsies were performed routinely on days 7, 28, and 360 following transplantation or if there was clinical suspicion of rejection.

At the time of publication, the one-year overall survival of 88% was equivalent in the two arms. Tacrolimus prophylaxis was associated with an 82% rate of graft survival at one year versus 79% in those receiving CsA-based regimens. Two different dose schedules of tacrolimus were administered during the course of the study, but the toxicity was not stratified for dose. Despite this being the registration trial for tacrolimus, the target dose level was higher than generally used today. The higher blood concentrations may have contributed to the toxicity noted (Table 1). The European FK506 Multicenter Liver Study Group conducted a similar trial comparing the use of tacrolimus versus CsA for prevention of graft rejection in liver transplant recipients (117). As in the U.S. trial, dosing of tacrolimus was adjusted downwards during the course of the study. Furthermore, as in the U.S. trial, CsA-based regimens were not standardized. One-year overall survival rates were similar between the two arms, with 77% of those receiving CsA-based regimens and 82% of those receiving tacrolimus alive at one year. Those receiving CsA for prophylaxis had higher rates of both acute and chronic graft rejection and were refractory to treatment. In contrast, episodes of rejection in those receiving tacrolimus were controlled with lower doses of corticosteroids, and as a result, tacrolimus-treated patients demonstrated a lower incidence of infectious complications. The results of both trials suggest that while CsA- and tacrolimus-based regimens were equivalent in terms of graft survival and overall survival, the incidence of both acute rejection refractory to treatment with corticosteroids and of chronic rejection were lower in those patients receiving tacrolimus. Whether the somewhat greater toxicity associated with administration of tacrolimus would have been attenuated by lower doses of tacrolimus was not analyzed.

Registration trials have also been performed in renal transplantation. Four hundred and twelve patients were enrolled in a randomized, multicenter, nonblinded prospective trial in which either CsA or tacrolimus was given to patients that received antilymphocyte globulin, corticosteroids, and azathioprine. In this trial, as with the trial of hepatic transplantation, the rate of patient and graft survival was equivalent, and secondary endpoints could not be evaluated. Five-year follow-up of the phase II U.S. Multicenter Trial in kidney transplantation has been reported (119). Crossover to the alternate treatment arm was allowed under defined conditions and an intent-to-treat analysis performed. At 5 years patient and graft survival remained comparable, but treatment failure (defined by crossover) was lower in the tacrolimus arm. Fewer medications for the control of hyperlipidemia and hypertension were required in the tacrolimus arm. Long-term, tacrolimus-based therapy resulted in decreased graft failure (if crossover is defined as graft rejection) without an increase in adverse events or infection. Furthermore, overall costs and quality of life are improved in a tacrolimus-based regimen (120,121).

Many smaller, nonrandomized studies have confirmed the utility of tacrolimus in cardiac, lung, pancreatic, and small bowel transplantation. Tacrolimus demonstrates equal, if not greater, efficacy than traditionally CsA-based regimens for both the prevention and treatment of allograft rejection. Indeed, a recent prospective randomized trial directly compared Neoral® cyclosporine with tacrolimus-based therapy on the development of renal allograft nephropathy and fibrosis (122). Use of tacrolimus was associated with decreased chronic allograft nephropathy, decreased total cholesterol, and serum low-density lipoprotein. Furthermore, in cases of acute rejection, early conversion from CsA to tacrolimus is suggested to reduce the risk of recurrent renal rejection (123). In addition, there appear to be several advantages to administering tacrolimus rather than CsA for maintenance of immunosuppression. The ability to quickly taper corticosteroid therapy has reduced the incidence of infectious complications in this patient population. Hypertension and hyperlipidemia may be decreased in tacrolimus-based regimens. The commonly observed side effects of hirsutism and gingival hyperplasia associated with CsA administration do not occur with tacrolimus. These improvements in therapy may translate to improved quality of life for patients following transplantation. These and other factors appear to contribute to the acceptance of tacrolimus as a first-line therapy following allograft transplantation.

VI. CALCINEURIN INHIBITORS IN STEM CELL TRANSPLANTATION

Both murine and canine animal models demonstrated the efficacy of tacrolimus in the prevention of GVHD (124,125). Early phase II studies suggested comparable safety and efficacy of tacrolimus and cyclosporine in the prevention and treatment of GVHD in stem cell transplantation (126–128). An open-label, randomized, multicenter, phase III study compared tacrolimus with cyclosporine, each combined with methotrexate, for prophylaxis of GVHD in HLA-identical sibling related BMT in patients with hematological malignancies (129). The incidence of grades II–IV acute GVHD was significantly lower in patients receiving tacrolimus than among patients receiving CsA (31.9% vs. 44.4%; $p = 0.01$), although the proportions of patients with grade III–IV GVHD were similar. There was a higher proportion of patients with clinically extensive chronic GVHD in the CsA-treated arm. In patients with nonadvanced disease, tacrolimus-based therapy was superior in the prevention of grade II–IV acute GVHD and prevention of chronic GVHD; in this subgroup, disease-free and overall survival was similar. Overall, for all patients, the relapse rates were similar. Randomly assigned, the tacrolimus-treatment arm had a significantly higher proportion of patients with advanced disease, resulting in diminished 2-year and overall survival. The imbalance of underlying risk factors for death was addressed by a case-control study performed by the International Bone Marrow Transplant Registry (130). This study demonstrated that the use of tacrolimus was not associated with an adverse effect on relapse or survival. Furthermore, additional studies found no increase in regimen-related toxicity or mortality in patients treated with tacrolimus (128,131–133).

A second phase III trial comparing tacrolimus with CsA in the presence of methotrexate or steroids for prophylaxis of GVHD confirmed the superiority of tacrolimus (134). The incidence of grade II–IV acute GVHD was lower in the tacrolimus group than the cyclosporine group (17.5% vs. 48%; $p < 0.01$), particularly in the subset of patients who received grafts from HLA-matched siblings (13.3% vs. 41.3%; $p = 0.015$). The difference was also noted in patients who received transplants from donors other than HLA-matched siblings (21.4% vs. 53.8%; $p = 0.0029$). The incidence of chronic GVHD, the leukemia-relapse rate, and the estimate of overall survival were all similar.

Additional studies have demonstrated the safety and efficacy of tacrolimus in the prevention of GVHD in unrelated donor transplantation. Early phase II studies (128,135) were followed by a phase III, open-label, multicenter trial performed for prophylaxis of acute GVHD in recipients of marrow transplantation from unrelated donors (136). Combined with a short course of methotrexate, tacrolimus, compared to CsA, improved the incidence of acute GVHD (56% vs. 74%; $p = 0.0002$) and decreased the use of glucocorticoids for treatment of GVHD (65% vs. 81%; $p = 0.019$). There was no difference in toxicity or rates of infection, and the overall and relapse-free survival rates at 2 years were similar.

Several studies have shown the utility of tacrolimus in mismatched unrelated donor marrow transplantation (137), in unrelated donor umbilical cord blood transplantation (138), and in non-myeloablative transplantation for various indications, including high-risk hematological malignancies (139), indolent lymphoma (140), severe aplastic anemia (141), in sickle cell anemia and β-thalassemia (142), in renal cell carcinoma (143), and in patients with breast and renal cell carcinomas (144).

While tacrolimus has been shown to be effective in GVHD prophylaxis, the utility of tacrolimus has been difficult to demonstrate in the treatment of refractory acute GVHD (145). Chronic GVHD has been successfully treated with tacrolimus, particularly if therapy is initiated early in the course of disease (146,147). The availability of a topical formulation of tacrolimus, a drug approved for patients with moderate to severe atopic dermatitis, has been shown to be valuable in cutaneous chronic GVHD (148,149).

Therapeutic blood monitoring of tacrolimus levels is critically important, although dosing must be based on clinical assessment of tolerability and efficacy. The relative risk of toxicity is increased with higher trough concentrations. Early studies demonstrated an increased incidence of nephrotoxity when the whole blood trough tacrolimus level exceeded 20 ng/mL (129,150,151). Generally, the trough concentration is not recommended to be above 20 ng/mL, and concentrations of 10 ng/mL may be sufficient. In pediatric patients in whom tacrolimus clearance varies with age (152), in patients with changes in medications that affect the cytochrome P450 system (Table 2) (153,154), and in patients early after transplantation (155), frequent monitoring is mandatory. In addition, tacrolimus clearance may be prolonged in patients with hepatic dysfunction (156). Guidelines for tacrolimus in the prophylaxis of GVHD have been developed (157). The dependence on CYP3A genotype and a weak dependence on P-glycoprotein genotype, which influences gastrointestinal absorption, was noted in renal transplants (158). In stem cell transplant patients, interindividual variability in tacrolimus pharmacokinetics may be explained, at least in part, by genetic polymorphisms in the metabolizing enzymes cytochrome P450 (CYP) 3A4 and 3A5, but not by genetic differences in the multidrug efflux pump P-glycoprotein (159). Of note, these genotyping determinants did not predict CsA concentrations, despite the commonality of CYP enzymes used for metabolism of the calcineurin inhibitors.

VII. THE BIOLOGICAL EFFECTS OF SIROLIMUS

A macrocyclic lactose, sirolimus is structurally similar to tacrolimus and binds to the same family of immunophilins, the FKBPs. As with CsA and tacrolimus, binding of sirolimus to

Table 2 Drugs That Alter Concentrations of CsA, Tacrolimus, and Sirolimus

Increase levels	Decrease levels
Calcium channel blockers	Anticonvulsants
Diltiazem	Carbamazepine
Nicardepine	Phenobarbital
Verapamil	Phenytoin
Antifungal agents	Antibiotics
Clotrimazole	Rifabutin
Fluconazole	Rifampin
Itraconazole	
Ketoconazole	
Other drugs	
Bromocriptine	
Cimetidine	
Clarithromycin	
Cyclosporin	
Danazol	
Erythromycin	
Methylprednisolone	
Metoclopromide	
Sirolimus	
Tacrolimus	

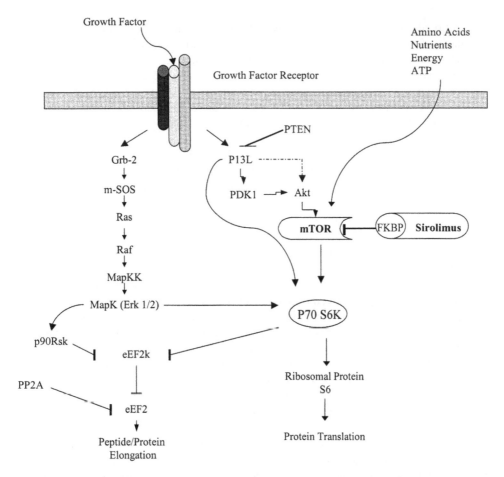

Figure 7 Molecular mechanism of sirolimus action. The mammalian target of rapamycin (mTOR) is the molecular target of the sirolimus-FKBP complex. The complex inhibits the kinase activity of mTOR, an enzyme that regulates the activity of p70 S6 kinase, involved in protein translation. In addition, mTOR regulates peptide/protein elongation factors eEF2 and others. mTOR is not only activated by growth factor stimulation but also regulated by amino acid and nutrient stores and by available ATP.

its intracellular receptor appears to be required for expression of its immunosuppressive effects. However, the target of sirolimus is not calcineurin, nor does sirolimus affect transcription of cytokine genes (66,68,70). Rather, it acts later in the cell cycle to interrupt growth factor mediated signaling pathways and prevent the $G_1 \rightarrow S$ phase transition (Fig. 7).

Response to stimulation by growth factors and other mitogenic stimuli (e.g., insulin) is inhibited in the presence of sirolimus. Ligation of many growth factor receptors results in rapid tyrosine phosphorylation of multiple substrates via protein tyrosine kinases (PTK) and the activation of mitogen-activated kinase (MAP) cascades. Phosphatidylinositol 3 kinase (P13K), PDK-1, and AKT-1 are all activated by growth factors. None of these events are affected by treatment with sirolimus. Phosphorylation of the 40S subunit of the S6 ribosome occurs later in growth factor signaling and promotes more efficient synthesis of proteins in cell cycle regulation. The S6 kinases, which catalyze 40S phosphorylation, have been divided into two distinct families, which differ in amino acid sequence and substrate specificity. While members of the p85-p90 S6 kinase family are not sensitive, the enzymatic activity of p70 S6 kinase family members is inhibited by sirolimus (160–164). Inhibition is not the result of direct interaction of drug with p70 S6 kinase (161,163). Rather, p70 S6 kinase is phosphorylated by another, upstream sirolimus-sensitive enzyme.

Sirolimus induces cell cycle arrest specifically in late G1 phase (165–168), and, therefore, a number of studies focused on cell cycle regulatory proteins as potential targets for drug action. The eukaryotic cell cycle is controlled by a series of regulatory cascades involving the cyclins and associated cyclin-dependent kinases (cdk) (169,170). In some cell systems, treatment with sirolimus inhibited the late rise in $p34^{cdc2}$ activity without affecting protein levels; inhibition was reversed in the presence of excess concentrations of tacrolimus (167). Other studies have shown decreased expression of cyclin A and, in nonhematopoietic cells, cyclin E in the presence of sirolimus during G1 phase (168). Sirolimus was shown to influence multiple proteins involved in regulation of the cell cycle, but no single protein controlled cell cycle progression, and the direct molecular target of the sirolimus/FKBP complex was not identified.

In *Saccharomyces cerevisiae* systems, two gene loci termed TOR1 (for target of rapamycin) (DRR1) and TOR2 (DRR2), were identified which, when mutated, conferred sirolimus resistance (171,172). Interestingly, the phenotypes of the two mutations differed. Genomic disruption of the TOR1 gene resulted only in a subtle growth defect (173), while mutation of the TOR2 gene was lethal, although it did not cause a cell cycle–specific arrest (174). Disruption of both TOR1 and TOR2 resulted in cell cycle arrest in G1 phase (173,174).

A number of independent groups identified a mammalian protein with homology to the yeast TOR proteins that appeared to bind selectively to the sirolimus/FKBP12 complex in vivo (175,176). The protein, referred to as mammalian (m)TOR (also termed RAFT1, FRAP, or RAPT1) is a 2549-amino-acid protein that bears significant homology to TOR1 and TOR2 (39 and 43%, respectively) (175,176). As in TOR1 and TOR2, the carboxy-terminal domain of mTOR contains a putative PI kinase domain, suggesting a role in intracellular signaling for this protein. Although mTOR is in many respects similar to the yeast proteins TOR1 and TOR2, it also contains unique sequences whose function are at present unknown. We now know that mTOR belongs to a family of phosphatidylinositol and serine/threonine protein-related kinases that regulate the cellular response to stress (e.g., nutrient deprivation, DNA damage, and cell cycle perturbations). mTOR itself is able to phosphorylate and regulate the activity of the ribosomal protein S6 kinase (S6K1) and to inhibit the eukaryotic initiation factor 4E–binding protein 1 (4E-BP1). Together these mTOR substrates control protein translational machinery in the cell (see Fig. 7). S6K1 and 4E-BP1 share a conserved TOR signaling (TOS) motif to which mTOR binds (177). mTOR itself is regulated by another adapter protein, raptor (178), and the mTOR/raptor protein complex functions as a nutrient sensor regulating cell growth (179). mTOR activity is controlled both by amino acid (nutrient) as well as energy (ATP) sources (180).

In certain tumor cells and cell lines, treatment with sirolimus leads to cell death by apoptosis. But only a subset of tumors and of cell types is sensitive to this effect of sirolimus (181). Recently, the mechanism for such sensitivity have been revealed. It correlates with prolonged hyperphosphorylation of JNK kinase only in cells that lack functional p53 (182). The class of tumors that lack p53 may be selectively sensitive to sirolimus and its analogues.

VIII. PHARMACOLOGY OF SIROLIMUS (RAPAMUNE)

Sirolimus is only available for oral administration. Sirolimus is rapidly absorbed (over an hour) in healthy subjects, and absorption increases if taken with a high-fat meal. The bioavailability of the tablet is higher than the oral suspension, but both are clinically equivalent. Nevertheless, dose adjustments may be needed. To minimize variability, the same formulation should be taken consistently with or without food.

Sirolimus is able to cross the cellular plasma membrane readily and is rapidly partitioned into formed blood cells. In the plasma, the drug is highly bound by plasma proteins. Sirolimus is a substrate for cytochrome P450 3A4 (CYP3A4), and, therefore, like CsA and tacrolimus, its administration may alter the bioavailability of other pharmaceutical agents (Table 3). In addition, it is a substrate of the multidrug efflux pump P-glycoprotein, the expression of which will affect gastrointestinal absorption and cellular levels. Sirolimus is extensively metabolized, but the metabolites are unlikely to be biologically active and cannot, at this time, be measured accurately (183). The vast majority (>90%) of sirolimus is excreted in feces.

FDA has approved sirolimus for prevention of organ rejection following renal transplantation, and it is recommended that it be given in combination with CsA and corticosteroids for this indication. Sirolimus therapy is initiated with a loading dose that is three times the maintenance dose, which, in adults, is 2 mg. A daily dose of 5 mg (and loading dose of 15 mg) of sirolimus was found to be safe and effective, but side effects were more frequent and there was no increase in efficacy. The dose is not often adjusted in adult populations, but patients <13 years old and <40 kg should be dose adjusted based on surface area to 1 mg/m^2/day with a loading dose of 3 mg/m^2/day. The dose is not changed for renal impairment. Whole blood trough concentrations of sirolimus are routinely measured only in pediatric patients, in patients with hepatic dysfunction, and in patients with concomitant administration of CYP3A4 or P-glycoprotein modifiers. Whole blood concentrations are most often measured by immunoassay but can be assessed by other methodologies such as high-pressure liquid chromatography (HPLC) or liquid chromatography/tandem mass spectroscopy (LC/MS/MS) (183,184). Because the results may differ depending on the method, the same laboratory should be used for repetitive comparisons to guide dose modifications (185).

Sirolimus is generally well tolerated, but certain side effects are common. Gastrointestinal side effects, including abdominal cramping, nausea, and constipation, can render the drug difficult to administer. In addition, hyperlipidemia and hypercholesterolemia are common, require monitoring, and may necessitate treatment. The long-term impact of sirolimus-associated dyslipidemias or cardiovascular events is unclear (186). Leukopenia and thrombocytopenia occur, and these potential adverse side effects led to initial concerns over use of sirolimus in stem cell transplant patients. A distinct advantage of sirolimus, however, is the lack of neurotoxicity, nephrotoxicity, and hypertension with continued use. The lack of overlapping toxicities enhanced the potential to combine sirolimus with the calcineurin inhibitors in novel immunosuppressive regimens in stem cell transplantation.

IX. SIROLIMUS IN STEM CELL TRANSPLANTATION

The use of sirolimus in clinical stem cell transplantation is limited (187,188). A single phase II trial has reported on the use of sirolimus in the prophylaxis of acute GVHD in alternative donor stem cell transplantation (189). In this study, 41 patients with hemato-logical malignances were treated with sirolimus added to a regimen of tacrolimus and low-dose methotrexate. Therapeutic blood levels were monitored and no significant toxi-city limited its use. The total rate of grades II–IV acute GVHD was 26%, which is signifi-cantly lower than historical controls for this high–risk population. Continued study was recommended. Importantly, the combination of sirolimus and tacrolimus was well toler-ated, despite the fact that both bind to FKBPs.

A single study utilizing sirolimus for the treatment of refractory acute GVHD has been reported. The toxicity and efficacy of sirolimus in the treatment of steroid-refractory acute GVHD showed some activity in this population (190). Of 18 patients who were able to receive six or more doses of sirolimus, 5 had complete and 7 had partial responses. Only 11 patients completed the intended 14-day course; toxicities included myelosuppression, thrombocytopenia, and dyslipidemias. Taken together, the utility of this agent seems to have not been adequately explored. Its use, in combination not only with calcineurin inhibitors but also with cell cycle inhibitors (e.g., mycophenolate mofetil, pentostatin, leflunomide), with tumor necrosis factor inhibitors (e.g., infliximab, etanercept), and with others requires further investigation.

X. SUMMARY

Studies of the mechanisms of action of CsA, tacrolimus, and sirolimus have furthered our understanding of T-cell signaling pathways. In order to exert their immunosuppressive effects, all three agents must bind to immunophilin receptors within the cell. Although not structurally similar, CsA and tacrolimus share a common molecular target, the ser-ine/threonine phosphatase calcineurin. Inhibition of calcineurin activity has been shown to correlate with decreased production of cytokines and chemokines and inhibition of T-cell proliferation. Sirolimus also inhibits T-cell proliferation, yet has no effect on cytokine production. Although tacrolimus and sirolimus are structurally similar and bind to the same intracellular receptors, sirolimus acts later in the cell cycle. mTOR is the molecular target of sirolimus. The TOR proteins function as phosphotidylinositol (PI) and serine/threonine kinases. These agents contributed to our scientific understanding of the mechanisms by which immune and other cells function.

The introduction of CsA into clinical transplantation in the early 1980s revolutio-nized the approach of solid organ and stem cell transplantation. Since that time, advances in surgical techniques and in the preservation of cadaveric organs have contributed to the improved outcome observed in solid organ transplantation. Similarly, improvements in supportive care, such as more effective antibiotics and improved manipulation of blood products, have decreased the morbidity associated with bone marrow transplantation.

Unfortunately, significant barriers still exist to the effective prevention and manage-ment of both graft rejection and, in the case of bone marrow transplantation, GVHD. CsA and tacrolimus have improved our ability to treat these conditions, and newer drugs are always being developed. However, their side effects are often prohibitive, leaving phys-icians with few options for maintenance of adequate immunosuppression in transplant recipients. As new agents become available, combination therapy using non–cross-reactive drugs may alleviate some of the associated toxicity while enhancing immunosuppressive efficacy.

REFERENCES

1. Amemiya H. 15-Deoxyspergualin. In: Kupiec-Weglinski JW, ed. New Immunosuppressive Modalities in Organ Transplantation. Austin, TX: R.G. Landes Company, 1994:75–91.
2. Nadler SG, et al. Interaction of the immunosuppressant deoxyspergualin with a member of the Hsp70 family of heat shock proteins. Science 1992; 258:484–486.
3. Nishikawa K, et al. Antitumor spectrum of deoxyspergualin and its lack of cross-resistance to other antitumor agents. J Antibiot (Tokyo) 1991; 44(10):1101–1109.
4. Nishikawa K, et al. The nature of in vivo cell-killing of deoxyspergualin, and its implication in combination with other antitumor agents. J Antibiot (Tokyo) 1991; 44(11):1237–1246.
5. Kawada M, et al. 15-Deoxyspergualin inhibits Akt kinase activation and phosphatidylcholine synthesis. J Biol Chem 2002; 277(31):27765–27771.
6. Lee JI, Burckart GJ. Nuclear factor kappa B: important transcription factor and therapeutic target. J Clin Pharmacol 1998; 38(11):981–993.
7. Karin M, Lin A. NF-kappa B at the crossroads of life and death. Nat Immunol 2002; 3(3):221–227.
8. Nemoto K, et al. Unique action of an immunosuppressive agent, deoxyspergualin, on hematopoiesis in mice. Exp Hematol 1997; 25(13):1339–1346.
9. Lebreton L, et al. Structure-immunosuppressive activity relationships of new analogues of 15-deoxyspergualin. 2. Structural modifications of the spermidine moiety. J Med Chem 1999; 42(23):4749–4763.
10. Ducoroy P, et al. LF 15-0195 immunosuppressive agent enhances activation-induced T-cell death by facilitating caspase-8 and caspase-10 activation at the DISC level. Blood 2003; 101(1):194–201.
11. Spencer DM, et al. Controlling signal transduction with synthetic ligands. Science 1993; 262:1019–1024.
12. Andolina M, et al. Etanercept in graft-versus-host disease. Bone Marrow Transplant 2000; 26(8):929.
13. Kobbe G, et al. Treatment of severe steroid refractory acute graft-versus-host disease with infliximab, a chimeric human/mouse antiTNFalpha antibody. Bone Marrow Transplant 2001; 28(1):47–49.
14. Chiang KY, et al. Recombinant human tumor necrosis factor receptor fusion protein as complementary treatment for chronic graft-versus-host disease. Transplantation 2002; 73(4):665–667.
15. Reimold AM. New indications for treatment of chronic inflammation by TNF-alpha blockade. Am J Med Sci 2003; 325(2):75–92.
16. Jacobsohn DA, Vogelsang GB. Novel pharmacotherapeutic approaches to prevention and treatment of GVHD. Drugs 2002; 62(6):879–889.
17. Salazar-Fontana LI, Bierer BE. T-lymphocyte coactivator molecules. Curr Opin Hematol 2001; 8(1):5–11.
18. Howland KC, et al. The roles of CD28 and CD40 ligand in T cell activation and tolerance. J Immunol 2000; 164(9):4465–4470.
19. Blazar BR, et al. Blockade of CD40 ligand-CD40 interaction impairs CD4+ T cell-mediated alloreactivity by inhibiting mature donor T cell expansion and function after bone marrow transplantation. J Immunol 1997; 158(1):29–39.
20. Blazar BR, et al. CD4(+) T cells tolerized ex vivo to host alloantigen by anti-CD40 ligand (CD40L:CD154) antibody lose their graft-versus-host disease lethality capacity but retain nominal antigen responses. J Clin Invest 1998; 102(3):473–482.

21. Taylor PA, et al. Analysis of the requirements for the induction of CD4+ T cell alloantigen hyporesponsiveness by ex vivo anti-CD40 ligand antibody. J Immunol 2000; 164(2):612–622.

22. Stuber E, von Freier A, Folsch UR. The effect of anti-gp39 treatment on the intestinal manifestations of acute murine graft-versus-host disease. Clin Immunol 1999; 90(3):334–339.

23. Quesenberry PJ, et al. Allogeneic chimerism with low-dose irradiation, antigen presensitization, and costimulator blockade in H-2 mismatched mice. Blood 2001; 97(2):557–564.

24. Williams JW, et al. Leflunomide. In: Kupiec-Weglinski JW, ed. New Immunosuppressive Modalities in Organ Transplantation. Austin, TX: R.G. Landes Company, 1994:65–73.

25. Carpenter PA, et al. A humanized non-FcR-binding anti-CD3 antibody, visilizumab, for treatment of steroid-refractory acute graft-versus-host disease. Blood 2002; 99(8):2712–2719.

26. Borel JF, et al. Biological effects of cyclosporin A: a new antilymphocytic agent. Agents Actions 1976; 6(4):468–475.

27. Borel JF. Pharmacology of cyclosporine (Sandimmune). IV. Pharmacological properties in vivo. Pharmacol Rev 1989; 41:260–272.

28. Kino T, et al. FK-506, a novel immunosuppressant isolated from a *Streptomyces* I. Fermentation, isolation, and physico-chemical and biological characteristics. J Antibiot 1987; 40(9): 1249–1255.

29. Kino T, et al. FK-506, a novel immunosuppressant isolated from a *Streptomyces* II. Immunosuppressive effect of FK-506 in vitro. J Antibiot (Tokyo) 1987; 40(9):1256–1265.

30. Vézina C, Kudelski A, Sehgal SN. Rapamycin (AY-22,989), a new antifungal antibiotic. I. Taxonomy of the producing streptomycete and isolation of the active principle. J Antibiot 1975; 28:721–726.

31. Sehgal SN, Baker H, Vezina C. Rapamycin (AY-22,989), a new antifungal antibiotic. II. Fermentatiion, isolation and characterization. J Antiobiot 1975; 28:727–732.

32. Fischer G, et al. Cyclophilin and peptidyl-prolyl cis-trans isomerase are probably identical proteins. Nature 1989; 337:476–478.

33. Siekierka JJ, et al. A cytosolic binding protein for the immunosuppressant FK506 has peptidyl-prolyl isomerase activity but is distinct from cyclophilin. Nature 1989; 341:755–757.

34. Harding MW, et al. A receptor for the immunosuppressant FK 506 is a cis-trans peptidyl-prolyl isomerase. Nature 1989; 341:758–760.

35. Walsh CT, Zydowsky LD, McKeon FD. Cyclosporin A, the cyclophilin class of peptidylprolyl isomerases, and blockade of T cell signal transduction. J Biol Chem 1992; 267(19):13115–13118.

36. Haendler B, Hofer-Warbinek R, Hofer E. Complementary DNA for human T-cell cyclophilin. EMBO J 1987; 6(4):947–950.

37. Price ER, et al. Human cyclophilin B: a second cyclophilin gene encodes a peptidyl-prolyl isomerase with a signal sequence. Proc Natl Acad Sci USA 1991; 88(5):1903–1907.

38. Hasel KW, et al. An endoplasmic reticulum-specific cyclophilin. Mol Cell Biol 1991; 11(7):3483–3491.

39. Arber S, Krause K-H, Caroni P. s-Cyclophilin is retained intracellularly via a unique COOH-terminal sequence and colocalizes with the calcium storage protein calreticulin. J Cell Biol 1992; 116(1):113–125.

40. Bram RJ, Crabtree GR. Calcium signalling in T cells stimulated by a cyclophilin B-binding protein. Nature 1994; 371:355–358.

41. Bram RJ, et al. Identification of the immunophilin capable of mediating inhibition of signal transduction by cyclosporin A and FK506: roles of calcineurin binding and cellular location. Mol Cell Biol 1993; 13(8):4760–4769.

42. Friedman J, Weissman I. Two cytoplasmic candidates for immunophilin action are revealed by affinity for a new cyclophilin: one in the presence and one the absence of CsA. Cell 1991; 66:799–806.

43. Bergsma DJ, et al. The cyclophilin multigene family of peptidyl-prolyl isomerases. J Biol Chem 1991; 266(34):23204–23214.

44. Kieffer LJ, et al. Cyclophilin-40, a protein with homology to the p59 component of the steroid receptor complex. J Biol Chem 1993; 268(17):12303–12310.

45. Anderson SK, et al. A cyclophilin-related protein involved in the function of natural killer cells. Proc Natl Acad Sci USA 1993; 90:542–546.

46. Marks AR. Ryanodine receptors, FKBP12, and heart failure. Front Biosci 2002; 7:d970–977.

47. Wehrens XH, et al. FKBP12.6 deficiency and defective calcium release channel (ryanodine receptor) function linked to exercise-induced sudden cardiac death. Cell 2003; 113(7):829–840.

48. Lehnart SE, et al. Immunophilins and coupled gating of ryanodine receptors. Curr Top Med Chem 2003; 3(12):1383–1391.

49. Nigam SK, et al. Localization of the FK506 binding protein, FKBP 13, to the lumen of the endoplasmic reticulum. Biochem J 1993; 294:511–515.

50. Jin YJ, Burakoff SJ. The 25-kDa FK506-binding protein is localized in the nucleus and associates with casein kinase II and nucleolin. Proc Natl Acad Sci USA 1993; 90:7769–7773.

51. Li TK, et al., Calcium- and FK506-independent interaction between the immunophilin FKBP51 and calcineurin. J Cell Biochem 2002; 84(3):460–471.

52. Pratt WB, Toft DO. Steroid receptor interactions with heat shock protein and immunophilin chaperones. Endocrine Rev 1997; 18(3):306–360.

53. Sykes K, Gething M-J, Sambrook J. Proline isomerases function during heat shock. Proc Natl Acad Sci USA 1993; 90:5853–5857.

54. Timerman AP, et al. Characterization of an exchange reaction between soluble FKBP12 and the FKBP-ryanodine receptor complex. J Biol Chem 1995; 270:2451–2459.

55. Cameron AM, et al. Calcineurin associated with the inositol 1,4,5-trisphosphate receptor-FKBP12 complex modulates Ca^{2+} flux. Cell 1995; 83:463–472.

56. Chen Y, Liu F, Massague J. Mechanism of TGFB receptor inhibition by FKBP12. EMBO J 1997; 16(13):3866–3876.

57. Yao D, Dore JJ Jr, Leof EB. FKBP12 is a negative regulator of transforming growth factor-beta receptor internalization. J Biol Chem 2000; 275(17):13149–13154.

58. Huse M, et al. The TGF beta receptor activation process: an inhibitor- to substrate-binding switch. Mol Cell 2001; 8(3):671–682.

59. Thali MB, A, et al. Functional association of cyclophilin A with HIV-1 virions. Nature 1994; 372:363–365.

60. Franke EK, Yuan HE, Luban J. Specific incorporation of cyclophilin A into HIV-1 virions. Nature 1994; 372(6504):359–362.

61. Liu J, et al. Calcineurin is a common target of cyclophilin- cyclosporin A and FKBP-FK506 complexes. Cell 1991; 66(4):807–815.

62. Fruman DA, et al. The complex of FK506-binding protein 12 and FK506 inhibits calcineurin phosphatase activity and IgE activation-induced cytokine transcripts, but not exocytosis, in mouse mast cells. J Immunol 1995; 154:1846–1851.

63. Fruman DA, et al. FK506 binding protein 12 mediates sensitivity to both FK506 and rapamycin in murine mast cells. Eur J Immunol 1995; 25:563–571.

64. Schreiber SL. Chemistry and biology of the immunophilins and their immunosuppressive ligands. Science 1991; 251:283–287.

65. Bierer BE, et al. Two distinct signal transmission pathways in T lymphocytes are inhibited by complexes formed between an immunophilin and either FK506 or rapamycin. Proc Natl Acad Sci USA 1990; 87:9231–9235.

66. Dumont FJ, et al. Distinct mechanisms of suppression of murine T cell activation by the related macrolides FK-506 and rapamycin. J Immunol 1990; 144(1):251–258.

67. Dumont FJ, et al. The immunosuppressive macrolides FK-506 and rapamycin act as reciprocal antagonists in murine T cells. J Immunol 1990; 144(4):1418–1424.

68. Bierer BE, et al. Probing immunosuppressant action with a nonnatural immunophilin ligand. Science 1990; 250:556–558.
69. Sigal NH, et al. Is cyclophilin involved in the immunosuppressive and nephrotoxic mechanism of action of cyclosporin A? J Exp Med 1991; 172:619–628.
70. Bierer BE, et al. Two distinct signal transmission pathways in T lymphocytes are inhibited by complexes formed between an immunophilin and either FK506 or rapamycin. Proc Natl Acad Sci USA 1990; 87:9231–9235.
71. Sigal NH, Dumont FJ. Cyclosporin A, FK-506, and rapamycin: pharmacological probes of lymphocyte signal transduction. Ann Rev Immunol 1992; 10:519–560.
72. Bierer BE, et al. FK506 and rapamycin: molecular probes of T-lymphocyte activation. Transplant Proc 1991; 23(6):2850–2855.
73. Schreiber SL, Crabtree GR. The mechanism of action of cyclosporin A and FK506. Immunol Today 1992; 13(4):136–142.
74. Fruman DA, Burakoff SJ, Bierer BE. Molecular actions of cyclosporin A, FK506, and rapamycin. In: Thomson AW, Starzl TE, eds. Immunosuppressive Drugs: Developments in Anti-Rejection Therapy. London: Edward Arnold, 1994:15–35.
75. Fruman DA, et al. Calcineurin phosphatase activity in T lymphocytes is inhibited by FK 506 and cyclosporin A. Proc Natl Acad Sci USA 1992; 89:3686–3690.
76. Fruman DA, et al. Correlation of calcineurin phosphatase activity and programmed cell death in T cell hybridomas. Eur J Immunol 1992; 22:2513–2517.
77. Dutz JP, et al. A role for calcineurin in degranulation of murine cytotoxic T lymphocytes. J Immunol 1993; 150(7):2591–2598.
78. Liu J, et al. Inhibition of T cell signalling by immunophilin-ligand complexes correlates with loss of calcineurin phosphatase activity. Biochemistry 1992; 31:3896–3901.
79. Aramburu J, Rao A, Klee CB. Calcineurin: from structure to function. Curr Top Cell Regul 2000; 36:237–295.
80. Klee CB, Ren H, Wang X. Regulation of the calmodulin-stimulated protein phosphatase, calcineurin. J Biol Chem 1998; 273(22):13367–13370.
81. Kincaid RL, et al. Cloning and characterization of molecular isoforms of the catalytic subunit of calcineurin using nonisotopic methods. J Biol Chem 1990; 265(19):11312–11319.
82. Hashimoto Y, Perrino BA, Soderling TR. Identification of an autoinhibitory domain in calcineurin. J Biol Chem 1990; 265(4):1924–1927.
83. Wang X, Culotta VC, Klee CB. Superoxide dismutase protects calcineurin from inactivation. Nature 1996; 383(6599):434–437.
84. Sommer D, et al. Differential susceptibilities of serine/threonine phosphatases to oxidative and nitrosative stress. Arch Biochem Biophys 2002; 404(2):271–278.
85. Clipstone NA, Crabtree GR. Identification of calcineurin as a key signalling enzyme in T-lymphocyte activation. Nature 1992; 357:695–697.
86. Nelson PA, et al. Immunosuppressive activity of (MeBm$_2$t)[1] -D-diaminobutyryl-8-, and D-diaminopropyl-8-cyclosporin analogues correlates with inhibition of calcineurin phosphatase activity. J Immunol 1993; 150(6):2139–2147.
87. Kissinger CR, et al. Crystal structures of human calcineurin and the human FKBP12-FK506-calcineurin complex. Nature 1995; 378(6557):641–644.
88. Griffith JP, et al. X-ray structure of calcineurin inhibited by the immunophilin-immunosuppressant FKBP12-FK506 complex. Cell 1995; 82(3):507–522.
89. Rao A. NFATp: a transcription factor required for the co-ordinate induction of several cytokine genes. Immunol Today 1994; 15(6):274–281.
90. Hogan PG, et al. Transcriptional regulation by calcium, calcineurin, and NFAT. Genes Dev 2003; 17(18):2205–2232.
91. Hoey T, et al. Isolation of two new members of the NF-AT gene family and functional characterization of the NF-AT proteins. Immunity 1995; 2(5):461–472.
92. Baeuerle PA, Henkel T. Function and activation of NF-κB in the immune system. Ann Rev Immunol 1994; 12:141–179.

93. Beg AA, Baldwin AS. The 1 κB proteins: multifunctional regulators of Rel/NF- κB transcription factors. Genes Dev 1993; 7:2064–2070.
94. Venkataraman L, Burakoff SJ, Sen R. FK506 inhibits antigen receptor-mediated induction of c-rel in B and T lymphoid cells. J Exp Med 1995; 181(3):1091–1099.
95. Frantz B, et al. Calcineurin acts in synergy with PMA to inactivate I kappa B/MAD3, an inhibitor of NF-kappa B. EMBO J 1994; 13(4):861–870.
96. Lilienbaum A, Israel A. From calcium to NF-kappa B signaling pathways in neurons. Mol Cell Biol 2003; 23(8):2680–2698.
97. Tian J, Karin M. Stimulation of Elk1 transcriptional activity by mitogen-activated protein kinases is negatively regulated by protein phosphatase 2B (calcineurin). J Biol Chem 1999; 274(21):15173–15180.
98. Nishi A, et al. Regulation of DARPP-32 dephosphorylation at PKA- and Cdk5-sites by NMDA and AMPA receptors: distinct roles of calcineurin and protein phosphatase-2A. J Neurochem 2002; 81(4):832–841.
99. Olyaei AJ, de Mattos AM, Bennett WM. Nephrotoxicity of immunosuppressive drugs: new insight and preventive strategies. Curr Opin Crit Care 2001; 7(6):384–389.
100. Fiedler B, et al. Inhibition of calcineurin-NFAT hypertrophy signaling by cGMP-dependent protein kinase type I in cardiac myocytes. Proc Natl Acad Sci USA 2002; 99(17):11363–11368.
101. Ritter O, et al. AT2 receptor activation regulates myocardial eNOS expression via the calcineurin-NF-AT pathway. FASEB J 2003; 17(2):283–285.
102. Cohen P, Cohen PTW. Protein phosphatases come of age. J Biol Chem 1989; 264:21435–21438.
103. Paterson JM, et al. Control of a novel adenylyl cyclase by calcineurin. Bioch Biophys Res Commun 1995; 214(3):1000–1008.
104. Antoni FA, et al. Ca^{2+}/calcineurin-inhibited adenylyl cyclase, highly abundant in forebrain regions, is important for learning and memory. J Neurosci 1998; 18(23):9650–9661.
105. Paterson JM, et al. Characterisation of human adenylyl cyclase IX reveals inhibition by Ca(2+)/calcineurin and differential mRNA polyadenylation. J Neurochem 2000; 75(4):1358–1367.
106. Coghlan VM, et al. Association of protein kinase A and protein phosphatase 2B with a common anchoring protein. Science 1995; 267:108–111.
107. Kashishian A, et al. AKAP79 inhibits calcineurin through a site distinct from the immunophilin-binding region. J Biol Chem 1998; 273(42):27412–27419.
108. Dell'Acqua ML, et al. Mapping the protein phosphatase-2B anchoring site on AKAP79. Binding and inhibition of phosphatase activity are mediated by residues 315-360. J Biol Chem 2002; 277(50):48796–48802.
109. Cristillo AD, Bierer BE. Identification of novel targets of immunosuppressive agents by cDNA-based microarray analysis. J Biol Chem 2002; 277(6):4465–4476.
110. Feske S, et al. Gene regulation mediated by calcium signals in T lymphocytes. Nat Immunol 2001; 2(4):316–324.
111. Aronow BJ, et al. Divergent transcriptional responses to independent genetic causes of cardiac hypertrophy. Physiol Genomics 2001; 6(1):19–28.
112. Tacrolimus (FK506) for organ transplants. Med Lett 1994; 36(931):82–83.
113. Reyes J, Tzakis A, Green M. Posttransplant lymphoproliferative disorders occurring under primary FK506 immunosuppression. Transplant Proc 1991; 23:3044–3046.
114. Cox KL, et al. An increased incidence of Epstein-Barr virus infection and lymphoproliferative disorder in young children on FK506 after liver transplantation. Transplantation 1995; 59(4):524–529.
115. Lake JR, et al. The impact of immunosuppressive regimens on the cost of liver transplantation—results from the U.S. FK506 multicenter trial. Transplantation 1995; 60(10):1089–1095.
116. Group TUSMFLS. A comparison of tacrolimus (FK506) and cyclosporine for immunosuppression in liver transplantation. N Engl J Med 1994; 331(17):1110–1115.

117. Group EFMLS. Randomised trial comparing tacrolimus (FK506) and cyclosporin in preven-
     tion of liver allograft rejection. Lancet 1994; 344:423–428.
118. Todo S, et al. One hundred ten consecutive primary orthotopic liver transplants under FK506
     in adults. Transplant Proc 1991; 23:1397–1402.
119. Vincenti F, et al. A long-term comparison of tacrolimus (FK506) and cyclosporine in kidney
     transplantation: evidence for improved allograft survival at five years. Transplantation 2002;
     73(5):775–782.
120. Neylan JF, et al. Assessment of the frequency and costs of posttransplantation hospitalizations
     in patients receiving tacrolimus versus cyclosporine. Am J Kidney Dis 1998; 32(5):770–777.
121. Shield CF III, McGrath MM, Goss TF. Assessment of health-related quality of life in
     kidney transplant patients receiving tacrolimus (FK506)-based versus cyclosporine-based
     immunosuppression. FK506 Kidney Transplant Study Group. Transplantation 1997;
     64(12):1738–1743.
122. Murphy GJ, et al. Randomized clinical trial of the effect of microemulsion cyclosporin and
     tacrolimus on renal allograft fibrosis. Br J Surg 2003; 90(6):680–686.
123. Briggs D, et al. Effects of immediate switch from cyclosporine microemulsion to tacrolimus
     at first acute rejection in renal allograft recipients. Transplantation 2003; 75(12):2058–2063.
124. Blazar BR, et al. FK506 inhibits graft-versus-host disease and bone marrow graft rejection in
     murine recipients of MHC disparate donor grafts by interfering with mature peripheral T cell
     expansion post-transplantation. J Immunol 1994; 153(4):1836–1846.
125. Yu C, et al. Tacrolimus (FK506) and methotrexate regimens to prevent graft-versus-host dis-
     ease after unrelated dog leukocyte antigen (DLA) nonidentical marrow transplantation. Bone
     Marrow Transplant 1996; 17(4):649–653.
126. Fay JW, et al. FK506 (Tacrolimus) monotherapy for prevention of graft-versus-host disease
     after histocompatible sibling allogenic bone marrow transplantation. Blood 1996;
     87(8):3514–3519.
127. Nash RA, et al. Tacrolimus (FK506) alone or in combination with methotrexate or methyl-
     prednisolone for the prevention of acute graft-versus-host disease after marrow transplan-
     tation from HLA-matched siblings: a single-center study. Blood 1995; 85(12):3746–3753.
128. Przepiorka D, et al. Tacrolimus and minidose methotrexate for prevention of acute graft-
     versus-host disease after matched unrelated donor marrow transplantation. Blood 1996;
     88(11):4383–4389.
129. Ratanatharathorn V, et al. Phase III study comparing methotrexate and tacrolimus (prograf,
     FK506) with methotrexate and cyclosporine for graft-versus-host disease prophylaxis after
     HLA-identical sibling bone marrow transplantation. Blood 1998; 92(7):2303–2314.
130. Horowitz MM, et al. Tacrolimus vs. cyclosporine immunosuppression: results in advanced-
     stage disease compared with historical controls treated exclusively with cyclosporine. Biol
     Blood Marrow Transplant 1999; 5(3):180–186.
131. Przepiorka D, et al. Allogeneic transplantation for advanced leukemia: improved short-term
     outcome with blood stem cell grafts and tacrolimus. Transplantation 1996; 62(12):1806–1810.
132. Uberti JP, et al. Tacrolimus and methotrexate for the prophylaxis of acute graft -versus-host
     disease in allogeneic bone marrow transplantation in patients with hematologic malignancies.
     Bone Marrow Transplant 1997; 19(12):1233–1238.
133. Devine SM, et al. The outcome of unrelated donor bone marrow transplantation in patients
     with hematologic malignancies using tacrolimus (FK506) and low dose methotrexate for
     graft-versus-host disease prophylaxis. Biol Blood Marrow Transplant 1997; 3(1):25–33.
134. Hiraoka A, et al. Phase III study comparing tacrolimus (FK506) with cyclosporine for graft-
     versus-host disease prophylaxis after allogeneic bone marrow transplantation. Bone Marrow
     Transplant 2001; 28(2):181–185.
135. Nash RA, et al. FK506 in combination with methotrexate for the prevention of graft-versus-
     host disease after marrow transplantation from matched unrelated donors. Blood 1996;
     88(9):3634–3641.

136. Nash RA, et al. Phase 3 study comparing methotrexate and tacrolimus with methotrexate and cyclosporine for prophylaxis of acute graft-versus-host disease after marrow transplantation from unrelated donors. Blood 2000; 96(6):2062–2068.

137. Przepiorka D, et al. Tacrolimus and minidose methotrexate for prevention of acute graft-versus-host disease after HLA-mismatched marrow or blood stem cell transplantation. Bone Marrow Transplant 1999; 24:763–768.

138. Przepiorka D, et al. Tacrolimus for prevention of graft-versus-host disease after mismatched unrelated donor cord blood transplantation. Bone Marrow Transplant 1999; 23:1291–1295.

139. Kobbe G, et al. Reliable engraftment, low toxicity, and durable remissions following allogeneic blood stem cell transplantation with minimal conditioning. Exp Hematol 2002; 30(11):1346–1353.

140. Khouri IF, et al. Nonablative allogeneic hematopoietic transplantation as adoptive immunotherapy for indolent lymphoma: low incidence of toxicity, acute graft-versus-host disease, and treatment-related mortality. Blood 2001; 98(13):3595–3599.

141. Murotani Y, et al. Non-myeloablative haematopoietic stem cell transplantation for severe aplastic anaemia with various complications. Clin Lab Haematol 2002; 24(5):303–306.

142. Iannone R, et al. Results of minimally toxic nonmyeloablative transplantation in patients with sickle cell anemia and beta-thalassemia. Biol Blood Marrow Transplant 2003; 9(8):519–528.

143. Rini BI, et al. Allogeneic stem-cell transplantation of renal cell cancer after nonmyeloablative chemotherapy: feasibility, engraftment, and clinical results. J Clin Oncol 2002; 20(8):2017–2024.

144. Ueno NT, et al. Rapid induction of complete donor chimerism by the use of a reduced-intensity conditioning regimen composed offiudarabine and melphalan in allogeneic stem cell transplantation for metastatic solid tumors. Blood 2003; 102(10):3829–3836.

145. Furlong T, et al. Clinical outcome after conversion to FK506 (tacrolimus) therapy for acute graft-versus-host disease resistant to cyclosporine or for cyclosporine-associated toxicities. Bone Marrow Transplant 2000; 26(9):985–991.

146. Carnevale-Schianca F, et al. Changing from cyclosporine to tacrolimus as salvage therapy for chronic graft-versus-host disease. Biol Blood Marrow Transplant 2000; 6(6):613–620.

147. Nagler A, Menachem Y, Ilan Y. Amelioration of steroid-resistant chronic graft-versus-host-mediated liver disease via tacrolimus treatment. J Hematother Stem Cell Res 2001; 10(3):411–417.

148. Choi CJ, Nghiem P. Tacrolimus ointment in the treatment of chronic cutaneous graft-vs-host disease: a case series of 18 patients. Arch Dermatol 2001; 137(9):1202–1206.

149. Elad S, et al. Topical tacrolimus—a novel treatment alternative for cutaneous chronic graft-versus-host disease. Transpl Int 2003; 16(9):665–670.

150. Wingard JR, et al. Relationship of tacrolimus (FK506) whole blood concentrations and efficacy and safety after HLA-identical sibling bone marrow transplantation. Biol Blood Marrow Transplant 1998; 4(3):157–163.

151. Przepiorka D, et al. Relationship of tacrolimus whole blood levels to efficacy and safety outcomes after unrelated donor marrow transplantation. Biol Blood Marrow Transplant 1999; 5(2):94–97.

152. Przepiorka D, et al. Tacrolimus clearance is age-dependent within the pediatric population. Bone Marrow Transplant 2000; 26(6):601–605.

153. Mignat, C. Clinically significant drug interactions with new immunosuppressive agents. Drug Saf 1997; 16(4):267–278.

154. van Gelder T. Drug interactions with tacrolimus. Drug Saf 2002; 25(10):707–712.

155. Woo M, et al. Toxicities of tacrolimus and cyclosporin A after allogeneic blood stem cell transplantation. Bone Marrow Transplant 1997; 20:1095–1098.

156. Jacobson P, et al. Factors affecting the pharmacokinetics of tacrolimus (FK506) in hematopoietic cell transplant (HCT) patients. Bone Marrow Transplant 2001; 28(8):753–758.

157. Przepiorka D, et al. Practical considerations in the use of tacrolimus for allogeneic marrow transplantation. Bone Marrow Transplant 1999; 24:1053–1056.

158. Macphee IA, et al. Tacrolimus pharmacogenetics: polymorphisms associated with expression of cytochrome p4503A5 and P-glycoprotein correlate with dose requirement. Transplantation 2002; 74(11):1486–1489.
159. Hesselink DA, et al. Genetic polymorphisms of the CYP3A4, CYP3A5, and MDR-1 genes and pharmacokinetics of the calcineurin inhibitors cyclosporine and tacrolimus. Clin Pharmacol Ther 2003; 74(3):245–254.
160. Calvo V, et al. Interleukin 2 stimulation of p70 S6 kinase activity is inhibited by the immunosuppressant rapamycin. Proc Natl Academy Sci USA 1992; 89:7571–7575.
161. Price DJ, et al. Rapamycin-induced inhibition of the 70 kilodalton S6 protein kinase. Science 1992; 257:973–976.
162. Kuo CJ, et al. Rapamycin selectively inhibits interleukin-2 activation of p70 S6 kinase. Nature 1992; 358:70–73.
163. Chung J, et al. Rapamycin-FKBP specifically blocks growth-dependent activation of and signaling by the 70 kd S6 protein kinases. Cell 1992; 69:1227–1236.
164. Terada N, et al. Failure of rapamycin to block proliferation once resting cells have entered the cell cycle despite inactivation of p70 S6 kinase. J Biol Chem 1993; 268(15):12062–12068.
165. Jayaraman T, et al. FK506 binding protein associated with the calcium release channel (ryanodine receptor). J Biol Chem 1992; 267(14):9474–9477.
166. Albers MW, et al. FKBP-rapamycin inhibits a cyclin-dependent kinase activity and a cyclin D1-cdk association in early G1 of an osteosarcoma cell line. J Biol Chem 1993; 266:22825–22829.
167. Morice WG, et al. Rapamycin-induced inhibition of p34^{cdc2} kinase activation is associated with G_1/S-phase growth arrest in T lymphocytes. J Biol Chem 1993; 268:3734–3738.
168. Morice WG, et al. Rapamycin inhibition of interleukin-2-dependent p33^{cdk2} and p34^{cdc2} kinase activation in T lymphocytes. J Biol Chem 1993; 268:22737–22745.
169. Norbury C, Nurse P. Animal cell cycles and their control. Ann Rev Biochem 1992; 61:441–470.
170. Sherr CJ. Mammalian G_1 cyclins. Cell 1993; 73:1059–1065.
171. Heitman J, Movva NR, Hall MN. Targets for cell cycle arrest by the immunosuppressant rapamycin in yeast. Science 1991; 253:905–909.
172. Cafferkey R, et al. Dominant missense mutations in a novel yeast protein related to mammalian phosphatidylinositol 3-kinase and VPS34 abrogate rapamycin cytotoxicity. Mol Cell Biol 1993; 13(10):6012–6023.
173. Helliwell SB, et al. TOR1 and TOR2 are structurally and functionally similar but not identical phosphatidylinositol kinase homologues in yeast. Mol Biol Cell 1994; 5:105–118.
174. Kunz J, et al. Target of rapamycin in yeast, TOR2, is an essential phosphatidylinositol kinase homolog required for G1 progression. Cell 1993; 73:585–596.
175. Brown EJ, et al. A mammalian protein targeted by G1-arresting rapamycin-receptor complex. Nature 1994; 369:756–758.
176. Sabatini DM, et al. RAFT1: a mammalian protein that binds to FKBP12 in a rapamycin-dependent fashion and is homologous to yeast TORs. Cell 1994; 78:35–43.
177. Nojima H, et al. The mammalian target of rapamycin (mTOR) partner, raptor, binds the mTOR substrates p70 S6 kinase and 4E-BP1 through their TOR signaling (TOS) motif. J Biol Chem 2003; 278(18):15461–15464.
178. Hara K, et al. Raptor, a binding partner of target of rapamycin (TOR), mediates TOR action. Cell 2002; 110(2):177–189.
179. Kim DH, et al. mTOR interacts with raptor to form a nutrient-sensitive complex that signals to the cell growth machinery. Cell 2002; 110(2):163–175.
180. Dennis PB, et al. Mammalian TOR: a homeostatic ATP sensor. Science 2001; 294(5544):1102–1105.
181. Huang S, Bjornsti MA, Houghton PJ. Rapamycins: mechanism of action and cellular resistance. Cancer Biol Ther 2003; 2(3):222–232.

182. Huang S, et al. Sustained activation of the JNK cascade and rapamycin-induced apoptosis are suppressed by p53/p21(Cip1). Mol Cell 2003; 11(6):1491–1501.
183. Gallant-Haidner HL, et al. Pharmacokinetics and metabolism of sirolimus. Ther Drug Monit 2000; 22(1):31–35.
184. Yatscoff RW, et al. Rapamycin: distribution, pharmacokinetics, and therapeutic range investigations. Ther Drug Monit 1995; 17(6):666–671.
185. Zimmerman JJ, Kahan BD. Pharmacokinetics of sirolimus in stable renal transplant patients after multiple oral dose administration. J Clin Pharmacol 1997; 37(5):405–415.
186. Chueh SC, Kahan BD. Dyslipidemia in renal transplant recipients treated with a sirolimus and cyclosporine-based immunosuppressive regimen: incidence, risk factors, progression, and prognosis. Transplantation 2003; 76(2):375–382.
187. Abo-Zena RA, Horwitz ME. Immunomodulation in stem-cell transplantation. Curr Opin Pharmacol 2002; 2(4):452–457.
188. Jacobsohn DA. Novel therapeutics for the treatment of graft-versus-host disease. Expert Opin Investig Drugs 2002; 11(9):1271–1280.
189. Antin JH, et al. Sirolimus, tacrolimus, and low-dose methotrexate for graft-versus-host disease prophylaxis in mismatched related donor or unrelated donor transplantation. Blood 2003; 102(5):1601–1605.
190. Benito AI, et al. Sirolimus (rapamycin) for the treatment of steroid-refractory acute graft-versus-host disease. Transplantation 2001; 72(12):1924–1929.

16

Prophylaxis and Treatment of Acute Graft-vs.-Host Disease

NELSON J. CHAO

Duke University, Durham, North Carolina, U.S.A.

ERNST HOLLER

University of Regensburg, Regensburg, Germany

H. JOACHIM DEEG

Fred Hutchinson Cancer Research Center and University of Washington, Seattle, Washington, U.S.A.

Graft-vs.-host disease (GVHD) remains one the major obstacles to successful allogeneic hematopoietic cell transplantation (HCT). GVHD is a major cause of morbidity and mortality even when recipient and donor are matched at the major histocompatibility complex (MHC) termed HLA in humans (1,2). In its acute and chronic forms, GVHD has an important impact on survival and the recipient's quality of life (3,4). The ability to prevent GVHD, i.e., the application of successful prophylaxis, is the cornerstone of success— treatment when prophylaxis fails is suboptimal. Previous chapters have dealt with the pathophysiology of GVHD, and based on insights from these important studies, investigators have attempted to develop effective preventive strategies.

I. PATHOPHYSIOLOGY-BASED PROPHYLAXIS

GVHD can be thought of as a process with an afferent and an efferent phase or as a continuous vicious cycle related to a "cytokine storm" triggered by the toxicity of the preparatory regimen with resultant tissue damage and endotoxemia (5). Steps along the way of this cascade present opportunities to block or attenuate the signals that lead to cytokine release, antigen presentation, T-cell activation, T-cell trafficking, recruitment and expansion of T cells, and other possible effector cells, including both pro-inflammatory and regulatory cells.

A. Step 1: Afferent Phase of Acute GVHD Before Infusion of the Graft

The stage for GVHD is set even before the donor cells are infused. The conditioning (or preparative) regimen plays an important role in the development of GVHD (6). Myeloablative regimens used to treat the patient's underlying disease and immunosuppress the host result in significant multiorgan damage, especially to the gastrointestinal mucosa. Damaged or activated cells from recipient tissues secrete many inflammatory cytokines, such as interleukin(IL)-1, tumor necrosis factor-alpha (TNFα), granulocyte-macrophage colony-stimulating factor (GM-CSF), and interferon-gamma (IFNγ) (6,7). Increased levels of these cytokines may lead to increased expression of adhesion molecules and MHC molecules leading to T-cell activation (6,8). A correlation between the intensity of the conditioning regimen and GVHD has been observed in animal models and in human recipients of stem cell transplantation (9–11). Furthermore, in some experimental and clinical studies, delaying the transfer of donor cells until well after conditioning results in a decreased risk of acute GVHD (12–14). Therefore, one method for decreasing the severity and possibly incidence of acute GVHD is to reduce the intensity of the conditioning regimen as is currently being investigated with the use of so-called non-myeloablative regimens.

More recently, cytokines, specifically TNFα and IL-1, have been implicated as the single most important components in the pathophysiology of acute GVHD in a murine model (15). In that model animals expressed MHC class I or II alloantigens on the antigen-presenting cells (APCs) but not on other tissues. The investigators demonstrated that acute GVHD developed in the usual target organs despite the absence of host MHC antigens. Moreover, neutralization of the two cytokines was sufficient to prevent GVHD. Two agents for neutralization of TNFα in humans are available: infliximab, a monoclonal antibody against TNF, and etanercept, a soluble TNF receptor. While these agents are being tested for their usefulness in the treatment of established acute GVHD, they have not been used for prophylaxis. Other available anticytokine molecules include dacluzimab, an anti–IL-2 monoclonal antibody, which has also been used for the treatment but not for prophylaxis of acute GVHD. Of note, an IL-1 receptor antagonist has been used for the prophylaxis of acute GVHD in allogeneic transplantation, but the use of this agent was not associated with a decrease in acute GVHD (16).

Another pretransplant component that may be important in the development of GVHD is the environment. Experimental data show that there is a reduction in the incidence of GVHD following HCT in gnotobiotic (pathogen-free) mice (17). Clinical studies also support this notion, suggesting that gut decontamination and isolation in laminar airflow rooms may decrease the incidence and severity of GVHD in selected allogeneic HCT patients (18,19).

Radiation and chemotherapy cause damage to the gut. That damage allows gut flora (i.e., bacteria) and endotoxins (lipopolysaccharide, LPS), well-known stimuli for TNF and other cytokines, to enter the circulation. Data supporting this explanation come from a trial that used monoclonal antibody against endotoxin and demonstrated protection of mice against GVHD (20). Increased serum TNF levels were found in patients who develop GVHD (21). Furthermore, the use of monoclonal antibodies against the TNFα receptors in patients with severe acute GVHD, refractory to conventional therapy, has resulted in a significant reduction in GVHD-related skin, liver, and intestinal lesions. However, GVHD recurred when therapy was discontinued (22). In another study, anti-TNFα antibody reduced the severity of skin GVHD lesions (23). Recent experimental data suggest that keratinocyte growth factor (KGF) may have a protective effect against GVHD while preserving a graft-vs.-leukemia (GVL) effect (24,25). The mechanism of action of KGF is thought to occur through the prevention of mucosal damage leading to prevention of bacterial and LPS translocation from gut to the circulation.

Another method of preventing GVHD via modification of the preparatory regimen is the inclusion of antithymocyte globulin (ATG). ATG is a polyclonal immunoglobulin prepared by injecting horses or rabbits with lymphocytes or thymocytes. Giving ATG is a form of in vivo T-cell depletion of the host and at the same time of the donor graft (since ATG is still present in the serum at the time of the infusion of the donor cells). ATG has been used as part of the preparatory regimen with the intent of decreasing the incidence of graft rejection and possibly preventing GVHD. Results have been varied (26,27). Recent data in unrelated donor transplants suggest that ATG is useful for the prevention of grades III–IV GVHD, however, this effect did not translate into lower treatment-related mortality because of an increase in the incidence of infections. Importantly, while survival was not different from that observed in patients not given ATG, the incidence of extensive chronic GVHD was markedly reduced and the quality of life improved in patients receiving ATG.

B. Step 2: Activation and Expansion of Donor T Cells

Most strategies of GVHD prophylaxis are aimed at the activation (induction)/expansion phase of donor T cells. This is a critical phase in the induction of the disease. Following the infusion of allogeneic cells, immunologically competent donor T cells, via their T-cell receptors (TCRs), recognize foreign antigens presented by APC in the context of the MHC. Although these events have been challenged recently in murine studies, it still represents the classical view of T-cell activation in GVHD. The APCs present the foreign antigens as peptides bound to their MHC molecules, thereby initiating the first step in the immune response. The peptides bound to the same MHC are derived from various proteins and serve as minor histocompatibility antigens (miH). It is these petide antigens in the context of MHC that serve as recognition targets of the donor T cells (28,29). Mismatches of miH antigens between donor and recipient in HLA-identical HCT may be associated with significant GVHD (30). Experimental model systems have targeted the interactions between the TCR and the MHC molecule as potential approaches to the prevention or treatment of GVHD. It has been shown that these interactions can be altered by the administration of a polymer that binds to the MHC molecule or a peptide modeled after the D1-CD4 domain (31,32), thereby suggesting new methods of interfering with the development of GVHD.

Donor T-cell activation requires multiple signaling events. TCR-peptide-MHC interactions provide the first signal (33,34). The second, a costimulatory signal, is provided by additional molecules on APCs and requires cell-to-cell contact (35,36). The outcome of the first signal is regulated by the second signal, resulting either in complete activation, partial activation, or anergy, i.e., a long-lasting state of antigen-specific unresponsiveness. Several costimulatory molecules have been identified, B7-1 (CD80) and B7-2 (CD86) being among the best characterized. CD28 and CTLA-4 are two T-cell surface receptors bound by B7 ligands. Normally, a signal from the TCR, a costimulatory signal from CD28, and an inhibitory signal from CTLA-4 determine the outcome of T-cell activation (37,38). In the absence of a CD28 costimulatory signal, signaling through the TCR complex results in events that lead to anergy. On the other hand, absence of CTLA-4 results in loss of the inhibitory signal, finally resulting in augmented and uncontrolled cytokine production and proliferation (37,38). CTLA4-Ig, a molecule created by fusion CTLA-4 with an immuno-globulin chain, blocks T-cell costimulation through the B7-CD28 signal pathway and, thus, induces a state of anergy (35,39,40). Therefore, one method for the prevention of GVHD would be the induction of a state of clonal anergy that is specific for the host allo-geneic antigens. In one clinical study of 12 patients who received one full haplotype-mismatched allogeneic HCT, incubation of donor cells with CTLA4-Ig was used to induce a state of anergy (41). All patients successfully engrafted, and only 3 patients developed GVHD. These results were encouraging and need to be confirmed with larger numbers of patients. Another molecule that may affect signaling through the CD28 molecule is siro-limus (rapamycin) (42,43). The mechanism of action of sirolimus is to inhibit specifically the progression of cells from G1 into the S phase, suggesting that it may interfere with the signaling that is critical for the cyclin-cdk complex required for cellular proliferation. Recent data using human peripheral blood T cells demonstrate that the block of G1 may be related to an increase in a species of titratable inhibitor of G1 cyclin-cdk (44,45). In addition to regulation of the cell cycle, sirolimus may also exert an effect in signal transduction pathways which mediates specific cytokine responses. For example, sirolimus has been shown to inhibit IL-1-driven IFNγ production (46). While the signal-ing through the TCR is not affected by sirolimus, the signaling through CD28 is inhibited by sirolimus (47). CD28 signaling leads to a sustained downregulation of the inhibitor I kappa B (IκB). CD28-mediated downregulation of IκBα is prevented by sirolimus. These data suggest that sirolimus affects the CD28 signaling pathway, which may be a sig-nificant mechanism of its action and distinct from other immunosuppressive drugs.

If a T cell engages its T-cell receptors and receives a costimulatory signal, T-cell activation ensues. Activation is a multistep process which involves calcium-dependent signal transduction pathways. Critical molecules in this pathway include calmodulin, cal-cineurin, and nuclear factor of activated T cells (NF-AT). The activation cascade follow-ing the first and second activation signals leads to calcium influx. The calcium binds to calmodulin, which in turn binds to calcineurin. The activated calcineurin triggers the dephosphorylation of the cytoplasmic unit of NF-AT. As a result, NF-AT translocates from the cytoplasm into the nucleus to form a competent transcriptional activator of the IL-2 gene. IL-2 is the critical survival and activation cytokine for T cells. T-cell activation via this pathway is prevented by cyclosporine or tacrolimus, which inhibit calcineurin.

Both of these calcineurin inhibitors are available as oral and intravenous prep-arations. They are currently the mainstay drugs for the prophylaxis of GVHD. Both drugs have been studied in phase III randomized trials, and both have been shown to be effective in the prevention of acute GVHD. Most commonly cyclosporine and tacrolimus are utilized in combination with methotrexate. The precise mechanism of action of meth-otrexate is not known; it acts as an anti-metabolite. Pharmacological prophylaxis of GVHD with methotrexate was adopted early in clinical studies after experimental evi-dence in dogs indicated that it decreased the incidence and severity of GVHD (1). Various combinations of methotrexate, cyclosporine, FK 506, and glucocorticoids have been widely used as GVHD prophylaxis. Pharmacological GVHD prophylaxis is generally administered in the immediate posttransplant period, gradually tapered off after 100 days, and stopped at 6–12 months after transplantation (if no GVHD is present).

The most widely utilized regimen is the combination of methotrexate and cyclosporine (48). Table 1 depicts standard two-drug regimen (cyclosporine/methotrexate) prophylaxis for acute GVHD. Dose adjustments are made according to the serum creatinine and bilirubin concentrations or on the basis of blood/plasma levels.

Immunosuppression with pharmacological agents such as cyclosporine or tacrolimus and methotrexate is more effective when drug combinations are used than it is with single agents (48–50). A survival advantage for those patients who received a combination of cyclosporine and methotrexate compared to either one of those drugs utilized alone has been demonstrated (51,52). Cyclosporine or tracrolimus are generally administered from day −2 or day −1. Both drugs are usually given intravenously for the first several weeks when patients are recovering from the side effects of the preparatory regimen; the oral mucosa and gastrointestinal tract are not healed yet so that oral cyclosporine or tacrolimus may be difficult to tolerate and may be erratically absorbed. While these drugs are administered to reach what are considered therapeutic target concentrations, studies to date have failed to show a clear correlation of blood drug levels and GVHD prevention. Nevertheless, the ability to deliver the target doses of cyclosporine is related to a better outcome with less GVHD. Since both cyclosporine and tacrolimus are nephrotoxic, other nephrotoxic drugs should be avoided, if possible, so that these calcineurin inhibitors can be delivered at the target doses.

Methotrexate is usually administered on days +1, +3, +6, and +11, and efforts should be made to administer the target doses. Urine alkalinization to a pH >7.0 with bicarbonate to aid in the excretion of methotrexate and hydration should be attempted to minimize methotrexate precipitation in the tubules, which can lead to acute renal failure. The dose of methotrexate is usually reduced in patients with hyperbilirubinemia or renal insufficiency (because of impaired clearance) and in patients with severe mucositis, which may be aggravated by methotraxate. Use of leucovorin rescue may be necessary in patients with severe side effects and in fact has been advocated as a standard measure by others, who have shown that such an approach does not increase the risk of GVHD (53).

A prospective study comparing a three-drug regimen [cyclosporine/methotrexate (three doses)/prednisone] to the standard two-drug regimen [cyclosporine/methotrexate (four doses)] was performed in order to investigate the potential benefit of prednisone used upfront for the prevention of acute and chronic GVHD. Results show that the addition of prednisone was associated with a somewhat lower incidence of early posttransplant

Table 1 A Commonly Used GVHD Prophylaxis Regimen

Cyclosporine			Methotrexate		
Day	Dose (mg/kg)	Route	Day	Dose (mg/m^2)	Route
−2 to +3	5	Iv qd over 20 h			
+4 to +14	3	Iv qd over 20 h			
+15 to +35	3.75	Iv qd over 20 h	+1	15	iv
+36 to +83	5	po bid	+3	10	iv
+84 to +97	4	po bid	+6	10	iv
+98 to +119	3	po bid	+11	10	iv
+120 to +180	2	po bid			
+181	Off				

464   Chao et al.

complications but did not have a positive impact on overall incidence of acute or chronic
GVHD, event-free or overall survival (54).

Several randomized studies have compared tacrolimus to cyclosporine (55–57) and
found tacrolimus to be superior for the prophylaxis of acute GVHD, but without a resulting
survival advantage. In a large multicenter trial, 329 recipients of HLA-identical marrow
transplants were randomized to receive a short course of methotrexate plus either tacrolimus or cyclosporine (55). Although a significantly greater proportion of patients with
advanced disease was randomized to tacrolimus, the incidence of grades II–IV acute
GVHD was significantly lower in patients who received tacrolimus (32% vs. 44% with
cyclosporine). This difference was largely due to a reduction in grade II disease. The incidence of chronic GVHD was similar in the two groups (56% and 49%, respectively),
but extensive chronic disease was more likely with cyclosporine. However, 2-year
survival was lower with tacrolimus (41% vs. 50% with cyclosporine), as was overall survival (47% vs. 57% with cyclosporine). These differences were mostly due to poorer
survival of patients with advanced disease (25% vs. 42% for tacrolimus and cyclosporine,
respectively).

In another clinical trial, 180 patients who underwent unrelated HLA-matched marrow transplantation were randomized for GVHD prophylaxis between tacrolimus and
cyclosporine combined with a short course of methotrexate (56). There was a significant
reduction in the severity of GVHD in patients who received tacrolimus plus methotrexate.
The incidence of grades II–IV GVHD was 56% in the tacrolimus arm versus 74% in the
cyclosporine arm ($p = 0.0002$). Moreover, the requirement for glucocorticoids for the
treatment of established GVHD was significantly lower with tacrolimus than with cyclosporine (65% vs. 81%, respectively; $p = 0.019$). However, there were no statistically significant differences in overall survival.

If patients are doing well and have no evidence of GVHD, cyclosporine or tacrolimus may be tapered at approximately day +90 and discontinued by the end of 6 months in
HLA-identical sibling transplants. In mismatched related or matched unrelated donor
transplants, the calcineurin inhibitors may need to be continued for much longer, sometimes even years. In addition, a slower taper may be preferable in older patients to prevent
the development of chronic GVHD, although this question requires further clarification. It
is important to follow patients carefully during the taper to recognize signs of incipient
chronic GVHD.

Another potentially useful drug during this phase of T-cell activation is mycophenolate mofetil (MMF). MMF is a morpholinoethyl ester of mycophenolic acid (MPA). MMF
inhibits the proliferation of T and B cells and the production of antibodies (58,59). Purines
are essential for the growth and survival of cells. T cells have two pathways to produce
purines: de novo and salvage pathways. Activated lymphocytes are highly dependent on
the de novo synthesis, while resting cells can utilize both. In the de novo pathway, the
ribose-phosphate portion of the purine nucleotide is derived from 5-phosphoribosyl-1-
pyrophosphate, which is derived from adenosine triphosphate and the sugar ribose-5-
phosphate. Therefore, 5-phosphoribosyl-1-pyrophosphate is an essential intermediary in
the synthesis of purines. Following T-cell stimulation, there is a brisk and sustained
increase in 5-phosphoribosyl-1-pyrophosphate, and guanosines and deoxyguanosines activate 5-phosphoribosyl-1-pyrophosphate synthetase (60). Therefore, depletion of guanosines would lead to a decrease in 5-phosphoribosyl-1-pyrophosphate synthetase and
inhibition of purine synthesis, which is required for T-cell activation. MPA action is
through the inhibition of inosine monophosphate dehydrogenase (IMPDH). This enzyme

catalyzes oxidation of inosine monophosphate to xanthine monophosphate. Xanthine monophosphate is a required intermediate metabolite in the synthesis of guanosine triphosphate. The enzyme IMPDH is a critical enzyme for the de novo biosynthesis of purine nucleotides, specifically guanosine monophosphate (GMP). Blockade of GMP synthesis leads to a negative feedback inhibition of 5-phosphoribosyl-1-pyrophosphate and prevention of T-cell activation. The therapeutic index of MMF depends on the lymphocytes reliance on de novo synthesis of purines, allowing for greater immunosuppressive activity with less toxicity.

Studies in a dog model of allogeneic transplantation by Storb et al. showed that the combination of MMF/cyclosporine was highly effective at the prevention of host-vs.-graft (rejection) and graft-vs.-host reactions following a nonmyeloablative (reduced intensity) conditioning regimen (61). Ongoing studies suggest that posttransplant immunosuppression with MMF is useful in establishing donor chimerism. Whether the incidence of GVHD is reduced by this approach is not certain.

C. Step 3: Effector Phase of Acute GVHD—Direct and Indirect Damage to Host Cells

Once T cells are activated and begin to proliferate, they and associated immune cells release a variety of pro-inflammatory cytokines. Cytokines are important in various steps of the graft-vs.-host reaction. As mentioned above, cytokines are important in the initial stimulation of T cells, but also in the maintenance of (stimulation) activation, the afferent phase, and the efferent phase, a period when toxicity (skin rash, diarrhea, and hyperbilirubinemia) is manifest (6).

There are at least two types of T-helper (TH) cells, TH1 and TH2, that play intricate roles in GVH reactions. This distinction is based on the cytokines, which these T cells generate, and the cytokines to which these T cells respond. TH1 cells produce IL-2 and IFNγ; in contrast, TH2 cells produce IL-4, IL-6, and IL-10. TH1 cells make and use IL-2 for their growth, TH2 cells produce IL-4 and require IL-1 or IL-4 for proliferation. A preponderance of TH1 cells could lead to activation of cytotoxic T lymphocytes (CTLs) and subsequent GVHD, compared to an abundance of TH2 cells, leading to a humoral response and prevention of GVHD (62,63). Therefore, if donor T cells are driven by IL-10 toward a TH2 phenotype prior to the transfer of these cells into the host, these cells have modified alloactivity and may not cause GVHD. Allogeneic T cells (CD4+) activated in the presence of IL-10 show a state of long-term anergy (64). Those observations have been confirmed by recent clinical studies (65). Although the donor T-cell dose in the transplant inoculum is higher in allogeneic peripheral blood precursor cells compared to unmobilized allogeneic marrow, this did not seem to result in an increased risk of acute GVHD. This protection from an increased risk of GVHD may be attributable to donor progenitor cell mobilization with G-CSF (or GM-CSF), which may polarize donor T cells towards IL-10–driven TH2-type cells (66). In addition, there is evidence that the function of CD14+ monocytes, which serve as antigen-presenting cells, is also altered. Although there is no significantly increased risk of acute GVHD with allogeneic PBSCT, there is a clear tendency toward increased chronic GVHD (67,68). The roles of TH1-type cytokines (such as IL-2 and IFNγ) are invoked in inducing GVHD and being deleterious, whereas TH2-type cytokines (i.e., IL-4 and IL-10) are considered as suppressive and protective of GVHD. That paradigm, however, may not be so clear-cut, and contradictory data also exist (69,70).

II. OTHER PROPHYLACTIC MEASURES

A. Immunoglobulin

Serum immunoglobulin (Ig) levels decrease significantly in the months after HCT. Serum IgA levels may remain low for up to 2 years (70,71). Initial studies of intravenous immunoglobulin (IVIG) following transplantation were performed with the goal of reducing the incidence and severity of cytomegalovirus infections. However, IVIG also seems to reduce the risk of acute GVHD. The potential benefit of this approach was illustrated in a randomized trial of 382 allogeneic bone marrow transplant recipients who were given IVIG (500 mg/kg weekly to day 90, then monthly to day 360) or no IVIG (72). Patients who were CMV+ and were given IVIG had a significantly lower incidence of interstitial pneumonia (13% vs. 22 %; $p = 0.02$), a lower risk of gram-negative septicemia (relative risk 0.38) and local infections, and among patients more than 20 years of age, a lower incidence of acute GVHD (34% vs. 51%; $p = 0.005$) than patients not given IVIG. Based on these findings, many groups utilize biweekly infusions of IVIG (500 mg/kg) until day 100 following allogeneic transplants.

B. Cellular Countermeasures: Regulatory Cells

As with most biological events, there are regulatory compensatory mechanisms in place to attenuate immune responses. Recent murine studies have identified subsets of T cells, which function in a regulatory capacity by suppressing the function of other T cells. It is believed that the physiological role of such regulatory T cells is to dampen immune responses against viruses, tumors, and self antigens (73,74). These regulatory T cells belong to the CD4+ subset and constitutively express CD25, the low-affinity IL-2–specific receptor (IL-2R), and CTLA-4 (CD4+CD25+). These regulatory T cells exhibit a partially activated phenotype but are hypo-responsive to activation and proliferation stimuli. Furthermore, they are antigen-specific in so far as their generation and activation to effector function (i.e., suppression of other T cells) require engagement of antigen and TCR signaling. However, their function does not appear to be antigen-specific. They appear to function in a locally restricted fashion, and they can inhibit both CD4 + and CD8+ T cells. The important role of CD4+CD25+ regulatory T cells in mice was shown in a model of GVHD where infusion of these cells led to the prevention of GVHD (75). Recently, researchers have identified a similar subset of regulatory T cells in humans. While clinical trials have not yet begun, there is considerable enthusiasm for cellular approaches to prevent acute GVHD.

Another cellular component that may prevent GVHD are natural killer (NK) cells. NK cells are innate immune lymphocytes critical to host defense against invading infectious pathogens and malignant transformation. NK cells act through elaboration of cytokines and cytolytic activity, which are regulated by specific receptors that recognize self antigens in the context of classical and nonclassical HLA class I molecules (76,77). Functionally, NK cells are an important source of innate immunoregulatory cytokines (e.g., IFNγ, TNFα, GM-CSF) that play an important role in immune responses. Recent murine experiments in stem cell transplantation across MHC barriers suggest that NK cells facilitate engraftment while at the same time preventing GVHD. In these murine experiments, pretransplant infusion of alloreactive NK cells into the recipient eliminated the need for high-intensity conditioning and reduced the incidence of GVHD. NK-cell alloreactivity could be exploited clinically to prevent GVHD. Recent studies by the Perugia group have demonstrated remarkable activity of these NK cells in recipients of haploidentical HCT. Patients with myeloid (but not lymphoid) leukemia had a marked difference in relapse if the donor NK cells could function in the recipient [mismatched killer inhibitory receptors (KIRs)], compared to those who where matched, and therefore the NK cells would not be activated (78).

III. TREATMENT OF ACUTE GVHD

Corticosteroids used for the treatment of established acute GVHD have remained first-line therapy (79). Corticosteroids are considered standard to the point that the term "steroid-refractory" has been used to describe patients requiring additional therapy. The broad effect of corticosteroids has been explained by cytotoxic or pro-apoptoic action on lymphocytes; however, there is clear evidence that anti-inflammatory activities resulting in suppression of cytokine production (80) or modulation of adhesion molecules also contribute significantly to the observed steroid effects in patients with GVHD.

A. First-Line Treatment with Corticosteroids

Despite the general acceptance of corticosteroids as first-line therapy, a broad spectrum of drug doses and schedules has been used (81). Doses between 1 and 20 mg/kg/day of methylprednisolone (MP) have been administered. In a randomized trial performed by an Italian group, 2 mg/kg vs. 10 mg/kg of MP were compared. There were minor advantages with regard to response rates for the high-dose regimen in young patients at the expense, however, of a higher rate of infections (82). Most widely used are initial doses of 2 mg/kg/day or 60 mg/m^{2}day. Corticosteroids are usually added to the prescribed prophylactic regimen consisting, for example, of cyclosporine or FK506 (tacrolimus) with or without methotrexate.

In general, acute GVHD of Glucksberg grade II is considered a clear indication for treatment, but again, the timing of treatment varies between centers and may differ for subgroups of patients. The same holds true for dose tapering after improvement of GVHD. A recent study (83) suggests that results with more rapid tapering are equivalent to those achieved with prolonged tapering in regard to flares of GVHD as well as long-term outcome. Whether differences in tapering or any distinct regimen translate into less severe long-term side effects of corticosteroid treatment (such as osteoporosis or osteonecrosis), however, is not clear and should be addressed in future trials. As the use of less intensive conditioning regimens allows an increasing number of older patients to be transplanted, consideration of long-term effects of corticosteroid treatment has become ever more important.

In large retrospective series (84,85) as well as in prospective trials, 25–35% of patients have shown complete resolution of GVHD, and an additional 15% have experienced improvement. A recent update shows these response rates to be independent of the initial grading system used (86).

In an attempt at improving these results, several agents with potential therapeutic efficacy have been added to corticosteroids in first-line treatment regimens. These include ricin A–conjugated anti-CD5 monoclonal antibodies (MAB) (87) or anti-CD25 MAB (88). However, those two trials failed to show clear superiority of long-term results in spite of somewhat higher initial response rates. In an attempt to accelerate the anti-inflammatory response, we have added a murine MAB-neutralizing TNFα (MAK195F) (80) to corticosteroid regimens in 32 patients. The response rate was 70%, but as with other trials, long-term survival was not significantly improved over that observed with corticosteroids alone. Other agents such as etanercept are now being investigated at several institutions. Some recent pilot trials suggest that the addition of polyclonal anti-thymocyte globulins might improve not only GVHD responses but also outcome. However, randomized studies (89) failed to show superiority.

These disappointing results with attempts aimed at improving results of first-line treatment of GVHD might reflect the clinical heterogeneity of patients with regard to prognosis and subsequent severity of GVHD. Early predictive parameters allowing for identification of high versus standard risk GVHD might help to custom tailor first-line immunosuppressive therapy of GVHD. Broadly used surrogate parameters would be most useful. The Genova group recently suggested to use ATG preemptively in patients with elevated bilirubin and blood urea levels at day +7 (90). Transplant-related mortality was reduced by this approach as compared to historical controls, and a prospective trial has been initated.

Another yet unresolved issue is whether GVHD manifestations should be treated in a more organ-specific manner. Data from animal models show that different effector molecules are involved in skin vs. gut vs. liver GVHD with a prominent role of TNFα in skin and gut GVHD and FAS/FAS-ligand in liver GVHD (91,92). Higher response rates of skin and gut GVHD as compared to liver GVHD with anti-TNF treatment might fit with this hypothesis. However, recent data from intestinal biopsies in patients with gastrointestinal symptoms suggest that both TNFα and FAS/FAS-ligand are relevant in human gut GVHD (93).

Improvement of results of first line treatment must be a priority, as the response to corticosteroids predicted long term results in almost all trials reported: 50-60% of patients achieving stable responses to first line treatment of GVHD survived, whereas long term survival was only 5–30% in patients with steroid-resistant GVHD.

B. Treatment of Steroid-Resistant GVHD

Clinically, two types of failure of corticosteroid treament of acute GVHD can be distinguished: true steroid resistance, i.e., progression of GVHD symptoms and manifestations while patients are receiving full dose corticosteroid treatment, and steroid dependence, i.e., reoccurrence (or flare) of GVHD during or after tapering of steroid treatment. In general, the prognosis with true steroid-resistant GVHD is worse than the prognosis of steroid-dependent patients. A comparison of trials dealing with steroid-resistant GVHD is hampered by variable inclusion of both patient groups in many of these trials.

A variety of agents has been tested, including chemical immunosuppressants such as MMF, broad (ATG, anti-CD3) anti–T-cell antibodies, as well as more specific agents directed against activation or adhesion molecules (anti-CD25, anti-CD147) or cytokines.

C. Chemical Immunosuppressants

A switch from cyclosporine to FK506 has been suggested by some authors for patients who fail to respond to cyclosporine. In a careful analysis from Seattle, only 2 of 20 patients with resistant GVHD responded to this approach (94). Also, substituting FK506 for cyclosporine did not improve manifestations of microangiopathic hemolytic anemia. Improvement was seen, however, in patients with cyclosporine-associated neurotoxicity. Based on promising results in the prophylaxis of GVHD, MMF has also been used for treatment of steroid-resistant GVHD. Response rates of 60–70% have been reported (95), albeit at the expense of a high rate of infectious complications. Similar response rates have been observed with the use of pentostatin (96), but long-term results are not yet available. Rapamycin (sirolimus) is another promising immunosuppressant with broad effects against cytokine responses and synergistic action with FK506 or cyclosporine. Treatment of steroid-resistant acute GVHD in a pilot study was associated with thrombocytopenia and leukopenia, requiring early discontinuation of treatment in several patients (97). However, favorable (including complete) responses were observed in evaluable patients. Further work is required to determine optimum dosing regimens. In another pilot study, interactions of cyclosporine, sirolimus, and azole antifungals were associated with a high rate of microangiopathic hemolytic anemia (Holler, E et al., unpublished).

D. Anti–T-Cell Antibodies with Broad Specificity

Both rabbit and horse ATG have been used for the treatment of steroid-resistant GVHD., but a survey (98) shows a lack of standardized approaches. In more recent trials, complete and partial response rates in the range of 30–70% have been reported (99–102). Severe infectious complications occurred in 80–90% of patients, and in general long-term survival ranged from 5% to 32%. Best results were obtained with early institution of treatment (103,104).

The broad anti-CD3 monoclonal antibody (MAB) OKT3 is active in acute GVHD (105). However, administration is associated with clinical toxicity due to early cytokine release, and there is a significant incidence of late infectious complications. More promising results have been reported with the use of visilizumab, a mutated humanized nonactivating anti-CD3 antibody that induces T-cell apoptosis. Among 6 patients given seven doses (0.25–1.0 mg/m^2) in a dose-escalation regimen, one had a complete and five had partial responses, but all patients died at a median of 87 days. Among 11 patients given a single dose of 3 mg/m^2, 9 were evaluable at day 42, and 6 of these had complete and 3 partial responses. At the time of reporting, 7 patients were alive at 260–490 days. While 2 of the first 7 patients developed a posttransplant lymphoproliferative disorder, none developed in the next 10 patients in whom rituximab was given prophylactically when EBV DNA titers rose (106).

E. Antibodies That Block Activation Molecules or Cytokines

Greater specificity and fewer side effects are expected with antibodies that target activation molecules. While murine MAB against the IL-2 receptor failed to induce sustained long-term responses, daclizumab, a humanized antiCD25 MAB, has been used with considerable success (response rates 50–70%, long-term survival 30–52%) (107,108). Data on infectious complications are contradictory, with a low rate in one and a rate of 80% in another trial. A novel activation-associated antigen not only on T, but also on B and NK cells, is targeted by the anti-CD147 MAB ABX-CBL. A response rate of 51% and a probability of 6-month survival of 44% have been reported (109). Myalgias but not infections were the dose-limiting toxicites. A randomized study comparing anti-CD147 MAB and equine ATG in patients with steroid-refractory GVHD has recently been completed. Results are pending.

Inflammatory cytokines are involved in almost all phases of GVHD, and numerous approaches using cytokine antagonists for the treatment of GVHD have been reported. Treatment with murine MABs that block TNFα (BC7, Mak195F) (22,110) and with

IL-1-receptor antagonist (111) resulted in rapid responses especially in patients with skin and gut GVHD (65–80% CR and PR). However, because of recurrent GVHD after cessation of treatment, initial responses did not translate into superior long-term outcome. Various combinations of TNF-blocking agents and murine anti–T-cell MABs were subsequently tested, but studies were not further pursued as humanized molecules such as MAB infliximab and the TNF receptor antagonist etanercept became available. Infliximab has been approved for the treatment of inflammatory bowel disease, and indeed, application of this MAB in patients with skin and especially gut GVHD gave very encouraging results (112,113). Due to its specific mechanism of action, infliximab not only blocks TNF but also eliminates TNF-positive cells (via ADCC and induction of monocyte apoptosis). Such a mechanism might explain the superior activity but might also be responsible for a high incidence of fungal infections (especially aspergillosis). Etanercept is a true TNF-blocking agent, and case reports on the treatment of acute and chronic GVHD suggest an activity comparable to infliximab (114,115). Etanercept might also be useful to prevent GVHD-associated pulmonary complications, as suggested by a recent report from Ann Arbor (116). Both infliximab and etanercept are presently being tested for efficacy as first-line treatment of GVHD.

F. Photopheresis

Since the first reports on successful treatment of chronic GVHD by extracorporal photopheresis (ECP), several immunological effects of ECP have been characterized (117–119). There is a modulation of antigen-processing cells and a shift from dendritic cell (DC)1 to DC2 resulting in diminshed alloresponses. In a recent meta-analysis of several trials, a response rate of 60–70% was reported (120). Of note, reponse rates were high not only in skin but also in liver disease. Moreover, 50–55% of patients receiving ECP became long-term survivors, a proportion that is superior to results observed with many other modalities (121,122). However, many trials enrolled primarily patients with skin GVHD. Further, patients with severe marrow suppression associated with early and severe GVHD were not given ECP. Thus, the high rate of success with ECP may in part be due to a bias in patient selection. Randomized trials and trials using ECP as first-line treatment are needed. In patients with isolated skin GVHD, administration of a psoralen preparation and direct exposure to UVA (PUVA) is often effective in inducing responses in some patients (123).

G. Other Supportive Approaches

Infections are the main cause of death in patients with steroid-refractory acute GVHD, and careful surveillance and control of infections is mandatory in patients with acute GVHD. Fungal infections, especially aspergillosis, are the leading complication. Prophylaxis and early aggressive treatment should be facilitated by the introduction of new agents such as voriconazole or echinocandins, which broaden therapeutic efficacy with acceptable toxicity.

A variety of further supplementary approaches have been suggested: massive diarrhea might be controlled by the use of octreotide (124). Substitution of factor XIII had a positive impact on gastrointestinal bleeding in one series in 21 of 23 patients (125). Milder intestinal GVHD might be controlled by addition of oral beclomethasone (or budesonide), as suggested by a randomized trial from Seattle (126,127). In skin GVHD, FAS-mediated apoptosis of keratinocytes is a major factor resulting in epidermolysis. Based on experience in patients with toxic epidermal necrolysis, treatment of this condition with high-dose immunoglobulins has been suggested (128).

H. Perspective

Although the repertoire of drugs to treat GVHD is steadily increasing, true progress, especially in the treatment of steroid-refractory GVHD, has been limited. New drugs such as deoxyspergulain, anti-CD52 antibody, or agents blocking CD40:CD40L pathways and TH1 responses will further broaden the available repertoire. However, qualitatively new approaches such as risk-adapted first-line treatment or preemptive therapy may be more likely to improve results; both require a better definition of predictive parameters. Endothelial cells have only recently been identified as important targets of GVHD (129), and agents modulating endothelial activation have not been tested so far. Finally, the increasingly recognized role of regulatory T cells such as CD4 + CD25 + T cells (130) or T-regulatory type 1 cells (131) suggests that strategies aiming at modulation of subpopulations or even cellular therapy using regulatory cells may be useful in the management of GVHD.

REFERENCES

1. Ferrara JLM, Deeg HJ. Graft-vs.-host disease (review). N Engl J Med 1991; 324:667–674.
2. Chao NJ, Schmidt GM, Niland JC, Amylon MD, Dagis AC, Long GD, Nademanee AP, Negrin RS, O'Donnell MR, Parker PM, Smith EP, Snyder DS, Stein AS, Wong RM, Blume KG, Forman SJ. Cyclosporine, methotrexate, and prednisone compared with cyclosporine and prednisone for prophylaxis of acute graft-vs.-host disease. N Engl J Med 1993; 329:1225–1230.
3. Socie G, Stone JV, Wingard JR, Weisdorf D, Henslee-Downey PJ, Bredeson C, Cahn JY, Passweg JR, Rowlings PA, Schouten HC, Kolb HJ, Klein JP. Long-term survival and late deaths after allogeneic bone marrow transplantation. Late Effects Working Committee of the International Bone Marrow Transplant Registry. N Engl J Med 1999; 341:14–21.
4. Sullivan KM. Graft-vs.-host-disease. In: Thomas ED, Blume KG, Forman SJ, eds: Hematopoietic Cell Transplantation, 2nd ed. Boston: Blackwell Science, 1999; p. 515–536.
5. Antin JH, Ferrara JLM. Cytokine dysregulation and acute graft-vs.-host disease. Blood 1992; 80:2964–2968.
6. Ferrara JL, Levy R, Chao NJ. Pathophysiologic mechanisms of acute graft-vs.-host disease (review). Biol Blood Marrow Transplant 1999; 5:347–356.
7. Xun CQ, Thompson JS, Jennings CD, Brown SA, Widmer MB. Effect of total body irradiation, busulfan-cyclophosphamide, or cyclophosphamide conditioning on inflammatory cytokine release and development of acute and chronic graft-vs.-host disease in H-2-incompatible transplanted SCID mice. Blood 1994; 83:2360–2367.
8. Hill GR, Krenger W, Ferrara JL. The role of cytokines in acute graft-vs.-host disease. (review). Cytokines Cell Mol Ther 1997; 3:257–266.
9. Clift RA, Buckner CD, Appelbaum FR, Bearman SI, Petersen FB, Fisher LD, Anasetti C, Beatty P, Bensinger WI, Doney K, Hill R, McDonald G, Martin P, Sanders J, Singer J, Stewart P, Sullivan KM, Witherspoon R, Storb R, Hansen J, Thomas ED. Allogeneic marrow transplantation in patients with acute myeloid leukemia in first remission: a randomized trial of two irradiation regimens. Blood 1990; 76:1867–1871.
10. Gale RP, Bortin MM, van Bekkum DW, Biggs JC, Dicke KA, Gluckman E, Good RA, Hoffmann RG, Kay HEM, Kersey JH, Marmont A, Masaoka T, Rimm AA, van Rood JJ, Zwaan FE. Risk factors for acute graft-vs.-host disease. Br J Haematol 1987; 67:397–406.

11. Hill GR, Crawford JM, Cooke KR, Brinson YS, Pan L, Ferrara JL. Total body irradiation and acute graft-vs.-host disease: the role of gastrointestinal damage and inflammatory cytokines. Blood 1997; 90:3204–3213.

12. Johnson BD, Truitt RL. Delayed infusion of immunocompetent donor cells after bone marrow transplantation breaks graft-host tolerance allows for persistent antileukemic reactivity without severe graft-vs.-host disease. Blood 1995; 85:3302–3312.

13. Xun CQ, Tsuchida M, Thompson JS. Delaying transplantation after total body irradiation is a simple and effective way to reduce acute graft-vs.-host disease mortality after major H2 incompatible transplantation. Transplantation 1997; 64:297–302.

14. Barrett AJ, Mavroudis D, Tisdale J, Molldrem J, Clave E, Dunbar C, Cottler-Fox M, Phang S, Carter C, Okunnieff P, Young NS, Read EJ. T cell-depleted bone marrow transplantation and delayed T cell add-back to control acute GVHD and conserve a graft-vs.-leukemia effect. Bone Marrow Transplant 1998; 21:543–551.

15. Teshima T, Ordemann R, Reddy P, Gagin S, Liu C, Cooke KR, Ferrara JL. Acute graft-vs.-host disease does not require alloantigen expression on host epithelium. Nat Med 2002; 8:575–581.

16. Antin JH, Weisdorf D, Neuberg D, Bressler S, Nicklow R, Lee SJ, Alyea E, McGarigle C, Soiffer R, Ferrara J. Interleukin-1 blockade does not prevent acute graft-vs.-host disease (GVHD). Results of a randomized, double blind, placebo-controlled trial of interleukin 1 receptor antagonist (IL-1RA) (abstr). Blood 1999. 94 (suppl 1):152a.

17. van Bekkum DW, Roodenburg J, van der Waaij D. Mitigation of secondary disease of allogeneic mouse radiation chimeras by modification of the intestinal microflora. J Natl Cancer Inst 1974; 52:401–404.

18. Storb R, Prentice RL, Buckner CD, Clift RA, Appelbaum F, Deeg J, Doney K, Hansen JA, Mason M, Sanders JE, Singer J, Sullivan KM, Witherspoon RP, Thomas ED. Graft-vs.-host disease and survival in patients with aplastic anemia treated by marrow grafts from HLA-identical siblings. Beneficial effect of a protective environment. N Engl J Med 1983; 308:302–307.

19. Beelen DW, Elmaagacli A, Muller KD, Hirche H, Schaefer UW. Influence of intestinal bacterial decontamination using metronidazole and ciprofloxacin or ciprofloxacin alone on the development of acute graft-vs.-host disease after marrow transplantation in patients with hematologic malignancies: final results and long-term follow-up of an open-label prospective randomized trial. Blood 1999; 93:3267–3275.

20. Shalaby MR, Fendly B, Sheehan KC, Schreiber RD, Ammann AJ. Prevention of the graft-vs.-host reaction in newborn mice by antibodies to tumor necrosis factor-alpha. Transplantation 1989; 47:1057–1061.

21. Holler E, Kolb HJ, Möller A, Kempeni J, Liesenfeld S, Pechumer H, Lehmacher W, Ruckdeschel G, Gleixner B, Riedner C, Ledderose G, Grehm G, Mittermüller J, Wilmanns W. Increased serum levels of tumor necrosis factor α precede major complications of bone marrow transplantation. Blood 1990; 75:1011–1016.

22. Hervé P, Flesch M, Tiberghien J, Wijdenes J, Racadot E, Bordigoni P, Plouvier E, Stephan JL, Bourdeau H, Holler E, Lioure B, Roche C, Vilmer E, Demcocq F, Kuentz M, Cahn JY. Phase I-II trial of a monoclonal anti-tumor necrosis factor α antibody for the treatment of refractory severe acute graft-vs.-host disease. Blood 1992; 79:3362–3368.

23. Piguet P.-F, Grau GE, Allet B, Vassalli P. Tumor necrosis factor/cachectin is an effector of skin and gut lesions of the acute phase of graft-vs.-host disease. J Exp Med 1987; 166:1280–1289.

24. Panoskaltsis-Mortari A, Lacey DL, Vallera DA, Blazar BR. Keratinocyte growth factor administered before conditioning ameliorates graft-vs.-host disease after allogeneic bone marrow transplantation in mice. Blood 1998; 92:3960–3967.

25. Krijanovski OI, Hill GR, Cooke KR, Teshima T, Crawford JM, Brinson YS, Ferrara JL. Keratinocyte growth factor separates graft-vs.-leukemia effects from graft-vs.-host disease. Blood 1999; 94:825–831.

26. Bacigalupo A, Lamparelli T, Bruzzi P, Guidi S, Alessandrino PE, Di Bartolomeo P, Oneto R, Bruno B, Barbanti M, Sacchi N, Van Lint MT, Bosi A. Antithymocyte globulin for graft-vs.-host disease prophylaxis in transplants from unrelated donors: 2 randomized studies from Gruppo Italiano Trapianti Midollo Osseo (GITMO). Blood 2001; 98:2942–2947.

27. Remberger M, Storer B, Ringden O, Anasetti C. Association between pretransplant thymo-globlulin and reduced non-relapse mortality rate after marrow transplantation from unrelated donors. Bone Marrow Transplant 2002; 29:391–397.

28. den Haan JM, Sherman NE, Blokland E, Huczko E, Koning F, Drijfhout JW, Skipper J, Shabanowitz J, Hunt DF, Engelhard VH, Goulmy E. Identification of a graft-vs.-host disease-associated human minor histocompatibility antigen. Science 1995; 268:1476–1480.

29. Chao NJ. Graft-vs.-host disease: the viewpoint from the donor T cell (review). Biol Blood Marrow Transplant 1997; 3:1–10.

30. Goulmy E, Schipper J, Pool J, Blokland E, Falkenburg JHF, Vossen J, Gratwohl A, Vogelsang GB, van Houwelingen HC, van Rood JJ. Mismatches of minor histocompatibility antigens between HLA-identical donors and recipients and the development of graft-vs.-host disease after bone marrow transplantation. N Engl J Med 1996; 334:281–285.

31. Jameson BA, McDonnell JM, Marini JC, Korngold R. A rationally designed CD4 analogue inhibits experimental allergic encephalomyelitis. Nature 1994; 368:744–746.

32. Schlegel PG, Aharoni R, Chen Y, Chen J, Teitelbaum D, Arnon R, Sela M, Chao NJ. A synthetic random basic copolymer with promiscuous binding to class II major histocompatibility complex molecules inhibits T-cell proliferative responses to major and minor histocompatibility antigens in vitro and confers the capacity to prevent murine graft-vs.-host disease in vivo. [erratum appears in Proc Natl Acad Sci USA 1996 aUG 6;93(16):8796.]. Proc Natl Acad Sci USA 1996; 93:5061–5066.

33. Sette A, Alexander J, Grey HM. Interaction of antigenic peptides with MHC and TCR molecules (review). Clin Immunol Immunopathol 1995; 76:S168–S171.

34. Sakihama T, Smolyar A, Reinherz EL. Molecular recognition of antigen involves lattice formation between CD4, MHC class II and TCR molecules (review). Immunol Today 1995; 16:581–587.

35. Yang Y, Wilson JM. CD40 ligand-dependent T cell activation: requirement of B7-CD28 signaling through CD40. Science 1996; 273:1862–1864.

36. June CH, Bluestone JA, Nadler LM, Thompson CB. The B7 and CD28 receptor families. Immunol Today 1994; 15:321–331.

37. Green JM, Noel PJ, Sperling AI, Walunas TL, Gray GS, Bluestone JA, Thompson CB. Absence of B7-dependent responses in CD28-deficient mice. Immunity 1994; 1:501–508.

38. Freeman GJ, Gribben JG, Boussiotis VA, Ng JW, Restivo VAJ, Lombard LA, Gray GS, Nadler LM. Cloning of B7-2: a CTLA-4 counter-receptor that costimulates human T cell proliferation. Science 1993; 262:909–911.

39. Blazar BR, Taylor PA, Panoskaltsis-Mortari A, Gray GS, Vallera DA. Coblockade of the LFA1:ICAM and CD28/CTLA4:B7 pathways is a highly effective means of preventing acute lethal graft-vs.-host disease induced by fully major histocompatibility complex-disparate donor grafts. Blood 1995; 85:2607–2618.

40. Durie FH, Foy TM, Masters SR, Laman JD, Noelle RJ. The role of CD40 in the regulation of humoral and cell-mediated immunity (review). Immunol Today 1994; 15:406–411.

41. Guinan EC, Boussiotis VA, Neuberg D, Brennan LL, Hirano N, Nadler LM, Gribben JG. Transplantation of anergic histoincompatible bone marrow allografts. N Engl J Med 1999; 340:1704–1714.

42. Vezina C, Kudelski A, Sehgal SN. Rapamycin (AY-22,989), a new antifungal antibiotic. I. Taxonomy of the producing streptomycete and isolation of the active principle. J Antibiot 1975; 28:721–726.

43. Martel RR, Klicius J, Galet S. Inhibition of the immune response by rapamycin, a new antifungal antibiotic. Can J Physiol Pharmacol 1977; 55:48–51.

44. Morice WG, Brunn GJ, Wiederrecht G, Siekierka JJ, Abraham RT. Rapamycin-induced inhibition of p34cdc2 kinase activation is associated with G1/S-phase growth arrest in T lymphocytes. J Biol Chem 1993; 268:3734–3738.

45. Nourse J, Firpo E, Flanagan WM, Coats S, Polyak K, Lee MH, Massague J, Crabtree GR, Roberts JM. Interleukin-2-mediated elimination of the p27Kip1 cyclin-dependent kinase inhibitor prevented by rapamycin. Nature 1994; 372:570–573.

46. Altmeyer A, Dumont FJ. Rapamycin inhibits IL-1-mediated interferon-gamma production in the YAC-1 T cell lymphoma. Cytokine 1993; 5:133–143.

47. Lai JH, Tan TH. CD28 signaling causes a sustained down-regulation of I kappa B alpha which can be prevented by the immunosuppressant rapamycin. J Biol Chem 1994; 269:30077–30080.

48. Storb R, Deeg HJ, Whitehead J, Appelbaum F, Beatty P, Bensinger W, Buckner CD, Clift R, Doney K, Farewell V, Hansen J, Hill R, Lum L, Martin P, McGuffin R, Sanders J, Stewart P, Sullivan K, Witherspoon R, Yee G, Thomas ED. Methotrexate and cyclosporine compared with cyclosporine alone for prophylaxis of acute graft-vs.-host disease after marrow transplantation for leukemia. N Engl J Med 1986; 314:729–735.

49. Herve P, Tiberghien P, Racadot E, Plouvier E, Cahn JY. Prevention and treatment of acute GvHD—new modalities (review). Bone Marrow Transplant 1993; 11(suppl 1):103–106.

50. Storb R, Deeg HJ, Farewell V, Doney K, Appelbaum F, Beatty P, Bensinger W, Buckner CD, Clift R, Hansen J, Hill R, Longton G, Lum L, Martin P, McGuffin R, Sanders J, Singer J, Stewart P, Sullivan K, Witherspoon R, Thomas ED. Marrow transplantation for severe aplastic anemia: methotrexate alone compared with a combination of methotrexate and cyclosporine for prevention of acute graft-vs.-host disease. Blood 1986; 68:119–125.

51. Ringden O, Klaesson S, Sundberg B, Ljungman P, Lonnqvist B, Persson U. Decreased incidence of graft-vs.-host disease and improved survival with methotrexate combined with cyclosporin compared with monotherapy in recipients of bone marrow from donors other than HLA identical siblings. Bone Marrow Transplant 1992; 9:19–25.

52. Mrsic M, Labar B, Bogdanic V, Nemet D, Pavletic Z, Plavsic F, Dobric I, Marusic M, Francetic I, Kastelan A, Kalenic S, Vrtar M, Markulin-Grgic L, Aurer I. Combination of cyclosporin and methotrexate for prophylaxis of acute graft-vs.-host disease after allogeneic bone marrow transplantation for leukemia. Bone Marrow Transplant 1990; 6:137–141.

53. Nevill TJ, Tirgan MH, Deeg HJ, Klingemann H.-G, Reece DE, Shepherd JD, Barnett MJ, Phillips GL. Influence of post-methotrexate folinic acid rescue on regimen-related toxicity and graft-vs.-host disease after allogeneic bone marrow transplantation. Bone Marrow Transplant 1992; 9:349–354.

54. Chao NJ, Snyder DS, Jain M, Wong RM, Niland JC, Negrin RS, Long GD, Hu WW, Stockerl-Goldstein KE, Johnston LJ, Amylon MD, Tierney DK, O'Donnel MR, Nademanee AP, Parker P, Stein A, Molina A, Fung H, Kashyap A, Kohler S, Spielberger R, Krishnan A, Rodriguez R, Forman SJ, Blume KG. Equivalence of 2 effective graft-vs.-host disease prophylaxis regimens: results of a prospective double-blind randomized trial. Biol Blood Marrow Transplant 2000; 6:254–261.

55. Ratanatharathorn V, Nash RA, Przepiorka D, Devine SM, Klein JL, Weisdorf D, Fay JW, Nademanee A, Antin JH, Christiansen NP, Van Der Jagt R, Herzig RH, Litzow MR, Wolff SN, Longo WL, Petersen FB, Karanes C, Avalos B, Storb R, Buell DN, Maher RM, Fitzsimmons WE, Wingard JR. Phase III study comparing methotrexate and tacrolimus (Prograf, FK506) with methotrexate and cyclosporine for graft-vs.-host-disease prophylaxis after HLA-identical sibling bone marrow transplantation. Blood 1998; 92:2303–2314.

56. Nash RA, Antin JH, Karanes C, Fay JW, Avalos BR, Yeager AM, Przepiorka D, Davies S, Petersen FB, Bartels P, Buell D, Fitzsimmons W, Anasetti C, Storb R, Ratanatharathorn V. Phase 3 study comparing methotrexate and tacrolimus with methotrexate and cyclosporine for prophylaxis of acute graft-vs.-host disease after marrow transplantation from unrelated donors. Blood 2000; 96:2062–2068.

57. Hiraoka A. Results of a phase III study on prophylactic use of FK506 for acute GVHD compared with cyclosporin in allogeneic bone marrow transplantation (abstr). Blood 1997; 90(suppl 1):561a.

58. Halloran P, Mathew T, Tomlanovich S, Groth C, Hooftman L, Barker C. Mycophenolate mofetil in renal allograft recipients: a pooled efficacy analysis of three randomized, double-blind, clinical studies in prevention of rejection. Transplantation 1997; 63:39–47.

59. Suthanthiran M, Morris RE, Strom TB. Immunosuppressants: cellular and molecular mechanisms of action (review). Am J Kidney Dis 1996; 28:159–172.

60. Hovi T, Allison AC, Allsop J. Rapid increase of phosphoribosyl pyrophosphate concentration after mitogenic stimulation of lymphocytes. FEBS Lett 1975; 55:291–293.

61. Storb R, Yu C, Wagner JL, Deeg HJ, Nash RA, Kiem H.-P, Leisenring W, Shulman H. Stable mixed hematopoietic chimerism in DLA-identical littermate dogs given sublethal total body irradiation before and pharmacological immunosuppression after marrow transplantation. Blood 1997; 89:3048–3054.

62. Mason DW. Subsets of T cells in the rat mediating lethal graft-vs.-host disease. Transplantation 1981; 32:222–226.

63. Fong TA, Mosmann TR. Alloreactive murine CD8+ T cell clones secrete the Th1 pattern of cytokines. J Immunol 1990; 144:1744–1752.

64. Groux H, Bigler M, de Vries JE, Roncarolo MG. Interleukin-10 induces a long-term antigen-specific anergic state in human CD4$^+$ T cells. J Exp Med 1996; 184:19–29.

65. Bensinger WI, Martin PJ, Storer B, Clift R, Forman SJ, Negrin R, Kashyap A, Flowers MED, Lilleby K, Chauncey TR, Storb R, Appelbaum FR. Transplantation of bone marrow as compared with peripheral-blood cells from HLA-identical relatives in patients with hematologic cancers. N Engl J Med 2001; 344:175–181.

66. Mielcarek M, Graf L, Johnson G, Torok-Storb B. Production of interleukin-10 by granulocyte colony-stimulating factor-mobilized blood products: a mechanism for monocyte-mediated suppression of T cell proliferation. Blood 1998; 92:215–222.

67. Blaise D, Kuentz M, Fortanier C, Bourhis JH, Milpied N, Sutton L, Jouet J.-P, Attal M, Bordigoni P, Cahn J.-Y, Boiron J.-M, Schuller M.-P, Moatti J.-P, Michallet M. Randomized trial of bone marrow vs. lenograstim-primed blood cell allogeneic transplantation in patients with early-stage leukemia: a report from the Société Française de Greffe de Moelle. J Clin Oncol 2000; 18:537–571.

68. Powles R, Mehta J, Kulkarni S, Treleavan J, Millar B, Marsden J, Shepherd V, Rowland JH, Sirohi B, Tait D, Horton C, Long S, Singhal S. Allogeneic blood and bone-marrow stem-cell transplantation in haematological malignant diseases: a randomised trial. Lancet 2000; 355:1231–1237.

69. Yang YG, Dey BR, Sergio JJ, Pearson DA, Sykes M. Donor-derived interferon gamma is required for inhibition of acute graft-vs.-host disease by interleukin 12. J Clin Invest 1998; 102:2126–2135.

70. Murphy WJ, Welniak LA, Taub DD, Wiltrout RH, Taylor PA, Vallera DA, Kopf M, Young H, Longo DL, Blazar BR. Differential effects of the absence of interferon-gamma and IL-4 in acute graft-vs.-host disease after allogeneic bone marrow transplantation in mice. J Clin Invest 1998; 102:1742–1748.

71. Sheridan JF, Tutschka PJ, Sedmak DD, Copelan EA. Immunoglobulin G subclass deficiency and pneumococcal infection after allogeneic bone marrow transplantation. Blood 1990; 75:1583–1586.

72. Sullivan KM, Kopecky KJ, Jocom J, Fisher L, Buckner CD, Meyers JD, Counts GW, Bowden RA, Petersen FB, Witherspoon RP, Budinger MD, Schwartz RS, Appelbaum FR, Clift RA, Hansen JA, Sanders JE, Thomas ED, Storb R. Immunomodulatory and antimicrobial efficacy of intravenous immunoglobulin in bone marrow transplantation. N Engl J Med 1990; 323:705–712.

73. Shevach EM. Certified professionals: CD4(+)CD25(+) suppressor T cells. J Exp Med 2001; 193:F41–F46.

74. Shevach EM, McHugh RS, Piccirillo CA, Thornton AM. Control of T-cell activation by CD4+ CD25+ suppressor T cells (review). Immunol Rev 2001; 182:58–67.
75. Taylor PA, Lees CJ, Blazer BR. The infusion of ex vivo activated and expanded CD4(+) CD25(+) immune regulatory cells inhibits graft-vs.-host disease lethality. Blood 2002; 99:3493–3499.
76. Ruggeri L, Capanni M, Martelli MF, Velardi A. Cellular therapy: exploiting NK cell alloreactivity in transplantation (review). Curr Opin Hematol 2001; 8:355–359.
77. Farag SS, Fehniger TA, Ruggeri L, Velardi A, Caligiuri MA. Natural killer cell receptors: new biology and insights into the graft-vs.-leukemia effect (review). Blood 2002; 100:1935–1947.
78. Ruggeri L, Capanni M, Urbani E, Perruccio K, Shlomchik WD, Tosti A, Posati S, Rogaia D, Frassoni F, Aversa F, Martelli MF, Velardi A. Effectiveness of donor natural killer cell alloreactivity in mismatched hematopoietic transplants. Science 2002; 295:2097–2100.
79. Thomas ED, Storb R, Clift RA, Fefer A, Johnson FL, Neiman PE, Lerner KG, Glucksberg H, Buckner CD. Bone-marrow transplantation. N Engl J Med 1975; 292:832–843, 895–902.
80. Holler E, Kolb HJ, Wilmanns W. Treatment of GVHD—TNF-antibodies and related antagonists (review). Bone Marrow Transplant 1993; 12(suppl 3):S29–S31.
81. Ruutu T, Hermans J, van Biezen A, Niederwieser D, Gratwohl A, Apperley JF. How should corticosteroids be used in the treatment of acute GVHD? EBMT Chronic Leukemia Working Party. European Group for Blood and Marrow Transplantation. Bone Marrow Transplant 1998; 22:614–615.
82. Van Lint MT, Uderzo C, Locasciulli A, Majolino I, Scime R, Locatelli F, Giorgiani G, Arcese W, Iori AP, Falda M, Bosi A, Miniero R, Alessandrino P, Dini G, Rotoli B, Bacigalupo A. Early treatment of acute graft-vs.-host disease with high- or low-dose 6-methylprednisolone: a multicenter randomized trial from the Italian Group for Bone Marrow Transplantation. Blood 1998; 92:2288–2293.
83. Hings IM, Filipovich AH, Miller WJ, Blazar BL, McGlave PB, Ramsay NK, Kersey JH, Weisdorf DJ. Prednisone therapy for acute graft-vs.-host disease: short- vs. long-term treatment. A prospective randomized trial. Transplantation 1993; 56:577–580.
84. Martin PJ, Schoch G, Fisher L, Byers V, Anasetti C, Appelbaum FR, Beatty PG, Doney K, McDonald GB, Sanders JE, Sullivan KM, Storb R, Thomas ED, Witherspoon RP, Lomen P, Hannigan J, Hansen JA. A retrospective analysis of therapy for acute graft-vs.-host disease: Initial treatment. Blood 1990; 76:1464–1472.
85. Weisdorf D, Haake R, Blazar B, Miller W, McGlave P, Ramsay N, Kersey J, Filipovich A. Treatment of moderate/severe acute graft-vs.-host disease after allogeneic bone marrow transplantation: an analysis of clinical risk features and outcome. Blood 1990; 75:1024–1030.
86. MacMillan ML, Weisdorf DJ, Wagner JE, DeFor TE, Burns LJ, Ramsay NK, Davies SM, Blazar BR. Response of 443 patients to steroids as primary therapy for acute graft-vs.-host disease: comparison of grading systems. Biol Blood Marrow Transplant 2002; 8:387–394.
87. Martin PJ, Nelson BJ, Appelbaum FR, Anasetti C, Deeg HJ, Hansen JA, McDonald GB, Nash RA, Sullivan KM, Witherspoon RP, Scannon PJ, Friedmann N, Storb R. Evaluation of a CD5-specific immunotoxin for treatment of acute graft-vs.-host disease after allogeneic marrow transplantation. Blood 1996; 88:824–830.
88. Cahn JY, Bordigoni P, Tiberghien P, Milpied N, Brion A, Widjenes J, Lioure B, Michel G, Burdach S, Kolb HJ. Treatment of acute graft-vs.-host disease with methylprednisolone and cyclosporine with or without an anti-interleukin-2 receptor monoclonal antibody. A multicenter phase III study. Transplantation 1995; 60:939–942.
89. Cragg L, Blazar BR, DeFor T, Kolatker N, Miller W, Kersey J, Ramsay M, McGlave P, Filipovich A, Weisdorf D. A randomized trial comparing prednisone with antithymocyte globulin/prednisone as an initial systemic therapy for moderately severe acute graft-vs.-host disease. Biol Blood Marrow Transplant 2000; 6:441–447.

90. Bacigalupo A, Oneto R, Lamparelli T, Gualandi F, Bregante S, Raiola AM, Di Grazia C, Dominietto A, Romagnani C, Bruno B, Van Lint MT, Frassoni F. Pre-emptive therapy of acute graft-vs.-host disease: a pilot study with antithymocyte globulin (ATG). Bone Marrow Transplant 2001; 28:1093–1096.

91. Hattori K, Hirano T, Miyajima H, Yamakawa N, Tateno M, Oshimi K, Kayagaki N, Yagita H, Okumura K. Differential effects of anti-Fas ligand and anti-tumor necrosis factor alpha antibodies on acute graft-vs.-host disease pathologies. Blood 1998; 91:4051–4055.

92. Stuber E, Buschenfeld A, von Freier A, Arendt T, Folsch UR. Intestinal crypt cell apoptosis in murine acute graft-vs.-host disease is mediated by tumour necrosis factor alpha and not by the FasL-Fas interaction: effect of pentoxifylline on the development of mucosal atrophy. Gut 1999; 45:229–235.

93. Daneshpouy M, Socie G, Lemann M, Rivet J, Gluckman E, Janin A. Activated eosinophils in upper gastrointestinal tract of patients with graft-vs.-host disease. Blood 2002; 99:3033–3040.

94. Furlong T, Storb R, Anasetti C, Appelbaum FR, Deeg HJ, Doney K, Martin P, Sullivan K, Witherspoon R, Nash RA. Clinical outcome after conversion to FK 506 (tacrolimus) therapy for acute graft-vs.-host disease resistant to cyclosporine or for cyclosporine-associated toxicities. Bone Marrow Transplant 2000; 26:985–991.

95. Basara N, Blau WI, Romer E, Rudolphi M, Bischoff M, Kirsten D, Sanchez H, Gunzelmann S, Fauser AA. Mycophenolate mofetil for the treatment of acute and chronic GVHD in bone marrow transplant patients. Bone Marrow Transplant 1998; 22:61–65.

96. Margolis J, Vogelsang G. An old drug for a new disease: pentostatin (Nipent) in acute graft-vs.-host disease (review). Semin Oncol 2000; 27:72–77.

97. Benito AI, Furlong T, Martin PJ, Anasetti C, Appelbaum FR, Doney K, Nash RA, Papayannopoulou T, Storb R, Sullivan KM, Witherspoon R, Deeg HJ. Sirolimus (rapamycin) for the treatment of steroid-refractory acute graft-vs.-host disease. Transplantation 2001; 72:1924–1929.

98. Hsu B, May R, Carrum G, Krance R, Przepiorka D. Use of antithymocyte globulin for treatment of steroid-refractory acute graft-vs.-host disease: an international practice survey. Bone Marrow Transplant 2001; 28:945–950.

99. Arai SM. Poor outcome in steroid-refractory graft-vs.-host disease with antithymocyte globulin treatment. Biol Blood Marrow Transplant 2002; 8:155–160.

100. Khoury H, Kashyap A, Adkins DR, Brown RA, Miller G, Vij R, Westervelt P, Trinkaus K, Goodnough LT, Hayashi RJ, Parker P, Forman SJ, DiPersio JF. Treatment of steroid-resistant acute graft-vs.-host disease with anti-thymocyte globulin. Bone Marrow Transplant 2001; 27:1059–1064.

101. McCaul K.G., Nevill TJ, Barnett MJ, Toze CL, Currie CJ, Sutherland HJ, Conneally EA, Shepherd JD, Nantel SH, Hogge DE, Klingemann H.-G. Treatment of steroid-resistant acute graft-vs.-host disease with rabbitt antithymocyte globulin. J Hematother Stem Cell Res 2000; 9:367–374.

102. Mollee P, Morton AJ, Irving I, Durrant S. Combination therapy with tacrolimus and anti-thymocyte globulin for the treatment of steroid-resistant acute graft-vs.-host disease developing during cyclosporine prophylaxis. [erratum appears in Br J Haematol 2001 Oct;115(1):235.]. Br J Haematol 2001; 113:217–223.

103. Graziani F, V. Treatment of acute graft-vs.-host disease with low dose-alternate day anti-thymocyte globulin. Haematologica 2002; 87:973–978.

104. MacMillan ML, Weisdorf DJ, Davies SM, Defor TE, Burns LJ, Ramsay NK, Wagner JE, Blazar BR. Early antithymocyte globulin therapy improves survival in patients with steroid-resistant acute graft-vs.-host disease. Biol Blood Marrow Transplant 2002; 8:40–46.

105. Hebart H, Ehninger G, Schmidt H, Berner B, Reuss-Borst M, Waller HD, Muller CA, Einsele H. Treatment of steroid-resistant graft-vs.-host disease after allogeneic bone marrow transplantation with anti-CD3/TCR monoclonal antibodies. Bone Marrow Transplant 1995; 15:891–894.

106. Carpenter PA, Appelbaum FR, Corey L, Deeg HJ, Doney K, Gooley T, Krueger J, Martin P, Pavlovic S, Sanders J, Slattery J, Levitt D, Storb R, Woolfrey A, Anasetti C. A humanized non-FcR-binding anti-CD3 antibody, visilizumab, for treatment of steroid-refractory acute graft-vs.-host disease. Blood 2002; 99:2712–2719.

107. Przepiorka D, Kernan NA, Ippoliti C, Papadopoulos EB, Giralt S, Khouri I, Lu JG, Gajewski J, Durett A, Cleary K, Champlin R, Andersson BS, Light S. Daclizumab, a humanized anti-interleukin-2 receptor alpha chain antibody, for treatment of acute graft-vs.-host disease. Blood 2000; 95:83–89.

108. Willenbacher W, Basara N, Blau IW, Fauser AA, Kiehl MG. Treatment of steroid refractory acute and chronic graft-vs.-host disease with daclizumab. Br J Haematol 2001; 112:820–823.

109. Deeg HJ, Blazar BR, Bolwell BJ, Long GD, Schuening F, Cunningham J, Rifkin RM, Abhyankar S, Briggs AD, Burt R, Lipani J, Roskos LK, White JM, Havrilla N, Schwab G, Heslop HE. Treatment of steroid-refractory acute graft-vs.-host disease with anti-CD147 monoclonal antibody, ABX-CBL. Blood 2001; 98:2052–2058.

110. Holler E, Kolb HJ, Hintermeier-Knabe R, Mittermüller J, Thierfelder S, Kaul M, Wilmanns W. Role of tumor necrosis factor alpha in acute graft-vs.-host disease and complications following allogeneic bone marrow transplantation. Transplant Proc 1993; 25:1234–1236.

111. Antin JH, Weinstein HJ, Guinan EC, McCarthy P, Bierer BE, Gilliland DG, Parsons SK, Ballen KK, Rimm IJ, Falzarano G. Recombinant human interleukin-1 receptor antagonist in the treatment of steroid-resistant graft-vs.-host disease. Blood 1994; 84:1342–1348.

112. Kobbe G, Schneider P, Rohr U, Fenk R, Neumann F, Aivado M, Dietze L, Kronenwett R, Hunerliturkoglu A, Haas R. Treatment of severe steroid refractory acute graft-vs.-host disease with infliximab, a chimeric human/mouse antiTNFalpha antibody. Bone Marrow Transplant 2001; 28:47–49.

113. Hahn J, Erdmann A, Grube M, Hildebrandt G, Schlottmann K, Andreesen R, Holler E. High incidence of invasive aspergillosis after treatment of acute GVHD with the combination of OKT3 and infliximab (abstr). Bone Marrow Transplant 2001; 27(suppl 1):S203.

114. Chiang KY, Abhyankar S, Bridges K, Godder K, Henslee-Downey JP. Recombinant human tumor necrosis factor receptor fusion protein as complementary treatment for chronic graft-vs.-host disease. Transplantation 2002; 73:665–667.

115. Andolina M, Rabusin M, Maximova N, Di Leo G. Etanercept in graft-vs.-host disease. Bone Marrow Transplant 2000; 26:929.

116. Cooke KR, Hill GR, Gerbitz A, Kobzik L, Martin TR, Crawford JM, Brewer JP, Ferrara JL. Tumor necrosis factor-alpha neutralization reduces lung injury after experimental allogeneic bone marrow transplantation. Transplantation 2000; 70:272–279.

117. Bladon JT. Extracorporeal photopheresis reduces the number of mononuclear cells that produce pro-inflammatory cytokines, when tested ex-vivo. J Clin Apher 2002; 17:177–182.

118. Gorgun G, Miller KB, Foss FM. Immunologic mechanisms of extracorporeal photochemotherapy in chronic graft-vs.-host disease. Blood 2002; 100:941–947.

119. Tambur AR, Ortegel JW, Morales A, Klingemann H, Gebel HM, Tharp MD. Extracorporeal photopheresis induces lymphocyte but not monocyte apoptosis. Transplant Proc 2000; 32:747–748.

120. Dall'Amico R, Messina C. Extracorporeal photochemotherapy for the treatment of graft-vs.-host disease (review) Ther Apher 2002; 6:296–304.

121. Furlong T, Leisenring W, Storb R, Anasetti C, Appelbaum FR, Carpenter PA, Deeg HJ, Doney K, Kiem H.-P, Nash RA, Sanders JE, Witherspoon R, Thompson D, Martin PJ. Psoralen and ultraviolet A irradiation (PUVA) as therapy for steroid-resistant cutaneous acute graft-vs.-host disease. Biol Blood Marrow Transplant 2002; 8:206–212.

122. Greinix HT, Volc-Platzer B, Kalhs P, Fischer G, Rosenmayr A, Keil F, Honigsmann H, Knobler RM. Extracorporeal photochemotherapy in the treatment of severe steroid-refractory acute graft-vs.-host disease: a pilot study. Blood 2000; 96:2426–2431.

123. Bonanomi S, Balduzzi A, Tagliabue A, Biagi E, Rovelli A, Corti P, Crippa D, Uderzo C. Bath PUVA therapy in pediatric patients with drug-resistant cutaneous graft-vs.-host disease. Bone Marrow Transplant 2001; 28:631–632.

124. Ely P, Dunitz J, Rogosheske J, Weisdorf D. Use of a somatostatin analogue, octreotide acetate, in the management of acute gastrointestinal graft-vs.-host disease. Am J Med 1991; 90:707–710.

125. Grothaus-Pinke B, Gunzelmann S, Fauser AA, Kiehl MG. Factor XIII replacement in stem cell transplant (SCT) recipients with severe graft-vs.-host disease of the bowel: report of an initial experience. Transplantation 2001; 72:1456–1458.

126. Bertz H, Afting M, Kreisel W, Duffner U, Greinwald R, Finke J. Feasibility and response to budesonide as topical corticosteroid therapy for acute intestinal GVHD. Bone Marrow Transplant 1999; 24:1185–1189.

127. McDonald GB, Bouvier M, Hockenbery DM, Stern JM, Gooley T, Farrand A, Murakami C, Levine DS. Oral beclomethasone dipropionate for treatment of intestinal graft-vs.-host disease: a randomized, controlled trial. Gastroenterology 1998; 115:28–35.

128. French LE, Tschopp J. Fas-mediated cell death in toxic epidermal necrolysis and graft-vs.-host disease: potential for therapeutic inhibition (review). Schweiz Med Wochenschr J Suisse Med 2000; 130:1656–1661.

129. Biedermann BC, Sahner S, Gregor M, Tsakiris DA, Jeanneret C, Pober JS, Gratwohl A. Endothelial injury mediated by cytotoxic T lymphocytes and loss of microvessels in chronic graft-vs.-host disease. Lancet 2002; 359:2078–2083.

130. Hoffmann P, Ermann J, Edinger M, Fathman CG, Strober S. Donor-type CD4(+)CD25(+) regulatory T cells suppress lethal acute graft-vs.-host disease after allogeneic bone marrow transplantation. J Exp Med 2002; 196:389–399.

131. Groux H. An overview of regulatory T cells (review). Microbes Infection 2001; 3:883–889.

17

Graft Manipulation to Prevent Graft-vs.-Host Disease

ROBERT J. SOIFFER

Dana-Farber Cancer Institute, Boston, Massachusetts, U.S.A.

I. INTRODUCTION

For the past 25 years, the effective prevention of graft-vs.-host disease (GVHD) has been the primary goal of laboratory and clinical investigators studying allogeneic hematopoietic stem cell transplantation (HSCT). GVHD, once established, can be difficult to treat. The survival of patients who develop moderate to severe GVHD is markedly inferior to that of patients with either mild or no GVHD (1–4). Mortality can result from direct organ damage or from opportunistic infections promoted by the use of immune-suppressive medications. Although the use of calcineurin inhibitors and methotrexate is somewhat effective as prophylaxis, GVHD remains a serious problem, particularly for patients receiving transplants from unrelated or HLA-nonidentical related donors. As the role of donor T cells in GVHD pathogenesis became established, efforts to limit the number of potentially allo-reactive T lymphocytes in the graft were undertaken in order to prevent GVHD. It was hoped that T-cell depletion (TCD) would improve the safety of and, consequently, survival after allogeneic HSCT (5). Most early trials documented that TCD substantially limited acute GVHD. However, these reductions in GVHD were counterbalanced by high rates of graft failure, immune deficiency, and disease recurrence (Table 1). Subsequent efforts have focused on ways of successfully manipulating allogeneic grafts without inducing these adverse complications.

II. T CELLS AND GVHD

T lymphocytes were first implicated as mediators of GVHD over 40 years ago (6). The role of T-cells became established with subsequent studies linking T-cell administration to

Table 1 Pros and Cons of T-Cell Depletion

Advantages	Disadvantages
Decreased incidence of acute and chronic GVHD	Higher incidence of graft failure
Reduced or no requirement for posttransplant immune suppression as GVHD prophylaxis	Loss of GVL activity (higher incidence of disease relapse, especially with CML)
Decreased organ toxicity	Delayed immune reconstitution
Lower early transplant–related mortality	Increased risk for posttransplant EBV-associated lymphoproliferative disorder

induction of GVHD. These observations suggested the potential benefits of removing T cells from the allograft.

Concepts of GVHD pathophysiology have evolved considerably during the past 30 years. The contributions of other factors (including the release of lipopolysaccharide from damaged tissues, elaboration of pro-inflammatory cytokines by mononuclear cells, and target antigen presentation by dendritic cells) appear to be critical in generating and maintaining graft-vs.-host reactions (7–9). Animal experiments in which these components and their pathways have been interrupted suggest that such approaches could be effective in preventing GVHD. As yet, however, efforts to block cytokine induction with agents such as interleukin (IL)-1 receptor antagonist or IL-11 have failed to reduce the incidence of GVHD in human studies (10,11). The only biological strategy that has successfully prevented GVHD in clinical studies has been the direct removal or disabling of donor T cells in the graft, either through pharmacological prophylaxis or through T cell depletion.

III. EARLY ANIMAL STUDIES OF GRAFT MANIPULATION

In the 1970s, investigators showed that both physical separation techniques and incubation of the donor graft with antibodies to target lymphocytes could prevent or reduce GVHD in animals. Infusion of spleen cells into irradiated mice after removal of lymphocytes permitted hematopoietic recovery without GVHD (12). Similar results were noted in mice that had received bone marrow and spleen cell suspensions pretreated with soybean and/or peanut agglutinin to deplete lymphocytes (13). Incubation of marrow with both antilymphocyte sera (ALS) or antithymocyte globulin (ATG) ex vivo depleted T cells and facilitated transplantation across major histocompatibility barriers while preventing GVHD in several animal systems (14–18). The development of monoclonal antibody technology permitted specific targeting of T cells and their subsets, expanding the potential of TCD as a strategy for GVHD prophylaxis (19).

IV. GRAFT MANIPULATION STRATEGIES

Most graft engineering strategies have relied upon the ex vivo removal of T cells or T-cell subsets from the donor cell inoculum (Table 2). Ex vivo removal of T cells from the donor graft can be accomplished either by negative selection of T cells or by positive selection of CD34+ stem cells. Examples of physical separation techniques include differential agglutination with lectins followed by rosetting with sheep red blood cells (20,21),

Table 2 Methods of T-Cell Depletion

Ex vivo negative selection
  Monoclonal antibodies $+/-$ complement
  Monoclonal antibody formulated as immunotoxin
  Monoclonal antibody bound to magnetic beads
  Soybean lectin agglutination
  Counterflow centrifugal elutriation
Ex vivo positive selection
  CD34+ immunoadsorption column
In vivo T-cell depletion
  Monoclonal antibody (e.g., alemtuzumab/Campath)
  Antithymocyte globulin preparations

counterflow centrifugal elutriation (22,23), and fractionation on density gradients (24). Monoclonal antibodies have been used alone (25–27), in conjunction with homologous or heterologous complement (28–34), as immunotoxins (35–37), or with immunomagnetic beads (38). Some methods may deplete components other than T lymphocytes.

The development of anti-CD34 antibody–coated columns to select hematopoietic progenitors provides an alternative. CD34 columns, initially developed to purge autologous grafts of tumor contaminants, will result in a reduction of the lymphocyte content in the infused product by as much as 4–5 log (39–43). Positive stem cell selection techniques can be followed by antibody–based negative selection to further deplete specific T-cell populations.

The availability of humanized anti-T-cell antibodies permit effective in vivo T-cell depletion. T-cell depletion with antithymocyte globulin preparations or humanized anti-T-cell antibodies such as Campath-1H (alemtuzumab) in vivo pre– and post–donor stem cell infusion can target recipient T cells that could mediate graft rejection and donor T cells that might induce GVHD (44–47). These antibodies have been particularly used for nonmyeloablative transplants as well as for haploidentical transplants.

V. T-CELL DOSE AND GVHD

The precise relationship between the number of T cells infused and the development of GVHD is not known. There is likely to be variability in the threshold T-cell GVHD dose between donor/recipient pairs depending on the degree of minor HLA antigen disparity and other polymorphisms (48). Most studies suggest that a minimum of 2 log-depletion of functional T cells from the marrow is necessary for effective GVHD prophylaxis with reduced or no posttransplant immune suppression. Limiting dilution analyses have suggested a threshold of approximately $2-3 \times 10^5$ T cells/kg for development of GVHD in recipients of HLA-identical bone marrow (49,50). Studies from recipients of HLA-matched CD34-selected mobilized peripheral blood indicate significantly higher rates of GVHD when the CD3+ T-cell count exceeds 1×10^5 T cells/kg (51). The extent of T-cell removal by different TCD techniques may vary from 2 to 5 log. It is therefore not surprising that the degree of protection against GVHD depends upon the method of T-cell depletion utilized. In general, the more exhaustive the T-cell depletion, the lower the risk of GVHD. However, it is likely that the relationship between T-cell number and the development of acute GVHD is not linear.

The degree of TCD necessary to prevent GVHD is greater for unrelated and HLA-mismatched transplants than for HLA-identical siblings. In patients receiving haplomismatched peripheral blood stem cells, acute GVHD incidence was low with extensive T-cell depletion (below $1-2 \times 10^4$ T cells/kg, a log lower than the GVHD threshold for recipients of peripheral blood stem cells from HLA-matched) (52). In a comparative analysis of CD6+ T-cell–depleted allogeneic bone marrow transplantation, the incidence of GVHD for recipients of unrelated marrow was more than twice as great as that observed in related marrow recipients (42% vs. 20%) despite an equivalent number of T cells infused (53).

VI. SPECIFICITY OF T-CELL DEPLETION

Graft-manipulation techniques also differ in the specificity of depletion. Some approaches may indiscriminately eliminate natural killer (NK) cells, immature thymocytes, B cells, and dendritic cells in addition to T cells. These cellular elements likely contribute to immune surveillance, graft facilitation, and elimination of minimal residual disease. It is also still not clear what contributions distinct T-cell subsets make to the pathogenesis of GVHD (54). It seems logical that the specificity of the TCD technique would have a significant effect on outcome.

T-cell–depletion techniques may have narrow or broad spectra of reactivity. Examples of narrow specificities include depletion with antibodies targeting mature T cells only, such as anti-TCR, anti-CD6, anti-CD8, and anti-CD5. Broad specificity depletion techniques include treatment with soybean lectin agglutination, Campath antibodies, which target the widely expressed CD52 antigen, and multiple antibody combinations. A study by the International Bone Marrow Transplant Registry (IBMTR) of unrelated donor transplantation found that depletion with narrow specificity anti-T-cell antibodies yielded superior leukemia-free survival than broad specificity approaches (55). The improvement in outcome was in part due to lower rates of disease relapse and infectious complications.

VII. T-CELL DEPLETION AND ACUTE GVHD

A. Matched Related Transplantation

Most of the commonly employed ex vivo TCD methods used for the past 15–20 years (i.e., soybean lectin agglutination, counterflow centrifugal elutriation, and antibody-based depletion) have been associated with reductions in the incidence of grades II–IV acute GVHD to less than 20–25% after matched sibling marrow transplantation (21,22,30–37,56–58). In many circumstances, a low incidence of GVHD is attained without additional immune suppression.

The ex vivos techniques described above do not lend themselves easily to processing the larger volumes of cells found in mobilized peripheral blood cell allografts. Consequently, newer methods, such as CD34+ selection and the use of high-density microparticles, have been explored in this setting. Studies of HLA-identical sibling PBSCT using CD34+ selection have reported wide variations in rates of acute GVHD (39–43). In these studies, the number of CD3+ cells infused, the number of

CD34+ cells infused, and the use of additional immune-suppressive agents appear to influence the incidence of GVHD (51). There is some question as to the influence of the type of CD34 selection device on GVHD development. However, a study comparing three products (CEPRATE, Isolex 300i, CliniMACs) found no apparent differences in allograft composition or outcome among the three, although ease of processing did differ among the units (59). Even easier than ex vivo engineering is administration of anti-T-cell antibodies in vivo. Treatment with humanized Campath-1H (alemtuzumab) or antithymocyte globulin preparations allows T-cell depletion to be performed in the absence of a cell-processing facility. Prevention of GVHD on a scale similar to other ex vivo TCD techniques has been achieved.

B. Transplantation from Unrelated Donors

Transplant from donors other than HLA-identical sibling donors carries a higher risk of GVHD. Consequently, there has been much interest in TCD in this setting. However, the incidence of acute GVHD is not as low after TCD unrelated donor (URD) transplantation as after TCD related donor transplantation. Graft engineering with anti-CD6 monoclonal antibody yielded an incidence of grades II–IV acute GVHD twice as high in URD marrow recipients as in patients receiving matched related donor marrow (53). Nonetheless, TCD does reduce the risk of acute GVHD after alternative donor transplantation. Reports from the NMDP and other sources indicate that the incidence of acute GVHD after unrelated TCD marrow transplantation is 20–50% (54,60–63), which compares favorably to the 40–75% incidence of acute GVHD observed in series of URD transplants without TCD. In the initial report from the NMDP involving 462 unrelated transplants, T-cell depletion was the most significant factor predicting freedom from severe (grade III–IV) acute GVHD (60). In a retrospective analysis from the IBMTR of 1868 leukemia patients who received allogeneic marrow transplants from donors other than HLA-identical siblings, the incidence of grade II–IV GVHD was 34–38% in the TCD group, as compared to 57% in the non-TCD group ($p < 0.0001$) (54). In the first large prospective randomized trial of T-cell depletion in unrelated marrow transplantation, 410 patients were randomized to receive either TCD with (monoclonal antibody $T_{10}B_9$ or soybean lectin agglutination) or immune suppression with cyclosporine/methotrexate. The incidence of grades III–IV acute GVHD was lower in patients receiving T-cell–depleted marrow plus cyclosporine compared with those receiving cyclosporine/methotrexate (15% vs. 27%; $p < 0.01$) (64).

C. Haploidentical Transplantation

T-cell depletion has permitted successful transplantation from fully haplotype-mismatched related donors. Despite the fact that early studies of TCD in HLA-mismatched related marrow transplants were complicated by high rates of graft failure, recent results are improved (65). In single institution studies, grade II–IV GVHD incidence has ranged from 20 to 40% in recipients of HLA-mismatched marrow (66,67). The most promising results have come from Perugia, where patients were given large numbers of CD34 + mobilized peripheral blood cells after rigorous CD34 selection. When the allograft contained less than 1×10^4 T cells/kg, haploidentical transplantation was performed with a low incidence of GVHD without the need for additional in vivo immunosuppression (52).

D. Nonmyeloablative Transplantation

Nonmyeloablative transplantation is based on the principle that the primary therapeutic benefit of allografting derives from allogeneic graft-vs.-leukemia effects (68,69). Conditioning is administered with chemotherapy or radiotherapy at doses adequate to permit engraftment of allogeneic hematopoietic stem cells, but likely not sufficient to kill significant numbers of tumor cells. Reduced intensity conditioning regimens have extended the potential eligibility for transplantation to those previously considered too fragile for conventional transplantation, including both older patients and patients with compromised organ function. Unfortunately, although reduced intensity regimens have been less toxic in the peri-transplant period, they have been associated with rates of acute GVHD equal to or greater than those noted after conventional ablative allotransplantation. T-cell depletion could be problematic in this setting as the reduced intensity conditioning delivered to the host might not be sufficiently immunosuppressive to prevent rejection of a T-cell–depleted graft.

Only a few attempts to reduce GHVD with ex vivo manipulation through CD34-positive selection or CD8-negative selection have been reported (70). It is in this setting that in vivo T-cell depletion with alemtuzumab or ATG preparations have been more intensely studied, as these antibodies serve the dual purpose of host immune suppression to prevent rejection and donor immune suppression to block GVHD. Phase 2 studies have suggested lower GVHD rates than those reported from series of nonmyelablative transplantation without any form of T-cell depletion.

E. Donor Lymphocyte Infusions

Donor lymphocyte infusions (DLI) can restore remissions in some patients who relapse after transplantation (71,72). Among patients with chronic myelogenous leukemia (CML), 70–80% achieve durable cytogenetic and molecular remissions with DLI in the absence of any chemotherapy. Lesser activity has been observed in patients with multiple myeloma, myelodysplasia, chronic lymphocytic leukemia, and other diseases. Unfortunately, DLI is often associated with GVHD, but remissions can be achieved in the absence of GVHD. Therefore, attempts to prevent GVHD without impacting GVL have been undertaken through selective T-cell depletion, most notably with anti-CD8 antibodies. Phase 2 trials of patients with relapsed hematological malignancies have yielded GVHD rates of 15–35%, lower than the 40–70% reported in a series of patients receiving unmanipulated DLI (70). In a small prospective randomized study for patients at high risk of relapse given prophylactic DLI, six of nine patients (67%) given conventional DLI developed GVHD compared to zero of nine (0%) receiving CD8-depleted DLI (73). No differences in relapse rates or immune reconstitution were noted.

In recent studies donor lymphocytes have been engineered so that the HSV–thymidine kinase is inserted into T cells (74). If GVHD develops after cell infusion, these donor T cells can be eliminated in vivo by subsequent exposure to ganciclovir, to which they have now been rendered susceptible.

VIII. CHRONIC GVHD

It has been more difficult to assess the effect of TCD upon chronic GVHD. Several TCD approaches in use for many years (e.g., soybean lectin agglutination, Campath antibodies, and anti-CD6 antibody + complement) have reported very low rates of chronic GVHD

($<15\%$) in matched sibling transplantation. The results in unrelated transplantation are less clear. In a small randomized trial of rabbit ATG 15 mg/kg in unrelated donor transplantation, patients receiving the ATG had a lower incidence of chronic GVHD than controls (39% vs. 62%; $p = 0.04$) (75). In contrast to these results, the recently reported randomized trial of TCD (using $T_{10}B_9$ or soybean lectin agglutination) plus cyclosporine versus cyclosporine/methotrexate demonstrated no significant difference in chronic GVHD (24% vs. 29%) (64).

IX. ORGAN DYSFUNCTION AFTER TCD TRANSPLANTS

Very few series have focused on the effects of TCD on organ toxicity. However, in several single institution studies, TCD was associated with less hepatic, renal, and pulmonary complications than conventional transplantation. The incidence of hepatic veno-occlusive disease (VOD) has been reported at 3.1% overall and 1.2% in patients receiving total body irradiation (TBI) as part of their conditioning (76). TCD has also been associated with decreased pulmonary complications posttransplant (77). In an analysis of 199 allogeneic transplants, the incidence of life-threatening pulmonary complications within the first 60 days was 8% among patients who received TCD as the sole form of GVHD prophylaxis, but 33% among those who received cyclosporine and methotrexate ($p < 0.0001$) (78). The protective effect of TCD was independent of the diagnosis of acute GVHD. Reductions in organ toxicity were also observed in a randomized trial of TCD plus cyclosporine versus cyclosporine/methotrexate. Pulmonary, hepatic, renal, central nervous system (CNS), and mucosal toxicity as determined by the Bearman toxicity scale revealed a significantly lower incidence and severity of organ damage in the TCD cohort (64). One possible explanation for the decrease in organ toxicity after TCD transplantation is the elimination of the need for pharmacological GVHD prophylaxis. Alternatively, decreases in allogeneic reactions after TCD transplanation could result in reductions in the levels of elaborated cytokines that could be damaging to hepatic, renal, or pulmonary parenchyma.

X. TRANSPLANT-RELATED MORTALITY

Since TCD protects against GVHD and reduces organ dysfunction, one would expect these benefits to translate into lower transplant-related mortality (TRM). Indeed, in several series, TRM after TCD transplants has been low—in some matched sibling TCD transplant series in the range of 2–15% (79–81). In a case-control study involving unrelated marrow recipients in Stockholm and Seattle, patients receiving in vivo TCD with rabbit ATG experienced less nonrelapse mortality than patients not given ATG (19% vs. 35%; $p = 0.005$) (82). However, other TCD studies have reported transplant-related mortality rates from 25 to 40% even after matched sibling transplants, with many deaths being secondary to infection EBV+ lymphoproliferative disorders (83–85). In the large randomized trial evaluating TCD in unrelated marrow recipients (see above), there was no difference in TRM between the groups, suggesting that elements other than GVHD, such as the intensity of conditioning, posttransplant immune suppression, graft failure, and immune reconstitution, play major roles in determining TRM. For TCD to be successful, it must do more than just protect against GVHD.

XI. COSTS AND QUALITY OF LIFE

Since TCD reduces the rates of GVHD and organ toxicity, it would seem that it should also improve overall quality of life (QOL) and reduce transplant-related costs. Few studies have been performed to assess costs. One series did suggest a decrease in inpatient early hospitalization costs in patients receiving TCD transplants, though no significant differences in overall QOL were detected (86).

XII. TCD AND GRAFT FAILURE

Many TCD transplant series in the 1980s and early 1990s reported higher incidences of graft failure than with transplantation of unmanipulated marrow (87–92). The IBMTR reported T-cell depletion to be associated with a ninefold increased risk for graft failure compared to unmanipulated marrow transplantation ($p < 0.0001$) (93). Graft failure can occur early (within the first few weeks) or late (several months after TCD transplant). Early graft failure after TCD transplantation appears to results primarily from immunological rejection by host lymphoid elements that have survived the conditioning process. Host T lymphocytes with donor-specific cytotoxic activity able to suppress donor CFU-GM and CFU-E proliferation in vitro have been identified from the blood of patients at the time of graft rejection (89,94–103). It is less likely that failure of initial engraftment is caused by injury to hematopoietic progenitors or auxiliary cells during marrow manipulation (104–106). The mechanism of late graft failure is poorly understood. No discrete host-derived cells with anti–donor cell activity have been isolated. It is possible that viral infections, such as cytomegalovirus (CMV) or human herpesvirus 6 (HHV-6), may contribute to late graft failure (107–110). However, although patients appear to have a higher risk of CMV reactivation after TCD transplant, (111–113), there is no direct clinical evidence linking these viruses to graft failure. The presence of mixed lymphoid and myeloid chimerism after TCD transplantation appears to be associated with graft failure, implying a state of immune tolerance between the graft and host (114–119). Graft failure may result when host lymphoid tolerance of the graft is broken.

Why T-cell depletion should lead to graft failure or rejection is still unclear. TCD or marrow manipulation removes cells that promote engraftment, perhaps by suppressing host-derived T lymphocytes or dendritic cells that could participate in the rejection process. Some murine models have suggested that NK cells are critical to engraftment (120), while others have implicated CD8+ T-cells (121). In a recent human trial using T-cell–depleted donor grafts with the addition of graded dose of CD4+ and CD8+ cells, it appeared that depletion of donor CD8+ cells, but not CD4+ cells, was associated with increased graft rejection (122).

Approaches to address the increased risk of graft failure associated with T-cell depletion have included increased myeloablation, increased host-directed immune suppression, modulation of T-cell removal, narrowing of the breadth of TCD, and infusion of increased numbers of hematopoietic precursors. Intensifying the conditioning regimen with additional chemotherapy may clear the host marrow more effectively, and thus increase "hematopoietic space" for the incoming donor graft, but the benefit of decreased graft failure may be offset by increased regimen-related toxicity (123–127). Increased immunosuppression with irradiation (total lymphoid or body irradiation), corticosteroids, or in vivo anti-T cell antibodies to target alloreactive T-cells has been reportedly successful in preventing graft rejection in phase 2 trials (45,84,91,128–133). T-cell add-back following marrow processing has yielded promising results in several settings, but this strategy can be problematic because of the potential for precipitation of GVHD (134,135). Selective removal of T cells appears to result in decreased graft failure rates when compared to broader methods. Studies using anti-CD5 immunotoxins, anti-CD6, and anti-TCR$\alpha\beta$ (T$_{10}$B$_9$) antibodies have all demonstrated low graft failure rates (1–3%) without compromising GVHD prophylaxis (12–20% GVHD) (34–37,55). The randomized trial of TCD in which T$_{10}$B$_9$ antibody was the predominant method used versus cyclosporine/methotrexate found no difference between groups with respect to neutrophil or platelet engraftment (64).

Dose escalation of CD34+ stem cells may be another effective way to overcome graft failure after TCD. Preclinical models have shown that mice given megadoses of TCD marrow engrafted despite sublethal doses of conditioning irradiation (136). In human studies, the addition of CD34+ cells to TCD marrow to augment stem cell dose has permitted reliable engraftment in leukemia patients despite full HLA haplotype mismatches (137). A subset of progenitor cells, called veto cells, may be responsible for the induction of tolerance in these high stem cell dose transplants (138). It is also possible that ex vivo T-cell depletion of mobilized peripheral blood progenitor cells may not carry the same risk of graft failure because of the increased number of CD34 cells infused with peripheral blood compared to bone marrow transplants. Recent experience with CD8 depletion of mobilized peripheral blood has been associated with no episodes of graft rejection, which contrasts with studies previously performed with CD8 depletion of bone marrow (57,139).

XIII. DELAYED IMMUNE RECONSTITUTION

Since TCD marrow contains fewer T cells than unmanipulated marrow grafts, delayed T-cell immune reconstitution is a concern after TCD (140–147). Total lymphocyte numbers are usually higher early after BMT in recipients of conventional marrow transplants compared to those who receive TCD grafts. Furthermore, the reconstituted T-cell compartment is predominantly of the CD8+ subset, and most TCD patients will have a deficit in CD4+ cells, with an inverted CD4+:CD8 + ratio for up to 2 years (141). The number of CD4+ cells normalizes at 7–9 months after conventional transplant, but this process is delayed after TCD (142). Functional recovery of T cells appears to be impaired after TCD. The proliferative response of peripheral blood mononuclear cells to exogenous IL-2 stimulation is abnormal for up to 6 months, compared to only 1 month for recipients of a conventional transplant (140). Similarly, the proliferative response of T cells to mitogenic stimulation can be impaired for over 18 months in recipients of TCD marrow (141). T lymphocytes from recipients of TCD transplants have restricted variability in their TCR repertoires (145,148). The T-cell compartment after transplantation is largely expanded from lymphocytes co-transfused with the marrow, and therefore recipients of TCD transplants would have much fewer precursors with which to reconstitute their repertoire than recipients of conventional transplants. CDR3 spectratyping has revealed that patients with persistent mixed chimerism after TCD have marked abnormal TCR repertoires, while others who had converted to full donor hematopoiesis possess a normal spectrum of TCR variability (148). Impairment of T-cell neogenesis as assessed by generation of T-cell receptor excision circles (TREC) has been noted after TCD and has correlated with increased risk of infection (149,150). The delayed reconstitution in numbers of CD4+ cells and impaired recovery of T-cell repertoire diversity have not been associated with an increased risk of bacterial or fungal infections after TCD transplantation. However, several studies have demonstrated a higher probability of reactivation for herpesviruses such as CMV (64,111–113,151,152).

XIV. POSTTRANSPLANT LYMPHOPROLIFERATIVE DISEASE

Posttransplant lymphoproliferative disease (PTLD), usually associated with Epstein-Barr virus, is uncommon after conventional transplantation. In contrast to recipients of unmanipulated marrow, PTLD is a concern after TCD, with an incidence as high as 20–30% in some circumstances (153,154). Recipients of TCD transplants using HLA-mismatched or unrelated donor marrow appear to be at particularly high risk, as are patients with severe GVHD and those treated with certain anti-T-cell monoclonal antibodies (153,155,156). PTLD is thought to arise from virally infected donor B cells, which have been co-transplanted with the allograft. If immune surveillance is compromised by the removal of donor EBV-specific cytotoxic T cells, then those B cells may proliferate in the host and develop into a polyclonal or monoclonal process.

Restoration of anti-B-cell immunity through the administration of unselected bulk DLI (157) or EBV-specific CTL cultivated in vitro from donor lymphocytes has proven to be effective treatment in many cases of PTLD (158–160). Recent data would suggest that it may not be necessary to resort to cellular therapy, and its potential for GVHD as anti-B cell antibodies, including the anti-CD20 monoclonal antibody rituximab, has induced durable remissions in a number of patients (161–163). Prevention of PTLD after TCD transplantation may be achieved by using methods of purging that also remove B-cells (e.g., Camapth antibodies or CD34+ cell selection) or by purging with B-cell monoclonal antibodies in addition to specific T-cell antibodies (164,165). Prophylactic administration of EBV-specific CTL has also been effective (160). Early detection of EBV reactivation with PCR-based methods may help to identify patients appropriate for preemptive therapy with either cellular or antibody-based modalities (166,167).

XV. TCD AND LEUKEMIA RELAPSE

An increased incidence of leukemia relapse associated with TCD was first reported in a randomized trial that included 40 patients with acute and chronic leukemia (32). Of the 20 patients randomized to the TCD arm, 7 had clinically apparent relapse, compared to only 2 in the control (non-TCD) arm. Multiple retrospective studies have subsequently demonstrated that disease relapse is more frequent after TCD, especially for CML (86,168–173). The increased rate of leukemia relapse after TCD has been linked, as least in part, to the reduction in GVHD and concomitant loss of the graft-vs.-leukemia (GVL) activity. Leukemia patients who develop clinically significant GVHD generally have a lower incidence of relapse than those without GVHD (174–176). More convincing evidence linking T cells and GVL comes from studies using donor lymphocyte infusions in patients with CML who have relapsed after transplantation, where complete response rates of 70–80% are achieved (71,72).

The effect of TCD on relapse has been less striking after unrelated transplantation (61,62,177–179). An analysis of unrelated transplant recipients from the EBMT indicated that TCD was associated with a significantly higher incidence of relapse in the univariate analysis, but not in the multivariate analysis (180). The prospective randomized trial of

TCD versus cyclosporine/methotrexate as GVHD prophylaxis (see above) did show a modestly increased relapse incidence (16% vs. 6%) in the TCD arm (64).

In contrast to CML, TCD has only a modest effect on the relapse rates of patients transplanted for acute leukemia (79,83,181–183). Retrospective data from the IBMTR show that TCD was associated with a 1.5- to 2.0-fold increased risk for recurrence in patients with acute lymphoblastic leukemia (ALL) in any phase and in patients with AML who were transplanted in relapse or in first complete remission (93). Acute myelogenous leukemia (AML) patients transplanted in second CR actually had a lower risk of relapse with T-cell depletion. In two separate randomized trials comparing TCD with methotrexate and cyclosporine as GVHD prophylaxis for leukemia patients undergoing HLA-identical related or unrelated transplantation, a higher relapse rate was observed after TCD only in patients with CML, but not in patients with acute leukemia (64,184).

The extent and specificity of TCD may influence its effect on relapse rates. An IBMTR analysis of 870 patients who underwent T-depleted unrelated or mismatched donor transplants for leukemia demonstrated that the relapse rates for patients whose grafts were T depleted with "narrow specificity" antibodies (e.g., anti-CD5, CD6, anti-TCR$\alpha\beta$) were significantly lower than those whose grafts had been T depleted with "broad specificity" antibodies (e.g., anti-CD2, ATG, Campath antibodies, elutriation, or lectin/SRBC agglutination) (55). The 5-year relapse rate in recipients of narrow specificity TCD was similar to that observed in recipients of unmanipulated transplants suggesting that, at least in the setting of unrelated or mismatched transplants, TCD using narrow specificity antibodies was not associated with loss of GVL activity.

It has long been hoped that distinct cellular subsets that mediate GVL and GVH could be identified so that those cells in the graft that cause GVHD could be eliminated while maintaining those responsible for GVL. The problem, of course, is identifying those subsets. In humans, CD8+ T cells have clearly been implicated; infiltrates of CD8+ T cells are often found in target organs of patients with GVHD. Also, the presence of high numbers of CD8+ T cells in peripheral blood early posttransplant has been associated with the development of GVHD (185). A small, randomized trial of patients receiving either CD8-depleted or unmanipulated marrow showed that those receiving CD8+-depleted marrow experienced significantly less grade II–IV GVHD. The leukemia relapse rate was similar between the two groups, suggesting that CD8+-depletion reduced GVHD without abolishing GVL (85). CD8-depleted DLI significantly reduces the incidence of GVHD, but retains important GVL activity with preserved clinical responses in patients with CML (186,187). A randomized study of CD8 depletion in patients receiving DLI showed a reduction in acute GVHD from 66% to 0% without loss of GVL activity (73). However, separating GVH from GVL is likely to be far more complicated.

The administration or manipulation of cytotoxic effectors cells after TCD-transplantation to reduce relapse rates is under investigation. Patients undergoing TCD related donor transplantation for CML using either anti-CD6 and anti-TCR antibodies and complement have similar disease-free survival after salvage therapy with DLI despite a comparatively high initial relapse rate (80,188). A retrospective analysis of CML patients receiving CD34+ peripheral blood cells with T-cell add-back demonstrated a lower rate of GVHD and superior 3-year survival (90%) compared with recipients of unmanipulated mobilized peripheral blood (68%; $p < 0.03$) or bone marrow (63%; $p < 0.01$) (189). Taken together, these results suggest that TCD transplants followed by posttransplant DLI at, or even before, disease relapse could be sa reasonable option for patients with CML.

For this strategy to be optimally effective, the TCD transplant itself must be of sufficiently low morbidity that patients are stable enough to receive DLI. Also, DLI must reduce relapse rates without inducing GVHD, perhaps by lowering the dose of lymphocytes infused, selectively depleting cell subsets from the lymphocyte pool, or by suicide gene insertion (74,186,187,190–192).

The success of DLI in salvaging CML patients after transplantation has led to investigation of T-cell infusions after TCD in other diseases. Twenty-four patients with myeloma who underwent a TCD transplant were given DLI at 6 months. Of the 11 patients who had persistent myeloma, 10 responses (6 CR, 4 PR) were observed after DLI. The 2-year-progression free survival for all 14 patients who received DLI was significantly improved compared to a comparable historical cohort who received TCD transplants without DLI (193).

The role of NK cells in preventing relapse after TCD transplantation has also been under study. The ability to expand or activate NK cells in vivo or ex vivo with cytokines such as IL-2 has prompted several clinical trials. Prolonged infusion of recombinant interleukin-2 (rIL-2) following TCD allogeneic transplants is well tolerated and results in a marked increase in cytotoxic NK cells with a suggestion that such treatment lowers the incidence of disease relapse relative to historical controls (194). The identification of killer immunoglobulin-like receptors (KIR) on NK cells has generated renewed interest in their role in controlling relapse. These receptors recognize groups of HLA class I (particularly HLA-Bx4 and HLA-C) alleles and, when engaged, will result in inhibition of NK reactivity. Absence of recognition of these alleles on a cell can trigger NK-cell destruction of that target. In an analysis of patients who received allografts mismatched at the HLA-C or Bw4 locus in the direction of GVHD, donor versus recipient alloreactive NK-cell clones could be isolated posttransplant in patients without evidence of GVHD (195). These alloreactive NK-cell clones could lyse pretransplant cryopreserved leukemia cells in vitro, suggesting that GVL activity mediated by NK cells exists in these patients without GVHD. In the setting of haploidentical transplantation under conditions of exhaustive T-cell depletion, donor NK activity appears to protect against relapse of AML without inducing GVHD, perhaps in part by eliminating host antigen-presenting cells (196,197). Such a role for NK cells may be limited to conditions of haploidentical transplantation and extensive TCD, as one analysis of KIR incompatibility as assessed by HLA-Bw4 and -C discrepancies in unrelated transplants showed no advantage in terms of relapse or GVHD (198).

XVI. ALTERNATIVE APPROACHES FOR GRAFT ENGINEERING

A. Functional T-Cell Depletion

Rather than focusing upon removal of anatomical subsets of T cells, some investigators have turned their attention to TCD techniques in which only alloreactive T cells are removed from the graft through either photoinactivation (199) or immunological purging. After priming by recipient mononuclear cells in vitro, alloreactive donor cells can be identified by expression of activation markers, such as CD25, CD69, CD71, or HLA-DR. These cells can then be separated from the remaining cells by immunomagnetic cell sorting (200–202). In one study, approximately 90% of the alloreactive component was purged while preserving >70% residual immunity as measured by third-party alloantigen response (200).

B. Induction of T-Cell Anergy

In experimental models, blockade of costimulatory pathways (e.g., CD28/B7, LFA-1/ICAM, CD40/CD40L) induces a state of alloimmune tolerance and thereby prevents the development of GVHD (203–205). In a small pilot series, patients were transplanted with HLA-mismatched bone marrow that had been treated in vitro with CTLA4-Ig in the presence of donor antigen-presenting cells (206). All patients engrafted and 3 of 11 patients were reported to have GVHD. If distinct targets for GVHD and GVL can be identified, it may ultimately be possible to induce GVHD-specific anergy while preserving the T-cell response to tumor antigens for a full GVL effect.

C. Suicide Gene Insertion

The insertion of herpes simplex thymidine kinase (HS-TK) gene into donor T lymphocytes renders them susceptible to destruction with ganciclovir. Recipients who develop GVHD after infusion can theoretically be treated systemically to eliminate the infused T cells (74,192,207). The use of "suicide" gene therapy may also be applicable in conjunction with TCD transplants. HS-TK gene modified T lymphocytes infused along with TCD marrow at the time of transplantation do not appear to interfere with engraftment (207). These gene-modified cells can be detected for months after infusion. In two of three patients who received engineered cells and who developed acute GVHD, a complete response was observed upon treatment with ganciclovir. Chronic cutaneous GVHD responsive to ganciclovir has also been reported in a patient who had received T cells bearing the HS-TK gene at the time of BMT (208).

D. Vaccine Strategies

As new leukemia antigens are identified that are potential targets for the GVL response, allogeneic tumor vaccines may be developed to stimulate specific antitumor activity without GVHD after TCD. In a murine model, mice that had undergone T-cell–depleted transplantation could mount a donor-cell–mediated antitumor response without GVHD after vaccination with irradiated tumor cells genetically engineered to secrete GM-CSF (209). It is not clear whether TCD will render human subjects immune incompetent so that they unable to respond to vaccination. Rather than vaccinating recipients, it may be possible to vaccinate donors in vivo or perhaps donor cells in vitro prior to graft infusion, thereby transferring immune effectors to the host. Still to be determined are the precise antigen and adjuvants needed for optimium immunization and whether TCD will completely eliminate transfer of protective effector populations.

E. T-Cell Modification

CD4 T cells can be divided into Th1 and Th2 subsets and CD8 T cells into Tc1 and Tc2 populations. The type 1 and 2 cells secrete different sets of cytokines—IL-2 and IFNY (type 1) and IL-4, IL-5, IL-10 (type 2). Animal data suggest that polarizing T-cell populations to the Th2 and Tc2 group may help suppress GVHD while preventing graft rejection (210,211). Clinical trials evaluating the additions of Th2 cells after nonablative transplantation are underway (212). In a similar manner, the recognition of CD4+ CD25+ cells with regulatory activity has prompted interest in isolating and expanding these cells for clinical use. Murine models show that these cells may play a role in reducing lethality due to GVHD (213–216).

XVII. CONCLUSIONS

Graft engineering to reduce the incidence of GVHD has been studied in clinical trials for over 20 years. There is no question that T-cell depletion can reduce the risk and severity of GVHD and in most cases reduce transplant-related mortality. However, it has yet to be definitively demonstrated that graft manipulation improves overall survival after transplantation. It is clear that T cells included in a marrow or peripheral blood graft serve many different functions. How to manipulate these grafts to minimize GVHD while preserving immunological integrity to fight infection and destroy residual tumor is an ongoing challenge. These questions will not be fully resolved until there is a better understanding of the pathogenesis of GVHD. Hopefully, the role of minor HLA antigens can soon be defined and antigen targets for GVHD and GVL can potentially be exploited through graft engineering. Separating GVH and GVL is critical for transplantation to emerge from the dark ages to enjoy widespread application in the future.

REFERENCES

1.   Ferrara JL, Levy R, Chao NJ. Pathophysiologic mechanisms of acute graft-versus-host disease Biol Blood Marrow Transplant 1999; 5:347–356.
2.   Martin PJ, Schoch G, Fisher L, Byers V, Anasetti C, Appelbaum F, Beatty P, Doney K, McDonald GB, Sanders JE. A retrospective analysis of therapy for acute graft-versus-host disease: initial treatment. Blood 1990; 76:1464–1472.
3.   Weisdorf D, Haake R, Blazar B, Miller W, McGlave P, Ramsay N, Kersey J, Filipovich A. Treatment of moderate/severe acute graft-versus-host disease after allogeneic bone marrow transplantation: an analysis of clinical risk features and outcome. Blood 1990; 75:1024–1030.
4.   Sullivan KM, Agura E, Anasetti C, Appelbaum FR, Badger C, Bearman S, et al. Chronic graft-versus-host disease and other late complications of bone marrow transplantation. Semin Hematol 1991; 28:250–259.
5.   Ho VY, Soiffer RJ. The history and future of T-cell depletion as graft-versus-host disease prophylaxis for allogeneic hematopoietic stem cell transplantation. Blood 2001; 98:3192–3204.
6.   Uphoff DE. Preclusion of secondary phase of irradiation syndrome by innoculation of hematopoietic tissue following lethal total body x-irradiation. J Natl Cancer Inst 1958; 20:625–631.
7.   Hill GR, Teshima T, Gerbitz A, Pan L, Cooke KR, Brinson YS, Crawford J, Ferrara JL. Differential roles of IL-1 and TNF-alpha on graft-versus-host disease and graft versus leukemia. J Clin Invest 1999; 104:459–467.
8.   Antin JH, Ferrara JLM. Cytokine dysregulation and acute graft-v-host disease. Blood 1992; 80:2964–2968.
9.   Hill GR, Crawford JM, Cooke KR, Brinson YS, Pan L, Ferrara JL. Total body irradiation and acute graft-versus-host disease: the role of gastrointestinal damage and inflammatory cytokines. Blood 1997; 90:3204–3213.
10. Antin JH, Lee SJ, Neuberg D, Alyea E, Soiffer RJ, Sonis S, Ferrara JLM. A phase I/II double-masked, placebo-controlled study of recombinant human interleukin-11 (rhIL-11) for mucositis and GVHD prevention in allogeneic transplantation. Bone Marrow Transplant 2002; 29:373–378.
11. Antin JH, Weisdorf D, Neuberg D, Nicklow R, Clouthier S, Lee SJ, Alyea E, McGarigle C, Blazar B, Sonis S, Soiffer SJ, Ferrara JLM. Interleukin-1 blockade does not prevent acute graft versus host disease. Results of a randomized, double blind, placebo-controlled trial of interleukin 1 receptor antagonist in allogeneic bone marrow transplantation. Blood 2002; 100:3479–3482.

12. Dicke KA, van Hoot JIM, van Bekkum DW. The selective elimination of immunologically competent cells from bone marrow and lymphatic cell mixtures. II. Mouse spleen cell fractionation on a discontinuous albumin gradient. Transplantation 1968; 6:562–568.

13. Reisner Y, Itzicovitch L, Meshorer A, Sharon N. Hematopoietic stem cell transplantation using mouse bone marrow and spleen cells fractionated by lectins. Proc Natl Acad Sci USA 1978; 75:2933–2936.

14. Trentin JJ, Judd KP. Prevention of acute graft-versus-host (GVH) mortality with spleen-absorbed antithymocyte globulin (ATG). Transplant Proc 1973; 5:865–868.

15. Rodt H, Kolb HJ, Netzel B, Rieder I, Janka G, Belohradsky B, Haas RJ, Thierfelder S. GVHD suppression by incubation of bone marrow grafts with anti-T-cell globulin: effect in canine model and application to clinical bone marrow transplantation. Transplant Proc 1979; 11:962–966.

16. Korngold R, Sprent J. Lethal graft-versus-host disease after bone marrow transplantation across minor histocompatibility barriers in mice. Prevention by removing mature T cells from marrow. J Exp Med 1978; 148:1687–1698.

17. Rodt H, Theirfelder S, Eulitz M. Antilymphocyte antibodies and marrow transplantation. III. Effect of heterologous anti-brain antibodies on acute secondary disease in mice. Eur J Immunol 1974; 4:15–19.

18. Kolb HJ, Rieder I, Rodt H, Netzel B, Grosse-Wilde H, Scholz S, Schaffer E, Kolb H, Thierfelder S. Antilymphocyte antibodies and marrow transplantation. VI. Graft-versus-host tolerance in DLA-incompatible dogs after in vitro treatment of bone marrow absorbed with antithymocyte globulin. Transplantation 1979; 27:242–245.

19. Vallera DA, Soderling CC, Carlson GJ, Kersey JH. Bone marrow transplantation across major histocompatibility barriers in mice. Transplantation 1981; 31:218–222.

20. Reisner Y, Kapoor N, Kirkpatrick D, Pollack MS, Dupont B, Good RA, O'Reilly RJ. Transplantation for acute leukemia with HLA-A and B nonidentical parental marrow cells fractionated with soybean agglutinin and sheep red blood cells. Lancet 1981; 2(8242):327–331.

21. Reisner Y, Kapoor N, Kirkpatrick D, Pollack MS, Cunningham-Rundles S, Dupont B, Hodes MZ, Good RA, O'Reilly RJ. Transplantation for severe combined immunodeficiency with HLA-A, B, D, DR incompatibility parental marrow cells fractionated by soybean agglutinin and sheep red blood cells. Blood 1983; 161:341–348.

22. De Witte T, Hoogenhout J, de Pauw B, Holdrinet R, Janssen J, Wessels J, van Daal W, Hustinx T, Haanen C. Depletion of donor lymphocytes by counterflow centrifugation successfully prevents acute graft-versus-host disease in matched allogeneic marrow transplantation. Blood 1986; 67:1302–1308.

23. Noga SJ, Donnenberg AD, Schwartz CL, Strauss LC, Civin CI, Santos GW. Development of a simplified counterflow centrifugation elutriation procedure for depletion of lymphocytes from human bone marrow. Transplantation 1986; 41:220–225.

24. Lowenberg B, Wagemaker E, van Bekkum DW, et al. Graft-versus-host disease following transplantation of "one log" versus "two log" T-lymphocyte depleted bone marrow from HLA-identical donors. Bone Marrow Transplant 1986; 1:133–140.

25. Prentice HG, Blacklock HA, Janossy G, Bradstock KF, Skeggs D, Goldstein G, Hoffbrand AV. Use of anti-T-cell monoclonal antibody OKT3 to prevent acute graft versus host disease in allogeneic bone marrow transplantation for acute leukemia. Lancet 1982; 1(8274):700–703.

26. Filipovich AH, McGlave PB, Ramsay NKC, Goldstein G, Warkentin PI, Kesey JH. Pretreatment of donor bone marrow with monoclonal antibody OKT3 for prevention of acute graft versus host disease in allogeneic histocompatible bone marrow transplantation. Lancet 1982; 1(8284):1266–1269.

27. Martin PJ, Hansen JA, Thomas ED. Preincubation of donor bone marrow cells with a combination of murine monclonal anti-T-cell antibodies without complement does not prevent graft-versus-host disease after allogeneic marrow transplantation. J Clin Immunol 1984; 4:18–22.

28. Waldmann HG, Polliak A, Hale G, Or R, Cividalli G, Weiss L, Weshler Z, Samuel S, Manor D, Brautbar C, et al. Elimination of graft-versus-host disease by in vitro depletion of alloreactive lymphocytes with a monoclonal rat anti-human lymphocyte antibody (Campath-1). Lancet 1984; 2(8401):483–486.

29. Martin PJ, Hansen JA, Buckner CD, Sanders JE, Deeg HJ, Stewart P, Appelbaum FR, Clift R, Fefer A, Witherspoon RP, et al. Effects of in vitro depletion of T cells in HLA-identical allogeneic marrow grafts. Blood 1985; 66:664–672.

30. Herve P, Cahn JY, Flesch M, Plouvier E, Racadot E, Noir A, Couteret Y, Goldstein G, Bernard A, Lenys R, et al. Successful graft-versus-host disease prevention without graft failure in 32 HLA-identical allogeneic bone marrow transplantations with marrow depleted of T cells by monoclonal antibodies and complement. Blood 1987; 69:388–393.

31. Trigg ME, Billing R, Sondel PM, Exten R, Hong R, Bozdech MJ, Horowitz SD, Finlay JL, Moen R, Longo W, Erickson C, Peterson A. Clinical trial depleting T lymphocytes from donor marrow for matched and mismatched allogeneic bone marrow transplants. Canc Treat Rep 1985; 69:377–386.

32. Mitsuyasu RT, Champlin RE, Gale RP, Ho WG, Lenarsky C, Winston D, Selch M, Elashoff R, Giorgi JV, Wells J, et al. Treatment of donor bone marrow with monoclonal anti-T-cell antibody and complement for the prevention of graft versus host disease. Ann Int Med 1986; 105:20–26.

33. Maraninchi D, Gluckman E, Blaise D, Guyotat D, Pico JL, Leblond V, Michallet M, Dreyfus M, Ifrah I, Bordigoni P. Impact of T-cell depletion on outcome of allogeneic bone-marrow transplantation for standard-risk leukaemia. Lancet 1987; 2(8552):175–178.

34. Soiffer RJ, Murray C, Mauch P, Anderson KC, Freedman AS, Rabinowe SN, Takvorian T, Robertson MJ, Spector N, Gonin R, Miller KB, Rudders RA, Freeman A, Blake K, Coral F, Nadler LM, Ritz J. Prevention of graft-versus-host disease by selective depletion of CD6-positive T lymphocytes from donor bone marrow. J Clin Oncol 1992; 10:1191–2000.

35. Laurent G, Maraninchi D, Gluckman E, Vernant JP, Derocq JM, Gaspard MH, Rio B, Michalet M, Reiffers J, Dreyfus F, et al. Donor bone marrow treatment with T101 Fab fragment-ricin A-chain immunotoxin prevents graft-versus-host disease. Bone Marrow Transplant 1989; 4:367–372.

36. Filipovich AH, Vallera D, McGlave P, Filipovich AH, Vallera D, McGlave P, Polich D, Gajl-Peczalska K, Haake R, Lasky L, Blazar B, Ramsay NK, Kersey J. T cell depletion with anti-CD5 immunotoxin in histocompatible bone marrow transplantation. Transplantation 1990; 50:410–414.

37. Antin JH, Bierer BE, Smith BR, Ferrara J, Guinan EC, Sieff C, Macklis RM, Tarbell NJ, Golan D, Lynch E, Reichert T, Blythman H, Bouloux C, Rappeport JM, Burakoff SJ, Weinstein HJ. Selective depletion of bone marrow T lymphocytes with anti-CD5 monoclonal antibodies: effective prophylaxis for graft-versus-host disease in patients with hematologic malignancies. Blood 1991; 78:2139–2144.

38. Vartdal F, Kvalheim G, Lea TE, Bosnes V, Gaudernack G, Ugelstad J, Albrechtsen D. Depletion of T lymphocytes from human bone marrow. Use of magnetic monosized polymer microspheres coated with T-lymphocyte-specific monoclonal antibodies. Transplantation 1987; 43(3):366–371.

39. Dreger P, Viehmann K, Steinmann J, Eckstein V, Muller-Ruchholtz W, Loffler H, Schmitz N. G-CSF-mobilized peripheral blood progenitor cells for allogeneic transplantation: comparison of T cell depletion strategies using different CD34 + selection systems or Campath-1. Exp Hem 1995; 23:147–154.

40. Finke J, Brugger W, Bertz H, Behringer D, Kunzmann R, Weber-Nordt RM, Kanz L, Mertelsmann R. Allogeneic transplantation of positively selected peripheral blood CD34+ progenitor cells from matched related donors. Bone Marrow Transplant 1996; 18:1081–1085.

41. Socie G, Cayuela JM, Raynal B, Esperou H, Fund X, Raffoux C, Devergie A, Ribaud P, Marolleau JP, Parquet N, Sigaux F, Brison O, Gluckman E. Influence of CD34 cell selection

on the incidence of mixed chimaerism and minimal residual disease after allogeneic unrelated donor transplantation. Leukemia 1998; 12:1440–1446.

42. Urbano-Ispizua A, Solano C, Brunet S, de la Rubia J, Odriozola J, Zuazu J, Figuera A, Caballero D, Martinez C, Garcia J, Sanz G, Torrabadella M, Alegre A, Perez-Oteiza J, Jurado M, Oyonarte S, Sierra J, Garcia-Conde J, Rozman C. Allogeneic transplantation of selected CD34+ cells from peripheral blood: experience of 62 cases using immunoadsorption or immunomagnetic technique. Bone Marrow Transplant 1998; 22:519–524.

43. Vij R, Brown R, Shenoy S, Haug JS, Kaesberg D, Adkins D, Goodnough LT, Khoury H, DiPersio J. Allogeneic peripheral blood stem cell transplantation following CD34+ enrichment by density gradient separation. Bone Marrow Transplant 2000; 25:1223–1228.

44. Hale G, Jacobs P, Wood L, Fibbe WE, Barge R, Novitzky N, Toit C, Abrahams L, Thomas V, Bunjes D, Duncker C, Wiesneth M, Selleslag D, Hidajat M, Starobinski M, Bird P, Waldmann H. CD52 antibodies for prevention of graft-versus-host disease and graft rejection following transplantation of allogeneic peripheral blood stem cells. Bone Marrow Transplant 2000; 26:69–75.

45. Henslee-Downey PJ, Parrish RS, MacDonald JS, Romond EH, Marciniak E, Coffey C, Ciocci G, Thompson JS. Combined in vitro and in vivo T lymphocyte depletion for the control of graft-versus-host disease following haploidentical marrow transplant. Transplantation 1996; 61:738–743.

46. Spitzer TR, McAfee S, Sackstein R, Colby C, Toh HC, Multani P, Saidman S, Weyouth DW, Preffer F, Poliquin C, Foley A, Cox B, Andrews D, Sachs DH, Sykes M. Intentional induction of mixed chimerism and achievement of antitumor responses after nonmyeloablative conditioning therapy and HLA-matched donor bone marrow transplantation for refractory hematologic malignancies. Biol Blood Marrow Transplant 2002; 6:309–315.

47. Perez-Simon JA, Kottaridis PD, Martino R, Craddock C, Caballero D, Chopra R, Garcia-Conde J, Milligan DW, Schey S, Urbano-Ispizua A, Parker A, Leon A, Yong K, Sureda A, Hunter A, Sierra J, Goldstone AH, Linch DC, San Miguel JF, Mackinnon S. Nonmyeloablative transplantation with or without alemtuzumab: comparison between 2 prospective studies in patients with lymphoproliferative disorders. Blood 2002; 100:3121–3127.

48. Goulmy E, Schipper R, Pool J, Goulmy E, Schipper R, Pool J, Blokland E, Falkenburg JH, Vossen J, Grathwohl A, Vogelsang GB, van Houwelingen HC, van Rood JJ. Mismatches of minor histocompatibility antigens between HLA-identical donors and recipients and development of graft-versus-host disease after bone marrow transplantation. N Engl J Med 1996; 334:281–285.

49. Kernan NA, Collins NM, Juliano L, Cartagena T, Dupont B, O'Reilly RJ. Clonable T lymphocytes in T cell-depleted bone marrow transplants correlate with development of graft-v-host disease. Blood 1986; 68:770–773.

50. Martin PJ, Hansen JA. Quantitative assays for detection of residual T cells in T-depleted human marrow. Blood 1985; 65:1134–1139.

51. Urbano-Ispizua A, Rozman C, Pimentel P, Solano C, de la Rubia J, Brunet S, Perez-Oteyza J, Ferra C, Zuazu J, Caballero D, Bargay J, Carvalhais A, Diez JL, Espigado I, Alegre A, Rovira M, Campilho F, Odriozola J, Sanz MA, Sierra J, Garcia-Conde J, Montserrat E. Risk factors for acute graft-versus-host disease in patients undergoing transplantation with CD34+ selected blood cells from HLA-identical siblings Blood 2002; 100:724–727.

52. Aversa F, Tabilio A, Velardi A, Cunningham I, Terenzi A, Falzetti F, Ruggeri L, Barbabietola G, Aristei C, Latini P, Reisner Y, Martelli MF. Treatment of high-risk acute leukemia with T-cell-depleted stem cells from related donors with one fully mismatched HLA haplotype. N Engl J Med 1998; 339:1186–1193.

53. Alyea EP, Weller E, Fisher DC, Freedman AS, Gribben JG, Lee S, Schlossman RL, Stone RM, Friedberg J, DeAngelo D, Liney D, Windawi S, Ng A, Mauch P, Antin JH, Soiffer RJ. Comparable outcome with T-cell-depleted unrelated-donor versus related-donor allogeneic bone marrow transplantation. Biol Blood Marrow Transplant 2002; 8:601–607.

54. Kawanishi Y, Passweg J, Drobyski WR, Rowlings P, Cook-Craig A, Casper J, Pietryga D, Garbrecht F, Camitta B, Horowitz M, Juckett M, Margolis D, Flomenberg N, Keever-Taylor CA. Effect of T cell subset dose on outcome of T cell-depleted bone marrow transplantation. Bone Marrow Transplant 1997; 19:1069–1074.

55. Champlin RE, Passweg JR, Zhang MJ, Rowlings PA, Pelz CJ, Atkinson KA, Barrett AJ, Cahn JY, Drobyski WR, Gale RP, Goldman JM, Gratwohl A, Gordon-Smith EC, Henslee-Downey PJ, Herzig RH, Klein JP, Marmont AM, RJ OR, Ringden O, Slavin S, Sobocinski KA, Speck B, Weiner RS, Horowitz MM. T-cell depletion of bone marrow transplants for leukemia from donors other than HLA-identical siblings: advantage of T-cell antibodies with narrow specificities. Blood 2000; 95:3996–4002.

56. Hale G, Cobbold S, Waldmann H. T-cell depletion with Campath-1 in allogeneic bone marrow transplantation. Transplantation 1988; 45:753–759.

57. Champlin R, Ho W, Gajewski J, Feig S, Burnison M, Holley G, Greenberg P, Lee K, Schmid I, Giorgi J, Yam P, Petz L, Winston D, Warner N, Reichert T. Selective depletion of CD8+ T lymphocytes for prevention of graft-versus-host disease after allogeneic bone marrow transplantation. Blood 1990; 76:418–423.

58. Wagner JE, Santos GW, Noga SJ, Rowley SD, Davis J, Vogelsang GB, Farmer ER, Zehnbauer BA, Saral R, Donneberg AD. Bone marrow graft engineering by counterflow elutriation: results of a phase I-II clinical trial. Blood 1990; 75:1370–1375.

59. O'Donnell PV, Myers B, Edwards J, Loper K, Rhubart P, Noga SJ. CD34 selection using three immunoselection devices: comparison of T-cell depleted allografts. Cytotherapy 2001; 3:483–488.

60. Kernan NA, Bartsch G, Ash RC, Beatty PG, Champlin R, Filipovich A, Gajewski J, Hansen JA, Henslee-Downey J, McCullough J, et al. Analysis of 462 transplantations from unrelated donors facilitated by the National Marrow Donor Program. N Engl J Med 1993; 328:593–602.

61. Soiffer RJ, Weller E, Alyea EP, Mauch P, Webb IL, Fisher DC, Freedman AS, Schlossman RL, Gribben J, Lee S, Anderson KC, Marcus K, Stone RM, Antin JH, Ritz J. CD6+ donor marrow T-cell depletion as the sole form of graft-versus-host disease prophylaxis in patients undergoing allogeneic bone marrow transplant from unrelated donors. J Clin Oncol 2001; 19:1152–1159.

62. Drobyski WR, Ash RC, Casper JT, McAuliffe T, Horowitz MM, Lawton C, Keever C, Baxter-Lowe LA, Camitta B, Garbrecht F, Pietryga D, Hansen R, Chitambar CR, Anderson T, Flomenberg N. Effect of T-cell depletion as graft-versus-host disease prophylaxis on engraftment, relapse, and disease-free survival in unrelated marrow transplantation for chronic myelogenous leukemia. Blood 1994; 83:1980–1986.

63. Marks DI, Bird JM, Vettenranta K, Hunt L, Green A, Cornish JM, Goulden N, Pamphilon DH, Steward CG, Oakhill A. T cell-depleted unrelated donor bone marrow transplantation for acute myeloid leukemia. Biol Blood Marrow Transplant 2000; 6:646–653.

64. Wagner JE, Thompson JS, Carter S, Jensen L, Kernan NA. Impact of graft-versus-host disease (GVHD) prophylaxis on 3-year disease-free survival (DFS): results of a multi-center, randomized phase II-III trial comparing T cell depletion/cyclosporine (TCD) and methotrexate/cyclosporine (M/C) in 410 recipients of unrelated donor bone marrow (BM). Am Soc Hematology, Orlando, 2002: Abstract 274.

65. Ash RC, Horowitz MM, Gale RP, van Bekkum DW, Casper JT, Gordon-Smith EC, Henslee PJ, Kolb HJ, Lowenberg B, Masaoka T, et al. Bone marrow transplantation from related donors other than HLA-identical siblings: effect of T cell depletion. Bone Marrow Transplant 1991; 7:443–452.

66. Soiffer RJ, Mauch P, Fairclough D, Alyea E, Anderson K, Fisher D, Freedman A, Bartlett-Pandite L, Robertson M, Schlossman R, Gollob J, Marcus K, Murray C, Kuhlman C, Freeman A, Nadler L, Ritz J. CD6+ T cell depleted allogeneic bone marrow transplantation from genotypically HLA nonidentical related donors. Biol Blood Marrow Transplant 1997; 3:11–17.

67. Henslee-Downey PJ, Abhyankar SH, Parrish RS, Pati AR, Godder KT, Neglia WJ, Goon-Johnson KS, Geier SS, Lee CG, Gee A. Use of partially mismatched related donors extends access to allogeneic marrow transplant. Blood 1997; 89:3864–3872.

68. Slavin S, Nagler A, Naparstek E, Kapelushnik Y, Aker M, Cividalli G, Varadi G, Kirschbaum M, Ackerstein A, Samuel S, Amar A, Brautbar C, Ben-Tal O, Eldor A, Or R. Nonmyeloablative stem cell transplantation and cell therapy as an alternative to conventional bone marrow transplantation with lethal cytoreduction for the treatment of malignant and nonmalignant hematologic diseases. Blood 1998; 91:756–763.

69. Niederwieser D, Maris M, Shizuru JA, Petersdorf E, Hegenbart U, Sandmaier BM, Maloney DG, Storer B, Lange T, Chauncey T, Deininger M, Ponisch W, Anasetti C, Woolfrey A, Little MT, Blume KG, McSweeney PA, Storb RF. Low-dose total body irradiation (TBI) and fludarabine followed by hematopoietic cell transplantation (HCT) from HLA-matched or mismatched unrelated donors and postgrafting immunosuppression with cyclosporine and mycophenolate mofetil (MMF) can induce durable complete chimerism and sustained remissions in patients with hematological diseases. Blood 2003; 101:1620–1629.

70. Baron F, Baudoux E, Frere P, Tourqui S, Schaaf-Lafontaine N, Greimers R, Herens C, Fillet G, Beguin Y. Nonmyeloablative stem cell transplantation with CD8-depleted or CD34-selected peripheral blood stem cells. J Hematother Stem Cell Res 2002; 11:301–314.

71. Kolb HJ, Schattenberg A, Goldman JM, Hertenstein B, Jacobsen N, Arcese W, Ljungman P, Ferrant A, Verdonck L, Niederwieser D, van Rhee F, Mittermüller J, de Witte T, Holler E, Ansari H. The European Group for Blood and Marrow Transplantation Working Party Chronic Leukemia. Graft-versus-leukemia effect of donor lymphocyte transfusions in marrow grafted patients. Blood 1995; 86:2041–2050.

72. Collins R, Shpilberg O, Drobyski W, Porter D, Giralt S, Champlin R, Goodman S, Wolff S, Hu W, Verfaillie C, List A, Dalton W, Ognoskie N, Chetrit A, Antin J, Nemunaitis J. Donor leukocyte infusions in 140 patients with relapsed malignancy after allogeneic bone marrow transplantation. J Clin Oncol 1997; 15:433–444.

73. Soiffer RJ, Alyea EP, Hochberg E, Wu C, Canning C, Parikh B, Zahrieh D, Webb I, Antin J, Ritz J. Randomized trial of CD8+ T-cell depletion in the prevention of graft-versus-host disease associated with donor lymphocyte infusion. Biol Blood Marrow Transplant 2002; 8:625–632.

74. Link CJ, Burt RK, Traynor AE, Drobyski WR, Seregina T, Levy JP, Gordon L, Rosen ST, Burns WH, Camitta B, Casper J, Horowitz M, Juckett M, Lawton C, Margolis D, Pietryga D, Rowlings P, Taylor C, Furtado M, Stefka J, Gupta-Burt S, Kaiser H, Vesole DH. Adoptive immunotherapy for leukemia: donor lymphocytes transduced with the herpes simplex thymidine kinase gene for remission induction. HGTRI 0103. Hum Gene Ther 1998; 9:115–134.

75. Bacigalupo A, Lamparelli T, Bruzzi P, Guidi S, Alessandrino PE, di Bartolomeo P, Oneto R, Bruno B, Barbanti M, Sacchi N, Van Lint MT, Bosi A. Antithymocyte globulin for graft-versus-host disease prophylaxis in transplants from unrelated donors: 2 randomized studies from Gruppo Italiano Trapianti Midollo Osseo (GITMO). Blood 2001; 98:2942–2947.

76. Soiffer RJ, Dear K, Rabinowe SN, Anderson KC, Freedman AS, Murray C, Tarbell NJ, Mauch P, Nadler LM, Ritz J. Hepatic dysfunction following T-cell-depleted allogeneic bone marrow transplantation. Transplantation 1991; 52:1014–1019.

77. Breuer R, Or R, Lijovetzky G, Naparstek E, Engelhard D, Lafair J, Weshler Z, Slavin S. Interstitial pneumonitis in T cell-depleted bone marrow transplantation. Bone Marrow Transplant 1988; 3:625–630.

78. Ho VT, Weller E, Lee SJ, Antin JH, Soiffer RJ. Prognostic factors for early severe pulmonary complications after hematopoietic stem cell transplantation. Biol Blood Marrow Transplant 2001; 7:223–229.

79. Soiffer RJ, Fairclough D, Robertson M, Alyea E, Anderson K, Freedman A, Bartlett-Pandite L, Fisher D, Schlossman RL, Stone R, Murray C, Freeman A, Marcus K, Mauch P, Nadler L, Ritz J. CD6-depleted allogeneic bone marrow transplantation for acute leukemia in first complete remission. Blood 1997; 89:3039–3047.

80. Drobyski WR, Hessner MJ, Klein JP, Kabler-Babbitt C, Vesole DH, Margolis DA, Keever-Taylor CA. T-cell depletion plus salvage immunotherapy with donor leukocyte infusions as a strategy to treat chronic-phase chronic myelogenous leukemia patients undergoing HLA-identical sibling marrow transplantation. Blood 1999; 94:434–441.

81. Hale G, Zhang MJ, Bunjes D, Prentice HG, Spence D, Horowitz MM, Barrett AJ, Waldmann H. Improving the outcome of bone marrow transplantation by using CD52 monoclonal antibodies to prevent graft-versus-host disease and graft rejection. Blood 1998;92: 4581–4590.

82. Remberger M, Storer B, Ringden O, Anasetti C. Association between pretransplant thymoglobulin and reduced non-relapse mortality rate after marrow transplantation from unrelated donors. Bone Marrow Transplant 2002; 29:391–397.

83. Papadopoulos EB, Carabasi MH, Castro-Malaspina H, Childs BH, Mackinnon S, Boulad F, Gillio AP, Kernan NA, Small TN, Szabolcs P, Taylor J, Yahalom J, Collins NH, Bleau SA, Black PM, Heller G, O'Reilly RJ, Young JW. T-cell-depleted allogeneic bone marrow transplantation as postremission therapy for acute myelogenous leukemia: freedom from relapse in the absence of graft-versus-host disease. Blood 1998; 91:1083–1090.

84. Hale G, Waldmann H. Control of graft-versus-host disease and graft rejection by T cell depletion of donor and recipient with Campath-1 antibodies. Results of matched sibling transplants for malignant diseases. Bone Marrow Transplant 1994; 13:597–603.

85. Nimer SD, Giorgi J, Gajewski JL, Ku N, Schiller GJ, Lee K, Territo M, Ho W, Feig S, Selch M, et al. Selective depletion of CD8 + cells for prevention of graft-versus-host disease after bone marrow transplantation. A randomized controlled trial. Transplantation 1994; 57:82–87.

86. Lee SJ, Zahrieh D, Alyea EP, Weller E, Ho VT, Antin JH, Soiffer RJ. Comparison of T-cell-depleted and non-T-cell-depleted unrelated donor transplantation for hematologic diseases: clinical outcomes, quality of life, and costs. Blood 2002; 100:2697–2702.

87. Wagner JE, Donnenberg AD, Noga SJ, Cremo CA, Gao IK, Yin HJ, Vogelsang GB, Rowley S, Saral R, Santos GW. Lymphocyte depletion of donor bone marrow by counterflow centrifugal elutriation: results of a phase I clinical trial. Blood 1988; 72:1168–1176.

88. Patterson J, Prentice HG, Brenner MK, Gilmore M, Janossy G, Ivory K, Skeggs D, Morgan H, Lord J, Blacklock HA, et al. Graft rejection following HLA matched T-lymphocyte depleted bone marrow transplantation. Br J Haematol 1986; 63:221–230.

89. Bordignon C, Kernan NA, Keever CA, Benazzi E, Small TN, Brochstein J, Cunningham I, Collins NH, Emanuel D, Laver J, et al. The role of residual host immunity in graft failures following T-cell-depleted marrow transplants for leukemia. Ann NY Acad Sci 1987; 511:442–446.

90. Martin PJ, Hansen JA, Torok-Storb B, Durnam D, Przepiorka D, O'Quigley J, Sanders J, Sullivan KM, Witherspoon RP, Deeg HJ, et al. Graft failure in patients receiving T cell-depleted HLA-identical allogeneic marrow transplants. Bone Marrow Transplant 1988; 3:445–456.

91. Delain M, Cahn JY, Racadot E, Flesch M, Plouvier E, Mercier M, Tiberghien P, Pavy JJ, Deschaseaux M, Deconinck E, et al. Graft failure after T cell depleted HLA identical allogeneic bone marrow transplantation: risk factors in leukemic patients. Leukemia Lymphoma 1993; 11:359–368.

92. Kernan NA, Bordignon C, Heller G, Cunningham I, Castro-Malaspina H, Shank B, Flomenberg N, Burns J, Yang SY, Black P, Collins NH, O'Reilly R. Graft failure after T-cell-depleted leukocyte antigen identical marrow transplants for leukemia: I. Analysis of risk factors and results of secondary transplants. Blood 1989; 74:2227–2234.

93. Marmont A, Horowitz MM, Gale RP, Sobocinski K, Ash RC, van Bekkum DW, Champlin RE, Dicke KA, Goldman JM, Good RA, Herzig RH, Hong R, Masaoka T, Rimm AA, Ringden O, Speck B, Weiner R, Bortin MM. T-cell depletion of HLA-identical transplants in leukemia. Blood 1991; 78:2120–2130.

94. Sondel PM, Hank JA, Trigg ME, Kohler PC, Finlay JL, Blank J, Meisner L, Borcherding W, Hong R, Steeves R, et al. Transplantation of HLA-haploidentical T cell-depleted marrow for leukemia: autologous marrow recovery with specific immune sensitization to donor antigens. Exp Hematol 1986; 14:278–286.

95. Bunjes D, Heit W, Arnold Schmeiser T, Wiesneth M, Carbonell F, Porzsolt F, Raghavachar A, Heimpel H. Evidence for the involvement of host derived OKT8-positive T cells in the rejection of T-depleted, HLA-identical bone marrow grafts. Transplantation 1987; 43:501–505.

96. Bunjes D, Theobald M, Wiesneth M, Bunjes D, Theobald M, Wiesneth M, Schrezenmeier H, Hoffmann T, Hertenstein B, Arnold R, Heimpel H. Graft rejection by a population of primed CDw52-host T cells after in vivo/ex vivo T-depleted bone marrow transplantation. Bone Marrow Transplant 1993; 12:209–215.

97. Kernan NA, Flomenberg N, Dupont B, O'Reilly RJ. Graft rejection in recipients of T cell depleted HLA-nonidentical marrow transplants for leukemia. Transplantation 1987; 43:842–847.

98. Bierer BE, Emerson SG, Antin J, Maziarz R, Rappeport JM, Smith BR, Burakoff SJ. Regulation of cytotoxic T lymphocyte-mediated graft rejection following bone marrow transplantation. Transplantation 1990; 49:714–71.

99. Bordignon C, Keever CA, Small TN, Flomenberg N, Dupont B, O'Reilly RJ, Kernan NA. Graft failure after T-cell-depleted leukocyte antigen identical marrow transplants for leukemia: II. In vitro analysis of host effector mechanisms. Blood 1989; 74:2237–2242.

100. Bosserman LD, Murray C, Takvorian T, Anderson KC, Freedman AS, Fitzsimmons J, Coral F, Nadler LM, Schlossman SF, Ritz J. Mechanism of graft failure in HLA-matched and HLA-mismatched bone marrow transplant recipients. Bone Marrow Transplant 1989; 4:239–245.

101. Voogt PJ, Fibbe WE, Marijt WA, Goulmy E, Veenhof WF, Hamilton M, Brand A, Zwann FE, Willemze R, van Rood JJ, et al. Rejection of bone marrow graft by recipient derived cytotoxic T lymphocytes against minor histocompatibility antigens. Lancet 1990; 335:131–134.

102. Fleischauer K, Kernan NA, O'Reilly RJ, Dupont B, Tang SY. Bone marrow-allograft rejection by T lymphocytes recognizing a single amino acid difference on HLA-B44. N Engl J Med 1990; 323:1818–1825.

103. Donohue J, Homge M, Kernan NA. Characterization of cells emerging at the time of graft failure after bone marrow transplantation from an unrelated bone marrow donor. Blood 1993; 82:1023–1029.

104. Gerritsen WR, Wagemaker G, Jonker M, Kenter MJ, Wielenga JJ, Hale G, Waldmann H, van Bekkum DW. The repopulation capacity of bone marrow grafts following pretreatment with monoclonal antibodies against T lymphocytes in rhesus monkeys. Transplantation 1988; 45:301–307.

105. Anderson KC, Anderson J, Soiffer R, Freedman AS, Rabinowe SN, Robertson MJ, Spector N, Blake K, Murray C, Freeman A, Coral F, Marcus KC, Mauch P, Nadler LM, Ritz J. Monoclonal antibody-purged autologous bone marrow transplantation therapy for multiple myeloma. Blood 1991; 77:712–720.

106. Freedman AS, Gribben JG, Neuberg D, Mauch P, Soiffer RJ, Anderson KC, Pandite L, Robertson MJ, Kroon M, Ritz J, Nadler LM. High dose therapy and autologous bone marrow transplantation in patients with follicular lymphoma during first remission. Blood 1996; 88:2780–2786.

107. Mutter W, Reddehase MJ, Busch FW, Buhring HJ, Koszinowski UH. Failure in generating hemopoietic stem cells is the primary cause of death from cytomegalovirus disease in the immunocompromised host. J Exp Med 1988; 167:1645–1650.

108. Steffens HP, Podlech J, Kurz S, Angele P, Dreis D, Reddehase MJ. Cytomegalovirus inhibits the engraftment of donor bone marrow cells by downregulation of hemopoietin gene expression in recipient stroma. J Virol 1998; 72:5006–5012.

109. Johnston RE, Geretti AM, Prentice HG, Clark AD, Wheeler AC, Potter M, Griffiths PD. HHV-6-related secondary graft failure following allogeneic bone marrow transplantation. Br J Haematol. 1999; 105:1041–1045.

110. Rosenfeld CS, Rybka WB, Weinbaum D, Carrigan DR, Knox KK, Andrews DF, Shadduck RK. Late graft failure due to dual bone marrow infection with variants A and B of human herpesvirus-6. Exp Hematol 1995; 23:626–630.

111. Couriel D, Canosa J, Engler H, Collins A, Dunbar C, Barrett AJ. Early reactivation of cytomegalovirus and high risk of interstitial pneumonitis following T-depleted BMT for adults with hematological malignancies. Bone Marrow Transplant 1996; 18:347–352.

112. Hertenstein B, Hampl W, Bunjes D, Wiesneth M, Duncker C, Koszinowski U, Heimpel H, Arnold R, Mertens T. In vivo/ex vivo T cell depletion for GVHD prophylaxis influences onset and course of active cytomegalovirus infection and disease after BMT. Bone Marrow Transplant 1995; 15:387–393.

113. Broers AEC, van der Holt R, van Esser JWJ, Gratama J-W, Henzen-Logmans S, VibekeK-B, Löwenberg B, Cornelissen JJ. Increased transplant-related morbidity and mortality in CMV-seropositive patients despite highly effective prevention of CMV disease after allogeneic T-cell-depleted stem cell transplantation. Blood 2000; 95:224–231.

114. Bertheas MF, Lafage M, Levy P, Blaise D, Stoppa AM, Viens P, Mannoni P, Maraninchi D. Influence of mixed chimerism on the results of allogeneic bone marrow transplantation for leukemia. Blood 1991; 78:3103–3111.

115. Offit K, Burns JP, Cunningham I, Jhanwar SC, Black P, Kernan NA, O'Reilly RJ, Chaganti RS. Cytogenetic analysis of chimerism and leukemia relapse in chronic myelogenous leukemia patients after T cell-depleted bone marrow transplantation. Blood 1990; 75:1346–1354.

116. Mackinnon S, Barnett L, O'Reilly RJ. Minimal residual disease is more common in patients who have mixed T-cell chimerism after bone marrow transplantation for chronic myelogenous leukemia. Blood 1994; 83:3409–3415.

117. van Leeuwen JEM, van Tol MJD, Joosten AM, Wijnen JT, Meera Khan P, Vossen JM. Mixed T-lymphoid chimerism after allogeneic bone marrow transplantation for hematologic malignancies of children is not correlated with relapse. Blood 1993; 82:1921–1928.

118. Butturini A, Seeger RC, Gale RP. Recipient immune-competent T lymphocytes can survive intensive conditioning for bone marrow transplantation. Blood 1986; 68:954–959.

119. Kedar E, Or R, Naparstek E, Zeira E, Slavin S. Preliminary characterization of functional residual host-type T lymphocytes following conditioning for allogeneic HLA-matched bone marrow transplantation (BMT). Bone Marrow Transplant 1988; 3:129–134.

120. Manilay JO, Sykes M. Natural killer cells and their role in graft rejection. Curr Opin Immunol 1988; 10:532–539.

121. Martin PJ. Donor CD8 cells prevent allogeneic marrow graft rejection in mice: potential implications for marrow transplantation in humans. J Exp Med 1993; 178:703–709.

122. Martin PJ, Rowley SD, Anasetti C, Chauncey TR, Gooley T, Petersdorf EW, van Burik JA, Flowers ME, Storb R, Appelbaum FR, Hansen JA. A phase I-II clinical trial to evaluate removal of CD4 cells and partial depletion of CD8 cells from donor marrow for HLA-mismatched unrelated recipients. Blood 1999; 94:2192–2199.

123. Ash RC, Casper JT, Chitambar CR, Hansen R, Bunn N, Truitt RL, Lawton C, Murray K, Hunter J, Baxter-Lowe LA, Gottschall JL, Oldham K, Anderson T, Camitta B, Menitove J. Successful allogeneic transplantation of T-cell-depleted bone marrow from closely HLA-matched unrelated donors. N Engl J Med 1990; 322:485–494.

124. Aversa F, Pelicci PG, Terenzi A, Carotti A, Felicini R, Mencarelli A, Donti E, Latini P, Aristei C, Martelli MF. Results of T-depleted BMT in chronic myelogenous leukaemia after a conditioning regimen that included thiotepa. Bone Marrow Transplant 1991; 7(suppl 2):24–26.

125. Schaap N, Schattenberg A, Bar B, Preijers F, Geurts van Kessel A, van der Maazen R, de Boo T, de Witte T. Outcome of transplantation for standard-risk leukaemia with grafts depleted of lymphocytes after conditioning with an intensified regimen. Br J Haematol 1997; 98:750–756.

126. Schattenberg A, Schaap N, Preijers F, van der Maazen R, de Witte T. Outcome of T cell-depleted transplantation after conditioning with an intensified regimen in patients aged 50 years or more is comparable with that in younger patients. Bone Marrow Transplant 2000; 26:17–22.

127. Guyotat D, Dutou L, Ehrsam A, Campos L, Archimbaud E, Fiere D. Graft rejection after T cell-depleted marrow transplantation: role of fractionated irradiation. Br J Haematol 1987; 65:499–500.

128. Burnett AK, Hann IM, Robertson AG, Alcorn M, Gibson B, McVicar I, Niven L, Mackinnon S, Hambley H, Morrison A, et al. Prevention of graft-versus-host disease by ex vivo T cell depletion: reduction in raft failure with augmented total body irradiation. Leukemia 1988; 2:300–303.

129. Bozdech MJ, Sondel PM, Trigg ME, Longo W, Kohler PC, Flynn B, Billing R, Anderson SA, Hank JA, Hond R. Transplantation of HLA-haploindentical T-cell-depleted marrow for leukemia: addition of cytosine arabinoside to the pretransplant conditioning prevents rejection. Exp Hematol 1985; 13:1201–1206.

130. Soiffer RJ, Mauch P, Tarbell NJ, Anderson KC, Freedman AS, Rabinowe SN, Takvorian T, Murray C, Coral F, Bosserman L, et al. Total lymphoid irradiation to prevent graft rejection in recipients of HLA non-identical T cell-depleted allogeneic marrow. Bone Marrow Transplant 1991; 7:23–33.

131. Ganem G, Kuentz M, Beaujean F, et al. Additional total lymphoid irradiation in preventing graft failure of T-cell depleted bone marrow transplantation from HLA-identical siblings. Transplantation 1987; 45:244–249.

132. Cobbold S, Martin G, Waldmann H. Monoclonal antibodies for the prevention of graft-versus-host disease and marrow graft rejection. The depletion of T cell subsets in vitro and in vivo. Transplantation 1986; 42:239–244.

133. Castro-Malaspina H, Childs B, Laver J, Shank B, Brochstein J, Gillio A, Flomenberg N, Young J, Boulad F, Black P, et al. Hyperfractionated total lymphoid irradiation and cyclophosphamide for preparation of previously transfused patients undergoing HLA-identical marrow transplantation for severe aplastic anemia. Int J Radiat Oncol Biol Phys 1994; 29:847–852.

134. Potter MN, Pamphilon DH, Cornish JM, Oakhill A. Graft-versus-host disease in children receiving HLA-identical allogeneic bone marrow transplants with a low adjusted T lymphocyte dose. Bone Marrow Transplant 1991; 8:357–362.

135. Barrett AJ, Mavroudis D, Tisdale J, Molldrem J, Clave E, Dunbar C, Cottler-Fox M, Phang S, Carter C, Okunnieff P, Young NS, Read EJ. T cell-depleted bone marrow transplantation and delayed T cell add-back to control acute GVHD and conserve a graft-versus-leukemia effect. Bone Marrow Transplant 1998; 21:543–551.

136. Bachar-Lustig E, Rachamim N, Li HW, Lan F, Reisner Y. Megadose of T cell-depleted bone marrow overcomes MHC barriers in sublethally irradiated mice. Nat Med 1995; 1:1268–1272.

137. Aversa F, Tabilio A, Terenzi A, Velardi A, Falzetti F, Giannoni C, Iacucci R, Zei T, Martelli MP, Gambelunghe C, et al. Successful engraftment of T-cell-depleted haploidentical transplants in leukemia patients by addition of recombinant human granulocyte colony-stimulating factor-mobilized peripheral blood progenitor cells to bone marrow inoculum. Blood 1994; 84:3948–3953.

138. Reisner Y, Martelli MF. Tolerance induction by 'megadose' transplants of CD34+ stem cells: a new option for leukemia patients without an HLA-matched donor. Curr Opin Immunol 2000; 12:536–541.

139. Soiffer RJ, Alyea EP, Kim H, Parikh B, Ho V, Hochberg E, Levin J, Fisher DC, Lee SJ, Antin JH. Engraftment, graft-vs-host disease (GVHD), and survival after CD8+ T cell depleted allogeneic peripheral blood stem cell transplantation (PBSCT). Proc Am Soc Hematology 2002: Abstract 1619.

140. Welte K, Keever CA, Levick J, Bonilla MA, Merluzzi VJ, Mertelsmann R, Evans R, O'Reilly RJ. Interleukin-2 production and response to interleukin-2 by peripheral blood mononuclear cells from patients after bone marrow transplantation: II. Patients receiving soybean lectin-separated and T cell-depleted bone marrow. Blood 1987; 70:1595–1560.

141. Soiffer RJ, Bosserman L, Murray C, Cochran K, Daley J, Ritz J. Reconstitution of T-cell function after CD6-depleted allogeneic bone marrow transplantation. Blood 1990; 75:2076–2084.

142. Keever CA, Small TN, Flomenberg N, Heller G, Pekle K, Black P, Pecora A, Gillio A, Kernan NA, O'Reilly RJ. Immune reconstitution following bone marrow transplantation: comparison of recipients of T-cell depleted marrow with recipients of conventional marrow grafts. Blood 1989; 73:1340–1346.

143. Ault KA, Antin JH, Ginsburg D, Orkin SH, Rappeport JM, Keohan ML, Martin P, Smith BR. Phenotype of recovering lymphoid cell populations after marrow transplantation. J Exp Med 1985; 161:1483–1488.

144. Parreira A, Smith J, Hows JM, Smithers SA, Apperley J, Rombos Y, Goldman JM, Gordon-Smith EC, Catovsky D. Immunological reconstitution after bone marrow transplant with campath-1 treated bone marrow. Clin Exp Immunol 1987; 67:142–148.

145. Roux E, Helg C, Dumont-Girard F, Chapuis B, Jeannet M, Roosnek E. Analysis of T-cell repopulation after allogeneic bone marrow transplantation: significant differences between recipients of T-cell depleted and unmanipulated grafts. Blood 1996; 87:3984–3990.

146. Roux E, Dumont-Girard F, Starobinski M, Siegrist CA, Helg C, Chapuis B, Roosnek E. Recovery of immune reactivity after T-cell-depleted bone marrow transplantation depends on thymic activity. Blood 2000; 96:2299–2305.

147. Small TN, Papadopoulos EB, Boulad F, Black P, Castro-Malaspina H, Childs BH, Collins N, Gillio A, George D, Jakubowski A, Heller G, Fazzari M, Kernan N, MacKinnon S, Szabolcs P, Young JW, O'Reilly RJ. Comparison of immune reconstitution after unrelated and related T-cell-depleted bone marrow transplantation: effect of patient age and donor leukocyte infusions. Blood 1999; 93:467–480.

148. Wu CJ, Chillemi A, Alyea EP, Orsini E, Neuberg D, Soiffer RJ, Ritz J. Reconstitution of T-cell receptor repertoire diversity following T-cell depleted allogeneic bone marrow transplantation is related to hematopoietic chimerism. Blood 2000; 95:352–359.

149. Lewin SR, Heller G, Zhang L, Rodrigues E, Skulsky E, van den Brink MR, Small TN, Kernan NA, O'Reilly RJ, Ho DD, Young JW. Direct evidence for new T-cell generation by patients after either T-cell-depleted or unmodified allogeneic hematopoietic stem cell transplantations. Blood 2002; 100:2235–2242.

150. Hochberg EP, Chillemi AC, Wu CJ, Neuberg D, Canning C, Hartman K, Alyea EP, Soiffer RJ, Kalams SA, Ritz J. Quantitation of T-cell neogenesis in vivo after allogeneic bone marrow transplantation in adults. Blood 2001; 98:2116–2121.

151. Engelhard D, Or R, Strauss N, Morag A, Aker M, Naparstek E, Breuer R, Ravid Z, Sarov I, Lijovetzky G, et al. Cytomegalovirus infection and disease after T cell depleted allogeneic bone marrow transplantation for malignant hematologic diseases. Transplant Proc 1989; 21:3101–3105.

152. Martino R, Rovira M, Carreras E, Solano C, Jorge S, De La Rubia J, Caballero MD, de Oteyza JP, Zuazu J, Moraleda JM, Ojeda E, Ferra C, Serrano D, De La Camara R, Urbano-Ispizua A, Brunet S. Severe infections after allogeneic peripheral blood stem cell transplantation: a

matched-pair comparison of unmanipulated and CD34+ cell-selected transplantation. Haematologica 2001; 86:1075–1080.

153. Zutter MM, Martin PJ, Sale GE, Shulman HM, Fisher L, Thomas ED, Durnam DM. Epstein-Barr virus lymphoproliferation after bone marrow transplantation. Blood 1988; 72:520–529.

154. Gerritsen EJ, Stam ED, Hermans J, van den Berg H, Haraldsson A, van Tol MJ, van den Bergh RL, Waaijer JL, Kroes AC, Kluin PM, Vossen JM. Risk factors for developing EBV-related B cell lymphoproliferative disorders (BLPD) after non-HLA-identical BMT in children. Bone Marrow Transplant 1996; 18:377–383.

155. Martin PJ, Shulman HM, Schubach WH, Hansen JA, Fefer A, Miller G, Thomas ED. Fatal Epstein-Barr virus associated proliferation of donor B-cells after treatment of acute graft-versus-host disease with a murine anti-T-cell antibody. Ann Intern Med 1984; 101:310–315.

156. Martin PJ, Hansen JA, Torok-Storb B, Moretti L, Press O, Storb R, Thomas ED, Weiden PL, Vitetta ES. Effects of treating marrow with a CD3-specific immunotoxin for prevention of acute graft-versus-host disease. Bone Marrow Transplant 1988; 3:437–444.

157. Papadapoulos EB, Ladanyi M, Emmanuel D, Mackinnon S, Boulad F, Carabasi MH, Castro-Malaspina H, Childs BH, Gillio AP, Small TN, Young JW, Kernan NA, O'Reilly RJ. Infusions of donor leukocytes to treat Epstein-Barr-associated lymphoproliferative disorders after allogeneic bone marrow transplantation. N Engl J Med 1994; 330:1185–1191.

158. Heslop HE, Brenner MK, Rooney C, Krance RA, Roberts WM, Rochester R, Smith CA, Turner V, Sixbey J, Moen R, et al. Administration of neomycin-resistance-gene-marked EBV-specific cytotoxic T lymphocytes to recipients of mismatched-related or phenotypically similar unrelated donor marrow grafts. Hum Gene Ther 1994; 5:381–388.

159. Rooney CM, Smith CA, Ng CY, Loftin S, Li C, Krance RA, Brenner MK, Heslop HE. Use of gene-modified virus-specific T lymphocytes to control Epstein-Barr-virus-related lymphoproliferation. Lancet 1995; 345:9–13.

160. Rooney CM, Smith CA, Ng CY, Loftin SK, Sixbey JW, Gan Y, Srivastava DK, Bowman LC, Krance RA, Brenner MK, Heslop HE. Infusion of cytotoxic T cells for the prevention and treatment of Epstein-Barr virus-induced lymphoma in allogeneic transplant recipients. Blood 1998; 92:1549–1556.

161. Fischer A, Blanche S, Le Bidois J, Bordigoni P, Garnier JL, Niaudet P, Morinet F, Le Deist F, Fischer AM, Griscelli C, et al. Anti-B-cell monoclonal antibodies in the treatment of severe B-cell lymphoproliferative syndrome following bone marrow and organ transplantation. N Engl J Med 1991; 324:1451–1457.

162. McGuirk JP, Seropian S, Howe G, Smith B, Stoddart L, Cooper DL. Use of rituximab and irradiated donor-derived lymphocytes to control Epstein-Barr virus-associated lymphoproliferation in patients undergoing related haplo-identical stem cell transplantation. Bone Marrow Transplant 1999; 24:1253–1257.

163. Kuehnle I, Huls MH, Liu Z, Semmelmann M, Krance RA, Brenner MK, Rooney CM, Heslop HE. CD20 monoclonal antibody (rituximab) for therapy of Epstein-Barr virus lymphoma after hemopoietic stem-cell transplantation. Blood 2000; 95:1502–1509.

164. Cavazzana-Calvo M, Bensoussan D, Jabado N, Haddad E, Yvon E, Moskwa M, Tachet des Combes A, Buisson M, Morand P, Virion JM, Le Deist F, Fischer A. Prevention of EBV-induced B-lymphoproliferative disorder by ex vivo marrow B-cell depletion in HLA-phenoidentical or non-identical T-depleted bone marrow transplantation. Br J Haematol 1998; 103:543–547.

165. Hale G, Waldmann H. Risks of developing Epstein-Barr virus-related lymphoproliferative disorders after T-cell-depleted marrow transplants. Blood 1998; 91:3079–3084.

166. Gustafsson A, Levitsky V, Zou JZ, Frisan T, Dalianis T, Ljungman P, Ringden O, Winiarski J, Ernberg I, Masucci MG. Epstein-Barr virus (EBV) load in bone marrow transplant recipients at risk to develop posttransplant lymphoproliferative disease: prophylactic infusion of EBV-specific cytotoxic T cells. Blood 2000; 95:807–813.

167. Rooney CM, Loftin SK, Holladay MS, Brenner MK, Krance RA, Heslop HE. Early identification of Epstein-Barr virus-associated post-transplantation lymphoproliferative disease. Br J Haematol 1995; 89:98–102.

168. Goldman JM, Gale RP, Horowitz MM, Biggs JC, Champlin RE, Gluckman E, Hoffmann RG, Jacobsen SJ, Marmont AM, McGlave PB, Messner HA, Rimm AA, Rozman C, Speck B, Tura S, Weiner RS, Bortin MM. Bone marrow transplantation for chronic myelogenous leukemia in chronic phase. Increased risk for relapse associated with T-cell depletion. Ann Intern Med 1988; 108:806–812.

169. Martin P, Clift RA, Fisher LD, Buckner CD, Hansen JA, Appelbaum FR, Doney KC, Sullivan KM, Witherspoon RP, Storb R, Thomas ED. HLA-identical marrow transplantation during accelerated-phase chronic myelogenous leukemia: analysis of survival and remission duration. Blood 1988; 72:1978–1984.

170. Marks DI, Hughes TP, Szydlo R, Kelly S, Cullis JO, Schwarer AP, Mackinnon S, Apperley J, Barrett AJ, Hows JM, et al. HLA-identical sibling donor bone marrow transplantation for chronic myeloid leukaemia in first chronic phase: influence of GVHD prophylaxis on outcome. Br J Haematol 1992; 81:383–387.

171. Wagner JE, Zahurak M, Piantadosi S, Geller RB, Vogelsang GB, Wingard JR, Saral R, Griffin C, Shah N, Zehnbauer BA, Ambinder R, Burns W, Jones R, May WS, Rowley S, Yeager A, Santos GW. Bone marrow transplantation of chronic myelogenous leukemia in chronic phase: evaluation of risks and benefits. J Clin Oncol 1992; 10:779–785.

172. Gratwohl A, Hermans J, Niderwieser D, Frassoni F, Arcese W, Gahrton G, Bandini G, Carreras E, Vernant JP, Bosi A, de Witte T, Fibbe WE, Zwaan FE, Michallet M, Tuutu R, Devergie A, Iriondo A, Apperley J, Reiffers J, Speck B, Goldman J. Bone marrow transplantation for chronic myeloid leukemia: long-term results. Bone Marrow Transplant 1993; 12:509–514.

173. Apperley JF, Mauro FR, Goldman JM, Gregory W, Arthur CK, Hows J, Arcese W, Papa A, Mandelli F, Wardle D, Gravett P, Franklin IM, Bandini G, Ricci P, Tura S, Iacone d, Torlontano G, Heit W, Champlin R, Gale RP. Bone marrow transplantation for chronic myeloid leukaemia in first chronic phase, importance of a graft-versus-leukaemia effect. Br J Haematol 1988; 69:239–244.

174. Weiden PL, Flournoy N, Thomas ED, Prentice R, Buckner CD, Storb R. Antileukemic effect of graft-versus-host disease in recipients of allogeneic-marrow grafts. N Engl J Med 1979; 300:1068–1074.

175. Sullivan KM, Weiden PL, Storb R, Witherspoon RP, Fefer A, Fisher L, Buckner CD, Anasetti C, Appelbaum FR, Badger C, Beatty P, Bensinger W, Berenson R, Bigelow C, Cheever MA, Clift R, Deeg HJ, Doney K, Greenberg P, Hansen JA, Hill R, Loughran R, Martin P, Neiman P, Petersen FB, Sanders J, Singer J, Stewart P, Thomas ED. Influence of acute and chronic graft-versus-host disease on relapse and survival after bone marrow transplantation from HLA-identical siblings as treatment of acute and chronic leukemia. Blood 1989; 73:1720–1727.

176. Horowitz MM, Gale RP, Sondel PM, Goldman JM, Kersey J, Kolb HJ, Rimm AA, Ringdén O, Rozman C, Speck B, Truitt RL, Zwaan FE, Bortin MM. Graft-versus-leukemia reactions after bone marrow transplantation. Blood 1990; 75:555–565.

177. Enright H, Davies SM, DeFor T, Shu X, Weisdorf D, Miller W, Ramsay NK, Arthur D, Verfaillie C, Miller J, Kersey J, McGlave P. Relapse after non-T-cell-depleted allogeneic bone marrow transplantation for chronic myelogenous leukemia: early transplantation, use of an unrelated donor, and chronic graft-versus-host disease are protective. Blood 1996; 88:714–721.

178. McGlave P, Bartsch G, Anasetti C, Ash R, Beatty P, Gajewski J, Kernan NA. Unrelated donor marrow transplantation therapy for chronic myelogenous leukemia: initial experience of the National Marrow Donor Program. Blood 1993; 81:543–549.

179. Hessner MJ, Endean DJ, Casper JT, Horowitz MM, Keever-Taylor CA, Roth M, Flomenberg N, Drobyski W. Use of unrelated marrow grafts compensates for reduced

graft-versus-leukemia reactivity after T-cell-depleted allogeneic marrow transplantation for chronic myelogenous leukemia. Blood 1995; 86:3987–3993.

180. Devergie A, Apperley JF, Labopin M, Madrigal A, Jacobsen N, Carreras E, Prentice HG, Jouet JP, Kolb HJ, Herstenstein B, Bacigalupo A, Evensen SA, Ljungman P, de Witte T, Reiffers J, Nagler A, Clark RE, Goldman JM, Gratwohl A. European results of matched unrelated donor bone marrow transplantation for chronic myeloid leukemia. Impact of HLA class II matching. Chronic Leukemia Working Party of the European Group for Blood and Marrow Transplantation. Bone Marrow Transplant 1997; 20:11–19.

181. Bunjes D, Hertenstein B, Wiesneth M, Stefanic M, Novotny J, Duncker C, Heit W, Arnold R, Heimpel H. In vivo/ex vivo T cell depletion reduces the morbidity of allogeneic bone marrow transplantation in patients with acute leukaemias in first remission without increasing the risk of treatment failure: comparison with cyclosporin/methotrexate. Bone Marrow Transplant 1995; 15:563–568.

182. Aversa F, Terenzi A, Carotti A, Felicini R, Jacucci R, Zei T, Latini P, Aristei C, Santucci A, Martelli MP, Cunningham I, Reisner Y, Martelli MF. Improved outcome with T-cell-depleted bone marrow transplantation for acute leukemia. J Clin Oncol 1999; 17:1545–1552.

183. Novitzky N, Thomas V, Hale G, Waldmann H. Ex vivo depletion of T cells from bone marrow grafts with CAMPATH-1 in acute leukemia: graft-versus-host disease and graft-versus-leukemia effect. Transplantation 1999; 67:620–626.

184. Remberger M, Ringden O, Aschan J, Ljungman P, Lonnqvist B, Markling L. Long-term follow-up of a randomized trial comparing T-cell depletion with a combination of methotrexate and cyclosporine in adult leukemic marrow transplant recipients. Transplant Proc 1994; 26:1829–1833.

185. Soiffer RJ, Gonin R, Murray C, Robertson MJ, Cochran K, Chartier S, Cameron C, Daley J, Levine H, Nadler LM, Ritz J. Prediction of graft-versus-host disease by phenotypic analysis of early immune reconstitution after CD6-depleted allogeneic bone marrow transplantation. Blood 1993; 82:2216–2223.

186. Giralt S, Hester J, Huh Y, Hirsch-Ginsberg C, Rondøn G, Seong D, Lee M, Gajewski J, Van Besien K, Khouri I, Mehra R, Przepiorka D, K''rbling M, Talpaz M, Kantarjian H, Fischer H, Deisseroth A, Champlin R. CD8-depleted donor lymphocyte infusion as treatment for relapsed chronic myelogenous leukemia after allogeneic bone marrow transplantation. Blood 1995; 86:4337–4343.

187. Alyea EP, Soiffer RJ, Canning C, Neuberg D, Schlossman R, Pickett C, Collins H, Wang Y, Anderson KC, Ritz J. Toxicity and efficacy of defined doses of CD4(+) donor lymphocytes for treatment of relapse after allogeneic bone marrow transplant. Blood 1998; 91:3671–3680.

188. Sehn LH, Alyea EP, Weller E, Canning C, Lee S, Ritz J, Antin JH, Soiffer RJ. Comparative outcomes of T-cell-depleted and non-T-cell-depleted allogeneic bone marrow transplantation for chronic myelogenous leukemia: impact of donor lymphocyte infusion. J Clin Oncol 1999; 17:561–570.

189. Elmaagacli AH, Peceny R, Steckel N, Trenschel R, Ottinger H, Grosse-Wilde H, Schaefer UW, Beelen DW. Outcome of transplantation of highly purified peripheral blod CD34+ cells with T-cell ad-back compared with unmanipulated bone marrow or peripheral blood stem cells from HLA-identical sibling donors in patients with first chronic phase chronic myeloid leukemia. Blood 2000; 101:446–453.

190. Mackinnon S, Papadapoulos EB, Carabasi MH, Reich L, Collins NH, Boulad F, Castro-Malaspina H, Childs BH, Gillio AP, Kernan NA, Small TN, Young JW, O'Reilly RJ. Adoptive immunotherapy evaluating escalating doses of donor leukocytes for relapse of chronic myeloid leukemia after bone marrow transplantation: separation of graft-versus-leukemia responses from graft-versus-host disease. Blood 1995; 86:1261–1268.

191. Dazzi F, Szydlo RM, Craddock C, Cross NC, Kaeda J, Chase A, Olavarria E, van Rhee F, Kanfer E, Apperley JF, Goldman JM. Comparison of single-dose and escalating-dose

regimens of donor lymphocyte infusion for relapse after allografting for chronic myeloid leukemia. Blood 2000; 95:67–71.

192. Munshi NC, Govindarajan R, Drake R, Ding LM, Iyer R, Saylors R, Kornbluth J, Marcus S, Chiang Y, Ennist D, Kwak L, Reynolds C, Tricot G, Barlogie B. Thymidine kinase (TK) gene-transduced human lymphocytes can be highly purified, remain fully functional, and are killed efficiently with ganciclovir. Blood 1997; 89:1334–1340.

193. Alyea EP, Weller E, Schlossman R, Canning C, Webb I, Doss D, Mauch P, Marcus D, Fisher D, Freedman A, Gribben J, Soiffer RJ, Ritz J, Anderson K. T cell depleted allogeneic bone marrow transplantation followed by donor lymphocyte infusion in patients with multiple myeloma: reduced transplant related toxicity with preservation of graft versus myeloma effect. Blood 2001; 98:934–939.

194. Soiffer RJ, Murray C, Gonin R, Ritz J. Effect of low-dose interleukin-2 on disease relapse after T-cell-depleted allogeneic bone marrow transplantation. Blood 1994; 84:964–971.

195. Ruggeri L, Capanni M, Casucci M, Volpi I, Tosti A, Perruccio K, Urbani E, Negrin RS, Martelli MF, Velardi A. Role of natural killer cell alloreactivity in HLA-mismatched hematopoietic stem cell transplantation. Blood 1999; 94:333–339.

196. Ruggeri L, Capanni M, Urbani E, Perruccio K, Shlomchik WD, Tosti A, Posati S, Rogaia D, Frassoni F, Aversa F, Martelli MF, Velardi A. Effectiveness of donor natural killer cell alloreactivity in mismatched hematopoietic transplants. Science 2002; 295:2097–2100.

197. Shlomchik WD, Couzens MS, Tang CB, McNiff J, Robert ME, Liu J, Shlomchik MJ, Emerson SG. Prevention of graft-versus-host disease by inactivation of host antigen presenting cells. Science 1999; 285:412–415.

198. Davies SM, Ruggieri L, DeFor T, Wagner JE, Weisdorf DJ, Miller JS, Velardi A, Blazar BR. Evaluation of KIR ligand incompatibility in mismatched unrelated donor hematopoietic transplants. Killer immunoglobulin-like receptor. Blood 2002; 100:3825–3827.

199. Chen BJ, Cui X, Liu C, Chao NJ. Prevention of graft-versus-host disease while preserving graft-versus-leukemia effect after selective depletion of host-reactive T cells by photodynamic cell purging process. Blood 2002; 99:3083–3089.

200. Koh MB, Prentice HG, Lowdell MW. Selective removal of alloreactive cells from haematopoietic stem cell grafts: graft engineering for GVHD prophylaxis. Bone Marrow Transplant 1999; 23:1071–1079.

201. Garderet L, Snell V, Przepiorka D, Schenk T, Lu JG, Marini F, Gluckman E, Andreeff M, Champlin RE. Effective depletion of alloreactive lymphocytes from peripheral blood mononuclear cell preparations. Transplantation 1999; 67:124–130.

202. Harris DT, Sakiestewa D, Lyons C, Kreitman RJ, Pastan I. Prevention of graft-versus-host disease (GVHD) by elimination of recipient-reactive donor T cells with recombinant toxins that target the interleukin 2 (IL-2) receptor. Bone Marrow Transplant 1999; 23:137–144.

203. Blazar BR, Taylor PA, Linsley PS, Vallera DA. In vivo blockade of CD28/CTLA4: B7/BB1 interaction with CTLA4-Ig reduces lethal murine graft-versus-host disease across the major histocompatibility complex barrier in mice. Blood 1994; 83:3815–3825.

204. Blazar BR, Taylor PA, Panoskaltsis-Mortari A, Gray GS, Vallera DA. Coblockade of the LFA1:ICAM and CD28/CTLA4:B7 pathways is a highly effective means of preventing acute lethal graft-versus-host disease induced by fully major histocompatibility complex-disparate donor grafts. Blood 1995; 85:2607–2618.

205. Blazar BR, Taylor PA, Panoskaltsis-Mortari A, Buhlman J, Xu J, Flavell RA, Korngold R, Noelle R, Vallera DA. Blockade of CD40 ligand-CD40 interaction impairs CD4+ T cell-mediated alloreactivity by inhibiting mature donor T cell expansion and function after bone marrow transplantation. J Immunol 1997; 158:29–39.

206. Guinan EC, Boussiotis VA, Neuberg D, Brennan LL, Hirano N, Nadler LM, Gribben JG. Transplantation of anergic histoincompatible bone marrow allografts. N Engl J Med 1999; 340:1704–1714 (see comments).

207. Tiberghien P, Ferrand C, Lioure B, Milpied N, Angonin R, Deconinck E, Certoux JM, Robinet E, Saas P, Petracca B, Juttner C, Reynolds CW, Longo DL, Herve P, Cahn JY. Administration of herpes simplex-thymidine kinase-expressing donor T cells with a T-cell-depleted allogeneic marrow graft. Blood 2001; 97:63–69.

208. Aubin F, Cahn JY, Ferrand C, Angonin R, Humbert P, Tiberghien P. Extensive vitiligo after ganciclovir treatment of GvHD in a patient who had received donor T cells expressing herpes simplex virus thymidine kinase. Lancet 2000; 355(9204):626–627.

209. Teshima T, Mach N, Hill GR, Pan L, Gillessen S, Dranoff G, Ferrara JL. Tumor cell vaccine elicits potent antitumor immunity after allogeneic T-cell-depleted bone marrow transplantation. Cancer Res 2001; 61:162–167.

210. Fowler DH, Gress RE. Th2 and Tc2 cells in the regulation of GVHD, GVL, and graft rejection: considerations for the allogeneic transplantation therapy of leukemia and lymphoma. Leuk Lymphoma 2000; 38(3–4):221–234.

211. Pan L, Delmonte J Jr, Jalonen CK, Ferrara JL. Pretreatment of donor mice with granulocyte colony-stimulating factor polarizes donor T lymphocytes toward type-2 cytokine production and reduces severity of experimental graft-versus-host disease. Blood 1995; 86:4422–4497.

212. Fowler DH, Gress RE. Th2 and Tc2 cells in the regulation of GVHD, GVL, and graft rejection: considerations for the allogeneic transplantation therapy of leukemia and lymphoma. Leuk Lymphoma 2000; 38:221–234.

213. Hoffmann P, Ermann J, Edinger M, Fathman CG, Strober S. Donor-type CD4(+)CD25(+) regulatory T cells suppress lethal acute graft-versus-host disease after allogeneic bone marrow transplantation. J Exp Med 2002; 196:389–399.

214. Cohen JL, Trenado A, Vasey D, Klatzmann D, Salomon BL. CD4(+)CD25(+) immunoregulatory T cells: new therapeutics for graft-versus-host disease. J Exp Med 2002; 196:401–406.

215. Taylor PA, Lees CJ, Blazar BR. The infusion of ex vivo activated and expanded CD4(+) CD25(+) immune regulatory cells inhibits graft-versus-host disease lethality. Blood 2002; 99:3493–3499.

216. Johnson BD, Konkol MC, Truitt RL. CD25+ immunoregulatory T-cells of donor origin suppress alloreactivity after BMT. Biol Blood Marrow Transplant 2002; 8:525–535.

18

Graft-vs.-Host Disease in Nonmyeloablative Transplant

DANIEL R. COURIEL and SERGIO GIRALT

The University of Texas M.D. Anderson Cancer Center, Houston, Texas, U.S.A.

I. INTRODUCTION

Myeloablative doses of chemotherapy and total body irradiation, typically used as preparative regimens in hematopoietic stem cell transplant (HSCT), are associated with a high rate of morbidity and regimen-related mortality. In this respect, graft-vs.-host disease (GVHD) continues to be one of the main limitations of allogeneic transplant (1,2). This has largely limited the use of myeloablative HSCT to life-threatening clinical indications in younger individuals without serious comorbidities (3).

However, hematological malignancies predominantly occur in older patients, usually with comorbidities, who are not considered eligible for this treatment. Nonmyeloablative preparative regimens have recently been developed as a means to reduce the morbidity related to hematopoietic transplantation (4–8). These reduced-intensity regimens provide sufficient immunosuppression to achieve engraftment of an allogeneic bone marrow or blood stem cell graft and allow the immune-mediated graft-vs.-malignancy effect to occur.

The syndrome of acute GVHD is in part related to cytokines produced in response to the toxicity of the preparative regimen (9–11). Intensive regimens can result in gastrointestinal (GI) mucosal injury, with increased permeability and endotoxemia, which stimulates and amplifies a cytokine cascade that is central in the pathophysiology of acute GVHD (9,12,13).

The increased morbidity and mortality associated with older age are the main reasons for not transplanting older or medically debilitated patients (14–17). In animal models the incidence of GVHD mortality and morbidity is related to the intensity of the preparative regimen, which in turn influences inflammatory cytokine expression and

511

release (18,19). Nonablative regimens in animal models have been developed that allow stable engraftment of donor stem cells (20–23). Thus strategies using less intensive preparative regimens (so-called nonablative or reduced-intensity conditioning regimens) have been developed to explore the efficacy of the graft-vs.-malignancy effect in patients with malignancies ineligible for high-dose chemotherapy or radiation because of age or concurrent medical conditions (4–8).

In addition to the toxicity and limitations of myeloablative conditioning regimens, there are other reasons to explore nonmyeloablative transplantation. These include the observations that:

1. Mixed chimerism can be achieved with nonmyeloablative regimens, and mixed chimerisms may protect against GVHD in both animal models and in humans (4–8,24–26).
2. Hematological and other malignancies can relapse despite intensive myeloablative regimens. Further modifications of the preparative regimens with current available agents are unlikely to improve results since decreases in relapse rates have always been offset by increases in nonrelapse mortality (27–29).
3. Induction of durable remissions can be achieved with donor lymphocyte infusions (DLI) in certain types of hematological malignancies that relapse after allogeneic transplant (30–36).

In this chapter the current experience with acute and chronic GVHD as it relates to nonmyeloablative regimens will be reviewed.

II. CLINICAL EXPERIENCE WITH NONMYELOABLATIVE TRANSPLANTATION

Current experience with nonmyeloablative stem cell transplantation (NST) has shown that engraftment can occur with immunosuppression and minimal myelosuppression (4–8). Optimal doses and agents required to achieve engraftment in different clinical situations have not been defined and will vary according to the immunocompetence of the recipient, the aggressiveness of the underlying malignancy, and the genetic disparity between donor and recipient (37).

A continuum of nonablative, reduced-intensity, and full ablative regimens has been used in the context of stem cell transplantation. Most nonmyeloablative regimens reported to date have been based on the use of either purine analogues or low-dose total body irradiation (TBI) (37) (Fig. 1). No randomized studies have yet compared different nonmyeloablative strategies or compared nonmyeloablative to conventional chemotherapy or to conventional myeloablative transplantation. Results of large retrospective series from a variety of institutions and registries are currently being reported. Myeloid leukemias and lymphomas are currently the most common indications for NST.

Table 1 summarizes the results of the largest series of patients receiving either truly nonablative or reduced intensity conditioning for acute myeloid leukemias (AML) or myelodysplastic syndromes (MDS) (4,38–41). The experience suggests that both reduced-intensity and truly nonablative regimens are feasible in older and infirm patients with AML and MDS. However, the results for patients with refractory disease are poor. Although nonrelapse mortality rates are relatively low in this setting, relapse rates are high, and salvage with immune manipulation is rarely successful (38,42). Thus, the optimal

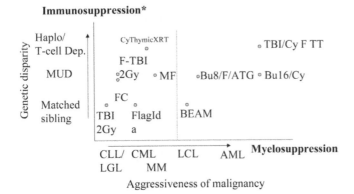

Figure 1 Commonly used nonablative and reduced intensity conditioning regimens graphed according to myelosuppressive and immunosuppressive potential. *Immunosuppression required depends on genetic disparity, immunocompetence, and sensitization of recipient.

application of NST for AML and high-risk MDS will depend on utilizing this therapy while patients are in remission or have chemosensitive disease.

The relevance of the intensity of conditioning in these diseases is underscored by the observation that disease control and treatment outcomes seem to be superior in patients with active disease when they receive a reduced-intensity conditioning regimen rather than a truly nonablative regimen (43).

Unrelated donor cells have been successfully engrafted after both reduced-intensity and truly nonablative regimens in patients with a variety of myeloid leukemias (38,44–46). However, the graft failure rate and GVHD rates are higher with unrelated donors. In the truly nonablative regimens with low-dose TBI, particularly in patients with chronic myelogenous leukemia (CML), the use of fludarabine in this setting has decreased the risk of graft failure (44). The use of alemtuzumab, a humanized anti-CD52 antibody, as well as pretransplant antithymocyte globulin have both been associated with lower risk of GVHD after NST from an unrelated or mismatched donor (46–49).

Results of the largest series of nonmyeloablative strategies for lymphoma are summarized in Table 2 (50–52). The data for lymphoid malignancies demonstrate the feasibility and tolerability of nonmyeloablative allogeneic transplantation in patients with either indolent or aggressive lymphomas. The high incidence of GVHD observed in these patients underscores the importance of limiting these therapies to centers with extensive experience with conventional allografting. Delayed graft-vs.-tumor responses may occur sometimes several months after the initial transplant. Further studies and comparative trials are warranted. Overall, patients with low-grade lymphomas and chemoresponsive disease appear to benefit the most from this approach.

III. GVHD IN NONMYELOABLATIVE TRANSPLANTATION

The impact of preparative regimen intensity on the incidence of acute and chronic GVHD has not been systematically addressed. At M.D. Anderson Cancer Center the influence of conditioning regimens on the occurrence of acute and chronic GVHD and nonrelapse mortality (NRM) in patients undergoing matched-related sibling transplants receiving the

Table 1 Results of Published Series of NST in AML/MDS

n	Age (yr)	CR1 + CR2 or RA	Regimen	Graft failure	GVHD II–IV (%)	NRM at 1 yr (%)	DFS at 1 yr (%)	Ref.
31	61 (21–74)	8/31	FAI/2CDA-arac	2	20	20	34	4
43	52 (22–70)	1/43	FM/2CDA-M	0	50	34	34	38
117	51 (3–60)	23/117	Fludarabine-based 98/149	11	43	47	40 AML	39
37	57 (22–66)	15/37	FB	0	20	5	62 MDS / 66	40
47	NS	41/47	F-TBI	4	37	15	46 Sib / 60 MUD	41

n, number; CR, complete remission; GVHD, graft-vs.-host disease; NRM, nonrelapse mortality; DFS, disease-free survival; FAI, fludarabine/ara-c/idarubicin; FM, fludarabine/melphalan; FB, fludarabine/busulfan; F-TBI, fludarabine/200 cGy; TBI, total body irradiation.

Table 2 Results of NST in Hodgkin's Disease and Non-Hodgkin's Lymphoma

Histology	n	Age (yr)	Chemosensitive (%)	Regimen	Graft failure	GVHD II–IV (%)	NRM at 1 yr (%)	DFS (%)	Ref.
Indolent	20	46 (27–65)	85	Various	0	20	10	84 at 2 years	50
Aggressive	15	55 (31–64)	75	PFA	2	10	27	40 at 1 year	51
Aggressive	62	43 (2–61)	73	Various	NS	NS	29	13 at 2 years	52
Hodgkin's	52	30 (15–53)	54	Various	NS	27	17	42 at 2 year	52

NRM, nonrelapse mortality; DFS, disease-free survival.

same GVHD prophylaxis has recently been evaluated. Results from 137 patients who received HSCT between June 1, 1996, and September 30, 2000, were analyzed. All patients received allogeneic hematopoietic transplantation from an HLA-identical sibling donor.

Regimens were classified as myeloablative if they resulted in severe myelosuppression, required stem cell support, and generally resulted in full donor chimerism. In this analysis the myeloablative regimens used consisted of busulfan 0.8 mg/kg IV every 6 hours on days -7 to -4 and cyclophosphamide 60 mg/kg on days -3 and -2 or fludarabine 25 mg/m^2 on days -6 to -2 and melphalan 90 mg/m^2 on days -3 and -2 (FM).

Nonmyeloablative regimens were defined by those regimens that have been routinely used without stem cell support and resulted usually in some degree of mixed chimerism. The nonmyeloablative regimens included in this analysis were: fludarabine 30 mg/m^2/day on days -6 to -3, idarubicin 12 mg/m^2/day on days -6 to -4, and cytarabine 2 g/m^2 on days -7 to -3 (Flag-Ida); cisplatin 100 mg/m^2 IV continuous infusion on days -6 to -3, fludarabine 30 mg/m^2 on days -4 and -3, cytarabine 500–1000 mg/m^2 on days -4 and -3 (PFA); and fludarabine 30 mg/m^2 on days -5 to -3 with cyclophosphamide 750 mg/m^2 on days -5 to -3 (FC) with or without rituximab.

Patient characteristics varied significantly according to the preparative regimen and are summarized in Table 3. The group receiving myeloablation was generally younger and had better prognosis disease than the nonmyeloablative group. Similarly, only a third of the patients receiving BuCy had serious comorbidities at the time of transplant compared with approximately half of the FM and nonmyeloablative groups ($p < 0.05$).

Table 3 Patients' Characteristics in the M.D. Anderson Cancer Center Experience

	Overall ($n = 137$)	Ablative ($n = 74$)	Nonmyeloablative ($n = 63$)	p-value
Gender M/F	85/52	47/27	38/25	NS
Age				
Median	53	45	59	
Range	(15–75)	(15–68)	(21–75)	<0.001
>40, n (%)	105 (77)	47 (63)	58 (92)	<0.001
Diagnosis, n (%)				
AML/MDS	61 (45)	42 (57)	19 (30)	
CML	36 (26)	30 (40)	6 (9)	
CLL	8 (6)	0	8 (13)	
NHL	32 (23)	2 (3)	30 (48)	<0.001
Cell source, n (%)				
PBSC	113 (82)	53 (72)	60 (95)	
BM	24 (18)	21 (28)	3 (5)	<0.001
Disease risk group, n (%)				
High risk	65 (48)	30 (40)	35 (56)	
Low risk	72 (52)	44 (60)	28 (44)	NS
Prior chemoregimens				
≤ 2	88 (64)	54 (73)	34 (54)	
> 2	49 (36)	20 (27)	29 (46)	0.02
Serious comorbidities, n (%)	63 (46)	29 (39)	34 (54)	NS

Patients in the nonmyeloablative and FM groups had similar characteristics except for the proportion receiving more than two chemotherapy regimens previously, which was significantly higher in the nonmyeloablative group ($p = 0.02$). The stem cell source was bone marrow in 36% of the BuCy group, compared with 17% and 5% of those receiving either FM or the nonmyeloablative regimens respectively ($p < 0.01$). Diagnoses were similar in the BuCy and FM groups, where over 95% were myeloid malignancies. The majority of patients in the nonmyeloablative group (61%) had lymphoid malignancies.

All patients received a common regimen of posttransplant immunosuppressive therapy as prophylaxis against GVHD. This included tacrolimus starting at day -2, with dose adjustment to maintain blood levels of $5-15$ ng/mL, and methotrexate 5 mg/ m^2 on days 1, 3, and 6. Bone marrow recipients received an additional dose on day $+11$. Tacrolimus was continued for at least 90 days in the absence of disease progression. Patients at low risk for relapse continued tacrolimus until $6-9$ months posttransplant. Those at high risk for relapse or minimal residual disease had immunosuppression withdrawal at 6 months posttransplant.

The occurrence of acute GVHD was evaluated within 100 days following HSCT. The staging and grading of acute GVHD was performed according to modified Glucksberg consensus criteria. Biopsies from involved tissues were obtained when possible. The incidence of grade $2-4$ acute GVHD in the myeloablative group was 36% (95% CI $24-48$), which was significantly higher than the 12% (95% CI $5-23$) incidence in the nonmyeloablative group (HR 3.6; 95% CI $1.5-8.8$)(Fig. 2). This effect was consistent when comparison was performed among patients older than 40 years of age, those who received PB stem cells, after adjustment for the number of prior chemotherapy regimens received, or the disease risk category. A total of 11 patients (8%) developed grade $3-4$ acute GVHD. The incidence of grade $3-4$ acute GVHD was higher in the ablative group (12%; 95% CI $7-25$) than in the nonmyeloablative group (4%; 95% CI $1-14$), but this was not statistically significant ($p = 0.2$).

Skin was the GVHD organ most frequently involved ($n = 18$, 15%), followed by the gastrointestinal tract ($n = 12$, 10%) and liver ($n = 5$, 4%) (Table 4). When individual

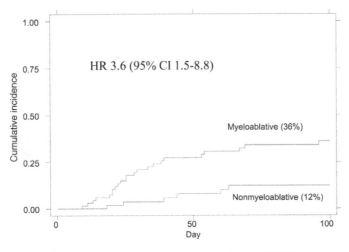

Figure 2   Actuarial incidence of grade $2-4$ acute GVHD.

Table 4 Acute GVHD Grade 2–4: Organ Involvement

	n	Skin, n (%)	GI, n (%)	Liver, n (%)
BuCy	41	8 (19)	3 (7)	3 (7)
FM	26	6 (23)	6 (23)[a]	1 (4)
NST	56	4 (7)[a]	3 (5)	1 (2)
Total	123	18 (15)	12 (10)	5 (4)

[a]Indicates a statistically significant difference in organ involvement in comparison with the other preparative regimens.

regimens were analyzed for organ involvement, there was a significantly higher proportion of skin involvement in the BuCy group ($p = 0.003$) and a higher proportion of GI involvement in the FM group ($p = 0.03$) compared with the other regimens. Only six patients with acute GVHD had liver involvement (4%). Liver was the single GVHD organ involved in three patients, all of whom were in the BuCy group. The pattern of organ involvement may relate to the tissue-specific toxicities of the preparative regimens.

Among patients receiving nonmyeloablative regimens, two patients (4%) of those with mixed chimerisms experienced grade 2–4 acute GVHD, compared to five patients with complete donor chimerism (16%); this difference was not statistically significant (HR 0.5; 95% CI 0.1–2.4).

The cumulative incidence of chronic GVHD was 40% for the myeloablative group and 14% for patients receiving nonmyeloablative regimens (Table 5). In the nonmyeloablative group there was a trend for a lower rate of chronic GVHD for patients with mixed chimerism compared to those with complete donor chimerism. This effect was not statistically significant: 4% ($n = 1$) of evaluable patients with mixed chimerism developed chronic GVHD compared with 20% ($n = 6$) of patients with complete donor chimerism (HR 0.3; 95% CI 0.03–2.4). The corresponding percentages for day 100 were 4% and 38%, respectively (HR 0.2; 95% CI 0.02–1.5).

The lower incidence of GVHD seen in the nonmyeloablative group increased in patients who had had immune manipulation (i.e., early withdrawal of immunosuppression, donor lymphocyte infusion, or both interventions) (Table 6). This observation must be interpreted with caution. Since the advent of nonmyeloablative strategies, new chemotherapeutic agents, and immunotherapeutic strategies such as DLI, the clinical

Table 5 Incidence of GVHD Before Immune Manipulation

	N[a]	AGVHD, N (%)	%KM (95% CI)	N[b]	CGVHD, n (%)	%CI[c] (95% CI)
Myeloablative	67	23 (34)	36 (26–49)	70	25 (36)	40
Non-myeloablative	56	6 (11)	12 (6–25)	55	7 (13)	14
Total	123	30 (24)		125	32 (25)	

[a]Patients with evidence of donor chimerism or aGVHD.
[b]Patients with evidence of donor chimerism or cGVHD.
[c]Cumulative incidence.

Table 6 Incidence of GVHD Occurring Before or After Immune Manipulation

	n	GVHD[a], n (%)	% KM (95% CI[b])	n	GVHD[c], n (%)	% CI[d] (95% CI)
BuCy/FM	67	23 (34)	35 (25–48)	70	30 (43)	47 (35–64)
NMA	56	10 (18)	18 (10–31)	55	19 (35)	36 (25–53)
Total		33			49	

[a]Up to day 90 posttransplant.
[b]Confidence interval.
[c]After day 90 posttransplant.
[d]Cumulative incidence at 18 months posttransplant.

characteristics of GVHD have changed. Some of the clinical features that differ from classic descriptions of acute and chronic GVHD include (a) delayed onset of acute GVHD, as noted in recent papers by the Fred Hutchinson Cancer Center and Ann Arbor groups in recent publications (54,55), (b) combined features of acute and chronic GVHD, and (c) organ involvement with GVHD conditioned by chemotherapy-specific toxicity (e.g., increased frequency of liver GVHD in patients receiving busulfan). For this reason the use of traditional classifications and grading systems for GVHD is somewhat problematic. In this part of our analysis, where patients undergoing immune manipulation are included, we analyzed all GVHD before and after the classical 100-day demarcation between acute and chronic GVHD. Before 90 days posttransplantation, the number of patients developing GVHD in the myeloablative group remained unchanged ($n = 23$) with a comparable incidence of 35% (95% CI 25–48). The myeloablative group continued to have a significantly higher incidence of GVHD within 90 days posttransplant (HR 2.3; 95% CI 1.1–4.8). Among patients who received nonmyeloablative regimens, four additional patients developed GVHD ($n = 10$), which increased the incidence of GVHD from 12 to 18% (95% CI 10–31). Beyond 90 days posttransplantation, seven and nine additional patients developed GVHD in the myeloablative ($n = 30$) and the nonmyeloablative groups, respectively ($n = 19$). Therefore, the cumulative incidence of GVHD beyond day 90 posttransplant increased to 47% for patients in the myeloablative group and to 38% in the nonmyeloablative group, making the GVHD risk similar among regimens (HR 1.2; 95% CI 0.7–2.2).

Mielcarek et al. (54) reported similar results in a smaller group of patients who received a variety of different regimens for GVHD prophylaxis. Nonmyeloablative transplants were associated with a lower incidence of grade 2–4 acute GVHD, with a tendency to more GVHD with acute features beyond day 100 posttransplant (54).

Acute and chronic GVHD affects the same target organs after both nonmyeloablative and ablative regimens. As mentioned above, distinct differences in the manifestations of GVHD are beginning to be observed (54,55). In our experience there may also be a tendency towards later manifestations of acute GVHD features.

IV. CONCLUSIONS

Nonablative preparative regimens have allowed the exploration of allogeneic bone marrow transplant (BMT) in older and debilitated patients. Most studies have shown that these regimens are well tolerated and can result in long term disease control in patients who otherwise would have not been considered eligible for allogeneic transplantation. In patients at M.D. Anderson Cancer Center, there appears to be a lower incidence of GVHD within the first 3 months posttransplantation. Nevertheless, acute and chronic GVHD still occur and represent important causes of morbidity and mortality in this patient population. Treatment of steroid refractory GVHD after nonablative transplantation is as ineffective as treatment of steroid-refractory GVHD after an ablative regimen. Whether the incidence of steroid-refractory GVHD is lower in recipients of nonablative vs. reduced-intensity conditioning regimens is a question requiring a randomized trial that controls for GVHD occurring after immune manipulation; in multiple trials such GVHD is as potentially lethal as GVHD occurring after a primary transplant. A role for various methods of T-cell depletion in the prevention of GVHD after nonablative transplantation will also require controlled trials, since retrospective analysis has shown that the incidence of GVHD is less, but overall survival does not seem to be positively affected.

An additional factor that complicates the characterization and prognosis of GVHD is the lack of adequate definitions and grading systems for this disease. As we recognize features such as late-onset acute GVHD or mixed manifestations of acute and chronic GVHD, the traditional classifications and grading systems for GVHD become increasingly difficult to apply. New grading criteria with a focus on type and degree of GVHD organ damage will need to be developed.

REFERENCES

1. Thomas E, Storb R, Clift R, et al. Bone marrow transplantation. N Engl J Med 1975; 292:832–842, 895–902.
2. Armitage JO. Bone marrow transplantation. N Engl J Med 1994; 330:827–838.
3. Popplewell LL, Forman SJ. Is there an upper age limit for bone marrow transplantation? Bone Marrow Transplant 2002; 29:277–284.
4. Giralt S, Estey E, Albitar M, et al. Engraftment of allogeneic hematopoietic progenitor cells with purine analog-containing chemotherapy: harnessing graft-versus- leukemia without myeloablative therapy. Blood 1997; 89:4531–4536.
5. Khouri I, Keating M, Korbling M, et al. Transplant lite: induction of graft versus malignancy using fludarabine based non ablative chemotherapy and allogeneic blood progenitor cell transplantation as treatment for lymphoid malignancies. J Clin Oncol 1998; 16:2817–2824.
6. Sykes M, Preffer F, McAfee S, et al. Mixed lymphohaemopoietic chimerism and graft versus lymphoma effects after non-myeloablative therapy and HLA- mismatched bone-marrow transplantation. Lancet 1999; 353:1755–1759.
7. Slavin S, Nagler A, Naparstek E, et al. Nonmyeloablative stem cell transplantation and cell therapy as an alternative to conventional bone marrow transplantation with lethal cytoreduction for the treatment of malignant and nonmalignant hematologic diseases. Blood 1998; 91:756–763.
8. Storb R, Yu C, Sandmaier BM, et al. Mixed hematopoietic chimerism after marrow allografts. Transplantation in the ambulatory care setting. Ann NY Acad Sci 1999; 872:372–375.
9. Hill GR, Crawford JM, Cooke KR, Brinson YS, Pan L, Ferrara JL. Total body irradiation and acute graft-versus-host disease: the role of gastrointestinal damage and inflammatory cytokines. Blood 1997; 90:3204–3213.
10. Ferrara J, Deeg H: Graft versus host disease. N Engl J Med 1991; 324:667–674.
11. Vogelsang GB, Wagner JE. Graft-versus-host disease. Hematol Oncol Clin North Am 1990; 4:625–639.

12. Fegan C, Poynton CH, Whittaker JA. The gut mucosal barrier in bone marrow transplantation. Bone Marrow Transplant 1990; 5:373–377.

13. Hill GR, Ferrara JL. The primacy of the gastrointestinal tract as a target organ of acute graft-versus-host disease: rationale for the use of cytokine shields in allogeneic bone marrow transplantation. Blood 2000; 95:2754–2759.

14. Gale R, Bortin M, Van Bekkum D, et al. Risk factors for acute graft versus host disease. Br J Haematol 1987; 67:397–406.

15. Ringden O, Horowitz MM, Gale RP, et al. Outcome after allogeneic bone marrow transplant for leukemia in older adults. JAMA 1993; 270:57–60.

16. Frassoni F, Labopin M, Arcese W, et al. The outcome of allogeneic hematopoietic stem cell transplantation (HSCT) for AML 1CR is significantly worse after 35 years. Implication for reducing the intensity of the conditioning regimen. Report of the acute leukemia working party of EBMT. Blood 2000; 96:393a.

17. Cahn J, Labopin M, Mandelli F, et al. Autologous bone marrow transplantation for first remission acute myeloblastic leukemia in patients older than 50 years: a retrospective analysis of the European Bone Marrow Transplant Group. Blood 1995; 85:575–579.

18. Holler E, Kolb H, Moller A, et al. Increased serum levels of tumor necrosis factor alpha precede major complications of bone marrow transplantation. Blood 1990; 75:1011–1016.

19. Xun C, Thompson J, Jenning C, et al. Effect of total body irradiation, busulfan-cyclophosphamide, or cyclophosphamide conditioning on inflammatory cytokine release and development of acute and chronic graft-versus-host disease in H-2-incompatible transplanted SCID mice. Blood 1994; 83:2360–2367.

20. Yu C, Storb R, Mathey B, Deeg HJ, Schuening FG, Graham TC, Seidel K, Burnett R, Wagner JL, Shulman H, et al. DLA-identical bone marrow grafts after low-dose total body irradiation: effects of high-dose corticosteroids and cyclosporine on engraftment. Blood 1995; 86:4376–4381.

21. McSweeney P, Storb R. Mixed chimerism preclinical studies and clinical applications. Biol Blood Marrow Transplant 1999; 5:192–203.

22. Sharabi Y, Sachs D. Mixed chimerism and permanent specific transplantation tolerance induced by a non lethal preparative regimen. J Exp Med 1989; 169:493.

23. Huang C, Fuchimoto Y, Scheier-Dolberg R, Murphy M, Neville D, Sachs D. Stable mixed chimerism and tolerance using a nonmyeloablative preparative regimen in a large-animal model. J Clin Invest 2000; 105:173–181.

24. Sykes M. Mixed chimerism and transplant tolerance. Immunity 2001; 14:417–424.

25. Sykes M, Sheard M, Sachs D. Graft versus host related immunosuppression is induced in mixed chimeras by alloresponses against either host or donor lymphohematopoietic cells. J Exp Med 1988; 168:2391–2396.

26. Mattson J, Uzunel M, Remberger M, Ringden O. T cell mixed chimerism is significantly correlated to a decreased risk of acute graft versus host disease after allogeneic stem cell transplantation. Transplantation 2001; 71:433–439.

27. Gale R, Aurer I. Are new conditioning regimens for transplants in acute myelogenous leukemia better? Bone Marrow Transplant 1999; 7:255–261.

28. Clift R, Buckner C, Appelbaum F, et al. Allogeneic marrow transplantation in patients with acute myeloid leukemia in first remission: a randomized trial of two irradiation regimens. Blood 1990; 76:1867–1871.

29. Bortin MM, Horowitz MM, Gale RP, et al. Changing trends in allogeneic bone marrow transplantation for leukemia in the 1980s. JAMA 1992; 268:607–612.

30. Antin JH. Graft-versus-leukemia: no longer an epiphenomenon. Blood 1993; 82:2273–2277.

31. Drobyski WR, Keever CA, Roth MS, et al. Salvage immunotherapy using donor leukocyte infusions as treatment for relapsed chronic myelogenous leukemia after allogeneic bone marrow transplantation: efficacy and toxicity of a defined T-cell dose. Blood 1993; 82:2310–2318.

32. van Rhee F, Lin F, Cullis JO, et al. Relapse of chronic myeloid leukemia after allogeneic bone marrow transplant: the case for giving donor leukocyte transfusions before the onset of hematologic relapse. Blood 1994; 83:3377–3383.
33. Kolb HJ, Mittermuller J, Clemm C, et al. Donor leukocyte transfusions for treatment of recurrent chronic myelogenous leukemia in marrow transplant patients. Blood 1990; 76:2462–2465.
34. Kolb HJ, Schattenberg A, Goldman JM, et al. Graft- versus-leukemia effect of donor lymphocyte infusions in marrow grafted patients. Blood 1995; 86:2041–2050.
35. Collins RH, Shpilberg O, Drobyski WR, et al. Donor leukocyte infusions in 140 patients with relapsed malignancy after allogeneic bone marrow transplantation. J Clin Oncol 1997; 15:433–444.
36. Slavin S, Naparstek E, Nagler A, Ackerstein A, Kapelushnik J, Or R. Allogeneic cell therapy for relapsed leukemia after bone marrow transplantation with donor peripheral blood lymphocytes. Exp Hematol 1995; 23:1553–1562.
37. Giralt S, Anagnostopoulos A, Shajahanan M, Champlin R. Non ablative stem cell transplantation for older patients with acute leukemias and myelodysplastic syndromes. Semin Hematol 2002; 39:57–62.
38. Giralt S, Thall PF, Khouri I, et al. Melphalan and purine analog-containing preparative regimens: reduced-intensity conditioning for patients with hematologic malignancies undergoing allogeneic progenitor cell transplantation. Blood 2001; 97:631–637.
39. Rezvani K, Lalancette M, Szydlo R, et al. Non-myeloablative stem cell transplant in AML, ALL, and MDS: disappointing outcome for patients with advanced phase disease. Blood 2000 96(suppl 1):479a.
40. Martino R, Caballero M, Perez-Simon J, et al. Evidence for a graft-versus-leukemia effect after allogeneic peripheral blood stem cell transplantation with reduced intensity conditioning in acute myelogenous leukemia and myelodysplastic syndromes. Blood 2002; 100:2243–2245.
41. Hegenbart U, Sandmaier B, Lange T, et al. Graft versus leukemia effect after related and unrelated allogeneic hematopoietic stem cell transplants (HSCT) in patients with acute myeloid leukemia following minimal conditioning. Blood 2001; 98(suppl 1):2814a.
42. Marks D, Lush R, Cavenagh J, et al. The toxicity and efficacy of donor lymphocyte infusions given after reduced-intensity conditioning allogeneic stem cell transplantation. Blood 2002; 100:3108–3114.
43. Shimoni A, Khouri I, Donato M, et al. Allogeneic transplantation with non-myeloablative or reduced intensity conditioning: the intensity of the conditioning regimen is related to the outcome in patients with active disease but not those in remission at the time of transplantation (abstr). Blood 2000; 96:199a.
44. Niederwieser D, Maris M, Shizuru J, et al. Low-dose total body irradiation (TBI) and fludarabine followed by hematopoietic cell transplantation (HCT) from HLA-matched or mismatched unrelated donors and postgrafting immune suppression with cyclosporine and mycophenolate mofetil (MMF) can induce durable complete chimerism and sustained remissions in patients with hematological diseases. Blood 2003; 101:1620–1629.
45. Nagler A, Aker M, Or R, et al. Low-intensity conditioning is sufficient to ensure engraftment in matched unrelated bone marrow transplantation. Exp Hematol 2001; 29:362–370.
46. Chakraverty R, Peggs K, Chopra R, et al. Limiting transplantation-related mortality following unrelated donor stem cell transplantation by using a nonmyeloablative conditioning regimen. Blood 2002; 99:1071–1078.
47. Perez-Simon J, Kottaridis P, Martino R, et al. Nonmyeloablative transplantation with or without alemtuzumab: comparison between 2 prospective studies in patients with lymphoproliferative disorders. Blood 2002; 100:3121–3127.
48. Michallet M, Bilger K, Garban F, et al. Allogeneic hematopoietic stem cell transplantation after nonmyeloablative preparative regimens: impact of pretransplantation and posttransplantation factors on outcome. J Clin Oncol 2001; 19:3340–3349.

49. Kroger N, Gottfried-Sayer H, Schwerdtfeger R, et al. Unrelated stem cell transplantation in multiple myeloma after a reduced intensity conditioning regimen with pretransplant anti-thymocyte globulin is highly effective with low transplant related mortality. Blood 2002; 100:755–760.

50. Khouri I, Saliba R, Giralt S, et al. Nonablative allogeneic hematopoietic transplantation as adoptive immunotherapy for indolent lymphoma; low incidence of toxicity, acute graft versus host disease, and treatment related mortality. Blood 2001; 98:3595–3599.

51. Khouri I, Giralt S, Saliba R, et al. 'Mini'-allogeneic stem cell transplantation for relapsed/refractory lymphomas with aggressive histologies. Proc Am Soc Clin Oncol 2000; 19:47a.

52. Robinson S, Goldstone A, Mackinnon S, et al. Chemoresistant or aggressive lymphoma predicts for a poor outcome following reduced intensity allogeneic progenitor cell transplantation: an analysis from the Lymphoma Working Party of the European Group for Blood and Bone Marrow Transplantation. Blood 2002; 100:4310–4316.

53. Couriel DR, Saliba RM, Giralt S, et al. Acute and chronic graft versus host disease after ablative and nonmyeloablative conditioning for allogeneic hematopoietic transplant 2004; 10:178–185.

54. Mielcarek M, Martin P, Leisenring W, et al. Graft versus host disease after nonmyeloablative versus conventional hematopoietic stem cell transplantation. Blood 2003; 102:756–762.

55. Levine JE, Uberti JP, Ayash L, et al. Lowered-intensity preparative regimen for allogeneic stem cell transplantation delays acute graft-versus-host disease but does not improve outcome for advanced hematologic malignancy. Biol Blood Marrow Transplant 2003; 9:189–197.

19

Adoptive Immunotherapy in Stem Cell Transplantation

DAVID L. PORTER

University of Pennsylvania, Philadelphia, Pennsylvania, U.S.A.

JOHN E. LEVINE

University of Michigan, Ann Arbor, Michigan, U.S.A.

HANS-JOCHEM KOLB

University of Munich, Munich, Germany

I. INTRODUCTION

It is of more than historical interest to recall that less than 50 years ago the earliest murine experiments first suggested that bone marrow transplantation (BMT) was successful because of immune mechanisms specific to the donor graft, independent of other antileukemia therapy (1). Within the next 10 years, allogeneic BMT was attempted in humans, rationalized by the hypothesis that the donor marrow graft "has a distinct value as an anti-leukemia agent" (2). It took an additional 25 years for sufficient clinical data to be generated, but through important clinical observations it became clear that allogeneic BMT in humans is also associated with a potent graft-vs.-leukemia (GVL) effect. It was further evident that the GVL reaction is mediated, at least in part, by mature donor T cells contained in the marrow graft and closely associated with graft-vs.-host disease (GVHD). It is a testament to clinical progress that in less than 5 decades, allogeneic BMT has become a powerful and successful method of adoptive immunotherapy for cancer.

Ultimately, it was the use of donor leukocyte infusions (DLI) to treat relapsed leukemia that provided the first direct evidence for a GVL reaction in the clinical setting. Numerous clinical trials of BMT and DLI have now provided the background to develop new therapies designed to manipulate and control the GVL activity of the donor immune system. Although many issues remain unsettled, the potential to harness the more general "graft-vs.-tumor" (GVT) activity of allogeneic donor cells may provide a new paradigm for the immunotherapy of cancer. Graft-vs.-tumor effects can be manipulated to both prevent and treat relapse and infections, and it is now possible to induce a direct GVT reaction without the need for intensive conditioning therapy. This chapter will review the role of allogeneic cell therapy as a method of adoptive immunotherapy to treat leukemia and other malignancies as well as relapse and infectious complications after allogeneic stem cell transplantation.

II. GVL EFFECTS IN EXPERIMENTAL MODELS OF TRANSPLANTATION

The importance of the GVL reaction has been suspected since some of the earliest BMT experiments in mice. One of the earliest studies by Barnes and colleagues determined that leukemic recipients of syngeneic marrow grafts treated with subtherapeutic doses of radiation were more likely to relapse than mice transplanted with allogeneic marrow grafts (3). They generated a remarkably insightful hypothesis that the allogeneic graft contained cells with "immune reactivity" capable of eradicating residual leukemia cells. They also observed that recipients of homologous or allogeneic grafts were most likely to be cured of leukemia, but died of a "wasting syndrome" now recognized as GVHD. Thus, in addition to describing the GVL properties in transplantation, they also identified the intricate relationship between a GVL response and GVHD. Since this early work, many murine models have studied the role of GVL induction in BMT. In model systems it is possible to explore various effector cell populations and target antigens and to design quantitative and qualitative experiments to understand GVL activity in detail. Much of this work as been reviewed in detail elsewhere (4–8) and is the subject of Chapter 6 in this volume.

While model systems are extremely useful, they also emphasize that GVL induction is a complex process, and direct application to clinical therapy must be made with caution. Conclusions about the magnitude of the GVL effect, the responsive tumor types, and the effector cells and their target antigens may all depend on the leukemia model studied, specific experimental conditions, and the degree of MHC variation between donor and host. In addition, in cases where murine leukemia is virally induced, there is always the concern that the observed antileukemic effect is due to specific antiviral immunity. Nevertheless, these important models help to define the role of specific cell subsets, cytokines, accessory molecules, antigen presentation, and other immunological properties necessary for GVL activity. Murine models will continue to form the basis for clinical trials and are necessary guides for the design of future studies.

III. GVL IN CLINICAL TRANSPLANTATION

The success of allogeneic stem cell transplantation in humans is at least partly dependent on the GVL properties of the donor graft, independent of the conditioning regimen. Initial evidence for GVL activity in clinical transplantation was first based on several important but indirect observations as outlined in Table 1. This clinical information also demonstrated that donor T cells are primary mediators of the GVL reaction. This evidence now provides the basis for newer and more rational approaches to adoptive immunotherapy designed to enhance and manipulate GVL effects for clinical benefit.

Table 1   Indirect Evidence of Graft-vs.-Leukemia Effect in Clinical Transplantation

Patients with leukemia who relapse after allogeneic stem cell transplantation may achieve complete
remission with a flare of graft-vs.-host disease or after withdrawal of immunosuppression.

Graft-vs.-host disease after allogeneic stem cell transplantation is protective against relapse.

The risk of relapse after syngeneic stem cell transplantation is significantly higher than the risk of
relapse after matched sibling stem cell transplantation.

T-cell depletion of the donor graft as GVHD prophylaxis increases the risk of relapse, especially for
patients with CML.

A.   Remission Induction Induced by a Flare of GVHD or Withdrawal of Immune Suppression

The association of GVHD with GVL activity was first suggested by several anecdotal case
reports describing patients with relapsed leukemia after BMT that reentered remission
associated with a flare of acute GVHD (9) or after discontinuation of immunosuppressive
therapy (10–12). The presence of a GVL reaction is now commonly reported based on
observations of response associated with GVHD. Furthermore, newer trials of adoptive
immunotherapy are typically designed to include withdrawal of immunosuppression to
enhance GVL activity.

B.   Association of Syngeneic Marrow Grafts with Increased Relapse Rates

Consistent with animal models of BMT, relapse rates after human syngeneic marrow
transplantation are higher when compared to transplant with matched sibling allogeneic
grafts. Data from the Seattle group showed that for patients with advanced leukemia,
the relapse rate was 62% for 785 recipients of allogeneic grafts compared to a relapse
rate of 75% for 53 recipients of syngeneic grafts ($p < 0.0001$) (13). In a subsequent multicenter analysis, the loss of GVL activity after syngeneic BMT was even more obvious for
patients with AML in first remission; 31 recipients of syngeneic marrow grafts had an
almost three-fold increase in relapse rate when compared with 339 recipients of allogeneic
grafts (actuarial probability of relapse $59 \pm 20\%$ vs. $18 \pm 4\%$) (14). Subsequent retrospective studies from the International Bone Marrow Transplant Registry (IBMTR) have confirmed these findings (15,16) (Fig. 1). These data also implied that the magnitude of the
GVL effect might depend on both the diagnosis and disease activity at the time of
BMT. For instance, a more recent update found that syngeneic transplantation was associated with higher relapse rates for patients with chronic myelogenous leukemia (CML) and
acute myelogenous leukemia (AML), but not for patients with acute lymphocytic leukemia (ALL) in first remission (15).

While loss of GVL activity after syngeneic BMT is now generally accepted, there
has been concern that the higher relapse rate after syngeneic BMT could be exaggerated by other confounding factors. For instance, while the conditioning regimens for
syngeneic and matched sibling BMT are often identical, recipients of non–T-cell-
depleted allogeneic marrow grafts often receive GVHD prophylaxis that includes methotrexate, while recipients of syngeneic grafts receive no GVHD prophylaxis. While it is

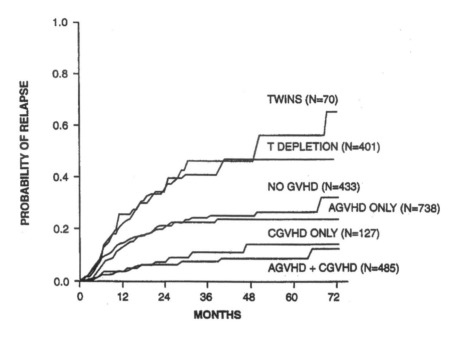

Figure 1 Probability of relapse after allogeneic bone marrow transplantation for 2254 patients from the International Bone Marrow Transplant Registry. (From Ref. 16.)

difficult to exclude the possibility that the GVHD prophylaxis contributes to the antileukemic effect of allogeneic BMT, the total dose of methotrexate is relatively low and is unlikely to be responsible for the significant differences in relapse rates. Another improbable concern is that recurrent leukemia arises from donor cells; these cells would be impossible to distinguish from the recipients' original leukemia in syngeneic twins.

C. Protective Effect of GVHD Against Relapse

There is now considerable evidence that GVHD after allogeneic BMT is protective against relapse. It was first observed that patients with advanced leukemia (AML or ALL in relapse, CML in accelerated phase or blast crisis, or patients in remission but at high risk of relapse) who develop acute and/or chronic GVHD had lower relapse rates than patients who have no GVHD (17–19). Similarly, GVHD was also protective against relapse for patients transplanted in early–stage leukemia (16,20). In the IBMTR analysis, the risk of relapse after BMT for over 2200 patients transplanted with "early leukemia" (AML or ALL in first remission or CML in chronic phase) who had acute and chronic GVHD was significantly lower when compared to patients who developed no GVHD (Fig. 1) (16). This report further emphasized that the magnitude of GVL activity is disease dependent. For instance, for recipients of unmanipulated donor marrow grafts, acute GVHD only was associated with less relapse in ALL, while the combination of acute and chronic GVHD was associated with lower relapse rates for patients with ALL, AML, and CML.

D. Increased Relapse Rates Following T-Cell Depletion of Donor Marrow Graft

GVHD is in large part mediated by alloreactive donor T cells contained in the marrow graft. T-cell depletion of the donor graft prior to stem cell transplant (SCT) has been one of the most successful means of limiting the incidence and severity of GVHD after allogeneic SCT (21–26). However, while it was initially anticipated that T-cell depletion would minimize transplant-related mortality and translate into improved survival rates, several studies show that despite less frequent and less severe GVHD, overall survival is not improved after T-cell–depleted BMT (23,27–30). This has been due in large part to a reciprocal increase in the rate of relapse and graft failure. The increase in relapse rate after T-cell–depleted BMT has been most dramatic in patients transplanted for CML, where the incidence of relapse is as high as 50% (16,27,30); the IBMTR analysis found that compared to recipients of unmanipulated marrow grafts who develop no GVHD, patients with CML receiving T-cell–depleted marrow have a relative risk of relapse of 6.91 (16). These results provide strong, though still indirect evidence that donor T cells possess important antileukemic properties that significantly influence the success of marrow transplantation.

IV. ADOPTIVE IMMUNOTHERAPY IN ALLOGENEIC STEM CELL TRANSPLANTATION

The indirect clinical evidence for GVL activity, taken together with animal experiments of bone marrow transplantation, strongly supports the important role of T cells for the control of leukemia relapse in CML patients. These data first encouraged the use of donor lymphocytes for the treatment of CML relapse in patients who had failed interferon-α (31). Three patients were treated in 1988 and 1989 with infusions of donor buffy coat cells, and all three are still in molecular remission. Subsequently, numerous reports have demonstrated the dramatic GVL potential of DLI for the treatment of relapsed CML (32–35). In earlier studies the response has been investigated by cytogenetic analysis and fluorescent in situ hybridization for BCR/ABL, but in recent years the quantitative analysis with RT-PCR has become standard; RT-PCR can detect up to 1 in 1 million cells containing the bcr-abl transcript (36).

In addition to many single-institution trials, two large retrospective studies of DLI were reported from Europe (37) and from North America (38) (Table 2). The EBMT study comprised patients with HLA-identical sibling donors, HLA-compatible unrelated donors, HLA-mismatched family donors, and identical twin donors. A GVL effect was observed in all groups with the exception of the group of identical twin donors (37). Best responses were seen in patients with chronic disease (hematological relapse) and in patients with cytogenetic and molecular evidence of the disease (Table 2). Responses were less frequent in patients with recurrent disease in accelerated and blastic transformation. Favorable factors other than type of relapse were T-cell depletion for prophylaxis of GVHD after stem cell transplantation and the absence of GVHD at the time of DLI. The presence of chimerism is necessary for a GVL response. In a single-center study the proportion of donor T cells present at the time of DLI was favorable for a GVL response (39).

In many patients with CML, the response to DLI is not immediate, but it may start only after several weeks or months. The time until a molecular remission is obtained is

Table 2 Response Rates to Donor Leukocyte Infusions
to Treat Relapse After Allogeneic Bone Marrow
Transplantation[a]

Disease	Response rate
CML chronic phase	76% (28/37) (38)
	79% (53/67) (37)
CML advanced phase	28% (5/18) (38)
	12% (1/8) (37)
AML	15% (6/39) (38)
	29% (5/17) (37)[b]
	36% (16/44) (69)
ALL	18% (2/11) (38)
	0% (0/12) (37)
	13% (2/15) (77)
MDS	40% (2/5) (38)
	25% (1/4) (37)
NHL	0/6 (0%) (38)
	2/2 (83)
	1/2 (82)
Multiple myeloma	50% (2/4) (38)
	31% (4/13) (137)
	22% (6/27) (87)
	9% (2/22) (86)[c]
	55% (6/11) (88)[d]

AML, acute myelogenous leukemia; ALL, acute lymphocyte leukemia; MDS, myelodysplasia; NHL, non-Hodgkin's lymphoma;
CML, chronic myelogenous leukemia; EBMT, European Group
for Blood and Marrow Transplantation.
[a]Representative response rates are illustrated from either registry
data or in some cases, larger series of DLI for a specific indication.
[b]All patients were pretreated with chemotherapy by design of the
protocol.
[c]A total of 25 patients were treated. An additional 3 patients
achieved a complete response after treatment with chemotherapy
before DLI.
[d]24 patients underwent T-cell–depleted allogeneic SCT and 11
received DLI for persistent disease.

between 4 and 6 months on average (Fig. 2), and it may take more than a year until the
leukemic clone is suppressed to undetectable levels. Fortunately most responses are durable and associated with improved survival (40,41); however, survival is dependent on the
stage of CML at the time of DLI (Fig. 3).

The major complications of DLI are myelosuppression and GVHD. Myelosuppression with thrombocytopenia, leukopenia, and/or reticulocytopenia occurred in 34% of
patients (37). It is more frequent in patients with hematological relapse than in those
with cytogenetic relapse, and in most cases it is transient. The lack of donor hematopoiesis
has been shown to predict myelosuppression after DLI (42). Persistent cytopenia may be
treated with recombinant human growth factors such as granulocyte colony-stimulating
factor (G-CSF) and erythropoietin. For persistent marrow aplasia, transfusion of donor

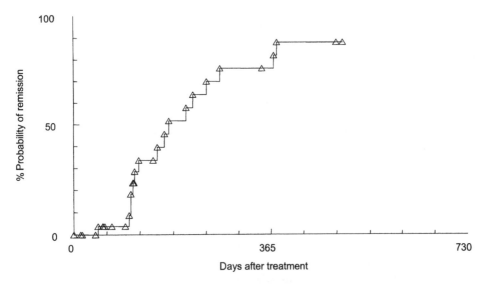

Figure 2 Time to molecular remission after DLI for CML (MUC-GH 03/01).

stem cells or bone marrow may lead to complete hematological restitution (32). Transfusion of G-CSF–mobilized donor blood cells instead of DLI has not been shown to decrease the risk of myelosuppression (43). In some patients pancytopenia is associated with chronic GVHD; neither hematopoietic growth factors nor transfusion of stem cells may help, but a trial with corticosteroids may be useful.

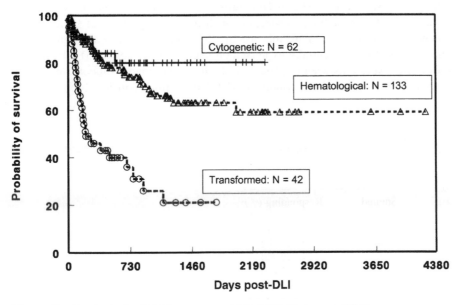

Figure 3 Survival after DLI for recurrent CML (EBMT, August 2000).

Grade II and higher acute GVHD was observed in 41% of patients treated with DLI reported to the EBMT (37). In the North American study 60% of patients treated with DLI developed acute GVHD (38). The GVL effect correlates with the presence of GVHD (Table 3). However, complete responses were seen in a significant proportion of patients without any sign of GVHD. The GVL effect in the absence of clinical GVHD provides further evidence for GVL activity separate from the GVH reaction.

The clinical picture of GVHD after DLI differs from that after stem cell transplantation in several aspects. In the North American study, the median time to onset of acute GVHD was 32 days (38) compared to a median time to onset of 16–20 days following myeloablative T-replete transplantation (44,45). Perhaps this difference is related to the absence of an acute inflammatory response induced by the conditioning treatment, a possibility supported by the finding that time to onset of acute GVHD is delayed following reduced-intensity transplantation (46). The target organs of acute GVHD following DLI are the same as those seen following stem cell transplantation, but the clinical manifestations may differ. A hepatitic variant of liver GVHD characterized by marked elevations of serum aminotransferase levels more than 10 times the upper limit of normal was observed in 11 of 73 (15%) patients who received DLI at Johns Hopkins University between 1998 and 2001 (47). Characteristic skin, liver, and intestinal acute GVHD manifestations can be seen following DLI, but their frequency and severity has not been well described. In a study of 81 patients who received DLI following reduced intensity HSCT, GVHD signs in the skin, liver, and intestinal tract developed in 26%, 8%, and 14% of patients, respectively (48). Likewise, characteristic findings of chronic GVHD can be seen following DLI (48), and on occasion both acute and chronic GVHD can manifest themselves simultaneously following DLI (49). Although various factors have been reported as predictive of the development of GVHD after DLI, including the number of infusions, the dose of CD3+ cells/infusion, the degree of HLA match, and levels of serum gamma glutamyl transferase (50–52), large, prospective clinical trials to validate these findings have yet to be performed.

The good response of CML to DLI throws light on the mechanism of adoptive immunotherapy with donor lymphocytes, although the primary target of the transfused T cells is not known. It may be leukemia specific (53,54) or directed against minor histocompatibility antigens differentially expressed on hematopoietic cells (55). The fact that responses to DLI were only seen in patients with allogeneic donors supports the role for histocompatibility antigens. Furthermore, mixed T-cell chimerism has been converted

Table 3   Graft-vs.-Leukemia Effect of Donor Lymphocyte Transfusions—EBMT Update

Grade of GVHD	No. of patients	
	Studied	Responding (%)
0	115	58 (50%)
I	40	30 (75%)
II	54	47 (87%)
III	22	19 (86%)
IV	9	6 (67%)

$p \leq 0.0001$.

to complete donor T-cell chimerism in patients treated with DLI (56), indicating a reaction against histocompatibility antigens rather than leukemia specific antigens. However, these findings do not exclude activity against antigens other than histocompatibility antigens. Cytotoxic T cells against a peptide of proteinase 3 were found in patients responding to interferon-α and in patients with a molecular response after allogeneic transplantation (57). Proteinase 3 is involved as a target protein in Wegener's granulomatosis. Another attractive target for donor T cells would be the BCR/ABL protein. Cytotoxic T cells directed against BCR/ABL have been found in CML patients (54), but vaccination with BCR/ABL fusion peptide did not induce cytotoxic T cells in CML patients (58).

The contribution of natural killer cells to GVL activity has not been elucidated in chronic phase CML. Natural killer (NK) cell activity may be more prominent in transformed phase rather than in chronic phase CML; in CML cells from patients with chronic phase, there is down regulation of co-stimulatory molecules and possibly also of HLA antigens. The Philadelphia chromosome has been identified by FISH analysis in dendritic cells of CML patients, supporting the hypothesis that CML is a good target for immunotherapy because mature dendritic cells develop from CML cells. Typically the fluorescent signal for bcr and abl co-localize in these patients. This stimulatory capacity of CML is poor in patients at diagnosis, when the majority of progenitor cells are DR negative (59). After treatment with interferon-α the majority of CD34+ progenitor cells disappear and the residual population of Philadelphia-positive cells is DR-positive. The combination of interferon-α and granulocyte-monocyte colony-stimulating factor (GM-CSF) has upregulated HLA-class I and class II antigens and co-stimulatory molecules CD80, CD86, and CD83, and CD40 on CML cells in culture (60), and it has improved the response to DLI in patients with advanced refractory disease.

V. DLI IN DISEASES OTHER THAN CML

The excellent response rates to DLI seen in the setting of early phase CML relapse have not been duplicated in other malignancies. In advanced relapse of other hematological malignancies, complete remissions after DLI are generally not seen in more than 20–25% of patients and can be seen in as few as 0% (Table 2). This is not surprising since available data suggest that GVL activity has disease specificity. For instance, depletion of T cells from the donor graft does not have a significant impact on the relapse rate of AML treated with allogeneic transplantation in first remission, unlike the situation for CML (16). Nevertheless, GVL activity is still observed in some patients with acute leukemia. For instance, syngeneic transplants carry a 2.5-fold higher risk of relapse than allogeneic transplants, and the occurrence of acute and chronic GVHD is associated with a significantly lower relapse risk after SCT for acute leukemia (15,16). In addition, one of the longest surviving recipients of DLI was treated for relapse of ALL and reportedly remained in remission more than 8 years after donor cell infusion (61). It was therefore logical to attempt GVL induction with DLI for patients with relapse of acute leukemia as well as CML.

A. DLI for Acute Myelogenous Leukemia

Initial reports demonstrated that DLI could induce complete responses in a small number of patients with relapse of AML or myelodysplastic syndrome (MDS) (62,63); multicenter data on the use of DLI for patients with AML showed that response rates of 15–29%

(37,38). One possible explanation for the relatively low response rate in acute leukemia to DLI may be that the rate of leukemia cell growth outstrips the cytotoxicity rate of the donor lymphocytes. The median time to remission following DLI in CML patients has been reported to be 2.8–4.1 months (Fig. 2) (38,64). The percentage of recipient cells present in the marrow at the time of DLI appears to correlate inversely with the lag time to response in CML patients (64,65), as might be predicted by the superior complete remission rates for patients treated in cytogenetic or molecular relapse compared to relapse in chronic phase or advanced phase (Table 2). This finding suggests that a heavy tumor burden in diseases with a high proliferative rate may contribute to failure to respond to DLI. The literature supports that conclusion. When patients with advanced leukemia are given cytoreductive chemotherapy prior to DLI, complete remissions are more common. A compilation of 79 reported cases in the literature of acute leukemia demonstrated that 52 patients (AML 25/35, ALL 19/32, not specified 6/9, CML 1/1, MDS 1/1, or non-Hodgkin's lymphoma 0/1), entered a complete remission for an overall complete response rate of 66% (38,66–68). For the 49 responders in whom duration of remission was reported, median disease-free survival was 26 months. These studies were retrospective in nature, and selection or reporting bias may have influenced the results.

Levine et al. reported results of a prospective study of 65 patients with hematological relapse of advanced myeloid malignancy after HLA-matched sibling BMT who were prospectively treated with cytarabine-based chemotherapy, then G-CSF–primed DLI (69). Twenty-seven of 57 (47%) assessable patients entered a complete remission. In this study, overall survival at 2 years was 19%. Treatment-related mortality (23%) was perhaps somewhat higher than the approximately 13% reported from other studies when DLI was given without chemotherapy (37,38). Predictably, patients with a complete response were more likely to survive, with 1- and 2-year survival rates of 51% and 41%, respectively, with a median follow-up of more than 2 years. The prognosis for non-responders was dismal, with 1-year survival of only 5%. A posttransplant remission lasting more than 6 months before relapse predicted a response rate and survival (Fig. 4) similar to the EBMT results. Survival at 1 year for patients with relapse within 6 months of transplant was 10% compared to 44% for patients who relapsed more than 6 months after transplant ($p < 0.001$) (69).

The use of chemotherapy prior to DLI in acute leukemia is not supported by all studies. In an initial EBMT survey, DLI in patients with recurrent AML and MDS after allogeneic transplantation induced complete remissions in 26% of patients not given chemotherapy or not responding to chemotherapy (Table 4). In this survey three groups of patients were identified: a group of 36 patients not given chemotherapy (group 1) and a group of 37 patients given chemotherapy; in the chemotherapy group 15 patients went into remission and were given DLI in addition (group 2), and in 22 patients remission was not achieved, and the patients were given DLI instead of further chemotherapy (group 3). The duration of the response was not different whether or not the remission was induced by chemotherapy. More recently, the outcome of DLI for relapsed AML and MIDS was evaluated in 108 of 120 patients reported to the EBMT (70). The response rate was 41%, including patients given chemotherapy; unfavorable factors were a short remission and the absence of GVHD after DLI. Notably the FAB subtype and the karyotype did not influence response and survival.

GVHD develops in the majority of patients (56%) who receive chemotherapy followed by DLI for relapse of advanced myeloid diseases (69). Interestingly, while GVHD has been reported to correlate with likelihood of achieving remission after

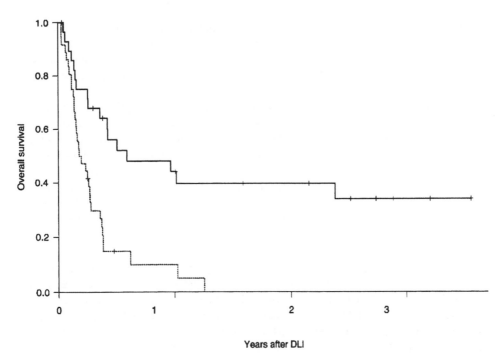

Figure 4   Overall survival for patients treated with chemotherapy and DLI for relapsed AML. Dashed lines, relapse after BMT within 6 months; solid lines, relapse after BMT after 6 months. [Source: Figure 2 from Levine JE, Braun T, Penza SL, et al. Prospective trial of chemotherapy and donor leukocyte infusions for relapse of advanced myeloid malignancies after allogeneic stem-cell transplantation. J Clin Oncol 2002; 20:405–412. Reprinted with permission from the American Society of Clinical Oncology (69).]

DLI (38), GVHD was not required for durable remission. Similarly, Porter et al. found that if a patient was in remission after DLI, acute GVHD was not predictive for subsequent relapse (41). Because the number of patients studied was small, one cannot rule out a possible protective effect of GVHD against relapse, nor eliminate the possibility that GVHD-related mortality affected the results. Nonetheless, this finding does suggest that clinically evident GVHD does not help sustain a remission established after DLI, consistent with

Table 4   Response to DLI for Recurrent AML/MDS After BMT—EBMT UPDATE

Chemotherapy	No. of patients in CR/number studied	Survival time (days)
No chemotherapy	9/36	112+, 155+, 291, 439, 503, 598+, 1007, 1014+, 2374
Chemotherapy—CR	14/15	60, 96, 159, 312+, 372+, 438+, 527, 646, 1173, 1245, 1416+, 1453+, 1463+, 1563+
Chemotherapy—no CR	6/22	152, 617+, 800, 977, 1234+, 1263+

prior observations that clinically evident GVHD is not a prerequisite for clinically evident antileukemia effect (16,71). While Porter did not find a survival benefit for the presence of chronic GVHD (41), Carlens et al. reported that chronic GVHD was associated with a survival advantage after DLI (72). Further studies will be needed to delineate the extent to which GVHD contributes to the durability of remission after DLI.

Not only are responses to DLI less common in patients with AML than with CML, relapse rates after DLI-induced remissions are high (37,38). Porter et al. reported long-term follow-up results for patients who achieved a complete remission following DLI (41). Eleven out of 27 (41%) patients without CML, mainly AML, MDS, or ALL, who were in remission after DLI relapsed at a median of 10 months later (range 1–37 months). Also affecting the durability of remission after DLI for acute leukemia has been the problem of extramedullary relapse, which have been reported in numerous anatomical sites, including those not usually considered sanctuary sites for leukemia (68,73,74).

Optimal dosing of DLI for advanced myeloid leukemia has not been established. In the prospective study of chemotherapy followed by DLI cited above, the targeted DLI dose was 1×10^8 CD3+ cells/kg of recipient body weight (69). A Japanese study of 100 patients reported that a DLI dose of 1×10^8 leukocytes/kg of recipient body weight appeared to be optimal (75). In that study, the minimal dose of leukocytes associated with developing fatal GVHD was 7×10^7 leukocytes/kg of recipient body weight, indicative of the difficulty in separating therapeutic effect from toxicity.

B.   DLI in ALL

The existence of a GVL effect in ALL is well established (16). In fact, one of the first recipients of DLI to treat relapse was a child with ALL (61), who remains in remission 15 years following the infusion (76). However, despite this particularly successful case, donor leukocyte infusions for ALL have generally been considered ineffective. Kolb et al. found little benefit for ALL patients in a European study, with no patients achieving remission from DLI alone, a median survival of less than 6 months after DLI, and a 100% probability of relapse at 15 months following treatment (37). A follow-up report from the same group 3 years later confirmed these findings (66). Collins et al. analyzed the efficacy of DLI in 44 patients with ALL reported to a North American registry database (77). Only 2 of 15 patients who received no pre-DLI chemotherapy achieved complete remissions, an equivalent result to that seen in Europe. Four patients received DLI as consolidation of remission induced by chemotherapy or immunosuppression-withdrawal, with one durable remission observed. Twenty of the remaining 25 patients who received DLI in the nadir after chemotherapy either failed to achieve remission or died within less than 30 days of the infusion. None of the five remissions lasted longer than 193 days. Second DLI were given to 7 of the 44 patients, with no durable remissions seen. Three-year overall actuarial survival was 13%.

The poor results for DLI in ALL have not been explained. It has been speculated that failure of DLI for ALL may be due to induction of T-cell anergy by ALL cells (78) or their inadequate expression of important co-stimulatory molecules or adhesion molecules (79,80). Likewise, ALL resistance to killing by NK cells has also been reported. Ruggeri et al. (81) found a 0% probability of relapse by 5 years for 20 AML patients whose donors had antirecipient NK cell clones following haploidentical T-cell–depleted transplantation. By contrast, the probability of relapse at 5 years for 14 ALL patients whose donors had antirecipient NK cell clones was 85%. These findings highlight the difficulty in generating effective strategies to employ immunotherapy against relapsed ALL.

C. DLI in Lymphoma and Myeloma

The DLI experience is more limited for hematological malignancies for which allogeneic transplant is not commonly performed either because of their rarity or because other treatments are traditionally preferred, such as autologous HSCT for lymphomas or multiple myeloma. Although Collins et al. (38) found no responses among 6 non-Hodgkin's lymphoma (NHL) patients who received DLI for posttransplant relapse, Bernard et al. reported two durable remissions following DLI for relapsed NHL (82). However, both patients relapsed more than 5 years after their transplant, so one must be especially cautious in extrapolating from the outcomes of these two patients to patients with earlier posttransplant relapse. Overall, DLI has not been well studied for lymphoma relapse after BMT. Case reports and small series demonstrate responses to DLI in patients with posttransplant relapses of low-grade lymphoma (83) and chronic lymphocytic leukemia (84), but more compelling evidence of a graft-vs.-lymphoma effect for these diseases has been demonstrated by studies of DLI to achieve remission after reduced intensity transplant. For example, Robinson et al. reported that 10 of 14 patients with relapsed or persistent lymphoma responded to DLI alone, including 6 complete responses (85). In two series comprising a total of 52 patients with multiple myeloma, complete responses to DLI with or without neoadjuvant chemotherapy were observed in 13 (25%) patients (86,87). Only 7 (13%) of the patients that were ongoing at 12 months following DLI had remissions. In other settings, such as prophylactic DLI following T-cell–depleted BMT (88) or reduced-intensity conditioning (89), a graft-vs.-myeloma effect has been reported. However, given the modest numbers of patients involved in these studies, the potential graft-vs.-myeloma benefit of DLI can only be estimated as moderate.

VI. UNRELATED DLI

Although the majority of data using DLI to treat relapse has been after matched sibling SCT, DLI has also been used after unrelated donor SCT. There was initial concern that unrelated DLI (U-DLI) might result in more frequent and severe GVHD than matched sibling DLI due to the higher degree of HLA disparity between recipient and donor. Furthermore, it was not known if U-DLI would provide similar, less, or even enhanced GVL activity compared to infusions from a matched sibling. Several initial studies describing the use of DLI for relapsed disease have included recipients of U-DLI (37,38,40,43,77,90–92), but it is difficult to draw conclusions about the toxicity or efficacy of this therapy since most trials include only small numbers of U-DLI recipients and data regarding the specific outcome after U-DLI is not always provided. Two larger retrospective studies have suggested, however, that outcome after U-DLI is similar to that of matched sibling DLI (37,38).

Two more recent analyses focused primarily on the role of U-DLI. In one study of patients with relapsed CML, outcomes after matched sibling DLI in 18 patients were compared directly to outcomes for 12 recipients of U-DLI. The median age for all patients was 42 years (range 19.5–58) and the median mononuclear cell (MNC) dose was similar in both groups (overall 2.5×10^8 MNC/kg). The incidence of cytogenetic remission was 73% after matched sibling DLI compared to 64% after U-DLI ($p = 0.71$). There was a trend toward more frequent grade II–IV acute GVHD in U-DLI recipients (58% vs. 39%), but this difference did not reach statistical significance ($p = 0.09$) possibly due to the small numbers of patients studied. The incidence of chronic GVHD was 49% for all patients and was not dependent on the donor source. The only factor associated with response was disease stage at the time of DLI, similar to other reports of matched sibling DLI (37,38) or U-DLI (93); patients treated in cytogenetic or molecular relapse were seven times more likely to respond when compared to patients treated in hematologic relapse. Remissions were durable without cytogenetic or hematological relapses at a median follow-up of 22 months.

In a larger retrospective analysis, 58 recipients of U-DLI were identified through the National Marrow Donor Program database. Patients received U-DLI for relapse of CML ($n = 25$), AML ($n = 23$), ALL ($n = 7$), or other diseases ($n = 3$). The median recipient age was 26 years (range 2–60), and donor and recipient were HLA-mismatched in at least 21% of cases. The median cell dose administered was 1.0×10^8 MNC/kg with 41% of patients receiving less than this amount. Complete remissions were achieved in 46% of patients with CML, 42% of patients with AML, and 2 of 4 evaluable patients with ALL. The incidence of grade II–IV acute GVHD was 25% and chronic GVHD occurred in 41% of patients, both in keeping with data from large series of matched sibling DLI. At a median follow-up of 66 weeks after U-DLI, 26% of patients were still in remission while 7 patients who achieved an initial CR relapsed and died of their original disease. The estimated probability of disease-free survival (DFS) at one year after CR was 65% for patients with CML, 23% for AML, and 30% for ALL (Fig. 5). As anticipated, overall

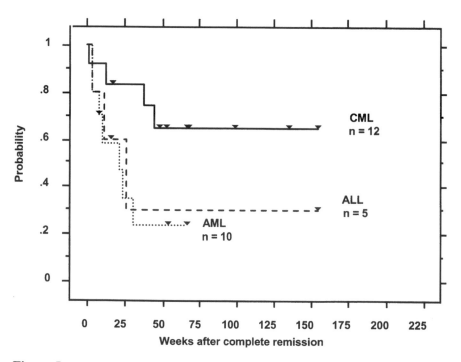

Figure 5   Disease-free survival after unrelated DLI for CML, AML, and ALL. (From Ref. 93.)

survival appeared superior for recipients of U-DLI for early-phase relapse of CML compared with patients with advanced-phase relapse.

Several other notable conclusions were drawn from this analysis. Induction chemotherapy prior to U-DLI in patients with AML or ALL did not appear to produce a
noticeable survival advantage. In addition, there was no association of mononuclear cell
dose with GVHD, response, survival, or DFS. Only a longer time interval from transplant
to relapse and transplant to U-DLI was associated with improved survival and DFS,
respectively. Although it is not possible to make direct comparisons to matched sibling
DLI from this retrospective study, toxicity was generally similar to that anticipated
after matched sibling DLI. For CML, response rates and remission durations were similar
to those reported for matched sibling DLI. Comparisons to matched sibling DLI for
patients with acute leukemia were more difficult, largely because of the small numbers
of patients studied and the relatively short follow-up. Given these reservations, the complete remission rates for recipients of U-DLI for acute leukemia appeared at least similar if
not higher than the 15–29% reported in matched sibling DLI studies (37,38).

The U-DLI analyses also failed to identify an association between acute and chronic
GVHD and disease response, in contrast to several (37,38,94), though not all (50), matched
sibling DLI studies that show a strong association between response and GVHD. Given
these data and the generally accepted poor outcome after relapse from unrelated donor
SCT, U-DLI appears to be a useful approach for patients who relapse with leukemia
after unrelated donor marrow grafting.

VII. ADOPTIVE IMMUNOTHERAPY FOR NONRELAPSE COMPLICATIONS AFTER ALLOGENEIC STEM CELL TRANSPLANTATION

The lack of adequate immune function after allogeneic SCT is directly responsible for several major and potentially life-threatening complications. It is therefore logical to suspect
that donor T-cell infusions would be effective therapy for both infectious and malignant
complications that develop due to insufficient reconstitution of cell-mediated immunity.
The best demonstration of this principle has been the effective use of DLI to treat
Epstein-Barr virus (EBV)–associated posttransplant lymphoproliferative disorders
(PTLD). PTLD is typically of donor origin and develops due to uncontrolled proliferation
of EBV-infected B cells in the absence of appropriate viral-specific immunity and T-cell
regulation. PTLD is most common when the donor stem cell graft is depleted of T cells as
GVHD prophylaxis. These lymphomas are usually aggressive and unresponsive to standard therapy, leading to a high mortality rate (95). After allogeneic SCT, T cells from a
donor who has had prior EBV exposure can be used to restore defective cellular immunity.
In fact, DLI will induce complete remission in the majority of patients with PTLD
occurring after allogeneic SCT (96,97). More recently, EBV-specific T cells have been
generated and expanded ex vivo and used effectively to both treat and prevent EBV-
related complications after allogeneic SCT. Since these cells have EBV specificity,
there is minimal risk for GVHD or other complications (98,99).

Donor leukocyte infusions may also be effective for prevention of other viral
complications after allogeneic SCT. For instance, cytomegalovirus (CMV) infections
are a frequent cause of life-threatening organ damage after SCT; in addition, both prophylaxis and therapy of CMV result in significant morbidity. Adoptive immunotherapy with
viral-specific T cells has the potential to restore CMV-specific immunity and prevent viral

reactivation. In one example of this principle, CD8+ T cells from CMV-seropositive marrow donors have been cloned and infused into transplant recipients (100,101). Transient survival of the T-cell clones was documented, and an increase in the circulating CMV-specific cytotoxic T cells was noted in most cases. Although these cells did not persist in patients with poor CD4+ helper function, no patient in this small cohort developed CMV viremia.

Donor leukocyte infusions have also been used to reverse acute life-threatening infections after allogeneic SCT caused by adenovirus (102) and respiratory syncytial virus (103). These examples further emphasize the broad potential application of this therapy to treat infections after allogeneic SCT. In the future, it is likely that allogeneic adoptive immunotherapy will have a wide range of clinical applications to both treat and prevent malignant and infectious complications after allogeneic cell transplantation.

It should be noted that the mechanism of response of PTLD or viral infections to DLI is likely to be qualitatively and quantitatively different than the GVL response. For instance, in donors with prior viral immunity, the frequency of precursor cytotoxic T lymphocytes (pCTL) with antiviral specificity will be much higher than the frequency of pCTLs with antileukemic specificity (97). It is therefore likely that the dose of donor T cells will be significantly less to treat viral complications than to treat relapse of leukemia. Hence, the effective cell dose may be lower than that required to induce GVHD. This has been noted in cases where DLI has been used to treat PTLD that occurred after allogeneic BMT for CML. DLI induced sustained and complete remission of the PTLD, but several patients relapsed with CML; this suggests that low numbers of donor T cells used to eradicate PTLD were insufficient to prevent relapse of CML (56,93). Qualitatively, these responses are also different from GVL induction. In most cases of PTLD and perhaps other viral complications, the desired antiviral effect is an autologous (donor-vs.-donor) immune reaction rather than an allogeneic response. In the case of PTLD, the donor T cells must interact with donor EBV-infected B cells.

VIII. NEWER APPROACHES TO DONOR LEUKOCYTE INFUSIONS

Several novel approaches have been used to improve outcomes after DLI (Table 5). Some strategies focus on minimizing toxicity, while others are aimed at enhancing GVL activity. One approach that appears to minimize GVHD involves administration of low-dose DLI with the intent of obtaining a threshold T-cell dose for GVL activity that does not cause GVHD. In initial studies, low doses of donor T cells were given to patients with CML; patients who did not respond received dose escalation of DLI (50). Complete remissions were achieved in 86% of patients with relapsed CML and only one patient developed acute GVHD. However, 41% of all patients developed chronic GHVD, which was more common in patients treated at the higher cell doses. In a recent analysis of 298 patients treated

Table 5   Newer Approaches to Donor Leukocyte Infusions

Low-dose DLI followed by dose escalation
CD8+ cell depletion or CD4+ cell selection
Transduction of suicide genes (i.e., HSV-TK) into donor T cells
Irradiated DLI
Generation of leukemia-specific T cells in vitro

in 51 European centers, a first dose of $\leq 2 \times 10^7$ donor lymphocytes per kg body weight predicted DLI-related toxicity and survival; the response rate was not lower than with higher initial doses (104). Doses were escalated in 61% of patients, in 27% of patients twice, and in 16% of patients three times. The interval between doses was 48 days on average. The treatment-related mortality at 3 years after the start of treatment was 5% with the low initial dose as compared to 20% with the higher initial doses. The escalating dose strategy may not be applicable to patients with relapse in an advanced phase and with rapid progression of the disease. The preferred strategy is observation of the patient with quantitative RT-PCR analyses at regular intervals of 3 or 6 months after the start of DLI with 1×10^7 T cells per kg body weight, with dose escalation if there is molecular or cytogenetic evidence of disease after discontinuation of immunosuppression for at least 3 months. Doses below 10^7 T cells/kg did not show any GVL effect in patients with HLA-identical family donors.

Low-dose DLI with dose escalation seems most appropriate for patients with minimal disease burdens. Patients with molecular and cytogenetic relapse are most likely to respond at lower T-cell doses, and patients with chronic phase disease appear to require higher cell doses and experience more GVHD. In addition, the time required for complete responses precludes sufficient control of advanced CML or rapidly progressing acute leukemia. The induction of molecular remission requires a median of 5 months, and some responses occur only after a year. Therefore, in more advanced relapses, DLI may be combined with Imatinib treatment, which has shown activity in patients not responding to DLI alone (105).

It is not completely clear why dose escalation of DLI minimizes GVHD. In some cases, there is likely an important effector−to−target cell ratio responsible for GVL induction; low doses of donor leukocytes may induce a GVL reaction against low numbers of leukemia cells, yet may be insufficient to induce clinical GVHD. However, protection from GVHD using dose escalation of DLI may not simply be due to infusion of lower cell doses. When a dose-escalation strategy was compared to infusions of similar T-cell doses given in one aliquot for relapsed CML, response rates were similar and the incidence of GVHD was lower using the dose-escalation strategy (106). It is possible that dose escalation permits similar doses of T cells to be given at progressively later times after the original transplant. T-cell infusions given soon after transplant are more likely to induce severe GVHD than when delayed from the initial transplant (107−109). However, a more intriguing explanation is that low doses of donor T cells may result in generation of suppressor cells (or induction of anergy) that inhibits GVHD; only subsequent higher doses of DLI would be sufficient to overcome this effect and induce a GVH reaction. This is supported by animal experiments showing that graft-vs.-host tolerance could not be abrogated by the transfusion of lymphocytes from the marrow donor unless the donor was immunized against the recipient (110). These dogs were chimeras for many years when donor lymphocytes were transfused. In dogs, experiments of transfusing donor lymphocytes at various time points after T-cell−depleted marrow transplantation showed that donor lymphocytes did not produce GVHD if transfused more than 2 months after transplantation (111). Mixed chimeras converted to complete chimeras after DLI without developing GVHD. Similarly, delayed transfusion of donor lymphocytes improved the resistance of marrow-transplanted mice to leukemia without producing GVHD (108).

Another approach that has been used to minimize toxicity after DLI has been depletion of effector cells suspected of causing GVHD. Given the preclinical and clinical evidence that the CD8+ T cells may be primary mediators of GVHD, CD8-depleted donor leukocyte products have been used to treat relapsed CML after allogeneic BMT (49,91).

Initial data suggest not only that GVL activity is retained and GVHD is minimized, but that the majority of responses have been sustained (112). The overall clinical impact of this approach will require additional testing and further follow-up.

Other strategies have been tested to minimize GVHD after DLI that involve methods to inactivate alloreactive T cells. In one nonspecific approach, irradiated donor T cells were given as DLI with the hypothesis that they would induce GVL effects at the time of infusion but could not proliferate in response to alloantigens; preliminary data suggest that these cells do retain GVL activity and result in minimal GVHD (113). A more specific approach designed to limit GVHD without altering GVL reactivity has been the use of genetically modified donor cells engineered to contain a suicide gene. Donor lymphocytes transduced with the herpes simplex thymidine kinase (HSV-TK) gene will be sensitive to treatment with ganciclovir (114). HSV-TK–modified T cells have successfully induced complete remissions in patients with PTLD. Acute GVHD that developed after DLI was treated with ganciclovir, which resulted in a decrease in the number and activity of alloreactive cells as well as a decrease in the number of cells containing the HSV-TK gene. Notably, after ganciclovir therapy, gene-modified circulating cells were still detectable for up to 12 months after infusion (115). This strategy is now being tested in larger clinical trials using DLI to treat relapsed disease after allogeneic BMT.

Several strategies are being tested to enhance response rates to DLI. For patients with AML, a remission rate of 67% was obtained using low-dose cytosine arabinoside, G-CSF–mobilized donor cells, and GM-CSF for 14 days after DLI (116). At 2 years the survival probability of responders was 37.5%; favorable factors of a durable response were response to low-dose cytosine arabinoside prior to DLI, an HLA-identical family donor, and chronic GVHD. Major complications were acute GVHD and infections; the nonrelapse mortality at 2 years was 25%. In most cases of AML the blasts do not express the co-stimulatory molecule CD80, and only a minority express CD86 necessary for activation of T cells (117). In 70% of cases AML blasts can be differentiated to dendritic-like cells in short-term cultures containing the recombinant human cytokines GM-CSF, interleukin-4 (IL-4), tumor necrosis factor-α (TNF-α) with or without stem cell factor (SCF) and FLT-3 ligand (118–120).

The most effective and efficient method of inducing GVL without GVHD would be to use leukemia-specific T cells. Donor T cells can be generated after selection for leukemia reactivity followed by in vitro expansion. Preliminary data in small numbers of patients demonstrate that this strategy is feasible and can induce complete remission for relapsed CML with minimal toxicity (121). Unfortunately, not only is this approach complicated and time consuming, for most all malignancies, tumor-specific antigens are unknown and this method is not yet applicable to the majority of patients. An alternative strategy is to use nonspecific activation and ex vivo expansion to enhance the antitumor potential of donor T cells and overcome possible in vivo suppression of T-cell activation (122). Donor T cells activated and co-stimulated by exposure to anti-CD3– and anti-CD28–coated beads are being tested for GVL activity in a variety of malignancies that historically do not respond well to DLI (123). These and other novel trials will continue to explore methods to improve the specificity, efficacy, and safety of DLI.

IX. NONMYELOABLATIVE ALLOGENEIC STEM CELL TRANSPLANT

The dramatic results of using DLI as adoptive immunotherapy after allogeneic SCT have led to a series of trials attempting to induce a direct graft-vs.-tumor (GVT) reaction without the need for intensive conditioning therapy. In a preliminary study, 18 patients with a variety of malignancies were treated with DLI from an HLA-matched sibling as primary therapy without the use of any conditioning (124). Sustained mixed chimerism (1–5% donor hematopoiesis) was achieved in 4 patients, and 3 patients had an antitumor response (2 had Hodgkin's disease, and one had myeloma). Mixed chimerism and/or a GVT response occurred in only 4 of the 18 patients who had relapsed disease after a prior autologous transplant. Therefore, these data suggested that donor cells could survive and induce a direct GVT reaction after primary adoptive immunotherapy, but only in the most heavily pretreated (and likely the most immunosuppressed) patients. Therefore, it was hypothesized that preinfusion immunosuppressive therapy would enhance engraftment and hence the likelihood of an antitumor response. Subsequent studies by many groups are exploring the role of nonmyeloablative therapy and allogeneic SCT (NST). It is clear that in some cases NST is effective and potent immunotherapy. Response rates have been impressive for some patients with non-Hodgkin's lymphoma and Hodgkin's I disease (125–128), multiple myeloma (129), and CML (130,131). The role of NST for patients with AML and ALL is less certain. Various regimens can induce a high rate of donor chimerism and even complete remission, but overall outcomes in several small trials have been poor, largely due to rapid relapse as well as other complications (132–134). In patients with AML, sustained remissions have been described primarily in patients receiving nonmyeloablative conditioned allogeneic SCT while in remission, (127,134–136).

The intensity of the conditioning regimens used in different trials is quite variable, and in many cases it is sufficiently intensive to provide significant antitumor activity. Therefore, in many of these trials, it is difficult to distinguish the immunological GVT reaction from direct activity of the conditioning therapy. Nevertheless, NST appears to hold significant promise for many patients who may benefit from alløgeneic adoptive immunotherapy but are not appropriate candidates for a conventional allogeneic SCT. Hopefully trials of NST will lead to future therapies that will cure malignancies with minimal conditioning regimen toxicity. A more detailed review of nonmyeloablative allogeneic SCT is provided in Chapter 18.

X. CONCLUSION

The rationale for allogeneic SCT has come full circle. It was first attempted with the hope that the suspected immunological features of the donor graft would destroy residual leukemia cells present after conditioning therapy. For a long period afterwards, attention was focused primarily on dose intensifying the conditioning regimen and using allogeneic donor cells to rescue myeloablation. In the past decade it has become increasingly clear that the original hypothesis was not only correct, but that the GVT effects in allogeneic cell therapy may be more potent, at least in some cases, than originally anticipated. Donor leukocyte infusions have provided a dramatic example of the potent GVT reaction, inducing complete and sustained remissions in many patients when all cytotoxic therapy has failed. Furthermore, DLI has been used as an extremely effective and safe method of adoptive immunotherapy to treat infectious and other non-relapse complications that develop after allogeneic SCT. New strategies are being developed to separate the GVT effects from GVHD, and important future trials will include adoptive immunotherapy using selective T-cell subsets for DLI, gene-modified donor lymphocytes to regulate

GVHD, donor T cells activated to enhance tumor cell killing, and development of tumor-specific donor lymphocytes to use as allogeneic cell therapy.

The potential to harness allogeneic GVT effects has led to a new paradigm in transplantation. Less intensive, nonmyeloablative conditioning therapy and allogeneic cell transplantation is now being used as primary tumor immunotherapy with exciting, though preliminary, clinical results. With this potentially safer strategy of transplantation, allogeneic immunotherapy can be applied to patients who are older or with comorbid diseases precluding conventional ablative conditioning regimens. The approach may also offer an innovative therapy for patients with solid tumors, genetic defects, and even autoimmune diseases who may benefit from donor cell transplantation and potent allogeneic immune therapy. The ultimate goal is to determine how allogeneic immune cells can be used as specific adoptive immunotherapy against many different tumor types without inducing GVHD or other complications.

ACKNOWLEDGMENTS

This work was supported in part by grants from the American Cancer Society (CRTG-00-089-01-LBC) and The Leukemia & Lymphoma Society (7000-02) (DLP), and the National Cancer Institute (CA088930) (JEL).

REFERENCES

1. Barnes D, Corp M, Loutit J, Neal F. Treatment of murine leukaemia with x-rays and homologous bone marrow. Preliminary communication. Br Med J 1956; 2:626–630.
2. Mathe G, Amiel J, Schwarzenberg L, Cattan A, Schneider M. Adoptive immunotherapy of acute Leukemia: experimental and clinical results. Cancer Res 1965; 25:1525–1531.
3. Barnes D, Loutit J. Treatment of murine leukaemia with x-rays and homologous bone marrow. Br J Haematol 1957; 3:241–252.
4. Truitt R, Johnson B, McCabe C, Weiler M. Graft Versus Leukemia. In: Graft-vs.-Host Disease. Ferrara JLM, Deeg HJ, Burakoff SJ, eds. New York: Marcel Dekker, Inc., 1997:385–424.
5. Porter D, Antin J. Graft-versus-leukemia effect of allogeneic bone marrow transplantation and donor mononuclear cell infusions. In: Winter J, ed. Blood Stem Cell Transplantation. Norwell, MA: Kluwer Academic Publishers, 1997:57–86.
6. Slavin S, Ackerstein A, Weiss L, Nagler A, Or R, Naparstek E. Immunotherapy of minimal residual disease by immunocompetent lymphocytes and their activation by cytokines. Cancer Invest 1992; 10:221–227.
7. Sykes M, Harty M, Szot G, Pearson D. Interleukin-2 inhibits graft-versus-host disease-promoting activity of CD4+ cells while preserving CD4- and CD8-mediated graft-versus-leukemia effects. Blood 1994; 83:2560–2569.
8. Truitt RL, Johnson BD. Principles of graft-vs.-leukemia reactivity. Biol Blood Marrow Transplant 1995; 1:61–68.
9. Odom L, August C, Githens J, Humbert J, Morse H, Peakman D, Sharma B, Rusnak S, Johnson F. Remission of relapsed leukaemia during a graft-versus-host reaction. A "graft-versus-leu kae mia reaction" in man? Lancet 1978; 2:537–540.
10. Collins R, Rogers Z, Bennett M, Kumar V, Nikein A, Fay J. Hematologic relapse of chronic myelogenous leukemia following allogeneic bone marrow transplantation: apparent graft-versus-leukemia effect following abrupt discontinuation of immunosuppression. Bone Marrow Transplant 1992; 10:391–395.

11. Higano C, Brixey M, Bryant E, Durnam D, Doney K, Sullivan K, Singer J. Durable complete remission of acute nonlymphocytic leukemia associated with discontinuation of immunosuppression following relapse after allogeneic bone marrow transplantation. A case report of a probable graft-versus-leukemia effect. Transplantation 1990; 50:175–177.
12. Sullivan K, Shulman H. Chronic graft-versus-host disease, obliterative bronchiolitis, and graft-versus-leukemia effect: case histories. Transplant Proc 1989; 21:51–62.
13. Fefer A, Sullivan K, Weiden P, Buckner C, Schoch G, Storb R, Thomas E. Graft versus leukemia effect in man: the relapse rate of acute leukemia is lower after allogeneic than after syngeneic marrow transplantation. In: Truitt R, Gale R, Bortin M, eds. Cellular Immunotherapy of Cancer. New York: AR Liss, 1987:401–408.
14. Gale R, Champlin R. How does bone-marrow transplantation cure leukaemia? Lancet 1984; 2:28–30.
15. Gale R, Horowitz M, Ash R, Champlin R, Goldman J, Rimm A, Ringden O, Veum Stone J, Bortin M. Identical-twin bone marrow transplants for leukemia. Ann Int Med 1994; 120:646–652.
16. Horowitz M, Gale R, Sondel P, Goldman J, Dersey J, Kolb H, Rimm A, Ringden O, Rozman C, Speck B, Truitt R, Zwaan F, Bortin M. Graft-versus-leukemia reactions after bone marrow transplantation. Blood 1990; 75:555–562.
17. Weiden P, Flournoy N, Donnall Thomas E, Prentice R, Fefer A, Buckner C, Storb R. Antileukemic effect of graft-versus-host disease in human recipients of allogeneic-marrow grafts. N Engl J Med 1979; 300:1068–1073.
18. Sullivan K, Weiden P, Storb R, Witherspoon R, Fefer A, Fisher L, Buckner C, Anasetti C, Appelbaum F, Badger C, Beatty P, Bensinger W, Berenson R, Bigelow C, Cheever M, Clift R, Deeg H, Doney K, Greenberg P, Hansen J, Hill R, Loughran T, Martin P, Neiman P, Peterson F, sanders J, Singer J, Stewart P, Thomas E. Influence of acute and chronic graft-versus-host disease on relapse and survival after bone marrow transplantation from HLA-identical siblings as treatment of acute and chronic leukemia. Blood 1989; 73:1720–1728.
19. Weiden P, Sullivan K, Flournoy N, Storb R, Thomas E. Antileukemic effect of chronic graft-versus-host disease. Contribution to improved survival after allogeneic marrow transplantation. N Engl J Med 1981; 304:1529–1533.
20. Goldman JM, Gale RP, Horowitz MM, Biggs JC, Champlin RE, Gluckman E, Hoffmann RG, Jacobsen SJ, Marmont AM, McGlave PB. Bone marrow transplantation for chronic myelogenous leukemia in chronic phase. Increased risk for relapse associated with T-cell depletion. Ann Intern Med 1988; 108:806–814.
21. Antin J, Bierer B, Smith B, Ferrara J, Guinan E, Sieff C, Golan D, Macklis R, Tarbell N, Lynch E, Reichert T, Blythman H, Bouloux C, Rappeport J, Burakoff S, Weinstein H. Selective depletion of bone marrow T lymphocytes with anti-0D5 monoclonal antibodies: effective prophylaxis for graft-versus-host disease in patients with hematologic malignancies. Blood 1991; 78:2139–2149.
22. Soiffer R, Murray C, Mauch P, Anderson K, Freedman A, Rabinowe S, Takvorian T, Robertson M, Spector N, Gonin R, Miller K, Rudders R, Freeman A, Blake K, Coral F, Nadler L, Ritz J. Prevention of graft-versus-host disease by selective depletion of CD6-positive T lymphocytes from donor bone marrow. J Clin Oncol 1992; 10:1191–1200.
23. Marmont A, Horowitz M, Gale R, Sobocinski K, Ash R, van Bekkum D, Champlin R, Dicke K, Goldman J, Good R, Herzig R, Hong R, Masaoka T, Rimm A, Ringden O, Speck B, Weiner R, Bortin M. T-cell depletion of HLA-identical transplants in leukemia. Blood 1991; 78:2120–2130.
24. Aversa F, Terenzi A, Carotti A, Felicini R, Jacucci R, Zei T, Latini P, Aristei C, Santucci A, Martelli MP, Cunningham I, Reisner Y, Martelli MF. Improved outcome with T-cell-depleted bone marrow transplantation for acute leukemia. J Clin Oncol 1999; 17:1545–1550.

25. Champlin R. T-cell depletion for allogeneic bone marrow transplantation: impact on graft-versus-host disease, engraftment, and graft-versus-leukemia. J Hematother 1993; 2:27–42.

26. Papadopoulos EB, Carabasi MH, Castro-Malaspina H, Childs BH, Mackinnon S, Boulad F, Gililo AP, Kernan NA, Small TN, Szabolcs P, Taylor J, Yahalom J, Collins NH, Bleau SA, Black PM, Heller G, O'Reilly RJ, Young JW. T-cell-depleted allogeneic bone marrow transplantation as postremission therapy for acute myelogenous leukemia: freedom from relapse in the absence of graft-versus-host disease. Blood 1998; 91:1083–1090.

27. Goldman J, Gale R, Horowitz M, Biggs J, Champlin R, Gluckman E, Hoffmann R, Jacobsen S, Marmont A, MoGlave P, Messner H, Rimm A, Rozman C, Speck B, Tura S, Weiner R, Bortin M. Bone marrow transplantation for chronic myelogenous leukemia in chronic phase. Ann Int Med 1988; 108:806–814.

28. Mitsuyasu R, Champlin R, Gale R, Ho W, Lenarsky C, Winston D, Seich M, Elashoff R, Giorgi J, Wells J, Terasaki P, Billing R, Feig S. Treatment of donor bone marrow with monoclonal anti-T-cell antibody and complement for the prevention of graft-versus-host disease. Ann Int Med 1986; 105:20–26.

29. Goldman J, Apperley J, Jones L, Marcus R, Goliden A, Batchelor R, Hale G, Waldmann H, Reid C, Hows J, Gordon-Smith E, Catovsky D, Galton D. Bone marrow transplantation for patients with chronic myeloid leukemia. N Engl J Med 1986; 314:202–207.

30. Apperley J, Mauro F, Goldman J, Gregory W, Arthur C, Hows J, Arcese W, Papa G, Mandelli F, Wardle D, Gravett P, Franklin I, Bandini G, Ricci P, Tura S, Iacone A, Torlontano G, Heit W, Champlin R, Gale R. Bone marrow transplantation for chronic myeloid leukaemia in first chronic phase: importance of a graft-versus-leukaemia effect. Br J Haematol 1988; 69:239–245.

31. Kolb H, Mittermuller J, Clemm C, Holler E, Ledderose G, Brehm G, Heim M, Wilmanns W. Donor leukocyte transfusions for treatment of recurrent chronic myelogenous leukemia in marrow transplant patients. Blood 1990; 76:2462–2465.

32. Porter D, Roth M, McGarigle C, Ferrara J, Antin J. Induction of graft-versus-host disease as immunotherapy for relapsed chronic myeloid leukemia. N Engl J Med 1994; 330:100–106.

33. Drobyski W, Keever C, Roth M, Koethe S, Hanson G, McFadden P, Gottschall J, Ash R, van Tuinen P, Horowitz M, Flomenberg N. Salvage immunotherapy using donor leukocyte infusions as treatment for relapsed chronic myelogenous leukemia after allogeneic bone marrow transplantation: efficacy and toxicity of a defined T-cell dose. Blood 1993; 82:2310–2318.

34. Helg C, Roux E, Beris P, Cabrol C, Wacker P, Darbellay R, Wyss M, Jeannet M, Chapuis B, Roosnek E. Adoptive immunotherapy for recurrent CML after BMT. Bone Marrow Transplant 1993; 12:125–129.

35. Hertenstein B, Wiesneth M, Novotny J, Bunjes D, Stefanic M, Heinze B, Hubner G, Heimpel H, Arnold R. Interferon-α and donor buffy coat transfusions for treatment of relapsed chronic myeloid leukemia after allogeneic bone marrow transplantation. Transplant 1993; 56:1114–1118.

36. Roth M, Antin J, Bingham E, Ginsberg D. Detection of Philadelphia chromosome-positive cells by the polymerase chain reaction following bone marrow transpant for chronic myelogenous leukemia. Blood 1989; 74:882–885.

37. Kolb H, Schattenberg A, Goldman J, Hertenstein B, Jacobsen N, Arcese W, Ljungman P, Ferrant A, Verdonck L, Niederwieser D, van Rhee F, Mittermueller J, de Witte T, Holler E, Ansari H. Graft-versus-leukemia effect of donor lymphocyte transfusions in marrow grafted patients. Blood 1995; 86:2041–2050.

38. Collins R, Shpilberg O, Drobyski W, Porter D, Giralt S, Champlin R, Goodman S, Wolff S, Hu W, Verfaillie C, List A, Dalton W, Ognoskie N, Chetrit A, Antin J, Nemunaitis J. Donor

leukocyte infusions in 140 patients with relapsed malignancy after allogeneic bone marrow transplantation. J Clin Oncol 1997; 15:433–444.

39. Schattenberg A, Schaap N, Van De Wiel-Van Kemenade E, Bar B, Preijers F, Van Der Maazen R, Roovers E, De Witte T. In relapsed patients after lymphocyte depleted bone marrow transplantation the percentage of donor T lymphocytes correlates well with the outcome of donor leukocyte infusion. Leukemia Lymphoma. 1999; 32:317–325.

40. Dazzi F, Szydlo RM, Cross NC, Craddock C, Kaeda J, Kanfer E, Cwynarski K, Olavarria E, Yong A, Apperley JF, Goldman JM. Durability of responses following donor lymphocyte infusions for patients who relapse after allogeneic stem cell transplantation for chronic myeloid leukemia. Blood 2000; 96:2712–2716.

41. Porter D, Collins R, Shpilberg O, Drobyski W, Connors J, Sproles A, Antin J. Long-term follow-up of patients who achieved complete remission after donor leukocyte infusions. Biol Blood Marrow Transplant 1999; 5:253–261.

42. Keil F, Haas QA, Fritsch G, Kalhs P, Lechner K, Mannhalter C, Reiter E, Niederwieser D, Hoecker P, Greinix HT. Donor leukocyte infusion for leukemic relapse after allogeneic marrow transplantation: lack of residual donor hematopoiesis predicts aplasia. Blood 1997; 89:3113–3117.

43. Flowers M, Leisenring W, Beach K, Riddell S, Radich J, Higano C, Rowley S, Chauncey T, Bensinger W, Sanders J, Anasetti C, Storb R, Wade J, Appelbaum F, Martin P. Granulocyte colony-stimulating factor given to donors before apheresis does not prevent aplasia in patients treated with donor leukocyte infusion for recurrent chronic myeloid leukemia after bone marrow transplantation. Biol Blood Marrow Transplant 2000; 6:321–326.

44. Ratanatharathorn V, Nash RA, Przepiorka D, Devine SM, Klein JL, Weisdorf D, Fay JW, Nademanee A, Antin JH, Christiansen NP, van der Jagt R, Herzig RH, Litzow MR, Wolff SN, Longo WL, Petersen FB, Karanes C, Avalos B, Storb R, Buell DN, Maher RM, Fitzsimmons WE, Wingard JR. Phase III study comparing methotrexate and tacrolimus (prograf, FK506) with methotrexate and cyclosporine for graft-versus-host disease prophylaxis after HLA-identical sibling bone marrow transplantation. Blood 1998; 92:2303–2314.

45. Nash RA, Pepe MS, Storb R, Longton G, Pettinger M, Anasetti C, Appelbaum FR, Bowden RA, Deeg HJ, Doney K, et al. Acute graft-versus-host disease: analysis of risk factors after allogeneic marrow transplantation and prophylaxis with cyclosporine and methotrexate [comment]. Blood 1992; 80:1838–1845.

46. Levine J, Uberti J, Ayash L, Reynolds C, Ferrara J, Silver S, Braun T, Yanik G, Hutchinson R, Ratanatharathorn V. Lowered-intensity preparative regimen for allogeneic stem cell transplantation delays acute graft-versus-host disease but does not improve outcome for advanced hematologic malignancy. Biol Blood Marrow Transplant 2003; 9:189–197.

47. Akpek G, Boitnott JK, Lee LA, Hallick JP, Torbenson M, Jacobsohn DA, Arai S, Anders V, Vogelsang GB. Hepatitic variant of graft-versus-host disease after donor lymphocyte infusion. Blood 2002; 100:3903–3907.

48. Marks DI, Lush R, Cavenagh J, Milligan DW, Schey S, Parker A, Clark FJ, Hunt L, Yin J, Fuller S, Vandenberghe E, Marsh J, Littlewood T, Smith GM, Culligan D, Hunter A, Chopra R, Davies A, Towlson K, Williams CD. The toxicity and efficacy of donor lymphocyte infusions given after reduced-intensity conditioning allogeneic stem cell transplantation. Blood 2002; 100:3108–3114.

49. Alyea E, Soiffer R, Canning C, Neuberg D, Schlossman R, Pickett C, Collins H, Wang Y, Anderson K, Ritz J. Toxicity and efficacy of defined doses of CD4+ donor lymphocytes for treatment of relapse after allogeneic bone marrow transplant. Blood 1998; 91:3671–3680.

50. Mackinnon S, Papadopoulos E, Carabasi M, Reich L, Collins N, Boulad F, Castro-Malaspina H, Childs B, Gillio A, Kernan N, Small T, Young J, O'Reilly R. Adoptive immunotherapy evaluating escalating doses of donor leukocytes for relapse of chronic

myeloid leukemia after bone marrow transplantation: separation of graft-versus-leukemia responses from graft-versus-host disease. Blood 1995; 86:1261–1268.

51. Raiola AM, Van Lint M, Valbonesi M, Lamparelli T, Gualandi T, Occhini D, Bregante S, di Grazia C, Dominietto A, Soracco M, Romagnani C, Vassallo F, Casini M, Bruno B, Frassoni F, Bacigalupo A. Factors predicting response and graft-versus-host disease after donor lymphocyte infusions: a study on 593 infusions. Bone Marrow Transplant 2003; 81:687–693.

52. Dazzi F, Szydlo RM, Goldman JM. Donor lymphocyte infusions for relapse of chronic myeloid leukemia after allogeneic stem cell transplant: where we now stand. Exp Hematol 1999; 27:1477–1486.

53. Bocchia M, Korontsvit T, Xu Q, Mackinnon S, Yang SY, Sette A, Scheinberg DA. Specific human cellular immunity to bcr-abl oncogene-derived peptides. Blood 1996; 87:3587–3592.

54. Clark RE, Dodi IA, Hill SC, Lill JR, Aubert G, Macintyre AR, Rojas J, Bourdon A, Bonner PL, Wang L, Christmas SE, Travers PJ, Creaser CS, Rees RC, Madrigal JA. Direct evidence that leukemic cells present HLA-associated immunogenic peptides derived from the BCR-ABL b3a2 fusion protein. Blood 2001; 98:2887–2893.

55. Voogt PJ, Goulmy E, Veenhof WF, Hamilton M, Fibbe WE, Van Rood JJ, Falkenburg JH. Cellularly defined minor histocompatibility antigens are differentially expressed on human hematopoietic progenitor cells. J Exp Med 1988; 168:2337–2347.

56. Mackinnon S, Papadopoulos E, Carabasi M, Reich L, Collins N, O'Reilly R. Adoptive Immunotherapy using donor leukocytes following bone marrow transplantation for chronic myeloid leukemia: is T cell dose important in determining biological response? Bone Marrow Transplant 1995; 15:591–594.

57. Molldrem JJ, Lee PP, Wang C, Felio K, Kantarjian HM, Champlin RE, Davis MM. Evidence that specific T lymphocytes may participate in the elimination of chronic myelogenous leukemia. Nat Med 2000; 6:1018–1023.

58. Pinilla-lbarz J, Cathcart K, Korontsvit T, Soignet S, Bocchia M, Caggiano J, Lai L, Jimenez J, Kolitz J, Scheinberg DA. Vaccination of patients with chronic myelogenous leukemia with bcr-abl oncogene breakpoint fusion peptides generates specific immune responses. Blood 2000; 95:1781–1787.

59. Schneider E, Chen Z, Ellwart J, Wilmanns W, Kolb H. Immune phenotype of chronic myelogenous leukemia progenitor cells. Bone Marrow Transplant 1996; 17:S69–319.

60. Chen X, Regn S, Raffegerst S, Kolb HJ, Roskrow M. Interferon alpha in combination with GM-CSF induces the differentiation of leukaemic antigen-presenting cells that have the capacity to stimulate a specific anti-leukaemic cytotoxic T-cell response from patients with chronic myeloid leukaemia. Br J Haematol 2000; 111:596–607.

61. Slavin S, Naparstek E, Nagler A, Ackerstein A, Samuel S, Kapelushnik J, Brautbar C, Or R. Allogeneic cell therapy with donor peripheral blood cells and recombinant human interleukin-2 to treat leukemia relapse after allogeneic bone marrow transplantation. Blood 1996; 87:2195–2204.

62. Szer J, Grigg A, Phillipos G, Sheridan W. Donor leucocyte infusions after chemotherapy for patients relapsing with acute leukaemia following allogeneic BMT. Bone Marrow Transplant 1993; 11:109–111.

63. Porter D, Roth M, Lee S, McGarigle C, Ferrara J, Antin J. Adoptive immunotherapy with donor mononuclear cell infusions to treat relapse of acute leukemia or myelodysplasia after allogeneic bone marrow transplantation. Bone Marrow Transplant 1996; 18:975–980.

64. Raanani P, Dazzi F, Sohal J, Szydlo RM, van Rhee F, Reiter A, Lin F, Goldman JM, Cross NC. The rate and kinetics of molecular response to donor leucocyte transfusions in chronic myeloid leukaemia patients treated for relapse after allogeneic bone marrow transplantation. Br J Haematol 1997; 99:945–950.

65. Baurmann H, Nagel S, Binder T, Neubauer A, Siegert W, Huhn D. Kinetics of the graft-versus-leukemia response after donor leukocyte infusions for relapsed chronic myeloid leukemia after allogeneic bone marrow transplantation [comment]. Blood 1998; 92:3582–3590 [erratum appears in Blood 1999 Mar 15; 93(6):2141].

66. Kolb HJ. Donor leukocyte transfusions for treatment of leukemic relapses after bone marrow transplantation. Vox Sanguis 1998; 74(suppl 2):321–329.

67. Mandanas RA, Saez RA, Selby GB, Confer DL. G-CSF-mobilized donor leukocyte infusions as immunotherapy in acute leukemia relapsing after allogeneic marrow transplantation. J Hematother 1998; 7:449–456.

68. Singhal S, Powles R, Kulkarni S, Treleaven J, Saso R, Mehta J. Long-term follow-up of relapsed acute leukemia treated with immunotherapy after allogeneic transplantation: the inseparability of graft-versus-host disease and graft-versus-leukemia, and the problem of extramedullary relapse. Leukemia Lymphoma 1999; 32:505–512.

69. Levine J, Braun T, Penza S, Beatty P, Cornetta K, Martino R, Drobyski W, Barrett A, Porter D, Giralt S, Horowitz M, Leis J, Johnson M, Collins R. Prospective trial of chemotherapy and donor leukocyte infusions for relapse of advanced myeloid malignancies after allogeneic stem cell transplantation. J Clin Oncol 2001; 20:405–412.

70. Schmid C, Alessandrino E, Bunjes D, Ferrant A, Frassoni F, Gluckman E, Holler E, Jacobsen N, Ljungman P, Schattenberg A, Verdonck L, Kolb HJ. Treatment of relapsed AML and MDS after allogeneic stem cell transplantation with donor lymphocyte transfusion—a retrospective analysis of EBMT results. Blood 2000; 96:477a.

71. Ringden O, Labopin M, Gorin NC, Schmitz N, Schaefer UW, Prentice HG, Bergmann L, Jouet JP, Mandelli F, Blaise D, Fouillard L, Frassoni F, Acute Leukemia Working Party of the European Group for B, Marrow T. Is there a graft-versus-leukaemia effect in the absence of graft-versus-host disease in patients undergoing bone marrow transplantation for acute leukaemia? Br J Haematol 2000; 111:1130–1137.

72. Carlens S, Remberger M, Aschan J, Ringden O. The role of disease stage in the response to donor lymphocyte infusions as treatment for leukemic relapse. Biol Blood Marrow Transplant 2001; 7:31–38.

73. Berthou C, Leglise MC, Herry A, Balcon D, Hardy E, Lessard M, Abgrall JF. Extramedullary relapse after favorable molecular response to donor leukocyte infusions for recurring acute leukemia. Leukemia 1998; 12:1676–1681.

74. Tringali S, Vasta S, Scime R, Catania P, Cavallaro AM, Majolino I. Testicular relapse of AML during chronic graft-versus-host disease induced by donor leukocyte infusion. Haematologica 1996; 81:339–342.

75. Shiobara S, Nakao S, Ueda M, Yamazaki H, Takahashi S, Asano S, Yabe H, Kato S, Imoto S, Maruta A, Yoshida T, Gondo H, Morishima Y, Kodera Y. Donor leukocyte infusion for Japanese patients with relapsed leukemia after allogeneic bone marrow transplantation: indications and dose escalation. Ther Apheresis 2001; 5:40–45.

76. Slavin S, Morecki S, Weiss L, Or R. Donor lymphocyte infusion: the use of alloreactive and tumor-reactive lymphocytes for immunotherapy of malignant and nonmalignant diseases in conjunction with allogeneic stem cell transplantation. Hematother Stem Cell Res 2002; 11:265–276.

77. Collins RH Jr, Goldstein S, Giralt S, Levine J, Porter D, Drobyski W, Barrett J, Johnson M, Kirk A, Horowitz M, Parker P. Donor leukocyte infusions in acute lymphocytic leukemia. Bone Marrow Transplant 2000; 26:511–516.

78. Cardoso A, Schultze J, Boussiotis VA, et al. Pre-B acute lymphoblastic leukemia cells may induce T cell anergy to alloantigen. Blood 1996; 88:41–48.

79. Galandrini R, Albi N, Zarcone D, Grossi CE, Velardi A. Adhesion molecule-mediated signals regulate major histocompatibility complex-unrestricted and CD3/T cell receptor-triggered cytotoxicity. Eur J Immunol 1992; 22:2047–2053.

80. Han P, Story C, McDonald T, Mrozik K, Snell L. Immune escape mechanisms of childhood ALL and a potential countering role for DC-like leukemia cells. Cytotherapy 2002; 4:165–175.

81. Ruggeri L, Capanni M, Urbani E, Perruccio K, Shlomohik WD, Tosti A, Posati S, Rogaia D, Frassoni F, Aversa F, Martelli MF, Velardi A. Effectiveness of donor natural killer cell alloreactivity in mismatched hematopoietic transplants [comment]. Science 2002; 295:2097–2100.

82. Bernard M, Dauriac C, Drenou B, Leberre C, Branger B, Fauchet R, Le Prise PY, Lamy T. Long-term follow-up of allogeneic bone marrow transplantation in patients with poor prognosis non-Hodgkin's lymphoma. Bone Marrow Transplant 1999; 23:329–333.

83. Mandigers CM, Raemaekers JM, Schattenberg AV, Roovers EA, Bogman MJ, van der Maazen RW, De Pauw BE, De Witte T. Allogeneic bone marrow transplantation with T-cell-depleted marrow grafts for patients with poor-risk relapsed low-grade non-Hodgkin's lymphoma. Br J Haematol 1998; 100:198–206.

84. Rondon G, Giralt S, Huh Y, Khouri I, Andersson B, Andreeff M, Champlin R. Graft-versus-leukemia effect after allogeneic bone marrow transplantation for chronic lymphocytic leukemia. Bone Marrow Transplant 1996; 18:669–672.

85. Robinson S, Goldstone AH, Mackinnon S, Carella A, Russell N, DeElvira R, Taghipour G, Schmitz N. Chemoresistant or aggressive lymphoma predicts for a poor outcome following reduced intensity allogeneic progenitor cell transplantation: an analysis from the Lymphoma Working Party of the European Group for Blood and Bone Marrow Transplantation. Blood 2002; 100:4310–4316.

86. Salama M, Nevill T, Marcellus D, Parker P, Johnson M, Kirk A, Porter D, Giralt S, Levine J, Drobyski W, Barrett A, Horowitz M, Collins R. Donor leukocyte infusions for multiple myeloma. Bone Marrow Transplant 2000; 26:1179–1184.

87. Lokhorst HM, Schattenberg A, Cornelissen JJ, van Oers MH, Fibbe W, Russell I, Donk NW, Verdonck LF. Donor lymphocyte infusions for relapsed multiple myeloma after allogeneic stem-cell transplantation: predictive factors for response and long-term outcome. J Clin Oncol 2000; 18:3031–3037.

88. Alyea E, Weller E, Schlossman R, Canning C, Webb I, Doss D, Mauch P, Marcus K, Fisher D, Freeman A, Parikh B, Gribben J, Soiffer R, Ritz J, Anderson K. T-cell–depleted allogeneic bone marrow transplantation followed by donor lymphocyte infusion in patients with multiple myeloma: induction of graft-versus-myeloma effect. Blood 2001; 98:934–939.

89. Badros A, Barlogie B, Morris C, Desikan R, Martin SR, Munshi N, Zangari M, Mehta J, Toor A, Cottler-Fox M, Fassas A, Anaissie E, Schichman S, Tricot G, Aniassie E. High response rate in refractory and poor-risk multiple myeloma after allotransplantation using a nonmyeloablative conditioning regimen and donor lymphocyte infusions. Blood 2001; 97:2574–2579.

90. Verdonck LF, Petersen EJ, Lokhorst HM, Nieuwenhuis HK, Dekker AW, Tilanus MG, de Weger RA. Donor leukocyte infusions for recurrent hematologic malignancies after allogeneic bone marrow transplantation: impact of infused and residual donor T cells. Bone Marrow Transplant 1998; 22:1057–1063.

91. Giralt S, Hester J, Huh Y, Hirsch-Ginsberg C, Rondon G, Seong D, Lee M, Gajewski J, Van Besien K, Khouri I, Mehra R, Przepiorka D, Korbling M, Talpaz M, Kantarjian H, Fischer H, Deisseroth A, Champlin R. CD8-depleted donor lymphocyte infusion as treatment for relapsed chronic myelogenous leukemia after allogeneic bone marrow transplantation. Blood 1995; 86:4337–4343.

92. Mehta J, Powles R, Treleaven J, Horton C, Meller S, Pinkerton C, Singhal S. Outcome of acute leukemia relapsing after bone marrow transplantation: utility of second transplants and adoptive immunotherapy. Bone Marrow Transplant 1997; 19:709–719.

93. Porter D, Collins R, Hardy C, Kernan N, Drobyski W, Giralt S, Flowers M, Casper J, Leahey A, Parker P, Mick R, Bate-Boyle B, King R, Antin J. Treatment of relapsed leukemia

after unrelated donor marrow transplantation with unrelated donor leukocyte infusions. Blood 2000; 95:1214–1221.

94. Porter D, Antin J. Adoptive immunotherapy in bone marrow transplantation. In: Burakoff S, Deeg H, Ferrara J, eds. Graft-versus-Host-Disease. New York: Marcel Dekker, 1997:733–754.

95. Shapiro R, McClain K, Frizzera G, Gajl-Peczalska K, Kersey J, Blazar B, Arthur D, Patton D, Greenberg J, Burke B, Ramsay N, McGlave P, Filipovich A. Epstein-Barr virus associated B cell lymphoproliferative disorders following bone marrow transplantation. Blood 1988; 71:1234–1243.

96. Porter D, Orloff G, Antin J. Donor mononuclear cell infusions as therapy for B-cell lymphoproliferative disorder following allogeneic bone marrow transplant. Transplant Sci 1994; 4:11–15.

97. Papadopoulos E, Ladanyi M, Emanuel D, Mackinnon S, Boulad F, Carabasi M, Castro-Malaspina J, Childs B, Gillio A, Small T, Young J, Kernan N, O'Reilly R. Infusions of donor leukocytes to treat Epstein-Barr virus-associated lymphoproliferative disorders after allogeneic bone marrow transplantation. N Engl J Med 1994; 330:1185–1191.

98. Rooney C, Smith C, Ng C, Loftin S, Li C, Krance R, Brenner M. Use of gene-modified virus-specific T lymphocytes to control Epstein-Barr-virus-related lymphoproliferation. Lancet 1995; 345:9–13.

99. Rooney C, Smith C, Ng C, Loftin S, Sixbey J, Gan Y, Srivastava D-K, Bowman L, Krance R, Brenner M, Heslop H. Infusion of cytoxic T cells for the prevention and treatment of Epstein-Barr virus-induced lymphoma in allogeneic transplant recipients. Blood 1998; 92:1549–1555.

100. Riddell S, Watanabe K, Goodrich J, Li C, Agha M, Greenberg P. Restoration of viral immunity in immunodeficient humans by adoptive transfer of T cell clones. Science 1992; 257:238–241.

101. Walter E, Greenberg P, Gilbert M, Finch R, Watanabe K, Thomas E, Riddell S. Reconstitution of cellular immunity against cytomegalovirus in recipients of allogeneic bone marrow by transfer of T-cell clones from the donor. N Engl J Med 1995; 333:1038–1044.

102. Hromas R, Cornetta K, Srour E. Donor leukocyte infusion as therapy of life-threatening adenoviral infections after T-cell-depleted bone marrow transplantation (lett). Blood 1994; 84:1690–1691.

103. Kishi Y, Kami M, Oki Y, Kazuyama Y, Kawabata M, Miyakoshi S, Morinaga S, Suzuki R, Mon S, Muto Y. Donor lymphocyte infusion for treatment of life-threatening respiratory syncytial virus infection following bone marrow transplantation. Bone Marrow Transplant 2000; 26:573–576.

104. Guglielmi C, Arcese W, Dazzi F, Brand R, Bunjes D, Verdonck LF, Schattenberg A, Kolb HJ, Ljungman P, Devergie A, Bacigalupo A, Gomez M, Michallet M, Elmaagacli A, Gratwohl A, Apperley J, Niederwieser D. Donor lymphocyte infusion for relapsed chronic myelogenous leukemia: prognostic relevance of the initial cell dose. Blood 2002; 100:397–405.

105. Kantarjian HM, O'Brien S, Cortes JE, Giralt SA, Rios MB, Shan J, Giles FJ, Thomas DA, Faderl S, De Lima M, Garcia-Manero G, Champlin R, Arlinghaus R, Talpaz M. Imatinib mesylate therapy for relapse after allogeneic stem cell transplantation for chronic myelogenous leukemia. Blood 2002; 100:1590–1595.

106. Dazzi F, Szydlo RM, Craddock C, Cross NC, Kaeda J, Chase A, Olavarria E, van Rhee F, Kanfer E, Apperley JF, Goldman JM. Comparison of single-dose and escalating-dose regimens of donor lymphocyte infusion for relapse after allografting for chronic myeloid leukemia. Blood 2000; 95:67–71.

107. Barrett A, Mavroudis D, Molldrem J, Read E, Carter C, Dunbar C, Young N. Optimizing the dose and timing of lymphocyte add-back in T-cell depleted BMT between HLA-identical siblings. Blood 1996; 88:460a.

108. Johnson B, Drobyski W, Truitt R. Delayed infusion of normal donor cells after MHC-matched bone marrow transplantation provides an antileukemia reaction without graft-versus-host disease. Bone Marrow Transplant 1993; 11:329–336.
109. Sullivan K, Storb R, Buckner D, Fefer A, Fisher L, Weiden P, Witherspoon R, Appelbaum F, Banaji M, Hansen J, Martin P, Sanders J, Singer J, Thomas ED. Graft-versus-host disease as adoptive immunotherapy in patients with advanced hematologic neoplasms. N Engl J Med 1989; 320:828–834.
110. Weiden P, Storb R, Tsoi M, Graham T, Lerner K, Thomas E. Infusion of donor lymphocytes into stable canine radiation chimeras: implications for mechanism of transplantation tolerance. J Immunol 1978; 116:1212–1219.
111. Kolb HJ, Gunther W, Schumm M, Holler E, Wilmanns W, Thierfelder S. Adoptive immunotherapy in canine chimeras. Transplantation 1997; 63:430–436.
112. Shimoni A, Gajewski J, Donato M, Martin T, O'Brien S, Talpaz M, Cohen A, Korbling M, Champlin R, Giralt S. Long-term follow-up of recipients of CD8 depleted donor lymphocyte infusions for the treatment of chronic myelogenous leukemia relapsing after allogeneic progenitor cell transplantation. Biol Blood Marrow Transplant 2001; 7:568–575.
113. Waller EK, Ship AM, Mittelstaedt S, Murray TW, Carter R, Kakhniashvili I, Lonial S, Holden JT, Boyer MW. Irradiated donor leukocytes promote engraftment of allogeneic bone marrow in major histocompatibility complex mismatched recipients without causing graft-versus-host disease. Blood 1999; 94:3222–3233.
114. Servida P, Rossini S, Traversari C, Ferrari G, Bonini C, Nobili N, Vago L, Faravelli A, Vanzulli A, Mavillio F, Bordignon C. Gene transfer into peripheral blood lymphocytes for in vivo immunomodulation of donor anti-tumor immunity in a patient affected by EBV-induced lymphoma. Blood 1993; 82:214a.
115. Bonini C, Ferrari G, Verzeletti S, Servida P, Zappone E, Ruggieri L, Ponzoni M, Rossini S, Mavilio F, Traversari C, Bordignon C. HSV-TK gene transfer into donor lymphocytes for control of allogeneic graft-versus-leukemia. Science 1997; 276:1719–1724.
116. Schmid C, Lange C, Salat C, Stoetzer O, Ledderose G, Muth A, Schleuning M, Roskrow M, Kolb HJ. Treatment of recurrent acute leukemia after marrow transplantation with donor cells and GM-CSF. Blood 1999; 94:668a.
117. Hirano N, Takahashi T, Ohtake S, Hirashima K, Emi N, Saito K, Hirano M, Shinohara K, Takeuchi M, Taketazu F, Tsunoda S, Ogura M, Omine M, Saito T, Yazaki Y, Ueda R, Hirai H. Expression of costimulatory molecules in human leukemias. Leukemia 1996; 10:1168–1176.
118. Woiciechowsky A, Regn S, Guenther C, Kolb HJ, Roskrow M. Dendritic cells generated in votro from patients with acute myeloid leukemia (AML) stimulate autologous and allogeneic, HLA-matched leukemia-specific cytotoxic T-lymphocytes. Blood 1999; 94:81a.
119. Brouwer RE, van der Hoorn M, Kluin-Nelemans HC, van Zelderen-Bhola S, Willemze R, Falkenburg JH. The generation of dendritic-like cells with increased allostimulatory function from acute myeloid leukemia cells of various FAB subclasses. Hum Immunol 2000; 61:565–574.
120. Choudhury BA, Liang JC, Thomas EK, Flores-Romo L, Xie QS, Agusala K, Sutaria S, Sinha I, Champlin RE, Claxton DF. Dendritic cells derived in vitro from acute myelogenous leukemia cells stimulate autologous, antileukemic T-cell responses. Blood 1999; 93:780–786.
121. Falkenburg JH, Wafelman AR, Joosten P, Smit WM, van Bergen CA, Bongaerts R, Lurvink E, van der Hoorn M, Kluck P, Landegent JE, Kluin-Nelemans HC, Fibbe WE, Willemze R. Complete remission of accelerated phase chronic myeloid leukemia by treatment with leukemia-reactive cytotoxic T lymphocytes. Blood 1999; 94:1201–1208.
122. Liebowitz D, Lee K, CH J. Costimulatory approaches to adoptive immunotherapy. Curr Opin Oncol 1998; 10:533–541.
123. Porter D, Bunin N, Laport G, Duffy K, Bennett P, Than T, Luger S, Schuster S, Grupp S, Stadtmauer E, June C Graft-vs-tumor induction with donor leukocyte infusions expanded ex vivo by activation with CD3/CD28 costimulation. Blood 2001; 98:404a.

124. Porter D, Connors J, VanDeerlin V, Duffy K, McGarigle C, Saidman S, Leonard D, Antin J. Graft-versus-tumor induction with donor leukocyte infusions as primary therapy for patients with malignancies. J Clin Oncol 1999; 17:1234–1243.

125. Khouri I, Keating M, Korbling M, Przepiorka D, Anderlini P, O'Brien S, Giralt S, Ippoliti C, von Wolff B, Gajewski J, Donato M, Claxton D, Ueno N, Andersson B, Gee A, Champlin R. Transplant-lite: induction of graft-vs-malignancy using fludarabine-based nonablative chemotherapy and allogeneic blood progenitor-cell transplantation as treatment for lymphoid malignancies. J Clin Oncol 1998; 16:2817–2824.

126. Porter D, Luger S, Duffy K, Stadtmauer E, Laport G, Schuster S, Orloff G, Tsai D, McDaid K, Kathakali A, Leonard D, Antin J. Allogeneic cell therapy for patients who relapse after autologous stem cell transplantation. Biol Blood Marrow Transplant 2001; 7:230–238.

127. Slavin S, Nagler A, Naparstek E, Kapelushnik Y, Aker M, Cividalli G, Varadi G, Kirschbaum M, Ackerstein A, Samuel S, Amar A, Brautbar C, Bel-Tal O, Eldor A, Or R. Nonmyeloablative stem cell transplantation and cell therapy as an alternative to conventional bone marrow transplantation with lethal cytoreduction for the treatment of malignant and nonmalignant hematologic diseases. Blood 1998; 91:756–763.

128. Anderlini P, Giralt S, Andersson B, Ueno N, Khouri I, Acholonu S, Cohen A, Korbling M, Manning J, Romaguera J, Sarris A, Rodriguez M, Hagemeister F, McLaughlin P, Cabanillas F, Champlin R. Allogeneic stem cell transplantation with fludarabine-based, less intensive conditioning regimens as adoptive immunotherapy in advanced Hodgkin's disease. Bone Marrow Transplant 2000; 26:615–620.

129. Badros A, Barlogie B, Siegel E, Cottler-Fox M, Zangari M, Fassas A, Morris C, Anaissie E, Van Rhee F, Tricot G. Improved outcome of allogeneic transplantation in high-risk multiple myeloma patients after nonmyeloablative conditioning. J Clin Oncol 2002; 20:1295–1303.

130. Bornhauser M, Kiehl M, Siegert W, Schetelig J, Hertenstein B, Martin H, Schwerdtfeger R, Sayer HG, Runde V, Kroger N, Theuser C, Ehninger G. Cooperative German Transplant Study G Dose-reduced conditioning for allografting in 44 patients with chronic myeloid leukaemia: a retrospective analysis. Br J Haematol 2001; 115:119–124.

131. Khoury H, Adkins D, Brown R, Pence H, Vij R, Goodnough LT, Westervelt P, Trinkaus K, Lin HS, DiPersio Y. Low incidence of transplantation-related acute complications in patients with chronic myeloid leukemia undergoing allogeneic stem cell transplantation with a low-dose (550 cGy) total body irradiation conditioning regimen. Biol Blood Marrow Transplant 2001; 7:352–358.

132. Devine SM, Sanborn R, Jessop E, StockW, HumI M, Peace D, Wickrema A, Yassine M, Amin K, Thomason D, Chen YH, Devine H, Maningo M, van Besien K. Fludarabine and melphalan-based conditioning for patients with advanced hematological malignancies relapsing after a previous hematopoietic stem cell transplant. Bone Marrow Transplant 2001; 8:557–562.

133. Giralt S, Estey E, Albitar M, van Besien K, Rondon G, Anderlini P, O'Brien S, Khouri I, Gajewski J, Mehra R, Claxton D, Andersson B, Beran M, Przepiorka D, Koller C, Kornblau S, Korbling M, Keating M, Kantarjian H, Champlin R. Engraftment of allogeneic hematopoietic progenitor cells with purine analog-containing chemotherapy: harnessing graft-versus-leukemia without myeloablative therapy. Blood 1997; 89:4531–4536.

134. Schlenk RF, Hartmann F, Hensel M, Jung W, Weber-Nordt R, Gabler A, Haas R, Ho AD, Trumper L, Dohner H. Less intense conditioning with fludarabine, cyclophosphamide, idarubicin and etoposide (FCIE) followed by allogeneic unselected peripheral blood stem cell transplantation in elderly patients with leukemia. Leukemia 2002; 16:581–586.

135. Bornhauser M, Thiede C, Schuler U, Platzbecker U, Freiberg-Richter J, Helwig A, Plettig R, Rollig C, Naumann R, Kroschinsky F, Neubauer A, Ehninger G. Dose-reduced conditioning for allogeneic blood stem cell transplantation: durable engraftment without antithymocyte globulin. Bone Marrow Transplant 2000; 26:119–125.

20

Clinical Spectrum and Therapeutic Approaches to Chronic Graft-vs.-Host Disease

GÖRGÜN AKPEK and CHARLES S. VIA

University of Maryland Medical System, Baltimore, Maryland, U.S.A.

GEORGIA B. VOGELSANG

Johns Hopkins University School of Medicine, Baltimore, Maryland, U.S.A

I. BACKGROUND

Hematopoietic stem cell transplantation (SCT) provides effective therapy for patients with lymphohematopoietic, immunological, metabolic, and other disorders. Current estimates of annual numbers of allogeneic SCT are 12,000–15,000 worldwide, with continuing growth rate of 10–20% per year (1). Transplant-related mortality at 1 year after HLA-identical sibling transplants is about 30% (2). Long-term survivors are at risk for late complications. In the early 1990s chronic graft-vs.-host disease (GVHD) was the most common late complication of allogeneic SCT, with reported incidences ranging from 30 to 80% (3). Although prevention and treatment of acute GVHD have improved over the past two decades, similar progress in chronic GVHD has remained elusive as it continuous to be the leading cause of late nonrelapse mortality following allogeneic SCT (4). Beneficial graft-vs.-leukemia/lymphoma (GVL) effect on survival was offset by the increased nonrelapse mortality secondary to infections and organ failure during the course of chronic GVHD. Not surprisingly, large observational studies identified chronic GVHD as the most common cause of nonrelapse deaths occurring more than 2 years posttransplant, and increasing severity of chronic GVHD is associated with higher mortality rates (5,6). In aplastic anemia and refractory anemia where the risk of relapse and death from the primary disease is low, chronic GVHD has a substantial adverse impact on survival that has not improved significantly over the past 30 years (7,8). Przepiorka et al.

555

recently reported a high rate of chronic GVHD after allogeneic peripheral blood stem cell transplantation (PBSCT), and the high incidence of chronic GVHD adversely affected the outcome (9).

Chronic GVHD is also associated with decreased quality of life, due to impaired functional performance, and continued need for immunosuppressive medications (6,10– 15). Chronic GVHD may cause abnormalities of growth and development in children, decreased general health status, sexual inactivity, and loss of employment in long-term survivors (3,15–19). This chapter provides updated information for clinicians to observe patients for what is probably the most important late complication of allogeneic SCT, chronic GVHD.

II. PATHOGENESIS

The pathophysiology of chronic GVHD remains poorly characterized. Although animal models of chronic GVHD exist, the most commonly used model (a parent-into-F1 hybrid model) produces extensive antibody-mediated damage that more closely resembles lupus with renal damage than chronic GVHD (20). Clinical studies have not been very revealing in understanding the underlying mechanism(s) of chronic GVHD. In the following section, we introduce the most common models studied in chronic GVHD.

A. Animal Models of Chronic GVHD

A major impediment to the study of human chronic GVHD has been the difficulty in establishing animal models that adequately mimic human disease. A large number of animal models of acute GVHD exist and are described in Chapter 2. Due to the high mortality associated with most acute murine GVHD models, it has not been feasible to study the few survivors for development of chronic GVHD. Data are emerging that indicate that the parent-into-F1 (P → F1) model of GVHD may exhibit many features of human chronic GVHD and possibly serve as an instructive model.

B. The P → F1 Model of GVHD

The injection of homozygous parental T lymphocytes into normal (unirradiated) F1 mice results in a graft-vs.-host reaction due to donor T-cell recognition of the H-2 alloantigens of the second parent expressed on F1 cells (reviewed in Refs. 20,21). Acute and chronic GVHD are observed in this model. However, as described below, this classification is somewhat misleading as effector mechanisms in both disease phenotypes are induced acutely.

Acute, lethal GVHD is characterized by lymphocytopenia, depressed in vitro T-cell function, weight loss, and increased mortality beginning as early as 10 days after donor cell transfer. The disease is induced by the injection of donor CD4+ and CD8+ T cells into an F1 recipient that differs from the donor by a fully allogeneic MHC I and II haplotype, e.g., C57Bl/6 (H-2^b) → B6D2F1 (H-$2^{b/d}$).

Chronic (autoimmune) GVHD is characterized by lymphoproliferation, B-cell hyperactivity, autoantibody production, and a lupus-like renal disease. Chronic GVHD is induced by selective activation of donor CD4+ T cells, e.g., injection of CD8-depleted C57Bl/6 spleen cells into B6D2F1 mice or injection of MHC class II only disparate donor cells (C57Bl/6 → B6 × B6^{bm12}F1). Surprisingly, chronic GVHD can also be induced in B6D2F1 mice following the injection of fully allogeneic DBA parental T cells. The mechanism relates to defective cytotoxic T lymphocyte (CTL) maturation of DBA CD8+ T cells combined with normal DBA CD4+ T-cell activation and maturation (see below).

C. Cellular Immunology of Acute and Chronic GVHD

1. GVHD Initiation

The initial step in both acute and chronic GVHD is activation of donor CD4+ T cells in response to allogeneic MHC class II molecules on F1 host cells (22–24) resulting in the production of cytokines interleukin (IL)-2, IL-4, and IL-10 (25–28). In both forms of GVHD, host B cells become activated and produce autoantibodies initially (26). Distinguishing features of acute and chronic GVHD in the parent-into-F1 model are summarized in Table 1.

2. Acute GVHD Requires Activation of Both CD4+ and CD8+ Donor T Cells

In addition to the ongoing Th2 cytokine production, acute GVHD mice also exhibit significantly increased production of the Th1 cytokine interferon (IFN)-γ (26–29) and Th1-promoting cytokines such as IL-12 (30), beginning at about day 5 after donor cell transfer and corresponding to the engraftment and expansion of donor CD8+ T cells. By day 7 of disease, acute GVHD mice exhibit striking elevations in serum IFN-γ levels reaching > 5 log higher than controls (31). As donor CD8+ T cells mature into CTL specific for allogeneic MHC class I on the F1 host cells, F1 lymphocytes (both T and B cells) are eliminated, and the profound immunodeficiency that characterizes acute GVHD ensues. Because of the elimination of host B cells, the initial humoral autoimmunity in acute GVHD is transient (32).

Chronic GVHD results from selective activation of donor CD4+ T cells in the absence of CD8+ T-cell activation. In contrast to acute GVHD, mice with chronic GVHD do not produce Th1 cytokines other than IL-2, donor CD8+ T cells do not become

Table 1 Summary of Essential Distinguishing Features of Acute and Chronic GVHD in the Parent-into-F1 Model

Parameter	Acute GVHD	Chronic GVHD
Mortality	Early (weeks)	Late (months)
Pathogenic mechanism	Immunodeficiency, lymphocytopenia	Immune complex, glomerulonephritis
Splenocyte count (vs. normal)[a]	Reduced ($\leq 50\%$)	Increased (≥ 125–200%)
Autoantibody production	Transient	Sustained
Donor cells engrafted	CD4+, CD8+	CD4+
Th1 cytokines produced	IL-2, IFN-γ (?IL-12)	IL-2, (minimal IFN-γ)
Th2 cytokines produced	IL-4, IL-10	IL-4, IL-10
Donor antihost CTL	Present	Not detectable
Fas/FasL on lymphocytes[a]	Strong upregulation	Low-level upregulation
Predominant antihost immune response	Cell mediated	Antibody mediated

[a]Compared to age- and sex-matched normal mice at 2 weeks after parental cell transfer.
Source: Refs. (20,21,26,39).

activated, donor-antihost CTL are not generated, and cells of the F1 host that express MHC class I, including host B cells, are not eliminated (26). Instead, the initial activation of donor CD4+ T cells persists and results in continued production of B-cell stimulatory (Th2) cytokines (26,33), delivery of cognate help to autoreactive B cells (34), production of autoantibodies, and the development of an SLE-like disease (20). Thus, chronic GVHD is driven solely by donor CD4+ T cells. Major distinguishing features between chronic and acute GVHD are the lack of CD8+ T-cell activation and lack of significant IFN-γ production in chronic GVHD. Although low-level elevations in serum IFN-γ can be detected in chronic GVHD (approximately two-fold), a functional role for this cytokine in chronic GVHD has not been demonstrated (31).

3. Acute GVHD Is Mediated by Donor-Derived CD8+ Antihost CTL, Not by Suppressor Cells

Original descriptions of the acute GVHD model maintained that Lyt2 + (CD8+) T cells mediated acute GVHD through suppressor activity (35,36). However antihost cytolytic activity, rather than suppressor activity, is the likely mechanism (37,38). Recently, antihost CTL in acute GVHD have been detected ex vivo (without an in vitro restimulation period) (26,39), and killing of host lymphocytes can be mediated by both perforin and Fas/FasL pathways (39). In addition, significant upregulation of Fas/FasL expression on donor and host cells as seen in acute GVHD (39) is not seen in chronic GVHD. Thus, not only does FasL upregulation on donor CD8+ T cells enhance their killing ability, but Fas upregulation on host B cells also enhances their recognition by CTL and promotes their elimination.

D. P → F1 GVHD: Investigational Utility

1. Chronic GVHD Strongly Resembles Human SLE

Chronic GVHD is characterized by high serum levels of IgG autoantibodies (antinuclear, anti–double-stranded DNA, antihistone, anti-RNP) typical of human SLE (40–42). Autoantibodies not characteristic of SLE (antithyroglobulin, anti-insulin) are not observed (41). Similar to human SLE, Ig is deposited along the dermal-epidermal basement membrane (43), and immune complex formation occurs with deposition in the renal glomeruli. This in turn leads to the development of immune complex glomerulonephritis and death from nephrotic syndrome and renal failure (43,44). Chronic GVHD in the parent-into-F1 model is, thus, an appropriate model for the study of immune mechanisms involved in lupus pathogenesis (Table 2).

2. Acute GVHD Allows Study of In Vivo CTL Maturation

As described above, acute GVHD is mediated by donor-antihost CTL, which eliminate host lymphocytes. Although preparative regimens in humans also eliminate host lymphocytes prior to transplant, acute GVHD in humans is mediated by effector T cells, typically CD8+ with CTL function. Thus, the value of the P → F1 model of acute GVHD is not that it necessarily models the clinical features of human acute GVHD, but that it models the in vivo development of alloreactive CD8+ effector CTL (Table 2). Elimination of host lymphocytes in this model serves as a surrogate marker for in vivo donor-antihost CTL function. As described below, long-term survivors of acute murine GVHD in the P → F1 model may mimic features of human chronic GVHD.

Table 2 P → F1 GVHD: Investigational Advantages

The GVHD model lends itself to hypothesis testing and mechanistic studies studying in vivo ag-specific T-cell responses for the following reasons:

1. The basic cellular immunology of GVHD is well defined and the ag-specific T cells driving SLE are identifiable (donor origin) and can be studied separately from the remainder of the T-cell pool (host origin).
2. Because the exact time of disease onset is known, defects in T-cell activation, maturation, or effector function can be distinguished.
3. A predominantly Th1/CMI response (acute GVHD) or Th2/ab-mediated response (chronic GVHD) can be uniformly induced in the same immunologically normal F1, thereby reducing potential variables.
4. Disease phenotype can be determined as early as 2 weeks after parental cell transfer, allowing experiments with a relatively short duration.

E. Utility of the DBA → F1 Model

1. Defects in Donor CD8+ T-Cell Activation Convert Acute GVHD to Chronic GVHD

It is not necessary for CD8+ T cells to be totally absent from the donor inoculum for chronic GVHD to result. For example, in the DBA → F1 model of chronic GVHD, donor CD8+ T cells engraft in small numbers but are defective in their ability to induce acute GVHD (21). Although adequate numbers of both CD4+ and CD8+ T cells are present in the donor inoculum and a fully allogeneic MHC I and II disparity exists, mice develop chronic GVHD rather than acute GVHD. The exact mechanism has not been fully clarified, but despite injecting numbers of donor CD8+ T cells sufficient for induction of acute GVHD in other P → F1 combinations, at 2 weeks donor CD8+ T-cell engraftment is barely detectable in DBA → F1 mice (26). Initially it was reported that DBA mice had no defect in their ability to generate in vivo CTL under non–rate-limiting conditions (35) and that a significant increase in the number of DBA donor cells would eventually convert chronic GVHD to acute GVHD (45). Other workers have shown that in DBA → F1 mice, there is preferential activation of CD4+ Th2 cells (46). As a result, DBA mice have been termed "Th2 prone" (46). Similarly, we have not observed differences in anti-FT CTL activity in DBA vs. B6 mice under non–rate-limiting conditions; however, under more stringent conditions differences are seen (37). Specifically, the anti-F1 pCTL frequency of unfractionated splenocytes from DBA/2 mice is approximately ninefold lower than that of C57Bl/6 mice (37) or B10.D2 (unpublished observations). Based on these results, it is likely that chronic GVHD in DBA → F1 mice is a result of defective CD8+ T-cell activation rather than an inherent predisposition of CD4+ T cells to become Th2 cells. Supporting this idea are studies in which DBA CD4+ T cells were supplemented with either DBA CD8+ T cells or H-2^d-identical B10.D2 CD8+ T cells. Acute GVHD was readily induced with B10.D2 CD8+ T cells, indicating that DBA CD4+ T cells were capable of providing adequate help for in vivo CTL maturation and arguing against their being Th2 prone. Moreover, B10.D2 CD8+ T cells were numerically more efficient in acute GVHD induction than were DBA CD8+ T cells (26). When DBA CD8+ numbers were increased to levels sufficient to result in engraftment at 2 weeks equal to that of B10.D2 CD8+ T cells, host B-cell elimination was still less efficient in

DBA → F1 mice vs. B10.D2 cells. These results argue strongly that in addition to possible quantitative defects there may be a qualitative defect in DBA CD8+ T cells. Taken together, these data indicate that chronic GVHD in DBA → F1 mice results from the combination of normal donor CD4+ T-cell activation combined with suboptimal activation of donor CD8+ T cells. The DBA → F1 model is, therefore, a useful model for testing agents that can enhance CD8+ T-cell effector function in vivo (see below).

2. Preclinical Evaluation of Agents That Induce Immunomodulation (Immune Deviation) Versus Immune Suppression

A major advantage of this GVHD model is that it allows the differentiation of agents, that globally inhibit T-cell function from agents, that selectively inhibit CD8+ CTL maturation. Specifically, global immune suppression blocks both forms of GVHD entirely, whereas the selective inhibition of CD8+ CTL modulates disease, converting acute GVHD to chronic GVHD. Conversely, agents that promote CTL function convert chronic GVHD to acute GVHD in the DBA → F1 model.

F. Results of In Vivo Immunomodulation in the GVHD Model

1. Agents That Globally Impair T-Cell Activation Prevent Both Acute and Chronic GVHD

Both acute and chronic GVHD can be completely inhibited by in vivo treatment with agents that globally prevent T-cell activation by blocking the delivery of a costimulatory signal. For example, administration of CTLA4 Ig, a fusion protein, which blocks both CD80 and CD86 (47,48), or combined anti-CD80/anti-CD86 mAb treatment (49) will completely block the acute and chronic GVHD phenotype if administered at the time of donor cell transfer. These results not only confirm the role of donor T-cell activation in mediating disease, but also demonstrate that despite the increasing number of costimulatory molecules recently described (50), only CD80 and CD86 are critical for in vivo naive T-cell activation and generation of a Th1 or Th2 response.

2. Agents That Promote CD8+ T-Cell Function and CTL Maturation Convert Chronic GVHD in DBA → F1 Mice to Acute GVHD

Interleukin-12 is a strong promoter of CTL effector function (51). Treatment of DBA → F1 mice with rIL-12 converts chronic GVHD to acute GVHD by strongly promoting donor CTL effector function (52). Although donor CD8+ T-cell engraftment is enhanced with rIL-12, it does not normalize to that typically seen for B6 → F1 acute GVHD mice. Anti-CD80 blockade in DBA → F1 mice also converts chronic GVHD to acute GVHD by enhancing donor CD8+ T-cell engraftment and CTL effector function. CD80 is the preferential ligand for CTLA4 and the delivery of a downregulatory costimulatory signal (53,54). A similar enhancing effect on donor CD8+ T cells has been reported with CTLA4 blockade (55). It is possible that the CD8-promoting activities of CD80 blockade result from blocking CTLA4 mediated down regulatory costimulation.

3. Actions That Selectively Impair CD8+ T-Cell Activation and CTL Maturation Convert Acute GVHD to Chronic GVHD

It is well recognized that depletion of CD8+ T cells from the donor inoculum induces chronic GVHD in P → F1 combinations that would otherwise result in acute GVHD, indicating a critical role for CD8+ T cells in acute GVHD pathology (20,37). Further studies have shown that selective inhibition of cytokines important in CTL maturation will also result in chronic GVHD in P → F1 combinations that would otherwise develop acute GVHD. For example, IL-2 is absolutely required for in vitro CTL generation (56). In vivo blockade with anti-IL-2 mAb in B6 → F1 mice converts acute GVHD to chronic GVHD by preventing the development of antihost CTL activity (57). Donor CD4+ T-cell help for B cells, however, is not inhibited, and chronic GVHD ensues. Similarly, in vivo TNF-α blockade in acute GVHD (B6 → F1) selectively inhibits the induction of CTL effectors and production of Th1 cytokines such as IFN-γ. TNF-α blockade does not inhibit Th2 cytokines and chronic GVHD ensues (31). Of note, TNF-α blockade need only be present in the first few days after parental cell transfer and was ineffective if given only after day 7, implying that TNF-α plays a critical role in CTL induction but not in CTL effector function and elimination of host lymphocytes. These results underscore the role of donor CD8+T cells in mediating acute GVHD and demonstrate that selective defects in donor CD8+ T-cell activation and maturation result in Th2-driven chronic GVHD.

4. Qualitative Defects in CTL Killing Impair Acute GVHD Induction and Over Time Result in Chronic GVHD

The use of perforin-deficient or FasL-impaired (gld) donor cells results in lessened acute GVHD induction and impaired elimination of host B cells by CTL relative to that of wild-type donor cells (58,59). In both instances this defect can be overcome by doubling the donor cell inoculum. Thus, qualitative defects in CD8+ CTL function can appear as quantitative defects in GVHD induction. Moreover, incomplete elimination of host B cells using perforin-deficient donor cells allowed the persistence of activated autoreactive B cells and the eventual evolution of the disease phenotype into chronic GVHD (58).

5. Summary

The P → F1 model is useful to study the immunopathogenesis of lupus. However, an emerging role for this model is its potential for defining and differentiating the elements important for in vivo CMI/Th1 or antibody-mediated/Th2 responses. Through the administration of mAb directed against cytokines or cell surface targets, their in vivo role can be delineated. Thus, the model can be viewed as a preclinical model for testing of potential immunomodulatory agents.

G. Human Chronic GVHD, Autoimmunity, and the P → F1 Model

Chronic GVHD in the P → F1 model mimics human lupus and not human chronic GVHD. Human GVHD patients can develop clinical features, that resemble scleroderma and Sjögren's syndrome with interstitial lung disease (60–62). Chronic GVHD is not identical to human scleroderma, particularly with regard to the autoantibody profile and collagen deposition patterns; however, it supports the idea that chimerism or persistence of allogeneic T cells in an irradiated recipient can mediate autoimmune diseases such as scleroderma and Sjögren's syndrome. In murine models, bone marrow transplantation across minor histocompatibility differences into irradiated recipients results in sclerodermatous features such as dermal T-cell infiltration and collagen deposition (63). Alloreactive T-cell clones can be isolated that produce cytokines that promote collagen deposition and fibroblast proliferation (64). Long-term survivors of acute (P → F1) murine GVHD have sclerodermatous features. Mice that do not succumb during the early stages of acute GVHD may eventually develop a chronic form of GVHD, which resembles several human autoimmune diseases including lupus, rheumatoid arthritis, Sjögren's syndrome, scleroderma, and some other collagen vascular diseases. For example, induction of GVHD in BALB/c → (BALB/c × A) F1 mice leads to the development of chronic progressive polyarthritis with juxta-articular manifestations, including perivascular infiltrates, peritendinitis, myositis, and inflammatory nodules (65). In addition, mice were noted to have Sjögren-like salivary gland lesions, hepatic lesions resembling sclerosing cholangitis, scleroderma-like skin lesions, and immune complex glomerulonephritis. These mice develop positive ANA, anti-dsDNA, antihistone, and low-titer anti-snRNP antibodies (66). The scleroderma-like changes require 9–12 months to develop (65).

1. Lessons from the P → F1 Model for the Immunopathogenesis of Chronic GVHD

The two disease phenotypes termed acute and chronic GVHD in this model are both acute in onset. Although major organ pathology in chronic GVHD (immune complex glomerulonephritis) and death due to renal failure are late occurrences, immunological surrogate markers are evident by 2 weeks after donor cell transfer and reliably distinguish acute GVHD from chronic GVHD. Chronic GVHD in this model does not require preceding acute GVHD (as generally seen in human GVHD). A second important observation comes from long-term survivors of acute P → F1 GVHD. This second form of chronic GVHD, which we will designate "acute GVHD survivors," implicates long-term immuno-dysregulation and preceding acute GVHD as having a possible role in its pathogenesis. Potential mechanisms include the stable chimeric state and thymic dysfunction. For example, maternal-fetal microchimerism (the presence in an individual of DNA or cells from the mother or offspring at low levels) has recently been shown to be a frequent occurrence in both normal individuals and patients with autoimmune diseases such as PSS (67,68). The presence of microchimerism in normal individuals combined with the relatively low incidence of PSS indicates that additional factors are likely required for disease development. It is known that the thymus is a target in acute P → F1 GVHD and is not able to subsequently provide appropriate thymic education for new T cells (69). The consequences of long-term T-cell dysregulation stemming from acute GVHD-related thymic damage have not been defined. However, the delay of many months before the development of connective tissue disease in acute GVHD survivors is consistent with the time required for the emergence of defective T cells from the bone marrow with pathological activities.

H. Autologous GVHD Model

The importance of autoreactivity and the thymus in the pathogenesis of chronic GVHD is suggested by clinical manifestations of chronic GVHD that frequently mimic those of autoimmune diseases. Since thymic epithelium is damaged by prior therapy, the preparative regimen, and prior acute GVHD, aberrant thymic education may play a significant role in the pathogenesis of chronic GVHD (70–73).

The T-cell precursors that undergo aberrant "thymic education" after SCT become self-reactive (or autoreactive) (70). Because of decreased negative selection, reduced extrathymic generation, or acceleration of the normal thymic aging process with chronic GVHD, patients have an increase in peripheral autoreactive T lymphocytes (74,75). These autoreactive T lymphocytes act with IFN-γ to produce the increased collagen deposition seen histopathologically in chronic GVHD (76). Autologous GVHD models have been described in detail elsewhere (77–79).

I. Endothelial Injury in Chronic GVHD

Recent evidence suggests that vascular endothelium is a target in acute and chronic GVHD, and this finding would explain the ulcerations we see in patients with scleroder-matous forms of chronic GVHD. Biedermann et al. (80) investigated eight patients with acute GVHD and 10 with chronic GVHD for signs of endothelial injury and microvessel loss by measurement of von Willebrand factor (vWF) in plasma and blood vessel density in biopsy samples taken from skin lesions. There was more extensive loss of microvessels in the skin of patients with GVHD (median 66 capillaries/mm^2) than in healthy controls (205 capillaries/mm^2; $p = 0.005$). Patients with GVHD had higher concentrations of vWF (238%) than did those without GVHD (102%; $p = 0.0005$). Perivascular CD8 T-cell infil-trates in skin correlated with vWF plasma concentrations in patients with GVHD ($p = 0.01$), and activated cytotoxic T lymphocytes and endothelial injury were present in the same samples. These data suggest that endothelial cells are targets of alloreactive donor cytotoxic T lymphocytes. As a consequence, impaired blood perfusion and tissue fibrosis, the hallmark of chronic GVHD, may occur (80).

III. INCIDENCE AND RISK FACTORS

A. Incidence

The overall incidence of chronic GVHD is about 60% after allogeneic SCT. It may range from 30 to 85% (81,82). In a recent review of 116 HLA-identical PBSCT recipients, lim-ited chronic GVHD occurred in 6%, and clinical extensive chronic GVHD in 71% (9). Data from the National Marrow Donor Program (NMDP) indicate that up to 70% of patients receiving alternative donor marrow grafts and survive beyond day 100 to develop chronic GVHD (83).

B. Risk Factors

Four clinical risk factors, including prior grade II–IV acute GVHD, HLA disparity, older recipient age, and use of allogeneic peripheral blood stem cell transplants (PBSCT), have been consistently identified as risk factors.

1. Previous Acute GVHD

The greatest risk factor is the occurrence of acute GVHD (84–86). This implies that risk factors for acute GVHD also apply to chronic GVHD or that the insult of acute GVHD sets the stage for the chronic form (9). In one study a history of acute GVHD and the use of corticosteroids at day 100 [relative risk (RR) = 3.9] had the strongest association with the development of chronic GVHD (87).

2. HLA Disparity Between Donor and Recipient

The use of HLA-matched unrelated donors and HLA-nonidentical (including haploiden-tical) related donors is increasing (88). HLA disparity is a predictive factor for an increased risk of developing chronic GVHD (84–86,89). While chronic GVHD occurs in about one third of patients receiving HLA-identical sibling transplants, 50% of patients undergoing HLA-nonidentical related SCT and about two thirds of those undergoing matched unrelated SCT develop chronic GVHD (3). For patients receiving HA-1 one-antigen mismatched unrelated marrow grafts, the cumulative incidence of chronic GVHD was not different from those receiving matched unrelated or haploidentical family donor grafts (90).

Among 215 HLA-A2–positive patients who received HLA-identical sibling SCT, 34 patient-donor pairs (15.8%) were mismatched for HA-1 antigen (restricted by HLA-A2). While grades II–IV acute GVHD occurred in 52% of the HA-1–mismatched pairs compared to 37% among HA-1–identical pairs [odds ratio (OR) = 2.96], no differences were observed for chronic GVHD (91).

3. Recipient and Donor Age

Chronic GVHD increases with age (84–86,92). Adult (>20 years) transplant recipients develop chronic GVHD more often (46%) than children <10 years of age (13%) (3). Allogeneic SCT in older high-risk patients even after reduced intensity conditioning resulted in a high incidence of acute and chronic GVHD (93). However, among recipients of unrelated marrow, the age association was less prominent, and even in the youngest age group the probability of chronic GVHD was 42% (3). The impact of donor age on chronic GVHD remains controversial (94,95).

4. Allogeneic Peripheral Blood Stem Cell Transplantation

The use of peripheral blood stem cells has been steadily increasing (96,97). The reason for this increase is multifactorial, including the beneficial effect of PBSCT on engraftment and the convenience for both stem cell donors and physicians. In contrast to early reports (98,99), recent prospective studies clearly show a higher incidence of chronic GVHD with PBSCT. Approximately 40–80% of survivors transplanted with G-CSF stimulated allogeneic PBSCT from HLA-identical donors have developed extensive chronic GVHD (9,100–105).

A meta-analysis of 16 studies (5 randomized controlled trials and 11 cohort studies) comparing the incidence of acute and chronic GVHD after PBSCT and marrow transplantation was recently presented (96). The relative risk of acute GVHD and for chronic GVHD and extensive chronic GVHD after PBSCT was statistically significantly higher than with traditional marrow transplants. The excess risk of chronic GVHD was explained by differences in the T-cell doses delivered with the graft; however, that difference did not reach statistical significance. There was a trend towards a decrease in the rate of relapse after PBSCT.

The French transplant society recently published long-term results on 101 patients (97) from their initial randomized trial (103). At a follow-up of 31–57 months, the 3-year cumulative incidence of chronic GVHD was 65% (extensive 44%) in the PBSCT group, and 36% (extensive 17%) in the marrow transplant group. Cutaneous and liver involvement was similar among marrow and PBSCT recipients, but ocular involvement was more frequent in PBSCT recipients. Chronic GVHD after PBSCT required multiple courses of immunosuppressive therapy in addition to cyclosporine and corticosteroids and for longer periods of time. Chronic GVHD after PBSCT was associated with an antileukemic effect that was at least as potent as after marrow, but there was no survival difference (97).

In a multicenter, phase III trial there was no significant difference in the cumulative incidence of chronic GVHD between allogeneic PBSCT recipients and those receiving marrow (105). A follow-up report (106) showed cumulative incidence of chronic GVHD at 3 years that was similar. However, similar to other trials, the number of successive treatments and the duration of glucocorticoid treatment required were significantly longer after PBSCT. Involvement of skin and female genital tract was more frequent in PBSC recipients than in marrow recipients (106). It is not clear whether PBSC further increase the risk of chronic GVHD beyond that seen with marrow (83,107,108).

Recent data suggest that high CD34+ counts may be an important factor driving the development of chronic GVHD, which did not correlate with CD3+ and CD14+ counts (109). In that particular analysis of results in 181 HLA-identical sibling PBSCT recipients, there was no association between transplant outcome (acute GVHD, overall survival, disease relapse) and the particular cell doses in the graft (CD34, CD3, or CD14 cell doses) or the CD14-to-CD3 ratio. However, higher doses of CD34 cells ($>8.0 \times 10^6$/kg) were associated with a significantly increased hazard of clinical extensive chronic GVHD hazard ratio (HR) = 2.3].

The use of granulocyte colony-stimulating factor (G-CSF) for stem cell collection per se does not appear to lead to more chronic GVHD (110). Morton et al. (111) randomized HLA-matched sibling donors to marrow or PBSC collection after both groups received G-CSF stimulation. Rates of chronic GVHD were higher in the PBSC arm (80% vs. 22%; $p < 0.02$); overall survival was the same.

5. Donor Lymphocyte Infusion

Currently many high-risk patientsare offered non-myeloablative transplants followed by DLI to achieve total donor chimerism or treat residual disease (112). DLI given after non-myeloablative SCT or for relapse is associated with a high incidence of acute and chronic GVHD (113). This may not be surprising because patients with recurrent or residual disease post-SCT are treated with repeated DLI until GVHD occurs [hoping to achieve a graft-vs.-leukemia (GVL) effect]. In a recent report by Collins et al., 60% of DLI recipients developed chronic GVHD, and the presence of GvHD was highly predictive of leukemia remission (114).

6. Positive Skin or Oral Biopsies at Day 70–120 Post-SCT

In a study by Loughran et al. (115) GVHD detected by skin biopsy or oral mucosal biopsy, despite the lack of clinically evident GVHD, or a history of acute GVHD, independently predicted a threefold relative risk for chronic GVHD. However, in a subsequent study from the same institution, the value of routine chronic GVHD screening studies including skin biopsy, oral exam, lip biopsy, Schirmer's test, serum alkaline phosphatase, aspartate transaminase, immunoglobulin level, and platelet count performed between 70 and 120 days after allogeneic marrow transplantation failed to show any predictive value (116). Also, there are no data to suggest that treatment of chronic GVHD in its subclinical stage would improve outcome. Furthermore, it is possible that the preemptive treatment would blunt the GVL effect. Nevertheless, patients identified by biopsy or by the other risk factors listed above should be carefully monitored for the development of overt chronic GVHD. Patients who receive corticosteroids at day 100 should be considered for clinical trials to determine the efficacy of new immunosuppressive agents in preventing overt chronic GVHD.

7. Viral Infections

The relationship between infection and subsequent chronic GVHD remains unclear. Latent herpesvirus in the marrow donor or recipient may be important for the development of acute and chronic GVHD (117–120). However, there is no compelling evidence for a connection between CMV infection and subsequent onset of chronic GVHD. A recent study suggested that active CMV infection before day 60 was associated with a high incidence of de novo chronic GVHD among 489 patients (121).

8. Duration of Cyclosporine Prophylaxis

Shorter duration cyclosporine administration was thought to increase the incidence of chronic GVHD (122–124). However, a recent study showed no statistically significant difference in the incidence of clinical extensive chronic GVHD between recipients randomly assigned to receive a 24-month and those who received a 6-month course of cyclosporine prophylaxis (125).

9. Second Transplant

Second transplants are also complicated by a high rate of acute and chronic GVHD (126).

10. Transfusion of Nonirradiated Donor Buffy Coat or Marrow Boosts

The notion that tranfusion shortly before HLA-matched marrow transplantation was associated with a decrease risk of chronic GVHD and that second marrow infusion after allo-SCT resulted in increased chronic GVHD (127,128) has not been substantiated.

11. Risk Factors for De Novo Chronic GVHD

In a recent retrospective study the majority of patients with de novo chronic GVHD had received marrow grafts from HLA-identical sibling donors (85%) and postgrafting immunosuppression with methotrexate and cyclosporine. Among 489 patients with either grade 0 or I acute GVHD, 33% developed chronic GVHD (de novo). Overall survival was 70%, and relapse-free survival was 63% at 8 years. Risk factors included viable donor buffy coat infusions among patients with aplastic anemia, patient-donor sex/parity combination, grade I acute GVHD, and active CMV infection before day 60. Among 45 patients aged < 19 years who had male donors, only 1 developed chronic GVHD. However, overall and relapse-free survival rates at 8 years were lower than in the entire cohort (121).

IV. DIAGNOSIS OF CHRONIC GVHD

Therapies for chronic GVHD are highly immunosuppressive and must be continued for a prolonged time. It is important, therefore, to confirm the diagnosis before initiating therapy. Conversely, subtle manifestations of chronic GVHD may go undiagnosed for months, and this delay may render successful treatment and rehabilitation difficult. For example, the diagnosis of fasciitis without skin changes may be difficult to recognize, but systematic assessment of range of motion of wrists and ankles may detect early signs before permanent disability. In addition, pulmonary function testing at 3 months and at one year after transplant may detect early signs of bronchioliis obliterans before symptoms become apparent.

The diagnosis of chronic GVHD is generally made on the basis of clinical and laboratory parameters, in particular biopsies of the affected areas. The diagnosis of chronic

GVHD is traditionally made after day 100 posttransplant, although there is no biological reason for this distinction, and this practice is being abandoned. Initial presentation of chronic GVHD after 500 days post-SCT is rare. In an early study the median time to diagnosis was day 201 after HLA-identical sibling transplant, day 159 after mismatched related transplant, and day 133 after unrelated donor transplants (3). In a recent IBMTR/NMDP analysis, the median time of diagnosis was 4.5 months after HLA-identical sibling transplant and 4 months after unrelated donor transplant, with only 5% of cases diagnosed after 1 year (83).

To establish the diagnosis of chronic GVHD early, high-risk patients should be followed closely, and treatment should be instituted promptly to prevent disability and mortality due to chronic GVHD. Regular follow-up is very important. However, while there is a tendency to assume that whenever a patient returns to the transplant center the problem is chronic GVHD, we found that frequently patients had inactive disease or no GVHD at all (133). There is no reliable laboratory indicator of the onset of chronic GVHD. A recent study from Japan evaluated the expression of OX40 and showed percentages of both OX40+CD4+ and OX40+CD8+ T cells to be significantly higher in patients with chronic GVHD than in those without ($p < 0.0001$ and $p = 0.001$, respectively). OX40+CD4+ T cells were elevated before the onset of chronic GVHD and closely correlated with the therapeutic response. CD25, CD69, and HLA-DR were detectable on OX40+ T cells (134). This area should provide fertile soil for innovative research.

V. CLINICAL MANIFESTATIONS OF CHRONIC GVHD

In HLA-identical marrow transplantation with primarily methotrexate-based prophylaxis, skin (65–80%), mouth (48–72%), liver (40–73%), and eye (18–47%) involvement are most commonly reported. Other involved organs include gastrointestinal tract (weight loss) (16–26%), lung (10–15%), esophagus (6–8%), and joints (2–12%) (3,83,86). Neuromuscular, genitourinary, and serosal involvements are even less common (135,136).

The spectrum and the incidence of certain clinical manifestations of chronic GVHD have somewhat changed with the introduction of modern immunosuppressive regimens (137). PBSC recipients show a similar time to onset and a comparable spectrum of organ involvement, as do patients transplanted with marrow (106). A comprehensive study on the current clinical spectrum of chronic GVHD, however, is lacking.

A. Immune System

Chronic GVHD causes profound immune dysfunction (138–141), and most chronic GVHD deaths are secondary to infection. Increased susceptibility to infection is attributable to both features of the disease and its treatment. The etiology of impaired immunity is multifactorial and includes disrupted mucosal barriers, thymic injury, hypogammaglobulinemia, and qualitative T-cell and B-cell abnormalities (142,143). Functional asplenia with an increased susceptibility to encapsulated bacteria is common. Patients must be monitored for bacterial, viral, and fungal infections, particularly invasive fungal infections and *Pneumocystis carinii* pneumonia (PCP). Therefore, antimicrobial prophylaxis is indicated until immunosuppressive regimens are discontinued.

B. Skin

The organ most commonly involved in chronic GVHD is skin (135,144). Rarely, patients develop oral or hepatic chronic GVHD without skin involvement. Patients with chronic GVHD usually present with lichenoid skin eruptions, an erythematous, shiny, papular rash that resembles lichen planus and has no typical distribution pattern as in acute GVHD. Inspection with side-angle lighting more clearly defines the raised, flat-topped lesions. In some patients, sun exposure can trigger the appearance of new skin lesions or the rapid progression of existing background erythema. Erythema may begin in the malar area but soon spreads to sun-exposed and other areas. The onset may also be insidious, with reticular mottling, perifollicular papules, and papullo-squamous plaques. Affected skin may become either hyperpigmented or hypopigmented. Skin biopsies are necessary to confirm the diagnosis of chronic GVHD and to rule out skin rashes secondary to drugs such as trimethoprim-sulfamethoxazole (TMP-SMX) and infections. Serial assessments should document the extent, type, and distribution of skin involvement.

As the disease progresses, the skin becomes more sclerodermatous with thickening, limitation of mobility as a result of fascial involvement, and loss of dermal appendages (hair and sweat glands). The skin findings clinically resemble systemic sclerosis (145). In an advanced stage, the skin is very thickened, tight bound (unable to move), and fragile with very poor wound-healing capacity likely because of capillary and lymphatic damage. In cases of severe ulceration, skin grafts from the donor have been successful, and the donor tissue remains healthy and uninvolved by chronic GVHD (146,147). However, skin grafting is not a common procedure. Ulcers usually heal by controlling chronic GVHD and appropriate skin care. In patients with localized lesions, epidermal atrophy and dense focal dermal fibrosis are noted in the absence of significant inflammation. Guttate lesions sometimes appear on the trunk as shiny indurated areas, or they can be localized to areas of pressure, trauma, prior irritation, injury, zoster, or irradiation. Rarely, the skin may become blistered from poor lymphatic drainage or ulcerated from minor trauma, a marker for the severity of cutaneous involvement (148). Generalized scleroderma, if severe enough, leads to join contractures and severe disability (135,145). Patients with sclerodermatous GVHD and restricted range of motion may benefit from a regular program of physical therapy to help in recovery and to provide functional recommendations for limited joints. Fascial involvement in sclerodermatous GVHD is usually associated with skin changes, but may develop with normal, albeit fixed overlying skin. Isolated fascial scleroderma presents with decreased mobility with normal-appearing skin. When the overlying skin is soft and subtle but exhibits peau d'orange characteristic, fascial involvement is the likely explanation. A deep tissue biopsy is required to document fascial involvement (149). Fasciitis often affects forearms and legs causing significant limitations in range of motion and joint contractures. Patients with restricted range of motion benefit from regular physical therapy including deep muscle-fascial massage. Serial assessments of joints should document the range of motion.

1. Histopathological Findings

The lichenoid form of chronic GVHD resembles idiopathic lichen planus, showing hyperkeratosis, acanthosis, dyskeratosis, and vacuolar alterations in the basal cell layer, together with monocytic and lymphocytic infiltrates in the papillary dermis (150). The lesions heal without dermal fibrosis or loss of elastic tissue. The sclerodermatous form of chronic GVHD shows sclerosis and thickening of the reticular dermis, loss of distinction between the papillary and reticular dermis, plus loss of rete pegs due to increased collagen deposition, and a mild perivascular lymphocytic infiltrate. Characteristically, the sweats glands are infiltrated with lymphocytes and melanophages. Donor-derived cytotoxic T lymphocytes are the effector cells responsible for lesions in the skin and other tissues (151). In scleradermatous GVHD, sclerosis is located in the superficial dermis, and collagen fibers of irregular diameter are seen in the subepidermal area. In systemic sclerosis, sclerosis is seen in the lower dermis and subcutaneous fatty tissue, and collagen fibers of irregular diameter are located in the deep dermis. Some collagen fibers are degenerative in the superficial dermis in sclerodermatous GVHD (152).

2. Dermal Appendages

Hair loss, nail loss, and destruction of the sweat glands are common. Hair loss in areas of affected skin may also persist after treatment. Brittle hair often precedes allopecia. Regrowth of body hair and return of sweat gland function usually herald disease improvement. Premature graying is often associated with chronic GVHD, even in children, and may affect hair and eyebrows. Nails develop vertical ridges and cracking and are very fragile. Nail problems may persist even after skin changes have resolved (153).

C. Liver

Hepatic disease is also common in chronic GVHD and typically presents as cholestasis. The correlation between the degree of hyperbilirubinemia and clinical outcome is not as linear as in acute GVHD (135). Recently, an unusual form of liver GVHD has been described. Strasser and colleagues reported their observation in 14 patients in whom chronic GVHD of the liver presented with marked elevations of serum aminotransferases, clinically resembling acute viral hepatitis (154). Isolated hepatic chronic GVHD is being seen with increased frequency with the use of DLI (113,155). Patients are usually asymptomatic until the advanced stage of liver GVHD. Portal hypertension, cirrhosis, and hepatic failure are rare (156,157). Primary biliary cirrhosis can mimic the similar bile duct damage and features of ocular and oral sicca (158). Liver transplantation has rarely been successfully performed for end-stage hepatic chronic GVHD (159).

A liver biopsy is required to confirm the diagnosis as viral infection, and drug toxicity may mimic GVHD. The portal triads have a dense, mixed infiltrate of lymphocytes, histiocytes, and often eosinophils and plasma cells. The infiltrate extends into the lobule with piecemeal hepatocellular involvement. The bile ducts usually show lymphocyte-associated necrosis of the epithelium and prominent periportal bile stasis. There is increased portal fibrosis, occasionally leading to micronodular cirrhosis. After long-standing disease, the bile ducts in the portal triads decrease in number (ductopenia) or completely vanish. It takes a long time for these ducts to regenerate despite effective treatment of chronic GVHD.

D. Mouth

Oral manifestations of chronic GVHD include xerostomia, leukoplakia, mucosal atrophy, erythema, and ulcers. In its earliest manifestations, patients may simply complain of dryness of the mouth or food sensitivity, and examination may reveal no more than mild erythema. As the disease progresses, however, a fine reticular pattern or whitish plaques may appear on the buccal mucosa or tongue that resembles lichen planus. On the tongue, this may be confused with oral thrush. Pseudomembranes—large, nonhealing ulcers—may be found anywhere in the mouth, including the tongue and palate, but are often along the bite lines. These lichenoid lesions may be extensive and sometimes evolve to frank ulceration causing odynophagia (pain on swallowing) (160). Some lesions are resistant to treatment with topical and systemic immunosuppressive medications. Ultraviolet A irradiation therapy with oral psoralen has been shown to be effective in treating these resistant lesions (161) (see Sec. VIII. F).

Secondary infection with viruses (especially herpes simplex and human papilloma virus) and yeasts (*Candida*) are almost universal. Herpes simplex must be ruled out if ulcerative lesions are seen at the time of presentation (153,160,162). Changes in symptoms with little change in exam may occur with local infections. Serial viral and fungal cultures should be obtained in any patient complaining of increased oral pain. Patients usually require antiviral or antifungal treatment as long as their oral disease persists or immuno-suppression is given.

Atrophy of the gums can occur, and this predisposes the patient to severe dental decay. Salivary glandular disease also contributes to the dryness, predisposing to dental disease. Both major and minor salivary gland dysfunction occurs (163). Fibrosis causing decreased oral range of motion is a very late manifestation. Patients with chronic GVHD undergoing dental work should receive antibiotic prophylaxis. Rarely, patients will have esophageal involvement without oral disease. Salivary gland and mucosal involvement can be demonstrated by biopsy. Histopathological features of lichenoid oral lesions are similar to those in the lichenoid form of cutaneous chronic GVHD. Fibrosing sialoadenitis, as seen in Sjögren sicca syndrome, may be present in minor salivary glands.

E. Eyes

Ocular GVHD is common in conjunction with oral disease. Patients usually present with irritation or dry eyes. Lymphocytic infiltration, fibrosis, and destruction of lacrimal glands result in decreased tear production and chemosis plus corneal scarring and ulceration. The pathological changes in lacrimal gland resemble those in the sicca syndrome of Sjögren. Irreversible destruction of the lacrimal glands results in keratoconjunctivitis sicca, manifested by dryness, photophobia, irritation, burning, and pain (162,164,165). If dry eye is left untreated, severe corneal damage may occur. Punctate keratopathy can range from minimal stippling to massive corneal erosions. All patients with chronic GVHD must be monitored for tear function with Schirmer's test even in the absence of symptoms because ocular damage may occur before symptoms are present. In patients with abnormal tear function (Shirmer's test, ≤5 mm wetting) artificial tear replacement (preservative-free) should be started, and the cornea should be examined on a regular basis by biomicroscopy with fluorescein staining. Conjunctival GVHD with hyperemia progressing to pseudomembranes is a rare manifestation of severe chronic GVHD and is associated with a poor prognosis (166). Use of prolonged corticosteroids in the treatment of chronic GVHD and pretransplant total body irradiation promote cataract formation. Cataract repair can be performed safely in patients with chronic GVHD even in the presence of ocular sicca.

F. Neuromuscular System

Peripheral neuropathy and myasthenia gravis have been reported in patients with chronic GVHD (167–170). Metabolic and infectious etiologies are common causes of posttransplant neurological impairment and should be considered in differential diagnosis. Sural nerve biopsy and autoantibody (acetylcholine receptor antibodies) studies may help in diagnosing these complications. Peripheral neuropathy may resolve after the initiation of immunosuppressive therapy (167). Myasthenia gravis usually responds to cholinesterase inhibitors and immunosuppressive drugs. There is no compelling evidence for central system involvement by chronic GVHD, although vasculitis and white matter changes have been described (170a,b). Polymyositis and myopathy have both been described in patients with chronic GVHD (135,171,172). Muscle weakness other than steroid myopathy may respond to corticosteroid therapy (173). Myositis may start as a proximal myopathy, but is rare. Treatment with cyclosporine or tacrolimus may induce complete and sustained remissions (174). Polymyositis can be associated with myasthenia gravis (175,176), and rarely, severe forms of polymyositis causing respiratory failure occur (177).

Muscle cramps are a common complaint in patients with chronic GVHD, although the pathophysiology is not understood. Myositis does not explain the frequent complaints of severe cramps (178). Patients may also have significant edema and myalgia in their extremities. Finally, a case of granulomatous myositis as a manifestation of chronic GVHD was described and treated successfully with immunosuppression (179).

G. Gastrointestinal Tract

Although intestinal involvement in patients with untreated chronic GVHD was described in early studies, it is now rarely seen. Most of the definition of chronic GI GVHD was based on histological findings at autopsy series (62,180). These histological findings included mononuclear cell infiltrates in lamina propria, shortening of villi, mucosal architectural (crypt) distortion, and hyperplasia. In severe cases, hyalinization of small venules and subserosal fibrosis/scarring were described (181). While rectal biopsy is a major diagnostic tool in acute GVHD (180), there is no established role for chronic GI GVHD (181,182).

The esophagus is the most common GI site of chronic GVHD. Presenting symptoms may include esophageal reflux, dysphagia, substernal pain, and weight loss. Abnormal motility ranging from aperistalsis to high-amplitude contractions, mucosal desquamation, and formation of webs or strictures may rarely occur in the esophagus (183). Radiographic findings include web formation, ring-like narrowing, and tapering structures in the upper or mid-esophagus (184). Periodic endoscopic dilations and antacid medications may help symptomatically. In clinical practice, physicians are often faced with chronic GVHD patients who also have a variety of GI symptoms, such as esophageal reflux, dysphagia, bloating, weight loss, abdominal cramping, and diarrhea (132,185). The etiology of these symptoms is often attributed to gastrointestinal involvement by chronic GVHD. However, many of these GI complaints are not related to GVHD.

The questions of GI involvement in chronic GVHD lead our group to examine 40 consecutive chronic GVHD patients with persistent GI symptoms who underwent endoscopic evaluation (186). Over half of the cases (59%) had ongoing acute GVHD, and an additional 27% had both acute and chronic GVHD. Chronic GVHD alone was found in only 14% of cases. Patients with ongoing acute GI GVHD had poor survival. This finding may explain the IBMTR risk factor of diarrhea as a poor prognostic factor (83). Fifteen (35%) patients developed persistent GI symptoms requiring endoscopic evaluation beyond 1 year after the diagnosis of chronic GVHD. Chronic diarrhea, weight loss, abdominal pain, and dysphagia were the most common GI symptoms among this "late-onset" group. GI GVHD was diagnosed in only 3 patients (20%), all of whom had histological features suggestive of chronic GI GVHD. The most frequent diagnoses were drug-induced gastritis (33%), GI dysmotility (27%), and pancreatic insufficiency (13%). Two of the patients with dysmotility also met histological criteria for chronic GI GVHD (186). As many of these problems are correctable, full evaluation of symptoms is important.

Gastroparesis was previously described as a motility disorder after bone marrow transplantation. In a recent study, 14 of 18 patients who underwent bone marrow transplantation had delayed gastric emptying, mostly responsive to prokinetic agents. Nine of these patients were also evaluated by upper GI endoscopy. GVHD on gastric biopsy was noted to be an uncommon finding and was mild when present (187). Pancreatic insufficiency with or without characteristic laboratory and radiographic findings may occur and responds to pancreatic enzyme supplementation (188). The clinical presentation and histological findings in the remaining 25 patients who developed GI symptoms within 1 year of diagnosis of chronic GVHD (early-onset) were different from the late-onset group. Development of chronic GVHD during the prolonged course of unremitting acute GVHD was associated with acute GI symptoms such as severe diarrhea, abdominal pain/cramps, and nausea/vomiting. GI bleeding and partial intestinal obstruction were also observed in this group. All 22 patients who had acute GVHD features on biopsy samples were in this "early-onset" group, as were all 7 patients who had GI infections and all 12 patients who expired during the course of follow-up (186).

A group of investigators from France recently presented results of intestinal biopsies from children with chronic GVHD ($n = 17$) and normal controls ($n = 21$; 10 nontransplant cases, 4 non-GVHD transplant cases, 7 acute GVHD). Chronic GVHD with intestinal involvement was usually multisystemic (88%) and preceded by acute GVHD in 88% of cases. The outcome was severe, with complete recovery in only 59% and death related to chronic GVHD in 18%. Histological features were characterized by (1) villous atrophy and (2) glandular lesions, mainly apoptotic with variable intensity, and (3) lamina propria infiltrates with cytotoxic T lymphocytes (CD3+, CD8+, TiA1+, granzyme B−), which were significantly increased compared to non-GVHD transplant and nontransplant controls (189).

Wasting in patients with chronic GVHD is common. Malnutrition was observed in 43% of patients, and severe malnutrition with body mass index less than 18.5 in 14% in a recent study (190). Patients with active, ongoing chronic GVHD had lower BMIs. Full nutritional evaluation and interventions are recommended, but many patients with active GVHD continue to lose weight despite adequate caloric intake. The mechanisms of wasting are not fully defined but may include increased catabolic rate due to elevated resting energy expenditure (191) and high cytokine levels, especially tumor necrosis factor (TNF). A recent study suggested that patients with chronic extensive GVHD show an increase in resting energy expenditure and alterations in fat and carbohydrate oxidation rates. These changes seemed to be the result of increased action of glucagon and norepinephrine (191). In a murine model, overexpression of TNF-α resulted in severe cachexia and skin changes that resembled GVHD (192).

H. Respiratory Tract

Bronchiolitis obliterans (BO) is a late and serious manifestation of chronic GVHD. Patients typically present with a progressive history of recurrent bronchitis, wheezing and cough not responsive to bronchodilator therapy (193). The etiology may be multifactorial (infection, reactive airway disease, fluid overload, cardiac disease, etc.), and a comprehensive evaluation is needed. Patients with severe sclerotic chest wall disease may have similar symptoms but have no intrinsic pulmonary disease. Chest radiographs and regular computed tomography (CT) may be normal or may show hyperinflation, bleb formation, interstitial pneumatosis, pneumothorax, or peneumomediastinum. Pulmonary function tests show new obstructive lung defects defined by marked decrease in the forced expiratory volume in 1 second ($FEV_1 < 80\%$ predicted) compared with the forced vital capacity (FEV_1/FVC by $>10\%$), decreased expiratory flow, reduced vital capacity, and increased residual lung volume within a period of less than 1 year, not explained by infection, asthma, or recurrent aspiration from the sinuses or from gastroesophageal reflux.

Unlike interstitial pneumonitis, which generally occurs during the first 100 days after transplantation, BO occurs later on. The frequency of BO was increased in patients with chronic GVHD who received a 102-day course of methotrexate as GVHD prophylaxis (194). In addition, patients with chronic GVHD and hypogammaglobulinemia or IgG subclass deficiencies appear to be at increased risk for late obstructive airway disease (195). However, a randomized trial of prophylactic immunoglobulin replacement did not decrease the incidence of BO (137). In the absence of chronic GVHD in any other organ, the diagnosis of BO requires negative microbiological tests from bronchoalveolar lavage, evidence of air trapping by high-resolution end-expiratory and end-inspiratory CAT scan of the lungs, or confirmation by lung biopsy showing granulation tissue and scarring obliterating the small airways. BO must be distinguished histologically from bronchiolitis obliterans with organizing pneumonia (BOOP) because the latter condition is responsive to prolonged corticosteroid treatment and does not carry the same grave prognosis as BO (153). Patients with BOOP should be carefully evaluated for the presence of chronic GVHD manifestations in other organs. Another consideration is pulmonary infections. Even without BO, pulmonary sicca and bronchiectasis lead to frequent infections and bacterial colonization, often with *Pseudomonas* species. In the absence of histological confirmation of BO, it is hard to interpret the treatment results of BO. Therefore, confirmation of the diagnosis of BO by adequate lung biopsy is mandatory.

Histopathological findings of BO are best detected in terminal bronchioles. Open lung biopsy is frequently required in order to obtain the tissue of interest. Lymphocytic and mononuclear cell infiltrates and hyperplasia of bronchiolar smooth muscle may be noted. Focal or transmural necrosis of bronchioles and bronchi is present. The most striking feature is the intraluminal accumulation of inflammatory cells and granulation tissue, which leads to partial or even complete occlusion of the bronchioles. Mucus plugging with atelectasis or emphysema of distal air spaces may be present. Hyperplasia of bronchial mucus glands and alveolar destruction as occur in COPD are absent in cases of BO. Mild focal interstitial inflammatory reactions may be seen.

Treatment of BO with conventional immunosuppressive agents and bronchodilator therapy has been largely unsatisfactory. Patients with BO show minimal response to therapy and have a very poor prognosis; serial pulmonary function tests can quantify the degree of respiratory compromise (193,195). The majority of patients who develop posttransplant obstructive lung disease had extensive, chronic GVHD. Cumulative mortality at 3 years was 65% after transplant in these patients, 44% ($p = 0.01$) among those who survived beyond 80 days and had normal pulmonary function (193). These mortality figures have remained essentially unchanged over the past decade. Novel treatments should be explored for this debilitating and mostly fatal condition. Double lung transplants have been reported to be effective in a small number of pediatric cases (196). Patients with chronic GVHD are also at risk for chronic sinopulmonary disease, which may be relatively asymptomatic. The sinuses should be considered as a potential fever source in any patient with chronic GVHD. CT of the sinuses should be obtained and otolaryngology consultation should be requested for patients with evidence of sinusitis since extensive debridement is usually indicated (153).

I. Hematopoietic System

Cytopenias are common in chronic GVHD. However, multiple mechanisms may play a role in poor graft function observed in patients with chronic GVHD.

The growth of hematopoietic progenitors may be suppressed in chronic GVHD (198). This may be due to stromal damage (199), but autoimmune neutropenia, anemia, and thrombocytopenia also occur (200,201). Thrombocytopenia at the time of chronic GVHD diagnosis carries a poor prognosis (201–204). Eosinophilia may be seen and may track with disease activity, but does not influence survival (204). Factor VIII deficiency due to inhibitor antibody formation has been reported in chronic GVHD (205).

J. Other Manifestations of Chronic GVHD

Women may have vaginal or vulvar lichenoid changes, ulcers, web formation and vaginal strictures due to chronic GVHD (206). These effects must be distinguished from those resulting from ovarian failure (hormone deficiency) induced by conditioning regimen. Topical corticosteroids can be effective treatment for vaginal chronic GVHD, and mechanical or surgical dilation may be necessary for relief of symptoms.

Recurrent sterile serosal effusions have been reported in patients with chronic GVHD (207). Pericardial and pleural effusions can cause compressive loss of function and may require drainage and sclerosis. A recent report described a boy transplanted from his HLA-identical sister who developed chronic GVHD with severe polyserositis and polyarthritis. The patient shared the HLA antigens HLA-A2, B51, and DQW6, which are associated with autoimmune diseases (208). Although pericardial effusions after allogeneic transplantation are often sterile and related to conditioning therapy or associated with chronic GVHD, infectious etiologies such as pneumococcal pericarditis should be ruled out (209). Anecdotal cases of chronic GVHD of the kidneys have been reported (210). Treatment of chronic GVHD with prolonged courses of corticosteroids increases the risk of cataract formation, avascular necrosis, and osteoporosis (211). Other rare manifestations associated with chronic GVHD are phimosis and Peyronie's disease (skin discoloration of penis with erectile dysfunction) (212,213).

VI. CLINICAL CLASSIFICATION OF CHRONIC GVHD

Chronic GVHD can be classified according to the type of onset, need for systemic immunosuppressive therapy, or mortality risk. Chronic GVHD may evolve directly from acute GVHD (progressive), which has a grim prognosis, or may follow a period of resolution (quiescent), with an intermediate prognosis. In addition, about 20–30% of patients develop chronic GVHD with no history of prior acute GVHD (de novo), and these patients have a relatively good prognosis (62,135). Based on data from the IBMTR, the distribution of chronic GVHD onset for HLA-matched siblings is 20–30% progressive, 30–40% quiescent, and 35% de novo. Data from the NMDP for unrelated donor recipients, where the incidence of acute GVHD is higher, show 19% progressive, 69% quiescent, and 12% de novo onset (83).

The most commonly employed clinical grading system is the "limited/extensive" classification proposed by Sullivan et al. in 1980 based on a retrospective clinical and pathological review of 20 patients with chronic GVHD (62). Although this classification is highly reproducible (214), it provides little information about prognosis and is of limited clinical utility (215) beyond separating patients needing treatment (extensive GVHD) from those who do not (limited GVHD) (83). Localized skin involvement with or without hepatic dysfunction (limited disease) was associated with less severe disease and fewer infections. Generalized skin involvement or limited disease plus eye involvement, oral involvement, hepatic dysfunction with abnormal liver histology, or involvement of any other target organ was classified as extensive disease and was associated with more frequent infections. However, review of data from HLA-identical sibling recipients reported to the IBMTR suggests that transplant centers are not applying the formal definitions accurately, perhaps in part because many patients are unclassifiable by the strict organ criteria (83).

The usefulness of a clinical classification or grading system is dependent both upon its reproducibility among centers and its ability to stratify patients into meaningful prognostic categories. From these perspectives, the current system of grading chronic GVHD as limited or extensive has severe limitations. A significant proportion of patients falls into the extensive chronic GVHD category, and there is great heterogeneity in manifestations of chronic GVHD and patient outcomes within this group. In this group, mortality correlated best with Karnofsky performance status (KPS <70%) (62). However, KPS alone cannot address the mortality differences among patients with KPS greater than 70%.

The Seattle group has developed revised clinical criteria for limited and extensive chronic GVHD to clarify ambiguities of the original definition. In the revised classification, prolonged treatment with systemic immunosuppression is indicated for patients with clinically extensive chronic GVHD or anyone with high-risk features (i.e., platelets count $<100 \times 10^9$/L, progressive onset, or receiving treatment with corticosteroids at the time of the diagnosis of chronic GVHD). Chronic GVHD has been poorly studied. The long course of therapy needed to treat these patients has hindered clinical trials, because many years are needed for trials to mature. Finally, the absence of a standard clinical staging/grading system, which separates the patients with different outcome, has rendered the interpretation of clinical results reported in therapeutic trials almost impossible.

Several investigators have tried to develop improved prognostic grading scales based on larger numbers of observed patients, with survival as the primary endpoint. Various clinical features have had prognostic significance in these studies, including "extensive" chronic GVHD (62,135), KPS (62,83,135), thrombocytopenia (<100,000 platelets/μL) (9,135,202,204,216), progressive-type onset (204,216,217), extensive (>50% of body surface area) skin involvement (204), lichenoid histology (217), elevated bilirubin (>1.2 or >2.0 mg/dL) (217,218), age ≥20 years (216), gastrointestinal involvement (216), no response to therapy at 6 months (216), diarrhea and weight loss (83), oral GVHD (83), and subjective measures of severity (83).

Thrombocytopenia was the first reported and most reproducible prognostic factor associated with shortened survival (9202–204). In a recent study, high-risk chronic GVHD as defined by thrombocytopenia had an adverse impact on overall mortality and treatment failure at 18 months with hazard rates of 6.6 and 5.2, respectively (9). Multivariate analysis of 85 patients with chronic GVHD treated in Baltimore revealed an increased risk of death in patients with progressive-type onset, elevated serum bilirubin levels, and lichenoid histology on skin biopsy (217). Six-year overall survival for all 85 patients was 42%, but survival in the 26 patients with progressive onset was only 10%. Among unrelated donor transplant recipients, more than 6 months of interferon given before transplant for the treatment of chronic myelogenous leukemia significantly increases the risk of mortality from refractory chronic GVHD (219).

The definition of risk status in patients with chronic GVHD has remained controversial. Because of limitations in the numbers of subjects studied, heterogeneity of patient populations, and variations in diagnosis and management of chronic GVHD, no prognostic factors except for thrombocytopenia and progressive-type onset have been validated by other investigators. Recently, we reported a new prognostic grading system for chronic GVHD that stratifies patients into risk categories according to whether or not extensive skin involvement (ESI), thrombocytopenia (TP), and progressive-type onset (PTO) are present at diagnosis (204). We studied 151 consecutive patients with chronic GVHD and chronic GVHD-specific survival (survival without recurrent malignancy). We confirmed that TP and PTO were independent risk factors for shortened survival with respective hazard ratios of 3.6 and 1.7. Skin involvement of greater than 50% of body surface area was another independent risk factor for survival (HR 7.0). A composite prognostic factor score was calculated for each patient by adding together the weighted averages of each of the risk factors stratified patients into distinct prognostic groups (Table 3). We also evaluated the prognostic factors at the time of primary treatment failure and found the above three risk factors plus a Karnofsky performance status of less than 50% to be significant predictors for survival (204).

More recently, the IBMTR reported another set of prognostic factors for survival based on data from 1827 HLA-identical sibling transplant recipients reported to the registry. Performance status, diarrhea, weight loss, and cutaneous and oral involvement were found to be independent prognostic variables, from which a grading scheme was

Table 3 New Clinical Grading and Calculation of the Prognostic Score (PS)

Grade (risk group)	Prognostic score (PS)	No. of risk factors	Hazard ratio (95% CIs)	Survival (3 yr)	p-value (2-sided)
I (favorable, $n = 54$)	0	0	1.00	92%	—
II (intermediate, $n = 47$)	0–2	1	3.7 (1.4, 9.3)	71%	0.007
III (high, $n = 50$)	≥2	>1[a]	25 (10.3, 60.5)	9%	<0.001

[a]Except thrombocytopenia plus progressive-type onset, which is a rare presentation and falls into the intermediate-risk category ($0 < PS < 2$).
Score calculation (rounded):

$$PS = [1.9 \times (\text{skin extent}^b)] + [1.3 \times (\text{platelet}^c)] + [0.5 \times (\text{type of onset}^d)]$$

[b]If the extent of skin involvement is >50% of BSA, put 1, otherwise put 0.
[c]If platelet count is <100.000 cells/μL, put 1, otherwise put 0.
[d]If chronic GVHD is progressive-type onset, put 1, otherwise put 0.
Source: Ref. 222.

generated. This scheme, the limited/extensive classification system, and a classification based on clinical impression of overall chronic GVHD severity (mild/moderate/severe) was assessed in a parallel analyses of 1092 HLA-matched sibling transplant recipients from the IBMTR and 553 recipients of unrelated donor marrow from the NMDP. Presence of chronic GVHD was associated with fewer relapses (RR 0.5–0.6) but more treatment-related mortality (RR 1.8–2.8) in the three analyses. No grading scheme correlated chronic GVHD severity with relapse rates, but all schemes predicted treatment-related mortality. Survival and disease-free survival of the most favorable chronic GVHD group in each scheme were similar, or better, than those of patients without chronic GVHD. Notably, an overall clinical summary scale of mild, moderate, or severe chronic GVHD was the best predictor of survival (83). However, formal definitions for the mild, moderate, and severe categories have not been established (220).

All models reported to date had limitations because of the differences in definitions, data-collection methods, diagnostic criteria used, and management of chronic GVHD. Factors found to be significant in one sample were not significant in another. The internal consistency and rigor of diagnosis is the strength of the Hopkins sample and a concern for the IBMTR study. As stated above, 65–67% of IBMTR subjects scored as limited reported organ involvement other than skin and liver, i.e., were incorrectly reported. The patients were not reclassified for the analysis. Thus, the data set is limited by the expertise of those evaluating the patients, and this may help explain several unexpected findings in this study, such as the significance of diarrhea (83).

Recently, we updated our results and redesigned a simple three-factor clinical grading system that predicted 10-year rates of survival without recurring malignancy ranging from 9% to 90% (221). The difference in survival at 10 years was 30% between favorable and intermediate-risk groups, and 50% between intermediate- and high-risk groups. This data set included many patients transplanted before 1990, and median follow-up was over 8 years. The univariate analysis identified significant prognostic factors consistent with those reported separately by other investigators. Extensive skin involvement, thrombocytopenia, and progressive-type onset remained independent risk factors. A new prognostic score was calculated for each patient using the weighted averages of these risk factors (Table 4). The probability of survival for 54 patients with prognostic scores of 0 was 92%, 47 patients with prognostic scores of less than 2 had 71%, and 50 patients with scores of 2 or greater had a 9% probability of survival at 3 years.

More recently, using multiple data sets that included a total of 1105 patients from the University of Nebraska ($n = 60$), the IBMTR ($n = 708$), the Fred Hutchinson Cancer Research Center ($n = 188$), and the University of Minnesota ($n = 149$), we tested the validity of (1) prognostic scoring model and (2) each of the three prognostic factors that constituted this model. Despite significant heterogeneity of the data, for each data set the proposed grading system identified three prognostic groups, each with distinct survival outcomes (222). While thrombocytopenia by itself was uniformly associated with higher risk of mortality across all test samples, extensive skin involvement and progressive onset showed statistically significant associations with mortality in one and two cohorts, respectively (222). The model was predictive of chronic GVHD-specific survival, but the mortality hazard associated with extensive skin involvement was lower in each of these test samples compared to the Hopkins sample. Nonetheless, clinical grading based on the model appears promising because of its utility across multiple independent data sets. This grading may help to improve clinical management, trial design, and communication among transplant centers while prospective validation is pending.

Table 4 Summary of Clinical Manifestations and Management of Chronic GVHD

Organ	Clinical manifestation	Evaluation	Intervention
Skin	Erythematous papular rash (lichenoid) or thickened, tight, fragile skin (sclerodermatous)	Clinical and biopsy to confirm the diagnosis of GVHD	Moisturize (petroleum jelly), treat local infections, protect from further trauma
Nails	Vertical ridging, fragile	Clinical	Nail polish may help to decrease further damage
Sweat glands	Destruction leading to risk of hyperthermia		Avoid excessive heat
Hair	Scalp and body hair is thin and fragile, can be partially or completely lost	Clinical	
Eyes	Dryness, photophobia, and burning. Progression to corneal abrasion	Regular ophthalmological evaluation including Schirmer's test	Preservative-free tears during the day and preservative-free ointment at night
Mouth	Dry, sensitivity to mint, spicy food, tomato. Whitish lace-like plaques in the cheeks and tongue identical to lichen planus. Erythema and painful ulcerations, mucosal scleroderma with decreased sensitivity to temperature can also happen	Regular dental evaluation (with appropriate endocarditis prophylaxis). Viral and fungal cultures at diagnosis and at any worsening	Avoid foods that are not tolerated. Regular dental care preceded by appropriate endocarditis prophylaxis
Respiratory tract	Bronchiolitis obliterans can manifest as dyspnea, wheezing, cough with normal CT scan and marked obstruction at pulmonary function tests. Chronic sinopulmonary symptoms and/or infections are also common.	Pulmonary function tests including FEV1, FVC, DLCO, and helium lung volumes. CT scan in symptomatic patients. With abnormal chest CT must rule out infections. Lung biopsy if clinically indicated.	Investigational therapy

System	Manifestations	Evaluation	Treatment
Gastrointestinal	Abnormal motility and strictures. Weight loss	Swallowing studies, endoscopy if clinically indicated. Nutritional evaluation	Systemic treatment of GVHD; endoscopical/surgical treatment of strictures. Nutritional intervention
Liver	Cholestasis (increased bilirubin, alkaline phosphatase). Isolated liver involvement needs histological confirmation	Liver function tests. Liver biopsy if clinically indicated	No specific therapy is proven superior. FK506 may concentrate in the liver
Musculoskeletal	Fasciitis. Myositis is rare. Osteoporosis may occur secondary to hormonal deficits, use of steroids, decreased activity	Periodical physical therapy evaluation to document the range of motion. Bone density evaluation especially in patients using steroids	Aggressive physical therapy program
Immune system	Profound immunodeficiency. Functional asplenia. High risk of pneumococcal sepsis, PCP, and invasive fungal infections. Variable IgG levels	Assume all patients severely immunocompromised and asplenic	PCP prophylaxis (until 6 months after no GVHD) and pneumococcal prophylaxis (lifetime). Delay vaccinations to 6 months after GVHD has resolved
Hematopoietic system	Cytopenias. Occasional eosinophilia	Counts. Bone marrow aspirate and biopsy, antineutrophil and antiplatelet antibodies when indicated	Systemic treatment of GVHD
Others	Virtually all autoimmune disease manifestations have been described in association with chronic GVHD	As clinically indicated	

VII. PREVENTION OF CHRONIC GVHD

Therapies that prevent acute GVHD have been largely unsuccessful for the prevention of chronic GVHD except for T-cell depletion (76) and use of umbilical cord blood as a stem cell source, since lower rates of both acute and chronic GVHD are observed with these approaches (223,224).

A. T-Cell Depletion

Because the occurrence of acute GVHD is a strong predictor of chronic GVHD, efforts to reduce acute GVHD may also decrease the occurrence of chronic GVHD (95). T-cell depletion has been associated with about 50% reduction in the incidence of chronic GVHD (225). Overall survival, however, was not improved. Chronic GVHD was still noted in 85% of long-term survivors who received T-cell–depleted marrow from unrelated donors (226).

B. Immunosuppressive Agents

In early trials, cyclosporine (CSP) containing GVHD prophylaxis reduced the incidence of acute GVHD without altering the rate of chronic GVHD (227,228). Modification of methotrexate (MTX) dose and schedule in GVHD prophylaxis did not appear to influence the development of chronic GVHD (229). In a trial of 103 patients who were given CSP/MTX prophylaxis, 60-day CSP was compared with 180 day CSP. There was no difference in the cumulative incidence of chronic GVHD. Although mortality in patients with no previous acute GVHD was not different between the groups, it was significantly higher in those with previous acute GVHD given CSP prophylaxis for 60 days (230). In a recent nonrandomized retrospective study on 196 allogeneic SCT recipients, CSP with a short course of MTX was compared with CSP and prednisone (CSP-PRED). Prophylaxis with CSP-PRED was significantly associated with a higher risk of development of chronic (extensive) GVHD with a relative risk of 3.5 (4.2) (231).

Extended CSP administration has initially been reported to reduce the incidence of chronic GVHD (123,124). Kansu et al. (125) reported on clinical extensive chronic GVHD and other transplant outcomes among recipients randomly assigned to receive a 24- or 6-month course of CSP prophylaxis after transplantation of marrow from HLA-identical siblings or alternative donors. Patients who did not have clinical manifestations of chronic GVHD on day 80 after transplantation were eligible for the study if they previously had acute GVHD or if a skin biopsy showed histological evidence of chronic GVHD. Clinical extensive chronic GVHD developed in 35 of the 89 patients (39%) in the 24-month group, and 37 of the 73 patients (51%) in the 6-month group. The hazard of developing chronic GVHD, transplantation-related mortality, survival, or disease-free survival were not significantly different between the two groups (125).

A phase II trial in matched unrelated marrow recipients who were given FK-506 (Tacrolimus) and MTX prophylaxis showed a cumulative incidence of chronic GVHD of 48% (232) compared to 64% observed in the past with CSP/MTX (3). In a series of 116 evaluable HLA-identical blood stem cell transplant recipients, GVHD prophylaxis with tacrolimus and MTX was associated with a three fold reduced risk of chronic GVHD by multivariate analysis (9). A phase III trial comparing FK-506 plus MTX and CSP plus MTX showed no difference in the incidence of chronic GVHD between the two groups (56% and 49%, respectively). However, there were significantly more patients in the CSP group who had clinical extensive chronic GVHD (130). A recent trial using a triple drug combination of tacrolimus, MTX, and methylprednisolone failed to reduce the incidence of chronic GVHD (233).

C. Intravenous Immunoglobulin

Although weekly administration of IV Ig through day 90 posttransplant reduced the incidence and mortality of acute GVHD (235), monthly immunoglobulin treatment between days 90 and 360 posttransplant had no impact on the development of chronic GVHD (236).

D. Interleukin-18

A recent report suggests that IL-18 is beneficial for the prevention and treatment of chronic GVHD in mice. IL-18 significantly decreased immunological parameters indicative of chronic GVHD, such as elevated serum IgG antinuclear antibodies, IgG1 and IgE levels, and host B-cell numbers and their activation. IL-18 treatment partially but significantly restored the production of Il-2 and IFN-γ. The data further suggested that IL-18–mediated therapeutic effects may be due to the induction of donor CD8+ CTL, the decrease in donor CD4+ T cell numbers, and a down-regulation of MHC class II expression on host B cells (237).

VIII. TREATMENT OF CHRONIC GVHD

A. Initial Evaluation

Once the diagnosis of chronic GVHD is confirmed, the extent of involvement must be ascertained. A comprehensive evaluation can be used as a baseline to assess progression of the disease or response to therapy. Elements of evaluation are shown in Table 4. As a baseline for all patients with chronic GVHD, we recommend ophthalmological examination with Schirmer's test, pulmonary function tests, dental examination, gynecological evaluation, liver function tests, and complete blood counts. Taking photographs if skin involvement is present is helpful to assess the extent of the disease. Evaluation of range-of-motion evaluation by a physical therapist and consultation with a social worker are essential in patients with skin or fascial chronic GVHD. A morbidity scale can be used to record the severity of manifestation of chronic GVHD at the time of diagnosis, whenever therapy is changed, and at yearly intervals if treatment continues or if manifestations of chronic GVHD persist (153).

Should the patient be unable to return to the transplant center, center physicians should be available to help in determining the cause of the patient's difficulties and in reviewing biopsies (153). Specially designed symptom questionnaires should be implemented in the care of patients with chronic GVHD. Lee et al. (15) recently developed a 30-item symptom scale with 7 subscales to capture the chronic GVHD-specific symptom burden. The symptom scale correlated highly with patients' self-assessed mild, moderate, and severe chronic GVHD manifestations in cross-sectional analysis. It was recommend that either the SF-36 or the FACT-BMT be combined with a chronic GVHD-specific symptom scale to measure the impact of chronic GVHD on patients' quality of life and that this endpoint be included in clinical trials testing chronic GVHD interventions.

B. Team Work

Treatment of patients with chronic GVHD is most successful with a systematic approach to diagnosis, evaluation, and coordinated management by a multidisciplinary team. In addition to bone marrow transplant physicians and nurses, team members should include dermatologists, ophthalmologists, dentists, pathologists, dieticians, physical and occupational therapists, and social workers. Because chronic GVHD can affect virtually any organ system, consultants in subspecialty areas such as rehabilitation medicine, gastroenterology, pulmonary medicine, neurology, and infectious diseases who have experience-with chronic GVHD are invaluable resources to the team (153).

C. Primary Treatment

1. Principles

Chronic GVHD is associated with a GVL effect, which contributes to improved survival in patients transplanted in advanced-stage leukemia (238,239), but less so in patients transplanted in remission (240). It is not clear whether the protective effect relies on the presence of overt chronic GVHD or is durable once chronic GVHD resolves (241,242). If the GVL effect is the only chance of surviving for a particular patient, one could consider not treating chronic GVHD aggressively and defer intensive treatment to the time of rapid progression.

Treatment of patients with chronic GVHD should include both immunomodulatory approaches and supportive measures. Agents with efficacy in the treatment of autoimmune disorders have been utilized as therapy for established chronic GVHD and show response rates of 20–80% (95). For patients with lichenoid lesions or hepatic disease, monitoring response to treatment is relatively straightforward. For patients with sclerodermatous disease or fasciitis, responses are harder to gauge. Patients with active sclerotic disease have progressive sclerosis, frequently with erythema at the leading edge. Responding patients have no erythema and no new areas of sclerosis. Range-of-motion studies should show stability or improvement. When tapering these patients off immunosuppression, frequent range-of-motion studies and documentation of the areas of sclerosis are helpful to detect flares.

2. Introduction of Modern Immunosuppressive Treatment in Chronic GVHD

Sullivan and colleagues in the early 1980s studied 52 patients among 175 (30%) survivors of allogeneic transplantation who experienced chronic GVHD (135). Five patients had limited disease, received no therapy, and did well. Among the 47 patients with extensive disease, 13 received no therapy and only 2 (18%) survived. Mortality resulted from infection. Another 13 patients received a brief course of rabbit antithymocyte globulin (ATG) or a prolonged course of corticosteroids late in their disease. Three (23%) of these patients survived without significant disability. The remaining 21 patients were treated early in the course of their chronic GVHD with a combination of prednisone (1 mg/kg every other day) and an alkylating agent or azathioprine. Sixteen (76%) of these patients survived. Combination therapy given as either primary or secondary treatment was associated with improved disability-free survival (85% and 62%, respectively) (243). Based on this initial work, modern immunosuppressive regimens were developed and tested in clinical trials.

3. Common Immunosuppressive Regimens for Treatment of Chronic GVHD

Prednisone Versus Prednisone and Azathioprine. In a double-blind randomized trial, Sullivan et al. (202) reported that prednisone alone was superior to prednisone plus azathioprine for primary treatment of standard-risk extensive chronic GVHD. Nonrelapse mortality was significantly higher (40 vs. 21%) in standard-risk patients randomized to prednisone plus azathioprine, due to an increase in fatal infections. Survival was 61% among patients randomized to prednisone and placebo. However, in patients classified as high-risk on the basis of platelet counts <100,000/μL, treatment with prednisone alone resulted in only 26% 5-year survival (202).

Cyclosporine and Prednisone. When a similar group of patients with thrombocytopenia was treated with alternating day CSP (6 mg/kg every 12 hours every other day) and prednisone (1 mg/kg/day every other day), 5-year survival exceeded 50% (203). Functional performance of long-term survivors was maintained near normal, and the incidence of disabling scleroderma was decreased from 43% to 6%. However, infections remained a major cause of morbidity and mortality. Subsequently most centers adopted this regimen for initial treatment of all patients with chronic GvHD not just those deemed at high risk (138).

Standard Regimen of CSP and Prednisone. Patients are initially treated with daily prednisone at 1 mg/kg/day and daily CSP at 10 mg/kg/day, divided into two doses based on ideal or actual weight, whichever is lower. If chronic GVHD is stable or improving after 2 weeks, prednisone is tapered by 25% per week to a target dose of 1 mg/kg every other day. Once the steroid taper has been completed without a flare in GVHD, CSP is reduced by 25% per week to alternate day dosing such that the patient takes CSP (10 mg/kg in 2 divided doses) one day and alternates with prednisone (1 mg/kg) the next day (153). A 3-month time frame for evaluation of response to a given therapy at our institution is based on our own observation that 90% of patients who are ultimately going to respond to therapy will show signs of response at that point (217). If the disease has completely resolved, patients are gradually weaned from medication, with dose reductions made approximately every 2 weeks. Patients who continue to respond (incomplete response) are kept on the same therapy and are reevaluated after another 3 months. Once patients reach their maximal response, therapy is continued for an additional 3 months (total of 9 months) and then weaned from both medications. For those who do not respond or progress, alternative salvage regimens should be instituted (153).

Cyclosporine Prednisone Versus Prednisone Alone. Although a regimen of alternating CSP and prednisone is widely employed for the treatment of high-risk extensive GVHD, until recently there were no data on its effectiveness in standard risk patients. Flowers reviewed the success of initial combination therapy for patients treated in the 1980s. She reported a nonrelapse mortality of 21% in standard-risk patients ($n = 126$) and 39% in high-risk ($n = 111$) patients, defined by progressive onset or thrombocytopenia. Successful discontinuation of all immunosuppressive medications eventually occurred for 60% of standard risk patients and 40% of high-risk patients (244). Koc et al. reported the results of a study comparing prednisone alone to prednisone plus CSP in patients without thrombocytopenia in 287 patients with extensive GVHD (245). Prednisone was administered initially at doses of 1.0 mg/kg/day orally, followed by a prolonged taper, and CSP was administered at 6 mg/kg orally twice daily every other day. The hazards of transplant-related mortality, overall mortality, recurrent malignancy, secondary therapy, and discontinuation of all immunosuppressive therapy were not significantly different between the two arms, but survival without recurrent malignancy was superior in the prednisone-only arm ($p = 0.03$). However, 18 (13%) of the 142 patients in the CSP plus prednisone arm developed avascular necrosis compared to 32 (22%) of the 145 patients in the prednisone arm ($p = 0.04$). Thus, there is no evidence that initial combination therapy improved control of chronic GVHD in patients with platelet counts greater than $100 \times 10^9/L$.

Thalidomide. Thalidomide has been studied in chronic GVHD based on its effect on TNF-α production (246). We have previously reported a 48% survival rate at 3 years using thalidomide as primary treatment of 21 patients with chronic GVHD (247). There appeared to be less infectious complications with this regimen. In another trial patients with extensive chronic GVHD were randomized to receive CSP and alternate-day prednisone or CSP, prednisone, and thalidomide (200–800 mg/day). There was no difference between the two groups in regards to response and survival (248).

Cyclosporine Plus Mycophenolate Mofetil Versus Tacrolimus (FK 506) Plus Prednisone. A multicenter trial is currently planned that will examine the addition of mycophenolate mofetil (MMF) to CSP or tacrolimus (FK-506) plus prednisone in the upfront treatment of patients with extensive chronic GVHD.

D. Secondary (Salvage) Immunosuppressive Therapies

Approximately one third of patients do not respond to initial steroid-based therapy (203,249). There is no standard approach for refractory patients. In several phase I/II trials in patients with relapsed/refractory chronic GVHD survival, rates of approximately 75% have been reported with alternating CSP/steroid or thalidomide (236,247). Steroid-refractory chronic GVHD is formally defined as either failure to improve after at least 2 months, or progression after one month of standard immunosuppressive therapy with corticosteroids with or without CSP (250,251). Several phase II trials of salvage regimens have reported success rates of 25–50% (247,250).

1. Pulse Steroid Treatment

Prognosis of patients who are not responsive to primary therapy (primary refractory) or those who flare after an initial response is poor (204). Responsiveness to further immunosuppressive therapy can often be predicted by a short course of high-dose (pulse) corticosteroids (252). If disease progression is not controlled, novel treatment modalities should be investigated. In a recent trial, 27 of 62 patients with refractory GVHD (48%) showed a major response to pulsed steroids, while 15 (27%) showed a minor response. Twenty-one of the 42 responders (50%) had subsequent progression (median time to progression 1.9 years). Ten of the 42 responders (24%) were able to discontinue all systemic immunosuppressive treatments. The treatment was well tolerated with no serious adverse events (252).

2. Tacrolimus (FK 506)

Among 17 patients with extensive chronic GVHD after failure of at least 2 months of first-line therapy, persistent disease, or adverse reactions to first-line medication, Tzakis et al.

observed an unequivocal beneficial response with FK 506 in 6 patients (253). We are currently studying, in a phase II trial, a combination of mycophenolate mofetil and FK 506. In 26 patients with refractory chronic GVHD this steroid-sparing combination was well tolerated, and nearly half the patients showed an objective response (254). Another study reported a modest response to tacrolimus (255). Infections were the most frequent adverse event. Nephrotoxicity occurred in 16 patients (41%). Seven patients had discontinued all immunosuppression at last contact, leading to an estimated 29% probability of stopping all immunosuppression by 3 years posttransplantation. Systemic use of tacrolimus was reported to improve dry eye symptoms (256).

3. Thalidomide

Thalidomide has immunosuppressive properties and is active against chronic GVHD, although side effects of sedation prevent many patients from continuing on the drug (247). In a phase II study Parker et al. treated 80 patients with steroid-refractory chronic GVHD with thalidomide, and 16 (20%) had sustained responses (9 complete, and 7 partial). Twenty-nine patients (36%) had thalidomide discontinued because of side effect (sedation, constipation, neuritis, skin rash, and neutropenia). Side effects were reversible with drug discontinuation (250). In a recent randomized, placebo-controlled, double-blinded trial, thalidomide or placebo together with glucocorticoids and either CSP or tacrolimus were administered as initial therapy for clinical extensive chronic GVHD. All patients had thrombocytopenia or progressive-type onset (high-risk). Thalidomide was given initially at doses of 200 mg orally per day, followed by a gradual increase to 800 mg/day if side effects were tolerable. Treatment was discontinued before resolution of chronic GVHD in 23 (92%) of the 25 patients because of neutropenia and neurological symptoms (257).

In a Minnesota study 37 patients with extensive chronic GVHD refractory to standard immunosuppressive therapy were given thalidomide in addition to standard immunosuppressive therapy. The response rate, mostly partial, was 38%. There were no deaths among the responders (251). An Italian group observed complete responses in 6 of 14 children (43%) with refractory or high-risk chronic GVHD. No increased incidence of infectious complications was observed. At the time of reporting 9 of 10 responding patients were alive at 49–111 months (258). Thalidomide should not be considered for patients with preexisting neuropathies.

4. PUVA

Patients with refractory lichenoid GVHD may also benefit from the addition of PUVA (8-methoxypsoralen plus ultraviolet A irradiation). This treatment modality has been used for treatment of steroid-resistant lichenoid chronic GVHD and in patients for whom steroids are contraindicated (153,259,260). In a review of 40 patients treated with PUVA, responses were observed in 31 including 16 complete responses (261). PUVA is very difficult to administer to sclerodermatous GVHD and does not have significant effect on disease resolution.

5. Photopheresis

Extracorporeal photopheresis, extracorporeal exposure of peripheral blood mononuclear cells to a photosensitizing compound and UVA light to selectively eliminate lymphocytes, is a another therapeutic intervention for acute and chronic GVHD (262–264). Clinical responses have been reported in skin and visceral GVHD. In a recent report of 15 patients with extensive chronic GVHD not responsive to CSP and steroids, most patients responded with major improvement in cutaneous, oral, and hepatic manifestations of chronic GVHD. Knee and elbow contractures showed partial improvement. No severe infections were observed (262). Similar results have been reported by others (265–267). Recent studies of patients undergoing a 6- to 12-month course of photopheresis showed normalization of inverted ratios of CD4 to CD8 cells, an increase in the number of CD3-CD56+ NK cells, and a decrease in CD80+ and CD123+ circulating dendritic cells (267). In addition, alloreactivity of effector T cells and antigen-presenting DC was altered (268). The proliferation of T cells was decreased in all patients by a mean of 84% after a 2-day cycle of photopheresis and longitudinally over the 12-month course of therapy. Nine of 10 patients demonstrated a shift from DC1 to DC2 (plasmacytoid) cells, a decrease in antigen responsiveness by DC, and a concordant shift from a predominantly Th1 (IL-2, IFN-γ) to Th2 (IL-4, IL-10) cytokine profile (268). A multicenter, randomized trial is currently being conducted.

6. Total Lymphoid Irradiation

Improvement was also reported in nine patients who received 100 cGy thoracoabdominal irradiation (269,270). Similar results were observed in a recent study of 40 patients with refractory chronic GVHD given a total dose of 100 cGy to the abdomen midline. Clinical responses were observed in 90% of patients at a median of 2 months. Complete resolution of chronic GVHD was observed in 21% of patients at 1 year. Most patients, however, continued to take immunosuppressive medications (271).

E. New Immunomodulatory Approaches

1. IL-2 Receptor Antagonists

Competitive inhibition of IL-2–dependent lymphocytes by an IL-2 receptor antagonist (daclizumab) demonstrates some beneficial effects in the treatment of acute GVHD (272). However, treatment was complicated by frequent infections (273).

2. Targeting TNF-α

The concept of TNF blockage was introduced in the early 1990s to treat steroid-refractory acute GVHD (274). The M.D. Anderson group recently evaluated the efficacy and safety of TNF-α inhibition by a chimeric human/murine antibody (infliximab). Twenty-six patients with steroid refractory patients received infliximab at doses of 10 mg/week for a median of 3 doses (range 1–8). The response rate was 70%, with the majority having complete responses. However, 80% of patients developed infectious complications, which were fatal in 63% (275).

Recombinant soluble TNF receptor (Enbrel) was given in 10 patients with steroid-dependent chronic GVHD. Eight patients finished the 8-week treatment course without adverse effects. Seven showed improvement. Steroid taper was initiated as early as 1 month. These preliminary results call for additional studies to optimize Enbrel as a potential therapeutic agent in the treatment of chronic GVHD (276).

3. Anti-CD 20 Monoclonal Antibody

Anti-CD 20 monoclonal antibody (rituximab) has been used to treat immune-mediated thrombocytopenia (277), and it has been suggested that this antibody may be useful in patients with chronic GVHD and thrombocytopenia.

4. Pentostatin

Pentostatin is currently being studied in several clinical trials (278). We have treated 17 patients with steroid refractory, biopsy-proven chronic GVHD with Pentostatin. The treatment regimen included Pentosatatin at a dose of 4 mg/m^2/day IV q 2 weeks for a total 12 doses in 6 months. All patients received antibiotic prophylaxis. All but one patient had failed at least 2 previous systemic immunosuppressive regimens. The study is still ongoing, but results to date are encouraging.

5. Sirolimus

The antifibrotic properties of Sirolimus make it particularly attractive for GVHD (279,280). In a recent study, 29 patients with steroid-refractory acute and chronic GVHD were treated with Sirolimus at a loading dose of 6 mg, followed by a maintenance dose of 2 mg/day. The dose adjustment was made to maintain serum Sirolimus trough concentration of 5–15 ng/mL. The overall response rate was 62%, with five complete responses. Six patients (75%) with scleradermatous chronic GVHD responded. Hypertriglyceridemia and hypertension were the major side effects observed (281).

F. Adjunctive Therapies in Chronic GVHD

1. Topical Therapy

Patients with symptomatic disease limited to the oral cavity may benefit from topical steroids, thus sparing them the effects of systemic immunosuppression. Decadron elixir (0.5 mg/5 mL) can be effective local therapy when the patient rinses the mouth with 10 mL for 2–3 minutes at least four times a day. Topical steroids such as Lidex (Syntex, Palo Alto, CA) are useful. CSP swishes can be orintraoral PUVA can be given (161,283).

2. Retionoids

Etretinate has been used to treat patients with sclerodermatous and fascial chronic GVHD (284). Among 27 patients completing a 3-month trial, 20 showed some improvement in skin lesions or range of motion. Etretinate is not currently commercially available, and acitretin, a more rapidly cleared derivative, has been used in its place. In patients responding to treatment, we usually add acitretin to the main immunosuppressive therapy to increase the cutaneous response.

3. Clofazimine

This antimycobacterial drug used to treat leprosy and *Mycobacterium avium* complex, has anti-inflammatory activity in a number of chronic autoimmune skin disorders. Clofazimine was studied in 22 patients with chronic GVHD (285). Over half of the patients with sclerodermatous disease showed improvement in skin involvement, flexion contractures, or oral manifestations. Because of relatively low toxicity profile, this agent may be used as adjunctive therapy during steroid taper.

4. Hydroxychloroquine

Plaquenil (hydroxychloroquine) is an antimalarial drug. It interferes with antigen presentation and cytokine production and is synergistic with CSP and tacrolimus in vitro (82). In patients who do not tolerate acitretin because of skin drying, flaking, or ulceration, Plaquenil (Sanofi Winthrop) is an alternative drug to add to the immunosuppressive regimen. Following initial encouraging results with 50% response rate (286), Gilman et al. (287) recently published updated results in a larger patient population. Forty patients with steroid-resistant or steroid-dependent chronic GVHD received hydrochloroquine 800 mg (12 mg/kg) per day. Three complete responses (at 4–24 weeks) and 14 partial responses were seen in 32 evaluable patients (53%). Responders tolerated a > 50% reduction in their steroid dose while receiving the drug. No hematological, hepatic, renal, or retinal toxicity was observed (287). A phase III trial for initial therapy of chronic GVHD [cyclosporine plus prednisone with or without Plaquenil (Sanofi Winthrop)] is underway through the Children's Oncology Group.

G. Supportive Therapy in Chronic GVHD

1. Infection Prophylaxis

Infection is the primary cause of death in patients with chronic GVHD (84,236). Patient education and infection prophylaxis are very important (153). All patients should receive antimicrobial prophylaxis for *Pneumocystis carinii* (such as TMP-SMX) and against encapsulated organisms including pneumococcus (such as penicillin).

Penicillin Prophylaxis.   Bacteremia and sinopulmonary infections due to *Streptococcus pneumoniae* and *Haemophilus influenzae* are frequent in patients with chronic GVHD (142). These patients also have lifelong splenic dysfunction and should receive prophylaxis against encapsulated bacteria for life. A recent study indicates that there is a significant long-term risk for pneumococcal infection and sepsis in patients who have undergone allograft transplantation, especially those with chronic GVHD, which can be minimized by penicillin prophylaxis (288). Patients should also receive antibiotic prophylaxis with dental and other invasive procedures according to the endocarditis prophylaxis recommendations of the American Heart Association.

Immunoglobulin G Replacement.   Chronic GVHD and HLA nonidentity contribute to the increased rate of infection in unrelated marrow recipients as does the frequent presence of hypogammaglobulinemia (236). Some centers administer intravenous IgG to patients with hypogammaglobulinemia (<400 mg/dL) (153).

Pneumocystis Carinii *Pneumonia Prophylaxis.*   Prophylaxis with trimethoprim-sulfamethoxazole (TMP-SMX) significantly reduces the incidence of late interstitial pneumonia from 28% to 8% in patients with chronic GVHD (289). The risk of *P. carinii* pneumonia probably decreases once immunosuppressive therapy is stopped (153).

Antifungal Prophylaxis.   Patients receiving topical steroid therapy for oral GVHD should be treated with clotrimazole troches or nystatin swishes. If thrush occurs despite this, systemic antifungal therapy is indicated (153).

Antiviral Prophylaxis. Patients should receive prophylactic acyclovir for prevention of VZV infection or reactivation during the first year after the transplant, and later if systemic immunosuppression is still needed to control chronic GVHD. Acute episodes of herpes infections should be treated without delay. Patients who were serologically positive to cytomegalovirus at transplantation should have frequent surveillance cultures or testing for CMV antigenemia. Chronic GVHD patients who are at risk for late CMV disease (receiving systemic corticosteroids) should also have CMV activity monitored closely and treatment initiated at reactivation. A positive antigenemia test should be treated pre-emptively with ganciclovir, and immunoglobulin infusions should be added to the treatment for those with evidence of pulmonary CMV disease. Additional protection may be provided by supplemental intravenous IgG therapy inpatients with low serum IgG levels and recurrent infections (153).

Vaccination Guidelines. Vaccination should be delayed until 1 year after completion of GVHD therapy; patients will not mount an immune response with active disease or while receiving immunosuppressive medications. Antibody titers can be used to check responses to vaccines that are typically given to patients after SCT, such as inactivated polio, diphtheria, and tetanus toxoid. Patients can also be immunized against polyvalent influenza, pneumococcus, and *Haemophilus influenzae* B at that time. Live virus vaccines such as measles, mumps, rubella (MMR); oral poliovirus; oral typhoid; and bacillus Calmette-Guérin (BCG) should not be given to immunocompromised hosts. Clinical studies suggest that MMR can be given 2 years after transplantation in individuals who are free of chronic GVHD (290). Posttransplant vaccination guidelines are available on the Centers for Disease Control and Prevention web site (www.cdc.gov/mmwr/mmwr_rr.html) (291).

2. Symptom Management in Chronic GVHD

Skin Care. Dry skin should be treated aggressively with moisturizer. Petroleum jelly offers excellent lubrication, but patients often complain about its messiness. Trauma should be avoided because many of these patients have frail skin that can easily be abraded. Severe dermal involvement may benefit from burn care management. Skin allografting from the marrow donor has been performed in some instances (292). Patients should avoid sunburn and should wear sunscreen with a skin protection factor of at least 15. Because of poorly functioning sweat glands, precautions must be taken to avoid overheating (153).

Management of Sicca Symptoms. For patients with ocular sicca syndrome, preservative-free artificial tears at least every 4 hours during the day and preservative-free ointment at night are helpful. Protective eye- and sunglasses and frequent lubrication can help symptomatically and prevent further damage. Placement of punctual plugs or cauterization may be of benefit to conserve corneal wetting. Moisture chamber eyeglasses (a prosthetic device coupled to the eyeglasses) can significantly relieve the symptoms of dry eyes (293). Ocular sicca has been treated with retinoic acid in few cases with some success (294). Systemic immunosuppressive therapy may improve the symptoms of dry eye (256). Careful ophthalmological follow-up is needed to prevent long-term damage to the eyes.

Artificial saliva may be used for dry mouth. Pilocarpin has been reported to be helpful in alleviating dry mouth symptoms in chronic GVHD (295,296). Topical analgesic products may be used, with caution, in patients with painful oral GVHD. Patients with dry mouth are at increased risk for dental caries, and close dental follow-up is essential.

Muscle Cramps. Muscular aches and cramps are common symptoms, but the cause of these cramps is unclear. Electrolyte imbalances should be corrected. If the cramps persist, quinine may be added (153). If the cramps are disabling, dantrolene may be helpful, but it must be used cautiously and monitored carefully because of the side effects of muscle weakness, drowsiness, diarrhea, abnormal liver function, and sun sensitivity. It should not be used in patients treated with PUVA. Clonazepam treatment has been reported to improve muscle cramping, aches, and carpal spasm (297).

Cholestasis. Cholestasis secondary to hepatic chronic GVHD has been improved in 30% of patients with ursodeoxycholic acid (UDCA) therapy (298).

Wasting. Wasting is common in these patients, and malnutrition may result. The cause of the wasting is probably multifactorial and includes increased caloric requirement, oral disease, dry mouth, altered taste, and side effects of drugs. Additionally, infections in the mouth or the esophagus may contribute to poor oral intake. Nutritional assessment and monitoring is important to maintain the patient's well-being. Patients who are unable to maintain adequate caloric intake by mouth may need parenteral nutrition or enteral feeds through surgically placed tubes (153).

Osteoporosis. For patients who are receiving long-term corticosteroid therapy, estrogen replacement in young women, calcium supplements, and biphosphonates should be considered individuals at risk for osteopenia and bone fracture (299,300).

Joint Contractures. A thorough physical therapy evaluation and an individually designed program of activities can be invaluable for maintaining and increasing strength, range of motion, and mobility. For patients with sclerodermatous chronic GVHD, range-of-motion exercises may preserve joint mobility and decrease the pain associated with joint contractures. Occupational therapy may be instrumental for maximizing functional capabilities in activities of daily living, employment opportunities, and sexual satisfaction. Support groups or individual therapy may benefit patients as they learn to cope with this chronic illness (153). Surgical intervention in the treatment of joint contractures resulting from chronic GVHD does not appear to improve functional status (301).

IX. CHRONIC GVHD IN CHILDREN

Only a few studies have specifically focused on children, and little information is available on the antileukemic effect of chronic GVHD and its impact on disease-free survival in children. Zecca et al. retrospectively analyzed results in 696 children given allogeneic SCT. Chronic GVHD developed in 173 children (25%) at a median of 116 days after SCT (302). Donor and recipient age, grade II–IV acute GVHD, female donor for male recipient, diagnosis of malignancy, and use of total body irradiation were risk factors. Cord blood transplants had a very low risk of chronic GVHD (RR = 0.07) (304). In patients with hematological malignancies, chronic GVHD was associated with reduced relapse probability and improved relapse-free survival. An antileukemic effect of chronic GVHD was observed mainly in patients with acute lymphoblastic leukemia. In a study from Japan, 55 of 265 children developed chronic GVHD 1–25 months after SCT, and the 5-year cumulative incidence of chronic GVHD was 22% (303). Risk factors were identical to those identified in other studies. These studies indicate that the incidence of chronic

GVHD in children is lower than that observed in adults. Growth arrest (runting) is a common feature of chronic GVHD in children (305). Controlling the disease and withdrawal of steroids usually reverse this complication.

X. ASSOCIATION OF SECONDARY MALIGNANCIES AND CHRONIC GVHD

No clear association of chronic GVHD with secondary malignancies was shown in an initial analysis of 2246 patients undergoing marrow transplantation (306). However, subsequent studies suggested that GVHD may contribute to the development of posttransplant lymphoproliferative disorders, solid tumors (in particular squamous cell neoplasms of the skin and buccal mucosa), and Hodgkin's disease (307–311).

XI. FUTURE DIRECTIONS

Chronic GVHD will continue to be a challenge as numbers of allogeneic SCT increase, particularly those involving donors other than HLA-identical siblings. Increased use of donor lymphocyte infusion and peripheral blood stem cells will likely further increase the burden of chronic GVHD-related morbidity and mortality. Efforts to prevent the development of chronic GVHD have been largely unsuccessful. While basic research efforts continue to improve our understanding of the pathogenesis of this disease and help with the development of new therapeutic approaches, well-organized, multicenter trials are needed to address and answer clinical questions.

New strategies, potentially using sequential therapies to turn off immunological and cytokine damage, should be developed. Potentially fruitful approaches for the treatment of chronic GVHD include new immunosuppressive agents such as pentostatin and combination of standard immunosuppressive agents with anticytokine or cytokine receptor antagonists such as daclizumab (soluble IL-2 receptor antagonist) and infliximab (an anti-TNF-α monoclonal antibody). As a novel immunosuppressive modality, anti-CD52 (Campath-1H) and high-dose cyclophosphamide can be tested in high-risk patients. New clinical grading schemes should be incorporated in every prospective clinical trial to for patient stratification. Transplant centers and referring physicians must partner to provide the complex care these patients require. For allogeneic SCT to fulfill its promise for many disorders, better ways to prevent and treat GVHD must be found.

ACKNOWLEDGMENT

This work was supported in part by National Institutes of Health Grant No. K24CA83804 (GV).

REFERENCES

1. Horowitz MM. Uses and growth of hematopoietic cell transplantation. In: Thomas ED, Blume KG, Forman SJ, eds. Hematopoietic Cell Transplantation. Massachusetts: Blackwell Science, 1999; 12–18.
2. Statistical Center of the International Bone Marrow Transplant Registry (IBMTR) and Autologous Bone Marrow Transplant Registry (ABMTR), unpublished data 1995.

3. Sullivan KM. Agura E. Anasetti C, et al. Chronic graft-versus-host disease and other late complications of bone marrow transplantation. Semin Hematol 1991; 28:250–259.
4. Socie G, Gluckman E. Allogeneic hematopoietic stem cell transplantation: current issues and future prospects. Ann Med Interne (Paris) 1999; 150:642–655.
5. Clark JG, Crawford SW, Madtes DK, Sullivan KM. Obstructive lung disease after allogeneic marrow transplantation. Clinical presentation and course. Ann Intern Med 1989; 111:368–376.
6. Socie G, Stone JV, Wingard JR, et al. Long-term survival and late deaths after allogeneic bone marrow transplantation. Late Effects Working Committee of the International Bone Marrow Transplant Registry. N Engl J Med 1999; 341:14–21.
7. Deeg HJ, Leisenring W, Storb R, et al. Long-term outcome after marrow transplantation for severe aplastic anemia. Blood 1998; 91:3637–3645.
8. Goerner M, Gooley T, Flowers ME, et al. Morbidity and mortality of chronic GVHD after hematopoietic stem cell transplantation from HLA-identical siblings for patients with aplastic or refractory anemias. Biol Blood Marrow Transplant 2002; 8:47–56.
9. Przepiorka D, Anderlini P, Saliba R, Cleary K, Mehra R, Khouri I, Huh YO, Giralt S, Braunschweig I, van Besien K, Champlin R. Chronic graft-versus-host disease after allogeneic blood stem cell transplantation. Blood 2001; 98:1695–1700.
10. Syrjala KL, Chapko MK, Vitaliano PP, Cummings C, Sullivan KM. Recovery after allogeneic marrow transplantation: prospective study of predictors of long-term physical and psychosocial functioning. Bone Marrow Transplant 1993; 11:319–327.
11. Duell T, Van Lint MT, Ljungman P, Tichelli A, Socie G, Apperley JF, Weiss M, Cohen A, Nekolla E, Kolb HJ. Health and functional status of long-term survivors of bone marrow transplantation. EBMT Working Party on Late Effects and EULEP Study Group on Late Effects. European Group for Blood and Marrow Transplantation. Ann Intern Med 1997; 126:184–192.
12. Sutherland HJ, Fyles GM, Adams G, Hao Y, Lipton JH, Minden MD, Meharchand JM, Atkins H, Tejpar I, Messner HA. Quality of life following bone marrow transplantation: a comparison of patient reports with population norms. Bone Marrow Transplant 1997; 19:1129–1136.
13. Chiodi S, Spinelli S, Ravera G, et al. Quality of life in 244 recipients of allogeneic bone marrow transplantation. Br J Haematol 2000; 110:614–619.
14. Heinonen H, Volin L, Uutela A, Zevon M, Barrick C, Ruutu T. Quality of life and factors related to perceived satisfaction with quality of life after allogeneic bone marrow transplantation. Ann Hematol 2001; 80:137–143.
15. Lee SJ, Cook EF, Soiffer R, Antin JH. Development and validation of a scale to measure symptoms of chronic graft-versus-host disease. Biol Blood Marrow Transplant 2002; 8:444–452.
16. Wingard JR, Curbow B, Baker F, Piantadosi S. Health, functional status, and employment of adult survivors of bone marrow transplantation. Ann Intern Med 1991; 114:113–118.
17. Andrykowski MA, Greiner CB, Altmaier EM, et al. Quality of life following bone marrow transplantation: findings from a multicentre study. Br J Cancer 1995; 71:1322–1329.
18. Marks DI, Gale DJ, Vedhara K, Bird JM. A quality of life study in 20 adult long-term survivors of unrelated donor bone marrow transplantation. Bone Marrow Transplant 1999; 24:191–195.
19. Socie G, Mary JY, Esperou H, et al. Health and functional status of adult recipients 1 year after allogeneic haematopoietic stem cell transplantation. Br J Haematol 2001; 113:194–201.
20. Gleichmann E, Pals ST, Rolink AG, Radaszkiewicz T, Gleichmann H. Graft-versus-host reactions: clues to the etiopathology of a spectrum of immunological diseases. Immunol Today 1984; 5:324–332.
21. Via CS, Shearer GM. T-cell interactions in autoimmunity: insights from a murine model of graft-versus-host disease. Immunol Today 1988; 9:207–213.
22. Rolink AG, Gleichmann E. Allosuppressor- and allohelper-T cells in acute and chronic graft-vs.-host (GVH) disease. III. Different Lyt subsets of donor T cells induce different pathological syndromes. J Exp Med 1983; 158:546–558.

23. Moser M, Sharrow SO, Shearer GM. Role of L3T4+ and Lyt-2+ donor cells in graft-versus-host immune deficiency induced across a class I, class II, or whole H-2 difference. J Immunol 1988; 140:2600–2608.

24. Morris SC, Cohen PL, Eisenberg RA. Experimental induction of systemic lupus erythematosus by recognition of foreign la. Clin Immunol Immunopathol 1990; 57:263–273.

25. Via CS. Kinetics of T cell activation in acute and chronic forms of murine graft-versus-host disease. J Immunol 1991; 146:2603–2609.

26. Rus V, Svetic A, Nguyen P, Gause WC, Via CS. Kinetics of Th1 and Th2 cytokine production during the early course of acute and chronic murine graft-versus-host disease. Regulatory role of donor CD8+ T cells. J Immunol 1995; 155:2396–2406.

27. Garlisi CG, Pennline KJ, Smith SR, Siegel MI, Umland SP. Cytokine gene expression in mice undergoing chronic graft-versus-host disease. Mol Immunol 1993; 30:669–677.

28. Allen RD, Staley TA, Sidman CL. Differential cytokine expression in acute and chronic murine graft- versus-host-disease. Eur J Immunol 1993; 23:333–337.

29. Garside P, Reid S, Steel M, Mowat AM. Differential cytokine production associated with distinct phases of murine graft-vs-host reaction. Immunology 1994; 82:211–214.

30. Williamson E, Garside P, Bradley JA, Mowat AM. IL-12 is a central mediator of acute graft-versus-host disease in mice. J Immunol 1996; 157:689–699.

31. Via CS, Shustov A, Rus V, Lang T, Nguyen P, Finkelman FD. In vivo neutralization of TNF-alpha promotes humoral autoimmunity by preventing the induction of CTL. J Immunol 2001; 167:6821–6826.

32. Via CS, Shearer GM. Murine graft-versus-host disease as a model for the development of autoimmunity. Relevance of cytotoxic T lymphocytes. Ann NY Acad Sci 1988; 532:44–50.

33. Doutrelepont JM, Moser M, Leo O, Abramowicz D, Vanderhaegen ML, Urbain J, Goldman M. Hyper IgE in stimulatory graft-versus-host disease: role of interleukin-4. Clin Exp Immunol 1991; 83:133–136.

34. Morris SC, Cheek RL, Cohen PL, Eisenberg RA. Autoantibodies in chronic graft versus host result from cognate T-B interactions. J Exp Med 1990; 171:503–517.

35. van Elven EH, Rolink AG, Veen FV, Gleichmann E. Capacity of genetically different T lymphocytes to induce lethal graft-versus-host disease correlates with their capacity to generate suppression but not with their capacity to generate anti-F1 killer cells. A non-H-2 locus determines the inability to induce lethal graft-versus-host disease. J Exp Med 1981; 153:1474–1488.

36. Rolink AG, Radaszkiewicz T, Pals ST, van der Meer WG, Gleichmann E. Allosuppressor and allohelper T cells in acute and chronic graft-vs-host disease. I. Alloreactive suppressor cells rather than killer T cells appear to be the decisive effector cells in lethal graft-vs.-host disease. J Exp Med 1982; 155:1501–1522.

37. Via CS, Sharrow SO, Shearer GM. Role of cytotoxic T lymphocytes in the prevention of lupus-like disease occurring in a murine model of graft-vs-host disease. J Immunol 1987; 139:1840–1849.

38. Rozendaal L, Pals ST, Melief CJ, Gleichmann E. Protection from lethal graft-vs.-host disease by donor stem cell repopulation. Eur J Immunol 1992; 22:575–579.

39. Shustov A, Nguyen P, Finkelman FD, Elkon KB, Via CS. Differential expression of Fas and Fas ligand in acute and chronic graft-versus-host disease: up-regulation of Fas and Fas ligand requires CD8+ T cell activation and IFN-gamma production. J Immunol 1998; 161:2848–2855.

40. Van Rappard-Van Der Veen FM, Kiesel U, Poels L, Schuler W, Melief CJ, Landegent J, Gleichmann E. Further evidence against random polyclonal antibody formation in mice with lupus-like graft-vs.-host disease. J Immunol 1984; 132:1814–1820.

41. Gleichmann E, van Elven EH, Van der Veen JP. A systemic lupus erythematosus (SLE)-like disease in mice induced by abnormal T-B cell cooperation. Preferential formation of autoantibodies characteristic of SLE. Eur J Immunol 1982; 12:152–159.

42. Portanova JP, Claman HN, Kotzin BL. Autoimmunization in murine graft-vs-host disease. I. Selective production of antibodies to histones and DNA. J Immunol 1985; 135:3850–3856.

43. van Elven EH, Agterberg J, Sadal S, Gleichmann E. Diseases caused by reactions of T lymphocytes to incompatible structures of the major histocompatibility complex. II. Autoantibodies deposited along the basement membrane of skin and their relationship to immune-complex glomerulonephritis. J Immunol 1981; 126:1684–1691.

44. Rolink AG, Gleichmann H, Gleichmann E. Diseases caused by reactions of T lymphocytes to incompatible structures of the major histocompatibility complex. VII. Immune-complex glomerulonephritis. J Immunol 1983; 130:209–215.

45. Van Rappard-Van Der Veen FM, Radaszkiewicz T, Terraneo L, Gleichmann E. Attempts at standardization of lupus-like graft-vs-host disease: inadvertent repopulation by DBA/2 spleen cells of H-2-different nonirradiated F1 mice. J Immunol 1983; 130:2693–2701.

46. De Wit D, Van Mechelen M, Zanin C, Doutrelepont JM, Velu T, Gerard C, Abramowicz D, Scheerlinck JP, De Baetselier P, Urbain J. Preferential activation of Th2 cells in chronic graft-versus-host reaction. J Immunol 1993; 150:361–366.

47. Via CS, Rus V, Nguyen P, Linsley P, Gause WC. Differential effect of CTLA4Ig on murine graft-versus-host disease (GVHD) development: CTLA4Ig prevents both acute and chronic GVHD development but reverses only chronic GVHD. J Immunol 1996; 157:4258–4267.

48. Hakim FT, Cepeda R, Gray GS, June CH, Abe R. Acute graft-versus-host reaction can be aborted by blockade of costimulatory molecules. J Immunol 1995; 155:1757–1766.

49. Lang TJ, Nguyen P, Peach R, Gause WC, Via CS. In vivo CD86 blockade inhibits CD4+ T cell activation, whereas CD80 blockade potentiates CD8+ T cell activation and CTL effector function. J Immunol 2002; 168:3786–3792.

50. Coyle AJ, Gutierrez-Ramos JC. The expanding B7 superfamily: increasing complexity in costimulatory signals regulating T cell function. Nat Immunol 2001; 2:203–209.

51. Mehrotra PT, Wu D, Crim JA, Mostpwski HS, Siegal JP. Effects of IL-12 on the generation of cytotoxic activity in human CD8$^+$ T lymphocytes. J Immunol 1993; 151:2444–2452.

52. Via CS, Rus V, Gately MK, Finkelman FD. IL-12 stimulates the development of acute graft-versus-host disease in mice that normally would develop chronic, autoimmune graft-versus-host disease. J Immunol 1994; 153:4040–4047.

53. Greene JL, Leytze GM, Emswiler J, Peach R, Bajorath J, Cosand W, Linsley PS. Covalent dimerization of CD28/CTLA-4 and oligomerization of CD80/CD86 regulate T cell costimulatory interactions. J Biol Chem 1996; 271:26762–26771.

54. Linksley PS, Greene JL, Brady W, Bajorath J, Ledbetter JA, Peach R. Human B7-1 (CD80) and B7-2 (CD86) bind with similar avidities but distinct kinetics to CD28 and CTLA-4 receptors. Immunity 1994; 1:793–801.

55. Sakurai J, Ohata J, Saito K, Miyajima H, Hirano T, Kohsaka T, Enomoto S, Okumura K, Azuma M. Blockade of CTLA-4 signals inhibits Th2-mediated murine chronic graft-versus-host disease by an enhanced expansion of regulatory CD8+ T cells. J Immunol 2000; 164:664–669.

56. Nabholz M, MacDonald HR. Cytolytic T lymphocytes. Ann Rev Immunol 1983; 1:273–306.

57. Via CS, Finkelman FD. Critical role of interleukin-2 in the development of acute graft-versus-host disease. Int Immunol 1993; 5:565–572.

58. Shustov A, Luzina I, Nguyen P, Papadimitriou JC, Handwerger B, Elkon KB, Via CS. Role of perforin in controlling B-cell hyperactivity and humoral autoimmunity. J Clin Invest 2000; 106:R39–47.

59. Via CS, Nguyen P, Shustov A, Drappa J, Elkon KB. A major role for the Fas pathway in acute graft-versus-host disease. J Immunol 1996; 157:5387–5393.

60. Lawley TJ, Peck GL, Moutsopoulos HM, Gratwohl AA, Deisseroth AB. Scleroderma, Sjögren-like syndrome, and chronic graft-versus-host disease. Ann Intern Med 1977; 87:707–709.

61. Graze PR, Gale RP. Chronic graft versus host disease: a syndrome of disordered immunity. Am J Med 1979; 66:611–620.

62. Shulman HM, Sullivan KM, Weiden PL, McDonald GB, Striker GE, Sale GE, Hackman R, Tsoi MS, Storb R, Thomas ED. Chronic graft-versus-host syndrome in man. A long-term clinicopathologic study of 20 Seattle patients. Am J Med 1980; 69:204–217.

63. Jaffee BD, Claman HN. Chronic graft-versus-host disease (GVHD) as a model for scleroderma. I. Description of model systems. Cell Immunol 1983; 77:1–12.

64. DeClerck Y, Draper V, Parkman R. Clonal analysis of murine graft-vs-host disease. II. Leukokines that stimulate fibroblast proliferation and collagen synthesis in graft-vs.-host disease. J Immunol 1986; 136:3549–3552.

65. Pals ST, Radaszkiewicz T, Roozendaal L, Gleichmann E. Chronic progressive polyarthritis and other symptoms of collagen vascular disease induced by graft-vs-host reaction. J Immunol 1985; 134:1475–1482.

66. Gelpi C, Martinez MA, Vidal S, Alguero A, Juarez C C, Hardin JA, Rodriguez-Sanchez JL. Different strains of donor parental lymphoid cells induce different models of chronic graft-versus-host disease in murine (Balb/cs × A/J)F1 hybrid hosts. Clin Immunol Immunopathol 1990; 56:298–310.

67. Nelson JL. Microchimerism and autoimmune disease. N Engl J Med 1998; 338:1224–1225.

68. Evans PC, Lambert N, Maloney S, Furst DE, Moore JM, Nelson JL. Long-term fetal microchimerism in peripheral blood mononuclear cell subsets in healthy women and women with scleroderma. Blood 1999; 93:2033–2037.

69. Fukuzawa M, Via CS, Shearer GM. Defective thymic education of L3T4+ T helper cell function in graft-vs-host mice. J Immunol 1988; 141:430–439.

70. Parkman R. Clonal analysis of murine graft-versus-host disease. I. Phenotypic and functional analysis of T lymphocyte clones. J Immunol 1986; 136:3543–3548.

71. Krenger W, Ferrara JL. Graft-versus-host disease and the Th1/Th2 paradigm [review]. Immunol Res 1996; 15:50–73.

72. Ferrara JL, Krenger W. Graft-versus-host disease: the influence of type 1 and type 2 T cell cytokines. Transfus Med Rev 1998; 12:1–17.

73. Ferrara JL, Antin JH. The pathophysiology of graft-versus-host disease. In: Thomas ED, Blume KG, Forman SJ, eds. Hematopoietic Cell Transplantation. Malden, Massachusetts: Blackwell Science, 1999:305–315.

74. Sullivan KM, Parkman R. The pathophysiology and treatment of graft-versus-host disease. Clin Haematol 1983; 12:775–789.

75. Weinberg K, Blazar BR, Wagner JE, et al. Factors affecting thymic function after allogeneic hematopoietic stem cell transplantation. Blood 2001; 97:1458–1466.

76. Parkman R. Chronic graft-versus-host disease. Curr Opin Hematol 1998; 5:22–25.

77. Hess AD, Horowitz L, Beschomer WE, Santos GW. Development of graft-versus-host disease-like syndrome in cyclosporine treated rats after syngeneic bone marrow transplantation. I. Development of cytotoxic T lymphocytes with apparent polyclonal ant-Ia specificity, including autoreactivity. J Exp Med 1985; 161:718–730.

78. Hess AD, Thoburn C, Chen W, Horowitz L. Autoreactive T-cell subsets in acute and chronic syngeneic graft-versus-host disease. Transplant Proc 2001; 33:1754–1756.

79. Hess AD, Bright EC, Thoburn C, Vogelsang GB, Jones RJ, Kennedy MJ. Specificity of effector T lymphocytes in autologous graft-versus-host disease: role of the major histocompatibility complex class II invariant chain peptide. Blood 1997; 89:2203–2209.

80. Biedermann BC, Sahner S, Gregor M, Tsakiris DA, Jeanneret C, Pober JS, Gratwohl A. Endothelial injury mediated by cytotoxic T lymphocytes and loss of microvessels in chronic graft versus host disease. Lancet 2002; 359:2078–2083.

81. Goerner M, Gooley TT, Flowers ME, et al. Morbidity and mortality of chronic GVHD after hematopoietic stem cell transplantation from HLA-identical siblings for patients with aplastic or refractory anemias. Biol Blood Marrow Transplant 2002; 8:47–56.

82. Al Gilman, Schultz KR. Treatment of chronic GVHD. Bone Marrow Transplant 2000; 26:460–462.
83. Lee SJ, Klein JP, Barrett AJ, et al. Severity of chronic graft-versus-host disease: association with treatment-related mortality and relapse. Blood 2002; 100:406–414.
84. Storb R R, Prentice RL RL, Sullivan KM, et al. Predictive factors in chronic graft-versus-host disease in patients with aplastic anemia treated by bone marrow transplantation from HLA-identical siblings. Ann Intern Med 1983; 98:461–466.
85. Atkinson K K, Horowitz MM MM, Gale RP, et al. Risk factors for chronic graft-versus-host disease after HLA-identical sibling bone marrow transplantation Blood 1990; 75:2459–2464.
86. Ochs LA, Miller WJ, Filopovich AH, et al. Predictive factors for chronic graft-versus-host disease after histocompatible sibling donor marrow transplantation. Bone Marrow Transplant 1994; 13:455–460.
87. Wagner JL, Flowers ME, Longton G, Storb R, Schubert M, Sullivan KM. The development of chronic graft-versus-host disease: an analysis of screening studies and the impact of corticosteroid use at 100 days after transplantation. Bone Marrow Transplant 1998; 22:139–146.
88. Marks DI, Cullis JO, Ward KN, Lacey S, Syzdlo R, Hughes TP. Allogeneic bone marrow transplantation for chronic myeloid leukemia using sibling and volunteer unrelated donors. A comparison of complications in the first 2 years. Ann Intern Med 1993; 119:207–214.
89. Godder KT, Metha J, Chiang KY, et al. Partially mismatched related donor bone marrow transplantation as salvage for patients with AML who failed autologous stem cell transplant. Bone Marrow Transplant 2001; 28:1031–1036.
90. Drobyski WR, Klein J, Flomenberg N, Pietryga D, Vesole DH, Margolis DA, Keever-Taylor C. Superior survival associated with transplantation of matched unrelated versus one-antigen mismatched unrelated or highly human-leukocyte antigen disparate haploidentical family donor marrow grafts for the treatment of hematologic malignancies: establishing a treatment algorithm for recipients of alternative donor grafts. Blood 2002; 99:806–814.
91. Gallardo D D, Arostegui JI, Balas A, Torres A, Caballero D, Carreras E, Brunet S, Jimenez A, Mataix R, Serrano D, Vallejo C, Sanz G, Solano C, Rodriguez-Luaces M, Marin J, Baro J, Sanz C, Roman J, Gonzalez M, Martorell J, Sierra J J, Martin C, de la Camara R, Granena A A. GvHD Subcommittee of the Grupo Espanol de Trasplante Hemapoyetico (GETH). Disparity for the minor histocompatibility antigen HA-1 is associated with an increased risk of acute graft-versus-host disease (GVHD) but it does not affect chronic GVHD incidence, disease-free survival or overall survival after allogeneic human leucocyte antigen-identical sibling donor transplantation. Br J Haematol 2001; 114:931–936.
92. Niederweiser D, Pepe M, Storb R, et al. Factors predicting chronic GVHD after HLA-identical sibling bone marrow transplantation for aplastic anemia. Bone Marrow Transplant 1989; 4:151–156.
93. Schetelig J, Kroger N, Held TK, et al. Allogeneic transplantation after reduced conditioning in high risk patients is complicated by a high incidence of acute and chronic graft-versus-host disease. Haematologica 2002; 87:299–305.
94. Kollman C, Howe CW, Anasetti C, et al. Donor characteristics as risk factors in recipients after transplantation of bone marrow from unrelated donors: the effect of donor age. Blood 2001; 98:2043–2051.
95. Ratanatharathorn V, Ayash L, Lazarus HM, Fu J, Uberti JP. Chronic graft-versus-host disease: clinical manifestation and therapy. Bone Marrow Transplant 2001; 28:121–129.
96. Cutler C, Giri S, Jeyapalan S, et al. Acute and chronic graft-versus-host disease after allogeneic peripheral-blood stem-cell and bone marrow transplantation: a meta-analysis. J Clin Oncol 2001; 19:3685–3691.
97. Mohty M, Kuentz M, Michallet M, Bourhis JH, Milpied N, Sutton L, Jouet JP, Attal M, Bordigoni P, Cahn JY, Boiron JM, Blaise D. Societe Francaise de Greffe de Moelle et de Therapie Cellulaire (SFGM-TC). Chronic graft-versus-host disease after allogeneic blood stem cell transplantation: long-term results of a randomized study. Blood 2002; 100:3128–3134.

98. Bensinger WI, Clift R, Martin P, et al. Allogeneic peripheral blood stem cell transplantation in patients with advanced hematologic malignancies: a retrospective comparison with bone marrow transplantation. Blood 1996; 88:2794–2800.

99. Schmitz N, Bacigalupo A, Labopin M, et al. Transplantation of peripheral blood progenitor cells from HLA-identical sibling donors. Br J Haematol 1996; 95:715–723.

100. Majolino I, Saglio G, Scime R, et al. High incidence of chronic GVHD after primary allogeneic peripheral blood stem cell transplantation in patients with hematologic malignancies. Bone Marrow Transplant 1996; 17:555–560.

101. Storek J, Gooley T, Siadak M, et al. Allogeneic peripheral blood stem cell transplantation may be associated with a high risk of chronic graft-versus-host disease. Blood 1997; 90:4705–4709.

102. Durrant ST, Morton AJ, Herston O. A randomized trial of filgrastim (G-CSF) stimulated donor marrow (BM) versus peripheral blood (PBC) for allogeneic transplantation: increased extensive chronic graft versus host disease following PBPC transplantation [abstr]. Blood 1999; 94(suppl 1):608a.

103. Blaise D, Kuentz M, Fortanier C, et al. Randomized trial of bone marrow versus lenograstim-primed blood cell allogeneic transplantation in patients with early-stage leukemia: a report from the Societe Francaise de Greffe de Moelle. J Clin Oncol 2000; 18:537–546.

104. Snowden JA, Nivison-Smith I, Atkinson K, et al. Allogeneic PBPC transplantation: an effect on incidence and distribution of chronic graft-versus-host disease without long-term survival benefit? Bone Marrow Transplant 2000; 25:119–20.

105. Bensinger WI, Martin PJ, Storer B, et al. Transplantation of bone marrow as compared with peripheral-blood cells from HLA-identical relatives in patients with hematologic cancers. N Engl J Med 2001; 344:175–181.

106. Flowers ME, Parker PM, Johnston LJ, Matos AV, Storer B, Bensinger WI, Storb R, Appelbaum FR, Forman SJ, Blume KG, Martin PJ. Comparison of chronic graft-versus-host disease after transplantation of peripheral blood stem cells versus bone marrow in allogeneic recipients: long-term follow-up of a randomized trial. Blood 2002; 100:415–419.

107. Remberger M, Ringden O, Blau IW, et al. No difference in graft-versus-host disease, relapse, and survival comparing peripheral stem cells to bone marrow using unrelated donors. Blood 2001; 98:1739–1745.

108. Elmaagacli AH, Basoglu S, Peceny R, et al. Improved disease-free-survival after transplantation of peripheral blood stem cells as compared with bone marrow from HLA-identical unrelated donors in patients with first chronic phase chronic myeloid leukemia. Blood 2002; 99:1130–1135.

109. Zaucha JM, Gooley T, Bensinger WI, Heimfeld S, Chauncey TR, Zaucha R, Martin PJ, Flowers ME, Storek J, Georges G, Storb R, Torok-Storb B. CD34 cell dose in granulocyte colony-stimulating factor-mobilized peripheral blood mononuclear cell grafts affects engraftment kinetics and development of extensive chronic graft-versus-host disease after human leukocyte antigen-identical sibling transplantation. Blood 2001; 98:3221–3227.

110. Korbling M, Anderlini P. Peripheral blood stem cell versus bone marrow allotransplantation: does the source of hematopoietic stem cells matter? Blood 2001; 98:2900–2908.

111. Morton J, Hutchins C, Durrant S. Granulocyte-colony-stimulating factor (G-CSF)-primed allogeneic bone marrow: significantly less graft-versus-host disease and comparable engraftment to G-CSF-mobilized peripheral blood stem cells. Blood 2001; 98:3186–3191.

112. Roush KS, Hillyer CD. Donor lymphocyte infusion therapy. Transfus Med Rev 2002; 16:161–176.

113. Akpek G, Boitnott JK, Lee LA, Hallick JP, Torbenson M, Jacobsohn D, Arai S, Anders V, Vogelsang GB. Hepatitic-variant of graft-versus-host disease after donor lymphocyte infusion. Blood 2002; 100:3903–3907.

114. Collins RH Jr, Shpilberg O, Drobyski WR, et al. Donor leukocyte infusions in 140 patients with relapsed malignancy after allogeneic bone marrow transplantation. J Clin Oncol 1997; 15:433–444.

115. Loughran TP Jr, Sullivan K, Morton T, et al. Value of day 100 screening studies for predicting the development of chronic graft-versus-host disease after allogeneic bone marrow transplantation. Blood 1990; 76:228–234.

116. Wagner JL, Flowers ME, Longton G, Storb R, Schubert M, Sullivan KM. The development of chronic graft-versus-host disease: an analysis of screening studies and the impact of corticosteroid use at 100 days after transplantation. Bone Marrow Transplant 1998; 22:139–146.

117. Gratama JW, Zwaan FE, Stijnen T, et al. Herpes virus immunity and acute graft-versus-host disease. Lancet 1987; 1:471–473.

118. Bostrom L, Ringden O, Sundberg B, et al. Pretransplant herpes virus serology and chronic graft-versus-host disease. Bone Marrow Transplant 1989; 4:547–552.

119. Bostrom L, Ringden O, Jacobsen N, Zwaan F, Nilsson BA. European multicenter study of chronic graft versus host disease: the role of cytomegalovirus serology in recipients and donors, acute graft-versus-host disease, and splenectomy. Transplantation 1990; 49:1100–1105.

120. Ljungman P, Niederweiser D, Pepe MS, Longton G, Storb R, Meyers JD. Cytomegalovirus infection after marrow transplantation for aplastic anemia. Bone Marrow Transplant 1990; 6:295–300.

121. Wagner JL, Seidel K, Boeckh M, Storb R. De novo chronic graft-versus-host disease in marrow graft recipients given methotrexate and cyclosporine: risk factors and survival. Biol Blood Marrow Transplant 2000; 6:633–639.

122. Ruutu T, Volin L, Elonen E. Low incidence of severe acute and chronic graft-versus-host disease as a result of prolonged cyclosporine prophylaxis and early aggressive treatment with corticosteroids. Transplant Proc 1988; 20:491–493.

123. Lonnqvist B, Aschan J, Ljungman P, Ringden O. Long term cyclosporine therapy may decrease the risk of chronic graft-versus-host disease. Br J Haematol 1990; 74:547–548.

124. Bacigalupo A, Maiolini A, Van Lint MT, et al. Cyclosporin A, and graft versus host disease. Bone Marrow Transplant 1990; 6:341–344.

125. Kansu E, Gooley T, Flowers ME, Anasetti C, Deeg HJ, Nash RA, Sanders JE, Witherspoon RP, Appelbaum FR, Storb R, Martin PJ. Administration of cyclosporine for 24 months compared with 6 months for prevention of chronic graft-versus-host disease: a prospective randomized clinical trial. Blood 2001; 98:3868–3870.

126. Tomonari A, Iseki T, Ooi J, et al. Second allogeneic hematopoietic stem cell transplantation for leukemia relapse after first allogeneic transplantation: outcome of 16 patients in a single institution. Int J Hematol 2002; 75:318–323.

127. de Gast GC, Beatty PG, Amos A. Tranfusions shortly before HLA-matched marrow transplantation for leukemia are associated with a decrease in chronic graft-versus-host disease. Bone Marrow Transplant 1991; 7:293–295.

128. Bolger GB, Sullivan KM, Storb R, et al. Second marrow infusion for poor graft function after allogeneic marrow transplantation. Bone Marrow Transplant 1986; 1:21–30.

129. Socie G, Clift RA, Blaise D, et al. Busulfan plus cyclophosphamide compared with total-body irradiation plus cyclophosphamide before marrow transplantation for myeloid leukemia: long-term follow-up of 4 randomized studies. Blood 2001; 98:3569–3574.

130. Ratanatharathorn V, Nash RA, Przepiorka D, Devine SM, Klein JL, Weisdorf D, Fay JW, Nademanee A, Antin JH, Christiansen NP, van der Jagt R, Herzig RH, Litzow MR, Wolff SN, Longo WL, Petersen FB, Karanes C, Avalos B, Storb R, Buell DN, Maher RM, Fitzsimmons WE, Wingard JR. Phase III study comparing methotrexate and tacrolimus (prograf, FK506) with methotrexate and cyclosporine for graft-versus-host disease prophylaxis after HLA-identical sibling bone marrow transplantation. Blood 1998; 92:2303–2314.

131. Atkinson K, Downs K. Omission of day 11 methotrexate does not appear to influence the incidence of moderate to severe acute graft-versus-host disease, chronic graft-versus-host disease, relapse rate or survival after HLA-identical sibling bone marrow transplantation. Bone Marrow Transplant 1995; 16:755–758.

132. Sullivan KM. Graft-versus-host disease. In: Thomas ED, Blume KG, Forman SJ, eds. Hematopoietic Cell Transplantation. Massachusetts: Blackwell Science, 1999:515–536.
133. Jacobsohn DA, Montross S, Anders V, Vogelsang GB. Clinical importance of confirming or excluding the diagnosis of chronic graft-versus-host disease. Bone Marrow Transplant 2001; 28:1047–1051.
134. Kotani A A, Ishikawa T, Matsumura Y, Ichinohe T, Ohno H, Hori T, Uchiyama T. Correlation of peripheral blood OX40+(CD134+) T cells with chronic graft-versus-host disease in patients who underwent allogeneic hematopoietic stem cell transplantation. Blood 2001; 98:3162–3164.
135. Sullivan KM, Shulman HM, Storb R, Weiden PL, Witherspoon RP, McDonald GB, Schubert MM, Atkinson K, Thomas ED. Chronic graft-versus-host disease in 52 patients; adverse natural course and successfull treatment with combination immunosuppression. Blood 1981; 57:267–276.
136. Deeg HJ, et al. Bone marrow transplantation: a review of delayed complications. Br J Hematol 1984; 57:185–189.
137. Sullivan KM, Storek J, Kopecky KJ, et al. A controlled trial of long term administration of intravenous immunoglobulin to prevent late infection and chronic graft-versus-host disease after marrow transplantation. Biol Blood Marrow Transplant 1996; 2:45–53.
138. Siadak M, Sullivan KM. The management of chronic graft-versus host disease. Blood Rev 1994; 8:154–160.
139. Storek J, Witherspoon RP, Webb D, Storb R. Lack of B cells precursors in marrow transplant recipients with chronic graft-versus-host disease. Am J Hematol 1996; 52:82–89.
140. Sherer Y, Shoenfeld Y. Autoimmune diseases and autoimmunity post-bone marrow transplantation. Bone Marrow Transplant 1998; 22:873–881.
141. Maury S, Mary JY, Rabian C, et al. Prolonged immune deficiency following allogeneic stem cell transplantation: risk factors and complications in adult patients. Br J Haematol 2001; 115:630–641.
142. Atkinson K, Farewell V, Storb R, et al. Analysis of the infections after human bone marrow transplantation: role of genotypic nonidentity between marrow donor and recipient and of nonspecific suppressor cells in patients with chronic graft-versus-host disease. Blood 1982; 60:714–720.
143. Lapp WS, Ghayur T, Mendes M, et al. The functional and histological basis for graft-versus-host-induced immunosuppression. Immunol Rev 1985; 88:107–133.
144. Shulman HM, Sale GE, Lerner KG, et al. Chronic cutaneous graft-versus-host disease in man. Am J Pathol 1978; 91:545–570.
145. Lawley TJ, Peck GL, Moutsopoulos HM, et al. Scleroderma, Sjögren-like syndrome, and chronic graft-versus-host disease. Ann Intern Med 1977; 87:707–709.
146. Graze PR, Gale RP. Chronic graft versus host disease: a syndrome of disordered immunity. Am J Med 1979; 66:611–620.
147. Knobler HY, Sagher U, Peled IJ, et al. Tolerance to donor-type skin in the recipient of a bone marrow allograft. Treatment of skin ulcers in chronic graft-versus-host disease with skin grafts from the bone marrow donor. Transplantation 1985; 40:223–225.
148. Hymes SR, Farmer ER, Burns WH, et al. Bullous sclerodermatous-like changes in chronic graft-versus-host disease. Arch Dermatol 1985; 121:1189–1192.
149. Janin A, Socie G, Devergie A, et al. Fascitis in chronic graft-versus-host disease—a clinicopathologic study of 14 cases. Ann Intern Med 1994; 120:993–998.
150. Farmer ER. The histopathology of graft-versus-host disease. Adv Dermatol 1986; 1:173–188.
151. Favre A, Cerri A, Bacigalupo A, Lanino E, Berti E, Grossi CE. Immunohistochemical study of skin lesions in acute and chronic graft versus host disease following bone marrow transplantation. Am J Surg Pathol 1997; 21:23–34.
152. Tabata H, Yamakage A, Yamazaki S. Electron-microscopic study of sclerodermatous chronic graft-versus-host disease. Int J Dermatol 1996; 35:862–866.

153. Vogelsang GB. How I treat chronic graft-versus-host disease. Blood 2001; 97:1196–1201.
154. Strasser SI, Shulman HM, Flowers ME, Reddy R, et al. Chronic graft-versus-host disease of the liver: presentation as an acute hepatitis. Hepatology 2000; 32:1265–1271.
155. Arai S, Lee L, Vogelsang G. A systematic approach to hepatic complications in hematopoietic stem cell transplantation. J Hematother Stem Cell Res 2002; 11:215–230.
156. Yau JC, Zander AR, Srigley JR, et al. Chronic graft-versus-host disease complicated by micronodular cirrhosis and esophageal varices. Transplantation 1986; 41:129–130.
157. Knapp AB, Crawford JM, Rappepart JM, Gollan JL. Cirrhosis as a consequence of graft-versus-host disease. Gastroenterology 1987; 92:513–519.
158. Epstein, Thomas HC, Sherlock S. Primary biliary cirrhosis is a dry gland syndrome with features of chronic graft-versus-host disease. Lancet 1980; 1:1166–1168.
159. Rhodes DF, Lee WM, Wingard JR, et al. Orthotopic liver transplantation for graft-versus-host disease following bone marrow transplantation. Gastroenterology 1990; 99:536–538.
160. Schubert MM, Sullivan KM, Morton TH, et al. Oral manifestations of chronic graft-v-host disease. Arch Intern Med 1984; 144:1591–1595.
161. Redding SW, Callander NS, Haveman CW, Leonard DL. Treatment of oral chronic graft-versus-host disease with PUVA therapy: case report and literature review. Oral Surg Oral Med Oral Pathol Oral Radiol Endod 1998; 86:183–187.
162. Gratwohl AA, Moutsopoulos HM, Chused TM, et al. Sjogren type syndrome after allogeneic bone marrow transplantation. Ann Intern Med 1977; 87:703–706.
163. Nagler R, Marmary Y, Krausz Y, Chisin R, Markitziu A, Nagler A. Major salivary gland dysfunction in human acute and chronic graft-versus-host disease (GVHD). Bone Marrow Transplant 1996; 17:219–224.
164. Tichelli A, Duell T, Weiss M, et al. Late-onset keratoconjunctivitis sicca syndrome after bone marrow transplantation: Incidence and risk factors. Bone Marrow Transplant 1996; 17:1105–1111.
165. Johnson DA, Jabs DA. The ocular manifestations of graft-versus-host disease. Int Ophthalmol Clin 1997; 37:119–133.
166. Jabs DA, Wingard J, Green WR, et al. The eye in bone marrow transplantation: III. Conjunctival graft-versus-host disease. Arch Ophthalmol 1989; 107:1343–1348.
167. Greenespan A, Deeg HJ, Cottler-Fox M, et al. Incapacitating peripheral neuropathy as a manifestation of chronic graft-versus-host disease. Bone Marrow Transplant 1990; 5:349–351.
168. Smith CIE, Aarli JA, Biberfeld P, et al. Myasthenia gravis after bone marrow transplantation. N Engl J Med 1983; 309:1565–1568.
169. Bolger GB, Sullivan KM, Spencer AM, et al. Myasthenia gravis after bone marrow transplantation: relationship to chronic graft-versus-host disease. Neurology 1986; 36:1087–1091.
170. Nelson KR, McQuillen MP. Neurologic complications of graft-versus-host disease. Neurol Clin 1988; 6:389–403.
170a. Padovan CS, Bise K, Hahn J, Sostak P, Holler E, Kolb HJ, Straube A. Angiitis of the central nervous system after allogeneic bone marrow transplantation? Stroke 1999; 30:1651–1656.
170b. Takatsuka H, Okamoto T, Yamada S, Fujimori Y, Tamura S, Wada H, Okada M, Takemoto Y, Nishimura H, Tachibana H, Kanamaru A, Kakishita E. New imaging findings in a patient with central nervous system dysfunction after bone marrow transplantation. Acta Haematol 2000; 103:203–205.
171. Reyes MG, Noronha RA, Thomas W Jr, Heredia R. Myositis of chronic graft-versus-host disease. Neurology 1983; 33:1222–1224.
172. Urbano-Marquez A, Estruch R, Grau JM, et al. Inflammatory myopathy, associated with chronic graft-versus-host disease. Neurology 1986; 36;1091–1093.
173. Parker P, Chao NJ, Ben-Ezra J, et al. Polymyositis as a manifestation of chronic graft-versus-host disease. Medicine 1996; 75:279–285.
174. Couriel DR, Beguelin GZ, Giralt S, De Lima M, Hosing C, Kharfan-Dabaja MA, Anagnostopoulos A, Champlin R. Chronic graft-versus-host disease manifesting as polymyositis: an uncommon presentation. Bone Marrow Transplant 2002; 30:543–546.

175. Tse S, Saunders EF, Silverman E, Vajsar J, Becker L, Meaney B. Myasthenia gravis and poly-myositis as manifestations of chronic graft-versus-host-disease. Bone Marrow Transplant 1999; 23:397–399.
176. Yanagihara C, Nakaji K, Tanaka Y, Yabe H, Nishimura Y. A patient of chronic graft-versus-host disease presenting simultaneously with polymyositis and myasthenia gravis. Rinsho Shinkeigaku 2001; 41:503–506.
177. Leano AM, Miller K, White AC. Chronic graft-versus-host disease-related polymyositis as a cause of respiratory failure following allogeneic bone marrow transplant. Bone Marrow Transplant 2000; 26:1117–1120.
178. Parker PM, Openshaw H, Forman SJ. Myositis associated with chronic graft-versus-host dis-ease. Curr Opin Rheumatol 1997; 9:513–519.
179. Kaushik S, Flagg E, Wise CM, Hadfield G, McCarty JM. Granulomatous myositis: a mani-festation of chronic graft-versus-host disease. Skeletal Radiol 2002; 31:226–229.
180. Sale GE, McDonald GB, Shulman HM, Thomas ED. Gastrointestinal graft-versus-host disease in man. Am J Surg Patholo 1979; 3:291–299.
181. Snover DC, Weisdorf SA, Vercelloti GM, et al. A histopathologic study of gastric and small intestinal GVHD following allogeneic BMT. Hum Pathol 1985; 16:387–392.
182. Snover DC. Graft-versus-host disease of the gastrointestinal tract. Am J Surg Pathol 1990; 14:101–108.
183. McDonald GB, Sullivan KM KM, Schuffler MD, et al. Esophageal abnormalities in chronic graft-versus-host disease in humans. Gastroenterology 1981; 80:914–921.
184. McDonald GB, Sullivan KM, Plumley TF. Radiographic features of esophageal involvement in chronic graft-versus-host disease. Am J Roentgenol 1984; 142:501–506.
185. Ferrara JLM, Degg HJ. Graft vs host disease. N Engl J Med 1991; 324:667–674.
186. Akpek G, Chinratanalab W, Lee LA, Torbenson M, Hallick JP, Anders V, Vogelsang GB. Gastrointestinal involvement in chronic graft-versus-host disease: a clinicopathologic study. Biol Blood Marrow Transplant 2003; 9:46–51.
187. Eagle DA, Gian V, Lauwers GY, Manivel JC, Moreb JS, Mastin S, Wingard JR. Gastroparesis following bone marrow transplantation. Bone Marrow Transplant. 2001; 28:59–62.
188. Akpek G, Valladares JL, Lee L, Margolis J, Vogelsang GB. Pancreatic insufficiency in patients with chronic graft-versus-host disease. Bone Marrow Transplant 2001; 27:163–166.
189. Patey-Mariaud de Serre N, Reijasse D, Verkarre V, Canioni D, Colomb V, Haddad E, Brousse N. Chronic intestinal graft-versus-host disease: clinical, histological and immunohistochem-ical analysis of 17 children. Bone Marrow Transplant 2002; 29:223–230.
190. Jacobsohn DA, Margolis J, Doherty J, Anders V, Vogelsang GB. Weight loss and malnu-trition in patients with chronic graftversus-host disease. Bone Marrow Transplant 2002; 29:231–236.
191. Zauner C, Rabitsch W, Schneeweiss B, Schiefermeier M, Greinix HT, Keil F, et al. Energy and substrate metabolism in patients with chronic extensive graft-versus-host disease. Trans-plantation 2001; 71:524–528.
192. Cheng J, Turksen K, Yu QC, Schreiber H, Teng M, Fuchs E. Cachexia and graft-vs.-host-dis-ease-type skin changes in keratin promoter-driven TNF alpha transgenic mice. Genes Dev 1992; 6:1444–1456.
193. Clark JG, Crawford SW, Madtes DK, Sullivan KM. Obstructive lung disease after allogeneic marrow transplantation. Clinical presentation and course. Ann Intern Med 1989; 111:368–376.
194. Clark JG, Schwartz DA, Flournoy N, Sullivan KM, et al. Risk factors for airflow obstruction in recipients of bone marrow transplants. Ann Intern Med 1987; 107:648–656.
195. Holland HK, Wingard JR, Beschorner WE, et al. Bronchiolitis obliterans in bone marrow transplantation and its relationship to chronic graft-versus-host disease and low serum IgG. Blood 1988; 72:621–628.

196. Boas SR, Noyes BE, Kurland G, et al. Pediatric lung transplantation of graft-versus-host disease following bone marrow transplantation. Chest 1994; 105:1584–1586.

197. Philit F, Wiesendanger T, Archimbaud E, Mornex JF, Brune J, Cordier JF. Post-transplant obstructive lung disease ("bronchiolitis obliterans"): a clinical comparative study of bone marrow and lung transplant patients. Eur Respira J 1995; 8:551–558.

198. Atkinson K, Norrie S, Chan P, et al. Hematopoietic progenitor cell function after HLA-identical sibling bone marrow transplantation: influence of chronic graft-versus-host disease. Int J Cell Clonning 1986; 4:203–220.

199. Hirabayashi N. Studies on graft-versus-host (GvH) reactions: I. Impairment of hematopoietic stroma in mice suffering from GvH disease. Exp Hematol 1981; 9:101–110.

200. Godder K, Pati AR, Abhyankar SH, et al. De novo chronic graft-versus-host disease presenting as hemolytic anemia following partially mismatched related donor bone marrow transplant. Bone Marrow Transplant 1997; 19:813–817.

201. Anasetti C, Rybka W, Sullivan KM, Banaji M, Slichter SJ. Graft-v-host diseasse is associated with autoimmune-like thrombocytopenia. Blood 1989; 73:1054–1058.

202. Sullivan KM, Witherspoon RP, Storb R, Weiden PL, Flournoy N, Dahilberg S, Deeg HJ, Sanders JE, Doney KC, Appelbaum FR, McGuffin R, McDonald GB, Meyers J, Schubert MM, Gauvreau J, Shulman HM, Sale GE, Anasetti C, Loughran TP, Strom S, Nims J, Thomas ED. Prednisone and azathioprine compared with prednisone and placebo for treatment of chronic graft-v-host disease: prognostic influence of prolonged thrombocytopenia after allogeneic marrow transplantation. Blood. 1988; 72:546–554.

203. Sullivan KM, Witherspoon RP, Storb R, Deeg HJ, Dahlberg S, Sanders JE, Appelbaum FR, Doney KC, Weiden PL, Anasetti C, Loughran TP, Hill R, Shields A, Yee G, Shulman HM, Nims J, Strom S, Thomas ED. Alternating-day cyclosporine and prednisone for treatment of high-risk chronic graft-v-host disease. Blood 1988; 72:555–561.

204. Akpek G, Zahurak ML, Piantadosi S, Margolis J, Doherty J, Davidson R, Vogelsang GB. Development of a prognostic model for grading chronic graft-versus-host disease. Blood. 2001; 97:1219–1226.

205. Seidler CW, Mills LE, Flowers ME, Sullivan KM, et al. Spontaneous factor VIII inhibitor occurring in association with chronic graft-versus-host disease. Am J Hematol 1994; 45:240–243.

206. Corson SL, Sullivan K, Batzer F, et al. Gynecologic manifestations of chronic graft-versus-host disease. Obstet Gynecol 1982; 60:488–492.

207. Seber A, Khan SP, Kersey JH. Unexplained effusions: association with allogeneic bone marrow transplantation and acute and chronic graft-versus-host disease. Bone Marrow Transplant 1996; 17:207–211.

208. Toren A, Nagler A. Massive pericardial effusion complicating the course of chronic graft-versus-host disease (chronic GVHD) in a child with acute lymphoblastic leukemia following allogeneic bone marrow transplantation. Bone Marrow Transplant 1997; 20:805–807.

209. Perez Retortillo JA, Marco F, Richard C, Conde E, Manjon R, Bureo E, Iriondo A, Zubizarreta A. Pneumococcal pericarditis with cardiac tamponade in a patient with chronic graft-versus-host disease. Bone Marrow Transplant 1998; 21:299–300.

210. Gomez-Garcia P, Herrera-Arroyo C, Torres-Gomez A, et al. Renal impairement in chronic graft-versus-host disease: a report of two cases. Bone Marrow Transplant 1988; 3:357–362.

211. Socie G, Selimi F, Sedel L, et al. Avascular necrosis of bone after allogeneic bone marrow transplantation. Clinical findings, incidence and risk factors. Br J Haematol 1994; 86:624–628.

212. Kami M, Kanda Y, Sasaki M, Takeda N, Tanaka Y, Saito T, Ogawa S, Honda H, Chiba S, Mitani K, Hirai H, Yazaki Y. Phimosis as a manifestation of chronic graft-versus-host disease after allogeneic bone marrow transplantation. Bone Marrow Transplant 1998; 21:721–723.

213. Grigg AP, Underhill C, Russell J, Sale G. Peyronie's disease as a complication of chronic graft versus host disease. Hematology 2002; 7:165–168.
214. Atkinson K, Horowitz MM, Gale RP, et al. for the Advisory Committee of the International Bone Marrow Transplant Registry. Consensus among bone marrow transplanters for diagnosis, grading and treatment of chronic graft-versus-host disease. Bone Marrow Transplant 1989; 4:247–254.
215. Lee SJ, Vogelsang G, Gilman A, et al. A survey of diagnosis, management, and grading of chronic GVHD. Biol Blood Marrow Transplant 2002; 8:32–39.
216. Arora M, Burns LJ, Davies SM, et al. Chronic graft versus host disease: a prospective cohort study [abstr]. Blood 2001; 98(suppl 1):1667a.
217. Wingard JR, Piantadosi S, Vogelsang GB, et al. Predictors of death from chronic graft-versus-host disease after bone marrow transplantation. Blood 1989; 74:1428–1435.
218. Pavletic S, Tarantolo S, Lynch J, et al. Chronic graft-versus-host disease after allogeneic blood stem cell or bone marrow transplantation: factors determining the onset and survival [abstr]. Proc Am Soc Clin Oncol 1999; 18(suppl):201a.
219. Morton AJ, Gooley T, Hansen JA, et al. Impact of pre-transplant interferon alpha (IFNα) on outcome of unrelated donor marrow transplants for chronic myeloid leukemia (CML) in first chronic phase [abstr]. Blood 1997; 90(suppl):123a.
220. Gaziev D, Lucarelli G, Polchi P, et al. A three or more drug combination as effective therapy for moderate or severe chronic graft-versus-host disease. Bone Marrow Transplant 2001; 27:45–51.
221. Akpek G. Clinical grading in chronic graft-versus-host disease: is it time for change? Leuk Lymphoma 2002; 43:1211–1220.
222. Akpek G, Lee SJ, Flowers ME, Pavletic SZ, Arora M, Lee S, Piantadosi S, Guthrie KA, Lynch JC, Takatu A, Horowitz MM, Antin JH, Weisdorf DJ, Martin PJ, Vogelsang GB. Performance of a new clinical grading system for chronic graft-versus-host disease: a multi-center study. Blood 2003; 102:802–809.
223. Kurtzberg J, Laughlin M, Graham ML, et al. Placental blood as a source of hematopoietic stem cells for transplantation into unrelated recipients. N Engl J Med 1996; 335: 157–166.
224. Gluckman E, Rocha V, Boyer-Chammard A, et al. Outcome of cord-blood transplantation from related and unrelated donors. Eurocord Transplant Group and the European Blood and Marrow Transplantation Group. N Engl J Med 1997; 337:373–381.
225. Marmont AM, Horowitz MM, Gale RP, et al. T-cell depletion of HLA-identical transplants in leukemia. Blood 1991; 78:2120–2130.
226. Ash RC, Casper JT, Chitambar CR, et al. Successful allogeneic transplantation of T-cell depleted bone marrow from closely HLA-matched unrelated donors. N Engl J Med 1990; 323:485–494.
227. Santos GW, Tutschka PJ, Brookmeyer R, et al. Cyclosporine plus methylprednisolone versus cyclophosphamide plus methylprednisolone as prophylaxis for graft-versus-host disease: a randomized double blind study in patients undergoing allogeneic marrow transplantation. Clin Transplant 1987; 1:21–28.
228. Storb R, Deeg HJ, Pepe M, et al. Graft-versus-host disease prevention by methotrexate combined with cyclosporine compared to methotrexate alone in patients given marrow grafts for severe aplastic anemia: long-term follow-up of a controlled trial. Br J Haematol 1989; 72:567–572.
229. Sullivan KM, Storb R, Witherspoon RP, et al. Deletion of immunosuppressive prophylaxis after marrow transplantation increases hyperacute graft-versus-host disease but does not influence chronic graft-versus-host disease or relapse in patients with advanced leukemia. Clin Transplant 1989; 3:5–11.
230. Storb R, Leisenring W, Anasetti C, et al. Mathotrexate and cyclosporine for graft-versus-host disease prevention: What length of therapy with cyclosporine? Biol Blood and Marrow Transplant 1996; 2:86–92.

231. Kumar S, Chen MG, Gastineau DA, Gertz MA, Inwards DJ, Lacy MQ, Tefferi A, Harmsen WS, Litzow MR. Prophylaxis of graft-versus-host disease with cyclosporine-prednisone is associated with increased risk of chronic graft-versus-host disease. Bone Marrow Transplant 2001; 27:1133–1140.

232. Nash RA, Pineiro LA, Storb R, et al. FK506 in combination with methotrexate for the prevention of graft-versus-host disease after marrow transplantation from matched unrelated donors. Blood 1996; 88:3634–3641.

233. Ogawa H, Soma T, Hosen N, Tatekawa T, et al. Combination of tacrolimus, methotrexate, and methylprednisolone prevents acute but not chronic graft-versus-host disease in unrelated bone marrow transplantation. Transplantation 2002; 74:236–243.

234. Chao NJ, Parker PM, Niland JC, et al. Paradoxical effect of thalidomide prophylaxis on chronic graft-versus-host disease. Biol Blood Marrow Transplant 1996; 2:86–92.

235. Sullivan KM, Kopecky KJ, Jacom J, et al. Immunomodulatory and antimicrobial efficacy of intravenous immunoglobulin in bone marrow transplantation. N Engl J Med 1990; 323:705–712.

236. Sullivan KM, Mori M, Sanders J, et al. Late complications of allogeneic and autologous marrow transplantation. Bone Marrow Transplant 1992; 10:127–134.

237. Okamoto I, Kohno K, Tanimoto T, Iwaki K, Ishihara T, Akamatsu S, Ikegami H, Kurimoto M. IL-18 prevents the development of chronic graft-versus-host disease in mice. J Immunol 2000; 164(11):6067–6074.

238. Weiden PL, Sullivan KM, Flournoy N, Storb R, et al. Antileukemic effect of chronic graft-versus-host disease. Contribution to improved survival after allogeneic marrow transplantation. N Engl J Med 1981; 304:1529–1533.

239. Brunet S, Urbano-Ispizua A, Ojeda E, et al. Favourable effect of the combination of acute and chronic graft-versus- host disease on the outcome of allogeneic peripheral blood stem cell transplantation for advanced haematological malignancies. Br J Haematol 2001; 114: 544–550.

240. Horowitz MM, Gale RP, Sondel PM, et al. Graft-versus-leukemia reactions after bone marrow transplantation. Blood 1990; 75:555–562.

241. Sullivan KM, Weiden PL, Storb R, et al. Influence of acute and chronic graft-versus-host disease on relapse and survival after bone marrow transplantation from HLA-identical siblings as treatment of acute and chronic leukemia. Blood 1989; 73:1720–1728 [published erratum appears in Blood 1989 Aug 15; 74(3):1180].

242. Pichert G, Roy DC, Gonin R, et al. Distinct patterns of minimal residual disease associated with graft- versus-host disease after allogeneic bone marrow transplantation for chronic myelogenous leukemia. J Clin Oncol 1995; 13:1704–1713.

243. Sullivan KM, Deeg HJ, Sanders JE, et al. Late complications after marrow transplantation. Semin Hematol 1984; 21:53–56.

244. Flowers MED. Traditional treatment of chronic graft-versus-host disease. Blood Marrow Transplant Rev 2002; 12:5–8.

245. Koc S, Leisenring W, Flowers ME, Anasetti C, Deeg HJ, Nash RA, Sanders JE, Witherspoon RP, Storb R, Appelbaum FR, Martin PJ. Therapy for chronic graft-versus-host disease: a randomized trial comparing cyclosporine plus prednisone versus prednisone alone. Blood 2002; 100:48–51.

246. Sampaio EP, Sarno EN, Galilly R, et al. Thalidomide selectively inhibits tumor necrosis factor alpha production by stimulated human monocytes. J Exp Med 1991; 173:699–703.

247. Vogelsang GB, Farmer ER, Hess AD, et al. Thalidomide for the treatment of chronic graft-versus-host disease. N Engl J Med 1992; 326:1055–1058.

248. Arora M, Wagner JE, Davies SM, Blazar BR, Defor T, Enright H, Miller WJ, Weisdorf DF. Randomized clinical trial of thalidomide, cyclosporine, and prednisone versus cyclosporine and prednisone as initial therapy for chronic graft-versus-host disease. Biol Blood Marrow Transplant 2001; 7:265–273.

249. Sullivan KM, Witherspoon RP. Cyclosporine treatment of chronic graft-versus-host disease following allogeneic bone marrow transplantation. Transplantation 1990; 22:1336–1338.

250. Parker PM, Chao N, Nademanee A, et al. Thalidomide as salvage therapy for chronic graft-versus-host disease. Blood 1995; 86:3604–3609.

251. Browne PV, Weisdorf DJ, DeFor T, Miller WJ, Davies SM, Filipovich A, McGlave PB, Ramsay NK, Wagner J, Enright H. Response to thalidomide therapy in refractory chronic graft-versus-host disease. Bone Marrow Transplant 2000; 26:865–869.

252. Akpek G, Lee SM, Anders V, Vogelsang GB. A high-dose pulse steroid regimen for controlling active chronic graft-versus-host disease. Biol Blood Marrow Transplant 2001; 7: 495–502.

253. Tzakis AG, Abu-Elmagd K, Fung JJ, Bloom NB, Greif F, Starzl TE. FK506 rescue in chronic graft-versus-host disease after bone marrow transplantation. Transplant Proc 1991; 23:3225–3227.

254. Mookerjee B, Altomonte V, Vogelsang G. Salvage therapy for refractory chronic graft-versus-host disease with mycophenolate mofetil and tacrolimus. Bone Marrow Transplant 1999; 24:517–520.

255. Carnevale-Schianca F, Martin P, Sullivan K, Flowers M, Gooley T, Anasetti C, Deeg HJ, Furlong T, McSweeney P, Storb R, Nash RA. Changing from cyclosporine to tacrolimus as salvage therapy for chronic graft-versus-host disease. Biol Blood Marrow Transplant 2000; 6:613–620.

256. Ogawa Y, Okamoto S, Kuwana M, Mori T, Watanabe R, Nakajima T, Yamada M, Mashima Y, Tsubota K, Oguchi Y. Successful treatment of dry eye in two patients with chronic graft-versus-host disease with systemic administration of FK506 and corticosteroids. Cornea 2001; 20:430–434.

257. Koc S, Leisenring W, Flowers ME, Anasetti C, Deeg HJ, Nash RA, Sanders JE, Witherspoon RP, Appelbaum FR, Storb R, Martin PJ. Thalidomide for treatment of patients with chronic graft-versus-host disease. Blood 2000; 96:3995–3996.

258. Rovelli A, Arrigo C, Nesi F, Balduzzi A, Nicolini B, Locasciulli A, Vassallo E, Miniero R, Uderzo C. The role of thalidomide in the treatment of refractory chronic graft-versus-host disease following bone marrow transplantation in children. Bone Marrow Transplant 1998; 21:577–581.

259. Hymes SR, Morison WL, Farmer ER, Waters LL, Tutschka PJ, Santos GW. Methoxsalen and ultraviolet A radiation in treatment of chronic cutaneous graft-versus-host reaction. Acad Dermatol 1986; 12:30–37.

260. Atkinson K, Weller P, Ryman W, Biggs J. PUVA therapy for drug resistant graft-versus-host disease. Bone Marrow Transplant 1986; 1:227–236.

261. Vogelsang GB, Wolf D, Altomonte V, et al. Treatment of chronic graft-versus-host disease with ultraviolet radiation and psorelen (PUVA). Bone Marrow Transplant 1996; 17:1061–1067.

262. Greinix HT, Volc-Platzer B, Rabitsch W, Gmeinhart B, Guevara-Pineda C, Kalhs P, Krutmann J, Honigsmann H, Ciovica M, Knobler RM. Successful use of extracorporeal photochemotherapy in the treatment of severe acute and chronic GVHD. Blood 1998; 92:3098–3104.

263. Child FJ, Ratnavel R, Watkins P, Samson D, Apperley J, Ball J, Taylor P, Russell-Jones R. Extracorporeal photopheresis (ECP) in the treatment of chronic graft-versus-host disease (GVHD). Bone Marrow Transplant 1999; 23:881–887.

264. Foss FM, Görgün G, Miller KB. Extracorporeal photopheresis in chronic graft-versus-host disease. Bone Marrow Transplant 2002; 29:719–725.

265. Owsianowski M, Gollinck H, Siegert W, et al. Successful treatment of chronic graft-versus-host disease with extracorporeal photopheresis. Bone Marrow Transplant 1994; 14: 845–848.

266. Rosetti F, Zulian F, Dall'Amico R, et al. Extracorporeal photochemotherapy as single therapy for extensive, cutaneous, chronic graft-versus-host disease. Transplantation 1995; 59:149–151.

267. Alcindor T, Görgün G, Miller KB, Roberts TF, Sprague K, Schenkein DP, Foss FM. Immunomodulatory effects of extracorporeal photochemotherapy in patients with extensive chronic graft-versus-host disease. Blood 2001; 98(5):1622–1625.

268. Görgün G, Miller KB, Foss FM. Immunologic mechanisms of extracorporeal photochemotherapy in chronic graft-versus-host disease. Blood 2002; 100:941–947.

269. Socie G, Devergie A, Cosset JM, et al. Low dose (one gray) total lymphoid irradiation for extensive, drug resistant chronic graft-versus-host disease. Transplantation 1990; 49:657–658.

270. Bullorsky EO, Shanley CM, Stemmelin GR, Musso A, Rabinovich O, Ceresetto J, Quiroga L. Total lymphoid irradiation for treatment of drug resistant chronic GVHD. Bone Marrow Transplant 1993; 11:75–76.

271. Guardiola P, Fernandez G, Girinski T, Socie G, Ribaud P, Esperou H, Gluckman E, Devergie A. Low-dose Thoracoabdominal irradiation for the treatment of refractory chronic GVHD [abstr]. Blood 2002; 100(suppl I):3341a.

272. Anasetti C, Hansen JA, Waldmann TA, Appelbaum FR, Davis J, Deeg HJ, Doney K, Martin PJ, Nash R, Storb R R, et al. Treatment of acute graft-versus-host disease with humanized anti-Tac: an antibody that binds to the interleukin-2 receptor. Blood 1994; 84: 1320–1327.

273. Willenbacher W, Basara N, Blau IW, Fauser AA, Kiehl MG. Treatment of steroid refractory acute and chronic graft-versus-host disease with daclizumab. Br J Haematol 2001; 112:820–823.

274. Herve P, Racadot E, Wijdenes J, Flesch M, Tiberghien, Bordigoni P, Holler E, Powles M, Bourdeau M, Wilmer E E, et al. Monoclonal anti TNF alpha antibody in the treatment of acute GvHD refractory both to corticosteroids and anti IL-2 R antibody [abstr]. Bone Marrow Transplant 1991; 7(suppl 2):149.

275. Couriel DR, Saliba R, Hicks K, Cohen A, Ippoliti C, Neumann J, Giralt S, de Lima MJ, Champlin R. TNF-Alpha inhibition for the treatment of chronic GVHD. Controlled prospective trials are needed to assess the role of anti-TNF antibody treatement in chronic GVHD [abstr]. Blood 2002; 100(suppl I):3343a.

276. Chiang KY, Abhyankar S, Bridges K, Godder K, Henslee-Downey JP. Recombinant human tumor necrosis factor receptor fusion protein as complementary treatment for chronic graft-versus-host disease. Transplantation 2002; 73:665–667.

277. Ratanatharathorn V, Carson E, Reynolds C, Ayash LJ, Levine J, Yanik G, Silver SM, Ferrara JL, Uberti JP. Anti-CD20 chimeric monoclonal antibody treatment of refractory immune-mediated thrombocytopenia in a patient with chronic graft-versus-host disease. Ann Intern Med 2000; 133:275–279.

278. Margolis J, Vogelsang G. Chronic graft-versus-host disease. J Hematother Stem Cell Res 2000; 9:339–346.

279. Vogelsang GB, Hess AD. Rapamycin effects on immunologic reconstitution. Transplant Proc 1993; 25:727–728.

280. Benito AI, Furlong T, Martin PJ, et al. Sirolimus (rapamycin) for the treatment of steroid-refractory acute graft-versus-host disease. Transplantation 2001; 72:1924–1929.

281. Couriel DR, Hicks K, Saliba R, Cohen A, Ippoliti C, Donato M, Paolo A, Giralt S, Khouri I, Hosing C, de Lima M, Andersson B, Neumann J, Champlin R. Sirolimus (rapamycin) for treatment of steroid-refractory chronic graft-versus-host disease. Blood 2002; 100(suppl I):3343a.

282. Arat M, Ilhan O, Iayan EA, Celebi H, Koc H, Akan H. Treatment of extensive chronic sclerodermatous graft-versus-host disease with high-dose immunosuppressive therapy and CD34+ autologous stem cell rescue. Blood 2001; 98:892–893.

283. Menillo SA, Goldberg SL, McKiernan P, Pecora AL. Intraoral psoralen ultraviolet A irradiation (PUVA) treatment of refractory oral chronic graft-versus-host disease following allogeneic stem cell transplantation. Bone Marrow Transplant 2001; 28:807–808.

284. Marcellus DC, Altomonte VL, Farmer ER, Horn TD, Freemer CS, Grant J, Vogelsang GB. Etretinate therapy for refractory sclerodermatous chronic graft-versushost disease. Blood 1999; 93:66–70.

285. Lee SJ, Wegner SA, McGarigle CJ, Bierer BE, Antin JH. Treatment of chronic graft-versus-host disease with clofazimine. Blood 1997; 89:2298–2302.

286. Gilman AL, Beams F, Tefft M, Mazumder A. The effect of hydroxychloroquine on alloreactivity and its potential use for graft-versus-host disease. Bone Marrow Transplant 1996; 17:1069–1075.

287. Gilman AL, Chan KW, Mogul A, Morris C, Goldman FD, Boyer M, Cirenza E, Mazumder A, Gehan E, Cahill R, Frankel S, Schultz K. Hydroxychloroquine for the treatment of chronic graft-versus-host disease. Biol Blood Marrow Transplant 2000; 6:327–334.

288. Kulkarni S, Powles R, Treleaven J, Riley U, Singhal S, Horton C, Sirohi B, Bhagwati N, Meller S, Saso R, Mehta J. Chronic graft versus host disease is associated with long-term risk for pneumococcal infections in recipients of bone marrow transplants. Blood 2000; 95:3683–3686.

289. Sullivan KM, Meyers JD, Flournoy N, Storb R, Thomas ED. Early and late interstitial pneumonia following human bone marrow transplantation. Int J Cell Clonning 1986; 4:107–121.

290. Ljungman P, Fridell E, Lonnqvist B, et al. Efficacy and safety of vaccination of marrow transplant recipients with a live attenuated measles, mumps, and rubella vaccine. J Infect Dis 1989; 159:610–615.

291. Guidelines for preventing opportunistic infections among hematopoietic stem cell transplant recipients. Biol Blood Marrow Transplant 2000; 6:659–713; 715; 717–727.

292. Knobler HY, Sagher U, Pled IJ. Tolerance to donor-type skin in the recipient of bone marrow allograft. Transplantation 1985; 40:223–225.

293. Hart DE, Simko M, Harris E. How to produce moisture chamber eyeglasses for the dry eye patient. J Am Optom Assoc 1994; 65:517–522.

294. Murphy PT, Sivakumaran M, Fahy G, et al. Successful use of topical retinoic acid in severe dry eye due to chronic graft versus host disease. Bone Marrow Transplant 1996; 18:641–642.

295. Singhal S, Powles R, Treleaven J, Rattenbury H, Mehta J. Pilocarpine hydrochloride for symptomatic relief of xerostomia due to chronic graft-versus-host disease of total body irradiation after bone marrow transplantation for hematologic malignancies. Leukemia Lymphoma 1997; 24:539–543.

296. Nagler RM, Nagler A. Pilocarpine hydrochloride relieves xerostomia in chronic graft-versus-host disease: a sialometrical study. Bone Marrow Transplant 1999; 23:1007–1011.

297. Adams F, Messner H. Neuropharmacologic therapy of the neuromuscular manifestations of graft-versus-host disease [abstr]. Proc Am Soc Clin Oncol 1987; 6:145.

298. Fried RH, Murakami CS, Fisher LD, Willson RA, Sullivan KM, et al. Ursodeoxycholic acid treatment of refractory chronic graft-versus-host disease of the liver. Ann Intern Med 1992; 116:624–629.

299. Stern JM, Chestnut CH III, Bruemmer B, et al. Bone density loss during treatment of chronic graft-versus-host disease. Bone Marrow Transplant 1996; 17:395–400.

300. Fink JC, Leisenring WM, Sullivan KM, Sherrard DJ, et al. Avascular necrosis following bone marrow transplantation: a case control study. Bone 1998; 22:67–71.

301. Beredjiklian PK, Drummond DS, Dormans JP, Davidson RS, Brock GT, August C. Orthopaedic manifestations of chronic graft-versus-host disease. J Pediatr Orthop 1998; 18:572–575.

302. Zecca M, Prete A, Rondelli R, Lanino E, Balduzzi A, Messina C, Fagioli F, Porta F, Favre C, Pession A, Locatelli F. AIEOP-BMT Group. Italian Association for Pediatric Hematology and Oncology-Bone Marrow Transplant. Chronic graft-versus-host disease in children: incidence, risk factors, and impact on outcome. Blood 2002; 100:1192–1200.

303. Kondo M, Kojima S, Horibe K, Kato K, Matsuyama T. Risk factors for chronic graft-versus-host disease after allogeneic stem cell transplantation in children. Bone Marrow Transplant 2001; 27:727–730.

304. Wagner JE, Barker JN, DeFor TE, et al. Transplantation of unrelated donor umbilical cord blood in 102 patients with malignant and nonmalignant diseases: influence of CD34 cell dose and HLA disparity on treatment-related mortality and survival. Blood 2002; 100:1611–1618.

305. Sanders JE. Graft-vs.-host disease. In: Burakoff SJ, Deeg HJ, Ferrara J, Atkinson K, eds. Effects of Chronic Graft-vs-Host Disease on Growth and Development. New York: Marcel Dekker, 1990: 665–680.

306. Witherspoon RP, Fisher LD, Schoch G, et al. Secondary cancers after bone marrow transplantation for leukemia or aplastic anemia. N Engl J Med 1989; 321:784–789.

307. Witherspoon RP, Storb R, Pepe M, Longton G, et al. Cumulative incidence of secondary solid malignant tumors in aplastic anemia patients given marrow grafts after conditioning with chemotherapy alone. Blood 1992; 79:289–292.

308. Deeg HJ, Socie G, Schoch G, et al. Malignancies after marrow transplantation for aplastic anemia and fanconi anemia: a joint Seattle and Paris analysis of results in 700 patients. Blood 1996; 87:386–392.

309. Curtis RE, Rowlings PA, Deeg HJ, et al. Solid cancers after bone marrow transplantation. N Engl J Med 1997; 336:897–904.

310. Gmeinhart B, Hinterberger W, Greinix HT, Rabitsch W, Kirnbauer R, Reiter E, Volc-Platzer B. Anaplastic squamous cell carcinoma (SCC) in a patient with chronic cutaneous graft-versus-host disease (GVHD). Bone Marrow Transplant 1999; 23:1197–1199.

311. Otsubo H, Yokoe H, Miya T, Atsuta F, Miura N, Tanzawa H, Sato K. Gingival squamous cell carcinoma in a patient with chronic graft-versus-host disease. Oral Surg Oral Med Oral Pathol Oral Radiol Endod 1997; 84:171–174.

21

Recent Advances and Future Directions

PAVAN REDDY, KENNETH R. COOKE, and JAMES L. M. FERRARA

University of Michigan Comprehensive Cancer Center, Ann Arbor, Michigan, U.S.A.

H. JOACHIM DEEG

Fred Hutchinson Cancer Research Center
and University of Washington, Seattle, Washington, U.S.A.

The final chapter of this volume has been compiled in an effort to present advances made in the area of graft-vs.-host disease (GVHD) and graft-vs.-leukemia (GVL) research while in production. The first section focuses on the experimental advances made with respect to the immunobiology of GVHD, the second on advances in understanding GVL activity, and the third section reviews relevant therapeutic and prognostic advances that have been made in clinical GVHD.

I. EXPERIMENTAL ADVANCES IN THE PATHOPHYSIOLOGY OF ACUTE GVHD

A. Costimulatory Pathways and Alloreactivity

As discussed in detail in Chapter 4, costimulatory signals are essential for many T-cell functions, since without these signals, T cells die or become unresponsive (1,2). Until recently, strategies to reduce GVHD by blocking costimulation of donor T cells have focused primarily on interactions between CD28/CTLA4–B7.1/B7.2 or between CD40–CD40L (3–6). Growing evidence suggests that several other members of the tumor necrosis factor receptor (TNFR) family including OX40 (CD134), 4-1BB (CD137), and CD27 are also important for the generation of T-cell responses (2). In contrast to CD28, the expression of these molecules is either rapidly (within hours) induced or greatly increased on the T-cell surface following recognition of antigen, and appears to provide signals that permit continued cell division and/or prevent excessive cell death. Thus, these molecules might control the absolute number of effector T cells generated at the peak of the immune response (2). Recent studies demonstrate that some of these costimulatory molecules play important roles in modulating acute GVHD.

OX40 (CD134) is expressed on activated T cells; its ligand, OX40 ligand (OX40L), is expressed on dendritic cells, B cells, and activated endothelial cells (7). Blazar and colleagues used an antagonistic anti-OX40L monoclonal antibody (mAb), donor deficient in OX40 and recipient deficient in OX40L, to interrupt OX40-OX40L interactions and observed less GVHD in MHC mismatched murine models (8). Blockade of OX40-OX40L interactions also reduced GVHD mortality when both Stat-6$-/-$ (Th2-defective) and Stat-4$-/-$ (Th1-defective) donors were used, indicating that the protection from GVHD by OX40 blockade did not require Stat-4 or Stat-6 signaling (8).

While the coreceptors OX40-OX40L transduce stimulatory signals in T cells, the programmed death-1 (PD-1) receptor has been shown to transduce negative or regulatory signals (9). Engagement of PD-1 with its ligand PD-L1 (B7-H1) or PD-L2 (B7-DC) recruits a *src* homology 2-domain–containing tyrosine phosphatase 2 (SHP-2) to the phosphorylated tyrosine residue in the cytoplasmic region of PD-1. Blockade of PD-1 pathway during GVHD was studied by Blazar and colleagues (10) utilizing three distinct approaches: PD-L1.Fc, anti-PD-1 mAb, and PD-1$-/-$ donor cells. They demonstrated that blockade of the PD-1 pathway increased the release of pro-inflammatory cytokines, particularly interferon-gamma (IFNγ) and accelerated GVHD mortality in multiple strain combinations. GVHD lethality was not dependent on perforin/FasL-mediated cytolysis. Coblockade of CTLA-4 and PD-1 augmented GVHD, indicating that these pathways were not fully redundant in modulating GVHD (10). These data thus suggest that ligation of the PD-1 receptor may represent a novel approach for preventing GVHD.

LIGHT is another T-cell costimulatory molecule that belongs to the TNF superfamily. Previous work has shown that lymphotoxin beta receptor-Ig (LTβR-Ig) can block LIGHT and ameliorate lethal GVHD in a B6 $\rightarrow$ B6D2F1 mouse model (11). A more recent study by Tamada and colleagues demonstrated that infusion of mAb against CD40 ligand (CD40L) increases the efficacy of LTβR-Ig, leading to complete prevention of GVHD (12). They also demonstrated that cytotoxic T lymphocytes (CTL) specific for alloantigen become anergic and persist in tolerized mice as a result of such costimulatory blockade.

B. Memory T Cells

Recent studies have illuminated the role of naïve and memory T-cell subsets in GVHD. Two groups independently studied the effect of CD62L+ (naïve) and CD62L$-$ (memory) T cells on acute GVHD after experimental allogeneic bone marrow transplant (BMT) (13,14). Both groups demonstrated that naïve (CD62L+) T cells were alloreactive in vitro and caused GVHD in vivo, but that the memory (CD62L$-$) T cells were neither alloreactive nor caused GVHD in multiple donor/recipient strain combinations. This effect was not due to the increased number of CD4+CD25+ regulatory T cells in the memory T-cell fraction, because depletion of CD25+ cells from the memory cell population did not result in GVHD. Memory T cells also contributed to T-cell reconstitution after BMT by peripheral expansion (14). Importantly, CD62L$-$ memory T cells from donors previously primed with a tumor cell line (BCL1) inhibited the growth of tumors in vivo, but did not induce GVHD in third-party recipients (14). Furthermore, memory T cells from a donor immunized to chicken γ-globulin (CGG) retained CGG-specific memory when the recipient of those memory T cells was immunized with CGG (13).

Together these studies suggest that elimination of naive cells and retention of memory cells in a donor graft may reduce GVHD while preserving donor specific immunity and GVL responses. An important caveat to these studies is that these experiments used naïve donor mice that had been housed in a pathogen-free environment and therefore possessed small numbers of memory T cells. By contrast, it is likely that the human donors will have been exposed to various antigenic stimuli and will possess a much larger repertoire of memory T cells that might cross-react to the recipient's alloantigens. It should also be noted that these data contradict other studies in solid organ transplant animal model systems, where memory T cells are resistant to tolerance induction (15). Furthermore, it is not known whether the behavior of human memory T cells parallels that of murine memory T cells in their migratory, functional, and cytolytic capabilities. Thorough evaluation of human memory T cell subsets and the potential suppression of undesirable memory responses will need evaluation prior to the initiation of clinical trials.

C. Regulatory T Cells

Several studies have demonstrated a critical role for donor CD4+CD25+ regulatory T (Treg) cells in the prevention of acute GVHD. The balance of donor-type CD4+CD25+ and conventional CD4+CD25− T cells can determine the outcome of acute GVHD (16–18). The ability of Treg cells to suppress GVHD after BMT depends in part on interleukin (IL)-10 production and/or CD28 expression, but the mechanisms that generate these cells in vivo are not known (16–18). Ex vivo expanded CD4+CD25+ regulatory T cells obtained after stimulation by allogeneic recipient-type antigen-presenting cells also modulate GVHD (6,19). Edinger and coworkers have investigated the effect of these cells on GVL responses in a series of experiments using a BALB/c into B6 allogeneic BMT model together with BCL1 ($H2^b$) and A20 ($H2^b$) tumor cell lines (20). They found that donor CD4+CD25+ regulatory T cells ($H2^d$) suppress the early expansion of alloreactive donor T cells and their capacity to induce GVHD without abrogating graft-vs.-tumor (GVT) effect or function against these tumors (20).

In a separate study Korngold and colleagues analyzed whether donor CD4+CD25+ regulatory T cells could control ongoing GVHD. Such an approach would provide an initial period of time during which antihost alloreactive responses occurred and thereby eliminated residual leukemia cells (21). Infusion of in vitro expanded donor CD4+CD25+ cells early after BMT (day +2) in the haploidentical C3H → B6 × C3HF1 model prevented GVHD mortality. Moreover, in a minor histocompatibility antigen-disparate model (B10.BR → CBA) of GVHD mediated by CD8 T cells, lethal disease was prevented by a single infusion of freshly isolated donor CD4+CD25+ cells administered as late as 10 days after BMT (21). Importantly, this infusion did not interfere with GVL response against MMCBA myeloid leukemia (21). Collectively, these observations suggest that cellular therapy with CD4+CD25+ Treg cells may be able to control GVHD and separate it from GVT activity.

Two recent studies have suggested the possibility that regulatory T cells of a different phenotype can also reduce GVHD. Brenner and colleagues demonstrated that activation of the Notch pathway generates T cells capable of regulating alloantigen responses (22). Activation of T cells by allogeneic antigen-presenting cells (APC) in the presence of Jagged (the ligand for Notch) induces regulatory T cells specific for alloantigen even though responses to other antigens are unaffected. These T cells regulated GVHD but retained activity towards infectious organisms; the effect on GVL was not evaluated. In another study, Chen et al. demonstrated that CD4+ T cells recovered from primary mixed lymphocyte reaction (MLR) cultures treated with IL-10 and transforming growth factor-beta (TGFβ) are regulatory and significantly reduce GVHD when injected together with naïve alloreactive CD4+ T cells into major histocompatibility class (MHC)II disparate recipients (23). Interestingly, depletion of CD25+ cells had no effect on generation of this regulatory activity (23).

While the aforementioned experimental studies have shown that CD4+CD25+ regulatory T cells can ameliorate GVHD following experimental allogeneic BMT, the activity of this cell population in the clinical setting is not known. A recent clinical study evaluated the relationship between donor CD4+CD25+ cells and GVHD in humans (24). The coexpression of CD25 on both CD4+ and CD8+ T cells was quantified in 60 matched sibling donor grafts, and the incidence of GVHD was evaluated in the recipients. In contrast to the murine studies, donor grafts containing larger numbers of CD4+ T cells coexpressing CD25 developed more GVHD than those with fewer CD4+25+ cells (9.26% vs. 2.22% $p = 0.004$). Furthermore, grafts containing fewer CD4+CD25+ and CD8+CD25+ T cells were less likely to cause acute GVHD, despite the fact that these donor-recipient pairs were similar to each other with respect to other relevant clinical variables (24). These data suggest that coexpression of CD4 and CD25 is insufficient to identify regulatory T cells in humans and show that an increased frequency and number of CD25+ T cells in donor grafts are associated with greater risks of GVHD after clinical BMT. It is likely that the precise role of regulatory T cells in clinical GVHD will depend upon better identification of these cells by specific molecular markers such as foxp3 and the ex vivo expansion of Treg in order to increase their number in the bone marrow inoculum.

D. Host Gamma/Delta T Cells

$\gamma\delta$ T cells are a subset of T lymphocytes that contribute to pathogen-specific immune responses (25). $\gamma\delta$ T cells are enriched in epithelial tissues, particularly the gastrointestinal (GI) tract and skin, and defects in $\gamma\delta$ T cells lead to organ-specific immunopathology (25). Leslie et al. demonstrated that the maturation of DCs by $\gamma\delta$ cells depends on cell contact and partially depends on TNF-α (26). Maeda et al. have observed that the absence of $\gamma\delta$ T cells in the host leads to a reduction in the severity of GVHD and to reduced T-cell activation in murine models across MHC barriers (27).

E. Dendritic Cells

Host-derived APCs are critical for the induction of GVHD (28,29). Dendritic cells (DC) are the most potent APC and are activated by pro-inflammatory cytokines, lipopolysaccharide (LPS), which enters the systemic circulation from a damaged intestinal mucosa, and necrotic cells that are damaged by recipient conditioning (30). These stimuli produce danger signals that cause maturation of DC and thereby facilitate subsequent T-cell activation (31). Sato et al. evaluated the role of immature DC in the regulation of GVHD (32). A single injection of immature DC with high levels of MHC molecules and extremely low levels of co-stimulatory molecules prevented donor T cells from inducing acute GVHD and preserved GVL effects, resulting in increased tumor-free survival. Immature DC also directly suppressed effector functions of in vivo primed allogeneic CD4+ and CD8+ T cells and blunted their responsiveness to restimulation in vitro. Furthermore, IL-10–producing CD4+CD25+ Treg cells were increased in immature DC-treated recipients. The depletion of CD25+ cells and the neutralization of IL-10, but not TGFβ, significantly impaired the ability of immature DC to prevent acute GVHD. Thus IL-10–producing CD4+CD25+ Treg cells were critical to the protective effect. Immature DC also induced tolerance more readily in CD4+ T cells compared to transplanted CD8+ T cells. The tolerized CD4+ T cells failed to cause acute GVHD, but maintained potent GVL effects (32).

Similar findings have recently been shown by Hill and colleagues, who found that progenipoiten-1 (a synthetic G-CSF and Flt-3 receptor agonist) and G-CSF expand a novel myeloid APC that is CD11b^{hi}Gr1^{lo} and induces profound tolerance to alloantigens via the generation of MHC class II-restricted, IL-10-producing, regulatory T cells (33). These cells are poor stimulators of allogeneic T-cell responses and differentiate into class II^{pos}, CD80/CD86^{pos}, CD40^{neg} APC during the induction of GVHD. Expansion of these cells was even greater when animals were treated with pegylated G-CSF, suggesting that mobilization of stem cells from healthy donors using agents like Neulasta may prove beneficial in reducing GVH reactions following allogeneic BMT.

Two human studies suggest that host APC might play a critical role in clinical GVHD. Munn et al. described a subset of human APC expressing indoleamine 2,3-dioxygenase (IDO) that inhibit T-cell proliferation (34). IDO suppresses T-cell activity by catabolizing the essential amino acid L-tryptophan (35–37). IDO expression may also play an important role in the prevention of fetal rejection by the placenta (34,35). Using RT-PCR, Steckel et al. compared IDO expression induced by interferon-gamma (IFNγ) on dendritic cells from patients who developed acute GVHD, pregnant women, and healthy volunteers (38). IDO expression was detected in all pregnant women, all volunteers, and 47 of 49 (96%) patients with a low-grade GVHD (grades 0–II) but in only 2 of 13 (16%) patients with grade III–IV GVHD. These data suggest that IDO expression by dendritic cells might be involved in the regulation of the severity of acute GVHD. In a separate study, Chan and colleagues observed that the persistence of host-type DC at day +100 post-BMT correlated with the development of severe acute and chronic GVHD ($p = 0.001$), suggesting that host APC may be critical for each of the processes (39).

F. Natural Killer Cells

Killer immunoglobulin-like receptors (KIR) on natural killer (NK) cells recognize groups of HLA class I alleles, and interaction between receptor and class I allele inhibits the activation of NK cells in a dominant fashion. Failure to recognize the appropriate KIR ligand on a stimulator cell leads to lack of the inhibitory signal and activates the NK cell, which eliminates the target cell (40). Donor NK1.1+ T cells have been shown to suppress GVHD in an IL-4–dependent manner (41,42). Strober and colleagues have now shown that noumyeloablative conditioning with total lymphoid irradiation (TLI) and anti-T-cell antibodies prevented acute GVHD in BALB/c mice recipients of allo BMT from allogeneic B6 donors (43). The reduction of GVHD was associated with a marked increase in the percentage of regulatory DX5+, NK 1.1+ T cells in the recipient spleen. The role of regulatory cells was confirmed using NK-cell–deficient CD1 (−/−) BALB/c hosts that were not protected from GVHD with this approach (43). These results suggest that conditioning regimens can be designed to reduce the severity of GVHD by inducing regulatory NK 1.1+T cells.

Studies of both clinical and experimental haploidentical hematopoietic transplants by Velardi and colleagues have shown a reduction of graft failure, GVHD, and relapse in those donor-recipient pairs with KIR ligand incompatibility in the GVH direction (44). A recent study by Giebel et al. made similar observations in 130 unrelated donor transplants (45). Four and half years after BMT, patients with KIR ligand incompatibility had higher probability of overall survival (87% vs. 48%; $p = 0.006$) and disease-free survival (87% vs. 39%; $p = 0.0007$) compared with those without KIR ligand incompatibility despite uniform GVHD prophylaxis between groups. Transplant-related mortality for the two groups was also significantly different (6% vs. 40%; $p = 0.01$). Relapse rates were 6% and 21% for patients receiving transplants with or without KIR ligand incompatibility, respectively ($p = 0.07$). All patients with myeloid malignancies receiving transplants from KIR ligand-disparate donors ($n = 13$) were alive and disease-free. Together, these data indicate that NK cell alloreactivity is associated with better outcome even after unrelated donor transplantation when (ATG) is used as part of GVHD prophylaxis.

A second by study Davies et al. also analyzed the effect of KIR ligand incompatibility in recipients of unrelated donor bone marrow transplants (46). One hundred and seventy-five patients were divided into those with and those without KIR ligand incompatibility, as described by Ruggeri et al. (44). Surprisingly, this study found no advantage for KIR ligand incompatibility. Several possibilities may account for these discrepant observations. The full haplotype-mismatched transplants reported by the Velardi and Giebel groups were performed using a high CD34+ cell dose for engraftment, combined with extensive T-cell depletion to prevent GVHD and no additional immunosuppression. Such transplants are typically associated with rapid recovery of NK cells and slow T-cell recovery. In contrast, the T-cell elutriation technique used in one third of the transplants in the study by Davies et al. typically yields only 2-log T-cell depletion, 100-fold less than the 4-log depletion achieved in the Velardi study. Because the donor grafts in the Davies study contained a larger number of T cells, the NK cell effects might have been obscured by donor T-cell effects and/or the immunosuppression necessary to prevent/control GVHD (46). Different kinetics of immune reconstitution might also have masked any potential role for NK-cell alloreactivity. Lastly, no functional assessment of the donor NK-cell repertoire was performed in the Davies study. It is therefore possible that stimulatory receptors, KIRs yet to be identified, or NK-cell receptors from other families (e.g., NKG2a/CD94 heterodimers) influenced the outcome of these unrelated donor transplants, superceding known KIR/KIR ligand interactions.

G. Cytokines

Th1 cytokines, particularly IFNγ, can amplify the "cytokine storm" of acute GVHD, but the role of Th1/Th2 polarization in acute GVHD is incompletely understood and controversial (47). In this regard, IL-18 is currently the only identified cytokine that can induce either Th1 or Th2 polarization depending upon the nature of the inflammatory stimulus and the immunological milieu (48). Using a parent $\rightarrow F_1$ ($p \rightarrow F_1$) murine BMT system wherein donor and host differ at both major and minor histocompatibility (H) complex antigens and in which GVHD is predominantly mediated by CD4+ T cells, administration of IL-18 early after BMT attenuated acute GVHD by enhancing Fas-dependent apoptosis of donor T cells (47,49). The mechanisms of apoptosis for CD4+ T cells are distinct from those of CD8+ T cells (50,51), and a study by Min et al. found divergent roles for IL-18 when GVHD is mediated only by CD4+ (MHC class II–disparate system) or by CD8+ cells (MHC class I–disparate system) (52). Three distinct approaches were tested: injection of IL-18, blockade of IL-18 by mAb, and transplantation IL18R$-/-$ donor T cells.

Consistent with previous work in the P → F$_1$ model mentioned above, IL-18 decreased the severity of GVHD in a CD4-mediated system. By contrast, the administration of IL-18 did not enhance apoptosis of donor CD8+ cells and instead exacerbated GVHD in the class I–disparate model regardless of Fas expression on donor T cells. These data underscore the importance of the diverse effects of a single cytokine in the biology of GVHD and indicate that cytokine manipulation strategies need to be carefully evaluated prior to clinical testing.

IL-7 is a pleotropic cytokine that has been studied extensively in murine BMT models with respect to its effects on immune reconstitution and GVHD. Work from one group has shown that the administration of IL-7 increases the homeostatic proliferation of non alloreactive T cells without amplifying GVHD (53,54) and suggests that IL-7 can promote peripheral T-cell reconstitution through its selective proliferative and antiapoptotic effects on nonalloreactive T cells (53,54). By contrast, work by Sinha and colleagues found that when administered after BMT, IL-7 worsened the severity of acute GVHD and substantially lowered the T-cell dose required to induce GVHD (54a). Although differences in the dose and schedule of IL-7 administration may explain these conflicting results, a recent study using IL-7 knockout (IL-7−/−) animals demonstrated that IL-7 is necessary for the induction of experimental GVHD because BMT recipients deficient in IL-7 did not develop GVHD unless they received exogenous IL-7. Moreover, IL-7 treatment enhanced the proliferation of activated (CD69+), donor-derived T cells in IL-7−/− mice and exacerbated the severity of GVHD when given to wild-type BMT recipients (55).

The inflammatory cytokines TNFα and IL-1β have been shown to contribute significantly to the pathophysiology of GVHD in both murine and human studies (29,56,57). The effects of TNFα in GVHD and GVL activity were recently evaluated using a monoclonal antibody directed against murine TNFα (CNTO2213) in strain combinations wherein the GVH responses were medicated by either CD4+ or CD8+ donor T cells (58). The neutralization of TNFα reduced the severity of GVHD in both systems, but such therapy had a greater effect on GVHD mediated by CD4+ T cells compared to CD8+ T cells. In these studies, the authors suggest that the administration of the anti-TNFα antibody did not impair GVL effects against a murine myeloid leukemia (58). These conclusions are limited by the following observations: (1) although mice treated with anti-TNFα mAb had improved survival, ultimately, all animals in this group died from their tumor burden, and (2) rapid and near complete mortality of the GVHD control group by day 20 precluded a true comparison of GVL activity between allogeneic groups. Furthermore, these findings contrast with work published earlier by Hill and colleagues, who evaluated the differential effects of TNFα. and IL-1 on GVHD and GVL and found that while blockade of either cytokine reduced the severity of GVHD in a P → F$_1$ model, neutralization of TNFα but not IL-1 also reduced GVL effects in that system (30).

H. Gene-Profiling Studies

Ichiba et al. studied the gene expression profiles of hepatic tissue during induction of GVHD using oligonucleotide microarrays (59). On day +35 after allogeneic BMT, genes related to cellular effectors and acute-phase proteins were upregulated, whereas genes related primarily to metabolism and endocrine function were downregulated. Before the development of histological changes (day 7) of GVHD, many genes were already upregulated including IFNγ-inducible genes, MHC class II molecules, and genes related to leukocyte trafficking (59). Increased expression of genes associated with the attraction and activation of donor T cells induced by IFNγ preceded the initiation of hepatic GVHD in this model. In another recent study, Fiscella et al. combined bioinformatic tools with high-throughput cell-based screening assays to identify novel factors involved in GVHD (60). They generated a library of cDNA that would encode both secreted and trans-membrane domain-containing proteins as predicted by the Human Genome Sciences cDNA database. Supernatants from mammalian cells transiently transfected with this library were incubated with primary T cells and T-cell lines. Using this strategy, they identified a novel T-cell factor, TIP (T-cell immunomodulatory protein). Treatment of primary human and murine T cells with TIP resulted in the secretion of IFNγ TNFα, and IL-β in vitro. Furthermore, intraperitoneal injections of TIP Fc had a protective effect in an unirradiated B6 $\rightarrow$ F$_1$ acute GVHD model (60). Thus, the combination of large cDNA databases, bioinformatic algorithms, and high-throughput screening was an effective approach to the discovery of novel proteins with therapeutic potential. The combination of microarray studies and functional genomics might also be an interesting approach to the identification of potential novel molecular targets for detection and treatment of acute GVHD.

I. GVHD and Minor Antigens

Minor histocompatibility antigens (miHA) are polymorphisms in cellular proteins that are presented as antigens in HLA molecules and are recognized by T cells (61). T-cell recognition of the miHA proteins expressed on recipient hematopoietic/malignant cells may result in GVL reactivity without concurrent GVHD if these miHA are not present in the GVHD target tissues (61–63). Therefore, characterization miHA that can generate tumor-specific immune responses could make GVL responses more specific and potent. Recently Murata and colleagues used cDNA expression cloning to identify a novel human miHA, UGT2B17. The protein is encoded by an autosomal gene in the multigene UDP-glycosyltransferase 2 family, and is selectively expressed in the liver and intestine and by dendritic cells and activated B cells (64). Unlike previously defined molecular mechanisms involved in the generation of miHA, the differential expression of UGT2B17 by donor and recipient cells was a consequence of the deletion of this gene in the donor. Gene deletion as a mechanism for generating miHA has broad implications for the identification of miHA that induce GVHD. For example, a number of enzyme families expressed solely in the gastrointestinal tract and liver could potentially become a target of GVHD if the donor, but not the recipient, is deficient for one of these enzymes and therefore expresses the protein in these tissues (65–68).

Another important issue is "dominant" minor H antigens that produce large responses. Choi and colleagues used a mouse model in which donor and recipient were incompatible at many minor histocompatibility antigens (miHAg) to track the CD8 T-cell response temporally and spatially through the course of GVHD. Donor CD8 T cells in the circulation, spleen, lung, and liver demonstrated virtually identical kinetics: rapid expansion and then decline prior to morbidity (68a). This contraction of the lymphoid compartment was accompanied by an increase in cells of myeloid lineage at the time of target organ damage, highlighting the biphasic nature of effector cell populations in GVHD. Remarkably, during lymphoid expansion up to fourth of the CD8 T cells were directed against a single minor antigen, H60. Extreme H60 immunodominance occurred regardless of sampling time, site, or genetic background. This study is the first to analyze the T cells participating in GVHD in "real time" and demonstrates the exceptional degree to which immunodominance of H60 can occur. These data also suggest that lymphocytes home to target organs not because of antigens specific to those targets, but due to expression of the dominant minor, histocompatibility antigen at those site most probably on antigen-presenting cells. The study also supports the notion that such superdominant histocompatibility antigens could be risk factors for GVHD.

II. ADVANCES IN UNDERSTANDING GRAFT-VS.-LEUKEMIA ACTIVITY

A. Mixed Chimerism and the GVL Effect

As detailed in Chapter 19, donor leukocyte infusions (DLI) represent an effective tool to induce remissions in several types of leukemia. Unfortunately, DLI can also result in significant GVHD. Mapara et al. recently investigated a strategy to separate GVL effects from GVHD after DLI using nonmyeloablative conditioning to establish mixed hematopoietic chimerism in a mouse BMT system (69). In these studies, administration of DLI on day 35 post-BMT caused conversion of mixed donor to full donor chimerism without causing GVHD. The authors observed a GVL effect against a host-type lymphoma (EL4) that had been injected 7 days later. But when these recipients were rechallenged with the same tumor dose 17 weeks later, the tumor caused 100% mortality (69). This study suggests that DLI after nonmyeloablative conditioning can mediate GVL, but only when mixed chimerim is present. Although the clinical translation of this study is difficult, it raises the intriguing possibility that host hematopoietic cells, perhaps APC may be critical for inducing GVL responses.

B. The Role of NK Cells in GVL Effects

As noted earlier in this chapter, NK cells are characterized by the expression of inhibitory and/or activating receptors specific for different MHC class I determinants (46,70). Experimental evidence shows that NK cells predominantly recognize the hematopoietic cells of the host and spare other GVHD target tissues (40). Studies in mice have demonstrated that allogeneic NK cells can mediate GVL in the absence of GVHD (40,71,72). Blockade of inhibitory receptors on NK cells is an effective means to purge leukemic cells from bone marrow, and transplantation of mice with bone marrow cells purged in this fashion resulted in long-term, relapse-free survival (73,74). Murphy and colleagues have extended these observations to assess the antitumor effects mediated by allogeneic NK cells (75). Several tumor cell lines were more susceptible to lysis by allogeneic NK cells than by syngeneic NK cells when comparable percentages of NK cells were used. Moreover, allogeneic NK cells more effectively removed leukemia cells from bone marrow prior to BMT compared to syngeneic NK cells and resulted in better survival without increasing GVHD (75). A longer co-culture period of NK cells and BM caused suppression of hematopoietic reconstitution, suggesting that allogeneic NK cells can mediate alloreactivity against both normal hematopoietic and leukemic cells under the right circumstances. These data underscore the narrow range of eliciting antitumor responses without compromising hematopoiesis.

C. The Role of Minor Antigens in GVL Effects

Marijt and colleagues recently demonstrated the clinical feasibility of utilizing cytotoxic T lymphocytes specific for miHA HA-1 or HA-2 to induce complete remissions of relapsed leukemia and myeloma (76). They treated three patients (two CML and one multiple myeloma) who were miHAg HA-1− and/or HA-2−positive and had relapsed after allogeneic BMT with DLI from their miHAg HA-1− and/or HA-2−negative donors. Using HLA-A2/HA-1 and A2/HA-2 peptide tetrameric complexes, they showed a profound increase in the number of CD8+ T cells specific for these miHAg in he blood of the recipients 5−7 weeks after DLI. This increase was followed by conversion to 100% donor chimerism and the disappearance of bcr/abl+ cells or of the M protein and myeloma cells. The cloned tetramer-positive T cells isolated during the clinical response specifically recognized HA-1 and HA-2 expressed on malignant progenitor cells of the recipient. Moreover, these T cells inhibited the growth of leukemic precursor (bcr/abl+) cells in vitro (76).

A large body of evidence supports the existence of separate T-cell clones that react with either normal or malignant cells (77). One strategy to amplify GVL would be to identify T-cell lines that are specific for leukemic blasts by amplifying the TCRβ CD3R sequences from T cells that lyse malignant (but not normal) targets. Michalek et al. recently attempted this approach (78). The authors performed MLR using donor peripheral blood mononuclear cells (PBMC) as responders and normal irradiated PBMC from the recipient as stimulators. The activated (i.e., GVHD-specific) CD4+CD25+ cells were sorted and then subsequently eliminated by an anti-CD25 immunotoxin. The remaining T cells were used in a secondary MLR with leukemia cells from the same recipient and the activated CD25+ subset (i.e., GVL-specific) was again sorted. The unique TCRβ CDR3 sequences from both the GVH- and GVL-specific T cells were then amplified by using an anchored RT-PCR technique. The amplified products contained all of the TCRβ CDR3 sequences present in donor CD4+ T-cell clones that were activated by either normal or malignant cells from the host. In HLA-mismatched pairs, a polyclonal alloresponse was observed due to the large number of histocompatibility differences between donors and recipients. However, in an HLA-matched pair, the alloresponse was oligoclonal. The donor cells specific for malignant targets showed different oligoclonal expansion of CD4+ T cells in both the HLA-mismatched and HLA-matched pairs. In a final experiment, the investigators constructed clone-specific primers and probes in order to monitor the frequencies of GVHD- or GVL-specific T cells in the peripheral blood of a patient with refractory acute myelogenous leukemia (AML) who received an HLA-matched allogeneic BMT. The patient engrafted 30 days after BMT but relapsed on day +52 and died on day +71. One of five CD4+ GVHD-specific clones initially identified from the MLR appeared at low levels in the peripheral blood and increased gradually even though the recipient showed no symptoms of GVHD. A leukemia-reactive clone, identified in the secondary MLR, appeared on day +28 and reached its peak on day 47 but decreased at the time of relapse and later became undetectable. Although the results of this study suggest that grafts depleted of allo-T cells could exert GVL effects without causing significant GVHD, it also demonstrates that identification of leukemic T-cell clones in vitro and in vivo may not translate into clinically relevant GVL responses.

Transplantation of stem cells from a female donor to a male recipient represents a special circumstance in which donor T cells specific for miHA encoded by genes on the Y chromosome might contribute to GVHD and GVL (61). Some H-Y antigens may be differentially associated with GVHD and GVL responses. Prior studies have shown that the male recipients of female HLA-matched donors experienced increased GVHD (79–81), but these studies did not examine whether such patients exhibit GVL independent of GVHD. In a recent study, Randolph et al. examined the contribution of donor/recipient gender to the risk of relapse and GVHD in 3238 individuals who received HLA-identical sibling BMT for hematological malignancies (82). Relative to other gender combinations, male recipients of female transplants had the lowest hazard of relapse and the greatest risk of GVHD. Female recipients with a male donor also had a higher likelihood of developing GVHD, albeit lower than that of the male recipients with a female donor. Of note, F → M transplants still exhibited a lower hazard of relapse compared with other gender combinations after controlling for GVHD as a time-dependent covariate, demonstrating a selective GVL effect distinct from that linked to systemic GVHD. The reduction in relapse after F → M BMT was observed in patients with chronic myelogenous leukemia (CML), AML, and acute lymphocytic leukemia (ALL). These findings are consistent with a previous study by Gratwohl et al., who also found lower relapse rates in CML patients after the F → M transplantation (81). Taken together, these data suggest that minor histocompatibility antigens encoded or regulated by genes on the Y chromosome contribute to a selective GVL effect (82). A careful search for Y-chromosome–encoded miHA may thus identify targets that can be exploited for selective GVL activity.

D. Novel Pharmacotherapeutic Strategies for Separating GVHD from GVL

Three recent studies have demonstrated the possibility of expanding the therapeutic options for GVHD without compromising GVL. Suberoylanilide hydroxamic acid (SAHA) is a histone deacetylase inhibitor that is currently undergoing clinical trials as an antitumor agent. At lower doses, SAHA reduces inflammation by reducing the production of proinflammatory cytokines. The effects of histone deacetylase inhibition on GVHD severity and GVL activity were recently studied using two well-characterized mouse models (83). Administration of SAHA from day +3 to day +7 after BMT reduced serum levels of TNFα IL-l, and IFNγ and decreased the intestinal pathology, clinical severity, and mortality associated with acute GVHD. SAHA had no effect on the proliferative and cytotoxic responses of donor T cells to host antigens in vivo or in vitro. Importantly, the administration of SAHA did not impair GVL activity and resulted in significantly improved leukemia-free survival in two different tumor and donor/recipient combinations (P815 and EL-4). These findings suggest that this class of pharmacological agents may provide a novel strategy to reduce GVHD while preserving GVL effects.

A second novel immune-suppressive drug, the sphingosine-1-phosphate receptor agonist, FTY720, was recently evaluated in murine models. Kim and colleagues hypothesized that FTY720 would prevent GVHD while permitting an alloresponse to proceed within the lymphohematopoietic system and thereby sustain a beneficial GVL effect (84). The administration of FTY720 markedly reduced GVHD in a haploidentical strain combination while permitting GVL effects against a T-cell lymphoma. Thus, FTY720 may also represent a pharmacological agent worthy of clinical investigation to control GVHD.

Murphy and colleagues recently demonstrated that PS-341, a proteasome inhibitor that has antitmor activity and acts via the NF-$\kappa\beta$ pathway could modulate the immune responses of donor T cells and separate GVL from GVHD. The study utilized the

MHC-mismatched lethally irradiated BALB/c → C57BL/6 murine BMT model of acute GVHD and found that recipient animals injected with PS-341 (15 mg/mouse/day) for the first 3 days after BMT exhibited significantly better survival. PS-341 treatment also reduced serum levels of IFNγ, IL-2, and TNFα and was associated with reduced donor CD4+ T expansion at early time points after BMT. Interestingly when recipient mice were injected with C1498 murine leukemic cells 7–13 days prior to BMT, treatment with PS-341 preserved GVL effect. Although these findings suggest that PS-341 can decrease GVHD and preserve the GVL effect, these beneficial effects were critically dependent on the timing of the PS-341 injection (85).

III. THERAPEUTIC AND PROGNOSTIC ADVANCES IN GVHD

A. Clinical Trials for the Prevention and Treatment of Acute GVHD

Strategies to reduce GVHD by immunosuppressive drugs have been the subject of numerous clinical trials over the past 25 years. As described in Chapter 15, sirolimus (rapamycin) is a newer agent that, like tacrolimus, binds to FKBP12 (86). The tacrolimus: FKBP12 complex inhibits calcineurin phosphatase and the dephosphorylation of NE-AT, thus preventing T-cell activation, IL-2 secretion, and cell cycle progression at the $G_0 \rightarrow G_1$ interface (87). In contrast, the sirolimus: FKBP12 complex binds to the mammalian target of rapamycin (mTOR), which blocks cytokine-mediated signal transduction pathways and prevents $G_1 \rightarrow S$ phase transition. Furthermore, sirolimus has synergistic immunosuppressive effects with tacrolimus (87,88). A recent clinical trial by Antin et al. took advantage of these synergistic interactions to try to prevent GVHD in high-risk recipients of matched unrelated or 5 of 6 related donors, adding sirolimus to tacrolimus and "minidose" methotrexate (89). Forty-one patients with hematological malignancies including AML, ALL, CML, non-hodykin's lymphoma (NHL) were conditioned with cyclophosphamide and total body irradiation. Sirolimus was administered as a 12 mg oral loading dose beginning on day −3, followed by 4 mg day orally in a single morning dose titrated for a target trough level of 3–12 ng/mL. All patients engrafted, and the toxicity attributable to sirolimus was manageable. The authors observed grade II–IV acute GVHD in 26% of the patients, whereas prior studies in this high-risk population typically show rates of 50–75%. There did not appear to be an increased risk of acute GVHD in a small number of patients with HLA mismatches. Furthermore, the risk of relapse was surprisingly low (24%) in the high-risk cohort included in the study (89).

This same group evaluated the ability of sirolimus to substitute for methotrexate (MTX) as GVHD prophylaxis after matched related allogeneic peripheral blood stem cell transplantation. Thirty patients with various hematological malignancies who received allografts from fully matched related donors were conditioned with cyclophosphamide and TBI. Sirolimus (target serum level 3–12 ng/mL) and tacrolimus (target serum level 5–10 ng/mL) were administered for GVHD prophylaxis. All of the patients tolerated the drugs well and engrafted neutrophils by 14 days (range 11–17) after BMT. Grade 0–I acute GVHD occurred in 27/30 patients (90%) and grade II GVHD occurred in 3 patients (10%), but no patient developed grade III–IV GVHD or idiopathic pneumonia syndrome. Chronic GVHD was observed in 4 patients (3 extensive, 1 limited), and disease relapse was seen in 6 patients with high-risk diseases (4 relapsed/refractory AML, 1 relapsed ALL, 1 relapsed Burkitt's NHL). No deaths attributable to GVHD or fungal infections were observed at a median follow-up of 204 days. These preliminary data suggest that tacrolimus and sirolimus without MTX are effective for GVHD prophylaxis, but this will need to be confirmed in larger studies (90).

A recent study by Finke et al. reported GVHD outcomes after matched and mismatched unrelated donor BMT when using high-dose rabbit ATG for GVHD prophylaxis (91). One hundred patients with hematological malignancies underwent transplantation during different phases of diseases with non-TCD bone marrow ($n = 87$) or peripheral blood–derived ($n = 13$) stem cells from HLA-A, HLA-B, HLA-DRB1, or HLA-DQB1 identical ($n = 75$) or mismatched (one antigen, $n = 21$; two to three antigens, $n = 4$) unrelated donors. In addition to cyclosporine and a short-course of MTX, GVHD prophylaxis included ATG administered before transplantation. The cumulative incidence of grades II–IV acute GVHD was 21% in HLA-matched and 30% after HLA-mismatched transplantations. The risk of relapse at 4 years was 17% for early disease and 43% for advanced disease patients. These results suggest that comparable outcomes could be obtained for GVHD in patients undergoing BMT from matched or 1 antigen mismatched unrelated donors when ATG is added to the standard GVHD prophylaxis (91).

Cytokine inhibition strategies have been used to treat GVHD in several recent studies. Anti-TNFα therapy for steroid-resistant GVHD using monoclonal antibodies appeared to be useful particularly if there was intestinal involvement (92). Couriel and colleagues reported that a weekly dose of 10 mg/kg infliximab in patients with steroid-refractory GVHD resulted in an 80% response rate in 37 patients with gastrointestinal involvement (93). Other centers have reported similar GVHD response rates in small series of patients (92,94).

Recently Uberti and colleagues reported on their experience using etanercept and steroids as primary therapy for GVHD. The endpoints of the study included safety of administration of etanercept and response rates of GVHD. Eligible patients had biopsy-proven clinical grade II–III acute GVHD. Etanercept was administered at 25 mg subcutaneously two times a week for 8 weeks and was started within 72 hours of the first dose of solumedrol. The study enrolled 20 patients (14 related and 6 unrelated transplants), and 15 patients (75%) responded to treatment (14 CRs and 1 PR). Only one GVHD flare was noted upon completion of therapy, and one patient developed disseminated zygomycosis infection. This study suggested that addition of etanercept to solumedrol resulted in better complete response rates with minimal toxicity. These exciting results will need to be further evaluated in larger number of patients (95).

A study by Marty et al. addressed the infectious risk when TNFα blockade with infliximab was used to treat severe grade III–IV GVHD (96). A retrospective analysis of patient records showed that 5 of 11 patients with severe GVHD treated with infliximab developed invasive noncandidal fungal infections (6.78 cases/1000 GVHD patient-days), compared with 5 of 42 patients with GVHD who did not receive infliximab (0.53 cases/ 100 GVHD patient-days). A time-dependent Cox regression analysis indicated that the adjusted invasive fungal infection risk hazard ratio of infliximab was 13.6 ($p = 0.004$; 95% CI) (96). These data underscore the protective role of TNFα against fungal infections and suggest that preemptive systemic antifungal therapy against molds should be considered in patients with several GVHD who are being treated with infliximab (96).

B. Prognostic Studies of GVHD

Several studies using mouse models have demonstrated that apoptosis of target cells mediated by TNFα and Fas plays a major role in the development of target organ

GVHD. A recent clinical study by Socie and colleagues was the first to document the in situ expression of TNFα and to demonstrate its association with GI tract GVHD in humans. This study reported a detailed pathological analysis of intestinal tissue that included quantification of the cellular infiltrates for TNFα, TNFR I, II, Fas expression and apoptosis (97). Ninety-five patients with a variety of underlying diseases and conditioning regimens were prospectively evaluated with gastroduodenal biopsies. Histological GI tract GVHD was found in 71 of the 95 patients. Of note, the gross appearance of the upper GI tract as seen by the endoscopist and the histological findings did not correlate with the diagnosis of pathological GVHD. Cellular staining of these biopsies showed neutrophils in the entire thickness of the lamina propria. Intense expression of TNF, TNFR I and TNFR II, and Fas was present in 100% of the biopsies with proven pathological GVHD. While Fas expression was widely observed, it failed to reach the criteria for specificity and sensitivity. In addition, this study demonstrated that the presence of apoptotic cells within the cellular infiltrate is a major factor associated with transplant-related mortality and suggested that neutrophils might play a hitherto unknown role in GVHD.

C. Genetic Polymorphisms and Acute GVHD

Polymorphisms in cytokine and other immune modulator genes can influence the inflammatory responses and tissue injury, and may therefore affect the outcome of GVHD after allogeneic BMT. Two recent studies have demonstrated a significant role for IL-10 promoter polymorphism in the recipients and the NOD2/CARD 15 polymorphisms in the donors/recipients, respectively, in GVHD severity and mortality after allogeneic BMT.

In a seminal study, Lin et al. analyzed single-nucleotide polymorphisms in the genes for IL-1β, IL-1R antagonist, IL-6, IL-10, and TNFα in 570 transplant recipients and their HLA-identical sibling donors. The genotypes were tested for an association with GVHD by multivariate analysis. A second cohort of 423 transplant recipients was then independently analyzed for the genotype associations identified in the first cohort. Analysis of all 993 transplant recipients from both cohorts showed that the IL-1β, IL-1Ra, TNFα, and IL-6 genotypes had no significant effect on the risk of GVHD, and only the IL-10$-$592A/A genotype was associated with a decreased risk of grade III or IV acute GVHD ($p = 0.02$) and death in remission ($p = 0.05$). But the impact of IL-10$-$592A allele on GVHD in unrelated or mismatched transplants has not yet been studied. Although this was a retrospective analysis, given the large number of patients analyzed and the clear association demonstrated by this study, evaluation of potential recipients of cells from matched sibling donors for the IL-10$-$592A allele marker might help in identification of patients with favorable GVHD outcome and allow for reduced immunosuppressive therapy after BMT (98,99).

In the second study, Holler and colleagues evaluated the impact of NOD2/CARD15 mutations in recipients and donors on GVHD-related mortality. The NOD2/CARD15 gene encodes for highly conserved proteins involved in intracellular recognition of microbial peptides and enables specialized epithelial cells of the ileum, monocyte/macrophages, and dendritic cells to respond to gut bacteria. These proteins then result in the activation of NF-κB and initiate an antimicrobial response. Single nucleotide polymorphisms (SNP 8, 12, and 13) in the NOD2/CARD15 gene located on chromosome 16 have been shown to increase the risk of Crohn's disease (100–102). Because of this association with GI tract inflammation, Holler and colleagues analyzed SNP of NOD2/CARD15 gene in 169 recipient/donor pairs of allogeneic BMT. Occurrence of these mutations in either the donor or the recipients was significantly associated with an increased risk of gastrointestinal and overall severity of GVHD. The incidence of severe GVHD was 20% and 77%, and the actuarial TRM was 32% and 100%, respectively, in donor recipient pairs without the NOD2/CARD15 mutation. Interestingly, this effect of NOD2/CARD15 mutations was observed in both HLA-matched related and unrelated donor transplants (E. Holler, personal communication). If these data are confirmed by analysis of larger cohorts of related and unrelated transplants, then NOD2/CARD15 typing might also be included in selection strategies for related and unrelated allogeneic transplants in the future.

D. Idiopathic Pneumonia Syndrome

Data in animal studies has led to the intriguing concept that the lung can be considered a target of acute GVHD (see Chapter 11). Several studies have reported the incidence of idopathic pneumonia syndrome (IPS) in the first 120 days after BMT to be 3% to 15% after allogeneic BMT with myeloablative conditioning (103,104). IPS results from a diversity of lung insults including immunological cell-mediated injury, inflammatory cytokines, toxic effects of myeloablative conditioning, and occult pulmonary infections (105,106). Fukuda et al. have recently compared the incidence and outcome of IPS among patients who underwent allogeneic BMT after nomnyeloablative ($n = 183$) and conventional ($n = 917$) conditioning (107). The cumulative incidence of IPS was significantly lower at 120 days after nonmyeloablative conditioning than conventional conditioning (2.2% vs. 8.4%; $p = 0.003$). However, once diagnosed, IPS progressed rapidly and was associated with a high mortality rate (75%) despite aggressive support in both subsets of patients. Grades III–IV acute GVHD remained prognostic for IPS after adjusting for other risk factors, confirming previous reports and supporting the hypothesis that the lung may be a target of graft-vs.-host reaction. Importantly, other risk factors are likely to be involved because acute GVHD occurred with similar frequency in the two study populations even though the incidence of IPS was lower after nonmyeloablative conditioning. In addition, greater patient age (>40 years) and diagnosis of acute leukemia or MDS were associated with significantly increased risks for IPS. Among the older patients with conventional conditioning, high-dose total body irradiation (TBI) was associated with an increased risk for IPS than were non–TBI-based regimens (16% vs. 5.8%; $p = 0.001$). Although there are limitations to the conclusions that can be drawn from this study the results suggest nonmyeloablative or targeted dose chemotherapy-based myeloablative regimens may reduce the risk of IPS in patients aged 40 years or older.

E. Chronic GVHD

Chronic GVHD is a major cause of morbidity and mortality in long-term survivors of allogeneic BMT (108), and the most important risk factor for chronic GVHD is a history of acute GVHD. Accordingly, strategies that prevent acute GVHD also decrease the risk of chronic GVHD (108), but no known pharmacological agents specifically prevent the development of chronic GVHD. Agents that have efficacy in acute GVHD and autoimmune diseases have been utilized as therapy for established chronic GVHD, but the response rate in extensive chronic GVHD is limited. One promising therapeutic strategy might be depletion of B cells with anti-CD20 monoclonal antibody as reported by Ratanatharathorn and colleagues (109). They described the clinical outcome of 8 patients with steroid-refractory chronic GVHD who received the anti-CD20 chimeric monoclonal antibody rituximab. All patients had extensive chronic GVHD with diffuse or localized sclerodermoid lesions and xerophthalmia. Other manifestations included cold agglutinin disease with Raynaud's phenomenon and restrictive or obstructive lung disease. Rituximab was given by intravenous infusion at a weekly dose of 375 mg/m^2 for 4 weeks. Four patients responded to treatment with ongoing resolution or improvement ranging from 265 to 846 days after therapy, despite recovery of B cells in 3 patients (109). Thus, rituximab seems to possess some activity in the treatment of refractory chronic GVHD, but larger studies are needed to confirm this potential effect.

IV. CONCLUSIONS AND FUTURE DIRECTIONS

Outstanding progress has been made on several research fronts in terms of the cellular interactions and networks that impact upon GVHD. Perhaps most striking is the number of "new" cell types, or rather subpopulations of previously known cells with "new" functions, that have been identified in these models. For example, regulatory T cells, regulatory dendritic cells, and allogeneic natural killer cells are three populations of "new" cells that have been shown to modulate or prevent GVHD in several experimental systems. The next few years will undoubtedly bring these heterogeneous cell types into greater focus so that we can identify and isolate them with greater precision and maximally exploit their potential.

On the clinical front, the increasingly widespread use of reduced-intensity BMT conditioning and donor leukocyte infusion has significantly altered the clinical spectra of GVHD; as the intensive conditioning regimens traditionally used in BMT give way to less toxic chemotherapy, the kinetics and manifestations of acute GVHD appear to be changing. Already the traditional day 100 endpoint used for this disease has become obsolete and is increasingly unsatisfactory as a marker to distinguish acute from chronic GVHD. Proposals for simplified grading systems are currently being considered.

In the next few years it is likely that many insights made at the bench will translate to the bedside, moving the clinical field of transplantation towards "component" cellular therapy. Cell populations will be isolated, expanded, purified, and administered for specific purposes, including the elimination of antigen-presenting cells and the suppression of alloreactive T-cell clones. It is also likely that new modulators of GVHD (cytokines, soluble receptors, etc.) will be definitively tested, although whether any single modulator will have clinical efficacy remains to be seen. Finally, the diagnostic modalities used for GVHD will improve. GVHD remains a clinical diagnosis, in large part because no standardized laboratory tests have been validated to diagnose, much less predict, the disease and its severity. Molecular medicine in the form of genomic and proteomic profiles is likely to find its clinical application in GVHD by the time the fourth edition of the textbook is written. Stay tuned.

REFERENCES

1. van der Merwe PA, Davis SJ. Molecular interactions mediating T cell antigen recognition. Annu Rev Immunol 2003; 21:659–684.
2. Davis SJ, Ikemizu S, Evans EJ, Fugger L, Bakker TR, van der Merwe PA. The nature of molecular recognition by T cells. Nat Immunol 2003; 4:217–224.
3. Blazar BR, Taylor PA, Linsley PS, Vallera DA. In vivo blockade of CD28/CTLA4: B7/BB1 interaction with CTLA4-Ig reduces lethal murine graft-versus-host disease across the major histocompatibility complex barrier in mice. Blood 1994; 83:3815–3825.

4. Blazar BR, Taylor PA, Panoskaltis-Mortari A, Gray GS, D.A. V. Co-blockade of the LFA1:ICAM and CD28/CTLA4:B7 pathways is a highly effective means of preventing acute lethal graft-versus host disease induced by fully major histocompatibility complex-disparate donor grafts. Blood 1995; 85:2607–2618.

5. Blazar B, Taylor P, Panoskaltsis-Mortari A, Buhlman J, Xu J, Flavell R, Korngold R, Noelle R, Vallera D. Blockade of CD40 ligand-CD40 interaction impairs CD4+ T cell mediated alloreactivity by inhibiting mature donor T cell expansion and function after bone marrow transplantation. J Immunol 1997; 158:29–39.

6. Taylor PA, Friedman TM, Korngold R, Noelle RJ, Blazar BR. Tolerance induction of alloreactive T cells via ex vivo blockade of the CD40:CD40L costimulatory pathway results in the generation of a potent immune regulatory cell. Blood 2002; 99:4601–4609.

7. Weinberg AD, Vella AT, Croft M. OX-40: life beyond the effector T cell stage. Semin Immunol 1998; 10:471–480.

8. Blazar BR, Sharpe AH, Chen AI, Panoskaltsis-Mortari A, Lees C, Akiba H, Yagita H, Killeen N, Taylor PA. Ligation of OX40 (CD 134) regulates graft-versus-host disease (GVHD) and graft rejection in allogeneic bone marrow transplant recipients. Blood 2003; 101:3741–3748.

9. Okazaki T, Iwai Y, Honjo T. New regulatory co-receptors: inducible co-stimulator and PD-1. Curr Opin Immunol 2002; 14:779–782.

10. Blazar BR, Carreno BM, Panoskaltsis-Mortari A, Carter L, Iwai Y, Yagita H, Nishimura H, Taylor PA. Blockade of programmed death-1 engagement accelerates graft-versus-host disease lethality by an IFN-gamma-dependent mechanism. J Immunol 2003; 171:1272–1277.

11. Tamada K, Shimozaki K, Chapoval AI, Zhu G, Sica G, Flies D, Boone T, Hsu H, Fu YX, Nagata S, Ni J, Chen L. Modulation of T-cell-mediated immunity in tumor and graft-versus-host disease models through the LIGHT co-stimulatory pathway. Nat Med 2000; 6:283–289.

12. Tamada K, Tamura H, Flies D, Fu YX, Celis E, Pease LR, Blazar BR, Chen L. Blockade of LIGHT/LTbeta and CD40 signaling induces allospecific T cell energy, preventing graft-versus-host disease. J Clin Invest 2002; 109:549–557.

13. Anderson BE, McNiff J, Yan J, Doyle H, Mamula M, Shlomchik MJ, Shlomchik WD. Memory CD4+ T cells do not induce graft-versus-host disease. J Clin Invest 2003; 112:101–108.

14. Chen BJ, Cui X, Sempowski GD, Liu C, Chao NJ. Transfer of allogeneic CD62L-memory T cells without graft-vs.-host disease. Blood 2003; 103:1534–1541.

15. Lakkis FG, Sayegh MH. Memory T cells: a hurdle to immunologic tolerance. J Am Soc Nephrol 2003; 14:2402–2410.

16. Johnson BD, Konkol MC, Truitt RL. CD25+ immunoregulatory T-cells of donor origin suppress alloreactivity after BMT. Biol Blood Marrow Transplant 2002; 8:525–535.

17. Hoffmann P, Ermann J, Edinger M, Fathman CG, Strober S. Donor-type CD4(+)CD25(+) regulatory T cells suppress lethal acute graft-versus-host disease after allogeneic bone marrow transplantation. J Exp Med 2002; 196:389–399.

18. Cohen JL, Trenado A, Vasey D, Klatzmann D, Salomon BL. CD4(+)CD25(+) immunoregulatory T cells: new therapeutics for graft-versus-host disease. J Exp Med 2002; 196:401–406.

19. Taylor PA, Lees CJ, Blazar BR. The infusion of ex vivo activated and expanded CD4(+) CD25(+) immune regulatory cells inhibits graft-versus-host disease lethality. Blood 2002; 99:3493–3499.

20. Edinger M, Hoffmann P, Ermann J, Drago K, Fathman CG, Strober S, Negrin RS. CD4(+) CD25(+) regulatory T cells preserve graft-versus-tumor activity while inhibiting graft-versus-host disease after bone marrow transplantation. Nat Med 2003; 9:1144–1150.

21. Jones SC, Murphy GF, Korngold R. Post-hematopoietic cell transplantation control of graft-versus-host disease by donor CD425 T cells to allow an effective graft-versus-leukemia response. Biol Blood Marrow Transplant 2003; 9:243–256.

22. Yvon ES, Vigouroux S, Rousseau RF, Biagi E, Amrolia P, Dotti G, Wagner HJ, Brenner MK. Over expression of the Notch ligand, Jagged-1 induces alloantigen-specific human regulatory T cells. Blood 2003; 102:3815–3821.

23. Chen ZM, O'Shaughnessy MJ, Gramaglia I, Panoskaltsis-Mortari A, Murphy WJ, Narula S, Roncarolo MG, Blazar BR. IL-10 and TGF-beta induce alloreactive CD4+ CD25 − T cells to acquire regulatory cell function. Blood 2003; 101:5076–5083.

24. Stanzani M, Martins SL, Saliba RM, St John LS, Bryan S, Couriel D, McMannis J, Champlin RE, Molldrem JJ, Komanduri KV. CD25 expression on donor CD4+ or CD8+ T cells is associated with an increased risk of graft-versus-host disease following HLA-identical stem cell transplantation in humans. Blood 2003.

25. Hayday A, Tigelaar R. Immunoregulation in the tissues by gamma delta T cells. Nat Rev Immunol 2003; 3:233–242.

26. Leslie DS, Vincent MS, Spada FM, Das H, Sugita M, Morita CT, Brenner MB. CD1-mediated gamma/delta T cell maturation of dendritic cells. J Exp Med 2002; 196:1575–1584.

27. Maeda Y, Reddy P, Min C, Liu C, Ferrara J. Host gamma delta T cells exacerbate acute GVHD by enhancing the allostimulatory capacity of host APCs. Blood 2003; 102:946a.

28. Shlomchik WD, Couzens MS, Tang CB, McNiff J, Robert ME, Liu J, Shlomchik MJ, Emerson SG. Prevention of graft versus host disease by inactivation of host antigen-presenting cells. Science 1999; 285:412–415.

29. Teshima T, Ordemann R, Reddy P, Gagin S, Liu C, Cooke KR, Ferrara JL. Acute graft-versus-host disease does not require alloantigen expression on host epithelium. Nat Med 2002; 8:575–581.

30. Hill GR, Teshima T, Rebel VI, Krijanovski OI, Cooke KR, Brinson YS, Ferrara JL. The p55 TNF-alpha receptor plays a critical role in T cell alloreactivity. J Immunol 2000; 164:656–663.

31. Matzinger P. The danger model: a renewed sense of self. Science 2002; 296:301–305.

32. Sato K, Yamashita N, Baba M, Matsuyama T. Regulatory dendritic cells protect mice from murine acute graft-versus-host disease and leukemia relapse. Immunity 2003; 18:367–379.

33. MacDonald K, Rowe V, Thomas R, Welply JK, Woulfe S, Ferrara JLM, Hill GR. Progenipoietin-1 and G-CSF expand a novel CD40neg APC that induces transplant tolerance through IL-10 producing regulatory T cells. Blood 2003; 102:191a.

34. Munn DH, Sharma MD, Lee JR, Jhaver KG, Johnson TS, Keskin DB, Marshall B, Chandler P, Antonia SJ, Burgess R, Slingluff CL, Jr., Mellor AL. Potential regulatory function of human dendritic cells expressing indoleamine 2,3-dioxygenase. Science 2002; 297:1867–1870.

35. Grohmann U, Fallarino F, Puccetti P. Tolerance, DCs and tryptophan: much ado about IDO. Trends Immunol 2003; 24:242–248.

36. Terness P, Bauer TM, Rose L, Dufter C, Watzlik A, Simon H, Opelz G. Inhibition of allogeneic T cell proliferation by indoleamine 2,3-dioxygenase-expressing dendritic cells: mediation of suppression by tryptophan metabolites. J Exp Med 2002; 196:447–457.

37. Mellor AL, Keskin DB, Johnson T, Chandler P, Munn DH. Cells expressing indoleamine 2,3-dioxygenase inhibit T cell responses. J Immunol 2002; 168:3771–3776.

38. Steckel NK, Kuhn U, Beelen DW, Elmaagacli AH. Indoleamine 2,3-dioxygenase expression in patients with acute graft-versus-host disease after allogeneic stem cell transplantation and in pregnant women: association with the induction of allogeneic immune tolerance? Scand J Immunol 2003; 57:185–191.

39. Chan GW, Gorgun G, Miller KB, Foss FM. Persistence of host dendritic cells after transplantation is associated with graft-versus-host disease. Biol Blood Marrow Transplant 2003; 9:170–176.

40. Parham P. Immunogenetics of killer-cell immunoglobulin-like receptors. Tissue Antigens 2003; 62:194–200.

41. Zeng D, Lewis D, Dejbakhsh-Jones S, Lan F, Garcia-Ojeda M, Sibley R, Strober S. Bone marrow NK1.1(−) and NK1.1(+) T cells reciprocally regulate acute graft versus host disease. J Exp Med 1999; 189:1073–1081.

42. Lan F, Zeng D, Higuchi M, Huie P, Higgins JP, Strober S. Predominance of NK1.1+TCR alpha beta+ or DX5+TCR alpha beta+ T cells in mice conditioned with fractionated lymphoid irradiation protects against graft-versus-host disease: 'natural suppressor' cells. Immunol 2001; 167:2087–2096.

43. Lan F, Zeng D, Higuchi M, Higgins JP, Strober S. Host conditioning with total lymphoid irradiation and antithymocyte globulin prevents graft-versus-host disease: the role of CD1-reactive natural killer T cells. Biol Blood Marrow Transplant 2003; 9:355–363.

44. Ruggeri L, Capanni M, Urbani E, Perruccio K, Shlomchik WD, Tosti A, Posati S, Rogaia D, Frassoni F, Aversa F, Martelli MF, Velardi A. Effectiveness of donor natural killer cell allo-reactivity in mismatched hematopoietic transplants. Science 2002; 295:2097–2100.

45. Giebel S, Locatelli F, Lamparelli T, Velardi A, Davies S, Frumento G, Maccario R, Bonetti F, Wojnar J, Martinetti M, Frassoni F, Giorgiani G, Bacigalupo A, Holowiecki J. Survival advantage with KIR ligand incompatibility in hematopoietic stem cell transplantation from unrelated donors. Blood 2003; 102:814–819.

46. Davies SM, Ruggieri L, DeFor T, Wagner JE, Weisdorf DJ, Miller JS, Velardi A, Blazar BR. Evaluation of KIR ligand incompatibility in mismatched unrelated donor hematopoietic transplants. Killer immunoglobulin-like receptor. Blood 2002; 100:3825–3827.

47. Reddy P, Ferrara JL. Immunobiology of acute graft-versus-host disease. Blood Rev 2003; 17:187–194.

48. Reddy P, Ferrara JL. Role of interleukin-18 in acute graft-vs-host disease. J Lab Clin Med 2003; 141:365–371.

49. Reddy P, Teshima T, Kukuruga M, Ordemann R, Liu C, Lowler K, Ferrara JL. Interleukin-18 regulates acute graft-versus-host disease by enhancing Fas-mediated donor T cell apoptosis. J Exp Med 2001; 194:1433–1440.

50. Zheng L, Fisher G, Miller R, Peschon J, Lynch D, Lenardo M. Induction of apoptosis in mature T cells by tumor necrosis factor. Nature 1995; 377:348–351.

51. Csencsits KL, Bishop DK. Contrasting alloreactive CD4+ and CD8+ T cells: there's more to it than MHC restriction. Am J Transplant 2003; 3:107–115.

52. Min C, Maeda Y, Liu C, Ferrara J, Reddy P. Differential effects of IL-18 on the severity of acute graft-versus-host disease mediated by CD4+ and CD8+ T cell subsets after experimental allogeneic bone marrow transplantation. Blood 2003; 102:409b.

53. Alpdogan O, Muriglan SJ, Eng JM, Willis LM, Greenberg AS, Kappel BJ, van den Brink MR. IL-7 enhances peripheral T cell reconstitution after allogeneic hematopoietic stem cell transplantation. J Clin Invest 2003; 112:1095–1107.

54. Alpdogan O, Schmaltz C, Muriglan SJ, Kappel BJ, Perales MA, Rotolo JA, Halm JA, Rich BE, van den Brink MR. Administration of interleukin-7 after allogeneic bone marrow transplantation improves immune reconstitution without aggravating graft-versus-host disease. Blood 2001; 98:2256–2265.

54a. Sinha ML, Fry TJ, Fowler DH, Mackall CL. Interleukin 7 worsens graft-versus-host disease. Blood 2002; 100:2642–2649.

55. Chung B, Dudl E, Toyama A, Barsky L, Weinberg K. IL-7 is necessary for induction of experimental graft-versus-host disease (GVHD). Blood 2003; 102:149a.

56. Reddy P, Teshima T, Hildebrandt G, Duffner U, Maeda Y, Cooke KR, Ferrara JL. Interleukin 18 preserves a perform-dependent graft-versus-leukemia effect after allogeneic bone marrow transplantation. Blood 2002; 100:3429–3431.

57. Brown GR, Lindberg G, Meddings J, Silva M, Beutler B, Thiele D. Tumor necrosis factor inhibitor ameliorates murine intestinal graft-versus-host disease. Gastroenterology 1999; 116:593–601.

58. Korngold R, Marini JC, De Baca ME, Murphy GF, Giles-Komar J. Role of tumor necrosis factor-alpha in graft-versus-host disease and graft-versus-leukemia responses. Biol Blood Marrow Transplant 2003; 9:292–303.

59. Ichiba T, Teshima T, Kuick R, Misek DE, Liu C, Takada Y, Maeda Y, Reddy P, Williams DL, Hanash SM, Ferrara JL. Early changes in gene expression profiles of hepatic GVHD uncovered by oligonucleotide microarrays. Blood 2003.

60. Fiscella M, Perry JW, Teng B, Bloom M, Zhang C, Leung K, Pukac L, Florence K, Concepcion A, Liu B, Meng Y, Chen C, Elgin EC, Kanakaraj P, Kaufmann TE, Porter J, Cibotti R, Mei Y, Zhou J, Chen G, Roschke V, Komatsoulis G, Mansfield B, Ruben S, Sanyal I,

Migone TS. TIP, a T-cell factor identified using high-throughput screening increases survival in a graft-versus-host disease model. Nat Biotechnol 2003; 21:302–307.

61. Riddell SR, Murata M, Bryant S, Warren EH. Minor histocompatibility antigens—targets of graft versus leukemia responses. Int J Hematol 2002; 76(suppl 2):155–161.

62. Goulmy E, Schipper R, Pool J, Blokland E, Falkenburg F. Mismatches of minor histocompatibility antigens between HLA-identical donors and recipients and the development of graft-versus-host disease after bone marrow transplantation. N Engl J Med 1996; 334:281–285.

63. Riddell SR, Berger C, Murata M, Randolph S, Warren EH. The graft versus leukemia response after allogeneic hematopoietic stem cell transplantation. Blood Rev 2003; 17:153–162.

64. Murata M, Warren EH, Riddell SR. A human minor histocompatibility antigen resulting from differential expression due to a gene deletion. J Exp Med 2003; 197:1279–1289.

65. Gaedigk A. Interethnic differences of drug-metabolizing enzymes. Int J Clin Pharmacol Ther 2000; 38:61–68.

66. Gaedigk A, Blum M, Gaedigk R, Eichelbaum M, Meyer UA. Deletion of the entire cytochrome P450 CYP2D6 gene as a cause of impaired drug metabolism in poor metabolizers of the debrisoquine/sparteine polymorphism. Am J Hum Genet 1991; 48:943–950.

67. Board P, Coggan M, Johnston P, Ross V, Suzuki T, Webb G. Genetic heterogeneity of the human glutathione transferases: a complex of gene families. Pharmacol Ther 1990; 48:357–369.

68. Board P, Tetlow N, Blackburn A, Chelvanayagam G. Database analysis and gene discovery in pharmacogenetics. Clin Chem Lab Med 2000; 38:863–867.

68a. Choi EY, Christianson GJ, Yoshimura, et al. Real-time T-cell profiling identifies H60 as a major minor histocompatibility antigen in murine graft-versus-host disease. Blood 2002; 100:4259–4265.

69. Mapara MY, Kim YM, Marx J, Sykes M. Donor lymphocyte infusion-mediated graft-versus-leukemia effects in mixed chimeras established with a nonmyeloablative conditioning regimen: extinction of graft-versus-leukemia effects after conversion to full donor chimerism. Transplantation 2003; 76:297–305.

70. Colucci F, Caligiuri MA, Di Santo JP. What does it take to make a natural killer? Nat Rev Immunol 2003; 3:413–425.

71. Farag SS, Fehniger TA, Ruggeri L, Velardi A, Caligiuri MA. Natural killer cell receptors: new biology and insights into the graft-versus-leukemia effect. Blood 2002; 100:1935–1947.

72. Velardi A, Ruggeri L, Alessandro, Moretta, Moretta L. NK cells: a lesson from mismatched hematopoietic transplantation. Trends Immunol 2002; 23:438–444.

73. Koh CY, Blazar BR, George T, Welniak LA, Capitini CM, Raziuddin A, Murphy WJ, Bennett M. Augmentation of antitumor effects by NK cell inhibitory receptor blockade in vitro and in vivo. Blood 2001; 97:3132–3137.

74. Koh CY, Raziuddin A, Welniak LA, Blazar BR, Bennett M, Murphy WJ. NK inhibitory-receptor blockade for purging of leukemia: effects on hematopoietic reconstitution. Biol Blood Marrow Transplant 2002; 8:17–25.

75. Koh CV, Ortaldo JR, Blazar BR, Bennett M, Murphy WJ. NK cell purging of leukemia: superior anti-tumor effects of NK cells H2-allogeneic to the tumor and augmentation with inhibitory receptor blockade. Blood 2003; 102:4067–4075.

76. Marijt WA, Heemskerk MH, Kloosterboer FM, Goulmy E, Kester MG, van der Hoorn MA, van Luxemburg-Heys SA, Hoogeboom M, Mutis T, Drijfhout JW, van Rood JJ, Willemze R, Falkenburg JH. Hematopoiesis-restricted minor histocompatibility antigens HA-1- or HA-2-specific T cells can induce complete remissions of relapsed leukemia. Proc Natl Acad Sci USA 100:2742–2747.

77. Falkenburg JH, van de Corput L, Marijt EW, Willemze R. Minor histocompatibility antigens in human stem cell transplantation. Exp Hematol 2003; 31:743–751.

78. Michalek J, Collins RH, Durrani HP, Vaclavkova P, Ruff LE, Douek DC, Vitetta ES. Definitive separation of graft-versus-leukemia- and graft-versus-host-specific CD4+ T cells by virtue of their receptor beta loci sequences. Proc Natl Acad Sci USA 2003; 100:1180–1184.

79. Flowers ME, Pepe MS, Longton G, Doney KC, Monroe D, Witherspoon RP, Sullivan KM, Storb R. Previous donor pregnancy as a risk factor for acute graft-versus-host disease in patients with aplastic anaemia treated by allogeneic marrow transplantation. Br J Haematol 1990; 74:492–496.

80. Atkinson K, Farrell C, Chapman G, Downs K, Penny R, Biggs J. Female marrow donors increase the risk of acute graft-versus-host disease: effect of donor age and parity and analysis of cell subpopulations in the donor marrow inoculum. Br J Haematol 1986; 63:231–239.

81. Gratwohl A, Hermans J, Niederwieser D, van Biezen A, van Houwelingen HC, Apperley J. Female donors influence transplant-related mortality and relapse incidence in male recipients of sibling blood and marrow transplants. Hematol J 2001; 2:363–370.

82. Randolph SS, Gooley TA, Warren EH, Appelbaum FR, Riddell SR. Female donors contribute to a selective graft versus leukemia effect in male recipients of HLA matched related hematopoietic cell transplants. Blood 2003; 103:347–352.

83. Reddy P, Maeda Y, Hotary K, Liu C, Reznikov LL, Dinarello C, Ferrara J. Histone Deacetylase inhibitor suberoylanilide hydroxamic acid reduces acute graft-versus-host disease and preserves graft-versus-leukemia effect. PNAS 2004; 101:3921–3926.

84. Kim YM, Sachs T, Asavaroengchai W, Bronson R, Sykes M. Graft-versus-host disease can be separated from graft-versus-lymphoma effects by control of lymphocyte trafficking with FTY720. J Clin Invest 2003; 111:659–669.

85. Sun K, Welniak LA, Wilkins D, A P-M, B B, Sayers TJ, Murphy W. PS-341 Administration inhibits acute graft-versus-host disease and preserves graft-versus-tumor after allogeneic BMT in advanced tumor-bearing mice. Blood 2003; 102:192a.

86. Kirken RA, Wang YL. Molecular actions of sirolimus: sirolimus and mTor. Transplant Proc 2003; 35:S227–230.

87. Dornan J, Taylor P, Walkinshaw MD. Structures of immunophilins and their ligand complexes. Curr Top Med Chem 2003; 3:1392–1409.

88. Huang S, Bjornsti MA, Houghton PJ. Rapamycins: mechanism of action and cellular resistance. Cancer Biol Ther 2003; 2:222–232.

89. Antin JH, Kim HT, Cutler C, Ho VT, Lee SJ, Miklos DB, Hochberg EP, Wu CJ, Alyea EP, Soiffer RJ. Sirolimus, tacrolimus, and low-dose methotrexate for graft-versus-host disease prophylaxis in mismatched related donor or unrelated donor transplantation. Blood 2003; 102:1601–1605.

90. Cutler C, Kim H, Micale E, Ho VT, Alyea E, Lee SJ, Fisher DC, Hochberg E, Soiffer RJ, Antin JH. Sirolimus and tacrolimus without methotrexate as graft-versus-host disease prophylaxis after matched, related peripheral blood stem cell transplantation: low transplant related morbidity and excellent GVHD control. Blood 2003; 102:242a.

91. Finke J, Schmoor C, Lang H, Potthoff K, Bertz H. Matched and mismatched allogeneic stem-cell transplantation from unrelated donors using combined graft-versus-host disease prophylaxis including rabbit anti-T lymphocyte globulin. J Clin Oncol 2003; 21:506–513.

92. Jacobsohn DA, Vogelsang GB. Novel pharmacotherapeutic approaches to prevention and treatment of GVHD. Drugs 2002; 62:879–889.

93. Couriel DR, Hicks K, Giralt S, Champlin RE. Role of tumor necrosis factor-alpha inhibition with inflixiMAB in cancer therapy and hematopoietic stem cell transplantation. Curr Opin Oncol 2000; 12:582–587.

94. Kobbe G, Schneider P, Rohr U, Fenk R, Neumann F, Aivado M, Dietze L, Kronenwett R, Hunerliturkoglu A, Haas R. Treatment of severe steroid refractory acute graft-versus-host disease with infliximab, a chimeric human/mouse antiTNFalpha antibody. Bone Marrow Transplant 2001; 28:47–49.

95. Uberti JP, Ayash L, Levine JE, Silver S, Reddy P, Becker M, Reynolds C, Cooke KR, Ratanatharathorn V, Ferrara JLM. Phase I/I trial on the use of Etanercept (Eubrel) and Solumefrol as primary treatment for acute graft-versus-host disease (aGVHD). Blood 2003; 102:243a.

96. Marty FM, Lee SJ, Fahey MM, Alyea EP, Soiffer RJ, Antin JH, Baden LR.Infliximab use in patients with severe graft-versus-host disease and other emerging risk factors of non-Candida invasive fungal infections in allogeneic hematopoietic stem cell transplant recipients: a cohort study. Blood 2003; 102:2768–2776.

97. Socie G, Mary JY, Lemann M, Daneshpouy M, Guardiola P, Meignin V, Ades L, Esperou H, Ribaud P, Devergie A, Gluckman E, Ameisen JC, Janin A. Prognostic value of apoptotic cells and infiltrating neutrophils in graft-versus-host disease of the gastrointestinal tract in humans: TNF and FAS expression. Blood 2004; 103:50–57.

98. Lin MT, Storer B, Martin PJ, Tseng LH, Gooley T, Chen PJ, Hansen JA. Relation of an interleukin-10 promoter polymorphism to graft-versus-host disease and survival after hematopoietic-cell transplantation. N Engl J Med 2003; 349:2201–2210.

99. Cooke KR, Ferrara JL. A protective gene for graft-versus-host disease. N Engl J Med 2003; 349:2183–2184.

100. Ogura Y, Bonen DK, Inohara N, Nicolae DL, Chen FF, Ramos R, Britton H, Moran T, Karaliuskas R, Duerr RH, Achkar JP, Brant SR, Bayless TM, Kirschner BS, Hanauer SB, Nunez G, Cho JH. A frameshift mutation in NOD2 associated with susceptibility to Crohn's disease. Nature 2001; 411:603–606.

101. Inohara N, Nunez G. NODs: intracellular proteins involved in inflammation and apoptosis. Nat Rev Immunol 2003; 3:371–382.

102. Sonwalkar SA, James RM, Ahmad T, Zhang L, Verbeke CS, Barnard DL, Jewell DP, Hull MA. Fulminant Crohn's colitis after allogeneic stem cell transplantation. Gut 2003; 52:1518–1521.

103. Crawford S, Longton G, Storb R. Acute graft versus host disease and the risks for idiopathic pneumonia after marrow transplantation for severe aplastic anemia. Bone Marrow Transplant 1993; 12:225.

104. Weiner RS, Mortimer MB, Gale RP, Gluckman E, Kay HEM, Kolb JJ, Hartz AJ, Rimm AA. Interstitial pneumonitis after bone marrow transplantation. Ann. Intern. Med. 1986; 104:168–175.

105. Cooke KR, Kobzik L, Martin TR, Brewer J, Delmonte J, Crawford JM, Ferrara JLM. An experimental model of idiopathic pneumonia syndrome after bone marrow transplantation. I. The roles of minor H antigens and endotoxin. Blood 1996; 88:3230–3239.

106. Cooke KR, Krenger W, Hill GR, Martin T, Kobzik L, Brewer J, Simmons R, Crawford JM, van den Brink MRM, Ferrara JLM. Host reactive donor T cells are associated with lung injury after experimental allogeneic bone marrow transplantation. Blood 1998; 92:2571–2580.

107. Fukuda T, Hackman RC, Guthrie KA, Sandmaier BM, Boeckh M, Maris MB, Maloney DG, Deeg HJ, Martin PJ, Storb RF, Madtes DK. Risks and outcomes of idiopathic pneumonia syndrome after nonmyeloablative and conventional conditioning regimens for allogeneic hematopoietic stem cell transplantation. Blood 2003; 102:2777–2785.

108. Ratanatharathorn V, Ayash L, Lazarus HM, Fu J, Uberti JP. Chronic graft-versus-host disease: clinical manifestation and therapy. Bone Marrow Transplant 2001; 28:121–129.

109. Ratanatharathorn V, Ayash L, Reynolds C, Silver S, Reddy P, Becker M, Ferrara JL, Uberti JP. Treatment of chronic graft-versus-host disease with anti-CD20 chimeric monoclonal antibody. Biol Blood Marrow Transplant 2003; 9:505–511.

Index

Milton Keynes UK
Ingram Content Group UK Ltd.
UKHW052030071024
449327UK00027B/2506